ESSENTIALS
of FAMILY
PRACTICE

Second Edition

Robert E. Rakel, M.D.

Professor
Department of Family and Community Medicine
Baylor College of Medicine, Houston, Texas

W.B. SAUNDERS COMPANY
A Division of Harcourt Brace & Company
Philadelphia / London / Toronto / Montreal / Sydney / Tokyo

W.B. SAUNDERS COMPANY
A Division of Harcourt Brace & Company

The Curtis Center
Independence Square West
Philadelphia, Pennsylvania 19106

Library of Congress Cataloging-in-Publication Data

Essentials of family practice / [edited by] Robert E. Rakel.—2nd ed.

p.   cm.

Includes bibliographical references and index.

ISBN 0–7216–5868–7

1. Family medicine.   I. Rakel, Robert E.
   [DNLM: 1. Family Practice.   WB 110 E783 1998]

RC49.E97   1998   610—dc21

DNLM/DLC   97-34009

ESSENTIALS OF FAMILY PRACTICE   ISBN 0–7216–5868–7

Printed in the United States of America

Last digit is the print number: 9   8   7   6   5   4   3   2   1

Contributors

Allan V. Abbott, M.D.
Professor of Family Medicine and Vice Chairman of Academic Affairs, University of Southern California School of Medicine, Los Angeles, California
Elbow Pain

Michael A. Altman, M.D.
Assistant Professor, Department of Family Practice and Community Medicine, University of Texas–Houston School of Medicine, Houston, Texas
Acne

Carol A. Baase, M.D.
Assistant Professor and Medical Director, Penn State–Good Samaritan Family Practice Residency Program of Penn State Geisinger Health System, Hershey; Medical Director—Lebanon Family Health Services, Lebanon, Pennsylvania
Amenorrhea

Mark M. Bajorek, M.D.
Assistant Professor, Oregon Health Sciences University, Portland, Oregon
The Abnormal Pap Smear

Alan Blum, M.D.
Associate Professor, Department of Family Medicine, Baylor College of Medicine; Attending Physician/Staff Member, St. Luke's Episcopal Hospital, Texas Children's Hospital, Methodist Hospital, and Park Plaza Hospital, Houston, Texas
Approaches to Patients Who Smoke

Karen M. Bolton, M.D.
Associate Professor, Department of Family Medicine, University of Tennessee, College of Medicine, Memphis, and University of Tennessee, Graduate School of Medicine, Knoxville; Staff, University of Tennessee Medical Center, Knoxville, Tennessee
Dysuria

James H. Bray, Ph.D.
Associate Professor, Baylor College of Medicine, Department of Family and Community Medicine; Consulting Staff, St. Luke's Episcopal Hospital;

Medical Scientist Staff, Methodist Hospital; Allied Health Staff, Park Plaza Hospital, Houston, Texas
Family Dynamics and Health

Baruch A. Brody, Ph.D.
Professor of Biomedical Ethics, Baylor College of Medicine, Houston, Texas
Ethics in Family Medicine

David E. Burtner, M.D.
Professor and Vice Chairman, Department of Family and Community Medicine, Mercer University School of Medicine, Macon, Georgia
Hypertension

Walter L. Calmbach, M.D.
Associate Professor, Department of Family Practice, University of Texas Health Science Center at San Antonio; Director, Family Practice Sports Medicine Fellowship, San Antonio, Texas
Lower Back Pain

Jon C. Calvert, M.D., Ph.D.
Professor, Department of Family Medicine, and Instructor, Department of Obstetrics and Gynecology, University of Oklahoma College of Medicine, Tulsa, Oklahoma
Menopause

Richard D. Clover, M.D.
Professor and Chairman, Department of Family and Community Medicine; Associate Vice President for Health Affairs/Primary Care, University of Louisville School of Medicine; Medical Staff, University of Louisville Hospital, Louisville, Kentucky
Immunizations; Nasal Congestion

Samuel T. Coleridge, D.O.
Professor and Chair, Department of Family Medicine, University of North Texas Health Science Center, Fort Worth, Texas
Eczema

Colleen Conry, M.D.
Associate Professor, University of Colorado School of Medicine and University of Colorado Health Sciences Center, Denver, Colorado
Breast Lump

Jane E. Corboy, M.D.
Assistant Professor of Family and Community Medicine, Baylor College of Medicine; Medical Director, The Health Channel, Baylor College of Medicine, Houston, Texas
Chest Pain

Louisa C. Coutts–van Dijk, M.D.
Assistant Professor, Department of Family and Community Medicine, Baylor College of Medicine; Medical Staff, St. Luke's Hospital, Texas Children's Hospital, Methodist Hospital, and Park Plaza Hospital, Houston, Texas
Contraception

Michael A. Crouch, M.D., M.S.P.H.
Associate Professor, Department of Family and Community Medicine, and Director, Family Practice Residency Program, Baylor College of Medicine, Houston, Texas
Family Dynamics and Health; Hypercholesterolemia

Daniel J. David, M.D.
Professor, Department of Family Medicine, and Residency Director, Johnson City Family Practice Residency Program, James H. Quillen College of Medicine, East Tennessee State University, Johnson City, Tennessee
Atrial Fibrillation

Richard W. Demmler, M.D.
Assistant Professor, Department of Family and Community Medicine, Baylor College of Medicine, Houston, Texas
Urinary Incontinence

Daniel J. Derksen, M.D.
Associate Professor, Department of Family and Community Medicine, University of New Mexico School of Medicine, Albuquerque, New Mexico
Vomiting and Low Back Pain

Jon Divine, M.D., M.S.
Assistant Professor, Department of Family and Community Medicine, Baylor College of Medicine, Houston, Texas
Knee Injury; Neck Pain

James E. Dunlap, M.D.
Assistant Professor of Family Practice, Michigan State University, East Lansing, Michigan
Shoulder Pain in a Recreational Athlete

Daniel T. Earl, D.O.
Clinical Associate Professor, Department of Family Medicine, and Clinical Instructor, Department of Pediatrics, James H. Quillen College of Medicine, East Tennessee State University, Johnson City, Tennessee
Abdominal Pain

John W. Ely, M.D., M.S.P.H.
Assistant Professor, Department of Family Medicine, University of Iowa School of Medicine, Iowa City, Iowa
Sinus Congestion

Jeanne M. Ferrante, M.D.
Assistant Professor, and Director, Predoctoral Education and Family Medicine Clerkship, Department of Family Medicine, University of South Florida College of Medicine; Medical Staff, Tampa General Hospital, Tampa, Florida
Dizziness

Daniel S. Fick, M.D.
Associate Clinical Professor, Department of Family Medicine, University of Iowa College of Medicine, Iowa City, Iowa
Ankle Injury

Richard E. Finlayson, M.D.
Consultant, Department of Psychiatry and Psychology and Department of Family Medicine, Mayo Clinic and Mayo Foundation; Associate Professor of Psychiatry, Mayo Medical School, Rochester, Minnesota
Memory Loss

Paul M. Fischer, M.D.
Senior Partner, Center for Primary Care, Augusta, Georgia
Interpreting Laboratory Tests

Scott H. Frank, M.D., M.S.
Associate Professor, Department of Family Medicine, and Director of Predoctoral Education, School of Medicine, Case Western Reserve University, Cleveland, Ohio
Alcoholism

Ernest Frugé, Ph.D.
Assistant Professor, Department of Family and Community Medicine, Baylor College of Medicine; Adjunct Clinical Assistant Professor, Department of Psychiatry and Behavioral Sciences, University of Texas Health Science Center; Board Member, Harris County Children's Protective Services and The Texas Center, A.K. Rice Institute (Fellow), Houston, Texas
Family Dynamics and Health

Rebecca H. Gladu, M.D.
Assistant Professor, Department of Family Practice and Community Medicine, University of Texas Medical School at Houston; Medical Director, UT/Hermann Center for Family Practice, Houston, Texas
Newborn Care

Eduardo C. Gonzalez, M.D.
Assistant Professor, Department of Family
Medicine, University of South Florida College of
Medicine, Tampa, Florida
Tremors

L. Kevin Hamberger, Ph.D.
Professor, Department of Family and Community
Medicine, Medical College of Wisconsin,
Milwaukee; Associate Residency Program Director,
Racine Family Practice Center, All Saints Health
Care System, Inc., Racine, Wisconsin
Domestic Violence

R. Brian Haynes, M.D., M.Sc., Ph.D.
Professor of Clinical Epidemiology and Biostatistics
and Medicine, McMaster University, Hamilton,
Ontario, Canada
Patient Compliance

Granvil L. Hays, D.D.S., M.S.
Associate Professor, Oral Diagnosis Section,
Department of General Dentistry, University of
Texas–Houston HSC Dental Branch, Houston,
Texas
Oral Leukoplakia

John M. Heath, M.D.
Associate Professor, Department of Family
Medicine, and Co-Director, Geriatrics Medicine
Fellowship Program, Robert Wood Johnson
Medical School, University of Medicine and
Dentistry of New Jersey, New Brunswick, New
Jersey
Joint Pain and Stiffness

Warren A. Heffron, M.D.
Professor, Department of Family and Community
Medicine, University of New Mexico School of
Medicine; Clinical Staff Member, University of New
Mexico Hospital, Albuquerque, New Mexico
Disease Prevention

Warren L. Holleman, Ph.D.
Assistant Professor, Department of Family and
Community Medicine, Baylor College of Medicine,
Houston, Texas
Ethics in Family Medicine

Glen R. Johnson, M.D.
Clinical Professor, Department of Family Medicine,
University of Miami Medical School; Senior Vice
President for Medical Affairs, Physician
Corporation of America, Miami, Florida
Managed Health Care

Jerry E. Jones, M.D., M.S.
Active Staff, Bessemer-Carraway Medical Center,
Bessemer, Alabama
Diarrhea

Michael G. Kavan, Ph.D.
Associate Dean for Student Affairs, Associate
Professor of Family Practice, and Associate
Professor of Psychiatry, Creighton University
School of Medicine, Omaha, Nebraska
Chronic Anxiety

Louis A. Kazal, Jr., M.D.
Clinical Associate Professor, Department of Family
and Community Medicine, Baylor College of
Medicine, Houston, Texas; Medical Director,
Navajo Health Foundation/Sage Memorial
Hospital, Ganado, Arizona
Laceration Repair

Sanford R. Kimmel, M.D.
Associate Professor, Department of Clinical Family
Medicine, Medical College of Ohio, and Associate
Residency Director, Medical College of Ohio;
Family Practice Residency, St. Vincent Mercy
Medical Center, Toledo, Ohio
Short Child

Isaac Kleinman, M.D.
Associate Professor, Department of Family and
Community Medicine, Baylor College of Medicine,
Houston, Texas
Blurring of Vision

Joseph C. Konen, M.D., M.S.P.H.
Clinical Professor, Department of Family Medicine,
University of North Carolina, Chapel Hill; Adjunct
Professor, Family and Community Medicine and
Public Health Sciences, Bowman Gray School of
Medicine, Wake Forest University, Winston-Salem;
Chairman, Department of Family Medicine,
Carolinas HealthCare System, Charlotte, North
Carolina
Nocturia

Greg L. Ledgerwood, M.D.
Associate Clinical Professor, Department of Family
Medicine, University of Washington School of
Medicine, Seattle, Washington; Speaker on Allergy
and Asthma, American Association of Family
Physicians
Wheezing

Walter D. Leventhal, M.D.
Clinical Associate Professor, Department of Family
Medicine, Medical University of South Carolina,
Charleston; Chief of Staff Elect, Columbia-Trident
Hospital System, North Charleston, South Carolina
Rash and Fever

Martin S. Lipsky, M.D.
Professor and Chair, Department of Family
Medicine, Northwestern University Medical School,
Chicago, Illinois
Type II Diabetes

John Lombardo, M.D.
Professor of Family Medicine, The Ohio State University; Medical Director, The Ohio State University Sports Medicine Center, Columbus, Ohio
Knee Injury

David P. Losh, M.D.
Associate Professor and Residency Program Director, Department of Family Medicine, University of Washington, Seattle, Washington
Selecting Radiographic Tests

Tomas G. Lumicao, Jr., M.D.
Assistant Professor, Department of Family and Community Medicine, Baylor College of Medicine; Active Staff, St. Luke's Episcopal Hospital, Methodist Hospital, Park Plaza Hospital, and Texas Children's Hospital, Houston, Texas
Obesity

Barbara A. Majeroni, M.D.
Assistant Professor, Department of Family Medicine, State University of New York at Buffalo School of Medicine and Biomedical Sciences; Director of Screening Services, Roswell Park Cancer Institute, Buffalo, New York
Weight Loss

Karl E. Miller, M.D.
Associate Professor, Department of Family Medicine, Chattanooga Unit, University of Tennessee College of Medicine, Chattanooga, Tennessee
Vaginal Discharge

Lawrence H. Miller, M.D.
Private practice, Kingsport, Tennessee
Hyperactivity; Eating Disorders

Susan M. Miller, M.D., M.P.H.
Associate Professor, Departments of Internal Medicine and The Center for Ethics and Health Policy, Baylor College of Medicine; Medical Director, Women's Health Initiative, Baylor College of Medicine, Houston, Texas
Weight Loss and Diarrhea

Carlos A. Moreno, M.D., M.S.P.H.
Professor, and Chairman, Department of Family Practice and Community Medicine, University of Texas–Houston Medical School; Chief of Family Practice, Hermann Hospital, Houston, Texas
Sore Throat

R. Michael Morse, M.D.
Professor of Family Medicine, University of Virginia School of Medicine; Director, Virginia Center for the Advancement of Generalist Medicine; Medical Director, University of Virginia

Health Services Foundation, Institute for Quality Health, Charlottesville, Virginia
Disease Prevention

Richard A. Neill, M.D.
Assistant Professor of Family Practice and Community Medicine, University of Pennsylvania School of Medicine, Philadelphia, Pennsylvania
Chronic Cough

George A. Nixon, M.D.
Associate Professor, Department of Family Medicine, Medical College of Georgia, Augusta, Georgia
Constipation

Kevin C. Oeffinger, M.D.
Associate Professor, Department of Family Practice and Community Medicine, University of Texas Southwestern Medical Center at Dallas, Dallas, Texas
Acute Bronchitis

John G. O'Handley, M.D.
Clinical Associate Professor of Family Practice, Ohio State College of Medicine; Program Director, Family Practice Residency, Mount Carmel Medical Center, Columbus, Ohio
Ear Pain

Paul M. Paulman, M.D.
Professor of Family Medicine, University of Nebraska College of Medicine, Omaha, Nebraska
Anemia

John G. Prichard, M.D., M.H.S.
Director, Internal Medicine, Ventura County Medical Center, Ventura; Associate Professor, University of California, Los Angeles, School of Medicine, Los Angeles, California
Fever and Chest Pain

Robert E. Rakel, M.D.
Professor, Department of Family and Community Medicine, Baylor College of Medicine; Attending Physician/Active Staff, St. Luke's Episcopal Hospital, Methodist Hospital, and Park Plaza Hospital, Houston, Texas
The Family Physician; The Consultation Process; The Problem-Oriented Medical Record; Terminal Cancer and Pain

Marc L. Rivo, M.D., M.P.H.
Medical Director, AvMed Health Plan, Miami; Clinical Professor, Department of Family Medicine and Community Health, University of Miami School of Medicine, Miami, Florida; Medical Editor, Family Practice Management; Senior Fellow, Center for the Health Professions, University of California, San Francisco, San Francisco, California
Managed Health Care

Shelley Roaten, Jr., M.D.
Professor and Chairman, Department of Family
Practice and Community Medicine, Southwestern
Medical School, Dallas, Texas
Skin Papule

William MacMillan Rodney, M.D.
Professor, Departments of Family Medicine and of
Emergency Medicine, University of Tennessee,
Memphis, College of Medicine, Memphis,
Tennessee
Heartburn; Fatigue and Anemia

John C. Rogers, M.D., M.P.H.
Professor, Department of Family and Community
Medicine, Baylor College of Medicine; Staff, St.
Luke's Episcopal Hospital and Methodist Hospital,
Houston, Texas
Problem Solving in Family Medicine

Dawn Schissel, M.D.
Associate Professor, University of Iowa College of
Medicine, Iowa City; Faculty Physician, Family
Practice Residency Program, Broadlawns Medical
Center, Des Moines, Iowa
Child with Fever and Lethargy

Thomas L. Schwenk, M.D.
Professor and Chair, Department of Family
Medicine, University of Michigan Medical Center,
Ann Arbor, Michigan
Sleep Disturbance

John W. Sellors, M.Sc., M.D.
Professor, Departments of Family Medicine and of
Clinical Epidemiology and Biostatistics, and
Director of Research, Department of Family
Medicine, McMaster University, Hamilton, Ontario,
Canada
Patient Compliance

Angela J. Shepherd, M.D.
Clinical Assistant Professor, Department of Family
Medicine, University of Texas Medical Branch,
Galveston, Texas
Postmenopausal Vaginal Bleeding

Patrick O. Smith, Ph.D.
Associate Professor, Department of Family
Medicine, University of Mississippi Medical School,
Jackson, Mississippi
Motor Vehicle Accident–Related Anxiety

Robert Smith, M.D.
Professor and Director Emeritus, Department of
Family Medicine, University of Cincinnati Medical
Center; Founder, Cincinnati Headache Center,
University Hospital, Cincinnati, Ohio
Headache

Stephen J. Spann, M.D.
Professor and Chairman, Department of Family
and Community Medicine, Baylor College of
Medicine; Chief of Service, Methodist Hospital,
Houston, Texas
Problem Solving in Family Medicine

Porter Storey, M.D.
Clinical Assistant Professor, Department of Family
and Community Medicine, and Clinical Associate
Professor, Department of Medicine, Baylor College
of Medicine; Consultant in Neuro-Oncology and
Adjunct Assistant Professor of Medicine, University
of Texas M.D. Anderson Cancer Center; Medical
Director, The Hospice at the Texas Medical Center,
Houston, Texas
Terminal Cancer and Pain

Amir Sweha, M.D.
Assistant Clinical Professor, University of
California, Davis; Medical Director, Mercy Family
Health Center, Mercy Family Practice Residency
Program, Mercy Healthcare, Sacramento,
California
Dyspnea

Thomas R. Terrell, M.D., M.Phil., FAAFP
Assistant Professor of Family Medicine, University
of Maryland; Co-Team Physician, University of
Maryland Athletics; Faculty, University of Maryland
Primary Care Sports Medicine Fellowship;
Physician, University of Maryland Hospital System
and Kerman Hospital, Baltimore, Maryland
Wrist and Hand Pain

Bruce T. Vanderhoff, M.D.
Associate Director, Grant Family Medicine
Residency; Director, Grant Family Practice–Grove
City; Physician, Grant/Riverside Methodist
Hospitals, Columbus, Ohio
Preschool Physical Examination

Steven C. Van Noord, M.D.
Private Practice, Metrosport Family Practice and
Sports Medicine, Grand Rapids, Michigan
Knee Injury

Stephanie Wiman Wells, M.D.
Assistant Professor, Department of Family and
Community Medicine, Baylor College of Medicine,
Houston, Texas
Shortness of Breath

Randy Wertheimer, M.D.
Associate Professor, Department of Family and
Community Medicine, University of Massachusetts
School of Medicine; Vice Chair, Department of
Family Medicine, Memorial Health Care; Chair,

Public Health Committee, Worcester District
Medical Society, Worcester, Massachusetts
Pregnancy

Jane V. White, Ph.D., R.D.
Professor, Department of Family Practice, Graduate
School of Medicine–Knoxville and College of
Medicine–Memphis, University of Tennessee,
Knoxville, Tennessee
Malnutrition in the Elderly

Lori Anne Whittaker, M.D., Ph.D.
Physician, Stevens Healthcare Birth and Family
Clinic, Edmonds, Washington
Hematuria

Hardy B. Woodbridge, Jr., M.D.
Professor Emeritus, Department of Family
Medicine, University of Mississippi Medical School;
Consulting Staff, St. Dominics Hospital and River
Oaks Hospital, Jackson, Mississippi
Basics of Prescription Writing

Preface

This second edition is designed, just as the first was, to serve as a resource for medical students and residents learning the essentials of our discipline. The format of this book is designed to supplement material presented in the *Textbook of Family Practice* and consists primarily of patient problems typical of those seen by family physicians.

Of the 83 chapters in this edition, 61 are new and the remaining 22 have been revised and updated. Twenty-four new cases have been added, giving a total of 71 clinical problems in this edition, compared with 47 in the first. The 19 chapters preceding the clinical cases in the first edition have been reduced to nine and three new chapters have been added. These are as follows: selecting radiographic tests, integrated health care systems, and the basics of prescription writing. New clinical problems include immunizations, ankle injury, elbow pain, terminal cancer, domestic violence, hematuria, and many more.

The first 12 chapters discuss the discipline of family medicine and present topics fundamental to family practice. Following this section are 71 clinical cases presented just as they are to the family physician. The cases are presented using the SOAP format, and a differential diagnosis is developed using problem-solving methods typical of those used in family practice. Discussion of each case focuses on which diagnosis is most appropriate, and the most appropriate management is presented as the patient is followed at subsequent visits. The intent is to illustrate for the student the variety of challenges that the family physician faces daily and the rewards of managing cases of this nature over time.

To ensure that the material in this book is relevant to practice, we have selected cases that represent the 20 most frequent problems encountered in practice as determined by the National Ambulatory Medical Care Survey conducted by the National Center for Health Statistics. These 20 most common diagnoses made by physicians in their offices are listed in Table 1–2, page 14, of the *Textbook of Family Practice,* fifth edition. Each problem on the list is represented by at least one clinical example, some by five or more.

The cases presented have been drawn from the practices of the authors, who are all family physicians, and I am indebted to them for sharing their experiences with us. Our goal is to show medical students the variety of challenges encountered in family practice and the rewards of being a patient's personal physician.

My special thanks to Ray Kersey and the excellent editorial staff at W.B. Saunders Company for their attention to detail and insistence on quality, and to Caroline Kosnik, my editorial assistant, who organizes the material and ensures that deadlines are met and that the book is published on time.

Robert E. Rakel, M.D.

Contents

Part I

FUNDAMENTALS

Chapter 1

The Family Physician

Robert E. Rakel, M.D.

The family physician provides continuing, comprehensive care in a personalized manner to patients of all ages and to their families, regardless of the presence of disease or the nature of the presenting complaint. Family physicians accept responsibility for managing an individual's total health needs while maintaining an intimate, confidential relationship with the patient.

Family medicine is the body of knowledge and the skills that constitute the medical discipline; when applied to the care of patients and their families, that discipline becomes the specialty of family practice. Family medicine emphasizes responsibility for total health care—from the first contact and initial assessment through the ongoing care of chronic problems. Prevention and early recognition of disease are essential features of the discipline. Coordination and integration of all necessary health services with the least amount of fragmentation, together with the skills to manage most medical problems, allow family physicians to provide cost-effective health care. The family physician personally takes care of 95 per cent of the patient's health needs; for the remainder of the patient's problems, the physician selects appropriate consulting physicians or other health professionals to assist in care.

Devotion to continuing, comprehensive, personalized care; to early detection and management of illness; to prevention of disease and maintenance of health; and to ongoing management of patients in a community setting uniquely qualifies the family physician to deliver primary care.

The curriculum for training family physicians is designed to represent realistically the skills and body of knowledge that they will require in practice. This curriculum relies heavily on an accurate analysis of the problems seen and the skills used by family physicians in their practices. Unfortunately, the content of residency training programs for the primary care specialties has not always been appropriately directed toward solving the problems most commonly encountered by physicians practicing in these specialties. The situation is changing, however, and future training programs should be more appropriately designed to meet the needs of the practicing physician. The almost randomly educated primary physician of previous years is being replaced by one specifically prepared to address the kinds of problems likely to be encountered in practice. For this reason, the "model office" is an essential component of all family practice residency programs.

THE JOY OF FAMILY PRACTICE

The rewards in family practice come largely from knowing patients intimately over time and in sharing their trust, respect, and friendship. The thrill of family practice is the close bond (actually friendship) that develops with patients. This bond is strengthened with each physical or emotional crisis in a person's life when he or she turns to the family physician for help.

It is especially rewarding when the family physician cares for a newly married couple, delivers their first baby, sees them frequently for well-child care, and provides ongoing care for the parents, the growing child, and subsequent children. No other medical specialty is so privileged. To participate in a family's life in such a close and intimate manner is uniquely rewarding.

The practice of family medicine involves the joy of greeting old friends in every examining room, and the variety of problems encountered keeps one professionally stimulated and perpetually challenged. In contrast, physicians practicing in narrow specialties often lose their enthusiasm for medicine after seeing the same problem hundreds of times. The variety of family medicine sustains the excitement and precludes boredom.

DEVELOPMENT OF THE SPECIALTY

In about 1923, Francis Peabody commented that the swing of the pendulum toward specialization had reached its apex and that modern medicine had fragmented the health care delivery system to too great a degree. He called for a rapid return of the generalist physician who would give comprehensive, personalized care.

Dr. Peabody's declaration proved premature; society and the medical establishment were not ready for such a proclamation. The trend toward specialization gained momentum through the 1950s, and fewer physicians entered general practice. In the early 1960s, leaders in the field of general practice began advocating a seemingly paradoxical solution to reverse the trend and end the scarcity of general practitioners—the creation of still another specialty. However, the physicians envisioned a specialty that embodied the knowledge, skills, and ideals that they knew as primary care. In 1966, the concept of a new specialty in primary care received official recognition in two separate reports published 1 month apart. The first of these was the *Report of the Citizens' Commission on Graduate Medical Education of the American Medical Association*, also known as the Millis Commission Report. The second report came from the Ad Hoc Committee on Education for Family Practice of the Council of Medical Education of the American Medical Association, also called the Willard Committee. Three years later, in 1969, the American Board of Family Practice (ABFP) came into being as the twentieth medical specialty board, thus giving birth to the specialty of family practice.

Much of the impetus for the Millis and Willard Reports came from the American Academy of General Practice, which was renamed the American Academy of Family Physicians (AAFP) in 1971. The name change reflected a desire to increase emphasis on family-oriented health care and to focus on the new specialty of family practice.

The ABFP has distinguished itself by being the first specialty board to require recertification (every 6 years) to ensure the ongoing competence of its members. In addition to the basic requirements for certification and recertification, the ABFP has included continuing education—the foundation on which the American Academy of General Practice had been built when organized in 1947. A diplomate of the ABFP must participate in 50 hours of acceptable continuing education each year (300 hours in 6 years) to be eligible for recertification. Once eligible, a candidate's competence is examined by performance evaluation and cognitive testing. The ABFP's emphasis on quality of education, knowledge, and performance has facilitated the rapid increase in prestige for the family physician in our health care system. The obvious logic of the ABFP's emphasis on continuing education to maintain required knowledge and skills has been adopted by other specialties and state medical societies. Now all specialty boards are committed to the concept of recertification in some form to ensure that their diplomates remain current with advances in medicine.

DEFINITIONS

FAMILY PRACTICE. Family practice is the medical specialty that provides continuing and comprehensive health care for the individual and the family. It is the specialty in breadth that integrates the biological, clinical, and behavioral sciences. The scope of family practice encompasses all ages, both sexes, each organ system, and every disease entity.

FAMILY PHYSICIAN. The family physician is a physician who is educated and trained in the discipline of family practice—a broadly encompassing medical specialty. Family physicians possess unique attitudes, skills, and knowledge that qualify them to provide continuing and comprehensive medical care, health maintenance, and preventive services to each member of the family regardless of sex, age, or type of problem, be it biological, behavioral, or social. These specialists, because of their background and interactions with the family, are best qualified to serve as each patient's advocate in all health-related matters, including the appropriate use of consultants, health services, and community resources (AAFP Congress, 1993).

The World Organization of Family Doctors (WONCA, world organization of national colleges, academies, and academic associations of general practitioners/family physicians) defines the family doctor in part as "the physician who is primarily responsible for providing comprehensive health care to every individual seeking medical care, and arranging for other health personnel to provide services when necessary. The family physician functions as a generalist who accepts everyone seeking care, whereas other health providers limit access to their services on the basis of age, sex, and/or diagnosis" (WONCA, 1991).

PRIMARY CARE. Primary care is that care provided by physicians specifically trained for and skilled in comprehensive first contact and continuing care for ill persons or those with an undiagnosed sign, symptom, or health concern (the "undifferentiated" patient) not limited by problem origin (biological, behavioral, or social), organ system, or gender.

Primary care includes, in addition to diagnosis and treatment of acute and chronic illnesses, health promotion, disease prevention, health maintenance, counseling, and patient education, in a variety of health care settings such as office, inpatient, critical care, long-term care, home care, and day care. Primary care is provided by a personal physician, utilizing other health professionals for consultation or referral as appropriate. Primary care promotes effective doctor-patient communication and encourages the role of the patient as a partner in health care.

Because many physicians deliver primary care in different ways and with varying degrees of preparation, the staff of ABFP has further clarified the definition:

Primary care is a form of delivery of medical care that encompasses the following functions:

1. It is highly personalized "first-contact" care, serving as a point-of-entry for the patient into the health care system;

2. It includes continuity by virtue of caring for patients over a period of time, both in sickness and in health;

3. It is comprehensive care, drawing from all the traditional major disciplines for its functional content;

4. It serves a coordinative function for all the health-care needs of the patient;

5. It assumes continuing responsibility for individual patient follow-up and community health problems; and

6. It is a highly personalized type of care.

PRIMARY CARE PHYSICIAN. A primary care physician is a generalist physician who provides definitive care to the undifferentiated patient at the point of first contact and takes continuing responsibility for providing the patient's care. Such a physician must be specifically trained for this task.

Primary care physicians devote the majority of their practice to providing primary care services to a defined population of patients. The style of primary care practice is such that the personal primary care physician serves as the entry point for substantially all of the patient's medical and health care needs—not limited by problem origin, organ system, gender, or diagnosis. Primary care physicians are advocates for the patient in coordinating the

use of the entire health care system to benefit the patient (AAFP Directors' Newsletter, 1994).

The American Board of Family Practice and the American Board of Internal Medicine have agreed on a definition of the generalist physician and that "providing optimal generalist care requires broad and comprehensive training that cannot be gained in brief and uncoordinated educational experiences." They define the generalist physician as one "who provides continuing, comprehensive, and coordinated medical care to a population undifferentiated by gender, disease, or organ system" (Kimball and Young, 1994).

Physicians who provide primary care should be specifically trained to manage the problems encountered in a primary care practice. Rivo and associates (1994) identified the common conditions and diagnoses that generalist physicians should be competent to manage in a primary care practice and compared these with the training of the various "generalist" specialties. They recommend that the training of generalist physicians should include at least 90 per cent of the key diagnoses. By comparing the content of residency programs they found that this goal was met by family practice (95 per cent), internal medicine (91 per cent), and pediatrics (91 per cent) but that obstetrics and gynecology (47 per cent) and emergency medicine (42 per cent) fell far short of this goal.

PERSONALIZED CARE

It is much more important to know what sort of patient has a disease than what sort of disease a patient has.

Sir William Osler

Family physicians do not just treat patients, they care for people. This caring function of family medicine emphasizes the personalized approach to understanding the patient as a person, respecting the person as an individual, and showing compassion for his or her discomfort. Compassion means co-suffering and reflects the physician's willingness somehow to share the patient's anguish and understand what the sickness means to that person. Compassion is an attempt to "feel" along with the patient. Pellegrino (1979) states that "we can never *feel* with another person when we pass judgment as a superior, only when we see our own frailties as well as his." Pellegrino goes on to comment that a compassionate authority figure is effective only when others can receive the "orders" without being humiliated. The physician must not "put down" the patients but must be ever ready, in Galileo's words,

to pronounce that wise, ingenuous, and modest statement—'I don't know.'

Compassion, practiced in these terms in each patient encounter, obtunds the inherent dehumanizing tendencies of today's highly institutionalized and technologically oriented patient care.

The physician should guard against thinking in terms of diseases and instead think in terms of patients who have problems needing attention. The whole-person approach to patient care is hampered by focusing primarily on the disease; specific diseases require specific treatments and tend to direct the physician's attention away from other needs of the whole patient.

Peabody (1930) noted that "the treatment of a disease may be entirely impersonal; the care of a patient must be completely personal." If an intimate relationship with patients remains our primary concern as physicians, high-quality medical care will persist, regardless of the way it is organized and financed. For this reason, family practice emphasizes consideration of the individual patient in the full context of his or her life, rather than the episodic care of a presenting complaint. The Millis Commission Report stresses that the family physician

. . . focuses not upon individual organs and systems but upon the whole man who lives in a complex social setting; and knows that diagnosis or treatment of a part often overlooks major causative factors and therapeutic opportunities.

It is generally recognized that medicine has become depersonalized, owing to the rapid rise of technology. In 1960 Theodore F. Fox wrote:

Nobody is going to persuade me that a nice receptionist, some good notes, and an internist keeping office hours adds up to a personal doctor who knows me and my home. Even if you throw in a psychiatric social worker, I still feel that I am being put off with a plastic substitute for the real thing.

Indeed, as Fox predicted, personalized care is returning to medicine, largely because of the advent of the specialty that provides family physicians who know patients in their home environment and who assess the psychosocial factors that exist within the family setting as well as the individual's problems.

Family physicians assess the illnesses and complaints presented to them, dealing personally with the majority and arranging special assistance for a few. The family physician serves as the patients' advocate, explaining the causes and implications of illness to the patients and their families, and serves as an advisor and confidant to the family—both individually and collectively. The family physician receives many intellectual satisfactions from this practice, but the greatest reward arises from the depth of human understanding and personal satisfaction inherent in family practice.

Patients have adjusted somewhat to a more impersonal form of health care delivery and frequently look to institutions rather than to individuals for their health care; yet, their need for personalized concern and compassion remains. Tumulty (1970) found that patients consider a good physician one who (1) shows genuine interest in them; (2) thoroughly evaluates their problem; (3) demonstrates compassion, understanding, and warmth; and (4) provides clear insight into what is wrong and what must be done to correct it.

The family physician's relationship with each patient should reflect compassion, understanding, and patience, combined with a high degree of intellectual honesty. The physician must be thorough in approaching problems but also possess a keen sense of humor. He or she must be capable of encouraging in each patient optimism, courage, insight, and the self-discipline necessary for recovery.

CHARACTERISTICS AND FUNCTIONS OF THE FAMILY PHYSICIAN

Attributes of the Family Physician

The following characteristics are certainly desirable for all physicians, but they are of greatest importance for the physician in family practice.

1. A strong sense of responsibility for the total, ongoing care of the individual and the family during health, illness, and rehabilitation.

2. Compassion and empathy, with a sincere interest in the patient and the family.

3. A curious and constantly inquisitive attitude.

4. Enthusiasm for the undifferentiated medical problem and its resolution.

5. An interest in the broad spectrum of clinical medicine.

6. The ability to deal comfortably with multiple problems occurring simultaneously in one patient.

7. A desire for frequent and varied intellectual and technical challenges.

8. The ability to support children during growth and development and during their adjustment to family and society.

9. The ability to assist patients in coping with everyday problems and in maintaining stability in the family and community.

10. The capacity to act as coordinator of all health resources needed in the care of a patient.

11. A continuing enthusiasm for learning and for the satisfaction that comes from remaining current through continuing medical education.

12. The ability to maintain composure in times of stress and to respond quickly with logic, effectiveness, and compassion.

13. A desire to identify problems at the earliest possible stage (or to prevent disease entirely).

14. A strong wish to maintain maximum patient satisfaction, recognizing the need for continuing patient rapport.

15. The skills necessary to manage chronic illness and to ensure maximal rehabilitation following acute illness.

16. An appreciation for the complex mix of physical, emotional, and social elements in holistic and personalized patient care.

17. A feeling of personal satisfaction derived from intimate relationships with patients that naturally develop over long periods of continuous care, as opposed to the short-term pleasures gained from treating episodic illnesses.

18. A skill for and commitment to educating patients and families about disease processes and the principles of good health.

The ideal family physician is an explorer, driven by a persistent curiosity and the desire to know more. The family physician is required to be part theologian, as was Paracelsus; part politician, as was Benjamin Rush; and part humorist, as was Oliver Wendell Holmes. At all times, however, the care of the patient—the whole patient—is the primary goal.

Continuing Responsibility

One of the essential functions of the family physician is the willingness to accept ongoing responsibility for managing a patient's medical care. Once a patient or a family has been accepted into the physician's practice, responsibility for care is both total and continuing. The Millis Commission chose the term "primary physician" to emphasize the concept of primary responsibility for the patient's welfare; however, the term "primary care physician" is more popular and refers to any physician who provides first-contact care.

The family physician's commitment to patients does not cease at the end of illness but is a continuing responsibility, regardless of the patient's state of health or the disease process. There is no need to identify the beginning or end-point of treatment, since care of a problem can be reopened at any time—even though a later visit may be primarily for another problem. This prevents the family physician from focusing too narrowly on one problem and helps maintain a perspective on the total patient in his environment. Peabody (1930) believed that much patient dissatisfaction results from the physician's neglecting to assume personal responsibility for supervision of the patient's care: "For some reason or other, no one physician has seen the case through from beginning to end, and the patient may be suffering from the very multitude of his counselors."

The greater the degree of continuing involvement with a patient, the more capable the physician becomes in detecting early signs and symptoms of organic disease and differentiating it from a functional problem. Patients with problems arising from emotional and social conflicts can be managed most effectively by a physician who has intimate knowledge of the individual and of his or her family and community background. This knowledge comes only from insight gained by observing the patient's long-term patterns of behavior and responses to changing stressful situations. This longitudinal view is particularly useful in the care of children and allows the physician to be more effective in assisting children to reach their full potential. The closeness that develops between physicians and young patients increases a physician's ability to aid the patient with problems that occur during later periods in life—such as adjustment to puberty, problems with marriage or employment, and changing social pressures. As the family physician maintains this continuing involvement with successive generations within a family, the ability to manage intercurrent problems increases with knowledge of the total family background.

By virtue of this ongoing involvement and intimate association with the family, the family physician develops a perceptive awareness of a family's nature and style of operation. This ability to observe families over time allows valuable insight that improves the quality of medical care provided to an individual patient. One of the greatest challenges in family medicine is the need to be alert to the changing stresses, transitions, and expectations of family members over time and to the effect that these and other family interactions have on the health of individuals.

Although the family is the family physician's primary concern, his or her skills are equally applicable to the individual living alone or to people in other varieties of family living. Individuals with alternative forms of family living interact with others who have a significant effect on their lives. The principles of group dynamics and interpersonal relationships that affect health are equally applicable to everyone.

The family physician needs to assess an individual's personality so that presenting symptoms can be appropriately evaluated and given the proper degree of attention and emphasis. A complaint of abdominal pain may be treated lightly in one patient who frequently presents with minor problems, but the same complaint would be investigated immediately and in depth in another individual who has a more stoic personality. The decision regarding which studies to perform and when is influenced by knowledge of the patient's lifestyle, personality, and previous response pattern. The greater the degree of knowledge and insight into the patient's background, which is gained through years of previous contact, the more capable the physician is in making an appropriate early and rapid assessment of the presenting complaint. The less background information the physician has to rely on, the greater is the need to depend upon costly laboratory studies and the more likely is overreaction to the presenting symptom. Families receiving continuing comprehensive care have fewer incidences of hospitalization, fewer operations, and fewer physician visits for illnesses compared with those having no regular physician. This is due, at least in part, to the physician's knowledge of the patients; seeing them earlier for acute problems and thus preventing complications that would require hospitalization; being available by telephone; and seeing them more frequently in the office for health supervision. Care is also less expensive, since there is less need to rely on x-ray, laboratory procedures, and visits to emergency rooms.

Collusion of Anonymity

The need for a primary physician who accepts continuing responsibility for patient care is emphasized by Michael Balint (1965) in his concept of "collusion of anonymity." In this situation, the patient is seen by a variety of physicians, not one of whom is willing to accept total management of the problem. Important decisions are made—some good, some bad—but without anyone's feeling fully responsible for them.

Francis Peabody (1930) examined the futility of a patient's making the rounds from one specialist to another without finding relief because he

> . . . lacked the guidance of a sound general practitioner who understood his physical condition, his nervous temperament and knew the details of his daily life. And many a patient, who on his own initiative has sought out specialists, has had minor defects accentuated so that they assume a needless importance, and has even undergone operations that might well have been avoided. Those who are particularly blessed with this world's goods, who want the best regardless of the cost and imagine that they are getting it because they can afford to consult as many renowned specialists as they wish, are often pathetically tragic figures as they veer from one course of treatment to another. Like ships that lack a guiding hand upon the helm, they swing from tack to tack with each new gust of wind but get no nearer to the Port of Health because there is no pilot to set the general direction of their course.

This statement is far more appropriate today than it was 70 years ago.

Chronic Illness

The family physician must also be committed to managing the common chronic illnesses that have no known cure but for which continuing management by a personal physician is all the more necessary to maintain an optimal state of health for the patient. It is a difficult and often trying job to manage these continuing, unresolvable, and progressively crippling problems, control of which often requires a remolding of the lifestyle of the entire family.

Quality of Care

Primary care provided by physicians specifically trained to care for the problems presenting to personal physicians and who know their patients over a span of time is of higher quality than that provided by other physicians. This has been confirmed by a variety of studies comparing the care given by physicians in different specialties.

Following a review of the literature on quality and cost of care, Boex and associates (1993) feel that "the quality of clinical outcomes of primary care practitioners is comparable to that of specialists or subspecialists in similar, clinically appropriate situations.... Practitioners working within their domains of practice have higher quality outcomes than those working outside their regular domains.... Physicians and advance practice nurse generalists trained in and practicing generalist competencies provide a higher quality of primary care to their patients than those whose domains of practice are by definition restricted to specialized areas."

McGann and Bowman (1990) compared the morbidity and mortality of patients hospitalized by family physicians and internists. They found that even though the family physicians' patients were older and more severely ill, there was no significant difference in morbidity and mortality. In addition, the total charges for their hospital care were lower.

The quality of our health care system is being eroded by physicians' being extensively trained at great expense to practice in one area and instead practicing in another, such as anesthesiologists practicing in emergency rooms and surgeons practicing as generalists.

Primary care, to be done well, requires extensive training specifically tailored to problems frequently seen by physicians in ambulatory care. These include the early detection, diagnosis, and treatment of depression; the early diagnosis of cancer (especially of the breast and colon); the management of gynecologic problems; and the care of those with chronic and terminal illnesses.

Cost-Effective Care

The physician who is well acquainted with the patient not only provides personal and humane medical care but also does so more economically than the physician involved only in episodic care. The physician who knows his or her patients well can assess the nature of their problems more rapidly and accurately. Because of the intimate, ongoing relationship, the family physician is under less pressure to exclude diagnostic possibilities by use of expensive laboratory and radiologic procedures and is more likely to use time as an ally in diagnosing a less urgent problem than is the physician who is unfamiliar with the patient.

The United States has the most expensive health care system in the world, with more than 14 per cent of the gross national product devoted to health care. Schroeder (1984) believes that this situation will continue as long as the system accepts a high concentration of specialists, fee-for-service payment, patient self-referral directly to specialists, practice of specialities by physicians who have not gone through the speciality certification process, and a high dependency on specialists for primary care.

Clearly, the increasing complexity of our health care system multiplies expense and wastefulness when a patient self-diagnoses his or her problems or selects his or her own specialist rather than developing a firm and ongoing relationship with a family physician. The most efficient and cost-effective system involves a single personal physician, who ensures the most logical and economical management of a problem. HMOs recognize this and have placed a high premium on hiring family physicians (see Table 1–4).

Medical care should be available to patients in the precise degree needed—neither too extensive nor too limited. This ensures that simple problems will not be magnified out of proportion. The more complex and involved a diagnostic process is, the more costly it becomes and the greater the potential for error. Specialists generally treat their patients more resource-intensively than do generalists, resulting in increased cost of care. Cherkin and associates (1987) showed that internists were 1.7 times more likely to hospitalize patients than family physicians and 1.3 times more likely to refer.

Family physicians order fewer tests than do specialists, perhaps because they know their patients well. MacLean (1993) compared the hospital care given by family physicians with that of all other specialties for patients with gastrointestinal bleeding, nonsurgical back pain, and nutritional, metabolic, or dehydration disorders. He found that the effectiveness of the care was comparable but that the cost of care provided by family physicians was less.

Comprehensive Care

The term "comprehensive medical care" spans the entire spectrum of medicine. The effectiveness with which a physician delivers primary care depends upon the breadth of problems encountered during training and practice. The family physician must be comprehensively trained to acquire all the medical skills necessary to care for the majority of patient problems. The greater the number of skills omitted from the family physician's training and practice,

the more frequent is the need to refer minor problems to another physician. A truly comprehensive
primary care physician adequately manages acute
infections, biopsies skin and other lesions, repairs
lacerations, treats musculoskeletal sprains and minor fractures, removes foreign bodies, treats vaginitis, provides obstetric care and care for the newborn
infant, gives supportive psychotherapy, and super-
vises or performs diagnostic procedures. The needs
of a family physician's patient will range from a
routine physical examination, when the patient feels
well and wishes to identify potential risk factors, to
a problem that calls for referral to one or more
narrowly specialized physicians with highly developed technical skills. The family physician must be
aware of the variety and complexity of skills and
facilities available to help manage patients and must
match these to the individual's specific needs, giving
full consideration to the patient's personality and
expectations.

Management of an illness involves much more
than a diagnosis and an outline for treatment. It
also requires an awareness of all the factors that
may aid or hinder an individual's recovery from
illness. This requires consideration of religious beliefs; social, economic, or cultural problems; personal expectations; and heredity. The outstanding
clinician recognizes the effects that spiritual, intellectual, emotional, social, and economic factors
have on a patient's illness.

Family practice is a comprehensive specialty involving varying depths of knowledge in many disciplines. A primary care physician requires knowledge
and skills of varying degrees in each specialty area,
depending upon the prevalence of problems encountered in everyday practice and the degree of
skills needed to become an excellent diagnostician.
A physician specializing in only one discipline, however, will have a much shallower base in comprehensive medicine and a much greater depth in the
chosen discipline. The subspecialist is an excellent
consultant but is not trained and cannot function
effectively as a primary generalist. The distribution
of his or her knowledge and skills is no more appropriate to that task than is the comprehensive
physician's competence in the esoteric nuances of a
limited discipline.

The family physician's ability to confront relatively large numbers of unselected patients with undifferentiated conditions and carry on a therapeutic
relationship over time is a unique primary care skill.
The skilled family physician will have a higher level
of tolerance for the uncertain than will his or her
consultant colleague.

Society will benefit more from a surgeon who

has a sufficient volume of surgery to maintain proficiency through frequent use of well-honed skills
than from one who has a low volume and who
serves also as a primary care physician. The early
identification of disease while it is in its undifferentiated stage requires specific training and is not a
skill that can automatically be assumed by someone
whose training has been mostly in hospital intensive
care units. It is unfortunate that when the demand
for complex technical procedures is inadequate to
fully occupy specialists trained to perform them, the
specialists' remaining time is spent providing care
(frequently primary care) in areas where training
was limited and often deficient.

Many physicians eventually enter a type of practice different from that which their residency prepared them for; the question remains whether
many, especially those entering primary care, will
undergo the difficult and costly retraining necessary
to do the job well.

The World Health Organization, United Nations, and other organizations sponsored a World
Conference on Medical Education in Edinburgh,
Scotland, in 1988, addressing the need for reform
in medical education. The meeting made a number
of recommendations to medical schools in its "Edinburgh Declaration":

1. Enlarge the range of settings in which educational programs are conducted, to include all health
resources of the community, not hospitals alone.

2. Ensure that curriculum content reflects national health priorities and the availability of affordable resources.

3. Ensure continuity of learning throughout
life, shifting emphasis from the passive methods so
widespread now to more active learning, including
self-directed and independent study as well as tuto-
rial methods.

4. Build both curriculum and examination systems to ensure the achievement of professional
competence and social values, not merely the retention and recall of information.

5. Train teachers as educators, not solely as experts in content, and reward education excellence
as fully as excellence in biomedical research or clinical practice.

6. Complement instruction about the management of patients with increased emphasis on promotion of health and prevention of diseases.

7. Pursue integration of education in science
and education in practice, also using problem-solv-

ing in clinical and community settings as a base for learning.

8. Employ selection methods for medical students that go beyond intellectual ability and academic achievement to include evaluation of personal qualities.

9. Encourage and facilitate cooperation between the Ministries of Health, Ministries of Education, community health services, and other relevant bodies in joint policy development, program planning, implementation, and review.

10. Ensure admission policies that match the numbers of students trained with national needs for doctors.

11. Increase the opportunity for joint learning, research, and service with other health and health-related professions, as part of the training for teamwork.

12. Clarify responsibility and allocate resources for continuing medical education.

Interpersonal Skills

One of the foremost skills of the family physician is the ability to effectively utilize the knowledge of interpersonal relations in the management of patients. This powerful element of clinical medicine is perhaps the specialty's most useful tool. Modern society considers the medical care system inadequate in those situations in which understanding and compassion are important to the patient's comfort and recovery from illness. Physicians are too often seen as lacking this personal concern and in being unskilled in understanding personal anxiety and feelings. There is an obvious need to nourish the seed of compassion and concern for sick people with which students enter medical school.

Our current health care system overvalues procedures at the expense of what has come to appear as old-fashioned medical compassion and concern, producing physicians who feel their task is to cure rather than care. We think of the body as a machine with replaceable parts and have forgotten that abdominal pain can come from life as well as from the gallbladder. The use of sympathy, tact, and gentleness in caring for a patient is as essential to quality medical care as are manipulative skills.

Good interpersonal skills enhanced by compassion enable the physician to dissect out the tangled mass of personal difficulties that so often form the core of functional disease or magnify the symptoms of an organic condition.

Family practice emphasizes the integration of compassion, empathy, and personalized concern to a greater degree than does a more technical or task-oriented specialty. Some of the earnest solicitude of the old country doctor and his untiring compassion for people must be incorporated as the effective yet impersonal modern medical procedures are applied. The patient should be viewed compassionately as a person in distress, who needs to be treated with concern, dignity, and personal consideration. He or she has a right to be given some insight into his or her problems, a reasonable appraisal of the potential outcome, and a realistic picture of the emotional, financial, and occupational expenses involved in his or her care.

To relate well to patients, a physician must develop compassion and courtesy, the ability to establish rapport and to communicate effectively, the ability to gather information rapidly and to organize it logically, the skills required to identify all significant patient problems and to manage these problems appropriately, the ability to listen, the skills necessary to motivate people, and the ability to observe and detect nonverbal clues.

Much of the family physician's effectiveness in interpersonal relationships depends upon his or her charisma. Charisma is a personal magic of leadership, a magnetic charm or appeal that arouses special loyalty or enthusiasm. The charismatic physician is most likely to engender maximal patient compliance and satisfaction. The physician must be aware of his or her own feelings, however, and their effect upon the patient. Charisma can be a useful therapeutic tool, but one must learn how and when to use it effectively, because it can also rebound with unfavorable consequences. The physician should be aware that the patient's needs are paramount. The temptation to take an ego trip is frequent and hazardous.

Accessibility

Just as charisma is therapeutic, so too is the mere *availability* of the physician. The feeling of security that the patient gains just by knowing that he or she can "touch" the physician, either in person or by phone, is in itself therapeutic and has a comforting and calming influence. Accessibility is an essential feature of primary care. Services must be available when needed and should be within geographic proximity. When primary care is not available, many individuals turn to hospital emergency departments. Emergency room care is, of course, fine for emergencies, but it is no substitute for the personalized, long-term, comprehensive care that a family physician can provide.

Diagnostic Skills—Undifferentiated Problems

Above all, the family physician must be an outstanding diagnostician. Skills in this area must be honed to perfection, since problems are usually seen in their early, undifferentiated state and without the degree of resolution that usually is present by the time patients are referred to consulting specialists. This is a unique feature of family practice, because symptoms seen at this stage are often vague and nondescript, with signs being either minimal or absent. Unlike the consulting specialist, the family physician does not evaluate the case after it has been preselected by another physician, and the diagnostic procedures used by the family physician must be selected from the entire spectrum of medicine.

At this stage of disease, there are often only subtle differences between the early symptoms of serious disease and those of self-limiting, minor ailments. To the inexperienced person, the clinical pictures may appear identical, but to the astute and experienced family physician, one symptom will be more suspicious than another because of the greater probability that it signals a potentially serious illness. Diagnoses are frequently made on the basis of probability, and the likelihood that a specific disease is present frequently depends upon the incidence of the disease relative to the symptom seen in the physician's community during a given time of year. Approximately one fourth of all patients seen will never be assigned a final, definitive diagnosis, since the resolution of a presenting symptom or a complaint may occur before a specific diagnosis can be made. Pragmatically, this is an efficient method that is less costly and achieves high patient satisfaction—even though it may be disquieting to the purist physician, who feels that a thorough work-up and specific diagnosis should always be obtained. Similarly, family physicians are more likely to use a therapeutic trial to confirm the diagnosis.

The family physician is an expert in the rapid assessment of a problem presented for the first time. He or she evaluates its potential significance, often making a diagnosis by exclusion rather than by inclusion, after making certain that the symptoms are not those of a serious problem. Once this is assured, some time is allowed to elapse. Time is used as an efficient diagnostic aid. Follow-up visits are scheduled at appropriate intervals to watch for subtle changes in the presenting symptoms. The physician usually identifies the symptom that has the greatest discriminatory value and watches it more closely than others. The most significant clue to the true nature of the illness may depend upon subtle changes in this key symptom. The family physician's effectiveness is often determined by his or her knack for perceiving the hidden or subtle dimensions of illness and following them closely.

The maxim that an accurate history is the most important factor in arriving at an accurate diagnosis is especially appropriate to family medicine, since symptoms may be the only obvious feature of an illness at the time it is presented to the family physician. Further inquiry into the nature of the symptoms, time of onset, extenuating factors, and other unique subjective features may provide the only diagnostic clues available at such an early stage. Above all, the family physician must be a skilled clinician with the ability to evaluate symptoms, verbal and nonverbal communication, and early signs of illness in order to choose those tests that are of greatest value in diagnosing a problem early.

The family physician must be a perceptive humanist, alert to early identification of new problems. Arriving at an early diagnosis may, in fact, be of less importance than determining the real reason that the patient came to the physician. The symptoms may be due to a self-limiting or acute problem, but anxiety or fear may be the true precipitating factor. Although the symptom may be hoarseness that has resulted from postnasal drainage accompanying an upper respiratory tract infection, the patient may fear that it is caused by a laryngeal carcinoma similar to that recently diagnosed in a friend. Clinical evaluation must rule out the possibility of laryngeal carcinoma, but the patient's fears and apprehension regarding this possibility must also be allayed. Similarly, a 42-year-old man with influenza and pleuritic chest pain may be anxious and apprehensive because his father died at age 45 of an acute myocardial infarction. (In fact, a frequent reason for a patient's requesting a complete checkup and electrocardiogram is the recent heart attack of an acquaintance at work.) Mild thrombophlebitis in a 35-year-old woman could bring her to the physician in a more anxious state than is warranted because her mother died from a pulmonary embolus; likewise, a housewife's anxiety about breast cancer may well stem from a friend's recent breast surgery.

Every physical problem has an emotional component, and although this factor is usually minimal, it can be extremely significant. A patient's personality, fears, and anxieties play a role in every illness.

THE FAMILY PHYSICIAN AS COORDINATOR

Francis Peabody, Professor of Medicine at Harvard Medical School from 1921 to 1927, was a man ahead of his time; his comments of 70 years ago remain appropriate today:

> *Never was the public in need of wise, broadly trained advisors so much as it needs them today to guide them through the complicated maze of modern medicine. The extraordinary development of medical science, with its consequent diversity of medical specialism and the increasing limitations in the extent of special fields—the very factors, indeed, which are creating specialists—in themselves create a new demand, not for men who are experts along narrow lines, but for men who are in touch with many lines.*

The family physician, by virtue of his or her breadth of training in a wide variety of medical disciplines, has unique insights into the skills possessed by physicians in the more limited specialties. The family physician is best prepared to select specialists whose skills can be applied most appropriately to a given case as well as to coordinate the activities of each so that they are not counterproductive.

As medicine becomes more specialized and complex, the family physician's role as the integrator of health services becomes increasingly important. The family physician not only facilitates the patient's access to the whole health care system but also interprets the activities of this system to the patient, explaining the nature of the illness, the implications of the treatment, and the effect of both upon the patient's way of life. The following statement from the Millis Commission Report concerning expectations of the patient is especially appropriate.

> *The patient wants someone of high competence and good judgment to take charge of the total situation, someone who can serve as coordinator of all the medical resources that can help solve his problem. He wants a company president who will make proper use of his skills and knowledge of more specialized members of the firm. He wants a quarterback who will diagnose the constantly changing situation, coordinate the whole team, and call on each member for the particular contributions that he is best able to make to the team effort.*

Such breadth of vision is important for a coordinating physician. He or she must have a realistic overview of the problem and an awareness of the many alternative routes in order to select the one that is most appropriate. A physician familiar with one form of treatment tends to rely on it excessively, whereas the family physician can select the best approach from all possible alternatives. As Pellegrino (1966) has stated:

> *It should be clear, too, that no simple addition of specialties can equal the generalist function. To build a wall one needs more than the aimless piling up of bricks, one needs an architect. Every operation which analyzes some part of the human mechanism requires to be balanced by another which synthesizes and coordinates.*

The complexity of modern medicine frequently involves a variety of health professionals, each with highly developed skills in a particular area. In planning the patient's care, the family physician, having established rapport with a patient and family and having knowledge of the patient's background, personality, fears, and expectations, is best able to select and coordinate the activities of appropriate individuals from the large variety of medical disciplines. He or she can maintain effective communication among those involved, in addition to functioning as the patient's advocate and interpreting to the patient and family the many unfamiliar and complicated procedures being used. This prevents any one consulting physician, unfamiliar with the concepts or actions of all others involved, from ordering a test or medication that would conflict with other treatment. J. E. Dunphy (1964a) has described the value of the surgeon and the family physician working closely as a team:

> *It is impossible to provide high quality surgical care without that knowledge of the whole patient which only a family physician can supply. When their mutual decisions . . . bring hope, comfort and ultimately, health to a gravely ill human being, the total experience is the essence and the joy of medicine.*

The ability to orchestrate the knowledge and skills of diverse professionals is a skill to be learned during training and cultivated in practice. It is not an automatic attribute of all physicians or merely the result of exposure to a large number of professionals. These coordinator skills extend beyond the traditional medical disciplines into the many community agencies and allied health professions as well. Because of his or her close involvement with the community, the family physician is ideally suited to be the integrator of the patient's care, coordinating the skills of consultants when appropriate, and involving community nurses, social agencies, the clergy, or other family members when needed. A knowledge of community health resources and a personal involvement with the community can be used to maximum benefit, not only for diagnostic and therapeutic purposes but also to achieve the best possible level of rehabilitation.

The Family Physician in Practice

The advent of family medicine has led to a renaissance in medical education involving a reassessment of the traditional medical education environment in a teaching hospital. It is now considered more realistic to train a physician in a community atmosphere, providing exposure to the diseases and problems most closely approximating those that he or she will encounter during practice. The ambulatory care skills and knowledge that most medical graduates will need cannot be taught totally within the tertiary medical center. The specialty of family practice emphasizes training in ambulatory care skills in an appropriately realistic environment, using patients representing a cross section of a community and incorporating those problems most frequently encountered by physicians practicing primary care.

The lack of relevance in the referral medical center also applies to the hospitalized patient. Figure 1–1, which is derived from data accumulated in the United States and Great Britain, places the health problems of an average community in perspective. In an adult population of 1000 people aged 16 years or older, 750 will experience at least one illness or injury during an average month. Most of these people will be managed by self-treatment, but 250 patients will consult a physician. Of these, five patients will be referred for consultation to another physician, and nine will be hospitalized—eight of them in a community hospital and one in a university medical center. It is obvious that patients seen in the medical center (the majority of cases used for teaching) represent atypical samples of illness occurring within the community. Students exposed only in this manner develop an unrealistic concept of the kinds of medical problems prevalent in society, and particularly those constituting primary care. It focuses their training on knowledge and skills of limited usefulness in later practice.

In a typical family practice that cares for 1500 to 3000 individuals, two thirds will be seen at least once each year. Family physicians who admit to hospitals average 13.7 hospital visits a week. Those in rural practice average more hospital visits per week (20.2) than do their colleagues in an urban setting (12.5) (AAFP, 1996).

Computers are contributing significantly to cost-

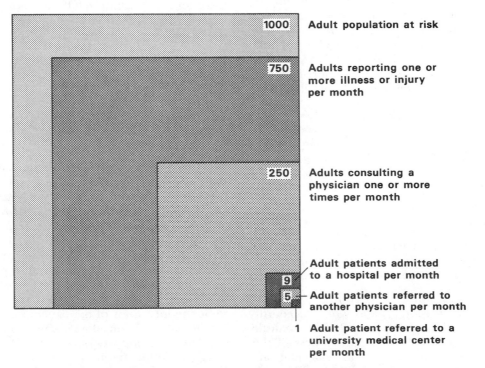

Figure 1–1. Number of persons experiencing illness or injury during an average month, per 1000 adult population. (From White KL, Williams F, Greenberg B. Ecology of medical care. N Engl J Med 1961; 265:885.)

effective, high-quality care in family practice. In May 1996, 70 per cent of office-based family physicians used a computer in their office, primarily for billing, accounting, electronic claims processing, word processing, and appointment scheduling. In addition, 85 percent had a personal or home computer and most of these (74%) were PC compatible. Of these, 81 percent had CD-ROM and 85 percent a modem (AAFP, personal communication, 1996).

PRACTICE CONTENT

The National Ambulatory Medical Care Survey conducted by the National Center for Health Statistics of the United States Department of Health and Human Services has, since 1975, annually reported the problems seen by office-based physicians (in all specialties) in the United States. A symptom classification was developed to document the complaints presented by patients to physicians in their offices. The National Ambulatory Medical Care Survey reverses the previous trend of evaluating the prevalence of disease after the fact (measuring causes of death) by evaluating the presenting complaints or symptoms. The 20 most common symptoms or reasons prompting office visits in 1991 are shown in Table 1–1. The principal diagnoses resulting from these visits are documented in Table 1–2.

In 1991, 12.7 per cent of patients of all ages were seen for high blood pressure and almost as many were seen for depression (6.1%) as for hypercholesterolemia (6.9%) (NCHS Advance Data, 1993).

OFFICE VISITS

Available data concerning primary care indicate that more people use this type of medical service than any other and that, contrary to popular opinion, sophisticated medical technology is not normally either required or overused in basic primary care encounters. Indeed, most primary care visits arise from patients requesting care for relatively uncomplicated problems, many of which are self-limiting but cause them concern or discomfort. Treatment is often symptomatic, consisting of pain relief or anxiety reduction rather than a "cure."

TABLE 1–1. The 20 Most Common Principal Reasons for Office Visits in the United States (1991)*

Rank	Principal Reason for Visit	Number of Visits in Thousands	Per Cent	Cumulative Per Cent
1	General medical examination	29,720	4.4	4.4
2	Cough	24,263	3.6	8.0
3	Routine prenatal examination	19,675	2.9	10.9
4	Symptoms referable to the throat	17,882	2.7	13.6
5	Postoperative visit	16,308	2.4	16.0
6	Earache or ear infection	13,404	2.0	18.0
7	Well-baby examination	13,276	2.0	20.0
8	Back symptoms	12,977	1.9	21.9
9	Skin rash	12,119	1.8	23.7
10	Stomach pain, cramps, and spasms	11,106	1.7	25.4
11	Fever	10,318	1.5	26.9
12	Headache, pain in head	10,128	1.5	28.4
13	Vision dysfunctions	10,011	1.5	29.9
14	Knee symptoms	9,522	1.4	31.3
15	Nasal congestion	8,444	1.3	32.6
16	Blood pressure test	7,645	1.1	33.7
17	Head cold, upper respiratory infection (coryza)	7,616	1.1	34.8
18	Neck symptoms	7,193	1.1	35.9
19	Depression	7,060	1.1	37.0
20	Low back symptoms	7,051	1.1	38.1
	Totals	**255,718**	**38.1**	**38.1**
	All other reasons	413,971	61.8	

*Total number of visits in thousands: 669,689.

Source: National Center for Health Statistics. (Schappert SM) 1991 Summary: National Ambulatory Medical Care Survey. Advance Data from Vital and Health Statistics of the Centers for Disease Control and Prevention. No. 230. DHHS pub. no. (PHS) 93-1250. Hyattsville, MD, Public Health Service, March 29, 1993.

TABLE 1–2. Rank Order of Office Visits by Diagnosis (1991)

Rank	Diagnosis	Per Cent	Cumulative Per Cent
1	Essential hypertension	3.5	3.5
2	Normal pregnancy	3.1	6.6
3	General medical examination	2.7	9.3
4	Health supervision of infant or child	2.6	11.9
5	Acute upper respiratory infections of multiple or unspecified sites	2.5	14.4
6	Suppurative and unspecified otitis media	2.4	16.8
7	Diabetes mellitus	1.9	18.7
8	Chronic sinusitis	1.7	20.4
9	Glaucoma	1.6	22.0
10	Acute pharyngitis	1.6	23.6
11	Bronchitis, not specified as acute or chronic	1.5	25.1
12	Diseases of sebaceous glands	1.4	26.5
13	Allergic rhinitis	1.4	27.9
14	Asthma	1.3	29.2
15	Cataract	1.1	30.3
16	Contact dermatitis and other eczema	1.1	31.4
17	Sprains and strains of other and unspecified parts of back	1.0	32.4
18	Special investigations and examinations	0.9	33.3
19	Neurotic disorders	0.9	34.2
20	General symptoms	0.9	35.1
	All other diagnoses	64.8	

Source: From National Center for Health Statistics. (Schappert SM) 1991 Summary: National Ambulatory Medical Care Survey. Advance Data from Vital and Health Statistics of the Centers for Disease Control and Prevention. No. 230. DHHS pub. no. (PHS) 93-1250. Hyattsville, MD, Public Health Service, March 29, 1993.

The greatest cost efficiency results when these patients' needs are satisfied, while the self-limiting course of the disease is recognized without incurring unnecessary costs for additional tests.

Each year 75 per cent of people in the United States make at least one visit to a physician. In 1991 the average was 2.7 office visits per person. Females accounted for 59.8 per cent of all visits (3.1 visits per person per year), and males had 2.2 visits per person per year. The annual visit rate ranged from 1.8 visits per person per year for young adults 15 to 24 years of age to 6.0 visits for patients 75 years and older. Approximately 25 per cent of all visits were to family physicians. Only 0.9 per cent of all physician visits made during 1991 ended in hospital admission, and only 3.3 per cent of office visits resulted in referral to another physician (NCHS Advance Data, 1993).

HOME CARE

Although the number of house calls being made by family physicians has declined significantly, home care by other health professionals is increasing because of the need resulting from shortened hospital stays and increased home care involving intravenous fluids, chemotherapy, and respiratory care that previously required hospitalization.

Adelman and associates (1994) surveyed primary care physicians and found that 63 per cent of family physicians made house calls compared with 47 per cent of general internists and 15 per cent of general pediatricians. Those who made house calls shared the belief that house calls are important for good comprehensive patient care and are satisfying for the physician as well as the patient. Reasons given for not making house calls are poor use of time, inadequate reimbursement, and the belief that they pose significant malpractice risks.

The house call continues to be a valuable tool used by family physicians to develop a thorough understanding of patients and their environment, and family practice residencies encourage house calls in their training programs. Family physicians who make house calls report an average of 1.6 per week (AAFP Facts, 1996).

Elderly patients, especially the frail elderly, often have considerable difficulty getting to and from the physician's office. The patient is more comfortable and under less stress at home, and more problems can be identified, leading to improved care. Ramsdell and coworkers (1989) have shown that home visit assessments reveal two new problems and up to eight new treatment recommendations when home visits follow physician office-based assessments. Home visits may be the only way to identify some environmental hazards and to accurately evaluate functional status. They may be the only way to detect neglect and overuse of prescription and over-the-counter medications. A physician who has a clear understanding of the home environment is in a better position to direct the home health care team.

Home visits are more considerate of patients who have impaired mobility, and these patients respond better and may improve more rapidly when cared for at home by health professionals and family members (Kavesh, 1986). Only 15 per cent of patients who need long-term supportive care in the home turn to available community resources; 85 per cent receive care entirely from family and friends.

Cauthen (1981) has described eight different types of house calls: the emergency house call; the acute illness house call; the chronic illness house call; the dying patient house call; the house call to pronounce death; the grief house call; the home management-versus-hospitalization house call; and the home visit house call. Some family physicians routinely visit patients in the home after a mother returns from the hospital with her new baby or after a patient is discharged following a serious illness.

GROUP OR SOLO PRACTICE

The majority of graduating family practice residents enter partnership or group practice. In 1996, 45.8 per cent entered family practice groups, 11.8 per cent joined multispecialty groups, and 8.8 per cent formed two-person practices (partnerships). Only 4.5 per cent of graduates entered solo practice (AAFP Survey, 1996).

Many graduates are attracted to group practice because of the opportunity to share calls. Such an arrangement allows physicians more time with their families and time to remain current with medical advances through continuing education. Many also select group practice because of the professional stimulation of working with colleagues. Group practices allow for overhead to be shared, and the cost of expensive equipment, such as x-ray machines and flexible sigmoidoscopes, can be spread over a wider financial base. Employment of paramedical personnel, such as a nutritionist, clinical pharmacist, or marriage and family counselor, is another luxury more easily borne by groups.

Group practice does, however, involve sacrificing some privacy and individuality, since each physi-

cian must adhere to the will of the majority. Solo practice, with the individual freedom it provides, is still alive and well in the United States. Solo physicians sacrifice the financial advantage of shared office space and more elaborate equipment for the privilege of being their own boss and making decisions unencumbered by the hassles and delays of group decision making.

Group practices are more likely to draw physicians into rural and inner city areas, where solo physicians are unlikely to want to practice "in isolation." Approximately 50 per cent of family physicians are located in towns of 10,000 population or less (Table 1–3).

PHYSICIAN SUPPLY

As the percentage of Americans who receive care from managed care networks continues to increase, the mix of specialties employed by those networks will increasingly determine the number of positions likely to be available to medical graduates. Weiner (1994) projects that by the year 2000, the number of primary care physicians needed will be about right, but specialists will exceed the demand by more than 60 per cent (165,000 more than are

TABLE 1–3. Population of Community in Which Primary Offices of Family Physicians Are Located, May 1995*

Population of Community	n = 2073 Percentage
Population under 5000, not within 25 miles of a major city	11.8
Population under 5000, within 25 miles of a major city	3.6
Population 5000–10,000, not within 25 miles of a major city	6.6
Population 5000–10,000, within 25 miles of a major city	5.6
Population 10,000–25,000, not within 25 miles of a major city	8.6
Population 10,000–25,000, within 25 miles of a major city	9.8
Population 25,000–100,000	20.8
Population 100,000–500,000	16.4
Population over 500,000	14.9
Not reported	2.0

*Includes only active member respondents of the American Academy of Family Physicians.
Source: American Academy of Family Physicians, Practice Profile II Survey, May 1995.
American Academy of Family Physicians. Facts About Family Practice, 1996.

needed). "The issue is not so much a primary care provider shortage as a specialty care surplus." Table 1–4 compares the number of physicians in different specialties who are employed by 16 HMO plans with the number practicing in the United States in 1992. It is clear that when the availability of most jobs is dictated by managed care plans, that physicians in the oversupplied specialties such as cardiology, anesthesiology, radiology, general surgery, pathology, neurology, and ophthalmology will have a difficult time finding employment. Many question whether

TABLE 1–4. Comparison of Selected HMOs' Specialty-Specific Physician Staffing Patterns with National Supply Levels*

Specialty	Staffing of 16 HMOs	1992 US Supply
Total	105.7	180.1
Primary care	49.6	65.7
Family/general practice	10.5	29.3
General internal medicine	25.0	23.3
Pediatrics	13.2	13.1
(% Primary care)	(46.8)	(36.0)
Medical subspecialties	12.5	17.8
Allergy	1.3	1.1
Cardiology	2.2	4.9
Dermatology	2.2	2.5
Endocrinology	0.8	0.8
Gastroenterology	1.5	2.4
Hematology/oncology	1.8	1.9
Infectious disease	0.6	0.6
Nephrology	0.7	1.1
Pulmonary disease	1.0	1.8
Rheumatology	0.6	0.9
Surgical specialties	29.7	43.8
Obstetrics/gynecology	10.4	11.4
General surgery	5.7	10.8
Neurosurgery	0.4	1.4
Ophthalmology	3.1	5.6
Orthopedics	4.2	6.5
Otolaryngology	2.5	2.7
Plastic surgery	0.5	1.7
Thoracic surgery	0.1	0.7
Urology	2.4	3.1
Hospital-based specialties	—	22.0
Radiology	5.3	8.6
Anesthesiology	4.4	9.2
Pathology	1.9	4.2
Other	—	—
Psychiatry	3.9	12.0
Emergency medicine	5.1	5.6
Neurology	1.5	2.7

*All figures represent full-time equivalent physicians per 100,000 population. Totals and subtotals may include some subspecialties not listed. HMO indicates health maintenance organization.
Source: Weiner JP. Forecasting the effects of health reform on US physician workforce requirement: Evidence from HMO staffing patterns. JAMA 1994;272:222–230.

physicians in these specialties can be adequately retrained to provide quality primary care.

In 1980 the Graduate Medical Education National Advisory Committee projected a surplus of 150,000 physicians in the United States by the year 2020. A recent study by the American Academy of Family Physicians estimates that by the year 2000, there will be an excess of 37,000 specialists and a need for 34,000 primary care physicians (AAFP Directors' Newsletter, Dec. 13, 1996).

Another federally convened group, the Council on Graduate Medical Education (COGME), projects a shortage of 80,000 generalists and a surplus of 120,000 specialists by the year 2020 (COGME Third Report, 1992). COGME appropriately feels that the medical profession has a responsibility to produce a physician workforce that meets the nation's needs. Until recently, academic health centers have not accepted this responsibility, and many remain slow to change. If the number of generalists being produced is to increase, residency positions must be based on societal and educational needs and not upon hospital service needs as in the past. In addition, disincentives must be removed and "the practice income of generalists would have to exceed that of specialists in order to overcome the specializing influences upon medical students of the educational milieu" (COGME, 1992). COGME considers the family physician, general internist, and general pediatrician as members of the generalist specialties, since these are the only physicians "trained to function as comprehensive primary care physicians for the undifferentiated problems of their patients" (COGME, 1992).

If the growth in physician supply continues, American Medical Association analysts warn that "soon some physicians might not have enough work to stay proficient, and the status of the profession might decline." Similarly, the quality of primary care will decline as physicians trained in a surplus subspecialty practice primary care without retraining. Rhee and associates (1981) showed that when physicians practice outside their specialty areas, the relative quality of their performance declines.

As much needed changes in the American medical system are implemented, it would be wise to keep some perspective on the situation regarding physician distribution. Paul Beeson commented in 1974:

I have no doubt at all that a good family doctor can deal with the great majority of medical episodes quickly and competently. A specialist, on the other hand, feels that he must be thorough, not only because of his training but also because he has a reputation to protect. He, therefore, spends more time with each patient and orders more laboratory work. The result is a waste of doctors' time and patients' money. This not only inflates the national health bill, but also creates an illusion of doctor shortage when the only real need is to have the existing doctors doing the right things.

REFERENCES

Adelman AM, Fredman L, Knight AL. House call practices: a comparison by specialty. J Fam Pract 1994;38:39–44.

Ad Hoc Committee on Education for Family Practice of the Council on Medical Education of the American Medical Association (Willard Committee). Meeting the Challenge of Family Practice (report), September 1966.

American Academy of Family Physicians. Congress Reporter, Oct. 5–7, 1993.

American Academy of Family Physicians. Directors' Newsletter, Dec. 13, 1996.

American Academy of Family Physicians. Facts About Family Practice, 1996.

American Academy of Family Physicians. Report on Survey of 1996 Graduating Family Practice Residents. Reprint No. 155V.

American Medical Association. Council on Long Range Planning and Development. The Future of Family Practice. Chicago, American Medical Association, 1988.

Balint M. The Doctor, His Patient and the Illness. New York, Pitman Publishing Corp., 1965.

Beeson PB. Some good features of the British National Health Service. J Med Educ 1974;49:43.

Bertakis KD. Cost-effectiveness of care by family physicians. J Am Board Fam Pract 1993;6:609–612.

Boex JR, Edwards J, Garg M, et al. Generalist and Specialist Practitioner: Analyses of Quality and Costs of Care. Report to the W. K. Kellogg Foundation, October 7, 1993.

Cauthen DB. The house call in current medical practice. J Fam Pract 1981;13:209.

Cherkin DC, Rosenblatt RA, Hart LG, et al. The use of medical resources by residency-trained family physicians and general internists: Is there a difference? Med Care 1987;25(6):455–469.

Citizens' Commission on Graduate Medical Education of the American Medical Association (Millis Commission). The Graduate Education of Physicians (report), August 1966.

Council on Graduate Medical Education. The Third Report of the Council. Washington, D.C., U.S. Dept. of Health and Human Services, Public Health Services, Bureau of Health Professions, 1992.

Darley W. We need a new specialty: Family practice. New Med Materia 1962;4(3):29.

Dunphy JE. Responsibility and authority in American surgery. Bull Am Coll Surg 1964a;49:9.

Dunphy JE. Role of the family physician in the medical care of the future. New Physician 1964b;13:331.

Family practice, a concept or a reality? JAMA 1963;185:208.

Fox TF. The personal doctor and his relation to the hospital. Lancet 1960;1:743.

Fry J. Common sense and uncommon sensibility. J R Coll Gen Pract 1977;27:9.

Geyman JP. Family Practice: Foundation of Changing Health Care. New York, Appleton-Century-Crofts, 1980.

Gonnella JS, Veloski JJ. The impact of early specialization on the clinical competence of residents. N Engl J Med 1982;306:275.

Graduate Medical Education National Advisory Committee (GMENAC). Final Report, v. 1. Hyattsville, MD, Health Resources Administration, September 1980 (DHHS pub. no. [HRA] 81-651).

Halsted JA. Personal care in medicine of the future. N Engl J Med 1962;267:1233.

James G. The general practitioner of the future. N Engl J Med 1964;270:1286.

Kavesh WN. Home care: Process, outcome, cost. Ann Rev Gerontol Geriatr 1986;6:135–195.

Kimball HR, Young PR. A statement on the generalist physician from the American Boards of Family Practice and Internal Medicine. JAMA 1994;271:315–316.

MacLean DS. Outcome and cost of family physicians' care: Pilot study of three diagnosis-related groups in elderly inpatients. J Am Board Fam Pract 1993;6:588–593.

Marsland DW, Wood M, Mayo F. Content of family practice. In Geyman JP (ed). A Statewide Study in Virginia with Its Clinical, Educational, and Research Implications. New York, Appleton-Century-Crofts, 1976.

McGann KP, Bowman MA. A comparison of morbidity and mortality for family physicians' and internists' admissions. J Fam Pract 1990;31:541–545.

McWhinney IR. An Introduction to Family Medicine. New York, Oxford University Press, 1981.

Mulhausen R, McGee J. Physician need: An alternative projection from a study of large, prepaid group practices. JAMA 1989;261(13):1930–1934.

National Center for Health Statistics. (Schappert SM) 1991 Summary. National Ambulatory Medical Care Survey. Advance Data from Vital and Health Statistics of the Centers for Disease Control and Prevention. No. 230. DHHS pub. no. (PHS) 93-1250. Hyattsville, MD, Public Health Service, March 29, 1993.

Osler W. Aequanimitas, with Other Addresses, 3rd ed. Philadelphia, The Blakiston Co., 1932.

Peabody FW. Doctor and Patient. New York, The Macmillan Co., 1930.

Pellegrino ED. The generalist function in medicine. JAMA 1966;198:541.

Pellegrino ED. Humanism and the Physician. Knoxville, University of Tennessee Press, 1979.

Ramsdell JW, Swart JA, Jackson JE, Renvall M. The yield of a home visit in the assessment of geriatric patients. J Am Geriatr Soc 1989;37(1):17–24.

Rhee S, Luke R, Lyons T, Payne B. Domain of practice and the quality of physician performance. Med Care 1981;19(1):14–23.

Rivo ML, Saultz JW, Wartman SA, DeWitt TG. Defining the generalist physician's training. JAMA 1994;271:1499–1504.

Schroeder SA. Western European responses to physician oversupply. JAMA 1984;252(3):373–384.

Steinwachs DM, Levine DM, Elzinga J, et al. Changing patterns of graduate medical education. N Engl J Med 1982;306:10.

Surgeon-General's Consultant Group on Medical Education. Physicians for a Growing America (Bane Report). Washington, D.C., U.S. Government Printing Office, 1959 (PHS pub. no. 709).

Tumulty PA. What is a clinician and what does he do? N Engl J Med 1970;283(1):20–24.

Tumulty PA. The Effective Clinician: His Methods and Approach to Diagnosis and Care. Philadelphia, W.B. Saunders Co., 1973.

Weiner JP. Forecasting the effects of health reform on US physician workforce requirement: Evidence from HMO staffing patterns. JAMA 1994;272:222–230.

White KL, Williams F, Greenberg B. Ecology of medical care. N Engl J Med 1961;265:885.

World Conference on Medical Education of the World Federation for Medical Education. The Edinburgh Declaration. Edinburgh, Scotland, August 12, 1988.

World Organization of National Colleges, Academies and Academic Associations of General Practitioners/Family Physicians (WONCA). The role of the general practitioner/family physician in health care systems. Victoria, Australia, 1991.

QUESTIONS

1. The most common problem (diagnosis) seen by family physicians in their offices is:
   a. Essential hypertension
   b. Normal pregnancy
   c. Otitis media
   d. Neurotic disorder
   e. Diabetes mellitus

2. COGME, the Council on Graduate Medical Education, estimates that by the year 2020, there will be a shortage of the following number of family physicians.
   a. 20,000
   b. 40,000
   c. 60,000
   d. 80,000

3. Match the following with the person who made the statement.
   a. William Osler
   b. J.E. Dunphy
   c. Oliver Wendell Holmes
   d. Francis Peabody
   e. Edmund Pellegrino

   (1) "The treatment of disease may be entirely impersonal, the care of a patient must be completely personal."
   (2) "It should be clear that no simple addition of specialties can equal the generalist's function."
   (3) "It is much more important to know what sort of patient has a disease than what sort of disease a patient has."
   (4) "It is impossible to provide high quality surgical care without that knowledge of the whole patient which only a family physician can supply."
   (5) "The secret of the care of the patient is in caring for the patient."

Answers appear on **page 603**.

Chapter 2

Ethics in Family Medicine

Warren L. Holleman, Ph.D.
Baruch A. Brody, Ph.D.

Economic, social, legal, and political factors have combined, in recent years, to effect major changes in medical practice and health care policy. Concern for patient rights and patient autonomy, as well as the demands of third-party payers, has transformed the practice of medicine. The ethical issues discussed in this chapter have taken on new dimensions as a result of this transformation.

MEDICINE AS A RELATIONSHIP AND AS A PROFESSION

At its most fundamental level, the practice of medicine should not be regarded as a science, an art, or a business, even though each of these elements is essential. The practice of medicine—particularly primary care medicine—is rooted, instead, in a relationship between the patient as person and the physician as professional (Smith and Churchill, 1986). Two problems currently threaten the quality of that relationship: a misunderstanding of patient autonomy and inappropriate third-party intervention.

When physicians respect the autonomy of their patients so that patients take control of their own health care, the physician is in danger of becoming a hired hand of the patient and the physician–patient relationship is in danger of degenerating into a purely commercial relationship. Patients "own" their bodies, but they should not "own" their physicians. Physicians have an obligation to practice within professional standards of care as well as a right to refrain from doing anything that would violate their own moral and religious conventions (Christie and Hoffmaster, 1986). Physicians must

respect the autonomy of their patients, but they also must avoid the temptation to shirk their own professional and moral responsibilities and must nurture a cooperative relationship with the patient. This is no easy task, but it is through cooperation that the physician and the patient can best work together toward a common goal—to maintain the health of the patient.

The physician–patient relationship also suffers when outside parties interfere inappropriately. When third-party payers set the standard of care, the physician is in danger of becoming a hired hand of the third party. The physician must balance competing loyalties between patients and third parties as well as between professional standards and personal beliefs. In this era of third-party payers, the physician–patient relationship can no longer be exclusive, but it must remain primary. In the remainder of this section we examine two areas in which these problems are particularly prominent: work-related visits and benefits-related visits.

Work- and School-Related Evaluations

Pre-employment examinations, work-release evaluations, school-absence excuses, and athletic physicals comprise a major component of many primary care practices. Inappropriate third-party interventions in this area challenge the primacy of the physician–patient relationship and the integrity of the medical profession. The following guidelines have been suggested (Holleman and Holleman, 1988; Holleman and Matson, 1991) and should help alleviate some of the problems most commonly associated with these evaluations.

The purpose of the pre-employment examination is to determine a person's fitness for work, to protect workers from illnesses and injuries, to protect employers from the costs of preventable job-related illnesses and injuries, and to collect baseline data for the future treatment of such illnesses and injuries. To enable the physician to make such an evaluation, the employer must provide the physician with a detailed job description, including physical requirements, psychological strains, and exposure to toxins. The physician should then tell the employer whether the prospective employee can perform the job without posing a risk to self or others. As discussed further on, the physician should not release any medical records to the employer but should keep them on file as baseline data. At the beginning of the evaluation, the physician should advise the patient of the investigative nature of the visit. The physician must warn the prospective employee regarding health risks of the particular occupation (e.g., toxins affecting pregnancies, stresses affecting hypertensive patients) and must tell him or her of any problems detected in the course of the evaluation, regardless of their effect on job performance.

Work-release evaluations, school-release evaluations, and athletic physicals should be performed in accordance with the same guidelines as pre-employment physicals, but they do present some additional problems of their own. Most work- and school-release evaluations involve short-term absences for minor problems for which there are few, if any, objective findings. Often workers and students present after their illness or injury has resolved. These absences often reflect personal, family, or job-related problems that are not strictly medical in nature. Investigating such problems for employers and school administrators damages the physician–patient relationship and discredits medicine as a healing profession. Patients will have difficulty trusting a physician who investigates on one occasion but offers therapy on another. We recommend that physicians encourage employers and school administrators to develop nonmedical strategies for policing casual absenteeism. Physicians who do perform these evaluations should minimize the harm to the physician–patient relationship and to the integrity of the profession by evaluating only in the context of treatment and by refusing to release confidential medical information to employers and school administrators.

Benefits-Related Evaluations

Many patients present to primary care physicians seeking to be certified as eligible for workers' com-

pensation, long-term disability, group or individual medical insurance, Medicare, Medicaid, and veterans' benefits. Many others have already been certified and are seeking proper care under the terms of these programs. Physicians must be familiar with the details of the various programs so as to enable their patients to benefit appropriately from them. Physicians also must be aware of the potential abuses of such programs so as to help protect those who legitimately qualify from being harmed by those who do not. For example, if a patient presents with an on-the-job injury but also requests treatment for some other problem, the physician should file separate bills so that the workers' compensation fund pays only for job-related illnesses and injuries. Physicians who detect intentional abuse should attempt to identify the reasons for the abuse, particularly in the case of habitual, long-term abusers. Long-term abuse of benefits programs can be prevented only if primary care physicians insist that patients receive continuing comprehensive care from one physician or from a small team of physicians who know the patient well.

SPECIAL PROBLEMS IN PRIMARY CARE SETTINGS

Having introduced the concept of medicine as a relationship and as a profession and having seen what this concept means in many primary care contexts, we turn in the next sections to problem areas that challenge our understanding of the physician–patient relationship and of the professional character of medicine.

Confidentiality

The principle of confidentiality is one of the most widely accepted and historically influential principles governing the patient–physician relationship in Western cultures. The Hippocratic Oath mandates that the physician not divulge "whatsoever I shall see or hear in the course of my profession as well as outside my profession in my intercourse with men, if it be what should not be published abroad." The 1980 Principles of Medical Ethics of the American Medical Association mandate that the physician "shall safeguard patient confidences within the constraints of the law."

Confidentiality is important as a way of encouraging patients to be frank in their communications with physicians, as a way of physicians keeping an implicit promise to patients that their confidence will be respected, and as a way of emphasizing the patient's right to privacy. In all these ways, preserving confidentiality strengthens the relationship between an autonomous patient and a professional physician.

As the delivery of health care has changed from the model of a single physician caring for individual patients to the model of a team of health care workers in an institutional setting providing care to a wide variety of patients, the mandate of confidentiality has changed. The emphasis has switched from physicians keeping secrets to information about patients being divulged only to those members of the health care team and those institutional employees who have a need for the information, either to provide appropriate care or to meet appropriate institutional needs (e.g., monitoring of quality of care or organizing reimbursement). The underlying theme remains that information should not be provided to anyone else without the patient's consent.

This last point deserves special emphasis because it structures the decision on when it is appropriate to provide information about the patient to insurance companies and to employers. Providing such information is perfectly appropriate if the patient consents; otherwise, it is not. For this reason, patients are commonly asked to authorize the release of information to particular individuals; the principle of confidentiality is not breached if information is provided pursuant to such a release (Bruce, 1984). However, the scope of information supplied and the persons to whom it is supplied are determined by the patient's instructions. Thus, if a patient requests a statement certifying that he or she is fit to return to work, it is not appropriate for the physician to provide to the employer a full account of the patient's illness and treatment; all that should be provided is the requested statement about the patient's fitness to return to work.

There are circumstances in which our society has judged that the need for information outweighs the principle of confidentiality; these are the circumstances in which the physician is required by law to disclose otherwise confidential information regardless of the wishes of the patient. The exact circumstances vary from jurisdiction to jurisdiction and are determined by state statutes and court decisions. Common circumstances include certain types of judicial proceedings, suspected abuse of dependent individuals such as children and the frail elderly, venereal and communicable diseases, and gunshot wounds (Bruce, 1984). In recent years, following the *Tarasoff* decision in California (Tarasoff, 1974), the concept has emerged that physicians are obligated to warn and/or to take measures to pro-

tect third parties threatened by the behavior of their patients, even if doing so involves a breach of confidentiality. The scope of that principle is far from clear; one obvious controversial example is whether physicians should warn the spouses or regular sexual partners of patients who test positively for the human immunodeficiency virus (HIV) about the threat this illness poses to them.

The principle of confidentiality extends to not providing information to family members of competent adult patients unless the patients want the information to be shared. Often, it will be clear that the patient has no concern about the sharing of information with his or her family. In cases of doubt, the patient should be consulted, especially if the information is of a sensitive nature or if there is evidence of family discord. An appropriate practice on admitting a patient to a hospital is to ask the patient to identify a particular family member, if any, to whom information should be provided for distribution to the family if the patient is not capable of fulfilling that role (e.g., in the immediate postoperative period).

Certain cases are particularly troublesome. Among the most troublesome are those involving teenage patients. Information about pediatric patients is, of course, provided directly to the parents of the patients and not to the patients themselves; information about adult patients is, of course, provided directly to the patient and not the patient's parents. What about teenage patients seeking abortions, contraceptive advice, or treatment for venereal diseases, substance abuse, or psychiatric problems? Unless confidentiality can be guaranteed, such patients may not seek out the care they need. If confidentiality is protected, such patients may not get the parental counseling and support from which they could also benefit. Considerable confusion exists about the morally appropriate and legally mandated approach to confidentiality of information involving adolescent patients (Morrissey et al., 1986). Equally troubling are cases involving elderly patients who are less than fully competent but far from totally demented. Families of such patients often ask physicians to provide them with information about the patient's condition, information that they may not want to share with the patient. Such a request may be perfectly appropriate for the clearly incompetent demented patient, whereas it is obviously inappropriate for normal geriatric patients. How to handle cases that fall in between these two extremes is unclear.

Informed Consent

The principle of informed consent is a much more recently articulated principle than the principle of confidentiality; the actual phrase "informed consent" first appeared in 1957 in the court case *Salgo* v. *Leland Stanford Jr. University Board of Trustees.* It has come, however, to be accepted as a fundamental principle governing the physician–patient relationship.

The principle's basic mandate is that a physician must obtain the free and informed consent of a patient, if the patient is competent to give that consent, or of the patient's surrogate, if the patient is not competent, before medical treatment is provided. Two exceptions are normally recognized. The first (the *emergency exception*) is invoked when emergency treatment is necessary to protect the patient's life or health and consent cannot be obtained in a timely fashion. The second (the *therapeutic privilege*) is invoked when there is strong reason to believe that the very attempt to obtain consent will be harmful to the patient because of the psychological impact of the information conveyed (Rozovsky, 1984).

Several complementary accounts of the significance of the principle of informed consent are available. One stresses the clinical benefits (in terms of building trust and obtaining compliance) from a therapeutic regimen begun as a result of a joint patient–physician decision rather than as a result of a unilateral physician decision. The other stresses the patient's right to control what happens to his or her body; the resulting obligation of the physician to obtain informed consent is the way in which the physician respects this right.

The standard practice in many institutions is to obtain written documentation of informed consent primarily (if not exclusively) in cases of invasive procedures. This practice should not be understood to mean that the principle of informed consent does not apply to other medical interventions; it applies to all of them. Signed consent forms are merely written evidence of the informed consent already obtained, and the practice reflects the prudent desire to obtain written documentation in cases in which potential liability is highest. Informed consent, as opposed to the written documentation of that consent, should be obtained in all cases, both as a way of obtaining clinical benefits and as a way of respecting patient's rights.

There has been considerable disagreement about the amount and type of information that must be supplied to the patient. Obviously, only a portion of the relevant information known by the physician can be conveyed to the patient. Moreover, any attempt to provide too much information may result in the physician overwhelming and confusing the patient. Some selection of information is required, and the disagreement centers around which principle of selection to adopt.

Two different proposals have been adopted by America's courts (Rozovsky, 1984). The first is the *professional practice standard*, which maintains that a consent is informed if the patient has been provided the information that reasonable medical practitioners would normally provide under similar circumstances. The second is the *reasonable person standard*, which maintains that a consent is informed if the patient has been provided the information that a reasonable person would need to have in order to make a decision about whether to undergo the therapy in question. The information to be provided would presumably fall under the categories shown in Table 2–1.

Most commentators have argued for the second standard, since it better corresponds to the goals of informed consent, but a majority of courts have adopted the usually less demanding professional practice standard (Rozovsky, 1984). Clinicians are, we believe, best advised to adopt the usually more stringent reasonable person standard, since it provides all the clinical and moral benefits of obtaining informed consent while firmly ensuring that the legal requirement of informed consent is satisfied. Clinicians also must be careful to provide that information using terminology that patients are likely to understand.

A very difficult problem arises when one is dealing with patients whose competency is impaired. Informed consent is obtained from the patient when the patient is clearly competent and from the patient's surrogate (a legally appointed guardian, if available, or the closest family member) if the patient is clearly incompetent. What, however, should one do when the patient's mental capacities are

TABLE 2–1. Elements of Informed Consent Under Reasonable Person Standard

---

Nature of the patient's condition (e.g., hypertension)
Description of the treatment proposed (e.g., particular medication)
Benefits of proposed treatment (e.g., control of hypertension and resulting lowering of risk of disease)
Risks of proposed treatment (e.g., side effects for that medication)
Alternatives (e.g., other medications, diet and exercise, no intervention)
Costs of proposed treatment

Source: From Rakel RE: Textbook of Family Practice, 4th ed. Philadelphia, WB Saunders, 1990.

clearly impaired but present to some degree? This problem is partially alleviated when one remembers that the assessment of the patient's competency is not an assessment of the patient's total ability to manage all his or her affairs; it is just the assessment of whether at this moment the patient can (1) receive the information relevant to giving or refusing informed consent for this particular treatment, (2) remember that information, (3) appropriately assess and use that information to make a decision, and (4) make a decision. Although no formal test exists to ensure that the patient has the capacity to perform items 1 to 4 in the list, a careful discussion with the patient will usually enable the physician to ascertain whether these criteria are satisfied. If doubt remains, one should obtain consent from both the patient and the surrogate.

A second difficulty involves teenage patients. Informed consent is obtained from parents before one treats children, but from patients once they become adults. How should physicians treat teenage patients? Most states have passed special laws allowing physicians to treat them after obtaining only their consent when (1) the treatment is for venereal disease, pregnancy or contraception, or drug-related problems, (2) they are living away from their parents and are responsible for their own affairs, or (3) they are married. Other cases (particularly abortion) are more problematic (Morrissey et al., 1986).

The "Noncompliant" Patient

Implicit in the principle of informed consent, the principle that medical treatment can only be provided after the patient has freely and knowingly consented to it, is the concept that a patient may choose not to comply with the physician's recommendations and that the choice not to comply must be respected. This concept can easily be misunderstood, however, leading to a quick and facile acceptance of a patient's noncompliance before its meaning is properly understood.

Most cases of noncompliance involve failures of communication, lack of trust due to previous bad experiences with the physician in question or others, and psychological and psychopathological factors. Only a minority of cases involve a true value difference between the physician and the patient. This finding has profound implications for the clinical management of noncompliance. Physicians confronting noncompliant patients need to assess the noncompliance, evaluate its cause, and react appropriately. Table 2–2 indicates how such a noncompli-

TABLE 2–2. Evaluation of Noncompliance

Cause	Clinical Response
Problem in communication	Patient should be reinformed about the need for treatment
Failure of trust	Address question of mistrust Involve other physicians who may be trusted
Psychological factors	Treat anxiety, depression, and so on
Value conflict	Respect patient wishes

Source: From Rakel RE: Textbook of Family Practice, 4th ed. Philadelphia, WB Saunders, 1990. (Reprinted with permission.)

ance assessment would proceed. In short, morality does not call on the physician to accept at face value every episode of noncompliance on the part of the patient. Doing so may in fact constitute a form of disrespect for the patient. What morality does call for is a full evaluation of the cause of the noncompliance, appropriate responses, where possible, to eliminate the cause, and respect for the patient's noncompliance only when it is an informed and competent refusal that is based on a difference between the patient's and the physician's values.

Even in those cases in which noncompliance represents an informed and competent refusal of the physician's recommendations because the patient's values differ, there may well exist alternative, second-best forms of treatment that could be mutually acceptable. Consider a patient who refuses to stay in a hospital for a full evaluation because the patient is concerned about the need to be home to handle personal problems. Such a patient should be scheduled for an outpatient evaluation, even if it is not as satisfactory as a full evaluation in the hospital. (More examples of such compromises are provided later.) Respecting patient values in cases of noncompliance is not a matter of letting the patient win a power struggle; it is, more often, finding a mutually acceptable (even though not necessarily optimal) course of action. A failure to seek out such alternatives may often represent a lack of respect for the patient.

A form of noncompliance that deserves special attention is the patient who does not fill the prescription the physician writes. This is sometimes due to the patient's financial condition. The optimal medication, from the physician's perspective, may cost too much from the patient's perspective. Particularly when dealing with patients who have high medication bills because they need so many drugs or with patients who have very limited means, physicians should raise the question of cost frankly and explore less expensive but satisfactory (even if not optimal) medications.

A similar problem often arises when one considers the question of side effects of various drugs. Different patients with different values and different tolerances may find certain side effects unacceptable. The physician should certainly not assume that a pattern of side effects that is acceptable to the physician will be acceptable to the patient. Taking the patient's values into account in deciding which medication to order is a far clearer example of respecting the patient's values than simply accepting a patient's noncompliance with a particular prescription.

SPECIAL PROBLEMS IN TERTIARY CARE SETTINGS

Quality of care can be improved by careful attention to the components examined thus far: the physician–patient relationship, medicine as a profession, confidentiality, informed consent, and the promotion of patient compliance. When the focus shifts from primary care provided by the family physician to care provided by subspecialists in tertiary care settings, new problems arise and old problems become even more complicated. The next two sections examine ways of resolving some of these problems.

Referrals

Decisions regarding referrals and consultations (see Chapter 12 of Rakel, *Textbook of Family Practice,* 5th edition, for the distinction between referrals and consultations) are often accompanied by great confusion. Referrals to subspecialists practicing in tertiary care institutions can provoke anxiety on the part of patients. The referring physician risks losing a patient and a substantial amount of money and is subject to embarrassment if a mistake is discovered. Referrals sometimes degenerate into power struggles between subspecialists and generalists. Because primary care is a community-based discipline, there is much debate and little consensus as to the primary care physician's role in the tertiary care setting (Christie and Hoffmaster, 1986). The following guidelines about appropriate referrals and about continuity through referrals are intended to help clarify these responsibilities and thus ease the tension and improve the quality of care.

Decisions to use consultants should be based on a realistic assessment of the potentialities and limitations of family medicine as a discipline, of oneself as a physician, and of the facilities available in one's geographic region. Unfortunately, a number of other factors (financial and institutional as well as medical) often cloud the decision-making process and disrupt relations between primary and tertiary care physicians.

Many subspecialists in oversubscribed areas have taken it upon themselves to practice primary care as a means of bolstering their incomes, despite their inadequate training in this area. Conversely, primary care physicians sometimes feel pressured to go beyond their areas of expertise for financial and professional reasons: They fear losing the patient and the income and fear that their seeking consultation might reinforce the misconception that primary care physicians are inferior.

Knowing when to use consultants requires courage and humility. Courage is the ability to act competently and wisely without being swayed by irrational fears. Some primary care physicians, motivated by unrealistic fears of mistakes and exposure, refer too early. Humility, on the other hand, is the willingness to recognize one's *actual* limitations and to act accordingly. Some primary care physicians, unaware of their limitations, refer too late. A proper combination of courage and humility, along with good working relationships with subspecialists, can prevent most of the problems involved in referring or seeking consultation too early or too late.

Even if the primary care physician does decide to refer the patient, he or she remains the patient's primary physician (Christie and Hoffmaster, 1986). Equipped with a strong knowledge of general medicine, of the patient's medical history, and of the patient's personal traits, and committed to treating the disease in the context of the person and the person in the context of the family, the primary care physician is ideally suited to manage the patient throughout the referral.

When initiating a referral, the primary care physician's responsibilities are to educate the patient on the reasons for referral, to recommend a subspecialist or treatment center best suited to the patient's medical and personal needs, to prepare the patient for what lies ahead, and to provide the specialist with data relevant to the patient's illness. Even after the referral, the primary care physician remains responsible for the quality of the patient's care. This may require translating medical jargon to patients or patient preferences to subspecialists and hospital staff, coordinating the activities of the various consultants, mediating disputes between consultants, ensuring that confidentiality is maintained by the health care team, and counseling patients and their families. The referral process is not complete until the subspecialist and the primary physician have discussed all findings, treatments, results, and recommendations and the patient has discussed these with the primary care physician (Christie and Hoffmaster, 1986).

Sometimes subspecialists disagree on how to manage a particular disorder. Consider the different way that surgeons and cardiologists may treat carotid artery disease. Or consider the range of approaches, within particular subspecialties, in treating certain disorders: differences among gynecologists regarding indications for a hysterectomy and differences among neonatologists in managing severely handicapped infants. This makes the referring physician's task a difficult and delicate one. The referring physician must be aware of the differences between subspecialties and between particular physicians within a subspecialty. The referring physician must know the patient and the patient's family well enough to recommend the appropriate subspecialist. In many cases, the principle of informed consent will mandate that the referring physician educate the patient and the family to the strengths and weaknesses of the available options. Primary care physicians should help their patients find a subspecialist who will be appropriate to both their medical needs and their personal preferences.

Financial Gatekeeping

The soaring costs of health care have led corporations and government agencies to develop prospective payment systems and capitation plans, with primary care physicians often serving as gatekeepers of the health care network. It is hoped that this will save money and streamline the referral process. On the other hand, this might drive a bureaucratic wedge into the physician–patient relationship, allow money to compete with quality in determining the standard of care, and inhibit the physician's freedom to practice an individualized style of medicine.

Prospective reimbursement systems (such as the Medicare diagnosis-related group [DRG] system) save money by limiting the reimbursement available to physicians, thereby encouraging them to do less. Designers of such systems have the legitimate right to require physicians to avoid wasteful procedures and referrals; this prevents unnecessary expenditures and ensures a more just distribution of health care expenditures. Such limitations do not, however, preclude the physician's responsibility to offer the patient the best possible care within the limitations set by those policies. When particular patients require care in excess of the normal level of reimbursement, the primary care physician confronts a major ethical dilemma.

Considerable controversy exists on whether physicians should do everything that they believe may benefit each patient without regard to costs or other societal considerations or whether physicians must not be allowed to ignore the bottom line. Traditionalists tend to ignore the fact that financial considerations have always limited the quality of care available to the poor. The question we are now confronting is whether these considerations may legitimately limit the quality of care available to everyone.

In caring for individual patients, physicians should distinguish between providing what the patient wants and what the patient needs. The controversy concerns whether all procedures and services likely to benefit the patient—as evidenced by outcome data—should be made available to the patient. When patients request unnecessary or marginally beneficial procedures and services, however, physicians must refuse.

It is often recommended that if societal costs necessitate that care be withdrawn from or limited for certain patients, these decisions must be made not at the bedside but at the policy level, prior to and apart from particular situations and applications. Such difficult policy decisions should not be made by physicians alone but should be negotiated at the policy level by the three major competing parties in the health care delivery system: institutional representatives, whose concern it is that the bills be paid; physicians, whose interest is professional integrity and personal income; and patients, who want the best care and the maximum choice at the lowest price. It is an open question whether these recommendations are reasonable, realistic, and appropriate.

THE PHYSICIAN AS HUMAN BEING

The medical profession has, in the past few decades, achieved truly impressive gains in the battle against sickness, suffering, and death. Diseases that killed their victims just a generation ago are now manageable, curable, or even preventable. Yet physicians seem remarkably inept at maintaining their own health and well-being; they suffer high rates of alcoholism, substance abuse, divorce, burnout, and suicide (Hilfiker, 1985). Why can't the healers heal themselves, and what can they do to get on the road to recovery? To deal with these problems, we recommend that physicians learn to distinguish between competence and perfectionism, dedication and "workaholism," and compassion and sentimentalism.

In medical school and residency, young doctors often learn to put their careers ahead of self and family (Gerber, 1983). This dedication is, in some ways, good. Young physicians want to do everything they can to help their patients. But this is often coupled with an unrealistic perception of their capabilities and those of their profession. They allow their egos to become too closely identified with their successes and failures. They become obsessed with insecurity (they are not good enough) and guilt (they do not work hard enough). They worry that they might have missed a diagnosis and fear that their patients will die or suffer unnecessarily. Physicians are not supposed to make mistakes, but they do. Their profession requires staying on top of an ever-expanding field of knowledge, adeptness at a wide range of techniques and skills, making the right decision when fatigued or hassled or angry, picking up on subtle clues or poorly articulated symptoms, and juggling a plethora of human needs at once. Mistakes are inevitable, but talking about them is taboo. The only place mistakes are openly discussed, it seems, is the courtroom (Hilfiker, 1985). To be more effective clinicians, physicians must learn to acknowledge their capacity to err and must learn to discuss errors in a constructive manner. Physicians who do not admit their mistakes are doomed to repeat them. Physicians who discuss their mistakes can learn from them and experience healing in the process.

The physician who takes the time to care for personal and family needs is a more effective clinician because he or she is better able to cope with the stresses and strains of a demanding profession. And, in the case of primary care physicians whose patients know them well, the physician will become a role model for personal health and fitness.

Another area in which physicians must learn to accept their humanity, and the humanity of their patients, is in the area of emotions. Clinicians must help patients recognize, express, and interpret their emotions. Clinicians must become aware of their own emotions, recognize their clinical value, and learn how to express and interpret them. The physician who ignores the emotions dehumanizes the physician–patient relationship. The primary care physician who improperly expresses, utilizes, or interprets emotional factors deprofessionalizes that relationship. Traditionally, physicians have been trained to maintain objectivity, affective neutrality, and clinical detachment. To be scientific, however, does not preclude recognizing the legitimacy of emotions or the necessity of empathy as a legitimate clinical and moral response to suffering. Sometimes a patient's feelings offer a clue to his or her symptoms. Sometimes a physician's feelings in response to a patient offer a clue to the patient's problem. Suffering patients need a physician who will suffer alongside them and who will help them to express and interpret their feelings. When their patients suffer, physicians suffer too. The physician who suffers alongside a suffering patient or family allows the opportunity for healing of self as well as of the patient or family. Many of the physician's feelings, however, cannot be expressed appropriately in the clinical encounter. To maintain personal well-being, therefore, the physician must find appropriate outlets for expression and interpretation.

THE SPECIAL CASE OF EUTHANASIA AND ASSISTED SUICIDE

No discussion of the ethics of family practice would be complete without examining euthanasia and assisted suicide, issues that have provoked considerable public debate and challenged long-standing notions of the physician–patient relationship and the nature of the medical profession. In the coming years, patients may turn increasingly to their family practice physicians for assistance in dying, and thus it is important for family practice physicians to be prepared to respond appropriately.

Some surveys indicate that most Americans favor legalization of some methods of ending the life of a seriously ill or impaired person. In November, 1993, 1254 adult Americans were asked: "Do you think that the law should allow doctors to comply with the wishes of a dying patient in severe distress who asks to have his or her life ended, or not?" Seventy-three per cent responded "Yes." Public support of assisted death has increased steadily over the past decade. In 1982, 53 per cent responded affirmatively to the same question, and in 1987, 62 per cent (Taylor, 1993).

Many fear that aggressive measures to keep them alive, administered against their will, might inflict more suffering and indignity than they wish to bear. Others worry that the pain and debilitation of the illness itself might become unbearable, and want the assurance that escape through euthanasia or assisted suicide is available. These are legitimate concerns: A recent study suggested that terminally ill patients frequently are overtreated against their will, and that physicians continue to undertreat pain despite advances in pain and symptom management (Solomon et al., 1993). Another study has shown that most terminal geriatric patients prefer palliative care but that these "patients . . . exert strikingly little influence in the making of the treatment decision" and frequently are misinformed regarding the terminal nature of their condition (Prigerson, 1992). A major factor, according to the study, is physicians' own discomfort with death. Physicians practicing in teaching hospitals were found to be particularly uncomfortable with death, less likely to disclose a terminal diagnosis, and more likely to provide curative treatment in the last months of life (Prigerson, 1992).

Some physicians have urged colleagues to take a more active role in helping patients who request assistance in dying (Brody, 1992). They regard such action as an acknowledgment of medical hubris and an expression of medical compassion and willingness to support the autonomous wishes of patients. The American Medical Association, however, and a number of prominent physicians and ethicists have opposed efforts to legalize euthanasia and physician-assisted suicide (Gaylin et al., 1988). Physician participation in euthanasia and assisted suicide would, in their view, violate the Hippocratic Oath and confuse patients, erode trust, and tarnish medicine's image as a healing profession.

The most widely publicized model of physician-endorsed euthanasia is found in the Netherlands, where the government does not prosecute physicians who abide by an agreed-on standard of care. The criteria for euthanasia are that the patient's suffering must be intolerable despite aggressive relief efforts; there must be a low probability of improvement; the patient must be rational and fully informed; the patient's requests for euthanasia must be voluntary and repeated consistently over a reasonable period of time; and two physicians must accede to the request.

Some patient advocacy organizations, most notably the Hemlock Society and Choice in Dying, urge the adoption of similar standards in the United States, with the government protecting physicians from criminal and civil litigation. These parties believe that aggressive attempts to prolong the lives of terminally ill persons are unnatural and torturous, and that euthanasia or assisted suicide are sometimes the most humane alternatives. Others, including many of the pro-life organizations, hold that the taking of a human life is what is unnatural and immoral, and that patients and physicians should always, in the words of the Hebrew scriptures, "choose life." They also express a practical concern that acceptance of this practice will lead to a slippery slope involving involuntary as well as voluntary euthanasia and euthanasia for patients who are not

terminally ill or not experiencing unbearable suffering. They point to an apparent erosion of standards in the Netherlands, where, for example, 1000 incompetent patients are euthanized per year. (Supporters respond that the percentage of life-terminating acts performed without the explicit request of the patient is relatively small, this percentage is stable or shrinking rather than growing, and that most of these cases represent patients who requested euthanasia prior to becoming incompetent.

Physician-assisted suicide, as opposed to euthanasia, has been proposed as a way to minimize the role of the physician in the action causing the death of the patient, while enabling the physician to provide expertise and, in some cases, the equipment necessary to make the death as painless as possible. The patient feels a greater sense of control, and the image of the medical profession is not tainted by a stigma of murder attached to the event. However, suicide also can carry a stigma. Moreover, many have suggested that the ethical distinction between euthanasia and assisted suicide may be more cosmetic than substantial, analogous to the now-obsolete distinction between withholding and withdrawing of treatment. Regardless of the methods, the motives and outcome are the same. Preoccupation with taints and stigmas reflects more concern for image than integrity, and also may indicate a lack of courage rather than a commitment to principle.

Another concern is that, in this era of cost containment, dying patients will feel unduly pressured to choose suicide rather than spend society's, and perhaps their family's, limited resources. This raises the question of whether such decisions ever can be truly autonomous and voluntary.

Hospice physicians, who have pioneered in the development of pain and symptom management for terminally ill persons, offer help to get beyond the impasse of those physicians who feel torn between wanting to relieve the suffering of the dying but not wanting to serve, directly or indirectly, as the cause of their patient's death. Hospice medicine has shown that the pain of dying persons usually can be palliated by aggressive pharmacologic treatment as well as by attention to "total pain," which includes all the physical, emotional, social, spiritual, and financial sources of the patient's suffering. The existence of this expertise, and the relative ease with which a family physician can master it, implies an obligation to utilize these methods and, when necessary, to seek consultation from palliative care specialists.

An ethical dilemma persists, however, in the occasional case of a patient whose pain or suffering remains unbearable despite the best care available and who requests assistance in dying (Brody, 1992). Patients with severe physical disabilities, such as those with amyotrophic lateral sclerosis, advanced Parkinson disease, or quadriplegia, also might request assistance in dying. Hospice care offers much less for these patients, and they may turn to their family practice physician for help. Many family physicians would like to assist such patients but fear legal repercussions. What should those physicians do?

It is disingenuous to deny assistance on the basis of pragmatic considerations, such as slippery slopes, outbreaks of mercy killings, and mistrust of white coats. Withholding and withdrawing treatment also could create slippery slopes and also have been opposed on the basis of inflated fears, but these concerns are now considered insufficient to justify a prohibition against these practices. Most Americans know the difference between the euthanasia-as-murder and the type of assisted dying currently being discussed, limited to patients suffering unbearably despite aggressive efforts to relieve physical and psychological pain, who request assistance voluntarily, and who receive voluntary, compassionate, competent assistance by their physicians. A review process should, of course, be established to assure that these criteria are met (Brody, 1992).

From an ethical perspective, the essential issue is whether the long-standing prohibition against killing, which many regard as absolute, should outweigh all other considerations, such as the patient's autonomy or the degree of pain and suffering. Or,

does the situation of unbearable pain and suffering pose a special situation that our society ought to regard as an exception to the general prohibition of killing, through granting certain types of patients the right to waive their right not to be killed? These two horns of the dilemma embody the crux of the issue, and all other concerns should be regarded as peripheral.

At the present time, assistance in dying is illegal in the United States and much of the world. Whether the legislatures and the courts should stand in the way of physicians who, with compassion and competence, are willing to assist this small category of patients is an issue that our society is in the process of resolving. The ethical obligation for family practice physicians remains to help patients live and die with as much dignity, control, and comfort as possible in light of whatever decision society makes.

CONCLUSION

The ethical questions faced by physicians have been transformed, in ways we have indicated, by changing economic, social, legal, and political factors. In the end, however, the ethics of medicine remains committed to a view of the physician–patient relationship as a relationship between two autonomous human beings—a patient who is suffering and seeks help and a physician who maintains his or her humanity as well as his or her professionalism.

REFERENCES

Brody H. Assisted death—a compassionate response to a medical failure. N Engl J Med 1992;327:1384–1388.

Bruce JA. Privacy and Confidentiality of Health Care Information. Chicago, American Hospital Association, 1984.

Christie RJ, Hoffmaster CB. Ethical Issues in Family Medicine. New York, Oxford University Press, 1986.

Gaylin W, Kass LR, Pellegrino ED, Siegler M. "Doctors must not kill." JAMA 1988;259:2139–2140.

Gerber LA. Married to Their Careers: Career and Family Dilemmas in Doctors' Lives. New York, Tavistock Publications, 1983.

Hilfiker D. A Physician Looks at His Work. New York, Pantheon Books, 1985.

Holleman WL, Holleman MC. School and work release evaluations. JAMA 1988;260:3628–3634.

Holleman WL, Matson CC. Preemployment evaluations: dilemmas for the family physician. J Am Board Fam Pract 1991;4:95–101.

Morrissey J, Hofmann A, Thorpe J. Consent and Confidentiality in the Health Care of Children and Adolescents. New York, Free Press, 1986.

Prigerson HC. Socialization to dying: Social determinants of death acknowledgment and treatment among terminally ill geriatric patients. J Health Soc Behav 1992;33:378–395.

Rozovsky F. Consent to Treatment: A Practical Guide. Boston, Little, Brown, 1984.

Smith HL, Churchill LR. Professional Ethics and Primary Care Medicine: Beyond Dilemmas and Decorum. Durham, N.C., Duke University Press, 1986.

Solomon MZ, O'Donnell LO, Jennings B, et al. Decisions near the end of life: Professional views on life-sustaining treatments. Am J Public Health 1993;83:14.

Tarasoff v. Regents of California 118 Cal. Rptr. 129 (1974).

Taylor H. Majority support for euthanasia and Dr. Kevorkian increases. The Harris Poll #63, 1993.

1. What does it mean to say that medicine is a "relationship" and a "profession"?

2. Why is respect for patient autonomy important, and how far should a physician go in respecting patient autonomy?

3. In what ways can third parties interfere with the physician–patient relationship, and what can the physician do to balance properly the relationship with the patient and competing third parties?

4. Why is it important to maintain confidentiality in the physician-patient relationship? Under what circumstances should the protection of confidentiality take a back seat to other concerns?

5. What are the two major exceptions to standard informed consent practices? Which two standards are usually invoked in determining how much information to tell the patient?

6. What are some of the major causes of noncompliance? What strategies should be used in caring for such patients?

7. What are the referring physician's responsibilities toward the patient after referral?

8. What are the advantages and disadvantages of prospective reimbursement systems, and what can the family physician do to mitigate the disadvantages?

9. What factors contribute to perfectionism, "workaholism," and alcoholism among physicians, and what can medical students, residents, and physicians do to maintain good physical, emotional, and spiritual health?

Answers appear on **page 603**.

Chapter **3**

Family Dynamics and Health

Ernest Frugé, Ph.D.

Michael Crouch, M.D.

James Bray, Ph.D.

In 1966 the American Medical Association produced *The Report of the Citizens' Commission on Graduate Medical Education*, which advocated the development of a new primary care specialty, Family Medicine. What came to be known as *The Mills Commission Report* characterized Family Medicine as a specialty that

> ... *focuses not upon individual organs and systems but upon the whole man (sic) who* lives in a complex social setting; and knows that diagnosis or treatment of a part often overlooks major causative factors and therapeutic opportunities (1966).

This systemic view considers patients to be unique and complex organisms existing in the context of larger systems such as families, workplaces, and communities. For most of us, the family is our most fundamental and enduring influential context—the ultimate source of genetic endowment, experience, learning, and values. Family physicians are trained to consider both the impact of family relationships on the development of health and disease and the impact of health and disease on subsequent family relationships. The systematic incorporation of this type of family data into diagnosis, treatment, and prevention efforts is a fundamental feature of Family Medicine.

The basic term "dynamics" refers to motion or change and the forces that produce this activity. When applied to human systems such as the family, dynamics refers to the driving forces (physical, emotional, intellectual) and the patterns of activity (growth, organization, communication, adaptation) within these systems. A complete definition of dynamics must also include a consideration of the conditions or constraints within which family systems must operate. This chapter will present an overview of how family physicians can apply an understanding of family dynamics to the care of patients. We begin with a brief review of research that links family factors to health and illness, followed by examples of the health-related functions of families as they are manifest in the basic developmental tasks of the family life cycle and the tasks of coping with illness. The final section presents ways of examining the dynamics of families that may interfere with the work of the family and the work of the family physician.

RESEARCH ON FAMILIES AND HEALTH

Following World War II the influence of cybernetics and general systems theory on biological and social sciences led to the theory that human systems are more than the sum of interacting individuals. As early as 1945, H. B. Richardson suggested that the patient was part of a larger, complex biopsychosocial system: the family (Richardson, 1945). From this perspective the lives of family members are interdependent, mutually influencing one another's experience and health in processes where causality is bidirectional or nonlinear rather than unidirectional or linear. Although there is as yet no unifying theory of family dynamics, researchers have begun to document the influence of family and social relationships in the development and maintenance of an individual's physical and emotional health (Doherty and Campbell, 1988). Examples of this line of research can be found in studies of family status and

studies of family process, affect, and support (Bray, 1995).

Family status measures include the makeup of the family (e.g., nuclear family, divorced family, stepfamily) and its membership (e.g., couple only, couple with children, single-parent family). Marital and family status are strongly related to morbidity, mortality, and health care utilization for both physical and psychological problems (Bray, 1995). For example, marital status is positively related to post–myocardial infarction survival time for both men and women (Chandra et al., 1983). Men's marital satisfaction was found to predict health at a 5-year follow-up (Gersten et al., 1976) while women's marital adjustment has been related to both health status and satisfaction with health (Sheldon and Hooper, 1969). Marital separation has been associated with increases in medical utilization in the 6 months before and 12 months after separation (Wertlieb et al., 1984). Kiecolt-Glaser et al. (1988) found several indices of depressed immune function in separated and divorced men. Parental remarriage is also associated with increased stress for both adults and children that may persist for many years (Bray and Berger, submitted for publication).

Family process, affect, and support measures reflect overt actions and interactions, including emotional expression and emotional responses, that characterize relationships (e.g., problem solving, communication, conflict, hostility, support). Examples of health-related research in this area include the finding that a lack of closeness to parents has been associated with an increased risk for lung cancer (Kissen, 1969). Lack of closeness in family relationships has also been related to suicide, mental illness, hypertension, coronary heart disease, and malignant tumor (Thomas & Duszynski, 1974). Parkerson et al. (1995) found that self-reported family stress (defined as stress caused by interactions with other family members) was associated with lower quality of life and functional health as well as higher rates of referral and/or hospitalization, more severe illness at follow-up, and higher follow-up service charges.

Research has also documented the alternate path of influence by demonstrating the effect of illness on the functioning of families. The impact is most clearly observable in chronic illnesses and has been well documented, whether the index patients are children, adults, or the elderly (Midence, 1994; Bernbaum et al., 1993; Given et al., 1992). Researchers have begun to investigate the mechanisms involved in the reciprocal pathways of influence, and promising evidence is accumulating from the study of bi-directional linkages between psychosocial factors and fundamental immune system function (Esterling et al., 1994; Maier et al., 1994). Practicing physicians also know that family dynamics can impact health in a variety of direct and indirect ways, from headaches associated with stressful marital interactions to patterns of secrecy that impair communication with health care professionals.

For the practicing family physician the pragmatic question is, "Do the dynamics of this particular family (organization, driving forces, and activities) support healthy lifestyles, development, and coping, or do they interfere with these tasks?" The next question is, "How can such dynamics be assessed in order to integrate them into comprehensive diagnostic and treatment plans?" The following sections will review examples of basic health-related family tasks as manifest in ordinary developmental challenges of the family life cycle and the general challenges families face in coping with illness. The final section will explore how one key dimension of family dynamics, the communication and management of anxiety, may impact these health-related tasks. This section also discusses how this family dynamic might be conceptualized, assessed, and incorporated into a physician's understanding of work with families.

HEALTH FUNCTIONS AND THE FAMILY LIFE CYCLE

There are a variety of legitimate answers to the question, "What is a family?" The stereotypic nuclear family, consisting of a breadwinner father, homemaker mother, and one or more nonadult biologic offspring, is present in only 7 per cent of all households in the United States. The range of answers to the question, "What is a family?" all include the idea that the family, regardless of its specific composition, is a biopsychosocial entity or organization that transcends the individuals involved. For example, in many families DNA and experience are joined, recombined, and passed along to new members. While individuals have finite life spans, families can have indefinite life spans. For purposes of discussion, we will talk about prototypic functions of the family as an enduring organization with bonds of attachment or loyalty and with a number of complex and interrelated tasks that impact health. We will also start from the premise that a primary, overarching task of the family is to support the healthy development of all of its members across their individual life spans.

In order to develop a comprehensive diagnosis the family physician should identify the relevant contexts of the clinical encounter. In terms of family dynamics this means articulating the developmental or adaptive challenges that face the family (e.g., birth of a child, coping with loss of function through illness or injury) and the internal and external factors that will make negotiating these challenges more or less difficult. This includes the family's unique combination of resources and burdens (e.g., educational and economic status, available supports, and vulnerabilities). Once the physician understands how the dynamics of each family help or hinder the family's primary health tasks, he or she may be able to formulate ways to help the family be more effective and adaptive.

Physicians can begin to understand the health-related dynamics of a particular family by exploring how the family has negotiated and is negotiating the typical developmental challenges and tasks predicted by the "family life cycle" (Korin et al., 1997). Where to begin the cycle is arbitrary, but each stage has its unique features. It is common to think of families as beginning when adults join for the purpose of creating a marriage or new family organization. This is typically a voluntary agreement between consenting adults. The principal task at this stage of family development is the negotiation between the prospective partners on how their interests may be allied without losing their sense of individuality. Successful negotiation of this task creates a family organization that is more adaptive and durable than the simple sum of its parts. The organizational and developmental challenge for the partners is to begin thinking about the health and welfare of the pair, rather than both individuals considering only their own personal interest.

The next major stage for many, but not all, families is the birth of children. Family factors influence the health of children even before they are conceived. Genetics, the parents' evolving health status, the environment (both internal and external to the family abode), and the resources and opportunities accessible to the parents are among the most influential elements. The arrival of children calls for a great deal of reorganization for the adult partners. The family tasks expand from those associated with a voluntary contract between consenting adults to tasks associated with assuming responsibility for new children. To accomplish this fundamental shift in task, the adult partners must reorient from the prevailing goals of mutual and individual gratification to a focused consideration of choices as they affect the best interest of the child.

From an evolutionary (Darwinian) perspective, a healthy family is one that simply survives long enough to reproduce itself. Success in the primary task of ensuring healthy development of all members across the life span, however, requires members of a family to continue helping one another adapt to expected and unexpected changes. Predictable developmental challenges beyond the childbearing years include the following: helping children separate and establish autonomous functioning; caring for aging grandparents; accommodating work, economic and physical changes in later life; the death of a partner and one's own death. These predictable developmental events are, of course, combined with unpredictable events, such as illnesses or economic dislocations. The features of each event form a context to which the family must adapt within the constraints of its resources.

Successful adaptation often requires family members to fundamentally change the way things are done or the way they relate to each other in order to successfully meet the challenges of the event. These challenges and the way the family manages these issues can have implications for the onset of illness and coping with it. For example, does a mother with young children have any time to devote to exercise? Is the sleeplessness of an older adult associated with the realities of retirement?

Illness itself is an important context for family functioning. Coping with illness occurs across all stages of the family life cycle and is an essential component of the larger task of supporting healthy development. When a family member becomes ill, the family is challenged to reorganize its activities to ensure that the illness is detected, accurately appraised, and appropriately managed within the family and with professional help if necessary. Each illness event has unique characteristics that shape the particular demands placed upon the family. These demands vary along a continuum of complexity and burden, depending on the particular features of the family member's condition. The tasks that families must cope with range from doing little or nothing (e.g., for a common cold) to exhausting commitments of time, labor, and money (e.g., managing home oxygen for chronic pulmonary disease) over extended periods of time.

Rolland (1994) has proposed a four-dimensional typology of illness that forecasts the type and degree of demands placed on patients and their families over the course of various chronic diseases. The first dimension is rate of onset, which ranges from acute to gradual. The course of an illness may be described as progressive, constant, or relapsing/episodic. Predictability is related to this dimension and affects the degree of ambiguity and anxiety that patients and families experience (e.g., sickle cell crises). The expectations of outcome, particularly

mortality, are a third dimension of an illness. Rolland's fourth dimension is the extent and type of incapacitation and timing of losses (e.g., cognitive, sensory, motor, stigma). Related issues are the severity of symptoms (e.g., pain levels), the nature of treatments (e.g., expense, time, and intrusiveness) and the patterning of these factors over time.

Again, a primary task of a family physician is to develop a comprehensive diagnosis, which means explaining the source of an illness and the implications for treatment in light of relevant contexts. Considering the context of family dynamics for this purpose means specifying the demands generated by the features of the illness event in the context of the current developmental stage of a family and its history of adaptation as well as current stressors, constraints, and resources. It also means determining what might impair the family's current adaptive capacity. Research and clinical experience support the view that the way emotions are experienced, expressed, and managed, particularly negative emotions such as anxiety and hostility, is a key dimension of family dynamics that can have a profound effect on the family's capacity for adaptation. The next section will present a framework for conceptualizing the family as an emotional system and methods for incorporating this type of analysis into the work of a family physician.

GENERAL OVERVIEW OF FAMILY DYNAMICS

All happy families are alike; every unhappy family is unhappy in its own way.

TOLSTOY

All happy families are more or less dissimilar; all unhappy families are more or less alike.

NABOKOV

While taking care of the same patients over long periods of time, physicians come to understand Tolstoy's and Nabokov's apparently contradictory observations. "Happy" families show some functional similarities and some healthy differences in how they manifest emotions, communicate, and make decisions about important family matters, including illness and disease. "Unhappy" families demonstrate some similar dysfunctional tendencies and some distinguishing variations in how they relate to each other as they try to accomplish the fundamental tasks of the family.

Happy/healthy families radiate a sense of integrity and caring. Their adult members live by clear human values, communicate effectively, and share power while negotiating decisions. Children, adolescents, and adults in healthy families are encouraged to develop their own life goals and emotional independence, while staying connected with the family as a whole. Such families cope relatively well with adversity, often coming out of a crisis stronger for the experience.

Unhappy families, in contrast, often manifest disorganization and rigidity. Their members behave in ways that indicate a high level of chronic underlying anxiety and regularly engage in negative, hostile, or critical exchanges. Unhappy families can be caring and considerate when life circumstances are calm. When stressed, members of unhappy families shift into counterproductive modes, avoiding responsibility by clinging, attacking, or escaping. When the level of anxiety rises, emotional reactions tend to override rational responses. Personal values may be adopted uncritically from authority figures, such as parents or clergy, or from friends and peers, without considering their logical and emotional consistency. Alternatively, values may be formed and behavior shaped by reacting in opposition to the espoused or actual values of influential people (teachers, bosses).

At one extreme, unhappy family members often express intense negative feelings. This style creates a hot, conflictual family atmosphere. At the opposite extreme, family members shut off, blunt, or hide their feelings, creating a cold, unfeeling atmosphere that masks an underlying emotional intensity. Communication in unhappy families tends to be disorganized, rigid, or sparse, paralyzing decision making or maintaining coercive power differentials between spouses.

Unhappy families tend to view individual differences and independence as disloyalty that threatens their precarious survival. They have great difficulty dealing with stress. Despite their numerous liabilities, many unhappy families have an admirable spirit of dogged persistence in the face of generations of trials and sorrow. The physician who appreciates this fortitude can be more helpful to such families and derive satisfaction from serving as a needed advocate and ally.

The foregoing discussion suggests that families can be validly sorted into two dichotomous categories. Various labels have been used for this purpose, including good versus bad, and functional versus dysfunctional. Reality is more complicated. Most families exhibit fluctuating mixtures of happy and unhappy features. Rather than stigmatize families with pejorative labels such as "dysfunctional," the family physician can be most effective by helping a family capitalize on its strengths and deal with its vulnerabilities in healthier ways.

THE FAMILY EMOTIONAL SYSTEM

In general, the more intense and precarious the family's struggle to meet basic needs, the less likely it is that family members will trust others and feel loved. Material and financial security do not, however, guarantee fulfillment of emotional needs. Emotional development is strongly influenced by learning and experiences in the family of origin during one's childhood. Since family members are powerfully influenced by each others' emotions, one useful way to view the family is as an emotional system (Bowen, 1978).

Family members experience two urges that create an ongoing dynamic tension. The desire to be emotionally close to one's spouse or lover, parents, and children derives from the reproductive urge and biological bonding as well as the survival advantages of the small group. On the other hand, the urge to be a separate and somewhat autonomous individual is a logical extension of the self-preservation instinct, seen in other animal species as territoriality and aggression. Exaggeration of either urge can unbalance the behavior of a given individual or family. In American society women have been socialized toward togetherness with their children and with other women, while men have been encouraged to seek separateness through work and competitive sports. The extreme outcome for the female is the "supermom," overinvested in her children and lacking societally valued job skills. The archetypal male is the workaholic, distant from his wife and children, who meets some togetherness needs by watching or playing sports or drinking with other men.

Human beings tend to have considerable difficulty integrating their rational thoughts with their feelings. This is especially true in difficult situations that evoke strong emotions. Some families appear better able to temper emotion with reason, even under stress. Members of these families have less chronic anxiety, and they tend to cope well with stress. Members of families with higher levels of anxiety for several generations become acutely anxious with less provocation and cope less well with stress.

Although acute anxiety commands more attention, chronic anxiety probably influences health more adversely in the long run. In this discussion the term "chronic anxiety" denotes a vague mental dissonance and uneasiness, of which the individual is often not aware. This definition, based on Bowen's family systems theory, differs from the conventional definition of anxiety. The physiologic alterations and pathophysiologic changes accompanying chronic anxiety are more subtle, unless they are compounded by overlapping acute anxiety or the development of a more tangible manifestation, such as peptic ulcer disease.

Family therapists have described numerous ways in which individuals and families experience and express chronic anxiety. Physicians see many people who develop physical and mental symptoms as manifestations of chronic anxiety about their home life and work situations. Depression, headaches, irritable bowel syndrome, sleep disorders, and chronic fatigue are among the most common stress-related health problems.

Difficulties with intimate relationships are another mode for expressing anxiety. Individuals tend to select partners whose levels of chronic anxiety and intellectual-emotional maturity are similar to their own. Individuals with higher levels of chronic anxiety tend to become overinvolved with each other emotionally. Their sense of self relies too much on the approval and reciprocal dependency of the partner.

Especially early in the history of a relationship, overinvolvement may look and feel quite positive ("being in love"). Each individual may overfunction in certain respects (work outside the home, domestic work, parenting) that benefit the partnership, while underfunctioning in other respects (mismanaging finances). Eventually one or both "fused" partners suffer from a lack of emotional breathing space. They may get into nonproductive conflict more quickly, more often, and more intensely. At the other extreme, some anxious persons go to great lengths to avoid conflict, because of a fear of being abandoned if they express negative feelings. In either event, important issues remain unresolved.

Distancing from others emotionally is another way of handling one's anxiety. Historically, men have been more likely than women to distance themselves from other family members, both while living in the household and by leaving the household through separation or divorce. Completely cutting off communication with one's parent, child, or sibling signals severe chronic anxiety, usually about particularly toxic family issues passed along for several generations.

Events and situations from a family's past continue to influence succeeding generations. Someone whose grandmother had diabetes mellitus with severe complications such as blindness, amputa-

tions, and kidney failure may be genetically predisposed to developing diabetes. Knowing about this risk often generates considerable fear about one's vulnerability to disability and early death. Patients who openly acknowledge their fear may make more conscientious efforts to avoid becoming overweight. Successfully maintaining a healthy weight status can, in turn, keep their level of anxiety down. In contrast, many patients who deny their vulnerability to diabetes become increasingly obese and develop a variety of somatic symptoms (back pain, headaches) that mask underlying depression. Physicians who focus on the somatic symptoms without exploring their meaning miss both the depression and the fear of getting diabetes. Astute physicians who explore patients' attitudes about personal health can pave the way for improved health care outcomes (e.g., better control of elevated blood pressure and prevention of stroke).

Psychosocial events in the past may also affect the health of subsequent generations. If a mother and her mother both became pregnant as unmarried teenagers, the mother may show ambivalence about her teenage daughter's emerging sexuality. Hypervigilance by the mother may actually increase the daughter's likelihood of repeating the family pattern of teenage pregnancy as well as her risk of acquiring sexually transmitted diseases or developing sexual dysfunction. Sexual and physical abuse often occur in successive generations of families as expressions of anxiety and troubled relationships. Women in unhappy marriages often visit physicians for minor somatic symptoms. Women abused first by their fathers or mothers, then by their husbands, have difficulty admitting the abuse to physicians and find it even harder to terminate abusive relationships. The prospect of divorce may be a toxic issue for families with strong religious values and no previous experience with marital dissolution, or for families with many failed marriages.

TRIANGULATION IN FAMILIES

Anxiety escalates when relationships are stressed by life circumstances. Sometimes anxiety is diminished or redistributed by involving a third person in a two-person relationship (triangling). A child may become a referee or peacemaker for the parents' conflictual marriage. In some families a child develops worsening symptoms of a physical illness such as asthma when conflict occurs, distracting attention from the marital issues. In more dysfunctional families a child may be blamed for the family's problems and treated harshly as a scapegoat. Another common form of triangling is the extramarital affair, which can restabilize a precarious family system or precipitate marital separation and divorce, depending on what the participants learn about themselves from the experience. Substance abuse may be a form of triangulation. The workaholic may use work as the third point of a triangle with the spouse.

ASSESSING FAMILY DYNAMICS

Family composition and structure can be elicited quickly with pertinent questions on a health history questionnaire or by doing a genogram (Crouch, 1987a). The genogram has the advantage of quickly eliciting and recording considerable information about family illnesses. The genogram also shows the clinician where the family is in its life cycle. Vulnerable life cycle phases include couple formation, childbearing, middle-aged parents with teenage children, adolescents leaving the home, and aging and dying grandparents.

A genogram can be drawn in skeletal form during one of the first few visits—ideally the first visit—then elaborated as indicated during subsequent visits. The genogram often reveals important family patterns of illness, disease, and psychosocial problems. The longevity of male and female members of previous and current generations gives clues to genetic vulnerability to life-threatening illness. Occurrences of heart disease, cancer, depression and anxiety disorders, alcohol and other substance abuse, and physical or sexual abuse are especially meaningful to the care of patients. A self-administered form of the genogram (Rogers, 1991) can save physician time. Because much of the value of the genogram derives from the doctor-patient communication process, however, using the self-administered form weakens its power to generate hypotheses and therapeutic attitudes. This disadvantage can be partially overcome by the physician's conducting a focused personal follow-up discussion.

Many primary care patients have family or work problems and would benefit from discussing them with their physician, but they seldom bring up these problems spontaneously. Screening for dissatisfaction with family life can be done efficiently by including questions from the Family APGAR (Table 3–1) and Work System APGAR (Table 3–2) (Smilkstein et al., 1982) on the intake questionnaire. Although some individuals will minimize or deny their problems, those under severe stress will

TABLE 3–1. Smilkstein's Family System APGAR Items

	Almost always	Some of the time	Hardly ever
1. I am satisfied that I can turn to my family for help when something is troubling me.	_____	_____	_____
2. I am satisfied with the way my family talks things over with me and shares problems with me.	_____	_____	_____
3. I am satisfied that my family accepts and supports my wishes to take on new activities or directions.	_____	_____	_____
4. I am satisfied with the way my family expresses affection and responds to my emotions, such as anger, sorrow, and love.	_____	_____	_____
5. I am satisfied with the way my family and I share time together.	_____	_____	_____

Source: Smilkstein G, Ashworth C, Montano D. Validity and reliability of a family APGAR as a test of family function. J Fam Pract 1982;15:303–311, with permission.

usually acknowledge their difficulties and discuss them.

THE FAMILY PHYSICIAN AS COUNSELOR/ THERAPIST

Most family physicians do informal counseling, usually with patients who are acutely anxious or depressed. Most of the family physicians who do formal counseling or psychotherapy obtain extra training in psychotherapy and/or family therapy. Such physicians often choose to improve their effectiveness by working collaboratively with a mental health professional, seeing patients together or discussing them in a consultative mode. This can be a source of intellectual and emotional support for both professionals, especially when working with difficult patients.

Unless the physician has formal training in psychotherapy or family therapy, patients with severe emotional or psychiatric problems should be referred to a mental health professional for evaluation and more intense therapy. Such a referral must be done in a careful, caring manner so that the patient

TABLE 3–2. Smilkstein's Work System APGAR Items

	Almost always	Some of the time	Hardly ever
1. I am satisfied that I can turn to a fellow worker for help when something is troubling me.	_____	_____	_____
2. I am satisfied with the way my fellow workers talk things over with me and share problems with me.	_____	_____	_____
3. I am satisfied that my fellow workers accept and support my new ideas or thoughts.	_____	_____	_____
4. I am satisfied with the way my fellow workers respond to my emotions, such as anger, sorrow, or laughter.	_____	_____	_____
5. I am satisfied with the way my fellow workers and I share time together.	_____	_____	_____
6. I am satisfied with the way I get along with the person who is my closest or immediate supervisor.	_____	_____	_____
7. I am satisfied with the work I do at my place of employment.	_____	_____	_____

Source: Smilkstein G, Ashworth C, Montano D. Validity and reliability of the family APGAR as a test of family function. J Fam Pract 1982;15:303–311, with permission.

does not feel rejected or labeled as "crazy." The primary care physician should stay in active contact with the patient about his or her therapy.

PHYSICIANS' UNDERSTANDING OF THEIR OWN FAMILY DYNAMICS

It is interesting and often useful to study your own family patterns and how they affect your functioning as a physician (Crouch, 1987b). You can start by doing your own genogram and looking for patterns of relationship, functioning, and illness. If you can learn to observe yourself in relation to your family patterns and history, you can develop strategies for changing your thoughts, feelings, and behavior with respect to problematic family issues.

By increasing your awareness of family patterns, you can develop a sense of humor about "losing it" and behaving counterproductively at times. You can develop new patterns and avoid repeating old ones so frequently or intensely when under greater stress. You can catch yourself sooner and recover more quickly when you repeat an old pattern. You can develop strategies such as taking a "time-out" to lower your anxiety when you sense it escalating. You can improve all your relationships with other people by responding more and reacting less in difficult situations.

Many physicians have benefited from discussing their most difficult patients with a relatively objective colleague. One structured format for doing this on a regular basis is a group process named for the British psychiatrist (Balint, 1957) who pioneered this area. The most difficult patients discussed in Balint Groups are generally the ones who strongly reactivate family patterns that are most touchy. Such patients can give valuable clues to the issues that we might most benefit from examining and working on. Physicians with personal problems or problematic family patterns often benefit greatly from getting individual and/or family therapy themselves.

FAMILY DYNAMICS AND MEDICINE

As Dr. Richardson (1945) noted, ". . . if the physician could control his impatience, . . . the study of the family context could be immensely helpful." He also recognized that "the consideration of the family in all its complexities would . . . add enormously to the physician's responsibilities." To the experienced clinician, however, the bare biomedical facts of routine health problems become straightforward and uninteresting. People, however, are seldom simple or dull. The infinite variety of family relationships, strengths, and problems adds spice to the practice of medicine. If you pause just long enough to enjoy the uniqueness of each person and each family, you will greatly enhance the help that you give and the joy that you receive as a physician.

REFERENCES

Balint M. The Doctor, His Patient, and the Illness. New York, International Universities Press, 1957.

Bernbaum M, Albert SG, Duckro PN. Personal and family stress in individuals with diabetes and vision loss. J Clin Psychol 1993;49 (5):670–677.

Bowen M. Family Therapy in Clinical Practice. New York, Jason Aronson, 1978, pp 337–387, 461–547.

Bray JH. Assessment of family health and distress: An intergenerational-systems perspective. In Conoley JC, Werth E (eds): Family Assessment. Lincoln, NE: Buros Institute of Mental Measurement, 1995, pp 67–102.

Bray JH, Berger SH. Length of remarriage, conflict, stress, and children's adjustment in stepfather families and nuclear families. Submitted for publication.

Chandra V, Szklo M, Goldberg R, Tonascia J. The impact of marital status on survival after an acute myocardial infarction: A population based study. Am J Gerontol 1983;117:320–325.

Citizen's Commission on Graduate Medical Education of the American Medical Association (Mills Commission). The Graduate Education of Physicians. Chicago, American Medical Association, 1966.

Crouch MA. Using the genogram clinically. In The Family in Medical Practice: A Family Systems Primer. New York, Springer-Verlag, 1987a.

Crouch MA. Working with one's own family issues. In The Family in Medical Practice: A Family Systems Primer. New York, Springer-Verlag, 1987b.

Doherty WJ, Campbell TL. Families and health. Beverly Hills, CA, Sage Publications, 1988.

Esterling BA, Kiecolt-Glaser JK, Bodnar JC, Glaser R. Chronic stress, social support, and persistent alterations in the natural killer cell response to cytokines in older adults. Health Psychol 1994;13(4):291–298.

Gersten JC, Friis R, Langer T. Life dissatisfaction and illness of married men over time. Am J Epidemiol 1976;103:333–341.

Given CW, Given B, Stommel M, et al. The caregiver reaction assessment (CRA) for caregivers to persons with chronic physical and mental impairments. Res Nurs Health 1992;15:271–283.

Kiecolt-Glaser JK, Kennedy S, Malkoff S, et al. Marital discord and immunity in males. Psychosomat Med 1988;50:213–229.

Kissen DM. Present status of psychosomatic cancer research. Geriatrics 1969;24:129–137.

Korin EC, Watson MF, McGoldrick M. Individual and family life cycle. In Mengel MB, Holleman WL (eds): Fundamentals of Clinical Practice: A Textbook on the Patient, Doctor, and Society. New York, Plenum Medical Book Company, 1997.

Maier SF, Watkins LR, Fleshner M. Psychoneuroimmunology. Am Psychologist 1994;49:1004–1017.

Midence K. The effects of chronic illness on children and their families: An overview. Genet Social Gen Psychol Monogr 1994;120(3):311–326.

Nabokov VA. A Family Chronicle. New York, McGraw-Hill, 1969.

Parkerson GR Jr, Broadhead WE, Tse CJ. Perceived family stress as a predictor of health-related outcomes. Arch Fam Med 1995;4:253–260.

Richardson HB. Patients Have Families. New York, Commonwealth Fund, 1945.

Rogers J. The self-administered genogram. In Rakel RE (ed). Textbook of Family Practice. Philadelphia, W. B. Saunders, 1991, pp 1732–1735.

Rolland JS. Families, Illness, and Disability: An Integrative Approach. New York, Basic Books, 1994.

Sheldon A, Hooper D. An inquiry into health and ill-health and adjustment in early marriage. J Psychosomat Res 1969; 13:95–101.

Smilkstein G, Ashworth C, Montano D. Validity and reliability of the family APGAR as a test of family function. J Fam Pract 1982;15:303–311.

Thomas CB, Duszynski KR. Closeness to parents and the family constellation in a prospective study of five states. Johns Hopkins Med J 1974;134:251–270.

Tolstoy LN. Anna Karenina. New York, Dodd, Mead & Co., 1966.

Wertlieb D, Budman S, Demby A, Randall M. Marital separation and health: Stress and intervention. J Hum Stress 1984; 10:18–26.

QUESTIONS

1. In the United States the stereotypic nuclear family, consisting of a breadwinner father, homemaker mother, and one or more nonadult biologic offspring, is present in approximately
   a. 12% of all households.
   b. 7% of all households.
   c. 25% of all households.

2. In general, health is more likely to be adversely affected by
   a. high levels of acute anxiety.
   b. overly concerned responses from caregivers.
   c. chronic anxiety.

3. Triangulation is a means of
   a. redistributing anxiety.
   b. determining the best course of action by including more family members in the decision.
   c. forming a coalition between the patient, the family, and the family physician.

Answers appear on **page 603**.

Chapter 4

Patient Compliance

John W. Sellors, M.D.
R. Brian Haynes, M.D.

[The physician] should keep aware of the fact that patients often lie when they state that they have taken certain medicines.

HIPPOCRATES

Although physicians have dispensed medicines and potions through the centuries in vast quantities, it is only in recent years that there has been systematic examination of whether patients actually take the treatment. It was perhaps to the patient's benefit in the past that little attention was paid to compliance, as poor compliance probably saved the patient's life on many occasions. Some treatments, especially the massive purges and bleeding of the eighteenth century and arsenic and hydrochloric acid of this century, certainly had lethal rather than therapeutic potential. Now our armamentarium of useful treatments is sizable and expanding rapidly; low patient compliance stands squarely in the way of achieving the full benefit of modern therapy.

The extent of poor compliance is distressing. Fifty per cent is a representative compliance figure for many long-term therapies. Only about two thirds of those who continue under care take enough of their prescribed medication to achieve adequate blood pressure control (Haynes et al., 1979). If we look at compliance with lifestyle changes, such as diets and smoking cessation, the figures are considerably more dismal (Best and Block, 1979).

Added to this, physicians—even family physicians—are not good at estimating compliance levels in patients (Gilbert et al., 1980). Physicians have a strong tendency to overestimate the compliance of their own patients and are usually unable to predict which patients will comply with treatment.

This chapter will review the practical methods of detecting poor compliance and strategies for improving it.

DEFINITIONS

The trend in medicine, and particularly in family medicine, is toward consumerism and a more democratic approach that involves the patient in medical decisions. The use of the word "compliance" has raised objections because it implies authoritarianism and anything but an equal relationship between physician and patient. Unfortunately, no better term has surfaced. Adherence and defaulting are probably the most common alternatives, but they still carry negative connotations. While we sympathize with the views of those who oppose the term, we will use compliance throughout this chapter because it is still the most widely used and recognized rubric.

Compliance has been defined as the extent to which a person's behavior (in terms of keeping appointments, taking medications, and executing lifestyle changes) coincides with medical advice (Sackett, 1976). Poor compliance is more difficult to define. What percentage of prescribed medication can a patient forget or omit before being classed as a poor complier? How are patients who take too much medication classified? One way of looking at the problem is to use patient outcomes as a guide. For instance, in hypertension studies, patients taking 80 per cent or more of prescribed medication were considered compliant because this amount of medication was found to produce systematic blood pressure reduction (Sackett et al., 1975). It makes sense that efforts directed at poor compliers should be concentrated on those not achieving therapeutic goals. This obviously makes for more efficient use of resources. However, some patients who respond to treatment may be doing so because of overprescribing rather than because of compliance. Should these patients be hospitalized or placed in some other situation in which compliance may be close to 100 per cent, they may well run into serious effects of overdose.

FACTORS INFLUENCING COMPLIANCE

Many approaches, ranging from complex psychological theories to simplistic or intuitive ideas, have been taken to explain compliance behavior. None is entirely satisfactory, and many are lamentably wrong (Leventhal and Cameron, 1987).

In looking at the many factors involved, there is a natural tendency for the physician to feel that poor compliance is the patient's fault—after all, it is the patient who must swallow the pill or keep the appointment. But many other factors leading up to the act of pill taking or returning for an appointment need to be considered. For instance, what about the disease or condition being treated: Is it symptomatic or asymptomatic, life-threatening, or purely a nuisance? What about the treatment itself: Is it unpleasant, inconvenient, or expensive? Is it efficacious? Is the medical environment conducive to regular follow-up? Does the physician inspire confidence in the treatment or do certain attitudes interfere with compliance? Only some of these factors have an important effect on compliance behavior.

The Patient

Attributes such as age, sex, marital status, education, intelligence, and economic status bear no consistent relationship to compliance. Two exceptions are the very young and the very old, whose compliance characteristics tend to conform to those of their caregivers. In a hepatitis B vaccine compliance trial, a lower education level was the strongest predictor of noncompliance, but fortunately these patients were also the most responsive to the intervention to improve compliance (Sellors et al., 1997).

Perhaps the most widely held theory of compliance behavior, probably because of its intuitive appeal, is the communications approach (Leventhal et al., 1984). In this model, it is proposed that patients generally do not know enough about their illness or treatment and that this ignorance leads to poor compliance. It follows that adequate instruction or message generation and reception, comprehension, and retention of the message should result in improved compliance. Although it appears that this is true for short-term treatments (less than 2 weeks in duration), knowledge bears little relationship to compliance with chronic disease regimens (Haynes, 1979).

Another popular theory looks at patient motivation and beliefs. Using the health belief model, Becker (1976) argues that the likelihood of an individual's undertaking a recommended health action depends on the perception of the level of personal susceptibility to the particular illness or condition; the degree of severity of the consequences of contracting the condition; the potential benefits or efficacy of the treatment in preventing or reducing susceptibility and/or severity; and the physical, psychological, financial, and other barriers or costs involved in initiating or continuing the treatment. The model also requires a stimulus or cue to action to trigger the appropriate behavior (compliance); this cue can be either internal (e.g., a symptom) or external (e.g., screening campaign or physician's advice). This model has been shown to have predictive value for some preventive and short-term therapeutic health actions, such as immunizations and medical regimens for acute disease, but the extent of its predictive value is modest at best (Janz and Becker, 1984).

The transtheoretical model maintains that behavior progresses through five stages—precontemplation, contemplation, preparation, action, and maintenance—and that there is a decisional balance between the pros and cons of the behavior (Prochaska and DiClemente, 1992). It follows that all patients may not be at the same stage of readiness for change in compliance. Although this has not been validated in a randomized clinical trial, assessment of the stage of change of a noncompliant patient should facilitate counseling that is appropriately tailored to move him or her toward action.

Other models have been studied, including the behavioral learning model, which is based on cognitive and social learning theory, and the self-regulating model. As yet, no model has been developed that adequately explains a person's compliance behavior or gives a clear rationale for modifying it (Haynes et al., 1982).

The Disease

With few exceptions, disease factors are relatively unimportant as determinants of compliance. Psychiatric patients with schizophrenia, paranoid features, and personality disorders are less compliant than other psychiatric patients—a fact that probably reduces the compliance of psychiatric patients as a whole below that of patients with nonpsychiatric disorders.

No relationship has been demonstrated between the severity of symptoms and compliance.

Surprisingly, the *more* symptoms a patient reports, the *lower* his or her compliance is likely to be. On the other hand, increasing disability produced by a disease appears to be associated with better compliance. Whether this is a result of increased severity of disease or specifically the result of the *increased supervision* that often accompanies increased disability has not been sorted out.

Chronic diseases requiring long-term treatment have been clearly shown to result in increasingly poor compliance. This fact is of great clinical importance in such potentially serious diseases as tuberculosis and hypertension and is more likely to be a function of the duration of the *treatment* regimen than the duration of the *disease* itself.

The Regimen

Generally speaking, the greater the behavioral demands of a treatment, the poorer the compliance. Regimens requiring changes in lifestyle, such as dieting, exercising, and stopping harmful habits, result in much poorer compliance than simply taking pills, because of the substantially greater behavioral changes needed.

Clearly, the greater the number of drugs or treatments prescribed for a patient, the greater the probability of poor compliance. This includes both errors of omission and commission. Although the frequency of pill taking is not so important, it has an effect in that patients are less likely to comply with a regimen requiring four or more doses a day than with one requiring one or two daily doses.

Alternative oral medications for the same condition do not appear to result in substantial differences in compliance, but there is a difference between different treatments for different problems. This ranges from 17 per cent compliance with antacids to 89 per cent with cardiac drugs (Closson and Kikugawa, 1975).

The injection of long-acting preparations, such as benzathine penicillin for acute streptococcal pharyngitis and rheumatic fever prophylaxis, long-acting phenothiazines for schizophrenia, and streptomycin for tuberculosis, have been shown to be acceptable to patients and more effective than oral preparations.

Another contradiction for intuitive reasoning is the fact that there is very little evidence that adverse effects of treatment are a major cause of poor compliance. Studies have shown that there is no difference in the reported frequency of adverse effects between compliers and noncompliers (Latiolais and Berry, 1969; Willcox et al., 1965). In studies in which patients were asked for reasons for their noncompliance, only 5 to 10 per cent implicated side effects (Glick, 1965; Rickels et al., 1964).

The cost of treatment is an important barrier to compliance for many people, although a complete understanding of the effect of cost is not as obvious as it might first appear. For instance, one study showed that hospital admissions *increased* among psychiatric outpatients given drugs at nominal cost compared with a group paying regular prices (Cody and Robinson, 1977).

The Physician

The physician is obviously in a key position to influence compliance. For example, if the frequency of dose affects compliance, then by the very act of prescribing a medication four times a day the physician is potentially reducing compliance below the level achievable with a single daily dose.

More complex than the mechanics of prescribing, however, is the interaction between physician and patient. Patients are more likely to comply with treatment if their expectations are met by the visit and if they are well satisfied with their care (Francis et al., 1969; Kincey et al., 1975). The concept of a personal physician or the feeling of knowing a physician well has also been associated with increased compliance (Ettlinger and Freeman, 1981). Dissecting the physician–patient relationship and measuring the factors that result in increased satisfaction are not easy. This is demonstrated in one study in which some patients felt that they knew their physician *well* after only one visit, whereas others felt that they still did not know their physicians after as many as *14* visits (Ettlinger and Freeman, 1981).

DETECTION OF POOR COMPLIANCE

Clinical Judgment

Most of us would like to believe that a good physician can detect poor compliance in patients; surely, this goes along with clinical judgment. Unfortunately, studies have shown that this is not the case: Using clinical judgment has been shown to be no better than flipping a coin as a detection method. The first studies demonstrating this were carried out in specialty settings and with physicians who did not have an ongoing relationship with patients. Unfortunately, the hope that family physicians with their ongoing relationships with their patients might be in a better position to make predictions has also been dispelled. Not only were family physicians unable to detect poor compliers among their patients, but also the length of time that they had known their patients had no effect on their ability to predict (Gilbert et al., 1980).

The emphasis on the inaccuracy of clinical judgment is important in that it serves to direct us to alternative approaches to detect poor compliance.

Monitoring Attendance

As mentioned previously, over 50 per cent of hypertensive patients stop visiting their physicians within a year of starting treatment, and those who do not appear for follow-up appointments are unlikely to be compliers with treatment. Many physicians are unable to detect this type of noncompliance because their appointment systems are inadequate or because the patients do not make a follow-up appointment.

It follows, then, that an important method of detecting poor compliance is to watch the appointment book and day sheet. While there is no guarantee that patients who keep appointments will comply with treatment, there is no doubt that those who do not appear for follow-up will not be in a position to comply with treatment. The importance of monitoring attendance cannot be overstressed: Dropping out of care is one of the most frequent and most severe forms of noncompliance (Stephenson et al., 1993).

Response to Treatment

Provided that the treatment prescribed is known to be efficacious, failure of a patient to respond to treatment can be used as a readily available indicator of compliance levels. However, this method of assessing compliance is not infallible. For example, patients who appear to respond to treatment may do so because they were misdiagnosed and do not have the condition of interest or because their physicians' overprescribing is compensating for their poor compliance. Nevertheless, from the compliance perspective at least, there is less need to be concerned about patients who have reached the therapeutic goal. On the other hand, patients not showing a response to treatment will include those who genuinely do not respond to therapy or who have been prescribed inadequate amounts and will also include a high proportion of poor compliers or noncompliers.

Asking the Patient

Although it is not always reliable, asking the patient directly about compliance can be a very valuable and practical way of determining the pattern of medication consumption (Table 4–1). When asked directly, about half of noncompliant patients will admit to missing at least some medication (Haynes et al., 1980; Stephenson et al., 1993). One can be assured that it is highly improbable that a *compliant* patient will admit to poor compliance, so patients admitting to missing medication have a very high likelihood of being poor compliers. The converse is not true, however, as even under optimal interview conditions about half of noncompliant patients will deny the fact. Patients who admit to missing medication generally overestimate the amount of medication they do take. In one study, the average overestimate was in the region of 20 per cent (Haynes et al., 1980).

It must be emphasized that the method of questioning is of paramount importance. Asking in a threatening or belligerent manner will result in reflex denial. Approaching the patient with a face-saving, nonthreatening, nonjudgmental question will yield a higher proportion of accurate responses. One way of doing this is to use an approach such as the following: "Many people find it difficult to remember to take medicines: During the past week, have you missed *any* of your pills?" Taking into account the tendency to overestimate compliance, admission of *any* noncompliance is associated with an average compliance rate of less than 80 per cent.

The methods of detecting low compliance described so far can be easily applied in any treatment setting and, if applied with care, will detect the

---

TABLE 4–1. A Simple Method to Detect Noncompliance

Asking the Patient
The easiest way to detect medication noncompliance is to ask the patient.
About 50 per cent of noncompliant patients will admit to missing at least some medication.
If patients admit to noncompliance, you can believe them.
Patients admitting to poor compliance are most responsive to attempts to improve compliance.
How to Ask
Use a matter-of-fact, nonjudgmental, nonthreatening manner.
Use an introduction that allows a patient to save face:
"Many people find it difficult to remember to take medicines: During the past week, have you missed *any* of your pills?"

---

majority of poor compliers. The following methods may be of help in detecting some of the remainder.

Counting Pills

As a quantitative estimate of compliance over a period of time, pill counts can be relatively reliable so long as they are carried out in the patient's home with strict attention to bookkeeping (Haynes et al., 1980). Unless the count can be carried out in such a manner that the patient is unaware of what is going on, it becomes a one-time-only procedure. It follows that while pill counts are very important research tools, they are not very practical for most clinical situations. It can be reasoned that using pill counts in the office or clinic will result in a bias in the direction of overestimating compliance, in that patients will consciously or unconsciously bring only *some* of their unused pills with them, giving the appearance that they have taken more of the medication than is actually the case. It is virtually impossible for the bias to go in the opposite direction unless the patient is receiving the same prescriptions from two or more physicians at the same time. In general, pill counts give higher estimates of compliance than quantitative drug assays and lower (but more accurate) estimates than patient self-reports.

Drug Levels

A laboratory test to detect the presence or absence of good compliance is an unrealistic dream in the case of most drugs. But for some drugs, especially those with long serum half-lives resulting in relatively steady serum levels, the measurement of serum levels can be an extremely useful indicator of compliance. The best examples of this are digoxin and phenytoin, for which plasma levels have been used successfully to both monitor compliance and improve it through feedback to the patient. Other drugs commonly measured in this way are phenobarbitone and other anticonvulsants, theophylline, tricyclic antidepressants, lithium, and a variety of cardiac drugs. The caution is, however, that there is a great deal of individual variation in drug absorption, metabolism, and excretion. In addition, serum levels of drugs with short half-lives indicate only how recently a dose was taken and give no information on long-term compliance.

Drug levels in urine have also been used as compliance indicators. For instance, the presence or absence of penicillin can be easily detected using inhibition of growth of a microorganism, *Sarcina*

lutea. While these methods and others involving inactive markers such as riboflavin and carbon-14 have been used in research, they are not practical methods for the clinician. What is more, as a measure of compliance, single qualitative assessments of urine samples have been shown to be inferior to simply asking the patient (Haynes et al., 1980).

PREVENTION AND TREATMENT OF POOR COMPLIANCE

Misconceptions

Before discussing prevention and treatment, it is worthwhile to re-examine some popular misconceptions about compliance. The first misconception is that a good clinician can identify poor compliers. In fact, *there is no stereotypic poor complier.* This is very important, because restricting prevention and treatment strategies to patients thought to be potentially poor compliers must result in neglect of a large number of patients who need attention as well as unnecessary attention to some patients who do not.

Another popular and important misconception is that all that stops patients from being near-perfect compliers is their ignorance of either the condition being treated or the treatment being used. While there is some evidence that written instructions help improve compliance for short-term regimens, even mastery learning, in which patients were given detailed step-by-step instruction on hypertension, had no beneficial effect on long-term compliance (Sackett et al., 1975). The belief that it is possible to scare a patient into complying with treatment has also been dispelled (Leventhal et al., 1967).

Logan (1978), in a survey of primary care physicians, has shown that the methods they employed to improve compliance were predominantly those that have been found lacking. Methods that *have* been shown to be effective were not generally applied. The transtheoretical model of readiness to change behavior can also be applied to a physician's own counseling behavior and predicts that unless realistic goals are set for improving compliance, the physician may become frustrated and slip into inaction (precontemplation) (Prochaska and DiClemente, 1992). Changing the long-term behavior of physicians to manage compliance successfully cannot be done by simply informing or instructing them about efficacious interventions (Evans et al., 1984; Haynes et al., 1984).

Prevention

The main thrust in the prevention of poor compliance is to remove barriers to compliance. Preventing patients from dropping out of care is of primary importance. Longer waiting times are associated with higher no-show rate's (Rockart and Hoffman, 1969), so that one aim is to keep patient waiting time to a minimum. Individual appointments at mutually convenient times help achieve this goal. Ensuring that patients leave the office with a *specific time* for a future appointment rather than with instructions to call for an appointment in, for example, 3 months, makes detection of those who do drop out much easier.

Simplifying the treatment regimen will remove another barrier to compliance. An essential element of this approach is to *eliminate unnecessary medications.* In addition, medications should be prescribed that need to be taken as few times daily as possible. The frequency of dosing with many drugs can be reduced below usually prescribed levels with no reduction in efficacy. For example, tricyclic antidepressants can be given as a single bedtime dose, thus reducing dosing frequency and timing side effects so that they occur mainly during sleep. A final strategy is titration to the least amount of medication necessary to achieve the therapeutic goal.

It has been shown that patients who feel that they are actively involved in their own care are better compliers than those who do not (Schulman, 1979). Studies have also shown that negotiating care with the patient rather than simply dictating or prescribing it results in better compliance (Eisenthal et al., 1979; Tracy, 1977). Encouraging patients to take greater responsibility for their care by asking more questions of their physicians results in improved attendance (Roter, 1977). It follows that encouraging patients to participate in and take more responsibility for their own care is another strategy for preventing poor compliance, and it not only makes scientific sense but also is consistent with trends in physician-patient relationships.

Treatment (Table 4–2)

Dropping out of care constitutes a *compliance crisis.* Mail and telephone reminders to increase attendance, at least in the short term, can help prevent dropout (Macharia et al., 1992). If the patient does fail to attend, it calls for prompt action by the receptionist or office nurse to reschedule (Takala et al., 1979). A simple method of identifying those

TABLE 4–2. Keys to Successful Compliance Management

Detection
Monitor attendance and achievement of the therapeutic goal.
Ask the patient.
Prevention
Make appointments convenient.
Simplify the regimen.
Give clear instructions, preferably written.
Make the patient an active participant.
Use telephone or mail reminders.
Treatment
Follow up nonattenders.
Increase attention and supervision.
Use cuing, feedback, and positive reinforcement.
Titrate frequency of visits to compliance need.
Involve spouse or other partner.
Maintain compliance interventions as long as compliance is desirable.

patients for whom compliance is important (e.g., the use of chart stickers or special symbols on the day sheet) may make the receptionist's task simpler. Personal contact by the physician and the use of outreach services such as public health nurses are other ways of "treating" persistent nonattendance.

Most successful compliance interventions have two features in common: increased supervision of, or attention to, the patient; and intentional reinforcement, reward, or encouragement of compliance (Haynes et al., 1987).

Low compliance is a chronic condition without a "one-shot" cure, so treatment of poor compliance must continue as long as the regimen of prescribed treatment. To make matters worse, none of the following has improved compliance when tested alone: special learning packages (Sackett et al., 1975) and pamphlets (Swain and Steckel, 1981); special unit dose reminder pill packaging (Becker et al., 1986); counseling about medication and compliance by a health educator (Levine et al., 1979) or by nurses (Shepard et al., 1979); visits to patients' homes (Johnson et al., 1978); provision of care at the worksite (Sackett et al., 1975); self-monitoring of blood pressure (Johnson et al., 1978; Shepard et al., 1979); tangible rewards (Shepard et al., 1979); and group discussions (Shepard et al., 1979). Although these tactics have not worked alone, many have been part of more complex interventions that have been successful; whether they are essential parts of these complex interventions or just along for the ride is difficult to say (Haynes et al., 1996).

A variety of inducements to comply have been used, including feedback of blood pressure response to hypertensive patients either by the provider (McKenney et al., 1973; Takala et al., 1979) or by patients' taking their own blood pressure (Haynes et al., 1976; Nessman et al., 1980); small tangible rewards for improved compliance and/or therapeutic response (Haynes et al., 1976; Shepard et al., 1979; Swain and Steckel, 1981); medication tailored to daily schedules to decrease forgetting and inconvenience (Haynes et al., 1976; Logan et al., 1979); encouragement of family support (Levine et al., 1979); stimulation of self-help through group support and discussion (Levine et al., 1979; Nessman et al., 1980); negotiation of a brief written contract with the patient to improve health behavior (Swain and Steckel, 1981); and calling back patients who miss appointments (Bass et al., 1986; Peterson et al., 1984; Takala et al., 1979; Sellors et al., 1997).

It is important to note here that there are many individuals other than physicians who have taken an effective part in this process. Nurses, pharmacists, health educators, a psychologist, and even an individual with no formal health training have played a key role in successful interventions.

In summary, the treatment of poor compliance involves many approaches. For short-term treatments, simple clear instructions are sufficient. For longer term treatments, there must be follow-up of nonattenders by telephone or mailed reminders. In addition, the practitioner must increase the attention paid to poor compliers and provide rewards or positive reinforcement for good compliance that could include simple praise and extending the time between appointments for those responding to treatment. Inui and colleagues (1976) have shown that such maneuvers can be successfully incorporated into regular practice by simply focusing on compliance for a few moments during each encounter, not only to emphasize the importance of following the regimen but also to tailor medication to daily routines. This can be accomplished without necessarily prolonging the visit. It is most important that all compliance interventions applied to noncompliers be maintained for as long as treatment is prescribed.

Ethical Issues

"Am I my brother's keeper?" (Genesis 4:9). This question highlights the dilemma in which physicians may find themselves when they are pressed to extend their compliance-improving strategies beyond a simple office visit.

The decision to apply tactics deliberately designed to change the compliance of patients should meet several ethical standards that apply to all therapeutic interventions (Levine, 1980). First, the diagnosis must be correct. Second, the therapy to be complied with must be of established efficacy. Third, neither the illness nor the proposed treatment should be trivial. Fourth, the patient must be an informed and willing partner in any attempt to maximize his or her compliance. Finally, the method employed to improve compliance must be of demonstrated effectiveness.

Having applied these standards and embarked upon a course of treatment, it makes no sense, ethically or otherwise, for the physician to abandon a patient at the first sign of poor compliance. Most physicians consider it *unethical* to withhold efficacious treatment from a patient with a serious physical disease. Why then should it be *ethical* to consider withholding treatment when the condition is *noncompliance?*

Future Trends

The advent of the personal computer has resulted in increasing use of microcomputers in physicians' offices. While initial applications have been for business purposes, the computerization of appointment systems and, increasingly, health records affords a potential for monitoring patient compliance and assisting in the implementation of reminder systems and the enhanced management of poor compliers (Johnston et al, 1994).

Computerized appointment systems make it possible to provide patients with appointment times for long periods ahead and can easily be modified to flag nonattenders and produce automatic reminders. The ability to record age, sex, and diagnoses makes it possible to design a system that can improve *provider* compliance with screening and preventive maneuvers (Bypass et al., 1988). Medication databases that store prescribing information can form the basis of a system that monitors whether patients are at least requesting prescription refills on time (Steiner et al., 1988). The potential is great, but it will require both effort and expenditure by physicians to make it work.

What of other advancements? The technology that brought us the efficacious treatments is also helping with compliance—drugs with long half-lives, long-acting parenteral preparations, conjunctival inserts, continuous transcutaneous absorption systems. The burgeoning use of high technology could result in an artificial pancreas that will not only dispense insulin but also adjust the dose according to blood levels. What is to stop the development of implanted arterial pressure sensors with automatic dispensing of parenteral antihypertensives? These thoughts make concerns about telephoning nonattenders seem trifling.

CONCLUSION

In dealing with compliance, we have consciously concentrated on compliance with medication, emphasizing long-term medications. This is not because we feel that compliance with short-term medications is inconsequential or that there is no problem of compliance with lifestyle or other behavioral changes. On the contrary, both these areas are very important and, in fact, noncompliance with lifestyle changes is a monster yet to be tamed.

It is our hope that we have raised the level of compliance consciousness in the reader. Awareness of the problem and the difficulties in detecting it is essential before any of these practical treatments can be instituted.

The past two decades have brought the therapist together with the patient, the family, and other members of the health care team in jointly working toward the full effectiveness of potent treatments. The rewards of this alliance are great—reduction of morbidity, disability, and preventable deaths. The family physician is in an ideal position to help create and share in these rewards.

REFERENCES

Bass MJ, McWhinney IR, Donner A. Do family physicians need medical assistants to detect and manage hypertension? Can Med Assoc J 1986;134:1247–1255. *A randomized trial of medical assistants in community-based family practice.*

Becker LA, Glanz K, Sobel E, et al. A randomized trial of special packaging of antihypertensive medications. J Fam Pract 1986;22:35–36. *A study of foil-backed blister packaging compared with regular medication vials. No significant difference in blood pressure control or compliance.*

Becker MH. Sociobehavioral determinants of compliance. In Sackett DL, Haynes RB (eds). Compliance with Therapeutic Regimens. Baltimore, Johns Hopkins University Press, 1976, pp 40–49.

Best JA, Block M. Compliance in the control of cigarette smoking. In Haynes RB, Taylor DW, Sackett DL (eds). Compliance in Health Care. Baltimore, John Hopkins University Press, 1979, pp 202–222. *An extensive review of strategies employed in attempting to modify smoking behavior.*

Bypass P, Hanlon PW, Hanlon LCS, et al. Microcomputer management of a vaccine trial. Comput Biol Med 1988;18:179–193. *A study involving a microcomputer for call and recall of infants due for vaccination in a trial of rotavirus vaccine in Africa.*

Closson R, Kikugawa C. Non-compliance varies with drug class. Hospitals 1975;49:89. *A study in a Veterans Administration population (San Francisco VA Hospital).*

Cody J, Robinson A. The effect of low-cost maintenance medication on the rehospitalization of schizophrenic outpatients. Am J Psychiatr 1977;134:73.

Eisenthal S, Emery R, Lazare A, et al. "Adherence" and the negotiated approach to patienthood. Arch Gen Psychiatry 1979;36:393.

Ettlinger PRA, Freeman GK. General practice compliance study: Is it worth being a personal doctor? Br Med J 1981;282:1192. *A general practice study involving two group practices. Compliance with antimicrobial prescription was assessed at an unannounced home visit and was found to be strongly associated with whether the patient thought that he knew the prescribing doctor well.*

Evans CE, Haynes RB, Birkett NJ, et al. Does a mailed continuing education program improve physician performance? Results of a randomized trial in antihypertensive care. JAMA 1984;255:501–504. *A population-based study of the effect of mailed continuing medical education material on hypertension treatment and control.*

Francis V, Korsch BM, Morris MJ. Gaps in doctor-patient communication. N Engl J Med 1969;280:535. *Pediatric patient population. The effects of doctor-patient communication on patient/parent satisfaction, reassurance, and compliance were assessed.*

Gilbert JR, Evans CE, Haynes RB, et al. Predicting compliance with a regimen of digoxin therapy in a family practice. Can Med Assoc J 1980;123:119. *This study involved 10 family physicians who were asked to predict the compliance of randomly selected patients on digoxin. Compliance was assessed by pill counts, serum levels, and patient report.*

Glick BS. Dropout in an outpatient, double-blind drug study. Psychosomatics 1965;6:44.

Haynes RB. Determinants of compliance: The disease and the mechanics of treatment. In Haynes RB, Taylor DW, Sackett DL (eds). Compliance in Health Care. Baltimore, Johns Hopkins University Press, 1979, pp 49–62. *A review of factors that have been studied in relation to their influence on compliance.*

Haynes RB, Davis DA, McKibbon A, et al. A critical appraisal of the efficacy of continuing medical education. JAMA 1984;251:61–64.

Haynes RB, Mattson ME, Chobanian AV, et al. Management of patient compliance in the treatment of hypertension. Hypertension 1982;4:415.

Haynes RB, McKibbon KA, Kanani R. Systematic review of randomized trials of interventions to assist patients to follow prescriptions for medications. Lancet 1996;348:383–386.

Haynes RB, Sackett DL, Gibson ES, et al. Improvement of medication compliance in uncontrolled hypertension. Lancet 1976;1:1265. *Report of a randomized control trial of a behaviorally oriented strategy for improving compliance, including blood pressure, self-monitoring, and tailoring treatment to daily habits.*

Haynes RB, Sackett DL, Taylor DW. Practical management of low compliance with antihypertensive therapy: A guide for the busy practitioner. Clin Invest Med 1979;1:175. *A "how to do it" review.*

Haynes RB, Taylor DW, Sackett DL, et al. Can simple clinical measurements detect patient non-compliance? Hypertension

1980;2:757. *A comparison of several methods of measuring compliance with antihypertensive medication, including pill counts, urine drug levels, patient self-reports, changes in uric acid and potassium, and blood pressure response.*

Haynes RB, Wang E, Gomes MD. A critical review of interventions to improve compliance with prescribed medications. Patient Educ Counseling 1987;10:155–166. *A review of scientifically sound investigations testing strategies intended to improve compliance.*

Inui T, Yourtee E, Williamson J. Improved outcomes in hypertension after physician tutorials. Ann Intern Med 1976;84:646. *Report of the effect of tutorials for physicians on the compliance of their hypertensive patients in a general medical outpatient clinic.*

Janz N, Becker M. The health belief model: A decade later. Health Educ Q 1984;11:1–47.

Johnson AL, Taylor DW, Sackett DL, et al. Self-recording of blood pressure in the management of hypertension. Can Med Assoc J 1978;119:1034.

Johnston ME, Langton KB, Haynes RB. A critical appraisal of research on the effects of computer-based decision support systems on clinician performance and patient outcomes. Ann Intern Med 1994;120:135–142.

Kincey J, Bradshaw P, Ley P. Patients' satisfaction and reported acceptance of advice in general practice. J R Coll Gen Pract 1975;25:558. *A general practice study evaluating patients' satisfaction with medical advice and the relationship between satisfaction and compliance.*

Latiolais CJ, Berry CC. Misuse of prescription medication by outpatients. Drug Intell Clin Pharmacy 1969;3:270–277.

Leventhal H, Cameron L. Behavioral theories and the problem of compliance. Patient Educ Counseling 1987;10:117–138. *An excellent review of behavioral theories related to compliance, outlining the strengths and deficiencies of each.*

Leventhal H, Watts J, Pagano F. Effects of fear and instructions on how to cope with danger. J Pers Soc Psychol 1967;6:313–321.

Leventhal H, Zimmersman R, Gutman M. Compliance: A self-regulation perspective. In Gentry D (ed): Handbook of Behavioral Medicine. New York, Pergamon Press, 1984, pp 369–434.

Levine DM, Green LW, Deeds SG, et al. Health education for hypertension patients. JAMA 1979;241:1700.

Levine RJ. Ethical considerations in the development and application of compliance strategies for the treatment of hypertension. In Haynes RB, Matteson ME, Engebretson TO Jr (eds): Patient Compliance to Prescribed Antihypertensive Regimens. Washington, D.C., U.S. Department of Health and Human Services, H.I.H. Publication No. 81-2102, 1980, pp 229–246.

Logan AS. Investigation of Toronto general practitioners' treatment of patients with hypertension. Toronto, Canadian Facts, 1978.

Logan AS, Milne BJ, Achber C, et al. Worksite treatment of hypertension by specially trained nurses: A controlled trial. Lancet 1979;2:1175.

Macharia WM, Leon G, Rowe BH, et al. An overview of interventions to improve compliance with appointment keeping for medical services. JAMA 1992;267:1813–1817.

McKenney JM, Slining JM, Henderson HR, et al. The effect of clinical pharmacy services on patients with essential hypertension. Circulation 1973;48:1104. *A controlled study of the use of clinical pharmacists who educated patients, monitored blood pressure control, and assisted in the management of questions and problems that arose.*

Nessman DG, Carnahan JE, Nugent CA. Improving compliance: Patient-operated hypertension groups. Arch Intern Med 1980;140:1427.

Peterson GM, McLean S, Millingen KS. A randomized trial of strategies to improve patient compliance with anticonvulsant therapy. Epilepsia 1984;25(4):412–417. *A randomized study of a combination of patient counseling, special medication containers, self-recording of medication intake and seizures, and mailed reminders to collect prescription refills and attend clinic appointments.*

Prochaska JO, DiClemente CC. Stages of change in the modification of problem behaviors. In Hersen M, Eisler RM, Miller PM (eds). Progress in Behavior Modifications. Sycamore, IL, Sycamore Press, 1992, pp 188–214.

Rickels K, Boren R, Stuart HM. Controlled psychopharmacological research in general practice. J New Drugs 1964;4:138.

Rockart JF, Hoffman PB. Physician and patient behavior under different scheduling systems in a hospital outpatient department. Med Care 1969;7:463. *A descriptive study of patient mean arrival time, waiting time, and no-show rate and of physician mean arrival time at several outpatient departments using different scheduling methods.*

Roter D. Patient participation in the patient-provider interaction: The effects of patient question asking on the quality of interaction, satisfaction and compliance. Health Educ Monogr 1977;5:281.

Sackett DL. Introduction. In Sackett DL, Haynes RB (eds). Compliance with Therapeutic Regimens. Baltimore, Johns Hopkins University Press, 1976, p 1.

Sackett DL, Haynes RB, Gibson ES, et al. Randomized clinical trial of strategies for improving medication compliance in primary hypertension. Lancet 1975;1:1205. *An evaluation of the effect on compliance of treatment at the worksite and of a special education program about new hypertensives.*

Schulman B. Active patient orientation and outcomes in hypertensive treatment. Med Care 1979;17:267.

Sellors J, Pickard L, Mahony JB, et al. Understanding and enhancing compliance with the second dose of hepatitis B vaccine: a cohort analysis and randomized trial. Can Med Assoc J 1997;157:143–148.

Shepard DS, Foster SB, Stason WB, et al. Cost-effectiveness of interventions to improve compliance with antihypertensive therapy. Prev Med 1979;8:229.

Steiner JF, Koepsall TD, Fihn SD, et al. A general method of compliance assessment using centralized pharmacy records: Description and validation. Med Care 1988;26(8):814–823. *A comparison of central pharmacy records with serum drug levels and patient outcomes.*

Stephenson BJ, Rowe BH, Haynes RB, et al. Is this patient taking the treatment as prescribed? JAMA 1993;269:2779–2781.

Swain MA, Steckel SB. Influencing adherence among hypertensives. Res Nurs Health 1981;4:213–218.

Takala J, Niemela N, Rosti J, Sivers K. Improving compliance with therapeutic regimens in hypertensive patients in a community health center. Circulation 1979;59:540. *A controlled trial of a very practical approach to improving compliance in primary care, including written directions, called-back nonattenders, and feeding back blood pressure levels at visits.*

Tracy J. Impact of intake procedures upon client attrition in a community mental health centre. J Consult Clin Psychol 1977;45:192.

Willcox DR, Gillan R, Hare EH. Do psychiatric outpatients take their drugs? Br Med J 1965;2:790.

1. What is the single most important compliance maneuver?

2. Name at least four special tactics that are helpful for

improving the compliance of patients with "lifestyle" changes.

Answers appear on **page 603**.

Chapter **5**

Disease Prevention

R. Michael Morse, M.D.
Warren A. Heffron, M.D.

ROLE OF THE FAMILY PHYSICIAN

The family physician has a special opportunity to be an effective force in disease prevention and health promotion. As the primary care provider for all ages in family units, the family physician has an inherent obligation to screen for a broad range of risk factors associated with preventable diseases and encourage appropriate preventive measures such as proper diet and exercise. To be most effective, many disease prevention and health promotion activities are applicable to the entire family unit and serve as the foundation for more age-specific recommendations and interventions for each individual family member.

Although other medical-surgical problem areas may occasionally require subspecialty consultation, the family physician is the specialist to whom patients and other specialists look for provision of this broad range of health promotion and disease prevention activities.

Disease prevention activities are traditionally classified according to the phase of the disease process in which intervention occurs: tertiary prevention (disease diagnosed and symptoms present); secondary prevention (disease present and diagnosable, but no symptoms present); and primary pre-

vention (no diagnosable disease or symptoms, but risk factors present).

The bulk of medical education focuses on the already ill patient (tertiary prevention); progressively less time is spent on secondary and primary prevention. This may lead medical students and physicians to provide evaluation and treatment primarily in "reaction" to patient symptoms, rather than in a "proactive" mode of care—that is, attempting to anticipate problems and prevent them.

Physicians may encounter a variety of obstacles to providing comprehensive preventive health services including heavy demands on the physician's time by patients already ill, lack of financial resources in the patient population, negative third-party attitudes toward reimbursement for preventive health care, and patients uninformed about the benefits of disease prevention. The advent of managed care, however, has placed family physicians in a position in which they now have the latitude to provide a full range of preventive health services.

EVALUATING PREVENTIVE HEALTH ACTIVITIES

Not all diseases lend themselves well to the shift from medical intervention at the tertiary level to prevention at the secondary or primary levels. Several parameters are used to determine the validity of such a shift for each disease and to determine the population group to whom the intervention should be applied. The general criteria are as follows:

1. Is the disease worth screening for? Does it have a significant impact on the quality or length of life, and is it of sufficient prevalence in the population to justify screening?

2. Is sufficient information available to accurately identify, using risk factors and screening tests, the individual or groups likely to develop the disease? Or using diagnostic tests, is it possible to identify those likely already to have the disease at a presymptomatic stage?

3. Are the tests for the screening or early detection satisfactory in terms of accuracy, morbidity, cost, and acceptability to the patient and physician?

4. If it is possible to predict the disease or diagnose it before the onset of symptoms, is there a known intervention that will significantly alter the course of the disease?

5. Is the intervention or treatment satisfactory in terms of proved effectiveness, risk, morbidity, cost, and patient acceptability.

Table 5–1 is a mortality table for the United States. From it one can begin to understand the relative impact of various diseases on death rates. The trend for the year 1993 and for the previous 14 years for each disease is shown, allowing the reader to assess the degree of progress in prevention and treatment. In particular, the decreases in mortality from heart disease, stroke, and accidents are highly encouraging and are due primarily to preventive health measures. On the other hand, the marked increases in human immunodeficiency virus, chronic pulmonary disease, pneumonia, and influenza are very frustrating when one considers how preventable these deaths are. Finally, careful examination of the consistent pattern of increased risk for males and blacks highlights a number of lifestyle risks in these groups.

As shown in Table 5–2, 50 per cent of the deaths in the United States are preventable and are directly attributable to environmental and behavioral issues, most of which are a result of individuals' lifestyle decisions.

INTERVENTIONS AND RECOMMENDATION. The 1996 recommendations of the U.S. Preventive Services Task Force are referred to in this chapter. The student should recognize that these recommendations are for preventive health activities for which there is a high level of proof of value. There are additional tests and interventions that are used by many physicians as a result of recommendations

TABLE 5–1. Ten Highest Age-adjusted Death Rates per 100,000 Population for 1993 with Per Cent Change from 1992 and 1979—United States

Rank Order*	Cause of Death	1993 Age-adjusted Death Rate	Per Cent Change, 1992–1993	Per Cent Change, 1979–1993	Male: Female	Black: White
1	Diseases of the heart	145.3	0.7	−27.7	1.9	1.5
2	Malignant neoplasm	132.6	−0.4	1.4	1.5	1.4
3	Cerebrovascular disease	26.5	1.1	−36.3	1.2	1.8
4	Chronic obstructive pulmonary disease	21.4	7.5	46.6	1.6	0.8
5	Accidents and adverse effects	30.3	3.1	−29.4	2.6	1.3
	Motor vehicle	16.0	1.3	−31.0	2.3	1.0
	All others	14.4	5.1	−26.5	2.9	1.6
6	Pneumonia and influenza	13.5	6.3	20.5	1.6	1.4
7	Diabetes mellitus	12.4	4.2	26.5	1.2	2.4
8	HIV infection	13.8	9.5	—	6.3	4.0
9	Suicide	11.3	1.8	−3.4	4.4	0.6
10	Homicide and legal intervention	10.7	1.9	4.9	3.8	6.8

*Listed in rank order according to total number of deaths.
HIV, Human immunodeficiency virus.
From Morbid Mortal Weekly Rep 45(8);Mar 1, 1996.

TABLE 5–2. Actual Causes of Death in the United States

Cause	Estimated No. of Deaths	Per Cent of Total Deaths
Tobacco	400,000	19
Diet/activity patterns	300,000	14
Alcohol	100,000	5
Microbial agents	90,000	4
Toxins	60,000	3
Firearms	35,000	2
Sexual behavior	30,000	1
Motor vehicles	25,000	1
Illicit drug use	20,000	<1
Total	**1,060,000**	**50**

From McGinnis JM, Foege W. Actual causes of death in the United States. JAMA 1993;270:2207–2212.

by other highly respected medical authorities and organizations.

PREVENTION APPLIED TO SPECIFIC DISEASES

Coronary Heart Disease

INCIDENCE. The yearly national incidence of myocardial infarction is estimated to be 1.5 million. The majority of individuals (67 per cent of men and 43 per cent of women) with coronary heart disease (CHD) have no warning of their disease and present with either an acute myocardial infarction or sudden death as their initial symptom.

PREVALENCE. It is estimated that 13.5 million people alive today have either a history of myocardial infarction or symptomatic CHD, and 1 to 2 million middle-aged men in the United States have asymptomatic, but significant CHD. The prevalence of CHD is estimated at 7.2 per cent of the population over the age of 20.

Autopsy studies have shown that by 20 to 24 years of age, about 44 per cent of white men, 34 per cent of black men, 11 per cent of white women, and 43 per cent of black women have raised lesions in their coronary arteries.

Although difficult, predicting the prevalence in *asymptomatic* adults is of importance to the physician if early aggressive intervention is to be targeted to the appropriate patients. These high-risk groups are identified by an analysis of the risk factors present for CHD.

COST AND IMPACT ON SOCIETY. It is estimated that the cost of medical treatment and lost productivity for all cardiovascular disease in the United States is $151.1 billion, of which $66.4 billion is due to heart disease.

MORBIDITY AND MORTALITY. One in every 4.6 deaths in the United States is due to CHD—489,970 per year or about one third of all persons suffering from a myocardial infarction. Of those who survive, about two thirds do not make a complete recovery, although 88 per cent of those under age 65 eventually return to work. In the 6 years following myocardial infarction, 13 per cent of men and 6 per cent of women experience sudden death, and 23 per cent of men and 31 per cent of women have another infarction.

IMPORTANT FACTS RELEVANT TO PREVENTION

1. A major focus for prevention of CHD is encouraging healthy lifestyles for all patients.

2. Risk factor identification and reduction will reduce the incidence of CHD, particularly when concentrated on blood cholesterol levels, hypertension, cigarette smoking, and a sedentary lifestyle.

3. Changing the American diet to a low–saturated fat, low-cholesterol diet will reduce the levels of serum cholesterol in the population.

4. No population in the world has been found with a combination of high total serum cholesterol levels and low CHD.

5. Regression of coronary lesions is possible with adequate treatment. Even a very low fat diet combined with exercise and meditation, but without medication, has been shown to be effective.

6. In patients with significantly elevated cholesterol, cholesterol lowering medications have proved effective in reducing the incidence and mortality of myocardial infarction in both symptomatic and asymptomatic persons.

SCREENING TEST RECOMMENDATIONS

For the General Population

1. Measure total and high-density lipoprotein

(HDL) cholesterol between 20 and 30 years of age and every 5 years thereafter. Patients found to be high risk based on screening values should obtain a complete fasting lipid panel (total, low-density lipoprotein [LDL] and HDL cholesterol plus triglycerides) to most accurately determine risk status. Generally, children do not need to be screened, but consideration should be made for those who have a parent with a high-risk lipid profile or a history of premature heart disease in a first-degree relative (less than age 55 for men and less than age 65 for women).

2. Measure blood pressure each office visit.

3. Update family history at least every 5 years.

4. Update smoking status:
   a. Every 5 years in previous nonsmokers.
   b. Yearly in previous smokers who have quit.
   c. Every visit in current smokers.

5. Monitor activity levels at least every 5 years for every patient for the recommended 30 to 40 minutes of aerobic activity three to four times weekly.

6. Evaluate for obesity (greater than 20 to 30 per cent over ideal body weight) yearly.

7. Monitor stress levels yearly (family, occupation).

8. Physicians may elect to measure fasting blood sugar every 5 years since the presence of diabetes is a major risk factor.

PREVENTIVE ACTIVITIES RECOMMENDATIONS. Current national guidelines for determining CHD risk according to LDL cholesterol levels are listed in Tables 5–3 and 5–4. All risk factors noted in Table 5–4 should be modified wherever possible.

Cholesterol Control. Physicians should prescribe a heart healthy diet for *all* patients regardless of age or risk. It is particularly important that children learn healthy eating habits early in life. For patients less likely or able to follow the more extensive dietary instructions of the Step 1 diet as published by the American Heart Association (AHA) (1994), Table 5–5 gives very general guidelines that most patients can easily implement in a progressive manner.

All patients should be screened for risk status. The presence of other risk factors is used to determine the type of intervention based on LDL levels. Table 5–3 shows these recommendations for intervention with diet and medications. A diet high in soluble fiber (oat bran products, legumes, and some fruits) has been shown in some studies to reduce

TABLE 5–3. National Cholesterol Education Program Guidelines for Reduction of Coronary Heart Disease (CHD) Risk Based on Low-Density Lipoprotein (LDL) Levels and Personal History of Coronary Heart Disease

Patient Category	LDL Intervention Levels (mg/dl)		LDL Treatment Goal (mg/dl)
	Dietary Therapy	Drug Treatment	
Without CHD and <2 risk factors	≥160	≥190	<160
Without CHD and ≥2 risk factors	≥130	≥160	<130
With CHD	>100	≥130	≤100

From the Expert Panel on the Detection, Evaluation, and Treatment of High Blood Cholesterol in Adults. Summary of the Second Report of the National Cholesterol Education Program (NCEP) Expert Panel on Detection, Evaluation, and Treatment of High Blood Cholesterol in Adults (Adult Treatment Panel II). JAMA 1993;269:3015–3023.

TABLE 5–4. Risk Factors for Coronary Heart Disease (CHD) in Addition to Low-Density Lipoprotein (LDL) Cholesterol Values and Personal History of Coronary Heart Disease

Positive Risk Factors
Age
   Male ≥45
   Female ≥55 or premature menopause without estrogen replacement therapy
Family history of premature CHD in a first-degree relative (<55 yr of age in males and less than 65 in females)
Cigarette smoker
Hypertension
HDL cholesterol <35 mg/dl
Diabetes mellitus

Negative Risk Factors
High HDL cholesterol (≥60 mg/dl)

Other Risk Factors to Consider
Elevated triglyceride levels
High-stress personality profile (probable)
Inactivity (probable)
Oral contraceptive use in smokers over age 35
Severe obesity (more than 30% overweight)
History of any occlusive vascular disease, peripheral or cerebrovascular

Positive and negative risk factors from the Expert Panel on the Detection, Evaluation, and Treatment of High Blood Cholesterol in Adults. Summary of the Second Report of the National Cholesterol Education Program (NCEP) Expert Panel on Detection, Evaluation, and Treatment of High Blood Cholesterol in Adults (Adult Treatment Panel II). JAMA 1993;269:3015–3023.

TABLE 5–5. Dietary Suggestions to Assist Patients in Reducing the Cholesterol and Fat in Their Diet

Foods to Reduce or Eliminate	Recommended Substitutions
Whole eggs	Egg whites (2 whites = 1 whole egg)
	Egg substitute
Cheese	Whey cheeses
	Low-fat cottage cheese
	Low-fat (part-skim) cheeses
	Nondairy nonfat cheese
Whole milk	Low-fat or skim milk
Butter and hard margarine	Soft margarines
	Powdered butter flavoring
Ice cream, sherbets	Nonfat "ice cream" and frozen yogurt
	Ice milks
	Sorbets or ices
Fatty meats, hot dogs, luncheon sausage, bacon, poultry skin, internal organ meats	Lean varieties of red meats
	Meats less often and in smaller (3 oz) portions
	Skinned chicken and turkey
	Fish
	Avoid frying
	Nonmeat meals
	Textured vegetable-based meat substitutes
	Reduced portions if used
Shellfish	Use lower-cholesterol varieties (crab, clams, scallops)
Chocolate	Fish-based mock crab legs
Highly refined prepared foods	Cocoa
High-fat prepared foods (bakery items, food prepared with coconut, palm, palm kernel, or hydrogenated vegetable oils or animal fat or lard)	Whole-grain varieties, fresh fruits and vegetables
	Homemade or prepared low-fat varieties using the unsaturated vegetable oils (soybean, canola or rapeseed, olive, corn or safflower, sesame, sunflower)

From Rakel RE. Textbook of Family Practice, 4th ed. Philadelphia, WB Saunders Company, 1990, with permission.

serum cholesterol, whereas nonsoluble fiber (present primarily in wheat, vegetables, and fruits) has consistently shown no effect on cholesterol.

Other methods of altering risk secondary to hypercholesterolemia include weight control, exercise, and drug therapy.

Control of Hypertension. Aggressive treatment of all patients with hypertension is essential. Risk is proportional to blood pressure even at diastolic levels between 80 and 90. In general, a systolic pressure greater than 140 or a diastolic pressure greater than 90 is used as the cutoff point for hypertension, but this cutoff point as well as a treatment goal must be individualized, particularly in the elderly.

Before institution of drug therapy for hypertension, nonpharmacologic methods should be considered. These include salt restriction, weight reduction, biofeedback, and regular aerobic exercise.

Smoking Cessation. Smoking may be the most correctable risk factor for CHD. It presents a serious risk not only for the smoker, but to all those exposed

to secondhand smoke, particularly in the home. Clinical practice guidelines from the Agency for Health Care Policy and Research recommend that each physician should have a plan for assisting patients and other family members in smoking cessation which includes the following elements:

1. Ask patients about their desire to quit and reinforce their intention.

2. Motivate patients who are reluctant to quit.

3. Help motivated smokers to set a quit date.

4. Prescribe or recommend purchase of nicotine replacement therapy.

5. Help patients resolve problems that result from quitting. Counseling may be helpful to some patients.

6. Encourage relapsed smokers to try quitting again.

The authors also recommend structured long-term follow-up with maximal support and encouragement from physician and office staff.

Other Preventive Activities. It is recommended that physicians assist all patients to avoid risk factor development through encouragement of healthy lifestyles, e.g., avoid smoking, promote physical activity, cope effectively with stress, maintain ideal body weight, and provide periodic preventive health care. The mechanism of risk reduction for many factors has not been clearly defined. For instance, some dietary factors such as vitamin E, an antioxidant in the diet, and intake of three or more servings of fish weekly have been associated with a decreased risk of CHD. Recently a strong association has been shown between serum homocysteine levels and the incidence of CHD. Homocysteine is elevated by increased intake of animal protein.

DISCUSSION. The incidence of CHD in the United States has been decreasing significantly as shown in Table 5–1 and Figure 5–1. Sixty per cent of this decline is due to lifestyle changes, especially diet modification and smoking cessation. This encouraging information alone provides physicians sufficient reason to pursue further aggressive risk factor prevention and modification on a population-wide basis. Although age-adjusted mortality *rates* are declining, the actual *numbers* of deaths continue to increase as the proportion of elderly in the population increases.

Although total cholesterol measurement may be appropriate for mass public screening, use of total or LDL plus HDL levels is more appropriate when determining risk for individual patients. Measuring the HDL increases the predictive power approximately 6 to 10 times that of measuring total cholesterol alone. A low level of HDL is a strong, independent predictor of CHD (see Table 5–4). Up to 20

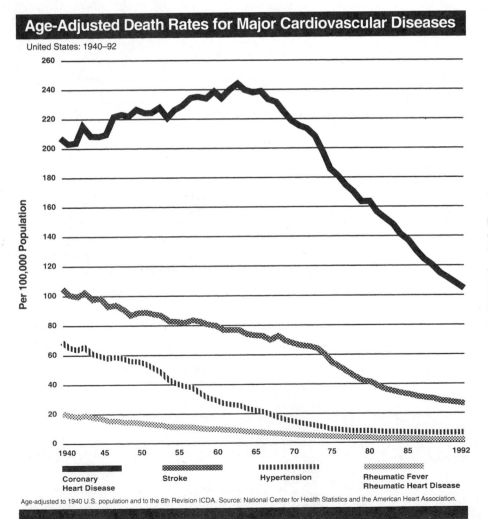

Figure 5–1. Cumulative per cent decline in age-adjusted death rates for coronary heart disease, (CHD), stroke, and total cardiovascular deaths, 1940–1992. (Reproduced with permission. Heart and Stroke Facts: 1996 Statistic Supplement, 1995. Copyright © American Heart Association.)

per cent of high-risk individuals are not identified using total cholesterol count alone.

Triglycerides can be important in determining risk. Women appear to be more affected than men by elevated triglycerides. In addition, there is a very high risk subpopulation with minimally elevated cholesterol and triglyceride levels and with an HDL under 40 mg/dl. Most authorities feel that use of the monounsaturated fats (olive oil, canola oil) should be emphasized in the total dietary fat allowance. This is based on epidemiologic studies and on the observation that these oils, when substituted for saturated fatty acids, reduce LDL cholesterol at least as much as the polyunsaturated fatty acids. Furthermore, they do not lower the HDL at the same time as do the polyunsaturated fats.

Recent data strongly suggest that sedentary lifestyle is a potent, independent risk factor that has an effect equal to the other major risk factors. The American Heart Association now recommends that sedentary lifestyle be included as a major independent risk for CHD. The effect of personality characteristics on CHD risk is poorly understood. Although type A personality has been traditionally implicated as a risk factor, studies are conflicting. There is general agreement that emotional status plays a significant role in CHD.

Assessing total risk for individual patients may be complicated by the presence of more than one risk factor. A model for visualizing this process is shown in Figure 5–2. In this figure one can better understand the effect of adding major risks to a baseline cholesterol of 200 mg/dl. However, it must be recognized that most major risk factors vary in impact as their values change. Figure 5–3 shows this variable effect using increasing cholesterol values. Using the concepts in these two figures, a valuable

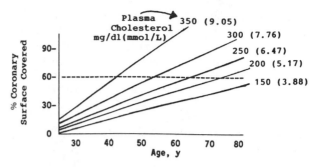

Figure 5–3. Relationship of coronary atherosclerosis (percentage of surface arteries covered with raised lesions) vs. age at different levels of plasma cholesterol. At 60% of coronary surfaces covered with lesions, patients enter zone of markedly enhanced risk for clinical coronary heart disease. (From Grundy, SM. Cholesterol and coronary heart disease: A new era. JAMA 1986;256:2848–2858, with permission.)

paradigm is presented for cardiovascular risk assessment.

IMPACT ON FAMILY UNIT. The lifestyles that are important for prevention of CHD cannot be easily implemented by an individual without due consideration of the person's family and environment. The chances of abstinence from smoking are dimmed considerably when there are other smokers in the home. Diet changes are especially difficult to implement for only one individual in a family unit. Major changes in knowledge, attitudes, and habits in the entire family are often required so that the desirable foods can be purchased, properly prepared, and consumed with an agreed-on common family goal of improved health. Anything less can lead to resentments, confusion, and outright rebellion.

When a family member needs dietary therapy, a family meeting at the beginning enhances the chances of long-term success. This meeting can be used to educate the family about risk and diet, enlist the cooperation and support of all family members, and make plans for flexibility to meet everyone's needs. Fortunately, the AHA diets are nutritionally well balanced and can be recommended to all, regardless of risk status. Helpful guidelines and educational materials for use in the office are available from the AHA through local and state chapters. Excellent cookbooks are widely available; one is available from the AHA.

Cerebrovascular Disease

INCIDENCE. Incidence of stroke is 500,000 people per year. The yearly incidence increases with age

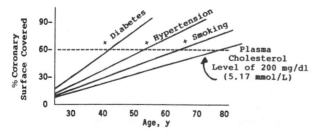

Figure 5–2. Relationship of coronary atherosclerosis (percentage of surface of coronary arteries covered with lesions) vs. age as modified by addition of risk factors. In absence of other risk factors, patient with cholesterol level of 200 mg/dl (5.17 mmol/L) should reach critical stenosis at about age 70 years. Addition of smoking reduces age to 60 years, and addition of more risk factors (i.e., hypertension and diabetes mellitus) reduces age further. (From Grundy, SM. Cholesterol and coronary heart disease: A new era. JAMA 1986;256:2848–2858, with permission.)

from 100 in 100,000 people for ages 45 to 54 to 1800 in 100,000 people at age 85. This translates into a 1 in 20 chance of having a stroke before age 70 for both men and women. Significant decreases have occurred in the last 25 years with recognition and management of risk factors and with lifestyle modification.

PREVALENCE. There are nearly 3.8 million living stroke victims in the United States. This does not include the millions of individuals with significant atherosclerotic cerebrovascular disease who are at an extremely high risk for stroke.

COST AND IMPACT ON SOCIETY. The yearly cost of stroke to society is estimated at $23.2 billion for medical costs and lost productivity.

MORBIDITY AND MORTALITY. Stroke is the cause of 1 in 15 deaths or 149,000 deaths per year and is the third leading cause of death in the United States after CHD and cancer. Thirty-one per cent of stroke victims die within 1 year.

In addition to the high mortality, stroke is the leading cause of long-term disability. Forty per cent of stroke survivors require special services and 10 per cent require total care.

IMPORTANT FACTS RELEVANT TO PREVENTION. The major risk factor for stroke is hypertension. The other risk factors for CHD are less predictive for stroke risk than is hypertension. However, the known presence of heart disease (CHD or atrial fibrillation) carries a high risk for emboli to the brain. Atrial fibrillation is responsible for 15 per cent of cerebral infarcts. Diabetes mellitus, even if mild, carries a significant increased risk for stroke. This risk rises dramatically if both hypertension and diabetes are present.

Transient ischemic attacks (TIAs) confer a high risk of subsequent stroke. One out of five stroke victims has had at least one of four major symptoms suggestive of TIA in the year previous: (1) temporary loss of vision (especially if in one eye), (2) unilateral numbness, (3) aphasia, and (4) focal weakness.

Patients with carotid bruits have a 1 to 3 per cent incidence of stroke per year. Although aspirin, anticoagulants, and surgery are commonly prescribed, the current data are not sufficient to show that these treatments effectively reduce the risk of stroke in patients with asymptomatic carotid bruits. Such studies are in progress and will provide further guidance in the future.

Other risk factors for stroke include family his-

tory of stroke, cigarette smoking, oral contraceptive use, hyperlipidemia, and elevated hematocrit.

SCREENING TEST RECOMMENDATIONS. Elevated blood pressure, systolic *or* diastolic, is the single greatest risk factor for stroke and should be evaluated at each office visit. Cigarette smoking is the other major modifiable risk factor for stroke. Other risk factors (similar to those for CHD) for atherosclerosis should be sought, as previously recommended in the discussion on coronary heart disease. Carotid bruits should be listened for every 5 years after age 40.

PREVENTIVE ACTIVITIES RECOMMENDATIONS. Prevention of stroke is aimed primarily at prevention and treatment of sustained, even mild, hypertension. Promotion of the healthy lifestyle habits discussed earlier for CHD are of likely, although unproved, benefit. Smokers, in particular, should be strongly advised to stop. Secondary prevention of completed stroke in patients with TIAs may include aspirin prophylaxis, anticoagulation, or carotid endarterectomy, depending on the clinical circumstances.

DISCUSSION. The most important reason to listen for carotid bruits is to document the existence of significant atherosclerosis in high-risk individuals and thus alert the physician to the need to more aggressively modify risk factors. There is a risk with this approach to initiating a process that includes angiography and endarterectomy, procedures that have no clear consensus as to their proper use in asymptomatic individuals.

IMPACT ON FAMILY UNIT. The common results of stroke—physical disability, intellectual disability, and depression—often cause a loss of independence. The family or friends are suddenly forced to help make parental-type decisions. Active participation in the rehabilitation and care of a stroke victim can create an enormous stress, financially and emotionally, on the family unit. Placement in a nursing home, however rational, requires a resolution of guilt within the family. The family physician plays a critical central role in the coordination of rehabilitation with the family and in helping the family to resolve conflicting feelings.

Substance Abuse, Alcoholism, and Other Drug Dependency

INCIDENCE. Difficulties in clearly identifying a point in time at which an individual becomes alcohol- or drug-dependent make incidence rates very difficult to determine reliably.

PREVALENCE. Estimates of the prevalence of alcohol abuse or dependence range up to 18 million Americans, or 7.5 per cent of the entire population. Among men estimates range from 17 to 24 per cent. In an ambulatory medical setting the prevalence of alcoholism is 10 to 20 per cent. The rates for dependency on other drugs is about 2 per cent. The rates of drug use and abuse in adolescents and young adults is particularly worrisome. After a decade of decline, drug use among 12- to 17-year-olds rose 78 per cent in just 3 years from 1992 to 1995 while there was no change among adults (Table 5–6).

COST AND IMPACT ON SOCIETY. The estimated yearly cost of alcohol abuse in the United States is $85.8 billion including $72.3 billion from lost employment and reduced productivity, and $13.5 billion in health care costs. The estimated total cost of illicit drug use is $58 billion. The social consequences of problem drinking, while nonquantifiable, may be as great as the costs of the medical consequences. Twenty per cent of alcohol abusers report problems with friends, family, work, or police which are secondary to drinking. Abusers have a higher rate of divorce, domestic violence, unemployment, and poverty.

MORBIDITY AND MORTALITY. Patients with alcoholism have 2.5 times the normal overall risk of mortality. Overall mortality is 30 to 38 per cent higher among men and more than doubled in women who drink more than six drinks a day. There are more than 100,000 deaths per year related to alcohol abuse and half of these are related to accidental deaths.

The morbidity for chemical dependency (alcohol and drug abuse) is substantial, ranging from the extremely high association with crime to cirrhosis, psychosis, depression, cardiomyopathy, peptic ulcer disease, overdose, cancer of directly exposed organs (lips, mouth, larynx, pharynx, esophagus, stomach, liver), pancreatitis, suicide, various infections (hepatitis, AIDS, endocarditis, pneumonia), fetal alcohol syndrome, and accidents of all types.

IMPORTANT FACTS RELEVANT TO PREVENTION. The most useful definition of chemical dependency is *the continued habitual use of a substance by a person despite resultant serious adverse effects on that person's life.* However, the majority of adverse consequences are a result of inappropriate use (abuse), not necessarily dependency. A helpful way of understanding the relationship between alcohol consumption and resultant problems is shown in Figure 5–4.

Measures to increase enforcement of drinking and driving laws, to increase prices for alcoholic beverages, and to increase the legal drinking age have been successful by reducing either alcohol consumption or the frequency of the legal consequences of drinking. Whether education can, in fact, reduce the rate of alcoholism is not known. Strong cultural biases (e.g., Orthodox Jews) against drunkenness substantially reduce the prevalence of dependency.

Children of alcoholics are at a three times greater risk of alcoholism, whether or not they are raised by their biological parents.

While spontaneous recovery from alcoholism is reported in up to 30 per cent of patients, treatment has been reported to result in a 61 per cent recovery rate. One must remember that studies use a variety of definitions of both alcoholism and of "recovery." It is unrealistic, dangerous, and delusional for an alcoholic ever to attempt controlled drinking.

SCREENING TEST RECOMMENDATIONS. All patients over 12 years of age should be screened regularly for alcohol and substance abuse. A yearly frequency of screening delivers a strong educational message to the patient.

Probably the single best screening is to ascertain through questioning, if the patient has ever had a health, legal, or personal problem as a result of drinking alcohol. Two positive responses for the CAGE questions (Table 5–7) are also highly suggestive of alcohol dependency and require further investigation. The MAST (Michigan Alcoholism

TABLE 5–6. Per Cent of Illicit Use of Drugs by 12- to 17-Year-Olds in 1995 and Per Cent Increase in 3 Years

Drug	1995, %	Per Cent Increase, 1992–1995
Use of illicit drugs past month	10.9	78
Use of drugs on a monthly basis	10.4	N/A
Monthly use of hallucinogens	1.7	183
Cocaine use	0.8	166
Marijuana use	37	105
Heroin use	0.7	133

From the National Household Survey on Drug Abuse.

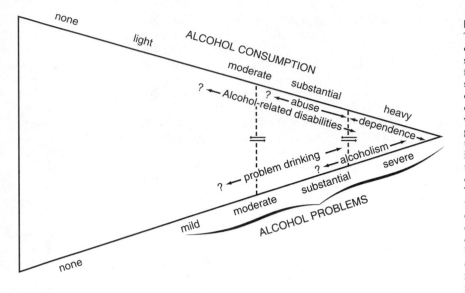

Figure 5–4. A terminological map. The triangle represents the population of the United States. The alcohol consumption of the population ranges from none to heavy (along the upper side of the triangle) and the problems experienced in association with alcohol consumption range from none to severe (along the lower side of the triangle). The two-way arrows and the dotted lines indicate that, both from an individual and a population perspective, consumption levels and the degree of problems vary from time to time. The scope of terms that are often used to refer to individuals and groups according to consumption levels and the degree of their problems is illustrated; question marks indicate that the lower boundary for many of the terms is uncertain. (Reprinted with permission from Broadening the Base of Treatment for Alcohol Problems. Copyright 1990 by the National Academy of Sciences. Courtesy of the National Academy Press, Washington, DC.)

Screening Test), as shown in Table 5–8, can also be helpful in the diagnostic evaluation.

The presence or absence of alcoholism in first-degree relatives should be a part of the family history. All patients, including children, should be asked yearly if there are any problems within the family that involve alcohol.

PREVENTIVE ACTIVITIES RECOMMENDATIONS. Literature concerning the warning signs of alcoholism and sources of help should be freely available in every medical office. If the subject of chemical dependency is dealt with openly there is an increased likelihood of seeking help through the family physician. All pregnant women should be advised against the use of alcohol and drugs during pregnancy and all users should be advised against driving and

performing other dangerous behaviors while intoxicated.

Patients with a family history of alcoholism should be counseled concerning their high-risk status and encouraged to become a member of Alanon or the Children of Alcoholics Foundation.

DISCUSSION. The same questions used for alcohol dependence may be equally applicable to drug abuse. Certain cues found in alcoholics and often in other drug-dependent patients help lead to the correct diagnosis: problems with children, separation, divorce, job changes, depression, anxiety, hypertension, macrocytosis of red blood cells, low resistance to infections, recurrent accidents, any trouble with legal authorities (including driving while intoxicated), upper gastrointestinal complaints, and abnormal liver enzymes.

IMPACT ON FAMILY UNIT. The family is at the epicenter of the alcoholic earthquake. As the rumblings of the disease progress, so does pathology within the family. Twenty-seven million American children live with an alcoholic parent and are at significant risk of serious physical and psychological consequences. Most prominent is the role of the "coalcoholic" or "enabler" who assumes the abnegated responsibilities of the alcoholic, covers for the alcoholic, and makes possible his or her continued drinking. This person is often the major focus of

TABLE 5–7.   CAGE Screening Test for Alcoholism

Any two positives are highly suggestive.

CAGE questions:
C utting down?
A nnoyed by criticism of your drinking?
G uilty about your drinking?
E ye opener ever?

From Rakel RE. Textbook of Family Practice, 5th ed. Philadelphia, WB Saunders, 1995, with permission.

TABLE 5–8. Michigan Alcoholism Screening Test

Question	Yes	No
Do you enjoy having a drink now and then?	0	—
Do you feel you are a normal drinker? (By normal we mean you drink less than or as much as most other people and you have not gotten into any recurring trouble while drinking)	—	2
Have you ever awakened the morning after some drinking the night before and found that you could not remember part of the evening?	2	—
Does either of your parents, or any near relative, or your spouse, or any girlfriend or boyfriend ever worry or complain about your drinking?	1	—
Can you stop drinking without a struggle after one or two drinks?	—	2
Do you feel guilty about your drinking?	1	—
Do friends or relatives think you are a normal drinker?	—	2
Are you able to stop drinking when you want to?	—	2
Have you ever attended a meeting of Alcoholics Anonymous? (AA)	5	—
Have you gotten into physical fights when you have been drinking?	1	—
Has your drinking ever created problems between you and either of your parents, or another relative, your spouse, or any girlfriend or boyfriend?	2	—
Has any family member of yours ever gone to anyone for help about your drinking?	2	—
Have you ever lost friends because of your drinking?	2	—
Have you ever got into trouble at work or school because of your drinking?	2	—
Have you ever lost a job because of drinking?	2	—
Have you ever neglected your obligations, your schoolwork, your family, or your job for 2 or more days in a row because you were drinking?	2	—
Do you drink before noon fairly often?	1	—
Have you ever been told you had liver trouble or cirrhosis?	2	—
After heavy drinking have you ever had severe shaking, or heard voices or seen things that really weren't there?	2 (5 DTs)	—
Have you ever gone to anyone for help about your drinking?	5	—
Have you ever been in a hospital because of drinking?	5	—
Have you ever been a patient in a psychiatric hospital or a psychiatric ward of a general hospital where drinking was part of the problem that resulted in hospitalization?	2	—
Have you ever been seen at a psychiatric or mental health clinic or gone to any doctor, social worker or clergy for help with any emotional problem, where drinking was a part of the problem?	2	—
Have you ever been arrested for drunk driving, driving while intoxicated, or driving under the influence of alcoholic beverages or any other drug? If yes, how many times? _____	2 each	—
Have you ever been arrested, or taken into custody even for a few hours, because of drunk behavior, whether due to alcohol or another drug? If yes, how many times? _____	2 each	—

Each response scores the number of points listed. A total of 0–3 points = probable normal drinker; 4 = borderline; 5–9 = 80% likelihood of dependence; 10 or more = 100% likelihood.

DTs = Delirium tremens.

From Selzer ML. The Michigan Alcohol Screening Test: The quest for a new diagnostic instrument. Am J Psychiatry 1971;127:1653, with permission.

the alcoholic's hostility. Treatment should include healing of the entire family.

Cancer

General Cancer Information

The incidence, mortality, and morbidity data for all cancers are summarized in this section and not necessarily repeated in the discussion on each type of cancer. The leading sites for new cancer cases and mortality for males and females are shown in Figure 5–5.

INCIDENCE. The number of estimated new U.S. cancer cases per year (excluding 800,000 carcinomas in situ and nonmelanotic skin cancers) is 1.36 million. The six most frequent cancers (excluding skin) are lung, colon-rectum, breast, prostate, urinary tract, and uterus. The chances of a female developing cancer in her lifetime is one in three; for males it is one in two.

PREVALENCE. There are over 10 million people alive today with a history of cancer. Seven million of these have survived more than 5 years since diagnosis and the majority of these are considered cured. No data

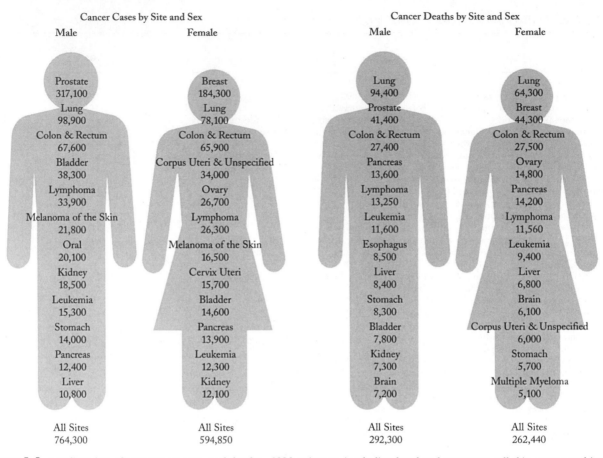

Figure 5–5. Leading sites of new cancer cases and deaths—1996 estimates (excluding basal and squamous cell skin cancer and in situ carcinomas except bladder). (From American Cancer Society. Cancer Facts and Figures—1996. Reprinted by the permission of the American Cancer Society, Inc.)

are available to indicate how many Americans have undiagnosed cancer at this time.

COST AND IMPACT ON SOCIETY. The estimated U.S. total cost of medical care for cancer is over $104 billion a year—$35 billion in medical costs and $69 billion in other costs to society. In comparison, screening programs account for only $3 to $4 billion of the total cost of medical services for cancer.

MORBIDITY AND MORTALITY. Cancer is second only to cardiovascular diseases as a cause of mortality in the United States and is responsible for one fourth of all deaths. The estimated yearly mortality for cancer is nearly 555,000. The eight leading causes of cancer death are lung, colon-rectum, breast, prostate, pancreas, urinary system, lymphoma, and leukemia.

From 1930 to 1992 the yearly U.S. mortality rate for cancer rose from 130 to 172 per 100,000 population. This rise has been primarily due to the continuing rise of mortality from cancer of the lung. The long-term trends and relative mortality of the major cancers for males and females are shown in Figures 5–6 and 5–7.

IMPORTANT FACTS RELEVANT TO PREVENTION. Thirty-five per cent of all cancer deaths are thought to be related to diet (including obesity). Obese individuals have increased risk of colorectal, breast, prostate, gallbladder, ovarian, and uterine cancers. High-fat diets are a risk factor for prostate, breast, and colon cancer. Foods rich in vitamins A (dark-green and deep-yellow vegetables and fruits) and vitamin C (citrus fruits, strawberries, and sweet peppers) and cruciferous vegetables (cabbage, broccoli, brussels sprouts, and cauliflower) are all thought to have protective effects for various cancers. Salt-cured, smoked, and nitrite-cured foods increase the risk of upper gastrointestinal cancers.

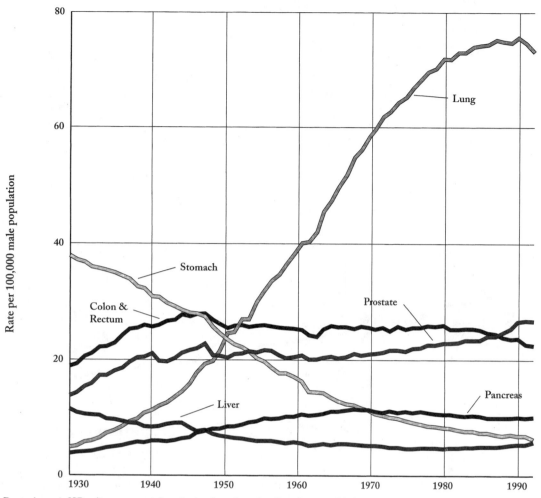

Note: Due to changes in ICD coding, numerator information has changed over time. Rates for cancer of the liver are particularly affected by these coding changes. Denominator information for the years 1930–1967 and 1991–1992 is based on intercensal population estimates, while denominator information for the years 1968–1990 is based on postcensal recalculation of estimates.

Source: Vital Statistics of the United States, 1995.

Figure 5–6. Age-adjusted cancer death rates per 100,000 population, males by site, United States 1930–1992. (From American Cancer Society. Cancer Facts and Figures—1996. Reprinted by the permission of the American Cancer Society, Inc.)

Smoking accounts for 30 per cent of cancer deaths (primarily lung, urinary bladder, mouth, throat, and larynx), while alcohol is responsible for approximately 3 per cent and occupational exposures for 5 per cent of cancer mortality.

Thus diet, smoking, alcohol, and occupational exposures may account for over 73 per cent of all cancer mortality. The American Cancer Society (ACS) estimates that if everything known about preventing cancer were applied, the occurrence rate of cancer would be reduced by two thirds. Many of these preventable causes are amenable to intervention by the family physician.

The ACS estimates that if their recommended screening programs for early detection of cancers of the breast, tongue, mouth, colon, rectum, cervix, prostate, testes, and of melanoma were fully implemented, the 5-year survival for these cancers would rise to 95 per cent—saving an estimated 115,000 lives each year. As shown in Figure 5–8, the stage at which cancer is discovered has a profound effect on the prognosis.

DISCUSSION. Family physicians must be prudent in determining whether to include new cancer screening tests in their preventive health screening program. In particular, the argument that a test detects cancers at an earlier, and therefore more curable,

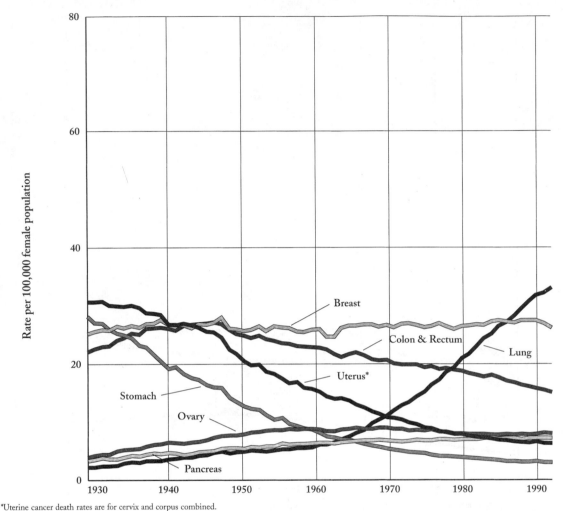

*Uterine cancer death rates are for cervix and corpus combined.

Note: Due to changes in ICD coding, numerator information has changed over time. Denominator information for the years 1930–1967 and 1991–1992 is based on intercensus population estimates, while denominator information for the years 1968–1990 is based on postcensus recalculation of estimates.

Source: Vital Statistics of the United States, 1995.

Figure 5–7. Age-adjusted cancer death rates per 100,000 population, females by site, United States 1930–1992. (From American Cancer Society. Cancer Facts and Figures—1996. Reprinted by the permission of the American Cancer Society, Inc.)

stage is not always validated when studied in a randomized, controlled trial. While awaiting such studies, physicians must make judgments based on the likelihood of a better outcome for patients versus the potential to cause harm, as well as the estimated cost-benefit ratio. The prevention of cancer takes on a new urgency when one considers the likely dramatic rise in incidence due to the increasing number of elderly and decreasing mortality from other causes.

Impact on Family Unit. For many cancers, a positive family history is a significant risk factor that can open the door for the physician to emphasize pre-

vention and early detection for these families. An increasing number of genetic screening tests for cancer risk will also become widely available. This entire preventive process must be approached very carefully as it may create a variety of behavioral problems within the family. Individual family members may experience hypochondriasis, depression, phobic disorders, generalized anxiety, and anger or hostility. These may be precipitated when issues of illness and death are being dealt with in the family.

Because of the great importance of lifestyle in the prevention of cancer, family health habits are the major source of successful cancer prevention. When one considers the fact that cancer strikes

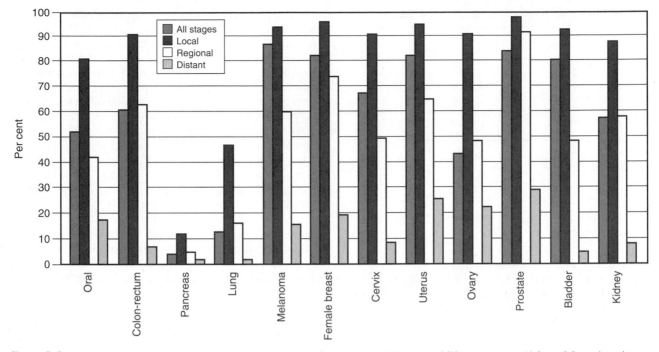

Figure 5–8. Five-year cancer relative survival rates by stage of diagnosis, adjusted for normal life expectancy. (Adapted from American Cancer Society. Cancer Facts and Figures—1996. Data from National Cancer Institute, Cancer Statistics Branch.)

three out of four families, the value of widely applied preventive health measures by every family physician becomes evident.

Colorectal Cancer

INCIDENCE. Colorectal cancer has the second highest incidence of all cancers. The incidence of colorectal cancer begins to rise after age 40, roughly doubling every 7 years after age 50. Ninety per cent occur in the population over age 50. The incidence is increased in younger people who have a family history of colon or rectal cancer.

MORBIDITY AND MORTALITY. The lifetime risk of dying of colorectal cancer is 2.6 per cent.

IMPORTANT FACTS RELEVANT TO PREVENTION. Colorectal cancer appears to arise over a period of 5 to 10 years almost exclusively from benign adenomatous polyps. However, only 20 to 30 per cent of polyps are adenomas, and only 5 to 10 per cent of adenomatous polyps become malignant. The appearance of adenomas begins primarily between ages 40 and 45 with a significant increase in colorectal cancer in those 5 to 10 years older.

When compared with pathologic findings on colonoscopy, stool guaiac specimens (stool samples daily for 3 consecutive days) were 52 per cent sensitive for carcinoma, 23 per cent sensitive for polyps greater than 1.0 cm, and 4.4 per cent sensitive for polyps less than 1.0 cm. A major prospective study (uncontrolled) of over 20,000 patients followed for up to 25 years and screened periodically with only a 25-cm sigmoidoscope showed a 50 per cent reduction in incidence of bowel cancers over that predicted. Although there has been a progressive change toward polyps occurring higher in the large bowel, over 60 per cent are still within reach of the 60-cm flexible sigmoidoscope.

Figure 5–8 shows the dramatic change in the survival rate with the stage of the cancer. Compared with the current 5-year survival rate of 61 per cent, it is estimated that potentially 80 to 90 per cent of all colon cancers could be prevented by screening stool for occult blood, sigmoidoscopy, and removal of adenomatous polyps found during further evaluation of positive screening tests.

Epidemiologically, 20 per cent of colorectal cancers can be attributed to a dietary cause, especially lack of fiber. High-fat diets have also been implicated. Risk factors for colorectal cancer are found in Table 5–9. Decreased incidence has also been associated with regular use of aspirin and other nonsteroidal anti-inflammatory drugs and with post-

TABLE 5–9. Risk Factors for Colorectal Cancer

Age >50
History of adenomas
Personal or family history of colorectal cancer or polyps
Ulcerative colitis
Crohn disease affecting colon
Personal or family history of genital or breast cancer in females
Physical inactivity

From Rakel RE. Textbook of Family Practice, 5th ed. Philadelphia, WB Saunders, 1995, with permission.

menopausal estrogen replacement therapy in women.

SCREENING TEST RECOMMENDATIONS. Patients should be offered a rectal examination and six slide fecal occult blood tests yearly as well as flexible sigmoidoscopy every 3 to 5 years starting by age 50. The American Cancer Society recommends annual digital rectal examinations commencing at age 40.

PREVENTIVE ACTIVITIES RECOMMENDATIONS. Risk factor analysis should be performed at least by 40 years of age. Preventive activities include the surveillance described earlier, looking for presymptomatic carcinomas and lesions with malignant potential (adenomas). All patients should be encouraged to eat a high-fiber, low-fat diet.

DISCUSSION. The most effective screening would be periodic colonoscopy on all high-risk persons. This is neither practical, cost-effective, or acceptable to patients. Some studies suggest that a screening interval of up to 10 years for flexible sigmoidoscopy may be equally effective as every 3 to 5 years.

IMPACT ON FAMILY UNIT. Since family history is a major risk factor, information obtained by the family physician should be used for family education concerning prevention.

Breast Cancer

INCIDENCE. The lifetime incidence of breast cancer for females is now one in nine. Thirty-one per cent of all new female cancers are breast cancers, compared with 13 per cent for lung cancer, the next most common cancer in females. In American women, the incidence of breast cancer increases with age as shown in Figure 5–9.

MORBIDITY AND MORTALITY. The mortality rate for breast cancer has been stable since 1930. This accounts for 17 per cent of all female cancer deaths—second to the 25 per cent of female cancer deaths caused by lung cancer. In situ breast cancer has a cure rate approaching 100 per cent. The 5-year survival rate today for localized breast cancer is 96 per cent, compared with 78 per cent in the 1940s. Five-year survival is 75 per cent for regional spread and 20 per cent for distant spread (Fig. 5–8). The survival rates at 5, 8, and 10 years were 88 per cent, 83 per cent, and 79 per cent for breast cancers diagnosed through screening in the Breast Cancer Detection Demonstration Project.

IMPORTANT FACTS RELEVANT TO PREVENTION. The major accepted risk factors are listed in Table 34–1, page 298. Despite evaluation of risk factors, 75 per cent of women with breast cancer have no risk factor other than their age. As already noted, the risk rises progressively with age.

Breast self-examination alone has an average sensitivity of 26 per cent (higher in young women and lower in the elderly), compared with an estimated 45 per cent for clinical breast examination and 71 to 75 per cent for mammography, and 75 to 88 per cent for a combination of mammography and clinical breast examination. Reported specificity of mammography ranges from 83 to 98.5 per cent. A definitive study showing a lowered mortality for those performing breast self-examination has not been done. Despite the lower sensitivity than mammography, clinical breast examination is thought to be useful. The Health Insurance Plan Trial estimated that two thirds of the effectiveness of its combined mammography and clinical breast examination screening was due to the clinical breast examination.

Overall, regular screening mammography results in a 20 to 35 per cent decrease in mortality in women 50 to 69 years of age. Although a number of randomized trials have included women ages 40 to 49 and 70 to 74, there is still inadequate statistical evidence to validate the value of mammography in these groups. However, a meta-analysis of seven randomized clinical trials has shown a statistically significant 24 per cent reduction in mortality for women, ages 40 to 49, screened with mammography (Smart et al., 1995). In most trials it appears that biennial mammography plus annual clinical breast examination may be as effective as doing both annually.

A number of factors have been shown *not* to alter the risk of breast cancer. These include breast trauma, fibroadenomas, fibrocystic breast disease of

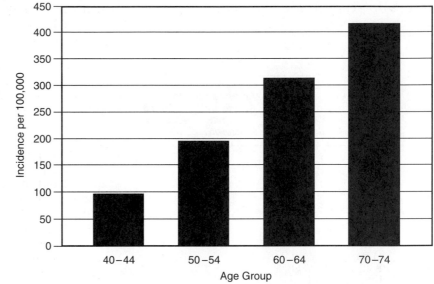

Figure 5–9. Annual incidence of breast cancer, American women, by age group. (From Ries LAG, Miller BA, Hankey BF, et al. [eds]. SEER Cancer Statistics Review, 1973–1991: Tables and Graphs. Bethesda, MD, National Cancer Institute, 1994.)

the nonproliferative type, caffeine consumption, mastodynia with negative mammographic and clinical examination, and breast feeding.

SCREENING TEST RECOMMENDATIONS. Table 5–10 outlines the official guidelines of the U.S. Preventive Services Task Force, the American Academy of Family Physicians, and the American Cancer Society. These recommendations range from conservative to aggressive. Each physician must decide the level of preventive care to implement in practice. The U.S. Preventive Services Task Force guidelines represent the minimum level of preventive health care expected of primary care physicians.

PREVENTIVE ACTIVITIES RECOMMENDATIONS. Very little has been proved concerning the primary prevention of breast cancer. Diet may have a significant role. Patients should be advised of the concern raised by the association of moderate alcohol ingestion, high-fat diets, and low-fiber diets with breast cancer. These dietary recommendations can be made on other grounds and are considered to be of general benefit. Therefore, physicians may wish to make these recommendations before a direct cause-and-effect relationship is firmly established.

Although of unproved benefit, breast self-examination is a logical, low-risk, no-cost activity. It should be taught to each woman at the time of her first gynecologic examination, and reviewed at each subsequent examination. Every woman should have an initial documented evaluation of risk factors for breast cancer at or before age 30 with updates every 3 to 5 years.

Secondary prevention (the early detection of disease before symptoms appear) is the focus of current major screening recommendations. All lesions of the breast should be promptly investigated. Any suspicious mass found on physician examination or mammography should be evaluated by needle aspiration, needle biopsy, or open excisional biopsy, depending on the clinical circumstances.

DISCUSSION. Environmental and lifestyle factors deserve more attention. The Japanese have a very low incidence of breast cancer. However, subsequent generations of Japanese immigrants to the United States have increasing incidence rates, eventually equaling the high U.S. levels.

Many factors may contribute to placing a girl or woman into the high-risk group. For instance, a mother and sister with premenopausal bilateral breast cancer imparts a 30 per cent lifetime risk.

The issue of screening with mammography from ages 40 to 49 remains controversial, although evidence of its value is increasing. Ironically, it appears that the most effective screening interval for ages 40 to 49 may be annually, whereas that for women over age 50 may be biennially.

A screening program that includes regular breast examinations and mammography produces a substantial reduction in breast cancer mortality, but up to 10 per cent of women have false-positive results and need to be evaluated with further diagnostic work-up, such as needle aspiration, needle biopsy, or open biopsy.

The costs of mammographic screening remain

TABLE 5–10. Official Recommendations for Breast Cancer Screening

| Age | Test | Interval | | |
		American Cancer Society	American Academy of Family Physicians	U.S. Preventive Health Services Task Force
20–34	BSE	Monthly		
	CBE	3 Yr		
35–39	BSE	Monthly		
	CBE	3 Yr		
	MAM			
40–49	BSE	Monthly		
	CBE	1 Yr	+	1 Yr*
	MAM	1–2 Yr	+	1 Yr*
50–59	BSE	Monthly		
	CBE	1 Yr	1–2 yr	1 Yr†
	MAM	1 Yr	1–2 yr	1–2 Yr
60–69	BSE	Monthly		
	CBE	1 Yr	1–2 yr	1 Yr†
	MAM	1 Yr	1–2 yr	1–2 Yr
70 +	BSE	Monthly		
	CBE	1 Yr		1 Yr†
	MAM	1 Yr		1–2 Yr†

*Consider for high risk.
†Elective at physician's discretion.
BSE = Breast self-examination; CBE = clinical breast examination; MAM = mammography.

a major concern. Even limiting mammography to those over age 50 would result in a 10-year cost of $3.3 billion at the current average cost of $100 per examination. This is by far the most expensive preventive health care activity recommended. However, in terms of cost per year of life saved, it compares favorably with screening recommendations for cervical and colorectal cancer.

The smaller the tumor when discovered, the better the prognosis. A review of several studies shows that nonpalpable cancers detected by mammography have a 13 to 20 per cent incidence of metastatic spread, whereas tumors found by palpation have positive lymph nodes 40 to 55 per cent of the time. It has been calculated that the average time between the ability of mammography to first detect the cancer and the ability to palpate the mass is 2 years, which may be of some value in estimating the optimal interval for mammography.

IMPACT ON FAMILY UNIT. The fear of breast cancer can produce substantial anxiety. This fear is heightened by a strong family history. As with other inher-ited risk for disease, the elements of guilt and resentment can have a profound effect on family functioning. Once a diagnosis of breast cancer is established a major concern is the patient's and husband's perceived loss of female identity. This can be allayed in part by a knowledgeable physician willing to discuss these issues openly and inform the patient and her husband of the variety of improved treatment alternatives now available. These include consideration of limited surgical procedures and radiation treatment. In addition, the family physician can play a critical role in preventing subsequent family dysfunction. The patient needs help in dealing with anger, helplessness, fear of recurrence, and the ill effects of treatments. Once cancer has been diagnosed, the emotional life of the family is changed forever. The family as a unit requires guidance and understanding.

Lung Cancer

INCIDENCE. Lung cancer now has the second highest cancer incidence for both males and females in the United States (see Fig. 5–5).

MORBIDITY AND MORTALITY. Lung cancer is the leading cause of cancer mortality for both males and females. Comparing the similarity of the incidence and mortality statistics, the grim nature of the prognosis is apparent—a 13 per cent 5-year survival rate.

IMPORTANT FACTS RELEVANT TO PREVENTION. Except for the minority of cases secondary to industrial exposure, the only known way to prevent lung cancers is to not smoke. Eighty-seven per cent of all lung cancer deaths are directly attributable to smoking. Reduction in environmental tobacco smoke (ETS) is an important public health measure. ETS is responsible for 3000 lung cancer deaths yearly in nonsmoking adults.

SCREENING TEST RECOMMENDATIONS. Although chest x-ray or sputum cytology studies may detect lung cancer at a presymptomatic stage, there is no study that shows a resultant improvement in the prognosis.

PREVENTIVE ACTIVITIES RECOMMENDATIONS. Patients at all ages should receive a strong health message from their physician concerning smoking: "It's addicting. Don't start. If you have started, stop." All preventive health examinations should have an inquiry concerning smoking.

DISCUSSION. It is ironic that lung cancer has the highest incidence and mortality rate of all cancers, and yet is one of the most preventable. Physicians can continue to have a major impact on the risk of this disease through community and patient intervention and education. Excellent support materials are available from the American Academy of Family Physicians, the American Cancer Society, and the American Heart Association. Physician recommendation has a great potential impact on patients' decisions to stop smoking.

IMPACT ON FAMILY UNIT. A single smoker in a family can be a source of secondary smoke exposure for the rest of the family. Angina, respiratory symptoms, and increased risk of lung cancer can result in those exposed. Children from households with smokers have a higher school absence rate as a result of increased incidence of respiratory illnesses and infections and of middle ear infections. Infants born to mothers who smoked during pregnancy are more likely to die from sudden infant death syndrome. Couples who smoke create a special problem for the physician who wishes to help. It is difficult to persuade one smoker to quit while the other continues, and it is equally problematic to bring two smokers to the point of wishing to stop at the same time. The withdrawal period is one of great stress and requires family education and support.

Carcinoma of the Cervix

INCIDENCE. The incidence of invasive cervical carcinoma is declining (see Fig. 5–7). The incidence rises steadily through age 50 and then remains steady. Worldwide, cervical carcinoma is the most common malignancy in women, while in the United States it is eighth.

MORBIDITY AND MORTALITY. The mortality for invasive carcinoma of the cervix is 4900 women per year. The preinvasive cancer lesion of cervical intraepithelial neoplasia (CIN III, or carcinoma in situ) has a 100 per cent cure rate with proper treatment, while localized cancer has a 91 per cent 5-year survival rate and with distant spread, a 39 per cent 5-year survival rate (see Fig. 5–8). Overall the 5-year survival rate is 68 per cent. The death rate has dropped 70 per cent in the last 40 years. This is primarily a result of Pap smear screening programs detecting this disease at earlier stages when cure rates are higher.

IMPORTANT FACTS RELEVANT TO PREVENTION. Squamous cell carcinoma of the cervix occurs almost exclusively in women who have had coitus. The mean time for progression from mild dysplasia (CIN I) to severe dysplasia/carcinoma in situ (CIN III) is 5.8 years, and the mean time for further progression to invasive carcinoma is an additional 10 years. The rate of progression for any one individual is unpredictable. CIN may regress spontaneously in 30 to 50 per cent of cases. At least 30 per cent of patients with CIN III have progression to invasive carcinoma.

Major risk factors are early age for first intercourse, multiple sexual partners, human immunodeficiency virus (HIV) infection, herpes simplex virus infection, history of condylomas (human papillomavirus, or HPV infection), smoking, and low socioeconomic status. Early sexual intercourse has an especially dramatic effect on risk. Females who have had coitus less than 1 year after menarche are 26 times more likely to eventually develop cervical carcinoma than the general population.

Fifteen to twenty per cent of American women do not undergo regular Pap tests, and they account for the majority of cases of carcinoma of the cervix. A single Pap smear is demonstrated to be 55 to 80 per cent sensitive (20 to 45 per cent of cases are missed). Specificity is reported to be 90 to 99 per cent (1 to 10 per cent are false-positive). Major variability in the effectiveness of the Pap smear as a screening tool depends on proper sampling and specimen handling and on the quality of the laboratory.

SCREENING TEST RECOMMENDATIONS. All women should begin having Pap smears when sexual activity begins. The American Cancer Society recommends that after at least three negative annual Pap smears, the frequency may be reduced to as little as every 3 years in low-risk populations at the discretion of the physician. For example, the 33 per cent incidence of CIN in patients with HPV infections may represent a high-risk subgroup needing more frequent monitoring. It is reasonable to consider discontinuing Pap smears in women over age 65 who have had consistently negative examinations. Suspicious Pap smears should be evaluated with colposcopy, a procedure that is increasingly available in the family physician's office.

PREVENTIVE ACTIVITIES RECOMMENDATIONS. Risk status should be re-evaluated at each preventive health visit, especially in groups who may have an increased likelihood of multiple sexual partners. Women should be advised of their risk status with emphasis on the importance of regular re-evaluation. Although barrier contraception has only theoretical benefit, it can also be strongly recommended to help prevent sexually transmitted diseases.

DISCUSSION. There are other good reasons to request many women to come in for an examination more often than every 3 years, such as monitoring use of birth control pills, dietary advice, contraceptive counseling, and pre-pregnancy counseling. It may be only a minority of women who need to visit their physician less often than once yearly. Women have been educated for many years that the yearly Pap test is essential, but *not* that there are other important issues to be dealt with during these visits.

IMPACT ON FAMILY UNIT. Invasive cervical cancer occurring during the childbearing years is usually treated surgically, ending chances of future pregnancy. This has a profound effect on a single woman's approach to possible marriage and on a married couple's plans and relationship. The family physician's role only begins with referral for appropriate treatment. Preventive counseling is necessary in these situations. Women past the childbearing years may still suffer a loss of identity, similar to, but not as intense as, the breast cancer victim.

Skin Cancer

INCIDENCE. There are 800,000 cases of basal and squamous cell skin cancer yearly plus an additional 38,300 malignant melanomas. This is over twice the cancer incidence of any other organ system. The incidence continues to rise dramatically.

MORBIDITY AND MORTALITY. Of the 9430 deaths each year, 7300 are from malignant melanoma.

IMPORTANT FACTS RELEVANT TO PREVENTION. The most important risk factor for all skin cancer is exposure to ultraviolet (UV) light. Major risk factors include severe sunburns as a child, fair complexion, multiple or atypical moles, a family or personal history of skin cancer, poor tanning ability, freckles, history of local treatment with ionizing radiation, and immunosuppression. Occupational exposures to coal tar, pitch, arsenic, radium, and creosote all increase risk.

SCREENING TEST RECOMMENDATIONS. During regular preventive health examinations, the skin should be thoroughly examined for suspicious lesions. All lesions suspicious for malignancy should be biopsied or prophylactically excised and submitted for pathologic interpretation.

PREVENTIVE ACTIVITIES RECOMMENDATIONS. For primary prevention, all patients at risk should be counseled in measures for UV wave avoidance (sun or artificial tanning), protection with higher sun protection factor (SPF) number sunscreens (15 or greater), and use of protective clothing. Secondary prevention includes regular self-examination. This is a logical activity, especially for patients with already existing melanotic nevi.

The physician should also be alert to actinic keratoses and treat these as appropriate with 5-fluorouracil or retinoic acid topical application when generalized or with local means such as cryocautery when localized.

Prostate Cancer

INCIDENCE. Prostate cancer is the most common noncutaneous cancer in men. Risk increases with age beginning at age 50. There were an estimated 317,100 new cases in 1996. It has recently increased 6 per cent per year probably secondary to increased detection efforts. African American men have the highest incidence of prostate cancer in the world—37 per cent higher than white men.

PREVALENCE. Prevalence increases with age. Some studies have found microscopic evidence of prostate cancer in 30 per cent of autopsies of men ages 30 to 49. Estimates of the prevalence in men over age 80 range up to 100 per cent.

MORBIDITY AND MORTALITY. Morbidity associated with progression of prostate cancer can result from widespread metastases with bone pain and urinary tract obstruction.

IMPORTANT FACTS RELEVANT TO PREVENTION. Only a small minority of men with microscopic evidence of prostate cancer ever have clinical evidence of their disease. Population studies have suggested that dietary fat may be related to increased risk of prostate cancer.

SCREENING RECOMMENDATIONS. The principal screening tests are digital rectal examination, serum tumor markers such as the prostate-specific antigen (PSA), and transrectal ultrasound. These tests have not been shown to prolong life and the sensitivity and specificity are difficult to calculate. Routine screening for prostate cancer is not recommended on a population basis, but physicians are advised to counsel all men over age 50 years of the availability, risks, and benefits of PSA testing.

Endometrial Cancer

INCIDENCE, MORBIDITY, AND MORTALITY. See Figures 5–5 and 5–7.

IMPORTANT FACTS RELEVANT TO PREVENTION. Endometrial cancer is primarily a postmenopausal disease. The major causative factor appears to be unopposed estrogen, whether physiologic or iatrogenic. The most important early warning sign is abnormal vaginal bleeding. Risk factors are obesity, prolonged treatment with estrogen alone, age, chronic anovulation, and increased number of years of menstruation (early menarche, late menopause, or no pregnancies). Hypertension and diabetes are associated with risk probably because of the prevalence of obesity in these patients.

SCREENING TEST RECOMMENDATIONS. Abnormal endometrial cells are occasionally found on Pap smear, but this is not an adequate screen. Any endometrial cells found on a postmenopausal Pap smear should be considered abnormal. All postmenopausal women with abnormal bleeding of any amount must have endometrial sampling performed.

PREVENTIVE ACTIVITIES RECOMMENDATIONS. Risk factors should be established at menopause and modified when possible. All women with an intact uterus who are treated with estrogen replacement therapy should also be prescribed a progestational agent.

In Brief: Screening for Other Cancers

TESTICULAR CANCER. Testicular cancer is quite rare with an annual incidence of 4 per 100,000 men. There were 7400 new cases and 370 deaths in 1996. Physician examination and self-examination of the testes has not been demonstrated to be effective enough to recommend mass screening. However, it is appropriate to examine the testes as part of an examination done for other reasons.

OVARIAN CANCER. Even though ovarian cancer is the fifth leading cause of death in women and has the highest mortality (see Fig. 5–5) of any of the gynecologic cancers, no screening measures are recommended by the U.S. Preventive Services Task Force. The potential screening measures of ultrasound, serologic tumor markers, or pelvic examination do not identify sufficient cases to be recommended.

PANCREATIC CANCER. Cancer of the pancreas is also a leading cause of death due to cancer in the United States (see Fig. 5–5). However, due to lack of evidence for effectiveness, screening in asymptomatic persons, using palpation, ultrasonography, or serologic markers, is not recommended.

ORAL CANCER. Primary care physicians are advised to include an oral examination during routine preventive health screening, particularly in high-risk persons. Physicians should advise all patients against the use of all forms of tobacco and against heavy use of alcohol.

BLADDER CANCER. There were over 52,900 new cases and 11,700 deaths in the United States in 1996. Routine screening for bladder cancer is not advised. However, patients who smoke tobacco double their risk and should be advised to stop.

THYROID CANCER. Thyroid cancer is rare, with only 14,000 new cases and 1000 deaths each year. Screening of asymptomatic patients is not recommended, but examination at intervals may be advised for those with an increased risk, such as those with a childhood history of head or neck irradiation.

OTHER PREVENTABLE DISEASES

Osteoporosis

INCIDENCE. The incidence of fractures secondary to osteoporosis is 1.3 million per year. Osteoporosis causes a fracture in more than half of all women after menopause usually in the hip, vertebral column, or distal forearm.

PREVALENCE. It is estimated that 15 to 20 million Americans have osteoporosis and are therefore at markedly increased risk for fractures.

COST AND IMPACT ON SOCIETY. The direct and indirect costs of caring for patients suffering fractures secondary to osteoporosis are $8 billion each year.

MORBIDITY AND MORTALITY. Between 12 and 20 per cent of hip fractures lead to death and 50 per cent lead to significant disability. Ultimately, the degree of osteoporosis is dependent on two major factors—the peak bone density at 20 to 30 years of age and the rate of bone loss thereafter.

IMPORTANT FACTS RELEVANT TO PREVENTION. In women bone loss abruptly increases to 2 to 3 per cent per year at menopause, and then gradually returns to premenopausal rates. Men follow a similar sequence, but without the accelerated phase. Total loss of bone mass in men is about two thirds that of females.

Before 30 years of age, adequacy of calcium intake affects the peak bone mass and after age 30 slows the rate of loss of bone mass slightly. All women and men need 1.0 gm of elemental calcium daily to maintain a zero calcium balance. In postmenopausal women not prescribed estrogen replacement therapy, increasing this amount to 1.5 gm still does not maintain zero calcium balance. There is an 80 per cent prevalence of inadequate calcium intake among females of all ages.

Estrogen replacement therapy is the most effective method of preventing the accelerated phase of bone mass loss after menopause and reduces fracture risk by 25 to 50 per cent. Discontinuation of estrogen results in a prompt return to accelerated bone loss. Other methods of maximizing peak bone mass and slowing bone mass loss include regular weight-bearing exercise. Actual gains in lumbar bone mass have been demonstrated in postmenopausal women placed on a weight-bearing exercise regimen. This effect was sustained as long as the exercise was continued.

There are many primary risk factors for osteoporosis plus multiple additional medical conditions that may place an individual at higher risk (Table 5–11). Contributing factors may be easily overlooked when an illness that may increase risk of osteoporosis consumes the focus of attention. A good example might be the elderly white woman in otherwise good health who develops polymyalgia

TABLE 5–11. Risk Factors for Osteoporosis

Positive family history
Advancing age
Female
Caucasian or Asian race
Early menopause (including surgical)
Underweight
Cigarette smoking
History of dietary calcium deficiency
Hypogonadism (males)
Sedentary lifestyle
Alcohol consumption
Subtotal gastrectomy
Hyperthyroidism
Hemiplegia
Chronic obstructive pulmonary disease
Glucocorticoid medications
Anticonvulsant medications

From Rakel RE. Textbook of Family Practice, 5th ed. Philadelphia, WB Saunders, 1995, with permission.

TABLE 5–12. Nutritional Sources of Calcium

Food	Serving Size	Calcium (mg)
Milk	1 cup	300
Cheese (low-fat)	1 oz	185
Yogurt (nonfat)	1 cup	450
Yogurt (whole milk)	1 cup	275
Cottage cheese (1%)	½ cup	70
Dark leafy greens	½ cup	150–180
Other vegetables	½ cup	30–100
Fruits	Average serving	<25

From Rakel RE. Textbook of Family Practice, 5th ed. Philadelphia, WB Saunders, 1995, with permission.

rheumatica. The attention required to make the diagnosis and treatment with corticosteroids become the major focus. It is easy to forget that such a person, 2 years later, may be free of polymyalgia symptoms but debilitated by vertebral fractures.

Obesity, due to increased endogenous estrogen levels, and thiazide diuretics, due to decreased calcium excretion, have a protective effect.

SCREENING TEST RECOMMENDATIONS. There is no screening test that can be recommended. Specifically, the role of densitometry has yet to be determined.

PREVENTIVE ACTIVITIES RECOMMENDATIONS. All patients, especially women, should be educated regarding the recommended intake of 1000 mg of dietary calcium. Postmenopausal women not receiving estrogens should increase calcium intake to 1500 mg plus supplemental vitamin D. Major nutritional sources of calcium are listed in Table 5–12. Dairy products should be low fat as part of the overall prudent diet. Women unable to meet minimal calcium needs through diet should be advised to use supplemental calcium.

Risk status should be determined for all females, preferably at menarche, and re-evaluated at the time of routine preventive health visits. Additional counseling concerning osteoporosis prevention should be given to those at higher risk.

Every woman should be thoroughly evaluated at menopause for risk factors and possible estrogen replacement therapy. In general, most white women with any other risk factors are candidates unless there are specific contraindications. All patients should be counseled to maintain regular aerobic weight-bearing activity as part of the overall program for general preventive health care. Although

50 to 60 minutes of exercise three times weekly has been shown to increase bone mass, the minimum levels necessary have not been determined.

DISCUSSION. When prescribing estrogen replacement therapy, a daily dosage equivalent to 0.625 mg of conjugated estrogen has been documented as being effective; 0.3 mg may be equally effective. It is desirable to add progesterone for at least part of the estrogen cycle to reduce the risk of endometrial cancer associated with unopposed estrogen therapy. Recent studies have shown increased benefit for bone density with a daily noncyclical combination of estrogen and progestin and persistence of the beneficial effect of hormone replacement therapy on the lipid profile. Medications that can protect or increase bone mass are being studied to determine their effect on reducing fracture incidence.

IMPACT ON FAMILY UNIT. Family eating patterns primarily determine the peak bone mass achieved. Therefore, counseling of women in the childbearing years should include recommendations for the entire family.

Elderly patients who are already at high risk create a dilemma for the family physician. The resulting impact of severe fractures is sudden loss of independence. In an elderly family member, this has great impact in both emotional and financial terms. The resulting major decisions that must be made often reverse the parent-child roles. Intimate knowledge of the elderly patient, his or her functional capacities, and the living situation place the family physician in a pivotal role in fracture prevention.

Sexually Transmitted Diseases

INCIDENCE. The peak incidence of sexually transmitted diseases (STDs) is in teenagers and young adults; teenagers alone account for 2.5 million cases. In 1994 there were 20,627 cases of syphilis reported. After two decades of increase, the incidence has decreased since 1990. The reported incidence of gonorrhea has dropped from a peak in 1974 to current levels of 420,000 cases in 1994, with over 60 per cent of the cases in those under age 25. The true incidence may be twice the actual reported incidence. The estimated yearly incidence for *Chlamydia* infection is an astounding 4 million cases at a cost of $2.4 billion. Each year 120,000 infants are infected with *Chlamydia* at birth. There are an estimated 500,000 new cases of herpes genitalis each year. There is marked clustering of STDs in large

cities, particularly in poor, minority communities, and in the rural Southeast.

PREVALENCE. Because of the long duration of infection, the two most prevalent STDs are herpes simplex virus (HSV) and human papillomavirus (HPV). The cumulative prevalence of genital HSV infection alone is 20 million cases. Because of the asymptomatic nature of many chlamydial infections, it is estimated that the prevalence in the general population is 5 per cent.

COST AND IMPACT ON SOCIETY. For pelvic inflammatory disease (PID) alone, the costs per year are $2.6 billion.

MORBIDITY AND MORTALITY. Over 200,000 women per year, one fifth of those with PID, become involuntarily infertile, and 50 per cent of all ectopic pregnancies are a result of PID. Twenty per cent of females with one episode of PID develop chronic pelvic pain.

IMPORTANT FACTS RELEVANT TO PREVENTION. All of the STDs have a high asymptomatic carrier rate making prevention of transmission very difficult. Therefore, the single biggest risk factor is multiple sexual partners. Only abstinence, monogamy, or condoms dramatically affect the risk.

SCREENING TEST RECOMMENDATIONS. No screening tests are recommended for the general population. Routine serologic tests for syphilis should be done for all pregnant women and persons at high risk for infection. High-risk groups should have a screening gonorrhea culture and direct fluorescent antibody test or enzyme-linked immunosorbent assay for *Chlamydia* performed at the time of routine pelvic examinations. Persons with multiple sexual partners should be examined yearly. All sexually active adolescent women should be screened for *Chlamydia* infection. High-risk women should be screened for gonorrhea during pregnancy. Screening of asymptomatic patients is not recommended for HSV.

PREVENTIVE ACTIVITIES RECOMMENDATIONS. Education should begin at least at, and preferably before, the onset of sexual activity. All sexually active patients should be encouraged to seek medical evaluation for even apparently minor genital tract symptoms.

DISCUSSION. Physicians must maintain a high index of suspicion for all STDs, since there is a very high percentage of asymptomatic and minimally symptomatic patients. In high-risk populations, presumptive treatment for *Chlamydia* infection, even with minimal signs or symptoms, is recommended by many experts. Current treatment recommendations for gonorrhea also include coverage for *Chlamydia* infection for all patients.

IMPACT ON FAMILY UNIT. The incrimination that can result when a husband or wife is diagnosed with an STD may lead to major family disruption. The physician plays the key role in interpreting the meaning of such an episode and bringing the couple to a mutual understanding. It is therefore critical that the physician know the natural course of the disease. For instance, 30 per cent of women with gonorrhea may be asymptomatic carriers (in some populations the percentage for men may be almost this high), 70 per cent of patients with genital herpes have no symptoms, and 70 per cent of female lower genital tract infections with *Chlamydia* are asymptomatic.

Human Immunodeficiency Virus Infections

INCIDENCE. The incidence of new cases of acquired immunodeficiency syndrome (AIDS) is rapidly increasing. There are now an estimated 40,000 to 80,000 new infections reported annually.

PREVALENCE. The Centers for Disease Control (CDC) estimates that 0.8 to 1.2 million persons are currently infected with the human immunodeficiency virus (HIV). Within 10 years of infection, 50 per cent of individuals develop AIDS and another 40 per cent develop associated clinical illnesses. The prevalence of diagnosed cases of AIDS is estimated to be 130,000 to 205,000 in 1995.

COST AND IMPACT ON SOCIETY. The cost of treatment alone has gone from $2.2 billion in 1988, to $13 billion in 1992, and to $15 billion in 1995.

MORBIDITY AND MORTALITY. Of the total of 476,899 patients reported to the CDC through June 1995, 62 per cent have died. HIV is the leading cause of death for men ages 25 to 44 and is among the top 10 causes of death for males and females ages 1 to 44.

IMPORTANT FACTS RELEVANT TO PREVENTION. The groups with the highest prevalence are hemophiliacs, homosexual men, intravenous drug users, individuals with multiple sexual partners, patients with multiple blood transfusions after 1977 and before blood screening in 1985, patients with other STDs, and babies born to infected mothers.

SCREENING TEST RECOMMENDATIONS. All patients should be screened for risk status with a careful sexual and drug use history. The frequency of screening varies depending on the patient population cared for. Patients in high-risk groups should be strongly encouraged to be screened for HIV antibodies. One major reason for screening, in addition to the benefit of early treatment, is to identify those individuals who are already infected so that intervention may be instituted to halt the further spread of the virus. This is particularly important during pregnancy; treatment has been shown to decrease vertical transmission to the newborn infant.

PREVENTIVE ACTIVITIES RECOMMENDATIONS. Education of patients is the number one priority for the family physician. At this time, the best chance for meaningful intervention is to prevent exposure to HIV-infected individuals. Children and teenagers in particular must be helped to understand the reality of the risks of sexual contact (especially if unprotected with condoms) and intravenous drug use (especially using shared needles or syringes). At-risk women in the childbearing years should be considered for yearly HIV antibody screening. Any of these women found to be HIV-positive should be strongly counseled against conception. Now that therapy is available during pregnancy that decreases vertical transmission, a case might be made to screen all pregnant women in addition to those with high-risk behaviors. Screening of infants born to high-risk mothers should be done if the maternal antibody status is unknown.

Within the office, the physician has a responsibility to employees and other patients to implement recommended measures to ensure protection from inadvertent transmission.

DISCUSSION. In addition to individual action, there is a need for continued and expanded aggressive public health measures. Secondary prevention becomes increasingly important as methods to stop or retard disease progression in its presymptomatic stages become more accessible and affordable.

Other Infectious Diseases and Immunizations

INCIDENCE. There are a number of infectious diseases that can be almost completely prevented by immunization. These diseases include measles, mumps, rubella, hepatitis A, hepatitis B, pneumococcal disease, influenza, pertussis, diphtheria, tetanus, poliomyelitis, and *Haemophilus influenzae* B disease. Many of these diseases have been public health scourges in the past and the source of great epidemics and even pandemics. As can be seen from Table 5–13, the development of immunizations has cut this incidence a hundredfold or even a thousandfold in some cases.

Another group of preventable infectious diseases are those usually encountered by international travelers. The most common are malaria and travelers' diarrhea. The physician should provide information about mosquito avoidance, prophylactic medication, and food and water consumption.

COST AND IMPACT ON SOCIETY. Although dollar values cannot be assigned for such a multiplicity of diseases, when the potential severe economic and health consequences of these diseases are compared with the marked efficacy of immunization, the cost-effectiveness is self-evident.

MORBIDITY AND MORTALITY. In the past, these diseases had highly significant morbidity and mortality. Measles (rubeola) can cause death during the acute phase, while rubella can have a tremendous impact by causing congenital damage to the babies of mothers infected during pregnancy. Hepatitis B has a low mortality rate of less than 1 per cent during the acute episode, but victims may develop a chronic infection with complications requiring extensive medical care. Although children under age 5 only account for 1 to 3 per cent of hepatitis B infections, the risk of developing chronic infection is highest in perinatal transmission (80 to 90 per cent), decreasing with age to less than 10 per cent of adults. Influenza and pneumococcal disease have had high incidences and mortality among the elderly.

IMPORTANT FACTS RELEVANT TO PREVENTION

1. Immunization against these diseases greatly decreases incidence, morbidity, and mortality.

2. Vaccines are available, relatively inexpensive, safe, and very cost-effective when compared with the costs associated with the morbidity and mortality of these diseases.

SCREENING TEST RECOMMENDATIONS

1. Each patient record should contain a flow-chart documenting the immunization status for each of these diseases, as well as rubella immune status for women in the childbearing years.

2. A quick review of the immune status should be made at each visit during the first 5 years of life and annually thereafter.

TABLE 5–13. U.S. Cases, Deaths, and Vaccination Rates of Vaccine-Preventable Infectious Diseases

Infection	Prevaccine Cases	Cases (1993)	Target Group Vaccination Rate (%)	Yearly Deaths
Measles	482,000	281	83	80–100 (estimated)
Hepatitis B	N/A	12,396	N/A	250 (immediate) 5000 (sequelae)
Pneumococcal disease	N/A	N/A	28	40,000
Influenza	N/A	N/A	55	10–40,000
Pertussis	74,700	6,335	83	1
Diphtheria	9490	0	83	1
Tetanus	601	43	83	16
Paralytic polio	18,300	4	72	0
Haemophilus influenzae B disease	1 per 200 children before age 5	N/A	N/A	N/A
Rubella	3900	195	80–90	0
Mumps	125,000	1640	N/A	2

N/A: Not available owing to lack of reliable data.

PREVENTIVE ACTIVITIES RECOMMENDATIONS

1. Each physician's office should be equipped to give needed immunizations when the screen reveals a need or be prepared to refer the patient to a facility that performs immunizations. A sample schedule of recommended immunizations is found in Table 5–14. Many older children have not received full immunization according to current guidelines. Specific makeup recommendations are:

   a. Tetanus and diphtheria toxoids—adult type (Td). Series of three immunizations for all not previously immunized.

   b. Measles-mumps-rubella (MMR) vaccine. One booster for all adolescent and young adults having only one shot as a child (original schedule). Administer to all persons born after 1956 without immunity from measles (immunization or disease), any nonpregnant woman of childbearing age without immunity to rubella, and any individual susceptible to mumps.

   c. Hepatitis B. All young adults not previously immunized and all adults in high-risk populations.

   d. Varicella vaccine. All individuals without history of immunization or disease.

2. All physicians should participate in community health education programs promoting public understanding of the need for appropriate immunizations.

DISCUSSION. Of all the activities carried out by physicians, the prevention of infectious diseases by immunization is the least expensive, takes less effort, and is the most efficient. The control of the major infectious diseases has been a marked success for preventive medicine in the twentieth century. However, there remain major deficiencies in the levels of immunization for pneumococcal disease and influenza. Health care workers in particular have an obligation to ensure that they personally have an adequate immunization status for hepatitis B.

IMPACT ON THE FAMILY UNIT. A particular challenge for the family physician is the family that refuses to immunize its children for religious reasons or out of neglect. Other parents fear the potential side effects of vaccines and rationalize that since most other children are immunized, the chances of their child's contracting the infection are near zero. Each physician should be aware of the relevant state laws and should have a strategy for dealing with these problems.

Moderate cost and occasional mild side effects such as fever, localized pain, or adenitis may cause some negative impact on the family. Although a disastrous complication may rarely occur, such as poliomyelitis in a nonimmunized family member, these are so unusual that they are far outweighed by the benefits to the general population. The ultimate impact of a proper immunization program is healthier and more productive families with fewer congenital anomalies and lost children, fewer paralyzed children and adults, and longer life spans for the elderly.

TABLE 5–14. Immunizations: Indications and Schedules

Immunization	Ages 0–15	Ages 16–64	Age ≥ 65
DTaP*	2, 4, 6, 15–18 mo and 4–6 yr		
Td	15 yr	Every 10 years	
IPV	2, 4 mo		
OPV	2, 4, 15–18 mo, 4–6 yr		
MMR	12–15 mo, 4–6 yr	College entrance‡	
Haemophilus B§	2, 4, 12 mo		
Influenza	Yearly if high risk	Yearly, high risk	Yearly
Pneumococcal	Once only when becomes high risk or at age 65		
Hepatitis B	Birth, 1–4 mo, 6–18 mo		
Varicella	12–18 mo		

*Vaccine containing acellular pertussis (DTaP) now approved and recommended for use in infants and children under 7 years of age.
‡Only if second dose not previously given.
§One manufacturer requires an additional injection at 6 mo.
  DTaP = Diphtheria toxoid, tetanus toxoid, and acellular pertussis vaccine; IPV = inactivated polio vaccine; MMR = measles, mumps, and rubella vaccine; OPV = oral poliovirus vaccine; Td = tetanus and diphtheria toxoids, adult type.

Accidents

INCIDENCE. The incidence of unintentional injuries is reflected in the fact that they result in 2.7 million hospitalizations, 34 million emergency room visits, and 62 million office visits per year. The highest rate is found in the 18- to 24-year-old age group. Motor vehicle injuries were the eighth leading cause of death in 1993.

COST AND IMPACT ON SOCIETY. An analysis of the estimated lifetime costs of injuries incurred in just one typical year (1995) is $182 billion.

MORBIDITY AND MORTALITY. There are over 89,000 deaths yearly from unintentional injuries. They are the fifth leading cause of death in the United States and the leading cause of death for persons ages 1 to 34. Almost half are secondary to automobile accidents. A distant second cause is falls, but these accidents are remarkable in that over 70 per cent occur in the over 65 age group and they are the most common type of nonfatal accident. The third most frequent cause of accidental death is drowning, followed by fire, poisoning, and unintentional firearm injuries. Nearly 1000 children under age 15 die each year from firearm injury.

IMPORTANT FACTS RELEVANT TO PREVENTION. Homes are the most common site of overall injury, whereas the automobile is the most common site for fatal injury. It is estimated that over half of all fatal automobile accidents involve a driver who has been drinking.

SCREENING TEST RECOMMENDATIONS. Screening for alcohol abuse is of top priority. Not only is it the major cause of traffic fatalities, it is also a major factor in all other types of traumatic accidents. Patients should be asked at the time of routine preventive health checks if they regularly use seat belts and have air bags in their vehicle.

PREVENTIVE ACTIVITIES RECOMMENDATIONS. The guidelines for prevention listed under alcohol abuse and osteoporosis should be followed. Parents should be encouraged to ensure that all children are taught to swim. Homes should be safety-proofed. All homes should have working fire alarms. Medications, poisons, toxins, and firearms should all be inaccessible when small children are in the home. When there are elderly within the home, specific measures should be taken to reduce the risk of falls. Use of seat belts and child restraint devices should be strongly encouraged. If available, air bags offer a significant additional degree of protection from automobile injury. Children should wear safety helmets when bicycle riding and, as appropriate, protective gear for other sports. Families should be counseled to place sleeping infants on their back to decrease the incidence of sudden infant death syndrome.

IMPACT ON FAMILY UNIT. In addition to the immediate trauma suffered, nonfatal accidents impact the individual and the family directly. An issue that must be confronted is the injured person's and the other family members' own mortality. Although some families grow closer at these times, others may distance as a defense mechanism. Fatal accidents present a special problem. The loss is unexpected and often occurs in those who are otherwise young and healthy. The process of grieving may become particularly difficult or pathologic.

Glaucoma

PREVALENCE. The prevalence of glaucoma rises from 0.5 per cent of persons under age 65 to 2 to 4 per cent of those over age 75. Glaucoma is four to six times more prevalent in African Americans than whites.

IMPORTANT FACTS RELEVANT TO PREVENTION. The ultimate result of untreated glaucoma is blindness. Primary open-angle glaucoma is the most common type of glaucoma and is asymptomatic until severe, often irreversible damage has occurred. The benefits of treatment have not been conclusively demonstrated.

The two major criteria for diagnosis are visual field defects and optic disc pallor and cupping. In glaucoma, the optic cup's diameter is 30 per cent greater than that of the disc. The funduscopic changes on direct ophthalmoscopy are best seen with the red filter. Patients with upper-normal intraocular pressure can have glaucoma and suffer from secondary blindness, yet only a minority of patients with elevated intraocular pressure develop glaucoma.

The risk factors for glaucoma are elevated intraocular pressure, family history, black race, diabetes mellitus, and age.

SCREENING TEST RECOMMENDATIONS. The value of screening for elevated intraocular pressure with the Schiotz tonometer is controversial. If the family physician elects to use this method, patients should be screened starting at age 40 and every 5 years thereafter until age 60, at which time the screening interval should be reduced to 2 to 3 years. Funduscopic evaluation by a well-trained physician at the time of tonometry increases the sensitivity of screening.

PREVENTIVE ACTIVITIES RECOMMENDATIONS. Although the treatment of elevated intraocular pressure is the standard of care, there are no proved primary or secondary preventive measures available.

DISCUSSION. Elevated intraocular pressure has less than a 30 per cent positive predictive value for developing glaucoma. In addition, up to 50 per cent of patients with glaucoma have normal intraocular pressure on a single random measurement. These facts make it important that high-risk patients have more extensive screening by an ophthalmologist, and that patients who are screened only with tonometry are advised that they are still at risk.

Diabetes Mellitus

Diabetes mellitus does not meet the criteria for mass screening, despite its high prevalence, high mortality, long presymptomatic stage, and ease of diagnosis. Early diagnosis and treatment have not been shown to alter the prognosis. Nevertheless, screening has been advocated because the presence of diabetes is a major risk factor for coronary heart disease.

There are rational, though unproved, reasons to screen some high-risk populations such as certain American Indian groups with a high prevalence of diabetes. The goal is to implement lifestyle changes already known to be of general benefit for other reasons (weight control, exercise, diet, smoking cessation).

Other Screening Recommendations

Routine screening for *thyroid disease* with laboratory tests is not recommended for asymptomatic children or adults. General screening for *iron deficiency anemia* is not recommended, but it is advised to screen during pregnancy as a high-risk state. Since *obesity* is such a common contributor to morbidity and screening during office visits is very inexpensive, it is recommended that weight be measured at each medical office visit. All children at increased risk should be screened for *lead levels* at least once at age 1. Very high risk children and children living in communities with a high prevalence of lead levels should be considered for subsequent testing.

Screening for *phenylketonuria* and *hypothyroidism* is recommended for all neonates.

Additional Preventive Activities

The family physician provides a large amount of general medical care and in the course of this care may easily identify patients who can benefit from individualized screening tests not recommended for the general population. These screening activities also include the discovery of patients who can benefit from lifestyle and other health-related counseling. These can include counseling to prevent tobacco use, to optimize physical activity, to achieve and maintain ideal weight, and to consume a healthy diet. Other helpful services include reviewing the home for prevention of accidents and accidental poisonings, providing information about safe sexual practices, and identifying potential occupational hazards. Older adults should be screened for hearing impairment at least by questioning about a deficit. Examples in the behavioral science area include screening for dementia, depression, suicide risk, family and youth violence, as well as drug and alcohol abuse in persons at risk.

Prevention of unwanted pregnancies is another important role for the family physician. An estimated 1 million teenage pregnancies occur each year and 30,000 are in girls under the age of 15. Family physicians are in a position to identify teenagers at risk for sexual activity, provide contraception for those who are sexually active, and assist with patient education.

Yet another area of disease prevention is in preconceptual obstetric risk assessment. Health promotion, patient education, and therapeutic intervention can reduce risk and improve outcome. Risk is associated with systemic disease, family history, genetics, demography, environment, and lifestyle. Regular supplementation of 0.4 mg of folic acid daily is recommended for all women who could become pregnant and of 1.0 mg daily once pregnancy has occurred. Identifying risks and providing appropriate counseling before conception may help formulate important health strategies and prevent morbidity while enhancing obstetric outcome.

A review of physical activity in children and a discussion of proper exercise for children is another counseling activity that is an important health promotional aspect of optimal health care.

LIFESTYLES FOR HEALTH

When one reviews the diseases discussed in this chapter, there is a strikingly common theme in their etiology and prevention: *An individual's lifestyle is the major modifiable determinant of health.*

Proper diet is of paramount importance to prevent the nation's number one killer, coronary heart disease; and it is estimated that 35 per cent of cancers, the nation's number two killer, are secondary to diet. Fortunately, the specific dietary recommendations for prevention of one disease are also beneficial in general. Therefore, it is possible to make broad, prudent nutritional recommendations as a basis on which all physicians and patients can build: (1) total calories to achieve and maintain ideal body weight; (2) fat less than 30 per cent of total calories; (3) saturated fat less than 10 per cent of total calories; (4) cholesterol less than 300 mg per day; (5) maximizing fiber levels in the diet with emphasis on soluble fiber sources; (6) calcium, minimum of 1000 mg daily; and (7) sodium chloride, minimize to less than 3 gm of sodium (7.5 gm salt). Dietary behaviors to accomplish these goals are outlined in booklets that can be made available in the physician's office (American Heart Association, 1994).

Cohort studies have shown a significant protective effect for all-cause mortality in both men and women engaging in even modest levels of exercise (Blair et al., 1996). Sedentary lifestyle imparts the same degree of increased risk for CHD as smoking and other major risk factors, i.e., 1.5 to 2 times. Weight-bearing exercises substantially reduce the risk of osteoporosis and its associated fractures. Anxiety and depression both appear to have lower incidence in those who exercise as well as benefiting individuals already suffering from these disorders. Hypertension, obesity, and non–insulin-dependent diabetes are all benefited by regular exercise. It is recommended that all patients be counseled as to the most appropriate types, amount, and intensity for their current health and risk status. General guidelines for all healthy adults are to engage in 30 to 40 minutes of moderate aerobic physical activity at least four to five times per week. This 30 to 40 minutes may be accumulated over the day. Adding additional exercise to increase muscle strength and joint flexibility is also recommended. Parents should ensure that their children engage in regular activities that involve vigorous exercise.

Another common prevention theme is the critical importance of avoiding toxins, especially the addictive substances nicotine and alcohol. Smoking accounts for 30 per cent of all cancer deaths as well as being a major factor in coronary heart disease. Each year 420,000 deaths can be directly attributed to cigarette smoking. It is estimated that each pack of cigarettes sold results in a cost of $2.17 in medical care and lost productivity. Four per cent of all cancer deaths in men and 2 per cent of all cancer deaths in women are due to alcohol. Alcohol is a major contributor to morbidity and mortality from accidents of all kinds, liver disease, suicide, and homicide.

Table 5–15 shows the major diseases discussed

TABLE 5–15.   Relationship Between Common Preventable Diseases and the Most Common Risk Factors

Risk Factor	Diet	Hyperlipidemia	Obesity	Hypertension	Smoking	Alcohol	Sedentary Lifestyle	Heredity	Stress and Depression	High Risk Sexual Behavior
Coronary heart disease	◆	◆	◆	◆	◆		◆	◆	◆	
Stroke	◆	◆	◆	◆	◆		◆	◆	◆	
Chemical dependence						◆		◆	◆	
Osteoporosis	◆				◆		◆			
Accident/suicide						◆	◆	◆	◆	
Sexually transmitted diseases and human immunodeficiency virus infection						◆				◆
Lung cancer					◆					
Breast cancer	◆					◆	◆	◆		
Colon cancer	◆						◆	◆		
Cervical cancer					◆					◆
Endometrial cancer			◆	◆						
Prostate cancer	◆							◆		

Adapted from Rakel RE. Textbook of Family Practice, 5th ed. Philadelphia, WB Saunders, 1995, with permission.

Flow Chart Instructions: Enter mo/yr test completed, D/E if done elsewhere, N/A if not applicable, add bars/tests as indicated by risk analysis.

AGE→	50	51	52	53	54	55	56	57	58	59
LIFESTYLE RISK ASSESSMENT	▬	▬	▬	▬	▬	▬	▬	▬	▬	▬
CHOLESTEROL	▬					▬				
STOOL GUAIAC X3	▬	▬	▬	▬	▬	▬	▬	▬	▬	▬
FLEXIBLE SIGMOIDOSCOPY	▬					▬				
IMMUNIZATIONS (Td,Flu,Pneumo)										
PAP	▬	◁▷	◁▷	▬	◁▷	◁▷	▬	◁▷	◁▷	▬
MAMMOGRAM with BREAST EXAM	▬	▬	▬	▬	▬	▬	▬	▬	▬	▬
ADVANCE DIRECTIVE	▬									

Flow Chart Key: ▬ = USPHTF Category A or B;or FM Dept.Policy ◁▷=Carefully consider per Risk Assessment

Risk Analysis Instructions: Circle items that are patient risk factors. Resolved risk factors add OK and mo/yr. Check items that are not risk factors. Unmarked items are assumed to have not been determined yet.

CHD Risk
+Family Hx
Elevated cholesterol
Tobacco
Hypertension
Diabetes mellitus
LVH
Sedentary

Colorectal Cancer
+Family Hx
High-fat/low-fiber diet
Hx polyps
Hx Ulcerative colitis

Suicide
Previous attempt
+ Family Hx
Depression

Breast Cancer
+Family Hx
Nulliparous
Primigravida >35 y/o
High risk biopsy

Alcohol/Substance Abuse
Felt like Cutting down
Annoyed by criticism
Guilty about drinking
Eye opener
+Family Hx
Previous problems
Cocaine/Opioids/THC
Prescription drugs:
    Opioids/Benzo's/Stimulants

Glaucoma
+Family Hx
Diabetes mellitus
African American
Hx Severe myopia

Sexually Transmitted Disease
Blood transfusions (1978–85)
Multiple sexual partners
Bisexual/homosexual
Presence of or exposure to STD
Hx of IV drug use

Cervical Cancer
Hx HPV/condyloma
Tobacco
Mult. sexual partners
Early first intercourse
Prior dysplasia

Osteoporosis
< 1 gm Ca/day
Sedentary
+Family Hx
Thin
White/Asian
Tobacco

Accident / Injury
Seat belts
Drink and drive
Firearms storage
Smoke detector

Notes:

Figure 5–10. *See legend on opposite page*

and the number of lifestyle issues implicated as risk factors for each one.

Developing a Preventive Health Care Flowsheet

A simple and flexible flowsheet is essential for the continuity and comprehensiveness of preventive health care. Such a form can be effectively used as a tool for educating patients concerning their preventive health care needs. Computer-based methods for health maintenance tracking are now available and may improve the family physician's ability to offer more preventive services in the future in cost-efficient manners.

Figure 5–10 shows examples of flowsheets that family physicians have found useful.

REFERENCES

American Cancer Society. Cancer Facts and Figures—1996. Atlanta, American Cancer Society, 1996.

American Heart Association. Step by Step: Eating to Lower Your Blood Cholesterol. Washington, DC, National Institutes of Health Publication No. 94-2920, August, 1994.

American Heart Association. Heart and Stroke Facts: 1996 Statistical Supplement. Dallas, American Heart Association, 1996.

Blair SN, Kampert JB, Kohl HW III, et al.: Influences of cardiorespiratory fitness and other precursors on cardiovascular disease and all-cause mortality in men and women. JAMA 1996;276:205–210.

Castelli WP. Epidemiology of coronary heart disease: The Framingham Study. Am J Med 1984;76:4–12.

Expert Panel on the Detection, Evaluation, and Treatment of High Blood Cholesterol in Adults. Summary of the second report of the National Cholesterol Education Program (NCEP) Expert Panel on Detection, Evaluation, and Treatment of High Blood Cholesterol in Adults (Adult Treatment Panel II). JAMA 1993;269:3015–3023.

Leininger LS, Finn L, Dietrich AJ, et al.: An office system for organizing prevention services: A report by the American Cancer Society Advisory Group on Preventive Health Care Reminder Systems. Arch Fam Med 1996;5:108–114.

McGinnis JM, Foege W. Actual causes of death in the United States. JAMA 1993;270:2207–2212.

Smart CR, Hendrick RE, Rutledge JH III, Smith RA. Benefit of mammography screening in women ages 40–49 years: Current evidence from randomized control trials. Cancer 1995;75:2788.

U.S. Preventive Services Task Force. Guide to Clinical Preventive Services. Baltimore, Williams & Wilkins, 1996.

U.S. Public Health Service. Cholesterol screening in children. Am Fam Phys 1995;51:1923–1927.

QUESTIONS

1. Which of the following has shown the *least* per cent reduction in mortality from 1979 to 1993?
   a. Diseases of the heart
   b. Cerebrovascular disease
   c. Chronic obstructive pulmonary disease
   d. Motor vehicle accidents
   e. Suicide

2. Which percentage of deaths are attributed to behavioral and environmental causes that are preventable?
   a. 10%
   b. 20%
   c. 30%
   d. 40%
   e. 50%

3. Which of the following is firmly established as a beneficial strategy in reducing alcohol consumption or the frequency of legal consequences of drinking? True or false for each.
   a. Strong cultural bias against drunkenness
   b. Alcohol education
   c. Reduction of alcohol content of beer
   d. Increased drinking age
   e. Increased prices for alcohol
   f. Strict enforcement of drinking and driving laws

Figure 5–10. Preventive health care and risk analysis flowchart. HPV = human papillomavirus; LVH = left ventricular hypertrophy; STD = sexually transmitted disease; THC = tetrahydrocannabinol. (From Department of Family Medicine, University of Virginia, Charlottesville.)

4. Match the type of cancer (excluding basal and squamous cell skin cancer) with each of the statements that follow the choices:
   a. Colon cancer
   b. Breast cancer
   c. Prostate cancer
   d. Lung cancer
   e. Cervix
   f. Pancreas
      (1) The most common cause of cancer death in the United States
      (2) Most common cause of cancer death in females in the United States
      (3) Highest number of *new* cancer cases in males in the United States
      (4) Most common cancer in women worldwide
      (5) Highest number of *new* cancer cases in U.S. females
      (6) Second most common cause of cancer and cancer mortality in the United States
      (7) The cancer with the most dramatic increase in mortality in the past 60 years

Answers appear on **page 603**.

Chapter **6**

The Consultation Process

Robert E. Rakel, M.D.

All physicians, regardless of their specialty, turn to other physicians at some time for advice. This process necessarily became formalized as physicians focused their training and limited their practice to a particular segment of medicine. The first specialty board, the American Board of Ophthalmology, was formed in 1917, and by 1996, there were 24 specialty boards and 74 subspecialties. The American Board of Family Practice was established in 1969 as the twentieth primary specialty.

It is a common misconception of medical students that less information needs to be mastered in a narrow subspecialty than in family practice or other primary care disciplines. The fact is that the amount of information required to practice each of the 98 specialties and subspecialties is clearly defined and is about the same. What varies is the degree of breadth and depth in each.

In addition to being trained in a wide variety of clinical areas, family physicians are also trained to coordinate the care of seriously ill individuals who require a variety of consultants, orchestrating the skills of each to achieve optimal patient care and satisfaction (see Chapter 1). "Every patient should have a primary care physician who not only sees him for first-contact care, but who actively participates in his secondary and tertiary care by arranging and coordinating his consultant needs, by providing continuity, and by taking the patient back" (Stephens, 1982).

The appropriate use of the consultation process is an art that contributes to improved patient care when utilized properly by family physicians. Although there is a definite distinction between consultation and referral, the terms are often used interchangeably. Consultation is by definition the practice of one physician asking another for an opinion or assistance, whereas referral is the transfer of responsibility to another physician for the care of a specific problem. Referral usually involves one physician requesting the services of another for a particular purpose and for a limited time, such as referral to a surgeon for a cholecystectomy or to a cardiologist for coronary angiography. In contrast, consultation is the process whereby one physician requests the opinion of a colleague regarding the diagnosis or management of a patient's problem. Regardless of this distinction, the physician initiating either process is spoken of as the *referring physician*, and the physician who is consulted or to whom the patient is referred is called the *consultant.*

In a study of patterns of consultation and referral, Geyman and associates (1976) found that 97 per cent of the exchanges between family physicians and other specialists were referrals and only 3 per cent were consultations. Because 46 per cent of graduates of family practice residency programs now join family practice groups of three or more family physicians, most early consultations are with colleagues in their group (see Chapter 1).

Fry (1971) notes with regret that consultation is no longer a deliberation between colleagues about diagnosis or proper treatment. He says, "We have come to view our specialist colleagues more as expert 'technicians' than as consultants." Although the system in the United Kingdom has been described as the specialist controlling the hospital and the general practitioner controlling the patient, this separation avoids much of the rivalry over patient care that occurs in the United States. Horder (1977) believes that, ". . . patients look to all of us for the same two things, technical competence and personal care. I believe that, at present, we have more cause to be concerned about the supply of personal care than technical competence."

Many consultations are discretionary; they can be divided into urgent or mandatory forms, in which the patient is likely to suffer harm if not referred, and an elective form, in which the patient is unlikely to suffer harm if not referred. Although only 3 to 4 per cent of patients seen by family physicians are referred, this rate may be reduced if the consultation requires review by colleagues. In a prospective review of nonurgent consultation requests Chao and colleagues (1993) used a committee of two faculty and two residents to review 930 nonurgent consultation requests during a 3-month period. Alternative management was recommended in 28 per cent, resulting in a decline of nonurgent consultations from 4.3 to 3.2 per cent. There were 71 urgent referrals that bypassed the committee and 166 nonurgent referrals that were reviewed. The specialties most frequently consulted, in rank order, were psychiatry, obstetrics-gynecology (ob-gyn), ophthalmology, orthopedics, general surgery, otolaryngology, dermatology, and urology (see Table 6–2). In a similar but retrospective study, Lawler (1987) found that half of all referrals were elective; the specialties receiving the highest proportion of urgent or mandatory referrals were ophthalmology and cardiology.

Family physicians see problems at their early, undifferentiated stage when it is most difficult to make an accurate diagnosis. The ability to make a diagnosis at this stage comes from experience and depends upon a high index of suspicion when key elements of a serious problem are present or suspected. The family physician's ability to make a diagnosis at this early stage is based on prior knowledge of the patient, previous care-seeking behavior of the patient (stoic or frequent complainer), the social situation, and risks based on family history and personal habits. Lawler and colleagues (1990) evaluated elective versus mandatory referrals in a rural family practice clinic. They found that half of all family practice referrals could be considered elective, and that a large number of referrals were made to assist in making or confirming the diagnosis when the disease was ill-defined.

WHEN TO REFER

Factors that influence a physician's decision to obtain a consultation or refer include potential cost to the patient, convenience to the patient, patient request for or expectation for referral, physician loss of income or self-esteem (admitting failure), quality of available consultants, and physician satisfaction with previous referrals.

It is wise to ask for a consultation whenever the patient or family expresses doubt or shows lack of confidence in the diagnosis or management. It is sometimes wise to obtain a second opinion for patients who have a life-threatening illness or a disease with a poor prognosis.

Consultation should also be considered when the family physician is dissatisfied with the patient's progress or is unsure of the diagnosis. Sometimes an agency or special unit has the capability of providing better service, such as in drug detoxification. Clinicians rarely get into trouble asking for help with a difficult problem, but every experienced physician can remember at least one case in which a consultation should have been obtained. A consultation should be promptly initiated any time patients or families request or hint that they would like to have one. The physician must be alert to subtle clues of doubt indicating the desire for another opinion. If these clues are recognized and acted upon, confidence in the family physician increases. If not recognized, patient dissatisfaction leading to malpractice litigation may result. When doubt is recognized, the patient or family member should be encouraged to discuss doubts openly; consultation is then often unnecessary.

An early consultation is much less likely to damage patient confidence than a delayed one. The confident and secure physician who considers patient welfare to be of the utmost importance is not threatened and freely utilizes consultants at the appropriate, sometimes early, stage of a problem, before it has progressed to serious proportions that are more difficult to manage.

The patient's family is more apt to display doubt regarding the management of a case than is the patient. The physician who communicates easily with members of the family and is aware of their feelings can detect this insecurity earlier than the physician who is familiar only with the patient. The patient is less likely than other family members to express doubt regarding a diagnosis or method of management for fear of offending the physician. Whenever doubt is noted among the family members, the physician should suggest that the opinion of another physician be obtained.

RESPONSIBILITIES OF THE REFERRING PHYSICIAN

The consultation process involves approximately 12 decision points, beginning with the family physician's decision to refer and concluding with the family physician's providing feedback to the consultant regarding the eventual outcome (Table 6–1).

Selection of the Consultant

The referring physician is responsible for the selection of the proper consultant for a particular pa-

tient. The family physician whose comprehensive training involves a broad range of disciplines has the insight needed to select the appropriate consultant for a specific problem. Care must be taken to select a consultant who has knowledge and skills appropriate to the patient's need, a personality compatible with that of the patient, availability, competency maintained by frequent use of the required skills, and the ability to work well with the referring physician. Compatibility of personalities is an especially important factor to be considered, if at all possible, when selecting a consultant. A surgeon who alienates the patient, no matter how skilled, is less effective than one who establishes good rapport and has the patient's confidence and cooperation.

Referrals to a psychiatrist sometimes pose special problems and can be among the most difficult because the family physician must avoid having the patient interpret the referral as rejection. Some patients resist such a referral, and the family physician may also feel uncomfortable making the suggestion. The patient frequently welcomes psychiatric help, however, and may be relieved by the recommendation. In a review of psychiatric problems encountered in hospitalized patients (Steinberg and colleagues, 1980), 50 per cent of the patients for whom psychiatric consultation would have been helpful did not receive it because of physician resistance or failure to recognize the psychiatric problem. In those patients who later received psychiatric care, most of them accepted it well.

Patients are likely to benefit more from a psychiatric referral if they enter into the consultation with a positive frame of mind. Once the need for a psychiatric referral has been determined, the patient should be told the reason in an honest, straightforward manner. Questions about psychosocial problems should be incorporated into the history from the beginning of an illness, because they are a part of every problem, rather than being avoided until organic possibilities have been exhausted.

Psychiatric referrals are also a problem because the referring physician is less likely to receive a letter or report from psychiatrists than from other consultants. This failure to communicate can be interpreted as the psychiatrist hiding behind patient confidentiality—a suspicion that would appear to be confirmed if no report is received.

A perceptive family physician—one having thorough knowledge of the patient's personality, lifestyle, and previous reaction to similar situations—can best select the consultant and clinical setting to which the patient will respond positively. Occasionally, it is necessary for the family physician to emphasize the consultant's excellent technical skills

---

TABLE 6–1.   The Consultation Process*

1. The decision is made to refer
2. Consideration is given to the patient's medical, emotional, cultural, and socioeconomic background
3. Selection of the appropriate discipline (specialty field)
4. Selection of the appropriate physician in that field
5. Preparation of both the patient and family for the consultation
6. Preparation of the consultant
7. The consultant provides feedback to the patient and family
8. The consultant provides feedback to the family physician
9. The family physician evaluates appropriateness of the consultant's recommendations
10. The family physician facilitates the patient's and the family's acceptance of recommendations
11. The family physician acts on the recommendations or selects another consultant in the same or a different field.
12. The family physician provides feedback to the consultant regarding eventual outcome.

*Modified from Barnett BL Jr, Collins JJ Jr. A new look at the consultation continuum. J Fam Pract 1977;5:665.

and forewarn the patient of possible personality differences or other idiosyncrasies. Patient and family confidence can play a major role in the effectiveness of that consultant. This confidence is enhanced if the referring physician shows respect for the consultant's skills and makes the recommendation with enthusiasm.

Adequate Transfer of Information

The referring physician must be sure that the referral contract is clearly understood by the consultant. If the referring physician wants help with a diagnosis but does not say so, the consultant may assume that the request is for help with management, leading to dissatisfaction and unwarranted charges of "patient stealing." The referring physician should state the reason for the request and the action desired so that the consultant knows clearly whether the request is for an opinion only or also for management.

The most common breakdowns of communication between referring and consulting physicians are the consultation request and the consultant's report. The referring physician must evaluate the problem adequately and transmit all necessary information to the consultant. Complete and accurate background information should avoid unnecessary duplication of diagnostic tests.

The process of information transfer varies with the nature of the problem. Some are straightforward, such as for a 67-year-old patient with a intertrochanteric fracture. If the patient has no medical problems and is a good surgical risk, the transfer report can be brief. Other problems may require a complete summary of the office record, such as in the referral of a 9-year-old patient for recurring fever that lasts approximately 1 week every month despite negative laboratory study results.

An outpatient consultation or referral note should be in the mail within 24 hours or, better still, carried by the patient to the consultant, accompanied by a copy of the problem list and other pertinent items from the data base, including recent progress notes, laboratory reports, and x-ray films. The problem-oriented medical record is ideally suited to this procedure, because it summarizes all major disorders affecting the individual and alerts the consultant to other past and potentially significant complications that should be considered in the management of the patient's current situation. An extensive referral note is not needed when adequate information is provided by the medical record.

Family physicians often complain that they do not receive reports from consultants, and consultants often complain that they do not receive adequate information from the referring physician. The two are probably related, with the quality of the consultant's report depending upon the adequacy of information supplied by the referring physician. Patient satisfaction with the consultant may also depend on the quality of this communication between physicians. Williams and Peet (1994) found that both the referring and consulting physicians prefer an initial verbal communication that is followed by a written report. They confirm the need for referring physicians to improve the quality of information provided to consultants. The facsimile (fax) machine is facilitating this process. The referring physician can send records to the consultant and receive a report almost immediately if the system is used properly.

Patient Preparation and Compliance

Ten to twenty per cent of all patients never keep the appointment with the consultant. Patient compliance may be improved if the patient feels more involved in the referral process. First, the referring physician should adequately inform the patient regarding the need for referral and ensure his or her understanding and cooperation. (The consent is particularly important if the patient is hospitalized, because almost half of the complaints to medical society grievance committees stem from patients receiving bills for hospital consultations that they had not authorized.) The informed patient understands what will occur and that the family physician will remain in charge or will resume responsibility at the conclusion of the referral. The understanding is important if the patient is to avoid feeling rejected or "sent away."

It is also likely that compliance will be increased if the patient is given some choice of consultants and control over the time of appointment. When the family physician recommends a consultation, the patient should be asked if a specific consultant is preferred. If not, qualified individuals should be suggested, with the positive features of each being identified. If the patient does not indicate a preference, the family physician should make the final decision. Hines and Curry (1978) encourage the patient to review the referral form and accompanying materials when carrying them to the consultant. They feel this process increases patient insight and cooperation, reducing "no shows" in the consultant's office.

Details about the appointment with the consultant may be difficult for the patient to remember; thus, providing a written note containing the consultant's name, address, and telephone number is helpful. It may also help to include directions to the consultant's office and to discuss with the patient what to expect during the visit, especially the amount of time it will take.

Contrary to previous belief, Lloyd and colleagues (1993) found that patient compliance with referrals was not related to the nature, severity, or duration of the problem or to the patient's perception of the need for referral. The researchers did find, however, that patients were less likely to follow through with the referral if they had been unable to adequately discuss their problem with their family physician, emphasizing the need to thoroughly address all of the patient's worries and concerns before referral to another physician.

Evaluation of Information

It is the family physician's responsibility to continue to interact with the physician to whom the patient is referred and to lend assistance in the management of the case to the degree that is necessary for the best care of the patient. Even referrals that are for specific surgical procedures require that the family physician remain involved to manage concomitant medical problems, especially if they require cooperation from other family members. Carson (1982) found that only 7.8 per cent of referrals were for the purpose of establishing a diagnosis. As in other studies, most referrals were for specific procedures, in this case to orthopedists, obstetricians, general surgeons, and dermatologists. Even when the consultation involves surgical or other technical skills, the family physician is responsible for ensuring that other aspects of the patient's medical background are not ignored and that the family is kept adequately informed.

Newly discovered information needs to be coordinated with that already recorded. When information is received from the consultant, the family physician must evaluate it within the context of the individual patient and the patient's family situation, work environment, expectations, and ability to comply. The family physician should also guide the consultant in the amount of information that should be given the patient and family, being aware of how much information the family can tolerate and how it should be provided to enlist maximal support. Continued involvement of the family physician improves compliance with the treatment program and facilitates long-term rehabilitation.

Feedback to Consultants

It may be of value to keep a log of all referrals. Such a log, containing the patient's name, name of consultant, and date of referral, can then be checked when the report is returned to ensure that the patient actually sees the consultant and that a report is received. The log also helps identify consultants who do not return information on patients. The log can be reviewed weekly and the consultant or patient contacted if no information is received after a specified time.

Family physicians should give feedback to the consultant regarding the outcome of an unusual case. Family physicians should not leave the consultant wondering whether the diagnosis was correct or the treatment successful. This communication is an especially appropriate courtesy if the consultant was prompt in reporting and in returning the patient. If the consultant has not provided information of value in managing the patient, a second consultation should be seriously considered. Clarfield (1980) found that referring physicians felt that one third of the time (31 per cent of consultations) they had learned nothing of value from the referral. It is also important to let the consultant know if the consultation was inadequate. Experienced family physicians can help young consultants improve their "art of consultation" and should accept this as a responsibility, because consultants are rarely taught this skill during residency training. Bates (1979) believes that "nothing better expresses the ideal fraternity of medicine than an older family doctor helping a young specialist with professional relationships."

Suspecting that faulty consultation practices may be learned during residency training, McPhee and colleagues (1984) studied the communication between 27 general internists at a university medical center and their subspecialty colleagues who practiced in the same building in San Francisco. Even in this close academic setting where the referral rate was 9.4 per cent, the referring physician did not receive a report 45 per cent of the time. The poorest responding consultants were ophthalmologists (no response 69 per cent of the time), obstetrics-gynecologists (61 per cent), orthopedists (57 per cent), and dermatologists (52 per cent). A response was most likely to be received if the referring physician personally contacted the consultant and if the patient had a return appointment.

RESPONSIBILITIES OF THE CONSULTANT

The consultant is expected to provide a prompt and concise report to the referring physician. The specific questions posed on the consultation request should be addressed and action limited to the amount of involvement requested. When the consultation involves a hospitalized patient, the consultant should see the patient promptly; provide an opinion and give therapeutic suggestions in a concise note on the consultation sheet; and, in general, avoid writing orders unless requested to do so by the referring physician.

The consultant has a responsibility to the patient and the referring physician to avoid unnecessary expense through duplication of studies recently obtained by the primary physician, unless there is good reason to doubt the results or deem sufficient need to repeat the test. Of course, the referring physician must have included the actual radiographs and adequate laboratory data as part of the referral document if such duplication is to be avoided. Adequate communication via the consultation request is essential, so that the consultant is made aware of the tests that already have been performed, methods used, and results obtained. The consultant's obligation is to build on this information, repeating procedures only when necessary to verify an abnormality or evaluate a change.

When a patient is referred for care, the consultant should remain in contact with the referring physician throughout the period of care and return the patient with a full written report when the problem is resolved or when no further involvement by the consultant is warranted.

A consultant should not refer patients to other consultants without the knowledge and consent of the primary physician, who should be coordinating or at least closely involved with this process.

The most common reason for discontinuing referrals to a particular consultant is failure to receive adequate reports or failure of the consultant to return the patient for continuing care. The latter occurs most frequently when the consultant also functions as a primary physician. The patient may "stay on" for continuing care if the consultant does not encourage the patient's return to the referring physician. Even though a specific request was made for follow-up information, Cummins and associates (1980) received a report from the consultant only 62 per cent of the time. Seventy-eight per cent of consultants who were in private practice responded, but only 59 per cent of those in university clinics did so. It was disappointing to note that the follow-up information was not better for patients who required continuing care by the family physician than for those with self-limiting problems. Although one university stressed to its staff the importance of providing such follow-up information, the faculty did so only 75 per cent of the time. It is distressing for the family physician who is responsible for continuing care of the patient to have the patient return after being hospitalized at a university center with no information having been sent regarding the treatment given or plans for follow-up. It is even more embarrassing to learn from a family member that a patient who was recently referred to a nearby medical center has died.

Curry and associates (1980) found that enclosing a return mailer with the consultation request (including a stamped, self-addressed envelope and a form specifically requesting feedback from the consultant) increased the percentage of consultant feedback from 39 to 60 per cent and increased the speed of the reply. These rates were significantly higher if the lack of reply from Veterans Administration hospitals was excluded. Even with the higher response rate, it is unfortunate that 40 per cent of the referrals resulted in no report to the referring physician.

Providing appropriate feedback to both patient and referring physician is a talent possessed by too few referral centers. The Mayo Clinic has an excellent reputation for providing good feedback to the referring physician. The Clinic also has a talent for maintaining or bolstering patients' respect for their family physician. Bates says, "The top notch consultant will render a report that informs without patronizing, educates without lecturing, directs without ordering and—sometimes most difficult of all—solves the problem without making the referring physician appear to be stupid. The real stars in this play are the consultants who discuss the differential diagnosis in such a way that they make a good case for the referring physician's previous diagnosis even when it was wrong."

The consultant's opinion should be weighed by the referring physician and the appropriate action taken, depending on the conclusions reached. The family physician may have already considered many of the recommendations the consultant makes but discarded them based on factors that may be unknown to the consultant.

Shortell and Anderson (1971) describe the rewards for both referring physician and consultant when their exchange is effective. For the referring physician, it is a positive and rewarding experience, knowing the patient has received proper treatment. It will be a negative experience if the patient does not return or is disappointed with the consultant. The consultant is flattered at being chosen as an expert and enjoys receiving a well-prepared, cooperative patient. This response can change to a negative feeling if the consultant receives an unpleasant problem patient because the family physician does not want to be "bothered" any longer (i.e., the "dumping syndrome"), or if the consultant is called upon to treat patients without having been provided adequate background information.

TABLE 6–2. Types and Rates of Referral for the United States

	Crump and Massengill	Dolezal et al	Geyman et al
Location	Alabama	South Dakota	California
Year conducted	1977 to 1985	1977 to 1978	1974
Length of study	9 years	1 year	2 months
Number of family physicians	161*	27*	8
Total number of patient visits during study period	177,838	15,609	6409 (office and hospital)
Referral rate (per cent)	1.4	1	1.6

Crump	Per Cent	Dolezal	Per Cent
ENT	13.4	Ortho.	17.9
Ortho.	13.3	OB-Gyn	17.3
OB-Gyn	12.2	Gen. Surg.	15.4
Gen. Surg.	12.1	ENT	13.0
Neurol.	8.0	Ophthal.	8.0

Ruane	Per Cent	Glenn	Per Cent
Gen. Surg.	22.0	Gen. Surg.	13.7
Ortho.	13.7	OB-Gyn	12.9
ENT	12.7	ENT	11.9
Univ. Hosp. Emerg. Dept.	10.8	Ortho.	10.5
		Ophthal.	
Ophthal.	8.8		7.9
Derm.	6.9		

Modified from Rakel RE. The consultation process. In Rakel RE. Essentials of Family Practice. Philadelphia, WB Saunders, 1993, p 147.
++ Number not specified.
*Residents and faculty.
†Residents, faculty, and nurse practitioners.

REFERRAL RATES

Rates of referral by family physicians in the United States and Canada average 2.7 per cent, with a range of 1.0 to 5.4 per cent, as shown in Tables 6–2 and 6–3. Referral rates are greater for women than men and are highest in 15- to 44-year-old people (Mayer, 1982). The National Ambulatory Medical Care Survey (1985) noted a 4.2 per cent consultation rate in general and family practice.

The largest study of outpatient consultation rates by family physicians has been conducted by Crump and Massengill (1988) at the University of Alabama in Huntsville. This was a 9-year study involving 177,838 patient visits to 143 residents and 18 faculty members. The overall consultation rate was 1.4 per cent; little year-to-year variation was noted (range 1.1 to 1.6 per cent). Most of the referrals were to specialists in otolaryngology and orthopedics, followed by obstetrics and gynecology, general surgery, neurology, and urology.

In pediatrics and internal medicine, the two other primary care specialties, referral rates are somewhat higher. Internal medicine has a referral rate of 2.2 to 18.2 per cent, and pediatrics a range of 1.0 to 9.5 per cent (Penchansky and Fox, 1970); however, the referral process in these specialties has not been studied in as much detail. It appears that this difference in rates can be explained by the less comprehensive nature of internists' and pediatricians' practices and their need for assistance in fields peripheral to areas of major emphasis in training. As noted in Table 6–2, most referrals are to a surgical specialty for a diagnostic procedure or specific therapy.

Ruane (1979) reviewed 108 consecutive refer-

Glenn et al	Mayer	Metcalfe and Sischy	Moscovice et al	Ruane	Schmidt	White
Missouri	Minnesota	New York	Washington	Vermont	Massachusetts	Illinois
1977 to 1979	1978	1973	1978	1978	1972 to 1973	1984
3 years	1 year	1.5 months	3 months	7 months	1 year	2 months
>20†	3	4	6 and 1 surgeon	*++	1	17
30,131	12,228	4604	6586	7220	5814 (office and hospital)	3975
1.65	3.85	2.2	2.4	1.5	3	2.97

Ranking of Top Five Specialties Consulted

Geyman	Per Cent	Metcalfe	Per Cent	Moscovice	Per Cent
Gen. Surg.	20.6	Gen. Surg.	25.5	Ortho.	21.2
Ortho.	15.8	OB-Gyn	10.8	Surg.	19.3
OB-Gyn	11.9	Ortho.	9.8	ENT	10.6
Ophthal.	11.1	ENT	9.8	Neurol.	7.5
Urology	7.9	Urology	7.8	Gynecol.	5.0

Mayer

Fee-for-Service	Per Cent	HMO	Per Cent	White	Per Cent
Gen. Surg.	17.3	Gen. Surg.	14.8	ENT	+ +
ENT	13.1	ENT	13.4	Surgery	+ +
Ortho.	12.5	Derm.	10.6	Neurol.	+ +
OB-Gyn	10.7	OB-Gyn	9.5	OB-Gyn	+ +
Derm.					
	8.9	Ortho.	8.1	Ortho.	+ +
				Ophthal.	+ +

rals in a family practice and found a 1.5 per cent referral rate. He noted that, "The well trained family physician provides definitive care for the vast majority (in this study 98.4 per cent) of patient encounters, contrary to the cherished beliefs of many medical school faculty." Twenty per cent of the referrals were for the specific treatment of clear-cut problems (usually surgery). Sixty-four per cent were for diagnostic tests not available to the primary care physician, such as allergy testing or arthrography. One family physician in his third year of practice found that less than one half of 1 per cent of patients were referred to a tertiary care center, and these referrals were usually for the management of uncommon problems such as leukemia, sepsis, bone tumor, or cardiac bypass rather than for diagnosis (Schmidt, 1977). Dixon (1976) studied a small rural community in Ontario (referral rate of 3.3 per cent) and found that referrals were primarily to specialists in general surgery, orthopedics, and obstetrics for specific surgical procedures such as appendectomy, cholecystectomy, and cesarean section.

Consultations in a rural practice have been documented according to the International Classification of Health Problems in Primary Care (Glenn and colleagues, 1983). By far, the most frequent problems requiring consultation involved the nervous system and sense organs. More than 86 per cent of these problems were referred to specialists in neurology, ophthalmology, or otolaryngology. The second most common problems that needed referral were those associated with the genitourinary system, requiring consultation from a urologist or gynecologist. Data of this type may assist residency directors in emphasizing those areas during graduate training, although most referrals will continue to be for specific subspecialty procedures.

When referral rates for fee-for-service patients were compared with those for members of a health maintenance organization (HMO) in Minnesota (Mayer) the fee-for-service patients had a lower referral rate (3.19 per cent) than the HMO patients (4.46 per cent). Although the percentages of referral differed, the rank order of specialties referred to

TABLE 6–3.   Types and Rates of Referral for Canada

	Brock	Dixon	Hines and Curry
Location	Ontario (London)	Ontario (Rainy River)	Ontario (Toronto)
Year conducted	1975	1975	1975 to 1976
Length of study	1 month	1 year	1 year
Number of family physicians	39 (8 private practice; 31 residents and faculty)	1.7 (1 full time; 1 for 8 months)	3 family practice teaching units 9 full time faculty 17 part-time faculty residents, and students
Total number of patient visits during study period	8616	6584 (estimated)	35,351
Referral rate (per cent)	5.4	3.3	5.3

Ranking of Top Five Specialties Consulted					
Specialty	*Per Cent*	*Specialty*	*Per Cent*	*Specialty*	*Per Cent*
OB-Gyn	18.0	Gen. Surg.	35.9	Ophthal.	12.1
Gen. Surg.	13.0	Ortho.	16.6	OB-Gyn	10.9
Ophthal.	13.0	OB-Gyn	13.8	Gen. Surg.	10.2
Int. Med.	11.0	Int. Med.	12.4	ENT	9.2
ENT	8.0	ENT	6.0	Ortho.	8.3

Modified from Rakel RE. The consultation process. In Rakel RE. Essentials of Family Practice. Philadelphia, WB Saunders, 1993, p 148.

was remarkably similar and matched the specialties referred to most commonly in other studies (see Table 6–2).

Referral rates in Europe are similar to those in North America. A study was conducted among 15 European countries to define and compare national referral patterns. Over 1500 general practitioners documented 44,134 referrals. The United Kingdom had the largest data set with 407 participating physicians referring 4.7 per cent of their patients to, in order of frequency, general surgery, gynecology, orthopedics, otolaryngology, obstetrics, and ophthalmology. The study also reviewed the percentage of referrals in each country that were thought to be influenced (requested) by the patient and the delay between specialist appointment and the first communication received by the referring physician. Reports were received within 2 weeks of the specialist appointment in 78 per cent of the referrals (European study of referrals).

That which is not clear is whether a low rate of referral indicates that the physician is competent and requires assistance infrequently or whether that physician is incompetent and does not recognize problems that require referral. Other factors may play a role as well; the practice may consist mostly of healthy young adults, or consultants may not be available and referral may be difficult.

PHYSICIAN SELF-REFERRAL

Physicians have come under considerable criticism when suspected of referring patients to colleagues or laboratories in which they have an interest or from which they derive some financial benefit as a result of the referral. Professional "kickbacks," in which the physician is paid for referring a patient, have long been unethical. Receiving or paying a kickback for referring a Medicare patient is now a felony in the United States. Although few physicians refer a patient to a poor-quality physician or laboratory purely because of a financial kickback, it is also clear that "anyone's judgment can be subtly influenced by financial interests" (Stark, 1989). Any time a physician referral is thought to be in the physician's best interest rather than the patient's, the profession of medicine is at risk of losing its valued place in society. Physicians must avoid any referral that involves personal gain, because this practice runs the risk of influencing decisions and affecting patient care.

THE TEACHER-PUPIL RELATIONSHIP

The consultation process works best when two physicians work together as colleagues to solve a difficult patient problem. Because the process is usually a learning opportunity for the referring physician, it is easy for the consultant to assume the role of teacher and the referring physician the role of pupil. The process is not a superior-inferior or teacher-pupil relationship, however, but rather that of two skilled physicians working together. The consultant has the responsibility to confirm the findings of the referring physician if no new information is detected. The consultant should not enter into a series of exotic tests merely because it is thought to be "expected" or because of fear that his or her prestige as a consultant will be jeopardized. The family physician may have requested another opinion primarily to confirm the diagnosis, perhaps wishing to obtain reassurance before telling the patient of a permanent and incurable disease.

If the referring physician places the consultant in the role of "teacher," the consultant may feel obliged to make comments or recommendations that may not be necessary. The "pupil" likewise feels obliged to follow these recommendations.

The referring physician is obliged to take only those actions that he or she feels are in the best interest of the patient. The family physician should accept full responsibility for interpreting and using the opinions of the consultant, in a manner similar to the evaluation of laboratory test results. The referring physician is as free to ignore the consultant's advice as to solicit it in the first place.

Balint (1964) feels that this teacher-pupil relationship interferes with patient care if the family physician is dissatisfied with the consultant's report but follows the advice solely out of respect for the consultant as the "expert." The consultant may have formed an opinion based on insufficient information or lacking total knowledge of the patient's emotional and medical background; or the opinion may have been generated, or even manufactured, as a result of having little additional information to offer. A good consultant admits that nothing further needs to be done and does not pursue unnecessary additional testing.

The consultation process is more successful when there is a personal interchange between two physicians rather than when communication is solely by letter. When the referring physician responds only to recommendations made in a report without the opportunity to discuss them with the consultant, inappropriate assumptions may be made. The more personal the interchange that occurs between the two physicians, the more effective the consultation.

COLLUSION OF ANONYMITY

A "collusion of anonymity" exists when neither the referring physician nor the consultant accepts responsibility for the patient (Balint, 1964). Inappropriate decisions regarding patient care can be made when neither physician accepts full responsibility. The problem is amplified when the family physician turns to various consultants for advice, yielding to each, with no one person accepting ongoing responsibility for the patient. The consultation process is not a ritual of "passing the buck" but an integral part of the family physician's continuing responsibility for patient care. If the consultant does not provide meaningful or useful information, then additional consultations must be obtained until the problem is satisfactorily resolved. The term *primary physician* implies primary responsibility for the patient, not just physician of first contact.

THE FAMILY PHYSICIAN AS A CONSULTANT

It is unfortunate that too much responsibility for primary care is burdening many subspecialists. Cardiologists who treat acne and general surgeons who remove ingrown toenails are wasting years of specialized training. Referrals to family physicians are frequently made by physicians in the surgical disciplines for the care of families when psychosocial problems are prominent, for geriatric care, for the long-term management of a chronic illness, and for medical emergencies. Pediatricians frequently refer teenagers or young adults who have outgrown their practice.

In a survey of family physicians from five midwestern states, Amundson and Vogt (1989) found that 35 per cent of the respondents received consultations and referrals from other generalist specialists and 28 per cent received them from subspecialists. The most common reason for the referral was that the patient did not have a family physician, but the second most common reason, when the referring physician was another generalist, was for a procedure such as flexible sigmoidoscopy or vasectomy. One of the most common reasons for referral overall was for the family physician to serve as a coordinator of care.

The family physician can be a valuable consultant when comprehensive and continuing health care is in the patient's best interest or when there is a need for a physician skilled in coordinating the care of multiple specialists.

REFERENCES

Amundson LH, Vogt HB. The consultant family physician. J Am Board Fam Pract 1989;2(1):34–36.

Balint M. The Doctor, His Patient, and the Illness. London, Sir Isaac Pitman and Sons, 1964.

Barnett BL Jr, Collins JJ Jr. A new look at the consultation continuum. J Fam Pract 1977;5:665.

Bates RC. The two sides of very successful consultation. Med Econ 1979;56:172.

Brock C. Consultation and referral patterns of family physicians. J Fam Pract 1977;4:1129.

Calman NS, Hyman RB, Licht W. Variability in consultation rates and practitioner level of diagnostic certainty. J Fam Pract 1992;35:31–38.

Carson ME. The referral process. Med J Aust 1982;1:180.

Chao J, Galazka S, Stange K, Fedirko T. A prospective review system of nonurgent consultation requests in a family medicine residency practice. Fam Med 1993;25:570–575.

Clarfield AM. A study of all referrals from a family practice unit. Can Fam Physician 1980;26:527.

Crump WJ, Massengill P. Outpatient consultations from a family practice residency program: Nine year's experience. J Am Board Fam Pract 1988;1(3):164–166.

Cummins RO, Smith RW, Inui TS. Communication failure in primary care: Failure of consultants to provide follow-up information. JAMA 1980;243:1650.

Curry RW Jr, Crandall LA, Coggins WF. The referral process: A study of one method for improving communication between rural practitioners and consultants. J Fam Pract 1980;10:287.

Dixon AS. Survey of a rural practice: Rainy River, 1975. Can Fam Physician 1976;22:693.

Dolezal JM, Amundson LH, Sinning NJ, et al. Pricare and ambulatory referrals. Cont Educ Fam Physician 1980;12:84–94.

European study of referrals from primary to secondary care: Report to the concerted action committee of health services research for the European community. Fleming, DM, project leader. Occasional paper 56. London, The Royal College of General Practitioners, 1992.

Everett GE, Parsons TJ, Christensen AL. Educational influences on consultation rates of house staff physicians in a primary care clinic. J Med Educ 1984;59:479–486.

Fry J. Hospital referrals: Must they go up? Changing patterns over 20 years. Lancet 1971;2:148.

Geyman JP, Brown RC, Rivers K. Referrals in family practice: A comparative study by geographic region and practice setting. J Fam Pract 1976;3:163.

Glenn JK, Hofmeister RW, Neikirk H, Wright H. Continuity of care in the referral process: An analysis of family physicians' expectations of consultants. J Fam Pract 1983;16:329–334.

Hines RM, Curry OJ. The consultation process and physician satisfaction: Review of referral patterns in three urban family practice units. Can Med Assoc J 1978;118:1065.

Horder JP. Physicians and family doctors: A new relationship. J R Coll Gen Pract 1977;27:391.

Lawler FH. Referral rates of senior family practice residents in an ambulatory care clinic. J Med Educ 1987;62:177–182.

Lawler FH, Purvis JR, Glenn JK, et al. Physician referrals from a rural family practice residency clinic: A pilot study. Fam Pract Res J 1990;10:19–26.

Lloyd M, Bradford C, Webb S. Non-attendance at outpatient clinics: Is it related to the referral process? Fam Pract 1993;10:111–117.

Ludke RL. An examination of the factors that influence patient referral decisions. Med Care 1982;20:782–794.

McPhee SJ, Lo B, Saika GY, Meltzer R. How good is communication between primary care physicians and subspecialty consultants? Arch Intern Med 1984;144:1265–1268.

Mayer TR. Family practice referral patterns in a health maintenance organization. J Fam Pract 1982;14:315.

Metcalfe DH, Sischy D. Patterns of referral from family practice. N Y State J Med 1973;73:1690.

Moscovice I, Schwartz CW, Shortell SM. Referral patterns of family physicians in an underserved rural area. J Fam Pract 1979;9:677.

National Center for Health Statistics: Unpublished data from 1985. National Ambulatory Medical Care Survey.

Nyma KC. Referral patterns in general practice. Aust Fam Physician 1973;2:173.

Penchansky R, Fox D. Frequency of referral and patient characteristics in group practice. Med Care 1970;8:368.

Phelps LA, Renner JH. The development of a "statement of policy regarding consultations." J Fam Pract 1977;5:979.

Price PB, Loughmiller GC, and Murray SL. Attributes of a good practicing physician. J Med Educ 1971;46:229.

Ruane TJ. Consultation and referral in a Vermont family practice: A study of utilization, specialty distribution, and outcome. J Fam Pract 1979;8:1037.

Saunders RC. Consultation-referral among physicians: Practice and process. J Fam Pract 1978;6:123.

Schmidt DD. Referral patterns in an individual family practice. J Fam Prac 1977;5:401.

Shortell SM, Anderson OW. The physician referral process: A theoretical perspective. Health Serv Res 1971;6:39.

Stark EH. Ethics in patient referrals. Acad Med 1989;64;146–147.

Steinberg H, Torem M, Saravey SM. An analysis of physician resistance to psychiatric consultations. Arch Gen Psychiatry 1980;37:1007.

Stephens GG. The Intellectual Basis of Family Practice. Tucson, AZ, Winter Publishing Company, 1982.

Tenney JB, White KL, Williamson JW. NAMC: Background and methodology. Vital and Health Statistics, Series 2, No. 61, DHEW Publication (HRA) 74-1335, 1974.

Tumulty PA. The Effective Clinician. Philadelphia, WB Saunders, 1973.

White FZ. Referral patterns among family practitioners. Ill Med J 1984;166(1):31–33.

Williams PT, Peet G. Differences in the value of clinical information: Referring physicians versus consulting specialists. J Am Board Fam Pract 1994;7:292–302.

1. In family practice, referrals are more common than requests for consultations. Of exchanges between family physicians and other specialists, what per cent are consultations?
   a. 5
   b. 15
   c. 25
   d. 35

2. Effective methods for ensuring that a report is received from the consultant are*
   a. Call the consultant personally
   b. Provide a written request including data already obtained
   c. Send Christmas gifts to favorite consultants
   d. Give the patient a return appointment after seeing the consultant
   e. Enclose a return mailer with the request

   _____
   *More than one answer may be correct.

3. The first specialty board was the American Board of
   a. Family Practice
   b. Internal Medicine
   c. Pediatrics
   d. Surgery
   e. Ophthalmology

4. Most referrals by family physicians are to
   a. Cardiology
   b. Orthopedic surgery
   c. Neurology
   d. Ophthalmology
   e. Urology

Answers appear on **page 603**.

Chapter **7**

The Problem-Oriented Medical Record

Robert E. Rakel, M.D.

A well-prepared medical record is among the most useful tools available to a family physician. When functioning effectively, it communicates the relevant facts regarding patient care to all health personnel involved and allows for the easy documentation and retrieval of information vital to the patient's ongoing care. The information should be organized in a systematic, logical, and consistent manner and should accurately reflect the patient's state of health. Orderly recording of data is vital to efficient care. Although the information should be simplified as much as possible, it must likewise be both complete and accurate.

Family medicine involves the care of patients over a prolonged period of time. Acute illnesses cannot be treated as totally isolated events but must be viewed in the total perspective of a person's or a family's long-term care. A pregnant woman, for example, may have a slightly elevated blood pressure, which should be compared with readings before and after pregnancy to assess its true importance. (Similarly, her smoking habits, alcohol intake, caffeine intake, weight, and other physiologic and psychological functions should be noted and followed.)

An office record system will maintain its usefulness and efficiency over time only if it is individually designed to match the objectives and the personality of the physician using it. The chart should be developed and organized based upon the individual physician's preferences and needs. Some enjoy using flow sheets frequently; others are put off by them. Some prefer, and are able to maintain, an adequate medication list; others may find it impossible to keep such a list current. The ideal record must also be kept simple and must not handicap or confine the busy physician's productivity by requiring unnecessary paper work.

The lengthy, illegible, and poorly organized office record of the past has developed into a logical, well-structured account that lends itself to quick and easy retrieval of information and ready assessment of the patient's present health care needs and potential health hazards. It also assists the physician in predicting the patient's potential future state of health by identifying significant risk factors.

THE PROBLEM-ORIENTED, OR PATIENT-ORIENTED, MEDICAL RECORD

The stimulus for change in record keeping came in 1969, when Weed developed the problem-oriented medical record (POMR). Although this innovative concept was originally applied to the hospital record, its principles have served as the nucleus for major changes in outpatient records as well. The "pure" form proposed by Weed has required some modification to be adapted to family practice, but its basic concepts serve as an excellent foundation for an efficient office medical record. The POMR has also been called the "patient-oriented medical record," because it helps to avoid depersonalization and emphasizes individuality of the patient by listing the specific problems unique to that person. Hence, the patient is not just another person with gallbladder disease but an individual with a unique combination of associated problems that identify him or her as different from other patients with gallbladder disease.

The POMR achieves its maximal potential in the hands of a family physician. It works especially well in the continuing care of patients with chronic illness and in complex cases involving multiple problems. Because these are areas in which family physicians are especially effective, it is no wonder that they are the greatest promoters of the POMR. Now that many patients who suffer from previously fatal illnesses are surviving, the family physician is involved in the continuing care of ever-increasing numbers of the chronically ill. Management of patients with these chronic illnesses requires a dynamic record that accurately reflects at all times the patient's present and past medical problems and assists the physician in remaining aware of other potential problems that can become significant at any time.

IMPROVED COMMUNICATION

As our society becomes more mobile and medical technology becomes increasingly complex, we need a well-organized medical record system that permits easy communication and transfer of information among health professionals, both within the same office and at separate sites. No longer can the record be a document understood only by the physician who places data in it. It must permit other physicians, as well as an increasing number of other health personnel, who also depend on the record, to readily assess the patient's condition, understand the plan of management, and recognize all elements important to the patient's ongoing care. As long as the record is able to communicate information in this manner, it serves as an effective tool for all members of the health care team.

The maintenance of a complete and well-organized medical record over a prolonged period of time contributes to high-quality care by permitting attention to be focused on preventive measures. The need for a uniform, organized collection of information in the office record will increase as more physicians practice in groups and a larger portion of costs is paid by third parties. Increased emphasis is being placed on the assessment of the quality of care, and outpatient records need to be organized in a manner that permits review, just as hospital records are reviewed. Terminology is also being influenced by third-party payers. The physician and other health professionals, such as the dentist, nurse, and therapist, are now called *providers*, and the office visit is an *encounter*. It is hoped that in family practice an encounter will remain a friendly interaction between physician and patient, rather than follow Webster's definition of "a meeting of adversaries or hostile persons to engage in conflict." It is no wonder that many physicians bristle at the use of this term to refer to their relationships with patients.

Improved patient care must remain the primary objective of any newly structured record system. As Murnaghan (1973) stated

> Data collection and information systems cannot be justified if they subvert the process of patient care and fail to benefit the patient and provider either directly or indirectly. The growth of public, as opposed to private, responsibility for personal health services means that more and more data requirements will be placed upon the providers of care.

Data collection must not be allowed to become threatening to either the patient or the physician but must be an obvious asset to the care and management of all problems related to patients.

THE COMPUTERIZED MEDICAL RECORD

Many commercial computerized systems are available for scheduling appointments, billing, and insurance processing, and about 80 per cent of medical offices now use one of these. Universal acceptance of the computerized medical record is just around the corner. An effective computerized system promotes better patient care by stabilizing costs, improves accessibility of information, and facilitates the demonstration of quality care.

As a result of the increased use of personal computers and their incorporation throughout industry, patient attitudes towards their use in medical record keeping are changing. Ornstein and Bearden (1994) found that patients felt that physicians using computerized patient records were using state-of-the-art technology, which can be interpreted as also practicing up-to-date medicine. Rather than be more concerned about confidentiality, some felt that information kept on a computerized record may be more secure than that on paper records.

Voice-activated systems will soon revolutionize the way family physicians document their care of patients. Many are already on the market, including VoiceMED for Primary Care marketed by Kurzweil Applied Intelligence of Waltham, MA, which was developed by family physicians. More are sure to follow as the technology improves.

PATIENT ACCESS TO MEDICAL RECORDS

Use of the computer in medical record keeping has focused more attention on confidentiality of the medical record. Access to medical records for management purposes is being given to more and more nonhealth care professionals who are neither sensitive to patients' concerns about confidentiality nor bound by strong ethical or professional codes of conduct regarding the use of such information. A fine balance between confidentiality and access will have to be struck.

The Federal Privacy Act of 1974 (Public Law 93-579) establishes the patient's right to obtain the medical record in federal institutions. A number of states also have statutes as well as precedent court decisions permitting direct access of patients to their medical records. Usually, physicians own the pieces of paper the medical record consists of, but the patient has the right to review the information contained in the record. For example, the Medical Practice Act of Texas states, "A physician shall furnish copies of medical records requested, or a summary or narrative of the record, pursuant to written consent for the release of the information."

Controversy still exists about the effect this disclosure will have on clinical care. Although there is no proof that sharing the record with the patient improves the quality of care, there is general agreement that it improves patient understanding and compliance. Dr. H. I. Schade, a family physician in Los Gatos, California, allows patients to keep their own complete medical record, and he maintains only a brief office record in note form. Patients thus have the record available if they are seen in an emergency room or by a consultant or when moving to a new area. He believes that making the records available to the patients not only enables them to develop a keen understanding of their medical problems and treatment but actually discourages rather than encourages the incidence of filing malpractice suits.

One survey of patients (Michael and Bordley, 1982) found that 80 per cent believed they should be permitted to see their medical record, but they were not convinced that possessing a copy was as important as reading it. Regardless of local law, the best policy is to allow patients to examine and copy their records upon request unless there is valid medical reason for refusing to do so. Tufo and colleagues (1977) gave patients copies of their medical records in an attempt "to provide a clear statement of problems and plans to emphasize self-help and patient responsibility." They believe that the patient's audit of the record provides feedback concerning the accuracy of the information and the level of patient understanding.

Fischback and associates (1980) promote the involvement of the patient; in developing their problem list and progress notes, they state, "The attitude that 'what you don't know won't hurt you' is proving unrealistic; it is what patients do not know, but vaguely suspect, that causes them corrosive worry."

Sharing the medical record with the patient certainly has its place and can be of value, yet discretion is called for because such disclosure can also be harmful. For example, some elderly patients may become depressed or confused by seeing a problem list containing 10 to 12 items and multiple medications. Patients with emotional problems may have difficulty understanding or coping with the content of progress notes.

INFORMATION RETRIEVAL

The medical record is rapidly becoming less the private property and sole responsibility of the physician and more the joint responsibility and common property of the physician, other health care providers, and patient. Information in the medical record should be highly visible, clear, and concise so that it can be retrieved easily to allow for effective and efficient use of time by the physician and other health professionals.

The use of facsimile (fax) transmission greatly facilitates the transfer of medical information including the electrocardiogram. In many ways, fax transmission is superior to telephone voice communication, express mail, and electronic mail. It can be especially useful in emergency care.

Transfer of Information

It is important that the family physician incorporate the patient's entire medical background into the record, so that the total comprehensive picture is constantly available to the physician and other health care personnel who have need of it. Valuable medical information is often scattered in a variety of locations and thus becomes relatively inaccessible or unavailable when needed.

When new patients are seen, a strong effort should be made to acquire all medical information from other physicians, government services, hospitals, and other health agencies previously involved in the patient's care. A great deal of unnecessary effort and expense results when each physician, in turn, must establish full medical data for every patient, because a variety of diagnostic tests and therapeutic trials must be needlessly repeated. When the transferred record is in the form of the POMR or some similarly concise system, putting it to use is a simple matter.

A well-organized record system, such as the POMR, also allows the referring family physician to communicate the patient's total health status more effectively to consulting physicians by submitting the problem list with the consultation request. This practice prevents the specialist from merely "treating his own disease" and ensures awareness of all of the patient's medical, social, and psychiatric problems, as well as the problems for which the consultation is being requested. When a cardiologist is asked to consult about a seriously ill patient in the coronary care unit, the problem list clearly illustrates other problems to be considered and managed and makes the need for continuing involvement by the family physician readily apparent. Subspecialists are prevented from concentrating on a single part to the detriment of the whole patient.

Legibility

Legibility is necessary if any data, no matter how systematically organized, are to be retrieved and collated in a rapid, accurate, and useful manner that will permit the quick review of a patient's total health status. The well-known illegibility of physicians' handwriting is an understandable product of conditioning during many years of rapid note-taking. This handicap, the greatest barrier to effective communication and good records, is now being removed as a rapidly increasing number of physicians turn to dictating their records to obtain clearly typed progress notes. Dictation directly into the computer is just around the corner. Improved legibility is an obvious advantage in group practices, in which more than one physician and several nurses or other health professionals are likely to depend upon the same record.

ORGANIZATION OF A RECORD SYSTEM

A record-keeping system, no matter how well organized, is of little value if the medical record cannot be found. Much time can be saved by using an efficient filing system.

Alphabetic Filing Systems

This is a popular method of record storage, especially for small practices. Records are filed alphabetically according to surname. Because of the similarity of many names, however, misfiling is common. Strong ethnic backgrounds in a community may lead to heavy concentrations of similar names. Family filing is also difficult with the alphabetic system, particularly when there are different surnames in the family.

Color coding of alphabetical filing systems limits misfiling and eases retrieval. Each letter has a distinctive color. Colored labels representing the first two letters of the patient's last name are fixed to the tab on each file. Misfiling is common however, when there are many charts filed under common family names such as Smith, Jones, and Young.

Numeric Systems

Terminal digit filing appears to be a more efficient system for family practice. Fewer charts are misfiled using this system, and it allows for a more rapid and accurate placement and retrieval of records. The only significant disadvantage is the need to maintain an alphabetic and numerical cross-reference index, but this is easily accomplished by computer because most offices now use computers for billing and for generating the encounter form.

Color Coding

Color-coded terminal digit filing largely eliminates the possibility of misfiling or at least limits it to a narrow area. Ten colors are used, one for each of the 10 Arabic numerals 0 (zero) to 9, as opposed to the large number of colors needed in alphabetic systems. This system permits ready recognition of visually distinct categories, especially when open shelving is used. Records are arranged according to the last two digits. Each number is keyed to a color on the record jacket edge. The two colors representing the two digits are easily recognized if the record is misfiled. Records with the same two terminal digits are then arranged in sequence according to the numbers preceding the two terminal digits. Thus, chart 00–00–13 is followed by 00–01–13, 00–02–13, and so on.

Open Shelving

Color-coded terminal digit filing works best with open-shelf filing, although it can be adapted to drawer files as well. Shelves are better than drawers, however, because they can be stacked higher. It is easier for more than one person to have access to them at a time.

Inactive Records

Purging of inactive records avoids burdening the record system with unused charts. To keep the unnecessary volume to a minimum, records of patients who have not been seen for 2 or 3 years should be considered inactive and removed from the active file. This weeding out can be a relatively simple process. A color-coded tab or mark corresponding to the year can be added to the margin of each chart. Each year the color is changed when a member of the family is seen so that the color represents the most recent year in which the patient or family was seen. If yellow was the color 3 years ago, it is an easy task to pull all charts with yellow tabs. For the system to work, however, the receptionist or nurse must check this tab each time the chart is pulled to make sure the color corresponds to the current year. A list of preprinted dates can also be stamped on the chart with check marks indicating the most recent year of chart use.

Family Charts

The physician's care of families is facilitated by a record system that focuses on the family. Family folders are filed under the name of the head of the household or the person responsible for the account. This is especially important when family members have different names. Sometimes the family is filed according to all persons living together in the same residence regardless of who is paying for the care. With the numeric filing system, there is only one possible shelf location for the family folder regardless of the variety of surnames involved. Even if surnames vary within a family because of children from previous marriages or because the wife's parents live with the family, each individual is identified by a one- or two-digit modifier within the family number.

The family folder usually consists of an outer file jacket containing selected family information as well as the individual charts of each family member. One of the first items in the family folder is the *family registration form* containing family demographic data that is usually obtained at the first office visit. The family registration form maintains a prominent location in the chart because it is a ready source of reference for the names and ages of all family members and includes occupational and insurance information. The purpose of the family chart is to provide the physician with as much information as possible relating to factors involving the entire family that can have an impact on the health of any individual member. It is important for the physician to note when the problems involving one family member influence the health of another.

It is useful to have a corner or prominent area in the chart to record events that are important occurrences in the patient's life so that these can be recalled and mentioned during subsequent visits. The patient is very impressed if the physician remembers important events such as the birth of a grandchild, move into a new home, or trip abroad. Patients are often amazed that the physician cared enough to remember items of such personal importance to them.

CHART ORGANIZATION

The organization of material within the chart varies with the type of chart selected, but in all cases the material should be organized in a consistent and predefined manner. If a folder is used, the problem list is usually the top sheet on the left, with the family registration record beneath it. The top sheet on the right contains the most recent progress notes, with previous progress notes beneath it, followed by the data base, electrocardiograms, and correspondence. If possible, each of these sections should be divided by tabs or by some other method to allow easy identification, perhaps by using different colors for each section. A more economical method than purchasing chart dividers is to cut away the edge of progress note pages to make the underlying data base accessible.

USING THE POMR

Weed describes four basic elements as the nucleus of the POMR: the data base, problem list, initial plan, and progress notes. Although his initial plan applies primarily to the complete work-up of a new office patient or the admission work-up of a hospitalized patient, most physicians prefer to incorporate it into ongoing patient care as a feature of the progress note (Fig. 7–1). The logical approach to record keeping, then, calls first for the establishment of a data base, after which a problem list is developed, initial plans are identified, and the patient's progress is monitored with continual updating of the data base and problem list.

PROBLEM LIST

Although the problem list is developed largely from information accumulated in the data base, it is the most important single ingredient of the POMR. A problem is anything that requires diagnosis or management or that interferes with quality of life as perceived by the patient. A problem can be a firm diagnosis, physical symptom, or social or economic problem. It is any physiologic, pathologic, psychological, or social item of concern to either the patient or the physician. A problem is any item that physicians believe they cannot afford to forget requiring ongoing concern or attention.

The problem list serves as a comprehensive overview of the patient's present and past state of health. It indicates whether the problems are active or have occurred in the past. The problem list is a reminder of that which has occurred so that the physician can be helped to remember that the patient had a cholecystectomy or hysterectomy and thus does not continue to ask about the function of the related organs while obtaining a history.

A special feature of the problem list is that each is unique to that individual. It is a "snapshot" of that person's health risks and current and past medical problems. Rarely would two persons have identical problem lists.

Problems can be any of the following:

1. Anatomic (hernia)

2. Physiologic (jaundice of unknown etiology)

3. A sign (hepatomegaly)

4. A symptom (dyspnea, fatigue)

5. Economic (financial difficulty)

6. Social (marital discord, alcoholic spouse)

7. Psychiatric (depression)

8. Physical handicap (paralysis, amputation)

9. Specific diagnosis (hypertension)

10. Abnormal laboratory test (elevated blood urea nitrogen, elevated sedimentation rate)

11. Risk factor (family history of diabetes mellitus or of cancer)

Each problem is numbered, and in the pure form of the POMR as developed by Weed, the progress notes are keyed by number to the appropriate problem on the list, thereby reflecting its present state of resolution. This degree of attention to detail, however, is not always followed in private practice.

The types of illness seen by a family physician are often more appropriately described as symptoms or undifferentiated problems than as diseases. *Disease* implies a full understanding of the pathology

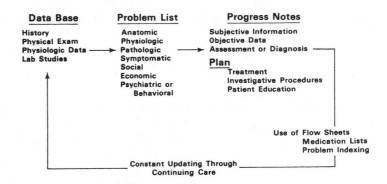

Figure 7–1. Basic elements of the problem-oriented medical record. (From Rakel RE. Textbook of Family Practice. 5th ed. Philadelphia, W. B. Saunders Company, 1995, p. 1618, with permission.)

and etiology of the illness, whereas many of the illnesses encountered by the family physician involve a varying degree of insight into the underlying etiology and a varying severity of the illness, which occasionally resolves while still in the undifferentiated state.

The problem list is a dynamic picture of the patient's health problems and is continually changed by updating, as new problems are added or old problems are carried to a greater degree of resolution. The list should contain all of the patient's continuing problems and should have a prominent position in the record, so as to constantly remind the physician to care for the whole patient and not limit attention to the problem that may be temporarily outstanding. One value of the problem list is that it continually "stares back at you" and prevents the physician from focusing on too limited an area to the exclusion of the patient's total health picture. With such a format, it is possible to rapidly orient oneself to the most important current problem without forgetting the others.

All problems can be kept in proper perspective. One physician on call for another can rapidly grasp the essential nature of a case by scanning the problem list and thereby can make a more rational decision regarding the acute presenting problem. To do this, however, the problems should be *printed* for ease of reading and rapid scanning. The POMR also allows for more efficient use of allied health personnel, by permitting the physician to effectively communicate an assessment of the patient's problems and their management.

The constant surveillance of the patient's state of health by the physician and allied health personnel and their efforts toward establishing effective health maintenance require constant monitoring of health hazards and risk factors. These risk factors should be identified on the problem list and should serve constantly to alert all health personnel to their presence.

It has been appropriately said that the main value of the POMR is not its structure but its honesty. The POMR demands that all problems be described straightforwardly and at their present stage of development and resolution, no matter how elementary the terms used to describe them may be. It insists that physicians list only what they *know* to be present, not what they *think* to be present. The principle to be followed is "record what is known, not what is supposed." The POMR discourages guesswork and demands an accurate listing of actual problems and observed facts. As Weed has said, "The problem list should not contain diagnostic guesses; it should simply state the problems at a level of refinement consistent with the physician's understanding, running the gamut from the precise diagnosis to the isolated, unexplained finding."

The POMR does not demand excessive compulsiveness but does require that all significant factors be displayed so that they cannot be ignored. Abnormal data should be placed on the problem list and accounted for. The logic behind clinical decisions is apparent in the POMR, and caution should be taken to avoid drawing conclusions prematurely.

Design of the Problem List

The problem list can be structured in a variety of ways. Physicians should select those components considered most desirable and arrange them in the manner most appropriate to their practice. Most practices design their own problem list, but a large variety of formats are available commercially. One example (Fig. 7–2) is that used at Baylor College of Medicine listing acute and chronic problems on the same page. Some programs use a separate problem list for acute, self-limited problems, because only chronic problems should be placed on the master problem list. The frequency of recurrence is indicated by dates of occurrence. In this manner, recur-

BAYLOR FAMILY PRACTICE CENTER
PROBLEM LIST
Please Print

Name _Bradford, James_   Date of Birth _7-13-32_

NO.	DATE	CHRONIC PROBLEMS AND RISK FACTORS	COMMENTS
1.	2/90	HEALTH MAINTENANCE	
	1986	Essential Hypertension	
	2/90	FH Colon Cancer	Father at age 66
	6/93	Allergic Rhinitis	
	5/94	BPH	
	8/94	Osteoarthritis	
	2/90	ADVANCE DIRECTIVE DISCUSSED	
		COPY IN CHART	

ALLERGIES	None

		ACUTE PROBLEMS	RECURRENCES									
	7/91	Acute Bronchitis	10/92									
	3/92	Low Back Pain										

Figure 7–2. Problem list, Baylor College of Medicine, Houston, Texas.

ring acute problems, such as otitis media or acute bronchitis, that can be potentially threatening to the patient's future health can be identified and transferred to the major problem list.

Many physicians believe that temporary prob-lems can be handled in the progress notes only and need not be identified on the problem list. This procedure simplifies the record system but runs the risk of failing to recognize recurring acute problems that deserve greater visibility and continuous monitoring. Most acute and temporary problems that are encountered, however, are self-limiting and usually do not recur with a frequency that requires their being placed on the master problem list.

Legibility is an important component of the problem list. Problems should be either typed or printed in large letters to support the major function of the list—that the problems be "visible at a glance."

Various methods can be used to illustrate the active or inactive status of each problem. Those problems that have been resolved but may have an impact upon the patient's future health must be retained on the problem list for continued visibility. A resolved problem can be identified by indicating the date of resolution under "comments" or in a separate column. A resolved problem can also be identified by drawing a line or arrow through it.

Family Problem List

Family problem lists are a method of depicting the problems of each family member on the same page, along with problems that involve the entire family unit. Many family physicians prefer to include this information as part of the family genogram instead of using a family problem list.

Whatever the method of organization, this comprehensive, visible, and concise overview of problems enables the physician to provide family-oriented care while keeping the ongoing problems of individual members in proper perspective. The only real disadvantage of a family problem list is the limited amount of space available and, thus, the limited amount of information that can be documented. If a family problem list is used, it should be prominently displayed in the family folder and should be the only place that master problems are listed. This prominence should force the physician to look at the family as a whole. Unfortunately, there is some risk that the physician may focus on the individual's record to the exclusion of information in the family folder.

The family problem list emphasizes the fact that no one in the family can have a problem without affecting other members in some manner; in fact, the problems of greatest importance are those that by their very nature affect each family member (Grace and colleagues, 1977). The family problem list gives the physician an awareness of the entire family's health problems. It serves as a reminder of the problems of other members who are not being seen but who may need attention or follow-up.

DATA BASE

The data base is the first step toward developing the problem list. It is the platform upon which the structure of the POMR depends for stability. The data base consists of the history (chief complaint, present illness, past history, systems review, and social history), physical examination, physiologic data, and baseline laboratory studies. The data base on each patient varies depending upon age, sex, and race. Each physician should define the minimum of data that will be collected on all patients in the practice so that office personnel can assist in ensuring that this minimum is accomplished. The collection of most elements of the data base can be assigned to allied health professionals who can obtain the information before the physician's involvement.

The data base serves as the groundwork for each patient's future care and should include those tests that are effective screening procedures for significant disease or are likely to be good reference points for future problems; for example, elevations of blood pressure can have a significant long-term detrimental effect, and a mild elevation may go undetected if an earlier baseline determination is not available for comparison. The data base should concentrate on the problem that cannot afford to be missed and should include those tests that are of greatest value in detecting these problems. Active debate continues regarding the need for various routine tests; the issue of which test is the most reliable indicator of potentially significant disease will be settled only by further research. Tests to be emphasized in the data base are those that detect disease at its earliest, presymptomatic phase so that the normal course of the disease can be interrupted and its impact minimized.

A complete data base is so essential to the success of the POMR that many physicians place "incomplete data base" as "Problem No. 1" on the list, where it remains until all required data have been obtained. A commitment should be made to obtain all of the data within a given period of time. If a complete history and physical examination cannot be obtained at one visit, information can still be collected bit by bit during a series of visits over a period of time. The visibility of an incomplete data base as Problem No. 1 serves as a constant reminder to continue accumulating the data, regardless of the nature of the episodic visit.

History

Various new methods for obtaining the medical history have been developed to save the physician time and still allow for an in-depth accumulation of valuable health history information. These health history questionnaires are available as printed forms for the patient to complete, either in the office waiting room or at home before the visit. A questionnaire can be either self-designed or commercially purchased.

When a complete history is being obtained, it is important to have available the records from the patient's previous physicians because the patient may have an unrealistic impression of the pathologic findings present. Accurate assessment of past problems is possible only by reviewing the actual records or a summary from the physicians involved. This history information should become a permanent part of the data base and should serve as a reference point for all present and future difficulties in the same areas.

Family History

Family background and family influences are not merely incidental items to be considered briefly during the care of the individual; they are essential to the continuing and comprehensive care of that individual and the risk factors unique to each patient. The family history has long been a major component of the medical record, because information concerning family background is a potential source of valuable diagnostic information. Too often, however, family data are treated superficially when the physician asks questions regarding the frequency of hereditary or transmissible problems within the family. This ritualistic inquiry is often no more than a recitation by the physician of diseases, such as tuberculosis and diabetes, for which a *yes* or *no* answer is requested, yielding data of only limited usefulness. The astute diagnostician delves into the patient's background more thoroughly, attempting to uncover subtle trends or relationships between significant past events and the present problem. The family physician usually accumulates a complete family history over a period of time, gradually adding items to the picture during a series of patient visits. In this way the patient, by asking other family members for additional data and clarification, is able to add more information at subsequent visits. Families usually enjoy developing a family genogram and cooperate in constructing one that not only reflects their lineage but also remains a dynamic picture that can be of medical value to future generations.

Physical Examination and Physiologic Data

One advantage of using a printed physical examination sheet is the ability to easily identify information that has been obtained in part but has yet to be completed. A highly structured "check-off" format is sometimes used. This format makes it possible to set a goal for completeness and to reveal when that goal has been reached or that which remains to be done. With a nonstructured, open-ended format, it is difficult to tell how much remains incomplete. Illustrations of body parts can be used in addition to the written report to depict abnormalities detected during a physical examination. Computer programs such as that described by Trace and associates (1993) allow the input of data by pointing and clicking at selections on input screens, many of which contain anatomic drawings to quickly and accurately describe variations noted during the physical examination.

Some practices insist upon a comprehensive data base for all new patients. They do not accept patients for treatment beyond the second visit for an episodic illness until the standard comprehensive examination is completed. Following the completion of this examination, the patient is sent a summary of the findings, including a problem list and the plans for following each problem. The patient is asked to review the material for accuracy and to keep it for a permanent record.

Laboratory Data

A valuable time-saving practice is to transfer all laboratory report slips to a single laboratory data sheet. This sheet is a beneficial feature of the computerized medical record. For those still using the paper method, a single sheet avoids the bulk and confusion that a mass of laboratory slips in a variety of colors and sizes contributes to the medical record. The significant amount of time saved in retrieving and comparing a sequence of laboratory information arranged side by side chronologically is well worth the time and effort involved. This ability to follow the variations of a single or multiple tests over time on a single page is of significant benefit in maintaining an accurate overview of the patient's laboratory data, especially when compared with the system of "shingling" laboratory slips that requires a variety of slips to be found and lifted if one is to follow a sequence of tests such as serum potassium, glucose, or cholesterol. Computers do this task quite well and can provide up-to-date documentation of a variety of tests in chronologic order on one summary page.

Such a summary sheet is also useful to document chronologically the dates and results of Papanicolaou smears, electrocardiograms, radiographic examinations, and other selected parameters. The actual report forms (if they contain a more detailed description of an abnormality) can be filed to the rear of the chart. Once complete information is transferred to the appropriate section of the data base form, the slip can be discarded.

The chronologic order of information in both the progress notes and the laboratory report is particularly useful in family practice because changes over time and frequency of involvement can be visualized and coordinated. When there is an abnormal laboratory or physiologic finding that cannot be explained by a disorder already on the problem list, the finding is included as a new problem and maintains that visibility until it is resolved by further diagnosis or treatment.

The data base should also identify all allergies and should include a summary of all immunizations, hospitalizations, and consultations. In this manner, the physician can note at a glance whether a patient has any allergies, has ever been hospitalized, or has ever required consultation by other physicians. Organizing data in this manner may take slightly longer, but the time saved in retrieval more than compensates for the effort.

PROGRESS NOTES

Well-organized and logically structured progress notes in combination with the problem list are the secret of the POMR's effectiveness in promoting continuing patient care. Progress notes are divided into four main components—subjective information, objective data, assessment, and plan (Fig. 7–3). These components correspond to the history, physical examination, diagnosis, and treatment sections of the traditional record. The acronym SOAP is used to describe the POMR format of a progress note and is a more descriptive and more easily pronounced term than is the acronym HPEDT.

An essential feature of any useful record is the organization of major components of the progress notes, placing the most important features in a consistent and readily identifiable position. The historical or subjective data should consistently occupy one specific position and the plan of management, or therapeutic data, another. The actual location is insignificant, as long as each maintains a separate, easily located, and readily visible identity.

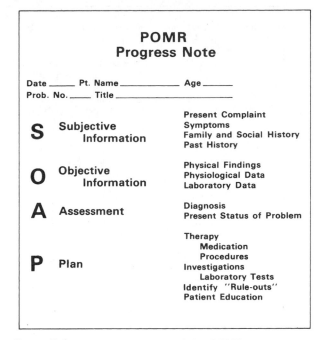

Figure 7–3. Major components of the POMR progress note. (From Rakel RE. Textbook of Family Practice. 5th ed. Philadelphia, W. B. Saunders Company, 1995, p. 1624, with permission.)

Every problem need not be described in a progress note at each visit. Comments need be made regarding only those problems that are pertinent to that visit and for which some change of status or new information is noted. Likewise, each item or component of the progress note need not be commented upon at each visit. If there is no change in status or no new information available, that section, whether it be the subjective, objective, assessment, or plan, should be omitted or a dash inserted to indicate "no need for comment." Meaningless terms such as "doing well" or "status quo" are of little value and should be avoided.

Narrative progress notes are usually long and the information is randomly arranged. Progress notes in the POMR format are in outline form and frequently contain more data, although fewer words (Fig. 7–4).

As new information is accumulated during each visit, the progress notes are used to provide feedback to continually update and modify the problem list.

Subjective Information

Subjective information includes the history of the problem and all descriptive information perceived

---

SOMR Progress Note
Milroy, John
11/21/75

Had recurrences of stomach pain 3 days ago similar to that of previous ulcer pain last year. Has been drinking again and not sticking to his diet. Has slight tenderness in epigastrium—denies tarry stools or change in bowel habits. Stool guaiac was negative. Wife says he won't stay on diet when at work or "out with the boys." Reinstructed on diet and need to stay away from alcohol and cigarettes. Rx—Maalox

73 words

POMR Progress Note

Milroy, John
11/21/75
Problem #3   Duodenal Ulcer
              S—Pain recurred 3 days ago—moderately severe—no melena—off diet and drinking
              O—Mild epigastric tenderness. Stool guaiac negative
              A—Duodenal Ulcer
              P—Maalox
                Instructed regarding diet
                DC alcohol and smoking
                    31 words

Figure 7–4. Comparison of volume and organization of POMR with narrative text.

as important by the patient, including symptoms and feelings. This is an interpretation of the problem from the patient's point of view.

Objective Data

This term refers to those items noted on examination by the physician or allied health personnel. These data include all measurements and factual information obtained by independent observers, and they represent the facts undistorted by bias. Information within this section should also be arranged consistently in the same order (e.g., data concerning blood pressure, temperature, pulse, and respiration).

Assessment

Assessment refers to either the diagnosis or the description of a problem at its present stage of resolution. Guesswork is not permitted, and only the degree of resolution that can be supported by data is described.

Problem-solving techniques are a fundamental component of traditional medical education. Problem recognition, however, is too often modified by a haste to play the academic game of one-upmanship and to establish a diagnosis rapidly and with the least amount of data. The POMR lays bare any attempt to short-cut the establishment of a sound diagnosis based on the logical acquisition of adequate data. This principle does not mean, however, that a differential diagnosis is to be avoided, since all "rule-outs" and potential causes for the problem should be reflected accurately in the record so that the problem can be pursed to a definite conclusion. A conclusion may be either the complete disappearance of the sign or symptoms without a final diagnosis ever being reached or the combining of various symptoms and signs into a definite diagnosis.

Plan

Plan refers to the diagnostic and therapeutic modalities used in the management of the problem. This section should include all present medications, laboratory tests, procedures (such as exercise or inhalation therapy), further diagnostic plans (such as radiographic studies), patient education (such as informative literature and diet instruction), counseling methods, and the use of consultants. The entire plan (or treatment) section is the most important portion of the progress notes and should be prominently located so that it can be easily found, because future evaluation requires the comparison of outcome with previous treatment plans to determine whether the results obtained match previous expectations. In this manner, the success or failure of earlier plans can be measured.

A well thought-out plan helps to maintain continuity of care and allows the physician to communicate the plans for the patient's management to an associate on call. Three major subdivisions constitute the execution of the plan:

1. *Diagnostic studies* should contain the "rule-outs" and the tests to be used in this process of differential diagnosis. Under the heading of diagnostic studies also are included the laboratory tests to be done at the next visit. The nurse or laboratory technician is then alerted to obtain these before the physician's involvement. The diagnostic studies category means that more information is needed, and the category has a list of tests to be conducted to assist in the future evaluation of a problem.

2. *Therapeutic measures* include medications and other treatment modalities.

3. *Patient education* consists of the factors necessary for patient understanding and compliance. Patient education, too, is often a neglected area and therefore warrants visibility by including it as a regular item in the progress notes. The patient education section is of greatest importance for patients with chronic problems, because treatment of one form or another is a constant feature throughout their lives. The patient should know what to expect from treatment, what side effects are possible, and how a specific medication may react with other drugs or foods. Unexpected events should be avoided as much as possible, so that maximal compliance is maintained. The patient also needs adequate insight into the problem to know when to seek help without further delay. When patient instruction is given, whether by the distribution of an American Heart Association booklet on hypertension or information about the hazards of smoking, instruction should be documented in the record so that other health personnel who share responsibility for continuing education of the patient remain informed.

Larimore and Jordan (1995) have suggested modifying the SOAP format to a SNOCAMP format to add documentation of severity and complexity of the visit to meet Medicare and other third-party documentation guidelines. The N refers to the nature of the presenting problem specified as minimal, self-limited or minor, low severity, moderate severity, and high severity. The C stands for counseling and/or coordination and documents the amount of time spent educating or counseling the patient about the condition, including items such as medications, the need to stop smoking, prognosis, and management options. The M stands for

medical decision making and designates whether the problem is straightforward, of low complexity, moderate complexity, or high complexity. These additional items justify the evaluation and management service code used by the physician when billing for the care given.

Hospital Discharge Summaries

These summaries should also be organized in the POMR format, with each problem being identified and numbered and the pertinent information "SOAP'd." The discharge summary is then incorporated into the office record at the appropriate chronological point to assist in the continuing care of the patient during future office visits.

AVOIDING LEGAL PITFALLS

Juries have a tendency to believe that if an event is not recorded it never occurred; therefore, a complete and accurate medical record is the physician's best defense in a malpractice suit. Often there is a 2- or 3-year delay before a case reaches court, and recall from memory is difficult. Therefore, an accurate and legible record is essential.

Every page of the medical record should bear the patient's name. Progress notes should be signed, dated, arranged chronologically, and typed or written in ink, never pencil.

Derogatory, trivial, or loose comments about patients or colleagues should not be recorded; they could prove embarrassing if publicized during a legal review. Similarly, vague and ambiguous statements, such as "the patient is feeling better" should be avoided.

Altering a Record

Adding to or changing a statement is no problem if it is done correctly and if no suit is pending. Altering the record after a suit has been filed, however, is the kiss of death. Altering records is considered tampering and arouses suspicions that are difficult to dispel. If it is necessary to change an entry in the chart because of an error, the inaccurate material should be crossed out with a single line so that the words remain legible. The change should be initialed and the date and time noted in the margin with a note explaining why the change was made.

Documenting Phone Calls

It is wise to document every telephone call received in the office. Requests for prescription refills should be documented in the medical record, as should any call involving medical advice or treatment.

Words to Avoid

Medical records are not privileged and confidential; the information belongs to the patient. Maligning or deprecatory remarks are certainly inappropriate. Words that should be avoided are *simple, routine,* and *uncomplicated,* because they suggest a guarantee or predict a good outcome. If the patient is described as uncooperative, the reasons should be documented. Similarly, if patients refuse to undergo certain diagnostic tests or procedures, refusal should be documented along with the reason for recommending the test. The fact that the patient was informed of the need for the test is also important. A suit has never been successfully brought because the physician gave the patient too much information.

FLOW SHEETS

Flow sheets are a useful adjunct to any medical record system, particularly when the POMR is used in conjunction with continuing patient care and management of chronic illnesses. It is sometimes difficult to review the course of a single problem over time using progress notes because a great deal of page turning is required to pick out that problem on successive visits. Placing the prolonged course of a single problem, or even selected multiple problems, on one flow sheet greatly facilitates comprehension and management. Flow sheets are also useful in any clinical situation requiring the monitoring of multiple laboratory and therapeutic parameters over a long period of time. Flow sheets present an overview of the illness, compressing events over time onto one page and allowing the physician to identify current values as well as observe trends in the course of a disease. Flow sheets permit speedy retrieval of data; they facilitate the ongoing analysis of the stage of chronic illness by indicating changing trends in response to therapy.

Once the parameters to be monitored have been identified, the flow sheet serves as a constant reminder to review these items. The flow sheet acts as an early warning system for potential problems by indicating variations from the previous pattern or baseline. Such sheets allow for a large amount of physiologic and management data to be accumulated in a compact area and observed at a glance.

The flow sheet permits ready comparison of all determinations of a single test; in addition, it permits physiologic and laboratory data to be monitored on the same time scale as therapeutic management. When material is categorized in this manner, physicians tend to write more concise and clearer notes, including fewer irrelevant details.

The time required to enter data on a flow sheet is much less than the time that is lost in sorting out disorganized information in the traditional record. A partially used flow sheet, however, can be more inefficient than none at all, because the physician is then required to search back and forth among the flow sheet, progress notes, and data base for the complete information.

The flow sheet can be a simple piece of graph paper, a self-designed form (Fig. 7–5), or a commercially printed form. In each instance, the left-hand column should contain the elements considered essential to the ongoing management of the problems being followed. Just as the data base must be individually designed for each practice, the flow sheet must be suited to the preferences of the physician and must be designed to measure those items considered most important in the management of the illnesses for which it is used.

Flow sheets serve as memory aids; they guard against the possibility of important aspects of a patient's continuing care being overlooked by the physician. For example, when monitoring the course of a diabetic patient, the physician may forget to regularly check the fundi or peripheral pulses for potential vascular change. Listing these as areas to be evaluated at prescribed intervals, along with the blood glucose level and other specific evaluations, serves as a reminder to all office personnel. The data-gathering activities of allied health personnel can easily be incorporated into the structure of the flow sheet by identifying those parameters to be measured at the next visit before the physician's examination. The flow sheet should monitor problems at intervals that reflect the degree of stability of the illness; the more acute and unstable the problem, the more frequently measurements are required. Items should be monitored often enough to ensure good care without undue expense. In an intensive care unit, the intervals between items are minutes or hours, whereas in the outpatient setting, they are days, weeks, or months.

The chart format of a flow sheet also minimizes problems caused by illegible handwriting. Effective use of flow sheets may obviate the need for progress notes when repeated visits are related only to the

BAYLOR COLLEGE OF MEDICINE
FAMILY PRACTICE CENTER
FLOW CHART

PROBLEMS

OBESITY

DIABETES MELLITUS

HYPERTENSION

HYPERURICEMIA

Patient ANDREWS, JASON

Chart No. 01-03-21

Physician H. AARON

TESTS   DATES

	1/3/94	2/22	3/24	6/13	9/15	10/7	11/30	12/12	1/31					
Weight	220	217	211	207	211	196	198	217	198					
Blood Pressure	140/96	130/84	126/80	110/80	138/100	150/80	138/82	140/96	130/84					
Glucose		259	151	133	111	109	132	151	128					
Creatinine		1.7	1.3	1.4	1.0	0.9	1.1	1.1	0.9					
Uric Acid		10.6	10.3	8.2	10.2	7.8	7.4	10.5	8.0					
Triglycerides		345	198	537	195	189	188	363	189					
HDL		22	27	21	30	35	36	22	29					
Glycohemoglobin			6.1	6.5	6.3	5.9	6.1	6.0	6.0					

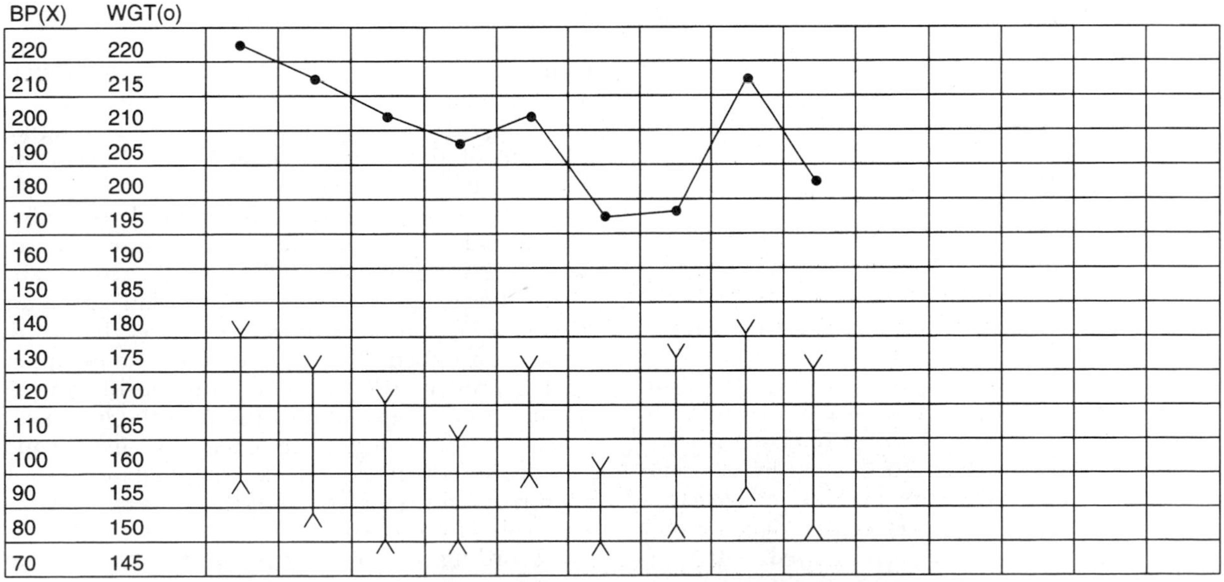

Figure 7-5. Flow sheet, Baylor College of Medicine, Houston, Texas.

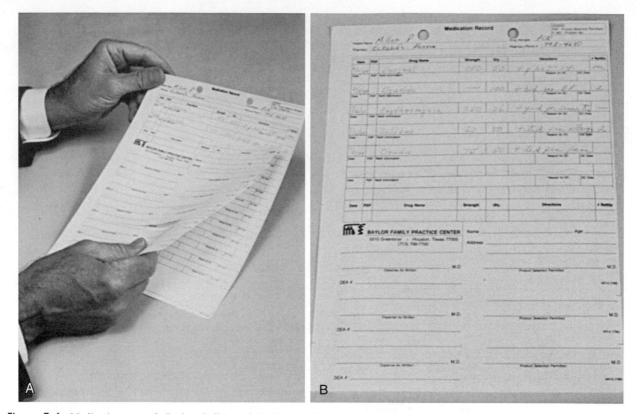

Figure 7–6. Medication record, Baylor College of Medicine, Houston, Texas. *A,* Shingled prescription forms attached along left margin overlying pressure-sensitive copy. *B,* Three of the six forms, containing up to two prescriptions each, have been used.

ongoing management of the chronic illnesses followed on the flow sheet. When progress notes are necessary, writing "see flow sheet" frequently suffices in lieu of entries in the objective and plan categories.

MEDICATION LISTS

Almost from the beginning, medication lists were a component of the POMR as it is used in family practice. Long-term medications are frequently documented below the problem list or in a similar prominent location. It is difficult, however, to keep these lists current. As soon as omissions occur, the list becomes more trouble than it is worth because it must be checked against the progress notes for accuracy. Various other methods are in use, the most accurate involving a direct copy of all prescriptions. Pressure-sensitive paper, upon which the prescription is placed when written, is used. Although redundancy occurs, the usefulness of this list lies in its accuracy. Problems arise only if prescriptions are written without being placed over the appropriate area on this sheet.

One way to avoid outmoded lists is to use a medication list such as that developed in the Department of Family Medicine at Baylor College of Medicine (Fig. 7–6). Prescriptions are fixed along the left side of the page by a perforation. An actual copy of the medication prescribed is left on the underlying pressure-sensitive sheet. Two medications can be written (one on each line) and the prescription form removed from the page, after which the patient's name and physician's signature are entered. If these names are entered before the prescription form is removed, the names appear on the pressure-sensitive sheet on top of the next prescription because the forms are shingled to save space. No loose prescription pads are used, which almost ensures an accurate record of all medications prescribed, plus their strength, quantity, instructions, and number of refills. Space is also allotted for recording the date and reason for discontinuing a drug.

REFERENCES

Ambulatory Medical Care Records: Uniform Minimum Basic Data Set. A report of the United States National Committee on Vital and Health Statistics, Lilienfield AM, chairman. US Department of Health, Education and Welfare, National Center of Health Statistics. Vital and Health Statistics Documents and Committee Reports, Series 4, No. 16, DHEW Publication No. (HRA) 75-1453, 1975.

Birtwhistle RV, Anderson JE. Transferring records when patients change family doctors. Can Fam Physician 1989;35:51–55.

Bjorn, JC, Cross HD. Problem Oriented Practice. Chicago, Modern Hospital Press, 1970.

Easton, RC. Problem-Oriented Medical Record Concepts. New York, Appleton-Century-Crofts, 1974.

Eggerstsen SC, Schneeweiss R, Bergman JJ. An updated protocol for pediatric health screening. J Fam Pract 1980;10:25–37.

Feldman WS. Pitfalls in documenting medical records. Med Aspects Hum Sex 1987; June:49–57.

Fischbach RL, Sionelo-Bayog A, Needle A, Delbanco TL. The patient and practitioner as co-authors of the medical record. Patient Counseling and Health Education, Excerpta Medica, Princeton, NJ, First Quarter 1980, pp 1–5.

Froom J, et al. An integrated medical record and data system for primary care (in eight parts). J Fam Pract 1977;4:951 to 5:1007.

Grace NT, Neal EM, Wellock CE, et al. The family-oriented medical record. J Fam Pract 1977; 4:91–98.

Hiller MD, Seidel LF. Patient care management systems, medical records, and privacy: A balancing act. Public Health Rep 1982;97:332–345.

Hurst JW, Walker HK. The Problem Oriented System. New York, Medcom, 1972.

Larimore WL, Jordan EV. SOAP to SNOCAMP: Improving the medical record format. J Fam Pract 1995;41:393–398.

Margolis CZ. The Pediatric Problem-Oriented Record. Pleasantville, NY, Docent Corp, 1977.

Michael M, Bordley C. Do patients want access to their medical records? Med Care 1982; 20:432–435.

Murnaghan JG. Ambulatory medical care data. Review of the conference proceedings. Report of a conference on ambulatory care records, Chicago, April 1972. Med Care 1973; 11[Suppl]:13.

Ornstein S, Bearden A. Patient perspectives on computer-based medical records. J Fam Pract 1994;38:606–610.

Recertification Handbook of Diplomates. American Board of Family Practice, Lexington, Kentucky, 1988.

Recertification Instruction Handbook. Application and Office Record Review, 1989 Recertification Examination. American Board of Family Practice, Lexington, Kentucky, 1989.

Ruth DH, Rigden S, Brunworth D. An integrated family-oriented problem-oriented medical record. J Fam Pract 1979;8:1179–1184.

Schade HI. My patients take their medical records with them. Med Economics, May 6, 1976, pp 75–81.

Schade HI. Office Policies Statement of the Schade Medical Clinic, Los Gatos, California, 1980.

Shapiro DM. A family data base for the family oriented medical record. J Fam Pract 1981; 13:881–887.

Sullivan RJ, Jr. Medical Record and Index Systems for Community Practice. Cambridge, MA, Ballinger, 1979.

Trace D, Naeymi-Rad F, Haines D, et al. Intelligent medical record — entry (IMR-E). J Med Systems 1993;17:139–151.

Tufo HM, Bouchard RE, Rubin AS, et al. Problem-oriented approach to practice: II. Development of the system through audit and implication. JAMA 1977; 238:502–505.

Walker HK, Hurst JW, Woody MF. Applying the Problem Oriented System. New York, Medcom, 1973.

Weed LL. Medical Records, Medical Education and Patient Care. Chicago, The Press of Case Western Reserve University, distributed by Year Book Medical Publishers, 1971.

Widmer RB, Cadoret RJ, North CS. Depression in family practice: Some effects on spouses and children. J Fam Pract 1980;10:45.

Yamamoto LG, Wiebe RA. Improving medical communication with facsimile (fax) transmission. Am J Emerg Med 1989;7:203–208.

QUESTIONS

1. The most important component of the Problem Oriented Medical Record is the
   a. Data base
   b. Problem list
   c. Progress notes
   d. Flow chart
   e. Filing system

2. Progress notes consist of which of the following?*
   a. Present complaint
   b. Genogram
   c. Diagnosis
   d. Patient education
   e. Flow sheet

3. When altering a record, which of the following should be included?*
   a. Initials of person making the change
   b. Date and time change was made
   c. Obliteration of wrong statement
   d. A note explaining why change was made

4. Flow sheets:
   a. Take more time but are worth it
   b. Monitor selected tests over time
   c. Work best in chronic illnesses
   d. Reduce the size of the progress note

Answers appear on **page 603**.

*More than one answer may be correct.

Chapter 8

Problem Solving in Family Medicine

John C. Rogers, M.D.
Stephen J. Spann, M.D.

Two decades ago medical educators began to emphasize the teaching and assessment of problem-solving skills. Teachers now assume that clinical skills include a set of reasoning strategies that students can learn and use to solve clinical problems successfully—even novel, complex ones. Research has shown, however, that problem-solving performance varies across different clinical domains, such as nephrology and gastroenterology, so that students need more than just a set of generic problem-solving skills for effective problem solving. They need specific biomedical knowledge as well. Thus, for effective problem-solving performance in primary care, students need specific knowledge about ambulatory problems (see later chapters about clinical problems) and a foundation of clinical reasoning steps, which this chapter provides.

Introduction to Clinical Medicine courses typically present students with one model for approaching clinical problems: the complete history and physical. This is the standard assessment performed when a patient enters the hospital. The assessment consists of the chief complaint, statement of the reliability of the patient as a historian, history of the present illness, past medical history, social history, family history, review of systems, complete physical examination, and laboratory test data followed by an impression and initial plans. Students rigorously follow this map for physician-patient encounters on internal medicine rotations when doing "complete work-ups" on their three to five admissions per week. Students also follow this general map on pediatrics, and in an abbreviated form on surgery and obstetrics-gynecology rotations, where a single problem is more typically the focus of the admission.

When students enter the ambulatory arena, they quickly realize that the complete history and physical format is not appropriate for most primary care physician-patient encounters. Although daily hospital visits are problem-focused like ambulatory visits, there are significant differences between daily hospital rounds and ambulatory visits:

1. The hospital patient's problems are reasonably well defined, whereas the ambulatory patient often presents undifferentiated, undiagnosed problems.

2. In the hospital, the physician has virtually total control, whereas in the ambulatory setting, the patient maintains most of the control.

3. The hospital-based physician has rapid access to laboratory tests, consultants, technology, and ancillary services, whereas the office-based physician has reduced access.

4. The hospitalized patient is conveniently available for re-evaluation, whereas the ambulatory patient leaves the office and is not readily available after the visit.

5. Physicians in hospital settings practice predominantly curative medicine, whereas primary care physicians provide considerable supportive care and practice preventive medicine.

In addition to these contrasts, ambulatory experiences provide students with two other challenges: the types of problems they confront and the stages of the diseases they encounter. First, outpatient medicine includes numerous conditions that are not seen or are ignored during hospital admissions and receive little attention in most medical curricula. Most medical students train in university medical centers, and, as noted in Chapter 1, these centers admit a very small fraction of patients seen in primary care. Hence, students do not see many of the illnesses patients present to primary care doctors. Second, the stages of diseases and appropriate therapeutic interventions differ considerably between hospital and ambulatory settings. For example, the Coronary Care Unit routines for unstable angina and "rule-out MI" bear little resemblance to the office management of stable exertional angina. Similarly, the treatment for diabetic ketoacidosis or the care of a patient with acute chronic obstructive pulmonary disease (COPD) exacerbation differs greatly from therapy for the patient with non-insulin-dependent diabetes or the patient who smokes and has early signs of obstructive lung disease on pulmonary function tests.

Three additional factors further complicate students' learning to care for patients in generalist ambulatory care settings. First, in family practice there are no limits on the types of patients or problems· students may see, as there are in narrowly focused specialties. Thus, students must be prepared to confront a broad range of problems. The top 30 diagnoses seen by office-based family physicians constitute only about two thirds of all problems seen in the outpatient setting. Even the three most common problems (general medicine examination, acute upper respiratory tract infection, and hypertension) are seen in only 1 of every 20 patients (Rosenblatt and colleagues, 1982). The next patient the student sees in the office can be of any age and either gender. The patient can have any of more than 100 problems involving virtually any organ system and any pathophysiologic process. Office-based family physicians also see a wide variety of clinical conditions in the hospital setting, where the 50 most common diagnoses constitute only 60 per cent of the hospital problems they treat (Rosenblatt and colleagues, 1982).

The second complicating factor is the amount of time dedicated to ambulatory visits. The mean time per encounter for the 25 most frequent diagnoses ranges between 9 and 17 minutes, with the bulk of the mean times between 10 and 14 minutes (Rosenblatt and colleagues, 1982). Not only must the students learn to deal with an extremely wide variety of problems, but they need to learn to do so in relatively short visits.

The third complicating factor differentiating ambulatory care from hospital care is the availability of the patient, especially for certain tests. In a hospital, the patient is virtually always "in the house" when the test is ordered, when it is done, and when the result is known. In the ambulatory setting, however, the patient is usually present in the physician's office when the test is ordered, virtually always gone when the test is done, especially if it is done in an outside laboratory or radiologist's office, and only sometimes present when the result becomes known. These contrasts between the hospital and ambulatory settings underscore the need for a systematic approach to the ambulatory visit.

If the "complete work-up" model from hospital-based practice does not fit well with office-based, generalist practice, what model does? Unfortunately, a single model probably does not work for all of the types of encounters family physicians have with patients: new patient visit, new problem visit, follow-up visit, preventive care visit, chronic illness visit, mental health visit, procedure visit. The "complete work-up" map works well for a new patient visit but not for the others. For example, at a chronic illness visit, the physician typically does several tasks—assesses control of the disease, asks about adherence with the treatment plan, checks for treatment side effects, seeks for evidence of end-organ damage, and scans for other risk factors for complications. At a well check-up visit, the physician covers several preventive medicine topics—cancer detection, coronary artery disease risk factors, immunizations and infectious disease risks, trauma prevention strategies, and metabolic disease risk and prevention. At each of the different types of ambulatory visits, primary care physicians attempt to complete specific tasks in a time-efficient way. This balance is one of the key skills in ambulatory generalist practice: how to efficiently accomplish a number of tasks that synthesize physicians' knowledge about that which constitutes good patient care. The educational challenge for students is to learn which tasks are important in what types of visits and then how to do those tasks.

During ambulatory experiences, students participate in all types of visits, but the new-problem visit represents the core educational goal, to learn how to evaluate and manage undifferentiated, undiagnosed problems. In this visit, the physician typically has five major tasks:

1. Construct a problem list

2. Assess the patient's expectations

3. Develop a therapeutic relationship

4. Negotiate a management plan

5. Learn from the encounter

In many ways, these tasks are relevant to nearly every type of visit. Together they could be seen as the general model for conducting ambulatory generalist visits. The remainder of this chapter covers these core problem-solving skills.

TASK 1: CONSTRUCT A PROBLEM LIST

The initial task is to construct a problem list (see Chapter 7). Most clinicians do this automatically. Students, however, may need more guidance, because a problem list can include more than the patient's biomedical diseases. Dr. I. R. McWhinney describes the difficulty in constructing problem lists:

1. The patient often presents more than one problem at the same visit.

2. The problems are often not presented in order of priority. The most serious problem may be left until last or not even mentioned at all.

3. The most sensitive problems may be expressed in indirect or metaphoric language.

4. The problem is not necessarily the same as the disease.

5. Much of the information presented by the patient is "noise," that is, it is not useful in solving the patient's present problems (Rakel, 1990).

Thus, a problem list may include a somatic complaint, an abnormal physical examination or laboratory finding for which a biomedical diagnosis has not been established, an emotional problem or significant social event that affects the patient's general health, or disease prevention and health promotion, in addition to established biomedical and/or psychiatric diagnoses.

INTRODUCTORY CASE HISTORY

A 25-year-old woman presents to her family physician complaining of epigastric pain of two weeks' duration. On her way into the examination room to see the patient, the physician glances at the nurse's notation on the chart: "chief complaint: epigastric pain × 2 wks; BP 120/70, P 70, R 12, T 98.6 °F." The physician immediately considers the following diagnostic hypotheses: reflux esophagitis, gastritis, duodenal ulcer, cholelithiasis, and pancreatitis. She enters the examination room, and finds a pleasant-looking young woman in no acute distress. The hypothesis of pancreatitis appears very unlikely. The physician asks the patient to describe the pain. "It's burning, food makes it better, and it has awakened me at night," the patient says, pointing to an area just below her xyphoid process to indicate the pain's location. The physician asks whether the patient has tried any antacids; the patient responds that chewing Rolaids relieves the discomfort. The doctor asks whether there has been any nausea, vomiting, hematemesis, or

melena; the patient denies any of these symptoms. The doctor asks if the patient is a smoker and how much alcohol and caffeine she consumes. The patient replies that she does not smoke, rarely drinks a glass of wine with dinner, and drinks one cup of coffee and one Diet Coke daily. The doctor asks if the patient has been under more stress than usual; she replies that she has been working hard on her PhD dissertation, which she has to defend next week. The physician's top diagnostic hypothesis is now duodenal ulcer; gastritis is second, esophagitis third. Cholelithiasis and pancreatitis are considered to be very unlikely. "What do you think might be causing your symptoms?" the doctor asks the patient. "I think that I have been under too much stress," the patient replies.

The doctor asks the patient to lie down on the examination table and palpates her abdomen. Mild tenderness to deep palpation is present in the mid-epigastrium. No right upper quadrant tenderness and no abdominal muscle guarding are present. A spun hematocrit is requested, and the result is 40%. "I think you probably have a duodenal ulcer," the doctor tells the patient. "Are you sure?" the patient asks. "About 80 per cent sure," the doctor replies. "Do you need to do some tests so that you can be absolutely sure?" the patient inquires. "No, I don't think so," the doctor replies. "The other possibilities include gastritis, which involves an irritation of the lining of the stomach, or esophagitis, which is an irritation of the lining of the esophagus. All of these problems respond to treatment with what we call H_2 blockers, which are drugs that decrease the acid secretion in the stomach. It is very unlikely to be anything else. I think that we should treat you with the H_2 blockers for 4 weeks, and see if you get better. If you don't improve, then we may need to do some additional tests."

The Hypotheticodeductive Model of Medical Decision Making

Patients usually visit their family physician because they have one or more symptoms that concern them. Although they often have an idea or explanation in mind of what they think could be causing their symptom—what Kleinman (1980) calls the patients' "explanatory model" of their illness—they really do not know the cause. They come seeking their doctor's explanation of the illness and advice on how to obtain relief. The symptoms are almost always *undifferentiated*, meaning that they are very general and can be associated with a number of different possible causes. Examples of common undifferentiated symptoms addressed by family physicians include headache, dizziness, shortness of breath, chest pain, abdominal pain, and back pain. The physician's task is to arrive at a diagnosis—an explanation of the cause of the patient's symptom—and a plan for managing or treating the problem.

How does the physician advance from an undifferentiated symptom to a specific diagnosis and management plan? The unsuspecting medical student learning physical diagnosis may have the impression that the physician gathers a large, standardized amount of data in the form of a complete history and physical examination, plus laboratory tests and diagnostic imaging study results, and out of this large amount of data falls the diagnosis. This scenario is an example of *inductive* reasoning but it is not the way things really happen. Elstein and coworkers (1978) have shown that practicing physicians use *deductive* reasoning. Very early in the encounter with the patient, the physician begins to develop diagnostic *hypotheses* about the cause of the patient's symptoms, based on a small number of diagnostic *cues* (items of meaningful information), such as the patient's chief complaint, vital signs, and general appearance. Physicians usually consider three to five hypotheses at a time, and never more than seven. Diagnostic hypotheses are usually rank ordered in the physician's mind. The rank ordering can be based on one of four methods: probability, seriousness, treatability, and curiosity value.

Ranking hypotheses based on probability involves ordering them by epidemiologic frequency, putting the most common problems at the top of the list. The aphorism "when we hear hoofbeats we think first of horses, and then zebras, except in Africa" describes probability-based ranking of diagnostic hypotheses. Ranking based on seriousness puts more serious diagnoses at the top of the list, even when they are less common. An example is ranking appendicitis at the top of the list of hypotheses considered in a 12-year-old presenting with right lower quadrant pain. Although viral gastroenteritis is a more common cause of right lower quadrant pain than appendicitis, the latter is a much more serious problem, which can have lethal consequences if missed. Ranking based on treatability gives priority in the ranking to diagnoses that are treatable. For example, a nonsmoker with a 2-day history of productive cough, no fever, recent upper respiratory infection, and expiratory rhonchi on pulmonary examination may have a viral bronchitis or a bacterial bronchitis. Because bacterial bronchitis is treatable, it is ranked higher on the hypotheses list. A diagnostic hypothesis that is serious and treatable is said to have a "high payoff" and is ranked high on the list of hypotheses, even if it is less probable than the other hypotheses. Sometimes physicians rank rare diseases high on their list, even though they know that these are unlikely. It appears that this ranking is done because of the "curiosity value" of the rare condition, which helps to keep physicians interested in the diagnostic process.

Once the doctor has developed and rank ordered the initial list of hypotheses, he or she then proceeds to explore the hypotheses through a *directed search* process, asking additional questions about history, performing certain physical examination maneuvers, and sometimes requesting certain diagnostic laboratory or imaging studies to refine the diagnostic hypotheses. As new cues are uncovered, they serve to strengthen some of the hypotheses, weaken others, or suggest new hypotheses not previously considered. The physician may also perform a *routine search*, such as a detailed review of systems, gathering data that are not necessarily pertinent to the working hypotheses, to uncover any new and unsuspected information that may change these hypotheses. The search process is cyclical, and it continues until the physician has gathered enough information to feel certain enough about the top diagnostic hypothesis that he or she is comfortable making a management decision. Diagnoses are always probabilistic and inherently uncertain. Management decisions have to be made, despite the uncertainty. Possible management decisions include doing nothing at the time and continuing to observe the patient, performing additional diagnostic tests, prescribing therapy, and referring the patient to another physician for additional diagnostic tests and/or for implementing therapy.

The Probabilistic Nature of Diagnosis

The physician is never absolutely sure that the patient has or does not have a given disease. Consider a patient who complains of chronic headaches that are bandlike and constricting in nature, and brought on by worry or stress, in a patient with a normal neurologic examination. The physician believes that these are most likely muscle contraction headaches. They can be common migraine headaches, however, and there is a very small chance that they can be the result of a brain tumor. Supposed that a brain computed tomography (CT) scan is ordered and reported as normal. Does that result absolutely rule out a brain tumor? A small chance always exists that there is a small tumor that was not revealed by the CT scan. Does a negative CT scan result make the diagnosis of muscle contraction headache absolutely certain? No, the headache can still be common migraine. Does the fact that the headaches improve with night-time doses of amitriptyline absolutely confirm that the headaches are of the muscle contraction type? No, some migraine headaches improve with amitriptyline, as well.

The probability of disease always lies somewhere between 0 and 1 (or 0 and 100 per cent). A *probabil-*

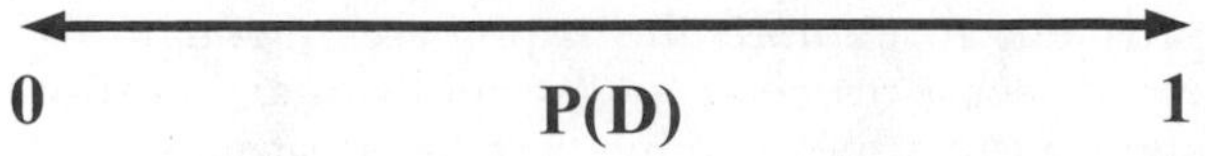

0   **P(D)**   **1**

Figure 8–1. The probabilistic nature of diagnosis.

ity line can be used to demonstrate this concept visually (Fig. 8–1).

How did the physician in the earlier case arrive at the estimate of an 80 per cent probability of peptic ulcer disease? Two methods are available for physicians to use to estimate disease probabilities. The first, and most common, is to base the estimate on their own experience. Physicians have to answer the question: "In my own experience with similar patients—patients of this age and sex, of the same socioeconomic background, with similar history, physical exam and laboratory findings—what proportion of them have had disease *x*?" The truth is that experienced physicians do this subconsciously and usually do not affix a specific numerical probability to their estimate. The thinking is more likely to be, "Most of the 25-year-old women whom I have seen who have burning epigastric pain which awakens them at night, and is relieved by food or antacids, who have mild epigastric tenderness on physical exam, have had a duodenal ulcer."

The second method is to base the probability estimate on information found in the medical literature. Medical textbooks typically describe the clinical findings for specific disease states. Although the books do not always give numerical probability estimates of disease, they usually describe the "typical" patient with the disease in question. If the patient being considered matches that description, then the physician estimates that the patient has a high probability of that disease. A word of caution is in order, however. Medical textbooks are typically written by medical school professors who are specialists and who typically see patients referred to tertiary care medical centers. These patients' characteristics can be very different from those of patients seen in a primary care setting. A better medical literature source for estimating disease probability is published epidemiologic studies. More and more studies are being published that link symptoms and results of physical examination and laboratory findings with the patient's diagnosis in a primary care setting.

The Purpose of Diagnostic Tests

What is the purpose of diagnostic tests? Physicians perform diagnostic tests to increase their diagnostic certainty regarding the diseases under consideration. Consider a patient who has malaise, fatigue, nausea, no jaundice, slight hepatomegaly, and mild right upper quadrant tenderness. The physician believes there is a "moderate" probability of viral hepatitis. He orders liver function tests. If these results are abnormal, his probability estimate of hepatitis increases to "high." If these results are negative, his probability estimate of hepatitis decreases to "low." Diagnostic tests change the *pretest* or *prior* probability estimate of disease. Abnormal test results increase the probability, and normal test results decrease the probability of the disease in question. Again, the probability line provides an excellent way to visualize this concept (Fig. 8–2).

What constitutes a diagnostic test? A diagnostic test is any maneuver that provides information that can change the probability estimate of disease. Asking a question in the medical history, such as "does your abdominal pain lessen when you take antacids?" constitutes a diagnostic test. Performing a physical examination maneuver, such as palpating the abdomen, is a diagnostic test. A laboratory test such as a serum amylase, or an imaging study such as an abdominal ultrasound, are diagnostic tests, as well.

Diagnostic Tests Are Imperfect

In the ideal world, all diagnostic tests are perfect. All diseased patients have abnormal or positive test results (true positives), and all nondiseased people have normal or negative test results (true negatives). But in the real world, tests are imperfect. Some diseased patients have normal or negative test results (false negatives), and some nondiseased people have abnormal or positive test results (false positives). This reality can be expressed graphically in a 2×2 table (Fig. 8–3).

A 2×2 table compares the results of a diagnostic test performed in a population of individuals

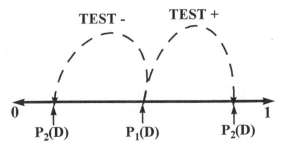

Figure 8–2. The effect of a diagnostic test on the probability of disease.

DISEASE

		+	−	
TEST	**+**	*TRUE POSTITIVES*	*FALSE POSITIVES*	*TOTAL POSITIVES*
	−	*FALSE NEGATIVES*	*TRUE NEGATIVES*	*TOTAL NEGATIVES*
		TOTAL DISEASE	*TOTAL NO-DISEASE*	*TOTAL TESTED*

Figure 8–3. The 2 × 2 table.

with their "true" state (diseased versus nondiseased), as defined by an independent reference or gold standard. For example, one could run stress echocardiograms (the test) in a population of patients with chest pain who had each undergone coronary angiography (the reference standard). One could then set up a 2 × 2 table to define the true positives, true negatives, false negatives, and false positives.

From the 2 × 2 table, we can define various terms and mathematical relationships. The *sensitivity* of a test, or *true positive rate*, is the probability that a diseased patient will have a positive test result:

Sensitivity = true positives/true positives + false negatives

The *specificity* of a test, or *true negative rate*, is the probability that a nondiseased person will have a negative test result:

Specificity = true negatives/true negatives + false positives

Sensitivity and specificity are characteristics of the test (often referred to as *test operating characteristics*), and do not change, so long as the test methods do not change. Test sensitivity varies according to the stage of the disease: the more advanced the disease, the more sensitive the test. For example, a Hemoccult test result is more likely to be positive in a patient with advanced colon cancer than in a patient with a small and early tumor.

For tests that yield results expressed as continuous variables, a *cutoff point* must be chosen to differentiate between a normal and an abnormal test result. The sensitivity and specificity of a test depend on the cutoff point chosen for defining abnormal. Consider the exercise stress electrocardiogram as a diagnostic test for coronary artery disease (CAD).

To interpret the test, one must decide on a cutoff point—the amount of ST depression necessary to call the test positive. If a low amount of ST depression, such as 1 mm, is chosen as the cutoff point, the test will be highly sensitive (it will detect the majority of patients with CAD); if a higher amount of ST depression, such as 2.5 mm, is chosen, the test will be less sensitive. Always there is a tradeoff between sensitivity and specificity: the higher a test's sensitivity, the lower its specificity. This tradeoff can be illustrated by plotting 1− specificity versus sensitivity for different test cutoff points; the resulting curve is called a *receiver operating characteristics* curve.

Interpreting Diagnostic Test Results

The clinician, however, usually does not know whether or not her patient has the disease in question; more typically, she has performed a diagnostic test and received the result, and wants to know the probability that this patient with this test result has (or does not have) the disease. The *predictive value positive* of a test is the probability that a patient with a positive test has the disease.

Predictive value positive = true positives/true positives + false positives

The *predictive value negative* of a test is the probability that a patient with a negative test result does not have the disease.

Predictive value negative = true negatives/true negatives + false negatives

The predictive values of a test are proportional to the pre-test probability of disease (the prevalence of disease in a population of patients identical to the patient tested). Predictive value positive is directly proportional to the probability of disease; in other words, the greater the clinician's suspicion that the patient has the disease before the test is performed, the greater the probability of disease if the test result is positive (and the more believable the positive test result). Conversely, predictive value negative is inversely proportional to the probability of disease; in other words, the greater the clinician's suspicion that the patient has the disease before performing the test, the lower the probability that the patient does not have the disease if the test result is negative (and the less believable the negative test result).

Bayes' formulas define the mathematical relationships between predictive value and test sensitivity and specificity, and pre-test probability (prevalence) of disease.

$$PV+ = \frac{Sensitivity \times prevalence}{Sensitivity \times prevalence + (1- specificity)(1- prevalence)}$$

$$PV- = \frac{Specificity \times (1- prevalence)}{Specificity \times (1- prevalence) + (1- sensitivity)(prevalence)}$$

Consider a 25-year-old female who presents with a two-day history of burning on urination, with urgency and increased frequency of urination. She denies chills, fever, back pain, or previous urinary tract infection (UTI). She denies vaginal discharge and has a stable monogamous marital relationship with her husband of two years. The physician's top hypothesis is that the patient has a lower UTI. Should she order a urinalysis? What will be the probability of lower UTI if the urinalysis shows pyuria? What will it be if it does not show pyuria?

To answer these questions, we need to know the probability of lower UTI in a patient with these historical characteristics, as well as the sensitivity and specificity of pyuria for UTI. In the literature, we find the following information:

Probability UTI = 0.80
Sensitivity pyuria = 0.80
Specificity pyuria = 0.95

By substituting the above values into Bayes' equations, we find the following:

PV+ = 0.98
PV- = 0.54

In other words, an abnormal test result takes us from 0.80 to 0.98 probability of UTI; a normal test result, however, still leaves a probability of UTI of 0.46 $(1-0.54)$; most physicians would probably treat the patient if they thought the probability of UTI was still 0.46. One may argue that in this case, performing a urinalysis would not be all that helpful, because physicians would not feel comfortable not treating the patient despite a negative urinalysis result.

Decision Making in Family Medicine

In family practice, management decisions are often made at relatively low levels of diagnostic certainty. Patients typically present undifferentiated symptoms, often with much "background noise" (many symptoms that may or may not be related to the patient's underlying problems, frequently related to the patient's psychosocial context). Patients often have self-limited problems, which are symptoms that cannot be attributed to an underlying disease process and that will, over time, resolve on their own. Many of the symptoms that patients present to their family physicians are due to underlying psychosocial problems and do not have a definable organic etiology. Many times the family physician needs to simply decide which one of two dichotomous categories best fits the patient: viral versus bacterial process; serious versus self-limited illness; acute abdomen versus nonacute abdomen; psychosocial versus organic etiology; and so on. Having chosen the best category for the patient, the physician can then move on to the management decision.

Decision making in family practice is, in many ways, different than it is in other medical specialties. A number of reasons are responsible for this. The epidemiology of illness and disease in primary care is quite different than it is in the tertiary care setting. White and colleagues (1961) described the illness and health care utilization patterns of 1000 adults whom they followed over a period of 1 month (see Fig. 1–1). Of these 1000 individuals, 750 experienced some type of symptoms or illness during the month. Of these, 250 consulted a primary care physician. Nine of these required hospitalization, and five of these required specialty consultation. One individual was sick enough to require transfer to a university medical center. Thus, it is apparent that the prevalence of various diseases is very different in a tertiary care medical center than it is in a family physician's office. For example, the prevalence of brain tumors in patients complaining of headaches is considerably higher in a tertiary care neurology practice than in a family practice. In family practice, common things are common, and the aphorism about hoofbeats, horses, and zebras is highly applicable.

Traditionally, the majority of medical education has taken place in university medical centers, which are "Africa" in the sense that they suffer from a patient referral bias and typically attract patients with rare "zebra" diagnoses. It is important that medical trainees have the opportunity to see patients with rare diagnoses, so that they will think of them in the future as they form diagnostic hypotheses and will recognize these rare diseases when they are in fact present. It is also important that medical trainees be exposed to the epidemiology of disease in the primary care setting, so that they can learn the prevalence of diseases associated with common presenting complaints. It is for this reason that most US medical schools now require student rotations in family practice as part of the curriculum.

Because of the relationship between the predictive value of a test and the probability of disease in the patient, family physicians frequently use different testing strategies than those used by other medical specialists. Consider a 30-year-old male who presents to his family physician with a 6-month history of chronic, band-like headaches, with no neurologic symptoms, who admits to being under significant life situational stress. His neurologic examination is normal. He is worried that he may have a brain tumor. Should the physician order a CT scan of the brain? The sensitivity of CT scan for brain tumor is 0.95, and the specificity is 0.93. According to a study performed in a family practice setting, the prevalence of brain tumor in patients who consult their family physicians with headache is 1 in 250 (0.04), at most. With these data, we can calculate that the predictive value positive of a CT scan in this patient would be only 0.05, whereas the predictive value negative would be 0.999. Whereas a negative test result slightly increases the confidence that the patient does not have a tumor (from 99.6 to 99.9 per cent), a positive CT scan result would most likely be a false positive, and it would launch a cascade of additional tests. Therefore, the patient should probably not have a CT scan.

Consider a 25-year-old male smoker who presents with a 2-day history of chills, fever, and cough productive of purulent sputum, following a 1-week history of cold symptoms. His physical examination shows rales and egophony at the right posterior lung base. In an emergency room (ER), the patient would probably have a complete blood count (CBC), chest radiograph, and sputum Gram stain and culture ordered before the prescription of treatment. In his family physician's office, he may simply be given a prescription for erythromycin, for treatment of a presumed community-acquired right lower lobe pneumonia, and may be told to return in 2 days for re-evaluation. Is one of these approaches correct and one incorrect? No, each setting is different, with a different epidemiology of disease. In the ER, there is a higher prevalence of complicated pneumonias, and the physicians neither know nor have a continuing, longitudinal relationship with the patient. The physician will probably see the patient only once, and thus a high level of diagnostic certainty is required. In the family physician's office, most patients with this clinical presentation have a community-acquired pneumonia. The patients are generally known to the physician, who can see them back in follow-up with ease. Thus, a management decision can be made at a lower level of diagnostic certainty, and a therapeutic trial with erythromycin is appropriate.

Experienced family physicians do not go through an analysis of sensitivity, specificity, and predictive value every time they evaluate hypotheses by interpreting clinical findings or ordering a test. They also often do not make their logic conscious and explicit unless they are explaining it to a patient or a student. This type of analysis, however, can lead to decision rules or standard operating procedures that are then routinely applied in common clinical situations. This analysis can also help the physician think through difficult or puzzling cases.

Experienced clinicians typically arrive at a diagnosis without being explicitly aware of having performed all of the steps required to construct a problem list during the clinical encounter. They are much like the tennis professional who concentrates on the strategy of the game and has little or no conscious awareness of the movements required for placing the serve or the forehand passing shot to take advantage of the opponent's weakness. A student is like a beginning tennis player who must learn the component parts of a forehand swing and practice them repeatedly alone, as well as with an instructor present. The task of constructing a problem list must be deliberately practiced many times over for the student to become a competent clinician.

TASK 2: ASSESS THE PATIENT'S EXPECTATIONS

Assessing patients' expectations can determine the need for and guide patient education. In addition, the process of learning patients' understanding or perceptions can be used in future encounters to negotiate the treatment plans with the patients and thus enhance compliance. Four key concepts are involved in this task: patients' goals, patients' requests, patients' explanatory model, and patients' prototypic experiences.

Patients' goals are the ends that they wish to achieve with regard to health, functional ability, or symptoms. Typically, patients do not make their goals explicit during the encounter and often cannot easily articulate them. Sometimes patients clearly state that they need to be well by a certain date because of some important event, such as a wedding or vacation or graduation. Others simply want to be rid of the symptoms, because they are uncomfortable. Others want to be reassured, because they are alarmed or concerned about bodily sensations. Still others wish to be able to perform certain levels of function for their job or personal satisfaction. Others may want to live long enough to see some critical personal event, at which time their lives can be complete. Attempting to identify as explicitly as possible a patient's goals can help form a strong alliance between the doctor and the patient, particularly if both are committed to achieving the goal.

As they go through medical training, physicians learn to work toward implicit goals of curing disease, relieving symptoms, and discovering causes of signs and symptoms. If at all possible, the primary goal is to cure disease. Usually clinicians settle for relieving symptoms until the cure removes the symptoms or the disease resolves itself or, in the case of chronic incurable diseases, function is maintained. The driving force for physicians, however, is finding an explanation for symptoms and signs, because the diagnosis provides the basis for providing cures and symptomatic relief.

These goals work well in most clinical encounters. Patients visit doctors wanting to be "fixed," returning to their normal state of health as soon as possible. If patients cannot be cured, usually they are satisfied with symptomatic relief until the condition resolves itself. When neither cure nor relief of symptoms is possible, knowing the cause of their troubles, with an understanding of how and maybe why they are ill, satisfies most patients. Sometimes, however, these goals lead to problems in the physician-patient relationship. Physicians may become so preoccupied with curing disease that they feel powerless when cure is impossible and caring and palliation are all they can offer. Physicians may not appreciate how important caring is to patients, perhaps more important than curing, and that patients certainly see caring as "doing something."

Another problem occurs when physicians are unable to find reasons for patients' symptoms or to relieve them. The search for the cause of the symptoms may escalate to more and more tests and more and more doctor visits, which is an expensive and potentially risky search that repeatedly finds "nothing wrong." For these patients, reassurances based on negative test results are often interpreted as, "The doctor said it was all in my head." In addition, if an explanation is not found, attempts to control the symptoms may repeatedly fail. In this case, attempts to achieve the implicit goals lead to frustration and a "stuck" feeling for both physicians and patients. One effective strategy is the opposite of the physician's usual "take charge" approach to clinical problems: "Don't just do something, stand there!" By altering the goal from finding an explanation for the symptoms to maintaining function despite persistent symptoms and no identifiable cause, the destructive spiral may be broken. After abandoning the fundamental goal, the physician can tell the patient that a cause will probably never

be found and the symptoms probably will never be resolved or even controlled, and that together the patient and the physician must focus on getting on with life (functional abilities) in the face of persistent, unexplainable problems. The patient may stay and strive to become optimally functional or may never return to the practice. Either way, the physician has not contributed to additional unwarranted testing or treatments, has minimized personal frustration from repeatedly thwarted goals, and may have weakened the patient's fixation on an unattainable goal. This strategy is useful whenever somatization is present and the patient's resistance to psychosocial exploration, much less psychogenic explanation for symptoms, is very high. Making patients' and physicians' goals explicit allows them to be validated, negotiated, or changed as needed to achieve the best outcome for both parties.

Patients' requests are their notions of the means needed to achieve their goals (Like and Zyzanski, 1986). Patients often want medical information about a problem, such as what it is called, what causes it, how long it is going to last, and which tests may be needed. At other times, patients want emotional assistance and are not seeking physical examination or laboratory testing. Very often in ambulatory care, patients simply want the physician to listen while they share their own perspective about the problems. Other patients want advice about general health matters such as diet and exercise. Patients often want some biomedical treatment such as medications or surgery for their physical discomfort. Patients sometimes are very explicit about what they expect the doctor to do, but often this opinion is only indirectly mentioned during the visit. By explicitly determining a patient's request for the visit, the clinician can address this issue and negotiate directly with the patient if there seems to be disagreement between the physician's recommended means of achieving the goal and the patient's desired means. This interaction, of course, presumes that both parties are working toward the same goal.

Typically, one source of patients' requests is their explanatory model. The concept of explanatory model comes from the anthropologic literature and refers to the theory about the disease (Kleinman, 1980). A number of available models exist about the causes of diseases, their prognosis, and appropriate treatments, such as the western biomedical model taught in allopathic and osteopathic schools of medicine, the chiropractic theory, and numerous others not typically taught in US medical schools, such as those followed by lay healers. In any community there may be specific cultural theories, which may follow the biomedical model but with misunderstandings, distortions, and unsubstantiated speculations. Nevertheless, the beliefs that patients hold often drive their requests and strongly influence what they expect of physicians and what they are willing to do for themselves to achieve their goals.

Another determinant of patients' requests is their prototypic experiences. Three main sources of these experiences are identified: personal experience with a problem, experience of a family member or friend, or reading or hearing about the issue through media such as magazines and television (Like and Steiner, 1986). Sometimes these sources of information, particularly significant family members or friends, have much more influence in patients' lives than do physicians. If strong experiences in these areas have led to a request that is contrary to the physician's recommendations, his or her plans for the patient may not produce the desired result unless this conflict and its source are addressed directly.

The task then is to gather information related to each of these four concepts before attempting to educate the patient or negotiate the management plan. This inquiry may reveal that there are no conflicts, no critical gaps in the patient's understanding, and no need for a long-winded discussion by the physician. Alternatively, the physician and patient may discover areas in which brief, focused education and dialogue can be very effective and satisfactory for both parties. This inquiry may even reveal major gaps or conflicts that perhaps can be resolved after serious negotiation or that may lead to the decision that the physician and patient cannot have a successful working relationship. This approach to clinical encounters is sometimes described as "patient-centered care" in contrast to the focus on diagnostic reasoning or "doctor-centered care" covered in task 1.

TASK 3: DEVELOP A THERAPEUTIC RELATIONSHIP

To be a healer and help solve patients' problems, the physician must foster a relationship of mutual trust and respect. In primary care, wherein a patient may be seen for many years, there are many opportunities to establish a workable therapeutic relationship. When the physician and patient do not have a long-standing interaction, however, a therapeutic relationship must be developed in a brief period of time.

Although a physician's nonverbal cues to the patient may be a major determinant in establishing an effective relationship, the direct questions can foster the desired relationship. Four areas the physician can ask about include: (1) the patient's family, work, and sociocultural context; (2) the patient's thoughts about the situation; (3) the patient's feelings in response to the context; and (4) the patient's efforts to cope with the context, thoughts and feelings (Stuart and Lieberman, 1986).

Gathering contextual information indicates to the patient that the physician is not interested simply in a diseased organ system or pathophysiologic process but is concerned about the person who is experiencing the illness. In addition to listening carefully and maintaining eye contact, asking a patient about work, family life, and social world demonstrates the physician's regard for the patient as a person. This conversation also allows the physician and patient to have a human connection on a basis other than the reporting of physical complaints and the prescribing of biomedical treatments.

By gathering information about the patient's thoughts, feelings, and coping efforts, the physician reinforces the view that the patient's physical complaints cannot be considered in isolation from the rest of the patient's life. This acknowledgment of the interaction of the patient's emotional life and physical well being also contributes to the development of a personal bond between physician and patient, which is necessary for an optimal healing relationship. Asking people questions about who is at home, what type of work they do, if they have a confidant or tangible social support or physical help, and what they think about that which is going on in their lives is relatively easy to do. Treading on emotional ground and asking people how they feel about their lives, however, takes more courage. Peoples' responses are unpredictable. The possibility of "opening Pandora's box" usually intimidates students, residents, and many practicing physicians, who feel they do not have enough skill to deal with strong emotions, especially negative ones. People usually do not expect the physician to solve these problems. Instead, most are very grateful that their physician has taken the time to ask and listen. Most importantly, verbally and nonverbally expressing empathy manifests the unconditional regard necessary in any therapeutic relationship (Stuart and Lieberman, 1986).

Asking how someone is coping with a situation is more straightforward and less difficult than asking about feelings. Coping mechanisms can be categorized into three types: (1) attempt to change the problematic situation itself; (2) change the attitude about the situation; and (3) decrease the stress from situations or attitudes that cannot be changed. By challenging a patient's restricted range of coping mechanisms and outlining alternatives that may not have been considered, the physician may expand the patient's repertoire of coping mechanisms. Patients also may gain specific coping skills through assertiveness training (type 1), cognitive restructuring (type 2), or stress management, specifically meditation, progressive relaxation, self-hypnosis, biofeedback, or exercise (type 3). Asking questions about the patient's context, thoughts, feelings, and coping skills goes beyond the biomedical model to the biopsychosocial model and may develop a therapeutic relationship that contributes to patients' lives in a meaningful manner.

TASK 4: NEGOTIATE A MANAGEMENT PLAN

Being a master diagnostician is often viewed as one of the higher levels of achievement in the medical art. The case studies in the New England Journal of Medicine provide challenges for those who aspire to become proficient diagnosticians. These cases illustrate how some of the best physicians perform the art. By observing their dialogue and reflecting upon their own approaches, physicians note how people may take different paths to arrive at a diagnosis. They also note how the process of diagnosing may be similar among practitioners, and finally, whether the selected hypothesis is the "correct diagnosis."

When it comes to management and discharge plans, however, the variability among practitioners is often even more dramatic than that observed for the diagnostic process. A "treatment of choice" or a series of "appropriate" treatments may be recognized, of which one may be "preferred." Even when the choice is limited to two or three different treatments, the process by which one course of action is selected is often unclear to the accomplished physician and even more obscure to the student.

Although it is not fully understood how experienced clinicians make management decisions, there are steps that at least help structure and define the decisions that must be made (Weinstein and colleagues, 1980). The first is to develop a decision tree that includes the therapeutic options and the outcomes that can result from each option. This structure outlines the treatment alternatives from which the physician and patient can choose, as well as the potential outcomes or consequences, both minor and major, of each selection. This step may be more difficult than it sounds; thus, just as patients may unconsciously restrict their range of coping responses, the clinician may unduly restrict the number of management options under consideration. Early in physicians' training this restriction may be due to lack of knowledge, but later it may occur because time pressure promotes automatic and unconscious judgment of options, which eliminates many from consideration even before they are mentioned to the patient. Always listing at least three treatment options prevents closed thinking about alternative choices.

Often, it is important to ask patients if they have any ideas, particularly if they know much about their disease or have had the problem previously. Stating several options to patients does not take much time and involves the patients in their own care. Sometimes by drawing the decision tree, both the physician and the patient can visualize and openly discuss the various options.

Just as three or more options are considered, three or more outcomes should be pondered. A clinician should know what the desired outcome is, those serious, even life-threatening complications that can occur, and those minor side effects that patients may experience. Patients want to know about all three to make an informed choice. Patients also may wish to know the likelihood of each of the outcomes.

The next step is to obtain the patient's preference with regard to the outcomes and the treatment alternatives. Unfortunately, clinicians often subtly, even nonverbally, reveal their biases at this step in the process. They typically "accentuate the positive and eliminate the negative" when discussing their preferred option, even when other options may be statistically equivalent. If the options are put in positive terms, patients tend to accept treatment. For example, if the physician states that the treatment has a 90 per cent chance of no serious complications, the patient tends to accept the treatment, but if the physician says that the treatment has a 10 per cent risk of serious complications, the patient tends to not accept the treatment. To truly inform rather than convince patients, the physician must give a balanced message using both phrases: 10 per cent chance of major complications or 90 per cent chance of no complications. Then, when the patient selects an option, the decision is informed, not skewed by the style of presentation, and it more accurately represents the patient's own values.

Physicians do not go through these processes explicitly during every encounter, because they do not have time, and because patients vary in their desire for direct involvement in medical decisions that affect them. In contrast, physicians may make their decisions informally and quite quickly in their heads. If, at a minimum, they share their thoughts with patients about three options and the major outcomes, patients are grateful. They know why the physician is recommending tests or treatments, feel more involved, and are more likely to comply with the suggestions or directions. In addition, such an approach takes a burden off the physician, because the patients now "own" and are more responsible for their health and the medical decisions that affect their health. This strategy permits real negotiation between physicians and patients about medical advice and what to do about their problems. By providing the patient with the options and eliciting an idea of the patient's preferences, the physician can usually quickly choose a course of action that is based on the best medical knowledge and the patient's values.

TASK 5: LEARN FROM THE ENCOUNTER

Learning from a patient encounter is a principal means by which physicians continue their education on a day-to-day basis. Reflecting on the encounter can help the physician determine ways in which the relationship with a particular patient and the management of that patient's problems can be improved as the care continues. Physicians can also develop a fuller understanding of the patient's problems in more general terms so that the care of other patients is improved.

Four key components are necessary for learning from the encounter: (1) identify the problem-solving method used or errors in the process committed during the encounter; (2) identify the type of doctor-patient relationship; (3) identify the decision policies, rules, or protocols used during the encounter, or at least those that are applicable to the clinical problems involved in the visit; and (4) declare an intention to improve.

Reviewing the processes by which a diagnosis was made and the management plan implemented can identify biases or pitfalls that may become habitual and may lead to misdiagnosis or inappropriate management decisions. Errors in problem solving cannot be completely avoided, but by reflecting upon encounters and noting when errors occur, clinicians may make these errors less frequently and may avoid the self-deception that all is well with their decision making.

One simple way of characterizing the type of doctor-patient relationship involves three different models: active-passive, guidance-cooperation, and mutual participation (Szasz and Hollender, 1956). In the active-passive relationship, the physician is presumed to know what is best for the patient in all ways, and the patient is presumed to be unable or unwilling to make independent decisions and assume responsibility for the consequences of those decisions. In this model, the physician is often very protective and directive of the patient. The patient in this model is passive and overtly or covertly says, "Tell me what to do, Doc."

The mutual participation model is more common as patients become very knowledgeable about their bodies, factors contributing to illness and health, and risks and benefits of available treatments. In this type of relationship, the physician shares decision making as equally as possible with a patient with the full understanding that it is the patient who must live with the consequences. The patient acknowledges this responsibility and works with the physician as he or she shares the uncertainty inherent in medicine by frankly discussing with the patient what could be wrong, diagnostic and therapeutic possibilities, and potential risks and benefits of these options. With the sharing of knowledge and responsibility between the partners, decisions are reached mutually and then implemented by those with the technical expertise required.

In between these two extremes is the guidance-cooperation model in which the patient is expected to follow the physician's advice but may assert some level of independent decision making. The physician provides information but believes that the patient is not entirely capable of autonomous adult decision making and acceptance of consequences. In this relationship there is a dynamic tension between the physician's desire to do what is in the best interest of the patient and the patient's need for independent decision making.

Individual physician-patient relationship models do not remain static over time but move among the three different types, depending upon the clinical problem, stage of the relationship over time, and clinical setting. The usefulness of classifying the physician-patient relationship in this way and reflecting upon it during an encounter is that models can be switched as needed to accomplish the mutual goals of the physician-patient encounter.

It also is useful to identify which decision policies, rules, or protocols are pertinent to the clinical encounter. Each physician develops policies regarding the diagnostic process and therapeutic management. Some of these policies may be related to the goals of diagnosis and therapy. For example, some physicians believe that they must rule out all organic problems before considering a psychosocial diagnosis; some believe that they should completely evaluate problems with diagnostic tests regardless of the cost; some focus diagnostic evaluation on treatable or serious conditions, with more unusual or less severe conditions receiving less priority. With regard to management, physicians develop policies for therapeutic goals, for example, "tight" versus "loose" diabetic control, aggressiveness regarding life-sustaining interventions, or emphasis on curative versus preventive care.

In addition to these goal-related policies, clinicians may adopt protocol-related policies developed by others, such as diagnostic protocols or algorithms that branch depending upon various test results. They may also adopt therapeutic protocols with standard duration and sequencing of interventions and standard evaluation procedures to monitor the effectiveness of therapy and to detect side effects or complications. In the treatment of hypertension, for example, step therapy and sequential monotherapy are alternative treatment protocols for this condition. Physicians have developed formal decision rules for determining obstetrical risk scores or diagnosing particular conditions (for example, Jones criteria for diagnosis of rheumatic fever). Sophisticated mathematical decision rules for diagnosing coronary ischemia or deciding whether or not to perform lymph node biopsy are also readily available (Pozen and colleagues, 1984, Slap and colleagues, 1986). These rules, however, contain a number of hidden assumptions, which may negate their applicability in certain situations.

By reflecting on the clinical encounter, the physician can determine whether any "standard operating procedures" were followed, whether the policies and protocols were appropriate in the particular clinical situation, and whether the procedures and rules may need to be revised in the light of new research and experience. A key learning task throughout the physician's career is to determine which clinical guidelines experts are recommending and how these recommendations are being revised on a continual basis. By reviewing the clinical encounter in these terms, the physician can determine whether his or her practice of medicine is state-of-the-art or behind the times.

Once this reflective self-assessment is completed, the physician must declare an intention for behavioral change—to improve. Consciously making a statement about intentions, whether general or specific, increases the likelihood that the physician will actually change.

SUMMARY: THE AMBULATORY ENCOUNTER CHECKLIST

These five general tasks—constructing a problem list, assessing the patient's expectations, developing a therapeutic relationship, negotiating a management plan, and learning from the encounter—provide a checklist to guide young clinicians through ambulatory generalist encounters. As noted earlier, these tasks are not the only ones that may need to be done during the different types of primary care visits, but they do include the core problem-solving activities for most encounters.

REFERENCES

Elstein AS, Shulman LC, Sprafka SA (eds). Medical Problem-Solving: An Analysis of Clinical Reasoning. Cambridge, Harvard University Press, 1978.

Griner PF, Panzer RJ, Greenland P. Clinical Diagnosis and the Laboratory—Logical Strategies for Common Medical Problems. Chicago, YearBook Medical Publishers, 1986.

Headache Study Group of The University of Western Ontario. Predictors of outcome in headache patients presenting to family physicians—a one year prospective study. Headache 26:285, 1986.

Kleinman A. Patients and Healers in the Context of Culture. Berkeley, University of California Press, 1980, p 106.

Kleinman A, Eisenberg J, Good B. Culture, illness and care: Clinical lessons from anthropologic and cross-cultural research. Ann Intern Med 1978; 88:251.

Like R, Steiner RP. Medical anthropology and the family physician. Fam Med 1986; 18:87–92.

Like R, Zyzanski S. Patient requests in family practice: A focal point for clinical negotiations. Fam Pract 1986; 3:216–227.

Pozen MW, D'Agostino RB, Selker HP, et al. A predictive instrument to improve coronary care unit admission practices in acute ischemic heart disease: A prospective multicenter clinical trial. N Engl J Med 1984; 310:1273–1278.

Rakel RE (ed). Textbook of Family Practice, 4th ed. Philadelphia, WB Saunders, 1990.

Rosenblatt RA, Cherkin OC, Schneeweis R, et al. The structure and content of family practice: Current status and future trends. J Fam Pract 1982, 15:681–722.

Sackett DC, Haynes RB, Tugwell P. Clinical Epidemiology—A Basic Science for Clinical Medicine. Boston, Little, Brown, 1985.

Schmidt HG, Norman GR, Boshuizen HPA. A cognitive perspective on medical expertise: Theory and implications. Acad Med 1990; 6S:611–621.

Slap GB, Conner JL, Wigton RS, Schwartz JS. Validation of a model to identify young patients for lymph node biopsy. JAMA 1986; 255:2768–2773.

Stuart MR, Lieberman JA. The Fifteen Minute Hour—Applied

Psychotherapy for the Primary Care Physician. New York, Praeger, 1986.

Szasz TS, Hollender MH. A contribution to the philosophy of medicine. The basic models of the doctor-patient relationship. Arch Intern Med 1956; 97:585–592.

Weinstein MC, Fineberg HU, Elstein AS, et al. Clinical Decision Analysis. Philadelphia, WB Saunders, 1980.

White RL, Williams F, Greenberg B. Ecology of medical care. N Engl J Med 1961; 265:885.

QUESTIONS

1. How many hypotheses should you consider at one time while formulating a differential diagnosis during a patient encounter?
   a. One to two
   b. Three to five
   c. Seven or eight
   d. More than ten

2. Sensitivity is
   a. TN/TN + FP
   b. TN/TN + FN
   c. TP/TP + FN
   d. TP/TP + FP

3. Positive predictive value is

   a. TN/TN + FP
   b. TN/TN + FN
   c. TP/TP + FN
   d. TP/TP + FP

4. Which of the following is not a type of coping mechanism?
   a. Change the problematic situation
   b. Decrease one's responsibility for the problem by blaming others
   c. Decrease the mental stress related to the problem if it cannot be changed
   d. Change one's attitude about the problem

Answers appear on **page 603**.

Chapter 9

Interpreting Laboratory Tests

Paul M. Fischer, M.D.

The diagnosis of disease is often easy, often difficult, and often impossible.

PETER MERE LATHAM (1789–1875)

Since the 1960s there has been an extensive change in how clinicians use laboratory tests. The 1960s were marked by an uncritical acceptance of "screening panels," which promised to diagnose disease before the patient became symptomatic. Multichannel chemistry analyzers made it possible to order large numbers of tests and to have the results back within a short time. Test ordering became simplified to just deciding the particular "panel" or "profile" that was needed.

During the 1970s and 1980s it became clear that few of the common tests were useful for screening asymptomatic individuals. This realization was the result of a better understanding of the limits of tests for predicting disease. Sophisticated decision analysis models were developed based on a test's sensitivity, specificity, and predictive value. *Sensitivity* refers to the rate at which a test is positive in a patient with disease. *Specificity* is the likelihood that the test will be negative in a patient without disease. *Predictive value* is the percent of patients with a positive test who actually have a disease.

Mathematical modeling based on test performance became a seductive area of research for academicians trying to characterize a "rational" way to order tests. The trend was further promoted by health care payers in an effort to eliminate unnecessary costs. Toward this end, the American College of Physicians and the Blue Cross/Blue Shield Association developed a text on the use and interpretation of common diagnostic tests (Sox, 1987). Just as the number of tests in a laboratory panel appeared to be a panacea for physicians during the 1960s, the complexity of these mathematical equations was touted as the panacea for rational test selection during the 1980s. Unfortunately, the promises of these mathematical models have not been realized. As explained later, the ambiguities of clinical practice make caring for patients a less precise science than mathematics. Furthermore, tests are used in many ways by clinicians. As George Lundberg (Editor, *JAMA*) has shown, physicians sometimes order tests merely because there is "nothing else to do" (Lundberg, 1983).

In the sections that follow, some of the issues that produce ambiguity for clinicians when ordering tests are highlighted. Common tests and outlines for using them in clinical practice then follow. The intent with these outlines is not to dictate how physicians should order tests but, rather, to help them interpret the test results that do not seem to make sense.

PROBLEM OF A "GOLD STANDARD"

Calculating a test's sensitivity and specificity requires a "gold standard." This standard is a reference test that can be considered definitive for characterizing a patient as either having a disease or being free of disease. Unfortunately, most gold standards for common tests are imperfect.

Coronary angiography is used as a gold standard for the presence of coronary artery disease; however, studies have shown that this test frequently misclassifies both the presence and the absence of significant coronary artery stenosis (Boyko et al.,

1988). For example, it does not indicate the presence of small-vessel coronary disease, which can produce ischemia. If a gold standard misclassifies individuals, both the sensitivity and specificity of a second comparison test are then artificially altered.

The inadequacy of reference tests is a problem for such common diseases as group A streptococcal pharyngitis and urinary tract infections. When diagnosing patients with sore throats, a throat culture has traditionally been used. More recently, rapid tests that detect group A streptococcal cell wall antigens have become available. Many microbiologists believe that these newer tests are inadequate because they have a 10 per cent false-negative rate compared to cultures (i.e., in 10 per cent of patients with negative antigen tests, group A streptococci grow on a throat culture). However, the colony count in these "false-negative" cases is often low. It is therefore not clear whether the patient is a noninfected carrier or an infected patient. The sensitivity of any group A streptococcal test can be discredited by employing more sophisticated culture techniques as reference methods, thereby recovering streptococci from a larger percentage of healthy individuals who carry group A streptococci in their throats but are not infected (DeNeef, 1987a).

Some have argued that a rise in streptococcal antibody titers (i.e., antistreptolysin O titers) should be used as the gold standard when determining who really has group A streptococcal pharyngitis. In one study looking at the clinical response to antibiotic therapy of individuals with a positive throat culture, patients with and without antibody response showed a clinical improvement with antibiotics compared to individuals with a negative throat culture (Gerber et al., 1988). This study raises significant questions about the appropriateness of using antibody response to identify who has a true streptococcal infection. There is to date no clear agreement on the gold standard for evaluating the common condition of streptococcal pharyngitis.

As another example, consider the diagnosis of urinary tract infections. Until recently it was not uncommon to tell a woman with urinary frequency, urgency, and dysuria that she "was not infected" because her urine culture grew only 50,000 organisms per milliliter. This judgment was based on the time-honored level of 100,000 colonies/ml of urine as a cutoff for "significant" bacteriuria. This diagnostic level failed to consider the patient's symptoms, how long the urine had incubated in the bladder, or the specimen's specific gravity. More recent studies have indicated that a colony count as low as 100/ml may indicate infection in a woman with dysuria. There is in fact no single level of bacteria that can be used as a gold standard for diagnosing a urinary tract infection.

The gold standard problem will become more complicated in the future because of the availability of DNA-based tests such as the polymerase chain reaction (PCR). These tests can amplify a single DNA chain to a level that permits detection. Whereas clinicians should have little difficulty making decisions about a single tuberculosis organism in a sputum specimen or a single gonorrhea organism in a cervical specimen, what will we do with a test that can identify a single group A streptococcus in a throat swab or a single *Escherichia coli* in a urine specimen?

Unfortunately, there is no precise way to adjust for the errors of an imperfect reference test. Clinicians should therefore be cautious when interpreting the performance characteristics of any test; they should always look to see what gold standard was used and then rely on their common sense.

PROBLEMS IN CONFIDENCE

A second problem is the great variability in reported test sensitivities and specificities. Pronouncements are made that a test has a "95 per cent sensitivity" as if it were for all times and all patient populations. The next month, an article using the same test reports "60 per cent sensitivity." No wonder clinicians have a difficult time putting these concepts to use. One reason for this variation is that the accuracy of the reported sensitivity and specificity depends on the size of the population studied. Many of these studies have few patients. If the numbers are low, there can be little certainty of the results.

It has been recommended that sensitivities and specificities be reported as a "confidence interval" (Heckerling, 1988). This interval is the range of values (usually ± 2 SD) supported by the data. For example, if a test is positive in 15 of 20 patients with a disease, the sensitivity is 75 per cent. The 95 per cent confidence limit for this sensitivity, however, would be 51 to 91 per cent, meaning that there is a 95 per cent chance that the true sensitivity is between 51 and 91 per cent and a 5 per cent chance that it is less than 51 per cent or greater than 91 per cent. This is a wide variation. If the same test is studied with a larger population, and 300 of 400 patients with the disease have a positive test, the sensitivity remains 75 per cent, but the 95 per cent confidence limits would be narrowed to between 70 and 79 per cent.

The lesson for the clinician should be to suspect all sensitivity and specificity values. Be especially cautious when there is great variation in the values reported for a single test.

SPECTRUM OF DISEASE

Traditional test performance models assume that either there is disease or there is not. This simplistic ideal is complicated by the concept of the spectrum of disease (Ransohoff and Feinstein, 1978), which is the range of features that characterize an illness (i.e., variation in chronicity and severity). Test results vary at different points in a disease. The usual pattern is that the test is more likely to be positive when the disease is of a longer duration or greater severity. Unfortunately, clinicians usually order tests early during the course of a disease, before the diagnosis is obvious. Many of the reported sensitivities and specificities from the literature are optimistically high because of the tendency of researchers to ignore the problem of disease spectrum.

An example is the literature on carcinoembryonic antigen (CEA) testing for colon cancer. The early studies indicated 90 per cent sensitivity for this test. Most of these studies were done on individuals with extensive disease. Later studies with more representative examples of colon cancer patients (i.e., some with localized disease and others with extensive disease) showed that the test was sensitive only in patients with extensive cancer.

Test specificity can be inaccurate because of the variety of nondiseased patients who are studied. Remember, specificity is defined as the percentage of individuals without the disease who have a negative test.) The early studies on CEA and colon cancer showed specificities of 90 per cent. The nondiseased individuals in these studies were healthy and asymptomatic. Later studies used a more appropriate spectrum of controls (i.e., individuals with other colon diseases or those with cancers other than of the colon). In these later studies, the specificity of CEA testing was greatly reduced. Not surprisingly, CEA can be elevated in colon diseases that mimic colon cancer.

PROBLEM OF PREVALENCE

Another concept used in the mathematical modeling for test interpretation is that of "disease prevalence." Prevalence is the number of individuals with the disease in a population at a given time. There are unfortunately almost no prevalence figures that can be easily "plugged into" a decision analysis formula for real clinical situations. The best that can usually be done to estimate the prevalence of a disease is to say whether it is common, uncommon, or rare.

There are typically two types of prevalence figures in the literature. The first type is derived from case-series seen in referral centers: What percentage of patients seen at a university urology clinic who have an elevated prostate-specific antigen (PSA) level also have prostate cancer? Such prevalence figures are notoriously inaccurate because of the problem of referral bias.

A second type of reported prevalence comes from population studies. With this type of research, a specified population is tested (i.e., PSA tests are done on all men over age 60 in a defined geographic region). Although this type of prevalence figure may help characterize the disease for the general population, it does not necessarily help the individual clinician deal with the symptomatic patient who presents for a diagnosis: What is the prevalence of prostate cancer in a 65-year-old man who complains of nocturia and a weak urinary stream and who has a large, smooth prostate by digital examination and a borderline high PSA value?

Another aspect of prevalence that is usually overlooked is that it varies from one practice to another and from month to month. Consider, for example, the differences in the prevalence of human immunodeficiency virus (HIV) disease in San Francisco compared with that in Omaha. Also consider the prevalence of influenza in February compared with July.

TREATMENT ASSUMPTIONS

It is often assumed that understanding a test's predictive value leads to clear, rational test ordering. However, even when clinicians can agree on the characteristics of a test, they may end up with different decisions on how to use the test. This point has been illustrated by DeNeef for testing to detect group A streptococcal pharyngitis (DeNeef, 1987b). DeNeef looked at 21 ways to evaluate and treat adults with pharyngitis. He included a wide range of treatment strategies including the empirical use of antibiotics, culturing all patients, or testing everyone with rapid tests. In the end, it was not the characteristics of the tests that determined the optimal clinical strategy but, rather, the physician's treatment goals. These goals could include minimizing the total test cost, minimizing adverse outcomes, or minimizing the cost of both adverse outcomes and unnecessary antibiotics. In the end, it was the

clinicians' assumptions about the optimal therapeutic goals, not the characteristics of the tests, that determined "appropriate" test ordering.

DECISION LEVELS

If clinicians cannot easily use sensitivity, specificity, or predictive value when making clinical decisions, then what do they use? It is our observation that when interpreting tests clinicians usually ask two questions:

1. Is the test result normal or abnormal?

2. If abnormal, is it a little abnormal or highly abnormal?

The degree of abnormality has been overlooked in many discussions about test interpretations (Statland, 1987). It is, however, what clinicians have intuitively used for a long time when deciding whether they should act on a test result. A serum calcium of 10.5 mg/dl, although outside the usual reference range, does not catch a clinician's attention. On the other hand, a level of 13 mg/dl is impossible to ignore.

The remainder of this chapter reviews many of the common tests that clinicians must learn to interpret. Each section includes background information about the test, common causes of abnormal results, and some of the common pitfalls in test interpretation. These rules should not be viewed as firm, but as clinically useful, guides. The information reflects my perspective based on work in primary care clinical settings.

Each section includes a table of "normal" values. This term has fallen out of favor with mathematical purists, who prefer the term "reference range." Although "reference range" may be statistically safer, it is not clinically useful. Most men would prefer a "normal" PSA to one that is "within the reference range." In the following sections, we have indicated, where appropriate, the differences between the normal values for adults and children, males and females. All values are given in both conventional units and Système International (SI) units. The U.S. medical community has flirted with adoption of SI units, but old habits die hard. Conversion factors (conventional units to SI units) are also given.

Despite the increasing interest in establishing rules for appropriate test ordering, the best that can be said is that there are a few instances when a test is clearly indicated, a few where it is clearly inappropriate, and many other instances that are open to debate. Clinicians live in a sea of uncertainty.

ALBUMIN

Albumin is produced by the liver and released into the plasma, where it accounts for 90 per cent of the intravascular oncotic pressure. A healthy adult liver is able to produce 12 to 14 gm of albumin per day (Table 9–1). This amount is reduced with advanced age, poor nutrition, or hepatic disease.

It is unclear how albumin is degraded in the body; only small amounts are normally lost through the urine or the gastrointestinal mucosa. When there is either a reduction in albumin synthesis or an increase in albumin loss, hypoalbuminemia develops, often associated with edema.

Serum albumin testing is not recommended for the general screening of healthy individuals. When such routine screening is done, most of the abnormal values are mildly elevated or decreased. These values represent the extremes of the normal distribution of values and can usually be ignored. The test is useful for evaluating patients with edema, liver disease, or suspected malnutrition.

An elevated albumin value is of no clinical significance. It is most commonly seen in the presence of dehydration.

TABLE 9–1.   Albumin

Diagnostic Units: gm/dl (gm/L)
SI conversion factor = 10
Normal: 4.0–6.0 gm/dl (40–60 gm/L)

Albumin Decreased (gm/dl)	Diagnoses to Consider	Actions to Consider
<4.0	Decreased synthesis	1. Dietary history
	Liver insufficiency	2. Urinalysis
	Malnutrition	3. 24-hour urine
	Malignancy	protein
	Increased loss	4. Bilirubin
	Nephrotic syndrome	5. Creatinine
	Extensive burns	6. Hemoglobin
	Protein-losing	
	enteropathy	
	Pregnancy	
	Inflammatory illness	

Values in parentheses are SI units.

TABLE 9–2.   Alkaline Phosphatase (ALP)

Diagnostic units: units/L
Normal: Adults 30–120
Children 50–400
Pregnant women: 30–200

ALP Increased (units/L)	Diagnoses to Consider	Actions to Consider
120–200	Nonfasting patient specimen	1. Repeat test with patient fasting
	Drug effect	2. Review patient medications
>200	Increased from bone	1. Review patient medications
	Paget disease	2. Serum bilirubin, GGT, and aminotransferases
	Osteomalacia	
	Bony metastasis	
	Hyperparathyroidism	3. RUQ abdominal ultrasonography
	Increased from liver	4. Pelvis or femur radiography
	Bile duct stone	
	Biliary cancer	5. Serum calcium
	Pancreatic cancer	6. Bone scan
	Pancreatitis	
	Liver infiltration (sarcoid)	
	Primary biliary cirrhosis	
	Viral hepatitis	
	Severe cirrhosis	
	Other causes	
	Drug effect	
	Heart failure	
	Hyperthyroidism	
	Lymphoma	
	Leukemia	

GGT = γ-glutamyl transferase; RUQ = right upper quadrant.

ALKALINE PHOSPHATASE

Alkaline phosphatase (ALP) is a family of enzymes found in nearly all body tissues but with no known function (Table 9–2). In normal adults about half of the measured serum ALP is produced by the liver and about half by bone. Children and adolescents have ALP levels two to four times that of a normal adult due to the rapid bone growth in this age group. Women in the third trimester of pregnancy also have an elevated ALP, due to production of this enzyme by the placenta. This level returns to normal by 1 month post partum.

Liver diseases are usually divided into those that are primarily hepatic and those that are cholestatic. Elevation in aminotransferase is the usual laboratory marker for direct hepatocyte insult. ALP, on the other hand, is the usual marker for a cholestatic illness, which includes any process that causes an obstruction in the bile ducts (i.e., stone, cancer, pancreatitis, primary biliary cirrhosis). In these illnesses, the ALP and conjugated bilirubin levels are moderately to markedly elevated, whereas the aminotransferase levels are normal or only mildly elevated. With illnesses that are directly hepatotoxic (i.e., viral hepatitis) the aminotransferase and conjugated bilirubin are greatly elevated, whereas the ALP may be normal or only mildly elevated. Although alcohol ingestion is often cited as a cause for an elevated ALP, it is rarely the case unless there is advanced cirrhosis or severe alcoholic hepatitis.

The ALP level is elevated in disorders associated with osteoblastic activity (i.e., new bone formation). Paget's disease of bone is the prototypical illness. Ninety per cent of these patients have an elevated ALP even though most are asymptomatic. Osteoporosis and fractures do not commonly lead to elevated ALP levels.

A γ-glutamyltransferase test (GGT) is useful for differentiating between biliary and bony sources of an elevated ALP. The GGT is usually elevated when the ALP is derived from the liver.

The ALP is not a useful screening test in asymptomatic individuals. Values less than the reference range are of no clinical significance. Because more than 200 medications can cause an elevated ALP, a good first step in anyone with an unexplained ALP elevation is a thorough medication review.

AMINOTRANSFERASES

The aminotransferases (or transaminases) are enzymes primarily located within hepatocytes. Alanine aminotransferase (ALT) was formerly referred to as serum glutamate pyruvate transaminase (SGPT). Aspartate aminotransferase (AST) was formerly referred to as serum glutamic-oxaloacetic transaminase (SGOT). Increased levels of the two enzymes are due to liver injury and the subsequent leaking of the enzymes from cells. In general, the level of the aminotransferases reflects the severity of hepatic injury (Table 9–3).

ALT is fairly specific for the liver. In contrast, AST is increased after injury to cardiac or skeletal muscle as well. This fact is useful clinically because if both enzymes are elevated a hepatic source is likely. With most illnesses the ALT value is greater than the AST. The only common exception to this rule is in patients with alcoholic hepatitis, in whom the AST is higher.

AST and ALT testing are not useful for screening healthy individuals. They are, however, useful

TABLE 9–3.   Aminotransferases

Diagnostic units: units/L
Normal: 0–35

Increased (units/L)	Diagnoses to Consider	Actions to Consider

35–400	ALT and AST elevated
	  Infectious hepatitis
	  Toxic hepatitis
	  Alcoholic hepatitis
	  Shock liver
	  Biliary obstruction
	Only AST elevated
	  Myocardial infarction
	  Hemolysis (in vivo)
	  Pulmonary infarction
	  Muscular dystrophy
		1. Review patient medication
		2. Review foreign travel, needle sticks, chemical exposures, transfusion history
		3. Alcohol history
		4. Serum bilirubin, alkaline phosphatase
		5. Test for viral hepatitis
		6. Peripheral smear for hemolysis

ALT = alanine aminotransferase; AST = aspartate aminotransferase.

for diagnosing and monitoring all forms of liver disease. They are also frequently used as screening tests in patients on medications that can produce liver injury (i.e., isoniazid).

Aminotransferase values less than the lower normal limit are infrequently seen and are of little clinical significance. The exceptions are advanced cirrhosis and fulminant hepatitis, where a normal or low level can indicate that the disease has progressed so far that few hepatocytes remain.

AMYLASE (SERUM)

There are few diseases that are diagnosed as regularly, based on a single test, as is pancreatitis after finding an elevated amylase level (Table 9–4). With few exceptions, an elevated amylase concentration indicates pancreatitis, and a normal level rules out the diagnosis. In addition to pancreatitis, patients with abdominal pain and an elevated amylase level should be evaluated for a perforated peptic ulcer or mesenteric infarction.

Amylase is produced by the pancreas, salivary glands, and some tumors (e.g., lung). Most of the amylase produced by the pancreas goes directly into the gut. A small fraction is absorbed into the circulation. Normally, about one third of serum amylase is pancreatic in origin, and two thirds is from the salivary glands. The amylase in the circulation is

TABLE 9–4.   Amylase

Diagnostic units: Somogyi units/dl (Units/L)
Normal: 50–150 (0–130)

Amylase Increased	Diagnoses to Consider	Actions to Consider
>150 Somogyi units/dl	Pancreatitis Alcoholic Gallstone Trauma Hyperlipidemia Infectious Drug-induced Familial After ERCP Perforating ulcer Mesenteric infarction Salivary gland disease Chronic renal failure Amylase-secreting cancer	1. Alcohol history 2. Abdominal examination 3. Complete drug history 4. RUQ ultrasonography 5. Urinary amylase 6. Amylase/creatinine clearance 7. Lipase or amylase isoenzyme

Values in parentheses are SI units.
ERCP = endoscopic retrograde cholangiopancreatography; RUQ = right upper quadrant.

excreted primarily by the kidneys. Modest elevations in serum amylase (i.e., two times normal) can therefore be seen in patients with chronic renal failure.

The degree of amylase elevation does not always correlate with the severity of pancreatic injury. In fact, pancreatitis without an elevation in amylase is seen in about 10 per cent of patients, especially those with recurrent disease or with a long duration of symptoms before testing. In such cases, a serum lipase assay, urinary amylase assay, or amylase/creatinine clearance ratio may be helpful.

For unexplained hyperamylasemia, serum lipase or amylase isoenzyme assays may be useful. Lipase is produced by the pancreas but not by salivary glands.

Low serum amylase levels are rarely of clinical significance.

BILIRUBIN (TOTAL)

Bilirubin is formed from the heme ring as senescent red blood cells are degraded. It is transported in blood attached to albumin and then delivered to the liver, where it is conjugated and excreted in the bile. The common causes for hyperbilirubinemia are increased red blood cell destruction, liver diseases, and biliary tract obstruction.

Laboratories measure the total bilirubin and conjugated (i.e., direct) bilirubin (Table 9–5). The

unconjugated bilirubin fraction (i.e., indirect) is then obtained by subtraction. For normal serum, less than 15 per cent of the total bilirubin is in the conjugated fraction. The various causes for hyperbilirubinemia have traditionally been divided into those associated with unconjugated bilirubin and those associated with conjugated bilirubin. In practice, many diseases are of a mixed form (i.e., elevation in both conjugated and unconjugated bilirubin).

With hepatic diseases, the bilirubin level is usually proportional to the level of hepatocyte injury. Jaundice is detectable only when the total bilirubin level exceeds 3.0 mg/dl. Low serum bilirubin levels are of no clinical significance.

TABLE 9–5.   Bilirubin

Diagnostic units: mg/dl (μmol/L)
SI conversion factor = 17.1
Normal: 0.1–1.0 (2–17)

Bilirubin Increased (mg/dl)	Diagnoses to Consider	Actions to Consider
Newborns 1.0–10	Direct <15% of total Physiologic Breast feeding ABO incompatibility Rh incompatibility Hemorrhage Maternal diabetes Direct >15% of total Sepsis TORCH infections Hepatitis Biliary atresia	1. Mother and infant blood type 2. Direct Coombs test 3. Hematocrit
10–20	Kernicterus possible	Phototherapy or exchange transfusion (base decision on days of age, weight, maturity)
Adults >1.0	Hepatic insufficiency Biliary obstruction Hemolysis Postoperative complications	1. Alcohol history 2. Complete drug history 3. Travel, dietary, and needle stick history 4. Peripheral blood smear 5. Conjugated bilirubin, AST, ALP 6. Reticulocyte count 7. Viral hepatitis tests 8. Direct Coombs test 9. RUQ ultrasonography

Values in parentheses are SI units.
ALP = alkaline phosphatase; AST = aspartate aminotransferase (SGOT); RUQ = right upper quadrant.

BLOOD UREA NITROGEN

The blood urea nitrogen (BUN) assay is commonly used to measure renal function. The serum creatinine is, however, a much more reliable indicator of the glomerular filtration rate (GFR). It is more reliable because in addition to GFR the BUN is affected by the nitrogen load, water intake, and urine flow. If you want to know about the kidney, order a creatinine assay.

The normal BUN is 8 to 26 mg/dl (2.9 to 9.3 mmol/L). The SI conversion factor is 0.357 (Table 9–6).

A rise in BUN is seen with renal insufficiency, but it is not a specific indicator of renal function. A more useful method is to calculate the BUN/creatinine ratio. This ratio can serve as a useful indicator of diseases that result in abnormalities of nitrogen load, urine flow, or water intake.

CALCIUM

Calcium is essential for maintenance of the skeleton and for normal neuromuscular function. The usual serum test for calcium measures the total calcium (Table 9–7). About half of the total calcium is bound to albumin. The rest is present in serum in the ionized form. The measurement of ionized calcium can also be specifically ordered.

TABLE 9–6.   Blood Urea Nitrogen/Creatinine Ratio

Normal 10:1 (BUN/Cr)

Ratio	Diagnoses to Consider	Actions to Consider
Increased >10	High nitrogen load Gastrointestinal bleeding High-protein diet High catabolism Low urine flow Dehydration Congestive heart failure	1. Examine for hydration status 2. Examine for congestive heart failure 3. Dietary history 4. Drug history (steroids) 5. Stool occult blood
Decreased <10	High urine flow Water intoxication SIADH Low-protein diet Protein malnutrition Liver insufficiency	1. Check serum and urine osmolality 2. Check serum sodium 3. Dietary history 4. Bilirubin

SIADH = syndrome of inappropriate antidiuretic hormone.

TABLE 9–7.   Calcium

Diagnostic units: mg/dl (mmol/L)
SI conversion factor = 0.2495
Normal: 8.8–10.3 (2.20–2.57)

Calcium (mg/dl)	Diagnoses to Consider	Actions to Consider
Increased 10.3–13.0	Hyperparathyroidism Metastatic cancer Thiazide diuretics Immobilization Vitamin D intoxication Milk-alkali syndrome Multiple myeloma Sarcoidosis Thyrotoxicosis	1. Repeat serum calcium 2. Complete diet and drug history 3. Ionized calcium, albumin, phosphorus, PTH, T_4 4. Chest radiograph 5. Hand radiographs 6. Evaluation for malignancy
>13.0	Hypercalcemic coma	1. Vigorous hydration 2. Furosemide 3. Close monitoring
Decreased 7.0–8.8	Hypoalbuminemia Chronic renal failure Hypoparathyroidism (neck surgery) Malnutrition Vitamin D deficiency Nutritional Anticonvulsants Malabsorption Liver disease Hypomagnesemia Pancreatitis	1. Serum albumin 2. Complete drug history 3. Alcohol history 4. Serum creatinine, phosphate, magnesium, PTH
<7.0	Hypocalcemic seizures Hypocalcemic arrhythmias	1. IV calcium gluconate 2. Serum ionized calcium 3. Serum magnesium

Values in parentheses are SI units.
IV = intravenous; PTH = parathyroid hormone; T_4 = thyroxine.

The serum level of calcium is under the complex control of parathyroid hormone (PTH) and calcitonin. These hormones and others control the rate at which calcium is absorbed from the gastrointestinal tract, excreted in the urine, and gained or lost to bone.

The most common laboratory abnormality seen is a low total calcium level in a patient with low serum albumin. It is primarily a disorder of serum albumin, not a problem with calcium, as the ionized calcium remains unchanged. In this setting it is possible to correct mathematically the calcium for the decreased albumin (1 gm/dl reduction in albumin leads to 1 mg/dl reduction in calcium).

Hypercalcemia is associated with fatigue, depression, constipation, polydipsia, ulcers, and hypertension. In the outpatient setting, the most common cause of hypercalcemia is hyperparathyroidism. Many of these patients are asymptomatic. Malignancies are the most common cause of hypercalcemia in the inpatient setting. The most common cancers that produce hypercalcemia are in the lung, breast, or kidney.

Hypocalcemia produces symptoms that result from neuromuscular excitability: carpopedal spasm, seizures, tetany, stiffness, fatigue, memory loss, and confusion.

There is debate about whether serum calcium is an appropriate screening test for asymptomatic individuals. It has frequently been included in screening chemistry panels. The rationale for its use as a screening test has been that hyperparathyroidism is frequently asymptomatic. This argument has come into question because of the uncertainty of whether asymptomatic hyperparathyroidism requires any specific therapy.

CHLORIDE

Chloride is the major extracellular anion in the body. Despite this fact, it is a relatively uninteresting analyte and is rarely clinically useful.

Most dietary chloride is absorbed. The level in the body is then controlled by renal excretion (Table 9–8). The primary cause for an abnormal chloride is in response to a shift in the serum carbon dioxide (CO_2) content. The CO_2 content decreases when there is a metabolic acidosis or metabolic compensation for respiratory alkalosis. In these situations, the chloride increases in response to the reduction in CO_2 content. CO_2 content is increased in cases of metabolic alkalosis or in a metabolic response to respiratory acidosis. In these settings, the chloride is reduced to compensate for the increased CO_2 content.

Chloride can be depleted by either gastrointestinal losses (vomiting) or renal losses (salt-losing renal diseases). In these circumstances, chloride depletion results in a persistent metabolic alkalosis.

The most frequent use of the chloride test is for determining the anion gap, which is calculated by subtracting the total measured anions (chloride + bicarbonate) from the total cations (sodium + potassium). The normal range for the anion gap is 16 ± 4 mEq/L. Increases in the anion gap indicate the presence of unmeasured anions such as ketoacids, lactic acids, methanol, and so forth.

TABLE 9–8.   Chloride

Diagnostic units: mEq/L (mmol/L)
SI conversion factor = 1
Normal 95–105 (95–105)

Chloride (mEq/L)	Diagnoses to Consider	Actions to Consider

Increased >105	Metabolic acidosis
	  Loss of bicarbonate
	  (HCO_3^-)
	  Production of
	  metabolic acids
	Respiratory alkalosis
	  with metabolic
	  compensation
	Dehydration
		1. HCO_3^-, Na, K, pH,
		  BUN, Cl
		2. Calculate anion gap

Decreased <95	Metabolic alkalosis
	  Hydrogen ion loss
	  HCO_3^- retention
	Respiratory acidosis
	  with metabolic
	  compensation
	Salt-losing renal disease
	Thiazide diuretics
		1. Urinalysis
		2. HCO_3^-, Na, K, pH,
		  BUN, Cl

Values in parentheses are SI units.
BUN = blood urea nitrogen.

CHOLESTEROL

The National Institutes of Health (NIH) has established a National Cholesterol Education Program. One goal of this program is to have all adults screened for hypercholesterolemia. Although there is considerable debate about which cholesterol levels require treatment and the optimal approach to treatment, most people now agree that the screening of adults is probably indicated (Table 9–9). Epidemiologic studies have shown that a 1 per cent decrease in total cholesterol is associated with a 2 per cent decrease in coronary heart disease (CHD) risk.

Considerable variation is often seen in repeated cholesterol values from the same patient. This variation is due to test inaccuracy ($\pm$ 3 per cent), test imprecision ($\pm$ 3 per cent), and day-to-day patient variation ($\pm$ 7 per cent). In addition, cholesterol has been shown to demonstrate a seasonal variation. Although the studies have been limited, there does not appear to be a variation in total cholesterol based on whether the patient is fasting. (Fasting is, however, essential when measuring triglycerides and the cholesterol lipoprotein fractions.)

Cholesterol measurements should be used to

TABLE 9–9.   Cholesterol

Diagnostic units: mg/dl (mmol/L)
SI conversion factor = 0.02586
Normal: <200 (5.2)

Cholesterol Increased (mg/dl)	Diagnoses to Consider	Actions to Consider

200–239	Borderline risk for CHD
	Familial hypercholesterol-emia
	High cholesterol diet
	Biliary obstruction
	Nephrotic syndrome
	Hypothyroidism
		1. Repeat cholesterol test
		2. Evaluate for CAD risks
		  a. Male sex
		  b. Smoking
		  c. Family history of CHD
		  d. Hypertension
		  e. Diabetes mellitus
		  f. Severe obesity
		  g. History of vascular disease
		  h. HDL less than 35 mg/dl
		3. If patient has known CAD or two or more risk factors, order lipoprotein analysis

≥240	High risk for CHD
	As above
		1. Repeat cholesterol
		2. Fasting lipoprotein analysis
		3. Classify based on LDL
		  a. <130 = desirable
		  b. 130–159 = borderline risk
		  c. ≥160 = high risk

Cholesterol Decreased (mg/dl)	Diagnoses to Consider	Actions to Consider
<140	Low risk for CHD Hyperthyroidism Hepatic insufficiency	1. Dietary history 2. Bilirubin 3. T_4, T_3U

Values in parentheses are SI units.
CAD = coronary artery disease; CHD = coronary heart disease; HDL = high-density lipoprotein; LDL = low-density lipoprotein; T_3U = triiodothyronine uptake; T_4 = thyroxine.

diagnose hypercholesterolemia much as blood pressure readings are used to diagnose hypertension. Several readings over time are required before a diagnosis can be made.

If the total cholesterol indicates that the patient is at risk for hypercholesterolemia, the NIH recom-

mends that a fasting lipoprotein profile be done. The total cholesterol, high-density lipoprotein (HDL) cholesterol, and triglycerides should be measured. The low-density lipoprotein (LDL) cholesterol can then be calculated by the formula: LDL cholesterol = total cholesterol − HDL cholesterol − triglycerides ÷ 5.

If the LDL cholesterol is 130 to 160 mg/dl, the patient is considered at borderline high risk for CHD. If the LDL cholesterol is higher than 160 mg/dl, the patient is considered at high risk for CHD. LDL values less than 130 mg/dl are desirable.

The NIH recommends that the decision to treat be based on a patient's risk factors for CHD and the LDL value. Total cholesterol measurements should be used only for case finding and to follow the response to therapy (NIH, 1985).

CARBON DIOXIDE CONTENT

The CO_2 content of blood is made up of bicarbonate, carbonic acid, and dissolved CO_2. Ninety-five per cent of the total CO_2 content is bicarbonate (HCO_3^-). Bicarbonate is the second most important anion in serum and is the most available base that is capable of buffering a metabolic acid load. This role in the body's acid-base balance is its principal clinical function. The two mechanisms for control of CO_2 content are respiratory elimination of CO_2 and renal reabsorption of filtered bicarbonate. Bicarbonate can also be lost pathologically through elimination from the gastrointestinal tract (Table 9–10).

The most common CO_2 content abnormality is a decreased level due to metabolic acidosis. In this setting it is useful to calculate the anion gap, which may provide a clue to the cause of the acidosis.

Metabolic alkalosis may be initiated by the loss of hydrogen ion, as is seen with nasogastric suction. Maintenance of the metabolic alkalosis requires that there be greater than normal reabsorption of bicarbonate by the kidneys. Therefore in patients with an elevated CO_2 content, look for diseases that affect the bicarbonate handling by the renal tubules.

CREATININE

Creatinine is released from skeletal muscle and is excreted unchanged in the urine. There are few factors other than renal function that affect its level in serum. It is therefore the best of the common tests for monitoring renal insufficiency. A rise in creatinine indicates a falling glomerular filtration rate.

TABLE 9–10.   Carbon Dioxide (CO_2)

Diagnostic units: mEq/L (mmol/L)
SI conversion factor = 1
Normal: 22–28 (22–28)

CO_2 (mEq/L)	Diagnoses to Consider	Actions to Consider

Decreased <22	Metabolic acidosis
	  Bicarbonate loss
	    Diarrhea
	    Renal tubular acidosis
	    Primary
	      hyperparathyroidism
	  Failure to reabsorb
	  bicarbonate
	    Triamterene,
	      spironolactone
	    Renal tubular acidosis
	  Production of metabolic
	    acids
	    Renal failure
	    Diabetic ketoacidosis
	    Lactic acidosis
	    Methanol
	    Ethylene glycol
	    Salicylates
	    Alcoholic ketoacidosis
	  Respiratory alkalosis with
	  compensation
	    Anxiety
	    Sepsis
	    Salicylates
	    CNS injury
		1. Full drug history
		2. Serum
		   electrolytes
		3. Blood gas
		4. Calculate anion
		   gap

Increased >28	Metabolic alkalosis
	  Volume contraction
	  Nasogastric suction
	  Vomiting
	  Potassium depletion
	  Furosemide
	  Cushing syndrome
	Chronic respiratory acidosis
	  with compensation
		1. Serum
		   electrolytes
		2. Blood gas
		3. Urine
		   electrolytes

Values in parentheses are SI units.
CNS = central nervous system.

The biggest problem with using creatinine as a measure of renal function is that it is a relatively insensitive marker of renal disease. A 50 per cent reduction in renal function from normal leads to a creatinine rise of from only 1 to 2.0 mg/dl (Table 9–11). Considerable early renal damage may therefore occur before it becomes apparent by a rising creatinine level.

A second problem with interpreting serum creatinine is that it is slow in reacting to sudden changes in renal function. For example, with sudden and severe renal failure (i.e., acute tubular necrosis following shock), the creatinine rises only 1 mg/dl per day—despite a creatinine clearance of zero.

Because creatinine is released by skeletal muscle, it is occasionally affected by total muscle mass. Small, elderly women may therefore have a normal creatinine level even with reduced renal function.

A patient's creatinine clearance can be estimated from the formula:

$$\text{Cr clearance} = [(140 - \text{age})(\text{weight in kg})]/(72 \times \text{Cr in mg/dl})$$

As a rough guideline, a creatinine level of 2 mg/dl is equivalent to a creatinine clearance of 50 ml/minute; a creatinine level of 4 mg/dl is equal to a creatinine clearance of 20 ml/minute; and a creatinine level of 6 mg/dl is equivalent to a creatinine clearance of 10 ml/minute.

TABLE 9–11.   Creatinine

Diagnostic units: mg/dl (μmol/L)
SI conversion factor = 88.4
Normal: 0.6–1.2 (50–110)

Creatinine Increased (mg/dl)	Diagnoses to Consider	Actions to Consider
1.2–1.6	Mild renal impairment Muscle injury	1. Repeat test 2. Urinalysis 3. Creatinine clearance

>1.6	Prerenal cause
	  Dehydration
	  Blood loss
	  Heart failure
	  Liver failure
	Intrinsic renal failure
	  Diabetes mellitus
	  Hypertension
	  SLE
	  Nephrotoxins
	  Glomerulonephritis
	  Acute tubular
	    necrosis
	Postrenal failure
	  Urethral
	    obstruction
	  Upper tract
	    obstruction
		1. Urinalysis
		2. Creatinine clearance
		3. Bladder
		   catheterization
		4. Renal imaging

>6.0	Severe renal failure	1. HCO_3^- (metabolic
		   acidosis)
		2. Serum potassium
		   (hyperkalemia)

Values in parentheses are SI units.
SLE = systemic lupus erythematosus.

The serum creatinine assay is a useful screening test for patients at risk of renal injury (i.e., those with hypertension or diabetes). It is not useful in asymptomatic patients without significant risk factors because of the low prevalence of chronic renal failure in the general population and the low sensitivity of the test. A low serum creatinine level is of no clinical significance.

FERRITIN

Ferritin is a protein produced by the reticuloendothelial system. It serves as the chief iron storage protein in the body. In general, the ferritin level (Table 9–12) is proportional to the total body iron storage level.

The most common uses for this test are to differentiate iron deficiency anemia from the anemia of chronic disease in patients with normal or low mean corpuscular volume (MCV) values; determine a patient's response to iron therapy; or evaluate for iron overload states, particularly in patients with hemolytic anemia.

In iron deficiency states, ferritin often decreases before anemia, microcytosis, a low iron, or an ele-

vated total iron-binding capacity (TIBC) appears. Therefore it is considered the most sensitive test for detecting iron deficiency. The levels are quickly responsive to iron therapy: They return to normal within days of initiating oral iron treatment even though total body iron stores may take months of therapy to restore.

Ferritin is less sensitive as a marker of iron overload than it is of iron deficiency. Therefore if iron overload is suspected, iron and TIBC assays are the preferred tests.

GLUCOSE

Interpreting glucose values can be difficult. The usual reasons for ordering this test are to diagnose diabetes, follow the course of diabetic treatment, or diagnose hypoglycemia (Table 9–13).

Two common reasons for abnormally elevated glucose tests are that (1) the specimen was obtained after a patient had eaten; and (2) the specimen was obtained from a vein above an intravenous infusion.

There are two types of hypoglycemia. The first is postprandial hypoglycemia, also referred to as reactive hypoglycemia. It is most commonly seen in patients with a history of gastric surgery, who therefore have rapid stomach emptying times. Their symptoms (i.e., sweating, weakness, anxiety, irritability) occur several hours after eating.

Fasting hypoglycemia is seen primarily in diabetics and alcoholics. Their symptoms (i.e., mental confusion, bizarre behavior, seizures) are more gradual in onset and more persistent. This form of hypoglycemia usually occurs only after a long period of fasting.

Other disorders associated with hypoglycemia are insulinoma, adrenal insufficiency, hypopituitarism, and drug-induced hypoglycemia (insulin, sulfonylureas, and salicylates).

It is essential to remember that not all glucose specimens are the same. A random specimen taken 2 hours after lunch should not be treated the same way as a fasting specimen. In addition, there are differences among whole blood, serum, and plasma values. Venous plasma and venous serum glucose values are 15 per cent higher than those in venous whole blood. Capillary whole blood values are 10 per cent higher than those measured in venous whole blood. Venous plasma and venous serum values are 5 to 7 per cent higher than those found in capillary whole blood. (The values given in Table 9–13 are for venous plasma or venous serum. Specimens other than these should be adjusted accordingly.)

TABLE 9–12.   Ferritin

Diagnostic units: ng/mL (mg/L)
SI conversion factor = 1
Normal: Adult male 20–300
Adult female 20–120

Ferritin (ng/ml)	Diagnoses to Consider	Actions to Consider
Decreased <20	Iron deficiency Hypothyroidism	1. Evaluate for GI blood loss 2. CBC 3. Dietary history 4. TSH

Increased >300	Iron overload
	  Hemochromatosis
	  Transfusion
	  Hemolytic anemia
	Liver disease
	Chronic
	  inflammation
	Malignancies
	Hyperthyroidism
		1. Iron, TIBC
		2. CBC
		3. ESR
		4. T$_4$, T$_3$U, TSH
		5. Bilirubin, albumin, AST

GI = gastrointestinal; CBC = complete blood count; TSH = thyroid-stimulating hormone. TIBC = total iron-binding capacity; ESR = erythrocyte sedimentation rate; T$_4$ = thyroxine; T$_3$U = triiodothyronine uptake; AST = aspartate aminotransferase.

TABLE 9–13.   Venous Glucose

Diagnostic units: mg/dl (mmol/L)
SI conversion factor = 0.05551

Screening Test: Fasting Glucose

	Normal	*Requires GTT*	*Diagnostic of Diabetes*
Adult	<115 (6.38)	115–140 (6.38–7.77)	>140 (7.7) on 2 occasions
Child	<130 (7.22)	130–140 (7.22–7.77)	>140 (7.77) on 2 occasions

Confirmatory Tests: Glucose Tolerance Tests (GTT)

Adult: 75 gm oral glucose dose

	Normal	*Impaired Glucose Tolerance*	*Diabetes*
Fasting	<115 (6.38)	<140 (7.77)	>140 (7.77)
30 min	<200 (11.1)		
60 min	<200 (11.1)	} 1 of 3 >200 (11.1)	} 1 of 3 >200 (11.1)
90 min	<200 (11.1)		
120 min	<140 (7.77)	140–200 (7.77–11.1)	>200 (11.1)

Child: 1.75 gm glucose per kg body weight up to 75 gm

	Normal	*Impaired Glucose Tolerance*	*Diabetes*
Fasting	<130 (7.22)	<140 (7.77)	>140 (7.77)
30 min	<200 (11.1)	<200 (11.1)	
60 min	<200 (11.1)	<200 (11.1)	} 1 of 3 >200 (11.1)
90 min	<200 (11.1)	<200 (11.1)	
120 min	<140 (7.77)	140–200 (7.77–11.1)	>200 (11.1)

Pregnancy

Screening: O'Sullivan screen
  Glucose 50 gm (patient can be nonfasting)
  "Positive" if ≥140 (7.77) at 1 hr
Confirmation: O'Sullivan 3-hr GTT
  Oral glucose 100 gm in a fasting patient
  Patient is positive for gestational diabetes if two or more of the values are:
    Fasting: ≥105 (5.79)
    1 hr: ≥190 (10.55)
    2 hr: ≥165 (9.16)
    3 hr: ≥145 (8.05)

Hypoglycemia

Males: <55 (3.05) at the same time as symptoms present.
Females: <40 (2.22) at the same time symptoms present.

Values in parentheses are SI units.

Table 9–13 differentiates screening tests from diagnostic tests. The usual screening test is a fasting glucose. The results of this test may indicate that the patient is normal, suggest that a diagnostic test (i.e., a glucose tolerance test) be done, or may be diagnostic of diabetes. Note that there are specific screening and diagnostic tests for gestational diabetes (i.e., O'Sullivan test).

GLYCOSYLATED HEMOGLOBIN

The glycosylation of hemoglobin occurs continuously during the life of a red blood cell and is directly related to the average glucose concentration. The measurement of glycosylated hemoglobin (HbA$_{1c}$) has therefore become a useful clinical test to assess the "average" glucose control in diabetic patients (Table 9–14). Increased percentages of glycosylated hemoglobin reflect increased hyperglycemia. Once glycosylated, hemoglobin remains as such throughout the life of the red blood cell. The test value can therefore be viewed as a measure of diabetic control for the previous 1 to 3 months.

Hyperglycemia is also associated with the glycosylation of other body proteins. This glycosylation may be the basis for some of the angiopathic and

TABLE 9–14.   Glycosylated Hemoglobin

Diagnostic units: % of total hemoglobin
Normal: 5–7% (varies by laboratory)

Glycosylated Hemoglobin Increased	Diagnoses to Consider	Actions to Consider
<7%	Good diabetic control (most glucose <200 mg/dl)	No change in therapy
7–9%	Average diabetic control (most glucose <300 mg/dl)	Home glucose monitoring
>9%	Poor diabetic control (i.e., persistent hyperglycemia)	Evaluate for causes of poor diabetic control

neuropathic changes seen with diabetes. Some clinicians therefore use this test as an assessment of a patient's risk for diabetic complications.

The HbA_{1c} value does not change with rapid hour-to-hour or day-to-day variations in serum glucose. It is therefore not appropriate to use this test when making decisions about insulin dosage in either the acutely ill hospitalized patient or ambulatory diabetics on insulin. Home glucose monitoring is a better source of data for these decisions.

There is wide variation between laboratories for both the "normal" range of values and the degree of elevation associated with various levels of hyperglycemia. It is therefore important to know the characteristics of your laboratory's test. The HbA_{1c} per cent may be falsely elevated with uremia, alcoholism, and aspirin use. The test may be falsely lowered in patients with anemia, hemoglobinopathies, or pregnancy.

HEMOGLOBIN AND HEMATOCRIT

Hemoglobin and hematocrit values are often used interchangeably in clinical practice to measure the oxygen-carrying capacity of a volume of blood (Table 9–15). It is important to remember that they are not measures of either the total blood volume or the red blood cell (RBC) mass.

Most modern hematology instruments directly measure the hemoglobin and calculate the hematocrit from the measured RBC and mean corpuscular volume (MCV). The hematocrit can also be measured by centrifugation of a microcapillary tube filled with whole blood. When this test is done, the hematocrit is defined as the per cent volume of RBCs after maximal packing has occurred. For most purposes, the hematocrit (Hct) and hemoglobin

(Hb) are convertible by a factor of 3 (i.e., Hct = 3 × Hb).

It is reasonable to use the hemoglobin and hematocrit interchangeably except for patients with abnormally shaped RBCs (i.e., sickled cells). In such patients, the measured hematocrit is artificially high because the RBCs fail to maximally pack. In such individuals, a hemoglobin is a better test to follow.

There is little evidence that the general population benefits from routine hemoglobin or hematocrit screening. Screening, however, may be indicated in groups at high risk for anemia, such as infants, pregnant women, the institutionalized elderly, or menstruating females. It is also customary to screen individuals undergoing a procedure that could be associated with blood loss and all hospitalized patients on admission.

The most common abnormal finding is a mild, unsuspected anemia that is usually asymptomatic. The importance of the finding is not based on the need to treat the anemia but, rather, the need to uncover the cause of the anemia. The cause is frequently a clinically important diagnosis (i.e., poor nutrition, menorrhagia, pernicious anemia, colon cancer).

In addition to screening, the hemoglobin or hematocrit is an essential test for any patient in whom anemia is suspected, in whom there is abnormal bleeding, or in whom polycythemia is part of the differential diagnosis.

The most common error when interpreting a hemoglobin or hematocrit value is to rely on it as an indicator of acute blood loss. These tests are not good measures of total blood volume. About 12 to 24 hours are required after an acute bleeding episode before fluid equilibration can occur. It is only then that the hemoglobin or hematocrit can be used to indicate the extent of blood loss.

TABLE 9–15.   Hemoglobin

Diagnostic units: gm/dl (gm/L)
SI conversion factor = 10.0

Age	Males	Females
Birth	18.5–21.5 (185–215)	18.0–21.0 (180–210)
1 mo	15.5–18.5 (155–185)	15.8–18.9 (158–189)
3 mo	13.5–16.5 (135–165)	13.3–16.4 (133–164)
6 mo	13.0–16.0 (130–160)	12.8–14.8 (128–148)
9 mo	12.0–14.0 (120–140)	11.7–13.9 (117–139)
1 yr	10.0–14.0 (100–140)	10.0–14.0 (100–140)
2 yr	10.5–14.2 (105–142)	10.5–14.2 (105–142)
4 yr	11.2–14.3 (112–143)	11.3–14.2 (113–142)
8 yr	12.0–14.8 (120–148)	11.5–14.5 (115–145)
14 yr	12.5–15.0 (125–150)	11.6–14.8 (116–148)
Adult	13.9–16.3 (139–163)	12.0–15.0 (120–150)

	Diagnoses to Consider	Actions to Consider

Increased
>16.5 (165)
	Dehydration
	Diuretic use
	Polycythemia vera
	Secondary polycythemia
	  High altitude
	  Pulmonary disease
	  Cardiac disease
	  Renal tumor
		1. Smoking history
		2. Check volume status
		3. Splenomegaly
		4. Urinalysis
		5. CBC
		6. Platelet count
		7. Alkaline phosphatase

>22 (220)	Severe polycythemia	Consider phlebotomy
Decreased <11 (110)	Blood loss Decreased blood cell survival Decreased marrow production RBC sequestration (spleen)	1. History of chronic disease 2. Menstrual history 3. Stool for occult blood 4. Splenomegaly 5. RBC indices 6. Reticulocyte count 7. Trial on iron therapy 8. Iron, TIBC, ferritin 9. Folate, vitamin B_{12}
<8 (80)	Severe anemia	Consider transfusion

Values in parentheses are SI units.
RBC = red blood cells; CBC = complete blood count; TIBC = total iron-binding capacity.

HUMAN CHORIONIC GONADOTROPIN

Human chorionic gonadotropin (hCG), a glycoprotein secreted by placental trophoblastic tissues, is essential for support of the corpus luteum during early pregnancy. With sensitive tests, hCG can be found in maternal serum within 24 hours of implantation. The levels then rise rapidly and peak at 10 weeks' gestation (Table 9–16). For the remainder of the pregnancy, levels continue at approximately one tenth of the peak level.

Qualitative and quantitative hCG tests are available. The most common are qualitative tests to be used on urine specimens to diagnose pregnancy. The sensitivity and specificity of these tests have greatly improved since they were introduced during the 1970s. Most are now sensitive at a level of 20 mIU/L, which means that they can detect pregnancy by the time of the missed menses.

If a patient is suspected to be pregnant but the hCG test is negative, it is best to repeat the test in 2 days with a concentrated, first-morning urine specimen. A quantitative serum test is not indicated in these cases, as serum tests are not more sensitive than current urine tests. Urine pregnancy tests are helpful for patients suspected of having ectopic pregnancy. Ninety-nine percent of these patients have positive urine pregnancy tests.

Quantitative serum hCG tests are most commonly used to evaluate the viability of "at risk" pregnancies, for example, a pregnant woman with bleeding. The standard practice is to perform quan-

TABLE 9–16. Human Chorionic Gonadotropin (HCG)

Diagnostic units: mIU/L
Normal: Males: <10

Nonpregnant females: <10
Normal pregnancy:

Gestational week	
1	<30
2	50–500
3	100–10,000
10	50,000–300,000
Second trimester	10,000–25,000
Third trimester	5,000–15,000

hCG (mIU/L)	Diagnoses to Consider	Actions to Consider
Increased >10	Pregnancy Hydatidiform mole After abortion (up to 2 wk) Choriocarcinoma Ovarian cancer Testicular cancer	1. Correlate with ultrasound findings 2. Repeat hCG to document trend

titative hCG serum tests 2 days apart. On average, there should be a 66 per cent rise in hCG between the first and second values, although there is great variability in hCG doubling times in normal pregnancies, ranging from 1.4 to 5.0 days. Clinicians should therefore be conservative when telling a patient that a pregnancy is nonviable.

The hCG doubling times are most useful up to the sixth gestational week. By week 9, cardiac activity detected by ultrasonography can be used reliably to determine fetal viability. Unfortunately, many women have bleeding between gestational weeks 6 and 9. There is no definitive test to establish viability during this time.

If the increase in hCG between two consecutive specimens is greater than expected, multiple pregnancy or a hydatidiform mole should be considered.

MEAN CORPUSCULAR VOLUME

The mean corpuscular volume (MCV) is the most important of the red blood cell (RBC) indices. In modern hematology instruments, this value is derived by the degree of impedance disturbance as cells pass between two electrodes. The magnitude of the disturbance indicates the size of the cell.

The primary use of the MCV is to differentiate anemias into macrocytic, normocytic, or microcytic types (Table 9–17). This differentiation is useful in theory but is often not helpful in practice. Most anemic patients are normocytic at the time of their diagnosis.

Reticulocytes and other young RBCs are macrocytic. A rapid marrow release of RBCs therefore produces an increased MCV. This condition should not be confused with the other causes of macrocytosis.

It is important to remember that the MCV is an average of all of the cell populations. Mixed populations of macrocytic and microcytic cells may therefore produce a normocytic MCV. This situation is seen during the early treatment of iron deficiency anemia (i.e., macrocytic reticulocytes plus microcytic cells) and in alcoholic patients who are both iron and folate deficient.

TABLE 9–17. Mean Corpuscular Volume (MCV)

Diagnostic units: cubic micrometers (fL)
SI Conversion factor = 1
Normal: 76–100 fL

MCV (fL)	Diagnoses to Consider	Actions to Consider
Increased 100–120	Reticulocytosis Folate deficiency Vitamin B_{12} deficiency Hypothyroidism Response to chemotherapy	1. Reticulocyte count 2. Serum vitamin B_{12} 3. Serum or RBC folate 4. T_4
>120	Folate deficiency Vitamin B_{12} deficiency	1. Serum vitamin B_{12} 2. Serum or RBC folate
Decreased 70–76	Iron deficiency Thalassemia Anemia of chronic disease Hereditary sideroblastic anemia Lead poisoning RBC fragmentation (burns)	1. Reticulocyte count 2. Peripheral smear 3. Serum iron, TIBC, or ferritin 4. Hb electrophoresis
<70	Severe iron deficiency Thalassemia	1. Reticulocyte count 2. Peripheral smear 3. Serum iron, TIBC, or ferritin 4. Hb electrophoresis

Hb = hemoglobin; RBC = red blood cells; T_4 = thyroxine; TIBC = total iron-binding capacity.

PLATELET COUNT

The normal adult platelet count ranges from 140 $\times$ 10^9 to 400 $\times$ 10^9/L. Counts below 140 $\times$ 10^9/L indicate thrombocytopenia. Counts greater than 400 $\times$ 10^9/L indicate thrombocytosis (Table 9–18).

Platelet counts are routinely reported on specimens sent for complete blood counts because most modern cell counters do an automated platelet count as a part of their routine testing. Hence the most common platelet count abnormality is a small increase or decrease from normal in an otherwise asymptomatic individual. There is usually no benefit derived from further evaluating or even repeating the platelet count in these cases.

There is little justification for ordering screening platelet counts on asymptomatic outpatients or as a part of the admission testing on hospitalized patients. The one exception is the individual who is admitted for a major surgical procedure. The platelet count is, however, useful for evaluating patients with abnormal bleeding, bruising, purpura, petechiae, or splenomegaly.

Thrombocytopenia can be caused by a reduc-tion in the marrow's production of platelets (due to marrow suppression or infiltration), increased destruction of platelets, or sequestration of platelets in the spleen. A platelet count is also a useful indicator of marrow sensitivity to cytotoxic medications in the treatment of cancer.

It should be remembered that platelets may be adequate in number but defective in function. Medications are the most common cause of abnormal platelet function (i.e., aspirin, other nonsteroidal anti-inflammatory drugs, alcohol, and penicillins).

POTASSIUM

Potassium is the major cation in the intracellular fluid. Ninety-eight per cent of total body potassium is contained within the cells. The kidneys are responsible for regulation of the extracellular potassium. Hypokalemia and hyperkalemia are principally due to renal disorders, medications, or abnormalities in the intake of potassium.

It is not useful to test healthy outpatients for

TABLE 9–18.   Platelet Count

Diagnostic units: platelets $\times$ 10^9/L
Normal: First week of life: 84–478
After first week of life: 140–400

Platelets ($\times$ 10^9/L)	Diagnoses to Consider	Actions to Consider
Decreased		
100–140	Response to viral illness	Repeat test
	Response to bacterial illness	
50–100 (may have bleeding with major surgery)	Thrombocytopenia purpura	History of all medications
	After transfusion	Alcohol history
	Spleen sequestration	Examine for splenomegaly
	Marrow infiltration (i.e., leukemia)	CBC
	Response to cytotoxic drugs	Trial off all medications
		Bone marrow biopsy
20–50 (may have bleeding with minor procedure)	Thrombocytopenia	Platelet transfusion from any procedure
	Marrow infiltration	
	DIC	
<20 (may have spontaneous GI or CNS hemorrhage)	Severe thrombocytopenia	Platelet transfusion
Increased	Splenectomy	
400–600	Infection	
	Blood loss	
	Inflammatory bowel disease	
	Collagen vascular disease	
600–100	Malignancy	Evaluate for malignancy
	Polycythemia vera	
>1000 (may have spontaneous thrombosis)	Severe thrombocytosis	Administer antiplatelet drugs

CBC = complete blood count; CNS = central nervous system; DIC = disseminated intravascular coagulation; GI = gastrointestinal.

this electrolyte. However, the test is useful for patients with renal disease, those on diuretics, and patients who complain of weakness (Table 9–19). It is also customary to determine the serum potassium for all acutely ill hospitalized patients. Disorders of potassium are common in hospitalized patients because of the frequent use of intravenous infusions and nasogastric suction.

The most commonly seen potassium disorder is a mild hypokalemia in patients on a thiazide or loop diuretic. These patients are often asymptomatic, and it is unclear whether such patients benefit from treatment. Mild hypokalemia can also be associated with vague complaints such as weakness, muscle cramps, and paresthesias. Severe hypokalemia may cause arrhythmias, a paralytic ileus, or paralysis. All hypokalemic patients on digoxin require treatment because of the increased risk for digoxin toxicity with even mild hypokalemia.

The most common cause of hyperkalemia is hemolysis of red blood cells during blood collection or processing. In some cases, these specimens have red serum. If in doubt, retest the patient before undergoing a long work-up for hyperkalemia associated with disease.

Hyperkalemia is associated with patient com-

TABLE 9–19.   Potassium

Diagnostic units: mEq/L (mmol/L)
SI conversion factor = 1
Normal: 3.5–5.0 (3.5–5.0)

Potassium (mEq/L)	Diagnoses to Consider	Actions to Consider

Increased 5.0–7.5	Hemolyzed specimen
	Drugs
	  Potassium-sparing diuretics
	  NSAIDs
	  ACE inhibitors
	  Potassium supplementation
	Decreased renal excretion
	  Acute renal failure
	  Chronic renal failure
	  Addison disease
	Acidosis
	Tissue destruction
		1. Repeat K on new specimen
		2. Drug and diet history
		3. Check ECG for peaked T
		4. Creatinine
		5. Serum electrolytes
		6. Urine electrolytes

>7.5	Hyperkalemic arrhythmias Paralysis possible	1. ECG for peaked T, wide QRS, absent P 2. Calcium gluconate 3. Glucose/insulin infusion 4. Bicarbonate 5. Ion-exchange resins

Decreased 3.5–2.5	Renal loss
	  Thiazide or loop diuretics
	  Renal tubular acidosis
	  Hyperaldosteronism
	Gastrointestinal loss
	  Vomiting
	  Diarrhea
	Inadequate dietary potassium
	Inadequate IV potassium
	Insulin therapy
	Metabolic alkalosis
		1. Drug and diet history
		2. Serum electrolytes
		3. Urine electrolytes
		4. ECG for ST sagging, T depression, and U waves
		5. Monitor for digoxin toxicity
		6. Administer oral potassium

<2.5	Hypokalemic arrhythmias	1. Monitor closely for arrhythmias and paralysis 2. Administer IV and oral potassium

Values in parentheses are SI units.
ACE = angiotensin converting enzyme; ECG = electrocardiogram; IV = intravenous; NSAIDs = nonsteroidal anti-inflammatory drugs.

plaints of weakness or paralysis. Severe hyperkalemia (potassium level higher than 8 mEq/L) is associated with bradycardia, hypotension, ventricular fibrillation, and cardiac arrest.

When there is suspicion of a laboratory error, a rapid, useful maneuver is to do an electrocardiogram (ECG). Clinically significant hyperkalemia or hypokalemia is usually associated with the ECG findings indicated in Table 9–19.

PROSTATE-SPECIFIC ANTIGEN

The prostate-specific antigen (PSA) assay has received wide acclaim as a prostate cancer screening test for older men. Elevated PSA values lead to lucrative urologic evaluations, and PSA testing has therefore been made available for free by some hospitals and urology groups. At this time, there is no agreement that screening provides any patient benefit. Using this test as a screening test does detect more prostate cancer, but it is not clear that detection and treatment of these cancers is better than no detection at all.

The PSA is produced by normal, hyperplastic, and cancerous prostate tissue (Table 9–20). Low serum levels are found in all adult men. These levels increase with most prostate diseases, including benign prostatic hyperplasia (BPH). In patients with BPH, the PSA level usually remains less than 10 ng/ml and is proportional to the volume of prostate tissue as detected by ultrasonography.

The PSA level in patients with prostate cancer increases with increased staging (stages A through E) and increased tumor mass. Therefore PSA can be used to stage patients with prostate cancer, confirm response to therapy, and detect recurrence. PSA

TABLE 9–20. Prostate-Specific Antigen (PSA)

Diagnostic units: ng/ml (µg/L)
SI conversion factor = 1
Normal: 0–4

PSA (ng/mL)	Diagnoses to Consider	Actions to Consider
Increased >4.0	BPH Prostate manipulation Prostatitis Prostate infarction Urinary retention Prostate cancer	1. Repeat PSA in 2 wk 2. Rectal examination 3. Prostate ultrasonography 4. Prostate biopsy

BPH = benign prostatic hyperplasia.

TABLE 9–21. Protein

Diagnostic units: gm/dl (gm/L)
SI conversion factor = 10.0
Normal: 6–8 (60–80)

Protein (gm/L)	Diagnoses to Consider	Actions to Consider

Decreased <6	Decreased synthesis
	  Liver insufficiency
	  Malnutrition
	  Malignancy
	Increased loss
	  Nephrotic syndrome
	  Extensive burns
	  Protein-losing enteropathy
	Inflammatory illness
	Myeloma
	Overhydration
		1. Dietary history
		2. Urinalysis
		3. 21-hr urine protein
		4. Bilirubin
		5. Creatinine
		6. Protein electrophoresis

Increased >8	Dehydration Multiple myeloma Sarcoidosis Monoclonal gammopathy Chronic inflammation	1. Creatinine BUN 2. Protein electrophoresis 3. Chest radiograph

Values in parentheses are SI units.
BUN = blood urea nitrogen.

levels can rise a year before clinically detectable prostate cancer metastases.

The PSA levels increase twofold with prostate massage and up to 50-fold following a prostate biopsy. The serum half-life of the antigen is 2 days. Therefore it is best to wait 1 to 2 weeks after prostate manipulation to perform a PSA assay.

There is no lower normal limit for PSA, and low normal values have no clinical significance.

PROTEIN (TOTAL)

The total protein measured by the laboratory includes albumin plus the various globulins (Table 9–21). Fibrinogen, another blood protein, is not measured because it is depleted when serum clots in a blood collection tube.

Decreased levels of total protein are seen in a wide variety of illnesses. In most cases, these diseases are better followed by albumin determination because it is the albumin fraction that is usually reduced. A reduction in albumin is also a better guide to edematous states, as it is responsible for 90 per cent of the oncotic pressure.

Increased levels of total protein are occasionally seen and usually lead to an evaluation for multiple myeloma. In fact, myeloma can be associated with increased, normal, or decreased total protein levels.

When there is a question about the interpretation of any abnormal total protein, it is useful to perform a protein electrophoresis. This test separates the albumin from the various globulins. The electrophoretic pattern may be diagnostically helpful. Immunologic typing should be done for any electrophoretic "spike" to further test for multiple myeloma.

PROTHROMBIN TIME

The prothrombin time (PT) is the only coagulation test commonly used in the outpatient setting (Table 9–22). It is the time required to initiate clotting when tissue thromboplastin is mixed with blood. The PT is a measure of both the extrinsic clotting system (i.e., factor VII) and factors common to the intrinsic and extrinsic systems (i.e., factor X, factor V, prothrombin, and fibrinogen).

The PT is not considered a useful screening test for asymptomatic patients, even those undergoing a surgical procedure. It is most commonly used to monitor the anticoagulation effects of patients on warfarin (Coumadin). It is also a useful test for evaluating any patient with abnormal bleeding. It is important to note that the PT is normal in patients

with classic hemophilia (i.e., factor VIII deficiency) and those with von Willebrand disease.

There has been a great deal of confusion about PT testing. A broad range of values has been called "normal" by different laboratories. In addition, there has been disagreement about appropriate therapeutic PT levels in patients on warfarin.

Many of these problems are due to the fact that the test relies on thromboplastin reagents that vary considerably in their clotting activity. Those used today are less responsive than those that were used in the early studies on therapeutic anticoagulation, which has led to some clinicians unknowingly over-anticoagulating their patients.

Prothrombin time results may be reported in seconds, as a ratio compared with normal controls, or as an international normalization ratio (INR). The INR is standardized to the World Health Organization's reference thromboplastin. It is essential that the clinician know which of these reporting systems is being used to ensure adequate anticoagulation without risking unnecessary bleeding.

SODIUM

Sodium is the major cation in extracellular fluid. To interpret the sodium assay properly it is necessary to think about it as a measure not of total body sodium but of the total body water and the effective circulatory volume (Table 9–23). In normal situations the serum osmolality is used by the body to adjust the serum sodium. When the osmolality in-

TABLE 9–22.   Prothrombin Time

	Seconds	Patient/control ratio (Rabbit brain thromboplastin)	INR
Normal	11–13	0.9–1.1	0.8–1.3
Anticoagulation therapy			
Treatment of deep vein thrombosis	15–18.5	1.3–1.6	2.0–3.0
Treatment of pulmonary embolism	15–18.5	1.3–1.6	2.0–3.0
Prevention of embolism in atrial fibrillation or tissue heart valves	15–18.5	1.3–1.6	2.0–3.0
Prevention of embolism in patients with prosthetic heart valves	18.5–21.0	1.6–1.8	3.0–4.5
Prevention of embolism in patients with recurrent emboli	18.5–21.0	1.6–1.8	3.0–4.5

Prothrombin Time	Diagnoses to Consider	Actions to Consider
Increased	Liver disease	1. Liver enzymes, bilirubin
	Malabsorption	2. PTT
	DIC	3. Clotting factor assays
	Warfarin therapy	4. Serum carotene
	Factor II, V, VII, X deficiency	5. 72-hr stool fat
	Vitamin K deficiency	6. Administer vitamin K

DIC = disseminated intravascular coagulation; INR = international normalization ratio; PTT = partial thromboplastin time.

TABLE 9–23.   Sodium

Diagnostic units: mEq/L (mmol/L)
SI conversion factor = 1
Normal: 135–147 (135–147)

Sodium (mEq/L)	Diagnoses to Consider	Actions to Consider
Increased		
>147	Fluid loss in excess of salt	1. Clinical assessment of fluid status
	Sweating	2. Serum electrolytes
	Diarrhea	3. Serum BUN/creatinine
	Diabetes mellitus (osmotic diuresis)	4. Serum glucose
	Diabetes insipidus	5. Urine specific gravity
	Hyperaldosteronism	6. Give oral fluids
	Reduced fluid intake	
	Altered mental status (unable to drink)	
	Vomiting	
	Excessive salt intake	
	Infant formula	
	Hypertonic nasogastric feeding	
	Salt poisoning	
>160	CNS symptoms if an acute change	Slow hydration with isotonic saline (reduce serum sodium no faster than 10 mEq/L/day)
Decreased		
<135	Excess water:	1. Clinical assessment of fluid status
	Psychogenic polydipsia	2. Urine/serum osmolality
	Excessive IV hydration	3. Urine protein
	Decreased effective circulatory volume:	4. BUN, creatinine
	Diuretic therapy	5. Urine specific gravity
	Congestive heart failure	6. Serum albumin
	Cirrhosis	7. Serum eletrolyte
	Nephrotic syndrome	8. Water restriction
	Dehydration with free water access	
	Inability to excrete water	
	Renal failure (Cr Cl <15)	
	SIADH	
	Sodium depletion:	
	Gastrointestinal loss	
	Excessive sweating	
	Adrenal insufficiency	
	Pseudohyponatremia	
<120	CNS symptoms are likely due to brain swelling	Administer hypertonic saline (3%) until sodium is 125 mEq/L

Values in parentheses are SI units.
Cr Cl = creatinine clearance; CNS = central nervous system; BUN = blood urea nitrogen; SIADH = syndrome of inappropriate antidiuretic hormone.

creases, thirst increases; more water is then taken in, and antidiuretic hormone (ADH) is secreted, resulting in less free water being lost by the kidneys. When osmolality decreases, thirst is turned off and ADH secretion is suppressed. In situations in which the effective circulatory volume is reduced (i.e., heart failure), the body may sacrifice a normal osmolality in an effort to maintain the circulatory volume. In this setting, the sodium concentration decreases as fluid is retained in an effort to maintain the circulation.

A serum sodium assay cannot be properly interpreted without a physical examination of the patient's volume status. In hypovolemic states there is an orthostatic blood pressure drop, decreased skin turgor, dry mucous membranes, and weight loss. Hypovolemia may be associated with either normal, increased, or decreased serum sodium. To a large extent it depends on the patient's access to free water. Hypovolemia leads to thirst. If it results in drinking fluids that are low in sodium, hyponatremia follows.

Heart failure, cirrhosis, and nephrotic syndrome are frequent causes of hypervolemia (i.e., edematous states). In each case the total body water is increased, but the effective circulating volume is decreased. Therefore ADH is stimulated and free water is retained. This situation leads to hyponatremia.

Pseudohyponatremia is seen with hyperglycemia, severe hyperlipidemia, or hyperproteinemia. In these situations, the presence of other solutes in the serum results in artificially low serum sodium values (if measured by flame photometry).

Testing for serum sodium is not useful for routine screening of healthy individuals. However, it is useful in patients with heart failure, liver disease, chronic renal failure, and other edematous states. All acutely ill hospitalized patients should be tested, as serum sodium is often altered by intravenous therapy or nasogastric suction. In addition, patients on lithium therapy should have their sodium evaluated because this drug can lead to nephrogenic diabetes insipidus.

THYROID-STIMULATING HORMONE (THYROTROPIN)

Thyroid-stimulating hormone (TSH), a glycoprotein secreted by the anterior pituitary, is responsible for increasing triiodothyronine (T_3) and thyroxine (T_4) secretion by the thyroid gland. TSH testing (Table 9-24) is used to diagnose hypothyroidism and to monitor drug therapy in patients taking levothyroxine. The first generation of TSH tests was not sensitive in the low range. Second- and third-generation tests have been developed that are sensitive below 0.5 µIU/ml. These newer tests are also useful for diagnosing hyperthyroidism. In patients with hyperthyroidism, TSH is suppressed. The more sensitive TSH tests can be used to screen for thyroid disease without the need for T_4 and T_3 uptake testing.

Most patients with hypothyroidism have primary hypothyroidism, which is due to thyroid gland failure. In such patients the TSH is elevated. A small number of hypothyroid patients have secondary (pituitary) or tertiary (hypothalamic) hypothyroidism. In this small group of patients, the TSH is low or normal.

The TSH assay is the most useful test for monitoring levothyroxine therapy. In general, patients can be considered euthyroid when the TSH level falls to normal. It is unnecessary to use other thyroid tests (i.e., T_4 assay) to regulate therapy. It is important to remember that it is best to treat the patient, not the test. Therefore even when using the TSH assay to determine levothyroxine dosage, evaluate the patient symptomatically.

Some hypothyroid patients have extremely high TSH values (100 µIU/ml). There is no direct correlation between the level of TSH and the severity of hypothyroidism. Patients with a TSH of 50 µIU/ml are not twice as hypothyroid as those with a TSH of 25 µIU/ml, whereas patients with a TSH of 10 µIU/ml can be profoundly symptomatic.

THYROXINE

Thyroxine (T_4) is the principal hormone secreted by the thyroid gland. It is almost completely bound to proteins in the circulation. Most of the binding is to thyroxine-binding globulin (TBG), but a small amount is also bound to albumin. The active form of the hormone is free thyroxine (i.e., thyroxine not bound to protein). Thyroxine is used in the body to regulate tissue metabolism.

The most common screening thyroid test is the serum thyroxine assay. Unfortunately, this test measures total thyroxine rather than just the active hormone (i.e., free T_4). Many of the abnormal results are therefore due to abnormal levels of thyroid-binding globulin instead of the active hormone.

The free T_4 level can be approximated by ordering a T_3 uptake test and calculating the free T_4 index (Table 9-25). This index approximates the free T_4. If it is increased, it suggests hyperthyroidism. If it is decreased, it suggests hypothyroidism.

When using the T_4 or the T_4 index as screening tests, there frequently remain cases in which the diagnosis is uncertain. If there is concern about hypothyroidism, a thyroid-stimulating hormone (TSH) test is usually helpful. If there is concern about hyperthyroidism, a free T_3 or sensitive TSH test is useful.

Tests for TBG and free T_4 are available but are rarely used diagnostically. In difficult cases, the response to thyrotropin-releasing hormone (TRH) can be used to sort out both hyperthyroid and hypothyroid diagnoses.

WHITE BLOOD CELL COUNT

Changes in the white blood cell (WBC) count are seen with many infectious, hematologic, inflamma-

TABLE 9–24.   Thyroid-Stimulating Hormone (TSH)

Diagnostic units: μIU/ml (mU/L)
SI conversion factor = 1
Normal: 0.4–6.0 μIU/ml (mU/l) (There may be slight differences in the normal range between laboratories, based on variations in test methods.)

TSH (μIU/mL)	Diagnoses to Consider	Actions to Consider
Increased >6.0	Primary hypothyroidism (i.e., thyroid gland failure) Thyroiditis Inadequate levothyroxine therapy	1. Drug compliance history 2. Physical examination 3. T_4, T_3 uptake 4. TRH stimulation test
Decreased <0.5	Hyperthyroidism Excessive levothyroxine intake Secondary hypothyroidism (i.e., pituitary failure) Tertiary hypothyroidism (i.e., hypothalamic failure)	1. Thyroid examination 2. Drug history 3. T_4, T_3U 4. TRH stimulation test

T_3U = triiodothyronine uptake; T_4 = thyroxine; TRH = thyrotropin-releasing hormone.

tory, and neoplastic diseases. This variety of diseases makes the WBC count a nonspecific test. It can, however, be a sensitive indicator of disease in some clinical situations. Its degree of increase or decrease

TABLE 9–25.   Thyroxine (T_4)

Diagnostic units: μg/dl (nmol/L)
SI conversion factor = 13.0
Normal: 5.5–12.5 (72–163)

	Diagnoses to Consider	Actions to Consider

Increased
>12.5
	Hyperthyroidism
	Elevated TBG
	  Birth control pills
	  Pregnancy
	  Estrogens
	Liver disease
	Drugs
	  Propranolol
	  Amphetamines
	  Contrast media
	  Amiodarone
	  Heparin
		1. Complete drug
		  history
		2. T_4 index
		3. Sensitive TSH
		4. Free T_3
		5. Thyroid uptake scan

Decreased
<5.5
	Hypothyroidism
	Decreased TBG
	  Malnutrition
	  Liver diseases
	  Nephrotic syndrome
	  Androgens
	  Glucocorticoids
	  Sick thyroid syndrome
		1. T_4 index
		2. TSH
		3. Albumin
		4. Urinary protein

Values in parentheses are SI units.
    T_3 = triiodothyronine; T_4 = thyroxine; TBG = thyroxine-binding globulin; TSH = thyroid-stimulating hormone.

often correlates with the severity of the disease process. Monitoring changes in the WBC count over time can therefore provide useful information about the course of an illness (Table 9–26).

Five types of WBCs are commonly counted in the WBC differential: neutrophils, lymphocytes, monocytes, eosinophils, and basophils. Changes in the relative percentages of these cells are recognized as useful patterns in many common illnesses (i.e., leukocytosis and a shift to the left in bacterial diseases).

Leukopenia, which usually indicates neutropenia, is defined as less than 2×10^9 neutrophils per liter in whites or 1.5×10^9/L in African Americans. In patients receiving chemotherapy, neutropenia of less than 0.5×10^9/L is often associated with severe infections. In patients with congenital neutropenia, at the same reduced neutrophil level there is usually no infection. This finding indicates that the patients have both a quantitative and a qualitative neutrophil defect.

Lymphopenia is defined as less than 1.5×10^9 lymphocytes per liter. It is frequently seen in association with a wide variety of physiologic stresses and is of no clinical significance. Reductions in monocytes, eosinophils, and basophils are occasionally seen and are not clinically useful.

An increased WBC count can be seen with a wide variety of diseases. The average WBC count tends to be higher in children than adults (see Table 9–26). Most elevated WBC counts are below 30,000 cells/mm³. Counts greater than 30,000/mm³ are usually due to leukemia or a leukemoid reaction. It is obviously important to differentiate between these two diagnoses.

TABLE 9–26.   White Blood Cell (WBC) Count

Diagnostic units: cells/mm³ (cells × 10⁹/L)
SI conversion factor = 0.001

	Age	Average	95% Range
Normal:	Birth	18,000	9,000–30,000
	12 hr	22,800	13,000–38,000
	24 hr	18,900	9,400–34,000
	1 wk	12,200	5,000–21,000
	2 mo	11,000	5,500–18,000
	1 yr	11,400	6,000–17,500
	2 yr	10,600	6,000–17,000
	6 yr	8,500	5,000–14,500
	10 yr	8,100	4,500–13,500
	20 yr	7,500	4,500–11,500
	Adult	6,500	3,200–9,800

	Diagnoses to Consider	**Actions to Consider**
Decreased 500–3200	Infections 　Severe bacterial infection 　Influenza 　Infectious mononucleosis 　Typhoid fever Drugs 　Cytotoxic 　Idiosyncratic Congestive splenomegaly Felty syndrome SLE Megaloblastic anemia Aplastic anemia Congenital neutropenia	1. Complete drug history 2. Peripheral smear 3. Platelet count 4. CBC 5. Mononucleosis test 6. ANA 7. Folate, vitamin B₁₂ levels 8. Bone marrow biopsy
<500	At risk for severe bacterial 　infections	1. Frequent examinations 2. Antibiotics for fever
Increased 9800–30,000	Physiologic reaction to stress Infection Tissue destruction Leukemia Cancer Hemorrhage Splenectomy	1. Symptom-directed physical examination 2. Peripheral smear
>30,000	Leukemia Leukemoid reaction	1. Peripheral smear 2. Examine for hepatomegaly and splenomegaly

Values in parentheses are SI units.
ANA = antinuclear antibody; CBC = complete blood count; SLE = systemic lupus erythematosus.

REFERENCES

Boyko EJ, Alderman BW, Barron AE. Reference test errors bias the evaluation of diagnostic tests for ischemic heart disease. J Gen Intern Med 1988;3:476.

DeNeef P. Evaluating rapid tests for streptococcal pharyngitis: the apparent accuracy of a diagnostic test when there are errors in the standard of comparison. Medical Decision Making 1987a;7:92.

DeNeef P. Selective testing for streptococcal pharyngitis in adults. J Fam Pract 1987b;25:347.

Gerber MA, Randolph MF, Mayo DR. The group A streptococcal carrier state: a reexamination. Am J Dis Child 1988;142:562.

Heckerling PS. Confidence in diagnostic testing. J Gen Intern Med 1988;3:604.

Lundberg GD. Using the Clinical Laboratory in Medical Decision Making. Chicago, American Society of Clinical Pathologists Press, 1983.

National Institutes of Health. Lowering blood cholesterol to prevent heart disease (consensus conference). JAMA 1985;253:2080.

Ransohoff DF, Feinstein AR. Problems of spectrum and bias in evaluating the efficacy of diagnostic tests. N Engl J Med 1978;299:926.

Sox HJ (ed). Common Diagnostic Tests, Use and Interpretation. Philadelphia, American College of Physicians, 1987.

Statland BE. Clinical Decision Levels for Lab Tests. Oradell, NJ, Medical Economics Books, 1987.

QUESTIONS

1. To differentiate between a bone or biliary source for an elevated alkaline phosphatase, the most useful test is:
   a. GGT
   b. Bone scan
   c. Hand x-ray studies
   d. Serum calcium
   e. Gallbladder ultrasound

2. If an otherwise healthy patient is found in routine testing to have a serum calcium of 12.2 mg/dl, the most common cause for this hypercalcemia is:
   a. Hyperparathyroidism
   b. Antacid abuse
   c. Lung cancer
   d. Vitamin D intake

3. The most sensitive test to identify iron deficiency is:
   a. Red cell MCV
   b. Hemoglobin
   c. Ferritin
   d. Serum iron
   e. Total iron-binding capacity

4. A man presents in your office with a 2-week history of epigastric pain and a 1-hour history of vomiting blood. His blood pressure is 105/72 and his pulse is 114. A stat hemoglobin is 14.1. Which of the following statements is most likely true?
   a. Since the hemoglobin is normal, the patient's elevated pulse is most likely due to anxiety.
   b. Of the information provided, the hemoglobin is the most useful indicator of intravascular volume.
   c. The patient is probably a smoker and had an increased hemoglobin before the gastrointestinal bleeding.
   d. Because of timing, the hemoglobin is an unreliable measure of the patient's overall condition.

5. In the average primary care population, the most common cause for a potassium of 6.3 mEq/L (normal 3.5 to 5.0 mEq/L) is:
   a. Excessive potassium supplementation
   b. Renal failure
   c. Addison disease
   d. Specimen hemolysis
   e. Acidosis

6. The most useful screening test in a patient complaining of fatigue, weight gain, and cold intolerance is:
   a. T_4
   b. T_3 uptake
   c. TSH
   d. Free T_3

Answers appear on **page 603**.

Chapter 10

Selecting Radiographic Tests

David P. Losh, M.D.

With the advent of sophisticated new equipment and computer technology, there have been remarkable advances in medical imaging. Computed tomography, magnetic resonance imaging, ultrasound, and sophisticated nuclear medicine studies have revolutionized the type and quality of information that can be obtained from medical imaging. The technology has provided the family physician with new choices for diagnostic imaging, some of which may be expensive or available only in larger centers. At the same time, physicians have been increasingly faced with the realities of practicing cost-effective medicine. It is therefore important for the family physician to effectively judge the cost:benefit ratio of a particular test and to select the most focused and effective imaging strategy for a particular clinical problem. Because the field of diagnostic imaging has become so technical, and has so many new and expensive techniques, the family physician is encouraged to regularly discuss cases and diagnostic dilemmas with the consulting radiologists. This chapter will provide background information on the most commonly available imaging studies and provide an imaging strategy for some common diagnostic problems encountered in family medicine.

BASIC TESTS AVAILABLE TO THE CLINICIAN

Standard Radiographic X-Rays and Contrast Material

Traditional x-rays are produced by an electric tube that generates electrons from a heated filament and accelerates them toward a rotating anode. The x-rays generated by this process are passed through the body and are partially absorbed by various densities of tissue. The x-rays remaining after passing through the body are recorded by a detector such as an x-ray film, a fluoroscope, or an analog-to-digital converter. Variations in the type of x-ray tubes and film allow for different types of images, such as mammograms. Tomograms are an application of standard x-rays in which the x-ray source and the detector are rotated to blur tissue above and below the desired level of examination. Standard x-rays have the advantage of being relatively inexpensive as well as portable for some applications at the bedside. The cost of standard x-rays varies according to the study. Examinations such as an upper gastrointestinal series, a barium enema, or an intravenous pyelogram cost about 2.5 to 3 times more than a standard chest x-ray. Standard x-rays are limited in their ability to detect small differences in tissue density and are often limited by the superimposition of other structures.

The Selection of Contrast Material

When ordering imaging studies, the family physician will be required to weigh the value of an examination requiring contrast and may need to decide what type of contrast material to recommend. High-osmolarity, ionic contrast medium is a water-soluble intravenous material containing iodine. It is frequently used in imaging of the urinary tract and in angiography. Contrast material is also used in enhanced CT applications, such as examinations of the head, chest, and liver. When used with CT, the contrast material is helpful in determining increased or decreased vascularity of an area, or in indicating a break in the blood-brain barrier. When receiving ionic contrast material, it is common for patients to feel a sense of heat, nausea, or flushing, and hives are not uncommon. Although fatal reactions occur in less than 1 in 100,000 doses, serious adverse reactions such as anaphylaxis, cardiovascular collapse, laryngospasm, and bronchospasm occur in about 1 in 500 to 1000 doses. The cause of the adverse reactions is unknown, but they may be related to the high osmolarity of the solution or may be true anaphylactic reactions. In addition, traditional contrast material must be used with great caution in patients with pre-existing renal disease, since it can cause potentially irreversible kidney failure in these individuals. Many of the adverse reactions may be avoided by the use of low osmolarity, non-ionic contrast materials. However, these newer agents are expensive and in some cases may double the cost of a procedure. Various approaches have been advocated to deal with potential adverse reactions to contrast material.

Prophylactic medication has provided good protection from anaphylaxis where there is a concern over the possibility of an allergic reaction to ionic contrast material. The following prophylactic regimen may be used: 50 mg prednisone orally 13, 7, and 1 hour(s) before the study, and 50 mg diphenhydramine 1 hour before the study. This regimen does not, however, protect against toxicity such as kidney damage. The American College of Radiology recommends the use of non-ionic contrast material in patients with a history of a previous adverse reaction to contrast material, a history of asthma or allergy, known cardiac dysfunction, generalized debilitation, or upon recommendation by the radiologist. In addition, others have recommended that the following additional patients be considered for non-ionic contrast material: children under age 2; patients with sickle cell disease; patients with renal failure (serum creatinine >2.5); patients with major trauma, including hypotension, shock, neurotrauma, or spinal precautions; and patients requiring angiography.

Computed Tomography

In computed tomography (CT) the x-ray beams are aimed through the patient from many different angles. Instead of striking film, the x-rays are detected by radiation detectors and the results are recorded as digital information in a computer. The computer is then able to produce images that may be manipulated and recorded on film. Standard CT images are axial cross sections through the body. For most studies, axial images are generated every 10 cm throughout the body. However, for some specialized studies, images may be obtained every 1 to 3 mm. The main advantage of CT scans is their ability to obtain cross-sectional images through the body without the superimposition of other structures. They are also able to detect much smaller differences in tissue density than are standard x-rays. Although CT scans offer much more detail, because of the complexity of the examination and the cost of the equipment, CT scans are more expensive than standard x-rays, and they are not portable. CT scans are generally in the cost range of 7 to 10 times the cost of a standard chest x-ray.

CT scans may be obtained with or without contrast. Ultrafast and spiral or helical CTs have recently been introduced. These new machines continuously scan as the patient is moved through them. They can obtain images in less than 1 second, and they allow for visualization of the vascular system without catheterization when intravenous contrast material is injected. They also allow an unlimited number of scans that may be used to create three-dimensional images, and they have eliminated the blur from breathing that is associated with standard machines.

Magnetic Resonance Imaging

Magnetic resonance imaging (MR or MRI) produces images by subjecting the body to a very strong magnetic field. Then, by exposing the body to pulses of radio-frequency energy, the MR computer is able to create a picture that can be obtained in any plane. The MR essentially images the distribution of hydrogen atoms and the surrounding molecular structure in the body. Since the magnetic field of an MR scanner is so strong, it will interfere with traditional pacemakers and defibrillators, and such devices are absolute contraindications to MR scans. Patients with any ferrous metal in their body should not receive MR scans. These include individuals with surgical clips, such as cerebral aneurysm clips. Although MR is expensive, it is particularly useful in evaluating the central nervous system (CNS) for masses and other abnormalities of the brain, spinal cord, and nerve roots. MR is also useful for evaluating the musculoskeletal system, including the joints and the spine, and is being used to evaluate the pelvis, retroperitoneum, mediastinum, and large vessels. The cost of an MR study may be in the range of 8 to 12 times the cost of a standard chest x-ray.

MR angiography (MRA) is a recently introduced technique of studying the blood vessels without the need for intravenous contrast. It is thought that this technique may eventually replace various types of traditional angiography.

Most MR machines are designed as a long tube that is open at both ends. The scans take several minutes to complete and require the patient to remain motionless. Although newer "open MR" design machines are now available, patients prone to claustrophobia may have problems with traditional MR machines. Recently introduced echo planar machines have reduced the imaging time to less than 1 second, thus reducing the problems with movement from breathing and allowing for imaging of the heart, lungs, and abdomen.

Ultrasound

Ultrasound (US) creates images by the use of a hand-held transducer that generates high-frequency sound waves. When the transducer is passed over a thin layer of gel on the surface of the body, it captures the returning sound waves, or "echoes," that bounce off the structures being imaged. The returned waves are then transformed into a picture by a computer.

Since US delivers no ionizing radiation, it is thought to be comparatively safe; it has been widely used in applications related to pregnancy, such as imaging of the fetus and uterine structures. However, US has limitations, especially since it cannot penetrate bone and gas. Bowel gas can interfere with the examination, and the technique cannot be used to image structures in the lung or brain. Many applications may be done at the bedside.

US has been found to be particularly useful in evaluation of structures such as the heart and the gallbladder. Doppler US is a technique used to assess organ perfusion and blood flow. It is particularly useful in cardiac applications and in identifying ischemic lesions such as testicular torsion. The cost of an ultrasound examination is in the range of three times that of a standard chest x-ray, although some examinations, such as echocardiography, may cost nearly twice that.

Nuclear Imaging

Nuclear imaging results from gamma rays emitted from isotopes that are administered to the patient, most often by the oral or intravenous route. The isotopes, such as technetium-99, are bound to different chemicals that determine the biodistribution of the compound. The gamma rays are then counted and turned into a picture by a gamma camera and computer. Nuclear imaging is particularly useful in making a functional assessment of certain organs or tissues. Applications that assess the function of the thyroid, lung, gallbladder, kidneys, and skeleton are particularly common. However, the detail of structures is less defined than with other techniques. Most nuclear imaging techniques deliver less radiation to the patient than do standard x-ray techniques. The cost of most nuclear imaging studies is in the range of 3 to 4 times that of a standard chest x-ray.

Single photon emission computed tomography (SPECT), a newer nuclear imaging technique, uses radionucleotides and generates thin-section views, much like a CT scan. This technique has increased the resolution and sensitivity of the examination but is nearly double the cost of standard nuclear imaging. Positron emission tomography (PET), another new technique for studying metabolic processes, generates thin-slice views showing the utilization of such substances as nitrogen, oxygen, and carbon. Because the radionucleotides are cyclotron-produced and are short-lived, PET is extremely expensive and available only at a relatively few large centers.

Selected Diagnostic Strategies for Common Clinical Problems

In this section, diagnostic imaging strategies are suggested in a numbered, stepwise fashion. Alternative choices are given in cases in which particular tests may not be widely available or are particularly expensive. It should be understood that as the costs of certain procedures change and certain studies become more widely available, these recommended approaches will change as well. In some cases a more expensive test is recommended first, because the test is so sensitive or specific that it may save the added expense of doing less focused tests first. Because of the limited scope of this discussion, only selected problems that either represent diagnostic controversy or that are thought to be most common in family medicine are addressed. The sources in *Suggested Reading* are highly recommended to the reader for other disease entities or symptom complexes. Table 10–1 gives an approximate comparison of the costs of various imaging studies and procedures.

Neurologic System

With a few exceptions, as noted below, MR and CT are the most useful examinations to study the CNS.

TABLE 10–1. Approximate Costs of Diagnostic Imaging and Procedures

Procedure	Approximate Relative Cost ($)*
CT	
Head	287
Chest	429
Abdomen	840
Pancreas	433
Spine	471
MR	750–1500
Head	845
Chest	1250–1350
Abdomen	1200–1400
Spine	1300–1475
Angiography, Cerebral	3000
ERCP	820
US	
Thyroid	350–400
Abdomen	300–350
Gallbladder	200
Renal	250–350
Nuclear Scan, Thyroid	350–700
HIDA	450–550
Cardiac Nuclear Scan	
(Thallium scan)	550–1250
V/Q Scan	
Ventilation	400–500
Perfusion	400–500
Liver/Spleen Scan	550–750
MUGA	500–1200
Chest X-Ray	135–150
Mammography	100–150
Plain X-Ray, Abdomen	150–200
Upper GI Series	300–425
Enteroclysis	500–575
Barium Enema	350–475
IVP	375–400

*Estimated ambulatory charge based on data in Grossman et al. Cost Effective Diagnostic Imaging. St. Louis, CV Mosby 1994, based on outpatient Physician Fees 1994, Practice Management Corp., Los Angeles, 1994. Charges may be significantly higher in some inpatient settings and may vary considerably from one institution to another.

EMERGENCIES. For head trauma and suspected subarachnoid hemorrhage, CT without contrast is performed first; MR is done if follow-up is required when symptoms remain unexplained. MR is inappropriate for the first-line examination in head trauma but may be useful in subacute or chronic conditions or in brain stem contusions.

STROKE. (1) CT can often differentiate between hemorrhagic and ischemic strokes, especially after 24 hours, and can exclude several problems that may act like a stroke, such as tumors or abscesses. (2) MR may be useful if CT does not explain the clinical findings or when a posterior fossa infarction is suspected. (3) Angiography may be considered when surgery is being considered for carotid or vertebral artery disease or when other vascular abnormalities are noted on CT or MR.

BACK PAIN AND SUSPECTED LUMBOSACRAL DISK HERNIATION AND NERVE ROOT COMPRESSION. The vast majority of patients with back pain respond to conservative therapy and do not require radiologic imaging.

Plain Lumbosacral Spine Films. Plain radiographs of the spine have low sensitivity and specificity but may be a rational starting point to rule out such abnormalities as fracture or metastases. They also can provide a correlation with further studies when they are needed.

CT Without Contrast or MR. These modalities may be used when disk herniation and nerve root compression are suspected. Controversy exists over whether CT or MR is the study of choice for suspected disk herniation and nerve compression. MR is preferred by many because of its ability to obtain views in multiple planes and because it shows excellent anatomic detail and avoids ionizing radiation. CT is also useful for detecting a herniated disk, but it is somewhat more limited for certain views by its one-plane image. However, large studies have not shown a significant difference in the diagnostic accuracy of these two studies for this application, and some advocate CT because of its cost advantage. CT is the study of choice for suspected spinal stenosis, degenerative disease of the facets, and spondylolysis in adults. Nuclear bone scans with SPECT are now being used in children suspected of spondylolysis because of its lower dose of radiation and its relatively high specificity in children.

HEADACHE. The majority of headaches presenting to the family physician may be diagnosed with reasonable accuracy by a careful history and physical examination. A CT with contrast should be considered when focal disease is suspected, when the pattern of the headaches changes significantly, or if other screening tests suggest the presence of an abnormality. Concerns for focal disease include aphasia, memory impairment, and focal sensory deficits.

SPINAL INJURIES. Plain x-rays are the first radiographic study. In most cases, a plain lateral film should be taken first. If no fracture is seen, further plain film studies (oblique, AP, open-mouth views) are obtained. If fracture is suspected but not definite, CT may be obtained, since it is particularly useful in evaluating for fracture. If plain views reveal no fracture and there is focal pain, flexion and extension views may be considered, or a CT may be done to clarify the diagnosis. If there is no focal pain, yet suspicions remain regarding cord trauma, then MR should be considered as step two.

CEREBRAL METASTASES. MR is the first choice. If MR is not routinely available, CT with contrast should be performed.

Cardiovascular System and Respiratory System

ANGINA PECTORIS AND SUSPECTED CORONARY ARTERY DISEASE. In a nonemergency situation, a resting ECG should be obtained as the first step. If the resting ECG does not show abnormalities that preclude valid exercise stress testing (left bundle branch block or ST segment changes), one should consider exercise stress testing. Controversy exists over whether to do an exercise stress test or to proceed directly to noninvasive imaging studies. Patients with good exercise capacity and a normal exercise ECG may avoid further, more expensive testing. An abnormal or equivocal exercise stress test is more likely to be a true reflection of disease in those patients at highest risk for coronary artery disease. However, these patients are the ones most likely to require further diagnostic studies, and it can be argued that the most effective approach is to proceed directly to noninvasive diagnostic studies.

Noninvasive Imaging Studies. Where it is available, stress echocardiography should be considered as the first choice. This test is based on the fact that poorly perfused myocardial tissue does not contract effectively when exercised. Wall motion abnormalities may be detected by echocardiography done within 1 minute of exercise. The test requires the patient to be free of advanced chronic obstructive pulmonary disease (COPD) or massive obesity and to be able to achieve 85 to 90 per cent of his or her maximal heart rate by exercising. In patients who cannot exercise, the heart may be stressed to obtain similar results by administering vasodilators (either dipyridamole or adenosine) or the sympathomimetic agent dobutamine.

Nuclear Myocardial Imaging Studies. These tests are helpful if stress echocardiography is unavailable or if the patient has significant COPD. The thallium stress test is based on the failure of areas of ischemic myocardium to take up the thallium radiopharma-

ceutical during exercise. Thallium-201 has been largely replaced by another radiopharmaceutical, technetium-99m sestimibi. SPECT images can now be used to yield highly sophisticated images. The sensitivities of SPECT nuclear imaging and of stress echocardiography are about the same. Stress echocardiography is generally less expensive (about $400) than nuclear imaging (about $650).

Coronary Angiography. When intervention is planned, it is necessary to proceed to coronary angiography, which yields the most information about the coronary artery anatomy as well as the exact location and degree of stenosis. Contrast injected into the ventricle allows study of the heart's contractility; in addition, direct measurements of the cardiac chamber are available. The cost of coronary angiography is in the range of $2000 to $4000.

Ultrafast "cine" CT scanners are now able to produce images of the coronary arteries following a peripheral injection of contrast material. It is thought that this technology may begin to supplement currently available imaging techniques in the evaluation of coronary artery disease.

PULMONARY EMBOLUS. Chest pain, dyspnea, tachypnea, or hemoptysis that is suspicious for pulmonary embolus raises the clinical question of whether anticoagulation is necessary. The physician is often faced with the dilemma of whether tests such as a ventilation/perfusion scan should be done on an emergency basis. If the symptoms are suspicious for pulmonary embolus, or if the patient has risk factors such as prolonged bed rest, recent surgery, myocardial infarction or heart failure, an indwelling venous catheter, or venous thrombosis of the pelvis or proximal lower extremities, then the first step should be a plain chest x-ray. The chest x-ray will usually be nonspecific or normal, but it is important to exclude other chest pathology and is helpful in interpreting the V/Q scan.

Nuclear Lung Scan (V/Q Scan). The V/Q scan consists of two parts. The perfusion portion is accomplished by intravenously administering technetium-labeled macroaggregated albumin, which lodges in the vascular bed of the lungs and is then scanned. In the ventilation portion of the study, the patient breathes radioactive-labeled xenon gas for a scan that determines the portion of the lung being ventilated. If the V/Q scan is normal, showing good perfusion, it virtually eliminates pulmonary embolus from the diagnosis. Areas of lung with poor alveolar ventilation also have resultant vasospasm. Therefore, the two areas of decreased uptake should "match." When perfusion and ventilation defects match, in the absence of other parenchymal disease, the scan will be read as "low probability." Clinical judgment will be required regarding anticoagulation, since there is about an 80 per cent chance that there is no embolus in this circumstance. "Indeterminate" scans are reported when there are multiple areas of poor perfusion and ventilation, making interpretation difficult, or when the ventilation-perfusion deficit is associated with a lung lesion of undetermined cause. The risk of embolus in indeterminate scans may range between 30 and 70 per cent. If the scan shows that there is normal ventilation of a segment but also a perfusion deficit, the scan is read as "highly probable," and there is enough certainty that the patient should be anticoagulated in the absence of other contraindications. A V/Q scan costs about $450.

Pulmonary Angiography. Pulmonary angiography is reserved for those patients with a high clinical suspicion of pulmonary embolus in the setting of a nondiagnostic or indeterminate V/Q scan. Pulmonary angiography is very sensitive and specific. It costs about $1500 and is associated with a mortality rate of between 0.5 and 1 per cent. Doppler examination of the lower extremities may be used as an adjunct in the evaluation of the patient with suspected pulmonary embolus, but it does not definitively diagnose the lung pathology.

OTHER CHEST PATHOLOGY. Aortic dissection is best diagnosed by first obtaining a chest x-ray and then proceeding to CT with and without contrast. If the patient cannot be given contrast, an MRI should be considered. In general, a plain x-ray, occasionally followed by CT when needed, is appropriate for the first two steps in many diagnoses related to the chest. This approach has been used with diseases such as lung abscesses, persistent atelectasis, asbestosis, blunt chest trauma, bronchiectasis, bronchogenic carcinoma, bronchopleural fistula, emphysema with recurrent pneumothoraces, empyema, pulmonary metastases, anterior and middle mediastinal masses, some cases of pneumonia, sarcoidosis, Wegener's granulomatosis, pneumothorax, and solitary lung nodules. Fiberoptic bronchoscopy may be useful after the chest x-ray in selected cases of hemoptysis, and CT may be needed if symptoms persist despite negative findings on bronchoscopy. A barium swallow may be indicated if esophageal pathology is suspected in the posterior mediastinum, and a thyroid nuclear scan may be indicated in the evaluation of a superior mediastinal mass.

CONGESTIVE HEART FAILURE. Following a plain chest x-ray, echocardiography should be considered. Echocardiography is useful in evaluating the size of the ventricular chambers, the motion and thickness of the ventricular walls, and the condition of the valves. The echocardiogram is useful in differentiating systolic failure from diastolic failure. Systolic failure is characterized by a decrease in contractility, with the heart usually dilated and an ejection fraction of less than 40 per cent. Diastolic failure, on the other hand, is associated with a normal or slightly hypertrophied heart size and a normal ejection fraction. Echocardiography is usually sufficient to estimate the cardiac ejection fraction. If a more precise measurement of ejection fraction is needed, consideration should be given to a nuclear ventriculogram displayed as a multi-gated acquisition (MUGA) study. A MUGA study is a series of images created by a computer as technetium-99m labeled red blood cells flow through the heart following intravenous injection.

Echocardiography is also useful in cases of cardiomyopathy, cardiac tumors, congenital heart disease, cor pulmonale, endocarditis, valvular heart disease, cardiac tamponade, and pericardial effusion. Echocardiography generally costs over $300.

ANEURYSMS. Ultrasound is the first choice when evaluating for suspected abdominal aortic aneurysm. CT should be considered if there is suspicion of a retroperitoneal hematoma secondary to a leaking aneurysm. Ultrasound with color Doppler is the modality for the initial assessment for peripheral aneurysms, although CT or MR may be required for subclavian artery aneurysms.

Gastrointestinal System

CHOLELITHIASIS. Ultrasound examination has largely replaced the oral cholecystogram as the study of choice for the detection of gallstones. Its sensitivity approaches 100 per cent when done by an experienced technician.

ACUTE CHOLECYSTITIS. The initial study, abdominal ultrasound examination, is particularly useful if the diagnosis is uncertain. This examination will localize the gallbladder and allow the ultrasonographer to confirm the area of pain (a sonographic Murphy sign). It will identify stones, gallbladder wall thickening, and fluid around the gallbladder. The finding of gallstones plus either a positive Murphy sign or gallbladder wall thickening is highly suggestive of acute cholecystitis. If only one of these findings is present, and the diagnosis is uncertain, one should proceed to nuclear technetium-99m-hepatobiliary iminodiacetic acid (HIDA) scan. This radioactive-labeled substance is rapidly excreted from the liver into the biliary system. The injection of intravenous morphine is used to constrict the sphincter of Oddi and to aid in the concentration of the HIDA in the gallbladder. HIDA is useful to determine whether or not the cystic duct is obstructed. If the gallbladder does not fill with HIDA, acute obstructive cholecystitis is highly likely. If the cystic duct is open, the likelihood of obstructive cholecystitis is virtually eliminated. Rare cases of acalculous cholecystitis are possible, especially after cardiopulmonary bypass surgery; however, the combination of HIDA scan and US is usually sufficient to make an appropriate clinical diagnosis. Abdominal ultrasound costs about $200, and HIDA is just slightly more expensive.

BILIARY TRACT OBSTRUCTION. A similar approach may be used in these cases. US will usually reveal dilated biliary and hepatic ducts, although occasionally these ducts can be normal early in the course of the obstruction. HIDA scan may be useful if obstruction is strongly suspected, but the ducts appear normal on ultrasound. CT may be necessary when the cause of the obstruction and ductile dilatation is not apparent or not revealed by ultrasound. CT can be helpful in locating tumors in the head of the pancreas. It may be necessary to resort to endoscopic retrograde cholangiopancreatography (ERCP) to further define the anatomy or location of the obstruction. This procedure involves cannulation of the duct with the use of an endoscope. Contrast material may be injected into the common bile duct, and sometimes an obstructing stone is able to be removed. Occasionally, percutaneous transhepatic cholangiography (PTC) is necessary as well. This procedure involves injecting an intrahepatic duct with contrast material through a thin (22 gauge) needle.

APPENDICITIS. Most of the time, the diagnosis of appendicitis may be made with reasonable certainty without imaging studies. However, when the diagnosis is uncertain, imaging studies may be helpful to establish the diagnosis. Groups of people who may present with atypical abdominal pain or uncertain findings include the elderly, infants and young children, women of childbearing age, and individuals with suspected appendiceal rupture. Initially, an abdominal plain x-ray film is helpful in ruling out other pathology, such as small bowel obstruction, a mass effect, or intra-abdominal air. However, an appendicolith is able to be seen only about 10 per cent of the time. The next step is to decide between US and CT. CT is the best choice in patients other than pregnant women, infants, and young children. It is especially useful when appendiceal rupture is suspected. CT is often able to detect an abnormal appendix or an appendicolith with surrounding inflammatory changes. US may be ordered as an alternative in pregnant women or in infants or young children. It is less sensitive at detecting a perforated appendix than is CT, and technical problems with loops of bowel, obesity, and retrocecal location may hamper the examination.

Other Gastrointestinal Problems

DYSPHAGIA. A barium swallow with fluoroscopy is a reasonable first step in the management of most cases. Its cost is about one-quarter that of endoscopy. This examination can be tailored to the specific type of dysphagia symptoms by giving various thicknesses of barium or barium-coated solids. This is especially important if the patient has dysphagia or suspected aspiration from a stroke or other neurologic problem. Endoscopy is usually required next if there is evidence of any strictures, ulcerations, tumors, or webs.

SMALL BOWEL OBSTRUCTION. This is best approached initially with plain x-ray films of the abdomen (supine, upright, and decubitus), which should be examined for air-fluid levels or evidence of air-filled bowel loops with decreased colonic gas. Barium studies are considered next. They are contraindicated if there is evidence of free air in the abdomen. If an obstruction is suspected in the distal small bowel or colon, it is generally preferable to proceed to a barium enema before an upper gastrointestinal (UGI) barium series. This is because barium may be difficult to evacuate when it is proximal to the lesion. Partial and intermittent obstructions can sometimes be better detected by a technique called enteroclysis. With this technique, a bolus of barium and methylcellulose is injected directly into the jejunum via an oral tube placed under fluoroscopic guidance. Finally, CT may have a role in the diagnosis of small bowel obstruction but should probably be reserved for those cases in which the barium studies are inconclusive.

ACUTE GASTROINTESTINAL BLEEDING. Endoscopy is indicated for evaluation. However, if endoscopy cannot locate the bleeding source, a technetium-99m red blood cell study may serve to document active bleeding before an angiogram is done. If active bleeding is present, the angiogram is very good at localizing duodenal or stomach bleeding but is rarely helpful in detecting bleeding from esophageal varices.

PANCREATIC TUMOR. Ultrasound should precede CT in the evaluation of the jaundiced patient with a suspected pancreatic tumor; however, CT may be the initial study in the nonjaundiced patient.

HEPATOMEGALY OR HEPATOSPLENOMEGALY. A nuclear liver/spleen scan can document these cases; however, CT may be needed if the cause of the enlargement is in question. Ultrasound is more cost-effective if there is a need to document *splenomegaly* alone.

HEPATIC METASTASES. CT with contrast is generally the study of choice. If contrast material is contraindicated, or if clinical suspicions continue despite a normal CT, an MRI is indicated. If MR is unavailable, an alternative is a nuclear liver/spleen scan with SPECT.

Endocrine System

THYROID NODULE. The dilemma for the practitioner when a thyroid nodule is identified is to confirm that the nodule is actually arising from the thyroid gland. Ultrasound of the thyroid gland region may be helpful in locating the nodule in this case. If the nodule is arising from the gland, the question becomes whether the nodule is benign or malignant. The best test to answer this question in euthyroid patients is fine-needle aspiration biopsy (FNAB) of the nodule. This test may be done without a radiologic imaging study. It yields usable material about 85 per cent of the time and has 95 per cent accuracy. A minority of nodules that do not yield diagnostic material may be repeated with US guidance if necessary.

A nuclear thyroid scan is reserved for situations in which an FNAB is unavailable, the FNAB yields inconclusive results, or the patient is hyperthyroid. If a thyroid scan is necessary, it will yield one of several results. If the scan reveals a solitary, nonfunctioning, "cold" nodule, the risk of malignancy is between 15 and 40 per cent. Although a US examination may be able to differentiate between cystic and solid lesions, some malignant lesions may have cystic components, and US cannot rule out malignancy with certainty. A functioning, or "hot," nodule, on the other hand, can generally be assumed

to be benign. Although multiple cold nodules are usually benign adenomas or cysts, malignancy cannot be ruled out, and a tissue diagnosis should be obtained. A tissue diagnosis must also be obtained for irregular cold areas. They may represent either a malignancy or benign lesions such as scars or an atypical adenoma.

THYROID GLAND ENLARGEMENT. The approach to a diffusely enlarged thyroid gland should be initiated by a nuclear thyroid scan with technetium-99m pertechnetate. When the results reveal an enlarged gland with multiple increased and decreased function areas, the diagnosis is usually a multinodular goiter. This condition is characterized by a gland with partial replacement by multiple cysts, poorly functioning normal tissue, and fibrosis. If a hard, growing, or dominant cold nodule is found in a multinodular goiter, it should be diagnosed by tissue biopsy. A diffusely enlarged homogeneous gland with increased uptake is suggestive of Graves disease, although it may rarely represent an organification defect in which iodine is trapped in the gland but not converted to thyroid hormone. An enlarged homogeneous gland with normal uptake may represent early Graves disease, a stage of Hashimoto or subacute thyroiditis, a multinodular goiter of fine consistency, or a normal variant. A large gland with poor uptake probably represents subacute thyroiditis and does not require further imaging.

OTHER ENDOCRINE ABNORMALITIES. Parathyroid adenomas may be visualized using a technetium-99m-sestimibi scan (MIBI) with SPECT. CT is the most common approach to adrenal masses. They must be done with very "thin" slices, since most adrenal tumors are less than 2 cm in diameter. CT is usually the first step for adenomas, aldosteronomas, and pheochromocytomas. However, I-131-iodocholesterol scans, I-131-metaiodobenzylguanidine (MIBG) scans, and adrenal vein sampling are available if the CT results are incongruous with the clinical findings or if further characterization of a nodule is necessary.

Skeletal System

FRACTURES. The majority of fractures can be detected adequately by plain x-ray films; however, there are several exceptions. When initial x-rays are negative and there remains a high suspicion of a fracture of a long bone or a bone such as the navicular in the hand, a repeat x-ray film done 10 to 14 days later may show resorption along the fracture line, or a periosteal reaction at the site of a fracture. In cases that cannot wait for this approach, either CT or MR should be ordered. CT can be used in most cases; however, MR is preferable for elderly patients with clinically suspected fracture of the femoral neck despite normal plain films. When the clinical diagnosis is unclear, a nuclear bone scan may be helpful in confirming the diagnosis of a stress fracture, since the plain x-ray films are often normal. Common areas for stress fractures include the tibia and fibula in runners and other athletes. Although the uptake of radionucleotide can result from a number of conditions, such as inflammation, trauma, neoplasm, and arthritis, these conditions are rarely confused when searching for a stress fracture, and a stress fracture is essentially ruled out by a negative scan.

OSTEOPOROSIS. Plain x-ray films are useful only late in the course of osteoporosis because at least 30 per cent of the bone must be lost before the loss is apparent on the plain x-ray. Therefore, x-ray absorptiometry techniques were developed to detect this problem in its earlier stages and to follow the progress of therapy. Among the more widely available techniques are dual-photon absorptiometry (DPA) and the faster and more reliable dual x-ray absorptiometry (DEXA). These techniques measure the absorption of x-rays or gamma rays through selected bones of the body, such as the hip and lumbar spine.

All pre- and postmenopausal women should be discussing ways to help prevent osteoporosis with their physicians. For the majority, the decision of whether or not to take estrogen replacement therapy is a clinical one, based on the patient's risk factors and the skeletal and cardioprotective effects of estrogen. Bone density measurement should be obtained only when the results would influence the physician's therapeutic recommendations or the patient's compliance, or when it is necessary to follow a patient's therapeutic progress. The cost of absorptiometry imaging is in the range of $100 to $200.

KNEE INJURY WITH MENISCAL TEAR. When the diagnosis of a meniscal tear is supported by history and physical findings following a knee injury, it is reasonable to first consider plain x-ray films of the knee. Although these do not show knee cartilage, they are useful as a first step to evaluate for joint effusion and other knee pathology, such as fracture. If a meniscal tear is suspected and it is not responding to conservative therapy or is interfering significantly with the patient's activity, the possibility

of arthroscopic surgery is raised. The family physician should confer with the intended arthroscopic surgeon to determine whether MR is indicated in the particular patient. If the symptoms are suggestive enough that surgery is likely, it may be most cost-effective to proceed directly to arthroscopic surgery, which costs around $3000.

An MRI is useful to determine the exact location and severity of meniscal and ligamentous injuries to the knee. It can be done at lower cost (about $900) than arthroscopy and is noninvasive. MR may be useful in identifying meniscal tears or cruciate ligament tears that are in locations difficult to visualize with the arthroscope. However, if arthroscopic surgery is ultimately required, MR can add significantly to the total expense. MR has largely replaced arthrography as the imaging study for the evaluation of meniscal tears.

Urinary and Reproductive Systems

OBSTRUCTIVE UROPATHY INCLUDING RENAL AND URETERAL STONES. A plain x-ray film of the abdomen should be the first imaging study when evaluating for renal or ureteral stones or other causes of obstructive uropathy. An intravenous pyelogram (IVP) should be considered next in patients who are producing adequate amounts of urine and who are free of severe renal disease. A renal ultrasound examination should take the place of the IVP if the patient is anuric, has severe renal disease, or is suspected to have obstruction from outside the urinary tract itself. The US examination is useful to define pelvis and calyceal enlargement. It often reveals both radiopaque and radiolucent stones and examines the kidneys regardless of their function. Antegrade and retrograde pyelograms, enhanced CT, or a voiding cystourethrogram may be needed if the cause and location of the obstruction remain obscure.

The renal US examination has several applications in addition to the detection of stones and obstructive uropathy. It is the main imaging method in the evaluation of *renal failure,* especially when obstruction is a possible cause. It is also one of the first imaging studies to consider when evaluating a *renal mass.* If the mass is cystic, the work-up often ends at that point. CT may be necessary when the mass is indeterminate or of solid character. When percutaneous guided needle aspiration or biopsy is needed, renal ultrasound is used to guide the needle.

TESTICULAR TORSION AND OTHER SCROTAL LESIONS. When it is available on an emergency basis, color Doppler ultrasound examination of the scrotum is becoming the preferred method to evaluate for possible torsion of the testicle. Because it is important to operate within hours of an acute testicular torsion, and because the clinical examination is frequently inconclusive, emergency imaging is necessary. An acceptable alternative when Doppler is unavailable is a nuclear scan. The scan does an excellent job of differentiating between decreased flow found in testicular torsion and increased flow found in epididymitis. Ultrasound imaging is also useful in the diagnosis of painful swelling arising from trauma and in differentiating mass lesions of the scrotum.

PROSTATE CARCINOMA. If a nodule is palpated, or if an unexplained high prostate-specific antigen (PSA) is obtained, biopsy is necessary and is usually done under US guidance. Transrectal ultrasound is the study of choice in this case. MR is beginning to have an important role in the evaluation of prostate cancer staging, since it is more effective than CT or US in evaluating local pelvic nodes or local spread.

Gynecology

BREAST. The diagnostic approach to a breast lump is addressed in Chapter 34. Screening for breast cancer is an important issue related to diagnostic imaging and the role of family physicians. The incidence of breast cancer has increased in North America, and there is justifiable public concern over this health problem. Breast cancer is the most common cancer diagnosed in women, accounting for approximately one third of all newly diagnosed cancers in women. The risk of developing breast cancer is age-dependent. For example, the risk of acquiring breast cancer is about 1:1000 for a woman in her forties and 1:500 for a woman in her fifties. Screening mammography has been shown to reduce the breast cancer mortality rate about 30 per cent for women above 50 years of age, although there is less evidence for a benefit under the age of 50. For this reason there has been a lack of consensus over when mammography screening should begin for the average-risk woman. The risk of radiation exposure with screening mammography has been judged to be negligible for women over age 40 when mam-

mographers use low-dose equipment and adhere to high-quality control standards. One of the problems with screening mammography is its relatively low positive predictive value, meaning that it results in a large number of benign biopsies. On the other hand, the physician must never be falsely assured about a palpable breast lump that is followed by a negative mammogram. A tissue diagnosis of a breast lump must be obtained regardless of the result of the mammogram. All women between ages 50 and 70 years should have an annual breast examination and mammography at least every 2 years. For average-risk women between 40 and 50 years of age who desire mammography, it should be made available yearly despite lack of strong evidence of its clinical efficacy; it should be available every 2 years for those over age 70 who desire it. High-risk women should have annual mammography starting at age 35, or 5 years before the age at which their first-degree relative developed cancer.

ECTOPIC PREGNANCY AND THE ADNEXAL MASS. Ultrasound examination is the preferred imaging study when diagnosing an adnexal mass. Imaging studies must always be preceded by an examination to confirm that the patient is in a stable condition and able to undergo the diagnostic evaluation. In most cases there is enough time to obtain a serum β human chorionic gonadotropin (βHCG), which will help exclude an ectopic or intrauterine pregnancy. When the βHCG is over 1800 IU/L, either abdominal US or transvaginal US may be used to confirm an intrauterine pregnancy. Transvaginal US is superior to the abdominal in detecting an ectopic pregnancy and is usually able to diagnose an intrauterine pregnancy when the βHCG is over 1000 IU/L. Beta-HCG levels below 1000 will warrant careful serial monitoring if the transvaginal US fails to detect an intrauterine pregnancy or other explainable pathology. Transvaginal US may also be useful when evaluating a suspected adnexal mass if there are equivocal findings or technical problems with the abdominal ultrasound. Many adnexal masses are nonspecific in their appearance and appear to have both cystic and solid components. When this is the case in postmenopausal women, or in premenopausal women without evidence of infection, a biopsy should be obtained to rule out malignancy. CT may be helpful in the staging process of ovarian cancer.

SUGGESTED READING

Carlson KJ, Eisenstat SA, Frigoletto FD, Schiff I. Primary Care of Women. St. Louis, CV Mosby, 1995.

Eisenberg RL, Margulis AR. Radiology Pocket Reference—What to Order When. Philadelphia, Lippincott-Raven, 1996.

Grossman ZD, Katz DS, Santelli ED, et al. Cost-Effective Diagnostic Imaging—The Clinician's Guide, 3rd ed. St. Louis, CV Mosby, 1995.

Guide to Clinical Preventive Services, 2nd ed, 1996. U.S. Preventive Services Task Force. Available through http://text.nlm.nih.gov/ or Williams & Wilkins, Baltimore, or International Medical Publishing, Alexandria, VA.

King DE. MRI or CT in CNS imaging. In Rakel RE (ed). Saunders Manual of Medical Practice. Philadelphia, W.B. Saunders, 1996, pp 1061–1062.

Juhl JH, Crummy AB. Paul and Juhl's Essentials of Radiologic Imaging. 6th ed. Philadelphia, JB Lippincott, 1993.

QUESTIONS

1. Contraindications to magnetic resonance (MR) imaging may include all except
   a. Patients with pacemakers
   b. Patients with surgical clips
   c. Patients with ferrous metal prostheses
   d. Patients with severe claustrophobia
   e. Patients with central nervous system disorders

2. The first imaging study of choice for head trauma with suspected subarachnoid hemorrhage is
   a. Skull plain x-ray films
   b. CT without contrast
   c. CT with contrast
   d. MR scan
   e. Angiography

3. In back pain with suspected lumbosacral disk herniation and nerve compression
   a. CT is clearly superior to MR
   b. MR is clearly superior to CT
   c. MR and CT have about the same diagnostic accuracy
   d. MR is limited by its one-plane image
   e. CT is limited in its ability to detect spondylolysis

4. Dual x-ray absorptiometry (DEXA) or dual-photon absorptiometry (DPA) should be ordered in
   a. All pre- and postmenopausal women
   b. In most women taking long-term estrogen replacement therapy
   c. In most women considering starting estrogen replacement therapy
   d. In cases in which the results would influence the decision to start estrogen replacement therapy
   e. In most obese women.

Answers appear on **page 603**.

Chapter 11

Managed Health Care

Glen R. Johnson, M.D., and
Marc L. Rivo, M.D., M.P.H.

Managed health care refers to a system for financing and delivering a specific set of health care services for a defined population, delivered through a specific network that is held accountable for controlling costs and improving health outcomes (Rakel, 1995). Over the years, the phrase *per capita reimbursement systems* was used synonymously with *managed health care*. The definition of managed health care transcends specific reimbursement methodology, however. Managed health care is defined by a variety of elements or building blocks, including the level of benefits or health care services that are offered to individuals for a certain premium; method by which physicians and other providers are paid; relationship among the physicians, providers, and facilities used; and management of health services delivered.

No single representative managed health care arrangement exists. Rather, one can best understand managed health care as representing a continuum of health care financing and delivery arrangements that range from least to most structured or managed. The traditional fee-for-service or indemnity system represents the least structured arrangement (Brown, 1996). Typically, patients had complete freedom of choice of physicians and services. The health care network consisted of any and all physicians and facilities; management of the utilization, quantity, and quality of health care services was nonexistent. In such a fragmented and open financing and delivery system, health care costs and quality are difficult if not impossible to manage. The classic prepaid staff or group model health maintenance organizations (HMO), such as Kaiser Health Plan or Group Health Cooperative of Puget Sound, represented the other end of the spectrum. In this highly managed arrangement, physicians are paid on a capitated basis, members receive their health care through a defined and limited network

of generalist physicians and specialist consultants as well as hospitals and other health care facilities. In this arrangement, the quality and cost of health care are carefully monitored and improved. The growth and popularity of managed care within the United States today reflect its potential to measure and deliver high quality and cost-effective health care within a finite budget to a defined population. The traditional, fragmented, and unmanaged fee-for-service system it has replaced was unable to deliver on this promise.

ORIGIN AND EVOLUTION OF MANAGED CARE

The origins of managed health care in the United States may be first traced to the 19th century. Early descriptions of managed health care may be found in the mid 1800s in Philadelphia and later on the West Coast (Mayer and Maye, 1985). It was not until the late 1930s and 1940s, however, that fully integrated and prepaid systems were developed to deliver comprehensive care under a fixed budget to defined populations. These early pioneers included Baylor Hospital in Texas, Ross-Loos and Kaiser Health Plans in California, the Farmer's Union Cooperative in Oklahoma, the Health Insurance Plan of Greater New York, and the Group Health Cooperative of Puget Sound in Washington State.

In the 1960s, public concerns about access to health care resulted in insurance reforms at the federal level, including the historic passage of Medicare and Medicaid legislation. Federal government–led health insurance reform opened the door for national legislation to expand and evaluate managed care. The Health Maintenance Organization Act of 1972 established a mechanism to standardize and distinguish HMOs from the traditional fee-for-service medical care system. Such HMOs had five basic characteristics: (1) the HMO assumed an explicit contractual responsibility for providing a stated range of health care services; (2) there was an enrolled, defined population; (3) subscribers voluntarily enrolled in the plan and providers voluntarily participated in it; (4) the HMO received a fixed periodic payment (a capitation per enrollee) from the subscribers, which was established independent of actual utilization by an individual subscriber; and (5) the HMO assumed financial risk for the capitated services. Physicians in these HMOs were either directly employed by the HMO (i.e., staff model HMO) or by a large, multispecialty group practice (i.e., group model HMO), which then entered into exclusive contract with that HMO for all physician services.

As HMOs became legitimized in the early 1970s, they opened the door for various alternative health care financing and delivery systems to emerge. All of these arrangements offered varying degrees of price discounts, defined provider networks, and management of the use of health care service (i.e., utilization management). Preferred provider organizations (PPOs), one popular enhancement to fee-for-service plans, represented a simple financial arrangement in which provider groups agreed to offer health services for discounted prices. Individuals covered by PPOs had greater health benefits and lower out-of-pocket costs if they chose PPO provid-

ers. The PPO arrangement differed from HMOs in that payments were not limited, so that neither health insurers nor providers were placed at financial risk for care provided.

Independent practice associations (IPAs) represented another popular variation from the staff and group model HMO. In this arrangement, the HMO contracted with a formal physician association, typically of primary care physicians in solo and small groups, who agreed to accept capitated payments for their services. In the IPA model, individual physicians did not have to give up their fee-for-service practice and continued to practice in the community.

ENROLLMENT GROWTH IN MANAGED CARE

In the 1980s, increasing concerns about rising health care costs in the private sector fueled a dramatic increase in employee enrollment in managed care plans. Group and staff model HMOs and IPA-type managed care plans offered significant price discounts to traditional indemnity insurance. As a result, enrollment in managed care plans was projected to skyrocket from 20 million to 60 million between 1986 and 1996 (Figs. 11–1 and 11–2).

In the 1990s, managed health care began to gain interest within government-funded Medicare and Medicaid programs. Medicaid enrollment is ex-

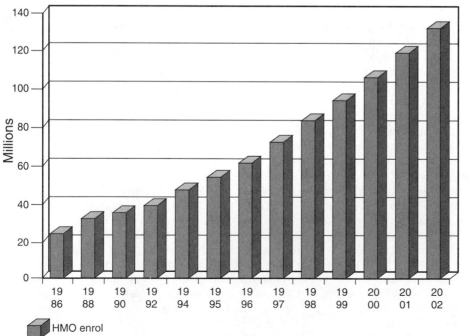

Figure 11–1. The growth of managed care. (From: InterStudy. Part II: Industry Report. St. Paul, MN, InterStudy, 1996.)

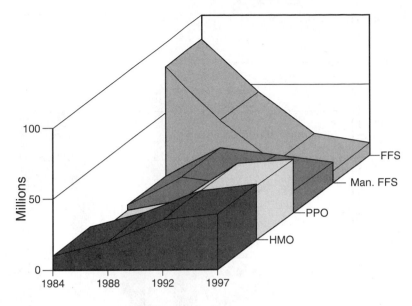

Figure 11–2. Managed health care and market penetration, private pay.

pected to grow from 18 per cent of eligibles in 1994 to over 40 per cent of eligibles, or 14 million enrollees by the year 2002 (Fig. 11–3). Primarily because of increased benefits in managed care, an estimated 80,000 Medicare members enroll monthly in managed care arrangements, driving projected enrollment to more than 12 million by the year 2000 (Fig. 11–4).

The approach toward managing a defined pop-

ulation within a fixed budget also is being integrated rapidly into worker's compensation programs. Under traditional worker's compensation programs paid on a fee-for-service basis, medical costs soared by 46 per cent between 1987 and 1993. In 1994, expenditures were $70 billion and were projected to double to $140 billion by the year 2000. Forty per cent of these costs was for health care services, whereas 60 per cent was for lost wages

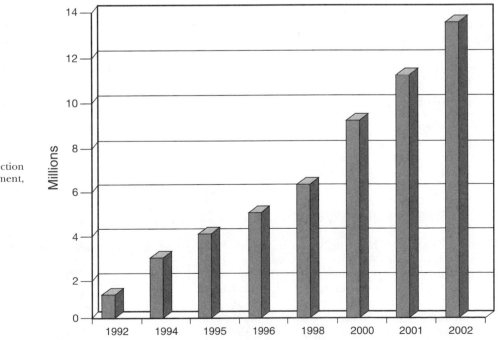

Figure 11–3. Growth projection for Medicaid HMO enrollment, 1992–2002.

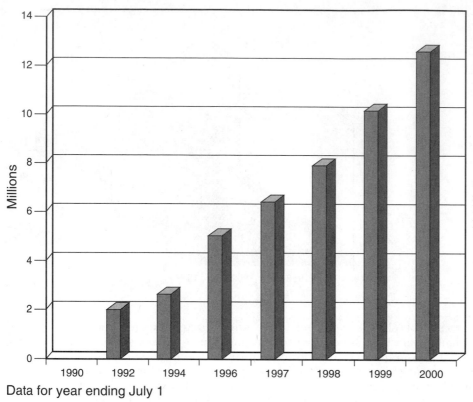

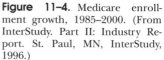

Figure 11–4. Medicare enrollment growth, 1985–2000. (From InterStudy. Part II: Industry Report. St. Paul, MN, InterStudy, 1996.)

Data for year ending July 1

and legal fees. In the 1980s, employers and public officials began exploring managed care alternatives to this traditional system, which encouraged overutilization of medical services and provided little incentive for prevention and rehabilitation. In 1991, 20 per cent of companies used managed worker's compensation programs. By 1993, 50 per cent of all companies used such approaches.

Although the health care financing and delivery system is in rapid evolution, managed care continues to both promote quality care and restrain costs. As managed health care evolves and matures in communities throughout the United States, a number of trends can be observed (Table 11–1). These trends are described in the following sections.

EVOLUTION IN REIMBURSEMENT STRATEGIES

Managed care fundamentally differs from traditional indemnity or fee-for-service medicine by its more sophisticated approach to controlling health care costs. Under fee-for-service plans, health insurance companies reimbursed health professionals and facilities for each unit of service performed. Fee-for-service reimbursement systems in medicine

were highly inflationary, however, because more services were rewarded with more reimbursement. Traditional approaches to cost management under fee-for-service plans included reducing benefits, increasing the sharing of costs among providers and consumers, and creative unit pricing. None of these, however, was able to restrain health care costs.

As managed care systems evolve, innovative reimbursement strategies are applied to assist in the management of medical costs. These include per capita reimbursement for both primary and consulting providers; innovative salary and compensation arrangements with a combination of base salary

TABLE 11–1. Trends Accompanying Growth of Managed Health Care

Evolution in reimbursement strategies
Evolution in managing health care utilization
Health system integration
Growing emphasis on improving and measuring quality
The new age of primary care, prevention, and wellness
The patient as educated consumer
Impact on the physician workforce and training

and incentives to control unnecessary hospital and specialty services; and, more recently, risk sharing and equity sharing relationships with provider groups. Although each of these mechanisms has been superior to fee-for-service reimbursement in controlling health care costs, each reimbursement system is associated with its unique problems that result from changes in physician behavior (Table 11-2).

Under capitation arrangements, physicians are paid a fixed amount for all professional services for each member under their care. Typically, payment is made on a per-member-per-month (PMPM) basis. The amount received varies depending on the age of patients and the type of insurance coverage they receive. For example, family physicians may receive $12 to $18 per working adult who obtains commercial health insurance through his or her employer and $35 to $45 per senior citizen over age 65 years on Medicare. The higher PMPM reimbursement for Medicare members is determined from actuarial analyses demonstrating that elderly members have more medical problems than younger adults and thus are more likely to need the services of the family physician. Capitation is superior to fee-for-service plans in restraining costs because the physician does not receive additional payments for each additional service he or she provides. Capitation may provide an incentive for services to be underutilized, however.

An alternative approach is for medical groups to place physicians on salary. Compared with fee-for-service plans, salaried providers cannot increase medical costs by providing additional services. Compared with capitation plans, providers cannot make additional money by withholding necessary care. Experience has shown that physician productivity may decline, however, as the incentive to work longer or more efficiently has been removed.

More recently, large provider groups have shown substantial interest in risk and equity sharing contractual relationships. Traditionally, most managed care organizations (MCOs or health plans) contracted with either individual physicians or groups and accepted financial risk only for the services they rendered. The MCOs managed the services provided by the group and retained whatever saving accrued from their management of medical costs.

Under risk and profit sharing contractual arrangements, large medical groups, IPAs, and networks accept full financial risk for all medical costs incurred by the members who are assigned to that group. These medical costs include primary care, consultant referral, emergency care, inpatient hospital, outpatient hospital, other medical services (e.g., home health, durable medical equipment), and pharmacy. Generally, a fixed percentage of the health care premium (averaging 75%–85%) is agreed upon, which represents the average cost for the medical services outlined earlier. If the group is able to efficiently manage the care so that their medical loss ratio (i.e., total medical costs/premium) is less than the budgeted amount, the group may retain all or a significant part of the savings.

EVOLUTION IN MANAGING HEALTH CARE UTILIZATION

Traditional health plan approaches to managing utilization have concentrated on changing provider behavior through precertification of referrals and hospital admissions, through daily review of hospital admissions to determine the need for continued stay (concurrent review), and through proactive planning for after-hospital care. These efforts were directed at the supplier of health care services—the physician or provider. Such "supply side" management strategies have been successful in reducing hospital admissions and length of stay, pharmacy cost, and referral rates to a very large degree.

Managed care has moved the provision of health services, when appropriate to do so, from the hospital to the community. The hospital is rapidly becoming a place for acutely ill and medically unstable patients. Patients whose conditions are not in danger of sudden deterioration but who require diagnostic or therapeutic care are now being managed in less intensive and expensive subacute or community-based settings. These community-based settings include outpatient surgical centers, nursing homes, rehabilitation centers, and hospices. Home health and custodial services are rapidly expanding. Nurses and social workers serve as case managers to coordinate many of these community-based services.

TABLE 11–2. Problems Associated with Reimbursement Strategies

Reimbursement Strategy	Associated Problem
Fee-for-service	Increasing costs
Capitation	Underutilization of services
Salary	Decreased productivity
Risk-sharing	Ethical issues

Risk identification and case management are other areas of expanded utilization management. Information systems help health plans identify and manage conditions that place members at increased risk for avoidable hospitalization. Many health plans develop programs for diabetes, congestive heart failure, asthma, hypertension, and other chronic diseases in which members identified with the condition are provided home visits, educational material, classes, and other support to help them stay healthy and in the community. Programs targeting pregnant women are also widespread; such programs offer prenatal education classes; high-risk case management; and incentives to obtain routine prenatal care and avoid use of alcohol and tobacco and other harmful behaviors.

More recent efforts to manage the utilization of health services have focused on patient demand, and therefore the term *demand-side management* was used. Demand management may be defined as the use of self-management and decision-support systems to enable, educate, and encourage people to improve their health and make appropriate use of medical care. The concept originated from the wellness and self-care programs of the early 1990s; it includes an array of approaches (Harmon, 1994):

- 24-hour nurse health counseling lines, in which members can call a 1–800 number for any health concerns and talk with a nurse who uses approved clinical protocols to evaluate and assist the members to manage their problems
- Health risk appraisal, in which individuals at risk for chronic illnesses are identified early in the course of the disease and a mutually-agreed-upon care plan is prepared and executed
- Wellness programs, directed at health promotion and lifestyle management
- Self-care programs, in which health information is provided to members to assist them in managing their own health problems and concerns

HEALTH SYSTEM INTEGRATION

Managed care is also driving practice, health plan, and health system integration. What used to be an independent patchwork of solo physicians, hospitals, pharmacists, dentists, and other providers and facilities is being replaced by expanding networks of care. The solo physician is being replaced by primary care, specialty, and multispecialty group practices and by larger IPAs and medical group or networks. Managed care penetration is accompanied by hospital, home care, pharmacy, oral health, mental health, and other health system mergers. For the first time, national health plans are being formed from the mergers of such managed care giants as Aetna and US Healthcare, United and Metra Health, and Pacificare with Family Health Plan. Health systems integration leads to greater administrative efficiencies, development of improved information systems, and a broader and better coordinated spectrum of care.

GROWING EMPHASIS ON IMPROVING AND MEASURING QUALITY

Efforts to improve the quality of clinical care and services to patients are greatly enhanced in a managed care system, which has a defined population not readily identified in the fee-for-service sector. As cost-control systems are being put in place, health plans and provider networks will be increasingly pressured by patients, employers, government, and the public to demonstrate their value and to differentiate themselves from their competitors on the basis of such measures as access to care, health outcomes, and patient satisfaction. In the 1980s and early 1990s, this growing movement began to call for the development of a common set of accreditation and performance standards from which to measure quality.

The primary organization that accredits managed care plans is the National Committee for Quality Assurance (NCQA). Health plans are evaluated on more than 50 standard and 200 total measures. The six major areas evaluated include quality management and improvement, credentialing, utilization management, member rights and responsibilities, medical records, and preventive health services. Although accreditation by NCQA or another recognized body is not yet a national requirement for health plans, a growing number of states' legislatures and large businesses are now requiring health plans to be accredited before they can do business.

In 1993, the NCQA released its first Health Plan Employer Data and Information Set (HEDIS 2.0), which resulted from a 4-year effort by employers, health plans, and consumers to define a set of health plan performance measures. In 1995, the NCQA released its first "report card" on 36 health plan performance measures, compiled from 21 health plans serving 10 million commercial members. The HEDIS project demonstrated that quality performance measures could be generated, carefully audited, and displayed in a common format to provide useful information on health plan performance. In 1997, HEDIS 3.0 was released, containing performance measures for the Commercial, Medicare, and Medicaid populations. The HEDIS 3.0 reporting set measures effectiveness of care (e.g., immunization, prenatal care, and smoking cessation rates); access and availability of care (e.g., appointment and telephone response time), member satisfaction with care; utilization of common ambulatory and hospital services; cost of care; and health plan stability. More than half of the over 500 health plans may be expected to devote significant resources to compiling HEDIS data to illustrate their impact on the health status of the population they serve.

This movement toward measuring and comparing quality performance data is in its infancy. Barriers that remain include inadequate information systems, lack of standardized performance measures, and overall cost of generating such quality-of-care data.

Furthermore, HEDIS only measures health plan performance, whereas consumers desire information on their own primary care physician, specialist, or health care network. In mature markets in Minnesota, California, and Massachusetts, however, such quality data on health care networks are becoming available, allowing consumers to make more informed choices among individual physicians and networks.

THE NEW AGE OF PRIMARY CARE, PREVENTION, AND WELLNESS

Primary care, prevention, and wellness are emphasized under managed health care financing arrangements. Under capitation, financial barriers to primary care services, such as copayment and deductibles, are substantially reduced or eliminated. Compared with traditional fee-for-service plans, managed care plans offer a wider range of basic covered benefits, such as immunizations, Pap smears, and mammograms for women, pharmacy, vision, and dental services. Typically, parents may bring in their children for only $5 to $10 and receive a complete examination, counseling, and immunizations. For a similar office visit charge, an adult woman may receive a yearly complete examination, Pap smear, and mammogram; and a senior citizen may receive home care services, eyeglasses, and all prescribed medications. In response to consumer demands, many health plans provide 24-hour nurse-staffed telephone call-in lines, wellness classes, expanded complementary medicine benefit packages (e.g., acupuncture, massage therapy), regular health publications, health-related videos, and a range of patient education materials available through the Internet.

Primary care physicians serve as the entry point and coordinators of care under managed health care systems. When members join a managed care plan, they are assigned to a primary care physician (e.g., usually a family physician, general internist, and pediatrician). In most health plans today, member referrals to specialty consultants for diagnostic and treatment services are approved by the primary care physician. As a result, the advent of managed care is widely seen as ushering in a new and central role of the primary care or generalist physician in the delivery system (Rivo and colleagues, 1995a).

THE PATIENT AS EDUCATED CONSUMER

The public is just beginning to understand and take advantage of the potential consumer benefits inherent in managed care systems. Managed care plans are required to make available and widely publicize member rights and responsibilities. Plans are required to have policies and procedures for responding to verbal complaints and written grievance and appeals from members who are unhappy with services provided or denied. Health plan performance data, such as HEDIS performance profiles or NCQA accreditation reports, are available to the public. In addition to conducting general member satisfaction surveys, many health plans and larger medical groups conduct similar surveys of their individual primary care physicians and even specialists. Today, however, the public generally is still unaware of this new consumer information, or sufficient standardized data are lacking to make informed decisions between health plans and between physicians or health care networks.

The absence of such information should not be interpreted as business-as-usual for health care in the 21st century. Increasingly, patients are demanding to be viewed as educated consumers and treated as informed partners in the health care system. Employers, government, and the public are demanding value (i.e., quality of care for amount spent) for their health care dollar and a standardized information set from which to judge the difference. Informed individuals are beginning to "shop" between individual physicians, health plans, and health care networks. In the 21st century, consumers will have such information to make educated decisions about what kind, how, where, and from whom to obtain their own health care.

TABLE 11–3. Stages in the Evolution of Managed Care

Stage 1	Stage 2	Stage 3	Stage 4
1970s	1980s	1990s	2000s
Emphasis on critical mass	Explosive growth	Accelerated enrollment	Growth in government programs
Era of discounts	High premiums	Capitation	Reduced premiums
	Capitation and discount contracts	Risk-sharing	
Micromanagement of medical care rationing	Strict gatekeeper	Management by use of guidelines	Disease management
	Rationing		
Hassle factor	Emphasis on supply side management	Equity sharing	Demand management
		Less restricted products	
Few affiliations	Loose provider networks	Strong networks	Provider-sponsored organizations
	Weak hospital affiliations	Affiliations	
High utilization			Low utilization

IMPLICATIONS FOR THE PHYSICIAN WORKFORCE AND TRAINING

Overall, the evolution of managed health care may be summarized as shown in Table 11–3.

The rapid changes in the health care system accompanying the growth of managed health care is widely seen as exacerbating the deficiencies in the physician workforce and training (Rivo and Satcher, 1993; Rivo and Kindig, 1996). In a managed care–dominated system and with the current production of doctors, the supply of physicians is expected to continue to outpace the growth of the population well into the early 21st century. Under various analyses, physician unemployment and underemployment may be expected in the United States at the turn of the century, for specialist physicians. In contrast, a modest need for more family physicians, general internists, and general pediatricians is projected during the upcoming decade (Council on Graduate Medical Education, 1996).

As importantly, the evolving health care is requiring a new physician for the 21st century equipped with a new set of managed care skills (Rivo and colleagues, 1995b). Physicians need to use clinical and management information systems to understand the health problems and needs of the entire population they serve; they must foster health promotion and disease prevention services and effectively involve patients and their families in decision making. They need to provide cost-effective care; work collaboratively with nurses, social workers, and other members of the health care team in coordinating care; and incorporate practice guidelines and other quality-improvement systems and techniques into their practice. The mission, curriculum, and sites of training for medical students and residents are changing rapidly as academic medical centers are attempting to respond to the new health care system.

Family medicine is evolving as well to remain responsive to the health needs of the public. The vast majority of family medicine clerkships for medical students take place in community-based physician office practices where the majority of medical care is provided, unlike internal medicine, pediatrics, surgery, and other clinical clerkships that still take place in highly specialized hospital settings. Similarly, family practice residents in most family medicine residency programs provide care to patients through managed care contracts, unlike their counterparts in other specialties. This exposure bodes well for the specialty in today's managed care environment; family practice is widely seen as the specialty in greatest demand in the United States. As managed care begins to expand around the world, the principles of family medicine and an adequate supply of family doctors are seen to be central to the achievement of quality, cost-effective, and equitable care to the world's population (World Health Organization and World Organization of Family Doctors, 1994).

REFERENCES

Brown A. Managed Care Industry Overview. February 20, 1996.

Council on Graduate Medical Education. Patient Care Physician Supply and Requirements: Testing COGME's Recommendations. Eighth Report to Congress and the Health and Human Services Secretary. Rockville, MD, Health Resources and Services Administration, 1996.

Crosby, PB. Quality Without Tears. New York McGraw-Hill, 1984.

Harmon RR. Demand Management and Self Care in the 1990s (manuscript). Fairfax, VA. United Health Care, 1994.

Health Market Survey—An Industry Report on HMO and Health Plan Markets, vol. XIII, no 6 and no 7, April 5, 1996. Washington, DC, Interpro Publications

Hedges D, et al: HMO Industry Profile, vol. 2. 1991.

InterStudy. Part II: Industry Report. St. Paul, MN, InterStudy, 1996.

Luft HS, Feder J, Holohan J, et al. Health Maintenance Organization. In Feder J, Holohan J, Marmor T (eds). National Health Insurance: Conflicting Goals and Policy Choices. Washington, DC, Urban Institute, 1980, pp 129–180.

Mayer TR, Maye GG. HMOs origins and development. N Engl J Med 1985;312:590.

Perkoff G. The History of Managed Care: The 'New' Problems Aren't. Presentation at the Generalist Physician Initiative Meeting sponsored by the Robert Wood Johnson Foundation, Key Biscayne, FL, 1996.

Rakel R. Textbook of Family Medicine, 5th ed. Philadelphia, WB Saunders, 1995, pp 1635–1647.

Rivo M, Altman D, Foss F (eds). Primary care and the education of the generalist physician: Coming of age. Acad Med 1995a;70[suppl]:S1–S116.

Rivo M, Kindig D. A report card on the physician workforce in the United States. N Engl J Med 1996;334:892–896.

Rivo M, Mays H, Katzoff J, Kindig D. Managed health care: Implications for the physician workforce and medical education. JAMA 1995b;274:712–715.

Rivo M, Satcher D. Improving access to health care through physician workforce reform: Directions for the 21st century. JAMA 1993;270:1074–1078.

Rivo M, Saultz J, Warman S, DeWitt T. Defining the generalist physician's training. JAMA 1994;271:1499–1504.

World Health Organization and World Organization of Family Doctors. Making Medical Practice and Education More Relevant to People's Needs: The Contribution of the Family Doctor. Working paper from the joint WHO-WONCA Conference. Ontario, Canada, 1994 (may be obtained from the American Academy of Family Physicians).

SUGGESTED READING

Council on Graduate Medical Education. Managed Health Care: Implications for the Physician Workforce and Medical Education. Sixth Report to Congress and the Health and Human Services Secretary. Rockville, MD, Health Resources and Services Administration, 1995.

Family Practice Management. (Monthly managed care journal of the American Academy of Family Physicians. Available with AAFP membership or through subscription.)

HEDIS 3.0 (Health Plan Employer Data Information Set). Washington, DC, National Committee for Quality Assurance, 1996.

QUESTIONS

1. Match the following terms with their definition
   a. Preferred provider organization (PPO)
   b. Independent practice association (IPA)
   c. Staff model HMO
   d. Group model HMO

   (1) Physicians who are directly employed by the HMO
   (2) Physicians who are directly employed by a medical group with an exclusive HMO contract
   (3) Solo or small groups of physicians who agree to accept capitated payments for their services
   (4) Groups that agree to offer health services for discounted prices

2. Paying primary care physicians $15 per member per month for all professional services for each member under their care is an example of
   a. Risk contract
   b. Fee-for-service
   c. Capitation
   d. Equity sharing
   e. Salary plus bonus compensation

3. A major problem associated with traditional fee-for-service reimbursement is
   a. Decreased productivity
   b. Underutilization of specialty care
   c. Underutilization of hospital care
   d. Increasing medical costs

Answers appear on **page 603**.

Chapter 12

Basics of Prescription Writing

Hardy B. Woodbridge, Jr., M.D.

A written prescription is that communication between a physician, or other licensed medical practitioner, and a pharmacist for the purpose of issuing a specific medication to a specific patient at a specific time and for a specific purpose. From primitive societies to tribal priestcraft eras and the mystery of the earliest apothecaries, practitioners were suspected of belonging to the world of spirits. Hippocrates helped to develop a more scientific basis for medicine, also introducing ethics into this mysterious field (Ansel, 1995). Fortunately, modern-day practitioners of pharmacy and medicine have developed less mysterious ways of using highly processed medication. There still exists a magical hope and trust by the patient in the use of modern drugs, as prescribed by the physician and checked and dispensed by the pharmacist.

The United States Congress passed the Federal Food, Drug, and Cosmetic Act of 1938 and created the Food and Drug Administration (FDA) to enforce this law. Every new drug must be approved by this agency before being promoted or distributed.

This chapter focuses on prescription (legend) drugs, and does not cover the myriad over-the-counter (OTC) drugs, which are considered safe enough to use for simple conditions and do not require prescriptions.

WHEN A PRESCRIPTION IS USED

The prescription evolves only when that part of a management plan requires the use of a prescription drug. This process follows the orderly sequence of performing a history and physical examination, interpreting laboratory work if used, establishing a diagnosis, and negotiating a management plan, or of following another version of problem-solving.

Medical prescriptions are used to order drugs when the prescriber and patient are in an outpatient setting or in a hospital or institutional setting. The outpatient prescription form is by far the more commonly used, inasmuch as most medical problems are seen and treated in an outpatient setting. In addition, the outpatient prescription is used for patients upon discharge from the hospital and in hospital clinic visits.

PRESCRIPTION FORM

A specific form is advocated for use in writing prescriptions for outpatients. Arrangement of names, addresses, and shape and style of the form vary among prescribers, but the classic components of a prescription are standard and follow in sequence. Hospitals and institutions use different forms to prescribe medications, which include other orders for diet, activity, and general care of the patient. Although the form and style of prescriptions differ for outpatient and inpatient settings, there are similarities. Both require that the name of a drug and its strength, quantity, and frequency and route of administration be given. Both result from the orderly decision-making process of using a specific drug for a specific problem in a patient. Outpatient prescriptions are written on a prepared form with printed information of the prescriber that aids the pharmacist with identification of the prescriber. The details of the drug and the other components are written on the form by the prescriber.

Pharmacists have their own forms for purposes of recording orders received verbally from prescribers. The prescriptions may be numbered to aid in the control and monitoring of prescription pads, and in particular, for detection of missing prescriptions. Prescription forms made in duplicate offer a convenient and accurate way of recording the information for the prescriber and pharmacist when questions arise.

COMPONENTS OF A WRITTEN PRESCRIPTION

(1) PRINTED NAME OF PRESCRIBER. (Fig. 12–1) The printed name of the prescriber, or the hospital, or both, is at the top of the prescription, providing legible identification of the name, address, and telephone numbers.

(2) INFORMATION ABOUT THE PATIENT. The patient's name, address, age, and weight (for pediatric ages) are designated on the prescription. This information identifies the patient for the pharmacist and helps to reveal possible dosing errors or medication known to have caused previous allergic reactions in the patient. This is particularly important in families when more than one person is taking medicine. Controlled drugs require this information (Table 12–1).

(3) DATE. The date the prescription is given to the patient by the prescriber is the date recorded on the prescription. The date is necessary for record-keeping purposes and alerts the pharmacist in recognizing delays in presentation of the prescription by the patient. With an unusual delay, the pharmacist determines if the intent of the prescriber can be met.

Prescriptions must be dated as required by federal law when written for controlled substances as listed in Schedule II, III, and IV of the 1970 Controlled Substances Act (see Table 12–1). When there is no date given for noncontrolled drugs some states allow the date of filling to be used as the prescribing date if the pharmacist thinks it appropriate.

(4) SUPERSCRIPTION OR ℞ SYMBOL. The symbol stems from the Latin *recipe* for "take thou" or "you take," and has evolved from ancient times. It is representative of the prescription and the pharmacy itself (Ansel et al, 1995).

(5) INSCRIPTION OR MAIN BODY OF THE PRESCRIPTION. Written at that area are the name of the drug or drugs, the drug form to be used, and the drug strength.

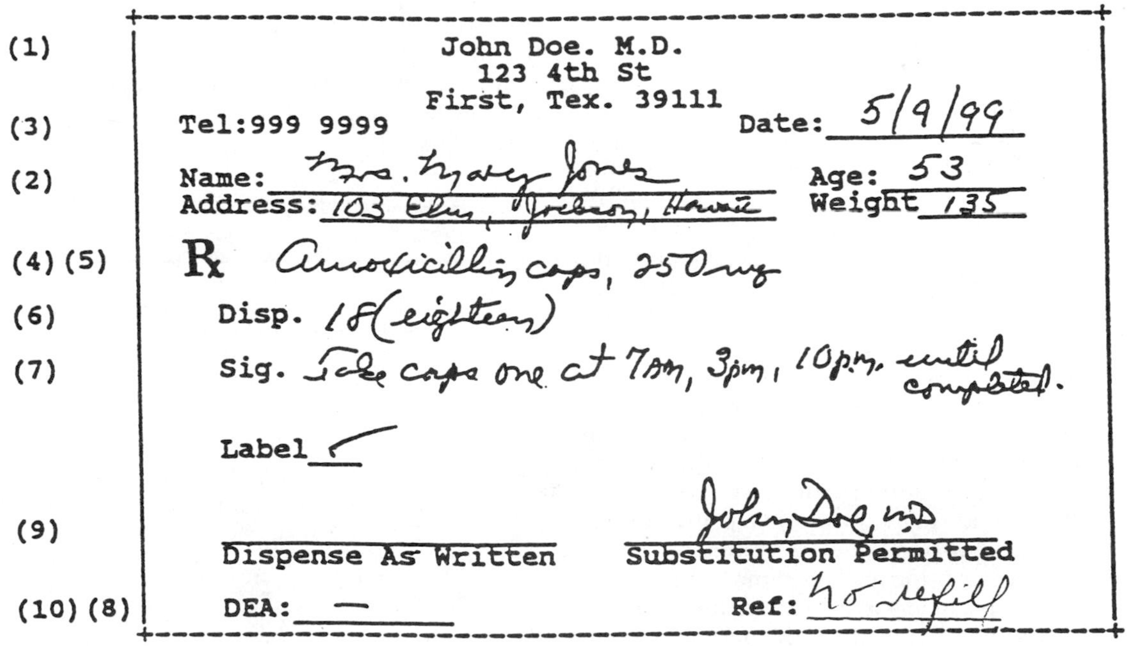
(1) John Doe. M.D.
123 4th St
First, Tex. 39111
(3) Tel:999 9999 Date: 5/9/99
(2) Name: Mrs. Mary Jones Age: 53
Address: 103 Elm, Jackson, Hawaii Weight 135
(4) (5) ℞ Amoxicillin caps, 250 mg
(6) Disp. 18 (eighteen)
(7) Sig. Take caps one at 7am, 3pm, 10pm. until completed.
Label ✓
(9) Dispense As Written John Doe, MD Substitution Permitted
(10) (8) DEA: — Ref: no refill

Figure 12–1. Example of a typical outpatient prescription. (Numbers in parentheses correspond to the respective components as described.)

TABLE 12–1. Scheduled Drugs

In 1970, the Comprehensive Drug Abuse Prevention and Control Act established a classification of drug substances that are subject to abuse in the public. Five schedules were created with decreasing levels of control, from schedule I through schedule V.

Schedule I
No accepted medical use in the United States and a high potential for abuse. Partial list includes LSD, heroin, marihuana, mescaline. Not for prescription use, but for research

Schedule II
Accepted medical uses, but high potential for abuse. May lead to physical or psychological dependence. Partial list includes opium, morphine, codeine, hydromorphone, methadone, meperidine, cocaine, dextroamphetamine, diphenoxylate, amobarbital, oxycodone

Schedule III
Less potential for abuse than in schedules I and II, and accepted medical uses, and may lead to low physical but high psychological dependence. Partial list includes nalorphine, benzphetamine, chlorphentermine, glutethimide, some barbiturates not included in other schedules

Schedule IV
Low potential for abuse and limited physical or psychological dependence. Accepted medical use. Partial list includes phenobarbital, barbital, 35 benzodiazepines, chloral hydrate, ethanamate, meprobamate, paraldehyde, propoxyphene

Schedule V
Less potential for abuse than schedule IV drugs and have accepted medical uses. May have limited quantities of opioids, for antidiarrheal or antitussive purposes. May be dispensed by pharmacist with limited amounts

---

The *name* of the drug is written in English, using the proprietary (manufacturer's brand name) or nonproprietary (generic) name, or both. If the proprietary name is designated, the pharmacist must use that specific preparation or determine whether the prescriber permits an acceptable nonproprietary drug substitute. The advantage of using a brand name is to ensure bioequivalency; the disadvantage may be a higher cost. When using the generic name, the pharmacist selects the appropriate drug to meet the intent of the prescription. An advantage of a generic drug may be less cost; a possible disadvantage may be less bioequivalency and efficacy than its brand counterpart.

Drug form is indicated by specifying the use of tablets, capsules, suspension, ointment, or other forms. If the prescription calls for more than one ingredient, the pharmacist compounds them, using each name and quantity of drug or inert substance as ordered by the prescriber.

Drug strength should be given using the metric system (Table 12–2). The apothecary system is still used by some prescribers, but the metric system is encouraged to conform more to international standards and generally is more accurate. Certain abbreviations may be misread and should be avoided. The symbol for microgram is easily misinterpreted for milligram, a difference of 1000. U for unit may be misread as a zero, producing a wrong amount. When using decimals, a leading zero should be used for any amount less than one (for example, 0.1, to avoid misinterpreting .1 as one). A decimal should not be used after a whole number, however, for example, 1.0, which may be read as 10 rather than one. Both examples represent 10-fold differences (Lofholm & Katzung, 1995).

(6) SUBSCRIPTION OR DIRECTIONS TO THE PHARMACIST. The term *dispense* is used to direct the pharmacist in the preparation of the medication. This serves to indicate the number or volume or size of medication to dispense and may include the use of an oral syringe, applicator, inhaler, or other measuring device. With two or more drugs, the direction may be to *mix* or *make*, as with a solution, capsules, or ointment. The Poison Prevention Packaging Act in 1970 resulted in safer packaging to prevent accidental poisoning in children by using child-resistant drug bottles and containers. The prescriber may request, however, that the pharmacist use a non–child-resistant container for those patients who have problems opening child-resistant drug containers, such as patients with arthritis or the elderly. Quantities of the drug, or drugs in compounded prescriptions, are also designated by the metric system (Benet, 1990). A potential problem in prescribing

TABLE 12–2. Metric-Apothecary Approximate Equivalents

Metric	Apothecary
1 gram (gm)	15 grains (rounded)
60 milligrams (mg)	1 grain
15 mg	¼ grain
7.5 mg	⅛ grain
1 mg	¹⁄₆₅ grain
30 milliliters (ml)	1 ounce
31.1 gm	1 ounce
500 (473.2) ml	1 pint
1000 (946.4) ml	1 quart
5 ml	1 teaspoon
15 ml	1 tablespoon
1 ml	20 drops (gtt)
1 drop	1 minim
1 kilogram (kg)	2.2 pounds (lb)

volume is the common use of teaspoons and tablespoons for dosages. These spoons vary in size, and some medications require more accurate measurement. Calibrated droppers, measuring caps, and oral syringes offer more accurate measurement for children and the elderly.

(7) TRANSCRIPTION OR DIRECTIONS TO THE PATIENT. *Signatura*, usually abbreviated to *Signa* or *Sig*, is the classic term and means from Latin "mark thou." The first word of direction should be to indicate how the drug is to be used, such as "take" for oral medication, "apply" for an ointment, "instill" or "place" for eyedrops, or "insert" for suppositories (Benet, 1990). Following the first word are directions for the amount of the drug to be used and when to use it, expressed in specific hours or referable to meals or activity. The last part of the direction states the purpose of the drug, such as for rash or relief of backache, or for whatever the medication is intended. The phrase "Take as directed" should not be used in place of specific times, amounts, and purposes stated. Latin words and abbreviations are frequently used in this part of the prescription. They were used in the past when Latin was the accepted language, and because of the easily written abbreviations the habit has carried over to modern day. Use of English words is preferred and helps to avoid misinterpretations by the pharmacist. Additional instructions by the pharmacist may remind the patient to "shake well" or "refrigerate" or "take on empty stomach," for example. The term *Label* is to ensure that the exact name and strength of the medication is stated on the label of the drug container. Many states now require this, so that the term *Label* is used by some prescribers in place of *Sig* in the transcription. *Sig* is still in use, however, and the term *Label* is designated with its own place on the prescription.

(8) REFILL DIRECTIONS. Definite indication to the pharmacist is made on the prescription as to the number of refills, if any. If *none* is indicated, no refill can be made. To ensure accuracy, a refill number should be spelled out rather than designated by an Arabic numeral. Long-term maintenance drugs can only be refilled up to 1 year in some states before requiring a new prescription. Schedule II drugs are not refillable without a new prescription, and some states require that they be filled within a specified time from the date of the prescription, for example, within a 48- or 72-hour period. Schedule III and IV drugs cannot be refilled more than five times and the prescription is invalid 6 months from the original date. The prescriber must be familiar with local and state laws that may impose more restrictions than the federal law on substance abuse drugs. The pharmacist may question a delay of refills of some medication, if not indicated within a time frame by the prescriber.

(9) SIGNATURE. A prescription is not official or legal until the prescriber signs it. The signature should be legible, for identification by the pharmacist. Preprinted prescriptions with the prescriber's name help to confirm the signature. For hospital or other institutional prescriptions, the name of the prescriber should be printed under the written name. Some states require that the signature be placed either in the right-hand space allowing for substitution by the pharmacist, or in the left-hand space, indicating that only the prescribed drug as written is to be dispensed.

(10) DRUG ENFORCEMENT AGENCY REGISTRY NUMBER (DEA NUMBER). For controlled drugs, the prescriber's signature must be written in ink and the DEA registry number must be given. This DEA number may be preprinted on the prescription form but is not encouraged because of the hazard of theft of prescription pads. Most prescribers prefer to write in the DEA number only when required for controlled substances. This number also serves as additional identification of the prescriber to the pharmacist.

HOSPITAL PRESCRIPTIONS

Hospital prescriptions are for drugs and other therapy for patients while in the hospital. The prescription is written on the hospital physician's order form as devised by a designated hospital committee. The form has the patient's name printed or stamped at the top. The date and time of the order are written; then the name of the medication, dose size, quantity, frequency, and route of administration are given (Fig. 12–2). The same guidelines for outpatient and hospital prescriptions are applicable regarding the use of directions and the language used.

In the hospital there may be an additional step in processing the prescription order. A copy of the physician's order may be sent directly to the hospital pharmacy in some hospitals. In others, however, the physician's order is transcribed from the order sheet by a nurse or ward clerk to the pharmacy, introducing a step of potential error. To prevent errors, many hospitals have a pharmacist present on the nursing unit who processes orders for medications

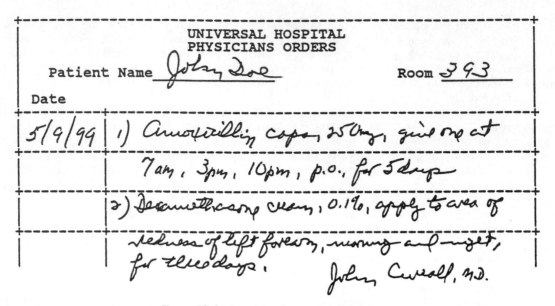

Figure 12–2. Example of a hospital order form.

and relays them to the pharmacy for dispensing, if not dispensing them from the floor. Prescriptions are also written for patients being discharged and for those seen in hospital outpatient clinics, but these prescriptions are written in the outpatient form, to be filled by a pharmacist of choice.

PRECOMPOUNDED AND COMPOUNDED DRUGS

With the development of precompounded drugs and drug combinations by pharmaceutical companies, physicians have largely discarded the former classic practice of ordering drugs that are compounded by the pharmacist and requiring individual ingredients with appropriate vehicles. Although some physicians still use this method, particularly with dermatologic preparations, the vast majority of prescriptions call for drugs and combinations compounded and prepared by pharmaceutical companies. Fixed combinations, however, do not allow for individual adjustment of dosage, whereas prescribing individual drugs permits adjustment of each to the predicted needs of the patient.

ERRORS AND NONCOMPLIANCE

Unfortunately, errors occur with prescriptions, beginning with the written order by the prescriber;

with the processing of the order by the pharmacist; with misinterpretation by the nurse in the hospital; and by the patient who does not understand the directions. One of the most common errors of concern is that of noncompliance by the patient. In addition to misunderstanding directions, patients fail to remember to take prescribed dosages or willfully misuse the prescribed drugs. The overuse or underuse of medication may result in serious consequences. Illegible writing by the prescriber to the pharmacist, in English or Latin terms, accounts for some errors (Table 12–3). Telephone prescriptions are another source of errors when misunderstandings occur between the prescriber and the pharmacist, or a nurse and the pharmacist. Involvement of more individuals in the transmission of an order increases the likelihood of error. When this custom is followed, the prescriber should determine that the assistant is thoroughly familiar with the skill of relaying the precise information to the pharmacist.

COMMUNICATION

The importance of communication between the prescriber and pharmacist is vital if potentially catastrophic problems or complications are to be avoided. It is equally important for the patient to understand the purpose and intent of the drug and when and how it is to be used. Understanding these

TABLE 12–3. Prescription Abbreviations of Latin and English Terms

Abbreviations	Latin	English Meaning
ac	ante cibos	Before meals
pc	post cibos	After meals
disp	dispense	Dispense
gtt	gutta	A drop
ml	milliliter	One-thousandth liter
cc	cubic centimeter	Approximately equal to an ml
hs	hora somni	At bedtime
q	quaque	Each
ss	semis	One half
tab	tabella	Tablet
caps	capsula	Capsule
IM	intramuscular	Intramuscular injection
IV	intravenous	Intravenous injection
SQ	subcutaneous	Subcutaneous injection
prn	pro re nata	When necessary
qid	quater in die	Four times a day
tid	ter in die	Three times a day
bid	bis in die	Two times a day
sig	signa	(You) write
gm	gram	Gram
gr	granum	Grain
mg	milligram	One-thousandth gram
mcg	microgram	One-millionth gram
mEq	millequivalent	One-thousandth gram equivalent weight

details is particularly important for the outpatient and is applicable to the hospital patient whenever possible. Once the prescriber has determined the drug to be ordered, there must be crystal clear and appropriate directions to the pharmacist, who must accurately prepare the drug ordered. The language used in this process, both written and verbal, is vitally important to ensure that the anticipated goal of the drug used is fulfilled. Thus, verbal communication should supplement written directions for the patient, given by the prescriber and the pharmacist. Estimates project that up to 20 per cent of adults are functionally illiterate, whereas others read at grade-school levels. It becomes the responsibility of the prescriber and pharmacist to make every attempt to clarify the directions for the patient.

SUMMARY

A prescription is a means of communication between a prescriber and a pharmacist for a specific drug for a specific patient. It is vital that there be legible writing of the directional part of the prescription to supplement the printed portion. Complete directions for a drug, its strength, quantity, and route and time of administration, will aid the pharmacist in ensuring that correct and appropriate written and verbal instruction is given to the patient to encourage compliance. Use of metric and English terms helps to avoid errors and assists in patient understanding. Coordinated effort by the physician and pharmacist plays a major role in the use of a drug as part of a treatment plan to be used in the wonderful art of healing.

REFERENCES

Ansel HC. The prescription. In Gennaro AR (ed). Remington: The Science and Practice of Pharmacy. Easton, PA, Mack Publishing, 1995, pp 1808–1821.

Ansel HC, Popovich NG, Allen LV. Pharmaceutical Dosage Forms and Drug Delivery Systems, 6th ed. Malvern, PA, Williams & Wilkins, 1995, pp 3–20.

Benet LZ. Principles of prescription order writing and patient compliance instructions. In Gilman AG, et al. (eds). Goodman and Gilman's the Pharmacological Basis of Therapeutics, 8th ed. Elmsford, NY, Pergamon Press, 1990, pp 1640–1649.

Lofholm PW, Katzung, BG. Rational prescribing and prescription writing. In Katzung BG (ed). Basic and Clinical Pharmacology, 6th ed. Norwalk, CT, Appleton & Lange, 1995, pp 969–976.

Dorfman JS. Pharmaceutical Latin. Philadelphia, Lea & Febiger, 1938, pp 100–105.

Padron VA, Hospodka RJ, DeSinone EM, Keefner KR. What the prescription should tell us. U.S. Pharmacist 1995;20:58–70.

Rogers JC, Biggs WS. Problem solving in family medicine. In Rakel RE (ed). Essentials of Family Practice. Philadelphia, WB Saunders, 1993, pp 206–220.

QUESTIONS

1. Similarities of content of prescriptions in outpatient and inpatient settings are
   a. Name of patient, address, age, weight
   b. Name of drug; its strength, quantity, frequency, and route of administration
   c. Printed forms, rectangular in shape, and lined for neatness
   d. Schedule II and III drugs always listed in Latin and apothecary method

2. Component parts of a prescription include
   a. Apothecaries, metrics, OTCs, pro re nata, granum, and milliequivalents
   b. Legend, schedule, errors, directions of form, directions of style, and adverse drug reactions
   c. Printed name of prescriber, patient's name, date, superscription, inscription, subscription, transcription, refill directions, signature
   d. Bioequivalencies, apothecaries, metrics, adverse drug reactions, legends, calibrations, container size, and schedules

3. Schedule II drugs
   a. Have no accepted medical use
   b. Have low potential for abuse
   c. May be dispensed by the pharmacist in limited amounts
   d. Have accepted medical uses but high potential for abuse

Answers appear on **page 603.**

Chapter 13

Immunizations

Richard D. Clover, M.D.

INITIAL VISIT

Patient Identification and Presenting Problem

Kristin C. is a 15-month-old girl who presents with a runny nose. Her mother states that Kristin was in her usual good health until approximately 3 days ago, when she developed a runny nose, nasal congestion, and a low-grade fever. Yesterday, Kristin's fever resolved, but her nasal congestion has persisted. Because of a past history of ear infections, Mrs. C. is concerned that Kristin may have another ear infection. Mrs. C. denies Kristin has had a cough, difficulty breathing, vomiting, or diarrhea.

PAST MEDICAL HISTORY. Kristin was a product of a term gestation to a 27-year-old white female. Pregnancy and delivery were uneventful. Kristin has been treated successfully three times previously for otitis media with amoxicillin. Growth and development have been normal. Her immunization record is as follows: hepatitis B (Hep B) at 2 days of age; diphtheria-tetanus-pertussis (DTP), *Haemophilus influenzae* type B (Hib), Hep B, and oral polio vaccine (OPV) at 7 weeks of age; DTP, Hib, and OPV at 4 months of age; and DTP, Hib, and Hep B at 6 months of age.

FAMILY HISTORY. Kristin's father, a physician, is in good health at age 28. Her mother, a teacher, is in good health. Her maternal grandmother died at age 32 from lymphoma. Her other grandparents are in their fifties with no major medical problems.

OBJECTIVE

Physical Examination

Kristin's vital signs are temperature of 37.3°C, respirations 20, heart rate 100, and weight 25 lb. Generally, Kristin was alert and active, although she was obviously nasally congested. Her tympanic membranes were normal. Her nose had clear rhinorrhea, and her throat was mildly injected but without exudate. Her neck was supple with small anterior cervical lymphadenopathy. Lung, heart, and abdominal examinations were within normal limits. Her neurologic examination was appropriate for her age. Her skin was without rashes.

ASSESSMENT

Working Diagnosis

1. Upper respiratory infection, probably viral in origin

2. Immunization-deficient. Kristin has had DTP × 3, Hib × 3, Hep B × 3, and OPV × 2 but has not received measles, mumps, rubella, and varicella immunizations.

Differential Diagnosis

1. Allergic rhinitis is usually associated with clear rhinorrhea, a more chronic history, and absence of

fever. In this case, the acute onset and initial fever makes an infectious etiology more likely.

2. Nonviral respiratory infection. Although multiple organisms may produce a respiratory infection, the improving course of this illness (i.e., resolved fever) makes a self-limited viral infection the most probable.

PLAN

Diagnostic

No diagnostic tests are appropriate at this time.

Therapeutic

1. Administration of the following vaccines: diphtheria, tetanus, acellular pertussis (DTaP), Hib, OPV, measles, mumps, rubella (MMR), and varicella

2. Symptomatic treatment for rhinorrhea (saline nasal spray)

Patient Education

1. Mrs. C. was advised that the child's symptoms should continue to improve.

2. The mother was advised of the potential side effects and adverse reactions to each of the vaccines and was given the appropriate vaccine information handouts. Acetaminophen may be given for fever and discomfort that accompany immunizations.

Disposition

Mrs. C. was asked to return with Kristin in 3 months for routine childhood examination or sooner if the child's condition does not improve or if it deteriorates.

DISCUSSION

Immunization programs have reduced the incidence of many childhood infections. By these initiatives, global eradication of smallpox has been accomplished, and polio has been eliminated from the Western hemisphere. Significant reductions in the incidence of other vaccine-preventable diseases have been accomplished. Varicella, hepatitis B, and hepatitis A have recently been added to the list of vaccine-preventable diseases. The re-emergence of measles from 1989 to 1992, however, reminds us of the importance of these programs.

Several factors are involved in children and adults not receiving age-appropriate vaccines. These factors include patient, provider, and system issues. Although this chapter reviews many of the indications, contraindications, and compliance issues as they exist at the time of publication, the readers are referred to the published recommendations of the Advisory Committee on Immunization Practices (ACIP) for a more detailed discussion.

The leading reasons for delayed or missing immunizations were failure of simultaneous administration, invalid contraindications, missed opportunities, missed appointments, parental concerns including vaccine safety, and religious beliefs. To raise the vaccination levels, the following Standards for Pediatric Immunization Practice were recommended by the National Vaccine Advisory Committee and approved by the United States Public Health Service.

- Immunization services are *readily available*
- There are *no barriers* or *unnecessary prerequisites* to the receipt of vaccines
- Immunization services are available *free* or at *minimal cost* in the public sector. In the private sector, charges should include the cost of the vaccine and a reasonable or the administration fee
- Providers utilize all clinical encounters to *screen and immunize* children when indicated
- Providers *educate* parents and guardians about immunization in general terms
- Providers *question* parents or guardians about *contraindications* and, before immunizing a child, *inform* them in specific terms about the risks and benefits of the immunizations their child is to receive. All public and private providers who administer MMR, polio vaccine, DTP, and tetanus and diphtheria toxoids (Td) are required to distribute a copy of the appropriate CDC-developed Vaccine Information Statement *every time* a patient is vaccinated. Providers are not required to obtain the signature of the parent or the child's legal representative to acknowledge receipt of the Vaccine Information Statement but must make a notation in the patient's permanent medical record that the information statement was provided at the time of vaccination
- Providers follow only true *contraindications*
- Providers administer *simultaneously* all vaccine doses for which a child is eligible at the time of each visit. If providers elect not to administer a needed vaccine simultaneously with others, they should document such actions and the reason why the vaccine was not administered
- Providers use accurate and complete *recording procedures* for *all* vaccines. Providers must record what vaccine was given, date the vaccine was given, name of the manufacturer of the vaccine, lot number, signature and title of the person who gave the vaccine, and the address where the vaccine was given. In addition, providers should record on the child's personal immunization record card what vaccine was given, date vaccine was given, and name of the provider
- Providers *co-schedule* immunization appointments in conjunction with appointments for other child health services
- Providers *report adverse events* following immunization promptly, accurately, and completely. All clinically significant events, including those required by law, should be reported to the Vaccine Adverse Event Reporting System, regardless of whether or not the provider believes the events are caused by the vaccines. Report forms and assistance are available by calling 1-800-822-7967
- Providers are encouraged to operate a *tracking system*
- Providers adhere to appropriate procedures for *vaccine management*. Vaccines should be handled and stored as recommended in the manufacturer's package inserts
- Providers are encouraged to conduct annual *audits* to assess immunization coverage levels and to review immunization records in the preschool patient populations they serve. A variety of methods may be used. CDC's Clinic Assessment Software Application (CASA) can be used in the private sector as well as the public sector, and staff of the Department of Health Services' Immunization Program may be requested to assist as resources allow. Another method is that of the Health Plan Employee Data and Information Set available through the National Committee for Quality Assurance (202-628-5788). Practitioners may devise their own audit method. Results of these audits may be helpful to providers in assessment of immunization coverage levels of their patient population
- Providers maintain up-to-date, easily retrievable *medical protocols* at all locations where vaccines are administered
- Providers operate with *patient-oriented* and *community-based* approaches
- Vaccines are administered by *properly trained* individuals

- Providers receive *ongoing education* and *training* on current immunization recommendations of the ACIP, AAP, and the AAFP

The frequent changes in the immunization schedules have produced uncertainties for providers. Tables 13–1 and 13–2 summarize the recommendations and schedules as published at the time of publication of this book. This schedule includes two relatively recent changes in the recommendations. The first is the use of DTaP (acellular pertussis) for the primary series in infants/children and the second is the use of inactivated poliovirus vaccine (IPV)/OPV sequential schedule, OPV alone, or IPV alone as the primary series for polio vaccination. Provider/patient choice is encouraged in the selection of the polio vaccine to be administered. This polio recommendation resulted from the fact that the only cases of paralytic polio that presently occur in the United States are vaccine (OPV)-associated. By using IPV (in a sequential dosing schedule or alone), the number of cases of vaccine-associated paralytic poliomyelitis (VAPP) should be decreased.

In special circumstances, the provider needs to alter the recommended schedule. In immunocompromised individuals, killed or inactivated vaccines do not represent a danger and generally should be administered as recommended for healthy children. Steroid therapy usually does not contraindicate administration of live virus vaccines (OPV, MMR, varicella vaccine) when such therapy is for a short term (less than 2 weeks); low to moderate dose; maintenance physiologic doses; or administered topically, by aerosol, or by intra-articular, bursal, or tendon injection. The use of a dose equivalent to 2 mg per kg of body weight or 20 mg per day of prednisone should raise concern about the safety of immunization with live-virus vaccines. Physicians should wait at least 3 months after discontinuation of therapy

TABLE 13–1. Immunization Indications

Agent	Route	Indication
Diphtheria, tetanus, pertussis (pediatric)	IM	All children starting at age 2 months, may be given up to the 7th birthday; DTaP (acellular) or DTP can be used, although DTaP produces fewer side effects
Diphtheria and tetanus (pediatric)	IM	Children <7 years who cannot take DTaP/DTP
Tetanus and diphtheria (adult)	IM	Every 10 years, all persons age 7 or over
Measles, mumps, and rubella	SQ	Children at age 12 to 15 months and again between 4 and 6 years or 11 to 12 years; adults (especially medical personnel, day care workers, college students, and international travelers) without prior immunization or uncertain immunizations born after 1957, 2 doses
Varicella	SQ	Children at age 12 to 18 months (1 dose), catch-up vaccination for children 18 months to 12 years without history of chickenpox (1 dose), vaccination approved for persons 13 years or older without history of chickenpox (2 doses), health care workers without a previous history of chickenpox
Polio	SQ, PO	All children starting at 2 months of age; adults previously immunized who will travel to areas where polio is prevalent; unimmunized adults should receive the inactivated IPV vaccine; polio vaccine options: OPV, IPV, or sequential (2 doses of IPV followed by 2 OPV doses)
Haemophilus influenzae type b	IM	All children starting at 2 months of age
Hepatitis B	IM	Infants (birth, 1 month, and 6 months of age); adolescents (age 11–12 years) who have not yet received the vaccine; adults—health care workers, laboratory personnel who may be exposed to the virus, intravenous drug users, male homosexuals, patients with a sexually transmitted disease
Pneumococcal	IM	All persons over age 65; all patients before splenectomy; patients with chronic liver, heart, lung, or renal disease; patients with diabetes mellitus, HIV, and asplenia
Influenza	IM	All persons over age 65; patients (>6 months of age) with chronic heart, lung, or renal disease; with diabetes mellitus, hemoglobinopathies, or immunosuppression; household members of these high-risk groups; children receiving long-term aspirin therapy; and health care workers
Hepatitis A	IM	Travelers to higher risk countries, patients with chronic liver disease, members of certain high-risk communities and ethnic groups (e.g., Native American/Alaskan, homosexual males, street drug users, laboratory personnel who may be exposed)

TABLE 13–2. Immunization Schedule*

Vaccines are listed under the routinely recommended ages. Bars indicate range of acceptable ages for vaccination. Shaded bars indicate immunizations for children not previously immunized as follows: Hepatitis B vaccine is recommended at 11–12 years of age for children not previously vaccinated; varicella zoster virus vaccine is recommended at 11–12 years of age for children not previously vaccinated and who lack a reliable history of chickenpox.

Vaccine	Birth	1 Month	2 Months	4 Months	6 Months	12 Months	15 Months	18 Months	4–6 Years	11–12 Years	14–16 Years
Hepatitis B†§	Hep B-1									HepB	
		Hep B-2				Hep B-3					
Diphtheria and tetanus toxoids and acellular pertussis¶			DTaP or DTP	DTaP or DTP	DTaP or DTP		DTaP or DTP¶		DTaP or DTP	Td	
Haemophilus influenzae type b**			Hib	Hib	Hib**	Hib**					
Poliovirus††			Polio††	Polio††		Polio††			Polio††		
Measles-Mumps-Rubella§§						MMR			MMR		
Varicella virus¶¶						Var				Var	

*This schedule indicates the recommended age for routine administration of currently licensed childhood vaccines. Some combination vaccines are available and may be used whenever administration of all components of the vaccine is indicated. Providers should consult the manufacturers' ' package inserts for detailed recommendations. Vaccines are listed under the routinely recommended ages. Bars indicate range of acceptable ages for vaccination. Shaded bars indicate catch-up vaccination: at 11–12 years, hepatitis B vaccine should be administered to children not previously vaccinated, and varicella virus vaccine should be administered to unvaccinated children who lack a reliable history of chickenpox.

†**Infants born to hepatitis B surface antigen (HBsAg)-negative mothers** should receive 2.5 μg of Merck vaccine (Recombivax HB) or 10 μg of SmithKline Beecham (SB) vaccine (Energix-B). The second dose should be administered >1 month after the first dose.

Infants born to HBsAg-positive mothers should receive 0.5 ml hepatitis B immune globulin (HBIG) within 12 hours of birth and either 5 μg of Merck vaccine (Recombivax HB) or 10 μg of SB vaccine (Engergix-B) at a separate site. The second dose is recommended at age 1–2 months and the third dose at age 6 months.

Infants born to mothers whose HBsAg status is unknown should receive either 5 μg of Merck vaccine (Recombivax HB) or 10 μg of SB vaccine (Energix-B) within 12 hours of birth. The second dose of vaccine is recommended at age 1 month and the third dose at age 6 months. Blood should be drawn at the time of delivery to determine the mother's HBsAg status; if it is positive, the infant should receive HBIG as soon as possible (no later than age 1 week). The dosage and timing of subsequent vaccine doses should be based on the mother's HBsAg status.

§Children and adolescents who have not been vaccinated against hepatitis B during infancy may begin the series during any childhood visit. Those who have not previously received three doses of hepatitis B vaccine should initiate or complete the series at age 11–12 years. The second dose should be administered at least 1 month after the first dose, and the third dose should be administered at least 4 months after the first dose and at least 2 months after the second dose.

¶Diphtheria and tetanus toxoids and acellular pertussis vaccine (DTaP) is the preferred vaccine for all doses in the vaccination series, including completion of the series in children who have received one or more doses of whole-cell diphtheria and tetanus toxoids and pertussis vaccine (DTP). Whole-cell DTP is an acceptable alternative to DTaP and may be administered as early as 12 months of age provided 6 months have elapsed since the third dose and if the child is considered unlikely to return at age 15–18 months. Tetanus and diphtheria toxoids (Td), absorbed, for adult use, is recommended at age 11–12 years if at least 5 years have elapsed since the last dose of DTP, DTaP, or diphtheria and tetanus toxoids. Subsequent routine Td boosters are recommended every 10 years.

**Three *H. influenzae* type b (Hib) conjugate vaccines are licensed for infant use. If PRP-OMP (PedvaxHIB[Merck]) is administered at ages 2 and 4 months, a dose at age 6 months is not required. After completing the primary series, any Hib conjugate vaccine may be used as a booster.

††Two poliovirus vaccines are currently licensed in the United States: inactivated poliovirus vaccine (IPV) and oral poliovirus vaccine (OPV). The following schedules are all acceptable by ACIP, AAP, and AAFP, and parents and providers may choose among them: 1) IPV at ages 2 and 4 months and OPV at age 12–18 months and at age 4–6 years; 2) IPV at ages 2, 4, and 12–18 months and at age 4–6 years; and 3) OPV at ages 2, 4, and 6–18 months and at age 4–6 years. ACIP routinely recommends schedule 1. IPV is the only poliovirus vaccine recommended for immunocompromised persons and their household contacts.

§§The second dose of measles-mumps-rubella vaccine is routinely recommended at age 4–6 years or at age 11–12 years but may be administered during any visit provided at least 1 month has elapsed since receipt of the first dose and that both doses are administered at or after age 12 months.

¶¶Susceptible children may receive varicella vaccine (Var) during any visit after the first birthday, and unvaccinated persons who lack a reliable history of chickenpox should be vaccinated at age 11–12 years. Susceptible persons aged ≥13 years should receive two doses at least 1 month apart.

Use of trade names and commercial sources is for identification only and does not imply endorsement by the Public Health Service or the U.S. Department of Health and Human Services.

From Advisory Committee on Immunization Practices (ACIP), American Academy of Pediatrics (AAP), and American Academy of Family Physicians (AAFP).

before administering a live-virus vaccine to patients who have received high-dose systemic steroids for 2 weeks or longer.

Children with human immunodeficiency virus (HIV) infection and those born to mothers with HIV infection should receive all routine vaccinations except OPV and varicella vaccine. Inactivated polio vaccine should be used for these infants. MMR, although indicated in the asymptomatic HIV-infected individual, should be withheld in the severely immunocompromised HIV-infected patient. In the case of severely immunocompromised (non–HIV related) children, they should receive all routine vaccinations except OPV, MMR, and varicella vaccine. It is recommended that children with HIV or those who are severely immunocompromised receive both pneumococcal and influenza vaccines. Varicella virus vaccine should not be given to individuals receiving immunosuppressive therapy except for children with acute lymphocytic leukemia in remission.

Contraindications

Providers' knowledge of relative and absolute contraindications is variable. Some of the most common invalid contraindications are mild illness, such as a low-grade fever, upper respiratory infection (URI), colds, otitis media, and mild diarrhea. Children with mild acute illnesses can and should be vaccinated. Several large studies have shown that young children with URI, otitis media, diarrhea, and/or fever respond as well to measles vaccine as those without these conditions. Furthermore, there is no evidence that mild diarrhea reduces the success of polio immunization of infants in this country. Low-grade fever by itself is not a contraindication to immunization. Other factors that are invalid contraindications to vaccination include concurrent antibiotic therapy, disease exposure or convalescence, pregnancy in the household, and breast feeding of the infant. The only family history that is relevant in the decision to vaccinate a child is immunosuppression.

TABLE 13–3.   Guide to Contraindications and Precautions to Immunizations

Vaccine	True Contraindications and Precautions		Not True (Vaccines may be given)
General for all vaccines (DTP/DTaP, OPV, IPV, MMR, Hib, HBV, VZV)	Anaphylactic reaction to a vaccine contraindicates further doses of that vaccine		Mild to moderate local reaction (soreness, redness, swelling) following a dose of an injectable antigen
	Anaphylactic reaction to a vaccine constituent contraindicates the use of vaccines containing that substance		
	Moderate or severe illnesses with or without a fever		Mild acute illness with or without low-grade fever
			Current antimicrobial therapy
			Convalescent phase of illness
			Prematurity (same dosage and indications as for normal full-term infants), except HBV
			Recent exposure to an infectious disease
			History of penicillin or other nonspecific allergies or fact that relatives have such allergies
DTP/DTaP	Encephalopathy within 7 days of administration of previous dose of DTP		Temperature of <40.5°C (105°F) following a previous dose of DTP
	Precautions*	Fever of >40.5°C (105°F) within 48 hrs after vaccination with a prior dose of DTP	Family history of convulsions**
		Collapse or shocklike state (hypotonic-hyporesponsive episode) within 48 hrs of receiving a prior dose of DTP	Family history of sudden infant death syndrome
		Seizures within 3 days of receiving a prior dose of DTP (see footnote** regarding management of children with a personal history of seizures at any time)	Family history of an adverse event following DTP administration
		Persistent, inconsolable crying lasting >3 hrs, within 48 hrs of receiving a prior dose of DTP	

Table continued on following page

TABLE 13–3. Guide to Contraindications and Precautions to Immunizations *Continued*

Vaccine	True Contraindications and Precautions	Not True (Vaccines may be given)
OPV***	Infection with HIV or a household contact with HIV	Breast feeding
	Known immunodeficiency (hematologic and solid tumors; congenital immunodeficiency; and long-term immunosuppressive therapy)	Current antimicrobial therapy
	Immunodeficient household contact	Diarrhea
	Precaution* Pregnancy	
IPV	Anaphylactic reaction to neomycin or streptomycin	
	Precaution* Pregnancy	
MMR***	Anaphylactic reactions to egg ingestion and to neomycin****	Tuberculosis or positive PPD
	Pregnancy	Simultaneous TB skin testing*****
	Known immunodeficiency (hematologic and solid tumors: congenital immunodeficiency; and long-term immunosuppressive therapy)	Pregnancy of mother of recipient
	Precaution* Recent IG administration	Immunodeficient family member or household contact
		Infection with HIV
		Nonanaphylactic reactions to eggs or neomycin
VZV	Anaphylactic reactions to neomycin	Pregnancy of mother of recipient
	Pregnancy	Immunodeficient family member or household contact
	Known immunodeficiency	Nonanaphylactic reactions to neomycin
	Infection with HIV	
	Precaution* Recent immune globulin administration	
Hib		
HBV	Anaphylaxis to baker's yeast	Pregnancy

*The events or conditions listed as precautions, although not contraindications, should be carefully reviewed. The benefits and risks of administering a specific vaccine to an individual under the circumstances should be considered. If the risks are believed to outweigh the benefits, the immunization should be withheld; if the benefits are believed to outweigh the risks (for example, during an outbreak or foreign travel), the immunization should be given. Whether and when to administer DTP to children with proven or suspected underlying neurologic disorders should be decided on an individual basis. It is prudent on theoretical grounds to avoid vaccinating pregnant women. However, if immediate protection against poliomyelitis is needed, OPV, not IPV, is recommended.

**Acetaminophen given prior to administering DTP and thereafter every 4 hours for 24 hours should be considered for children with a personal or with a family history of convulsions in siblings or parents.

***There is a theoretical risk that the administration of multiple live virus vaccines (OPV and MMR) within 30 days of one another if not given on the same day will result in a suboptimal immune response. There are no data to substantiate this.

****Persons with a history of anaphylactic reactions following egg ingestion should be vaccinated only with extreme caution. Protocols have been developed for vaccinating such persons and should be consulted (J Pediatr 1983;102:196–9, J Pediatr 1988;113:504–6).

*****Measles vaccination may temporarily suppress tuberculin reactivity. If testing cannot be done the day of MMR vaccination, the test should be postponed for 4–6 weeks.

This information is based on the recommendations of the Advisory Committee on Immunization Practices (ACIP) and those of the Committee on Infectious Diseases (Red Book Committee) of the American Academy of Pediatrics (AAP). Sometimes these recommendations vary from those contained in the manufacturers' package inserts. For more detailed information, providers should consult the published recommendations of the ACIP and the AAFP, and the manufacturers' package inserts.

OPV should not be given to a child with a personal or family history of immunosuppression, because the vaccine virus could spread to the immunosuppressed contact.

Nonspecific allergies and nonsevere allergies are frequently observed invalid contraindications. Infants and children with nonspecific allergies, duck or feather allergy, allergy to penicillin, relatives with allergies, and children taking allergy shots can be immunized. Children with egg allergies that are not anaphylactic in type should be vaccinated in the usual manner with MMR vaccine. Table 13–3 summarizes the true and invalid contraindications.

TABLE 13–4. Schedule of Accelerated Immunizations for Children Under Age 7

Visit	1	2	3	4	
Timing	≥ or = to 4 mo of age	1 mo after first visit	1 mo after second visit	≥6 mo after third visit	Age 4–6 yrs
Vaccines					
Diphtheria Tetanus Pertussis	DTaP/DTP[a]	DTaP/DTP[a]	DTaP/DTP[a]	DTaP/DTP[a]	DTaP/DTP[a,b]
Haemophilus influenzae type b	Hib[a,c]	Hib[a,c]	Hib[a,c]	Hib[a,c]	
Hepatitis B	HepB-1	HepB-2		HepB-3	
Polio (OPV)	OPV	OPV	OPV		OPV[b]
Polio (IPV)	IPV[e]	IPV[e]		IPV[e]	
Measles Mumps Rubella	MMR (if child is greater than 12 months)				MMR (second dose may be given at 11–12 years)
Varicella zoster	VZV[d] (if greater than 12 months)				

[a]Two DTP and Hib combination vaccines are available (DTP/HbOC(TETRAMUNE); and PRP-T (ActHIB, OmniHIB), which can be reconstituted with DTP vaccine produced by Connaught). DTaP preparations are currently recommended only for use as the fourth and/or fifth doses of the DTP series among children 15 months through 6 years of age (before the 7th birthday). DTP and DTaP should not be used on or after the 7th birthday.

[b]If the fourth dose of DTP or DTaP or the third dose of OPV is given after 4 years of age, this booster dose is not indicated.

[c]The recommended schedule varies by vaccine manufacturer. For information specific to the vaccine being used, consult the package insert and ACIP recommendations. Children beginning the Hib vaccine series at age 2–6 months should receive a primary series of three doses of HbOC (HibTITER) (Lederle-Praxis), PRP-T (ActHIB) (Pasteur Merieux; SmithKline Beecham; Connaught), or a licensed DTP-Hib combination vaccine; or two doses of PRP-OMP (PedvaxHIB) (Merck, Sharp, and Dohme). An additional booster dose of any licensed Hib conjugate vaccine should be administered at 12–15 months of age and at least 2 months after the previous dose. Children beginning the Hib vaccine series at 7–11 months of age should receive a primary series of two doses of an HbOC, PRP-T, or PRP-OMP-containing vaccine. An additional booster dose of any licensed Hib conjugate vaccine should be administered at 12–18 months of age and at least 2 months after the previous dose. Children beginning the Hib vaccine series at ages 12–14 months should receive a primary series of one dose of an HbOC, PRP-T, or PRP-OMP-containing vaccine. An additional booster dose of any licensed Hib conjugate vaccine should be administered 2 months after the previous dose. Children beginning the Hib vaccine series at ages 15–59 months should receive one dose of any licensed Hib vaccine. Hib vaccine should not be administered after the fifth birthday except for special circumstances as noted in the specific ACIP recommendations for the use of Hib vaccine.

[d]VZV vaccine should be given as soon as child is 12–18 months of age. Omit dose if child is greater than 18 months of age and has a history of chickenpox. Children under age 13 years should receive a single 0.5-ml dose.

[e]IPV is used for polio immunization; the interval between the first two doses should be at least 4 weeks, but preferably 8 weeks. The third dose should follow in at least 6 months, but preferable nearer to 12 months.

Accelerated Schedules

A common problem for providers is determining which vaccinations children need when they are behind schedule. Table 13–4 is the recommended accelerated immunization schedule for infants at least 4 months of age and children younger than 7 years of age who start the series late or who are more than 1 month behind in the immunization schedule (i.e., children for whom compliance with scheduled return visits cannot be ensured). Table 13–5 is the recommended immunization schedule for children older than 7 years of age not vaccinated at the recommended time in early infancy.

TABLE 13–5. Schedule of Accelerated Immunizations for Children over Age 7

Visit	1	2	3	Additional Visits
Timing		4–8 wks after first visit	6 mo after second visit	

Vaccines

	1	2	3	Additional Visits
Tetanus	Td[a]	Td[a]	Td[a]	Td (repeat every 10 yr throughout life)
Diphtheria				
Polio (OPV)	OPV[b]	OPV[b]	OPV[b]	
Polio (IPV)	IPV	IPV	IPV	
Measles	MMR[c]	MMR[c]		
Mumps				
Rubella				
Hepatitis B	HepB-1	HepB-2	HepB-3	
Varicella zoster	VZV[d]			

[a]The DTP and DTaP doses administered to children <7 years of age who remain incompletely vaccinated at age ≥7 years should be counted as prior exposure to tetanus and diphtheria toxoid (e.g., a child who previously received two doses of DTP needs only one dose of Td to complete a primary series for tetanus and diphtheria). Td is tetanus and diphtheria toxoid for use among persons ≥7 years of age.

[b]When polio vaccine is administered to previously unvaccinated persons ≥18 years of age, inactivated polio virus vaccine (IPV) is preferred. See specific ACIP statement on the use of polio vaccine.

[c]The ACIP recommends a second dose of measles-containing vaccine (preferably MMR to assure immunity to mumps and rubella for certain groups. Children with no documentation of live measles vaccination after the first birthday should receive two doses of live measles-containing vaccine not less than 1 month apart. The second dose may be given at 11–12 years of age.

[d]Varicella zoster virus vaccine (VZV) is recommended for children who lack a reliable history of chickenpox. Children under 13 years of age should receive a single 0.5-ml dose; persons 13 years of age and older should receive two 0.5-ml doses 4–8 weeks apart.

SUGGESTED READING

American Academy of Pediatrics, Committee on Infectious Diseases. 1994 Red Book: Report of the Committee on Infectious Diseases, 23rd ed. Elk Grove Village, IL, American Academy of Pediatrics, 1994.

General recommendations on immunization. Recommendations of the Advisory Committee on Immunization Practices (ACIP). MMWR 1994;43:1–38.

Immunization of adolescents. Recommendations of the Advisory Committee on Immunization Practices (ACIP). MMWR November 22, 1996;45.

Prevention of varicella. Recommendations of the Advisory Committee on Immunization Practices (ACIP). MMWR July 12, 1996;45.

Standards for pediatric immunization practices. Recommended by the National Vaccine Advisory Committee. Approved by the U.S. Public Health Service. MMWR April 23, 1993; 42.

Update: Vaccine side effects, adverse reactions, contraindications, and precautions. Recommendations of the Advisory Committee on Immunization Practices (ACIP). MMWR Sept. 6, 1996;45.

Zimmerman RK, Clover RD. Adult immunizations: A practical approach for clinicians. Parts I and II. Am Fam Physician 1995;51(4):859–867 and 51(5):1139–1148.

QUESTIONS

1. Which of the following vaccines is contraindicated in a 15-month-old with asymptomatic HIV infection?
   a. MMR
   b. DTaP
   c. OPV
   d. Conjugated Hib

2. A 2-month-old presents to your office for a routine well-baby visit in December. The infant has received no prior immunizations. The infant was a product of a term gestation that was uncomplicated. Upon taking the family history, you discover that the mother's father is living in the household and is undergoing chemotherapy for lymphoma. Which of the following combination of vaccines would you administer to the infant?
   a. Hep-B, DTaP/Hib, IPV
   b. Hep-B, DTaP/Hib, OPV
   c. Hep-B, DTaP/Hib, IPV, influenza
   d. Hep-B, DTaP/Hib, OPV, influenza

3. During the 1990s, paralytic poliomyelitis in the United States
   a. Occurred in contacts of individuals importing the disease from India
   b. Occurred in individuals living along the Texas/Mexico border from endemic wild-type virus
   c. Occurred in household contacts of recipients of OPV
   d. All the above

4. A true contraindication to receiving MMR is
   a. Immunocompromised family member
   b. A positive PPD result
   c. Pregnancy
   d. Nonanaphylactic reactions to eggs

Answers appear on **page 603.**

Part II

CASE STUDIES

Chapter 14

Weight Loss and Diarrhea

Susan M. Miller, M.D., M.P.H.

INITIAL VISIT

Subjective

PATIENT IDENTIFICATION. Robert is a 36-year-old divorced white attorney who has come to the office for a new patient visit because of a change in his group insurance policy.

PRESENTING PROBLEM. Robert had been in good health until 3 months ago, when he noticed unintentional weight loss, persistent diarrhea, and fatigue.

PRESENT ILLNESS. After a camping trip to Colorado Springs, Robert experienced crampy, watery diarrhea four to five times a day. His diarrhea was not melanotic, and it was not exacerbated by eating. He has not experienced incontinence, nausea, vomiting, or abdominal pain. The stool is semisolid to watery, malodorous, and not relieved with bismuth subsalicylate (Pepto-Bismol) or over-the-counter loperamide (Imodium A-D). He complains of a dry mouth, halitosis, and soreness of the tongue when he drinks orange juice. He estimates that he has lost 15 lb in the last 6 weeks, although his appetite is ravenous. He notes early satiety.

For the last month he has had to take a nap when he arrives home from work. Instead of sleeping 6 hours per night, he now needs 8 to 10 hours to feel rested the next morning.

PAST MEDICAL HISTORY. Robert had an appendectomy at age 11. At age 24 he was in a motor vehicle accident and underwent a splenectomy. He also sustained multiple rib fractures without pneumothorax. He received 4 units of blood. He does not remember his last tetanus immunization, nor does he remember a pneumococcal vaccination after his splenectomy. He is allergic to sulfa drugs (rash). He takes multiple vitamins and denies using laxatives or cathartics routinely. He received treatment for syphilis and gonorrhea 10 years ago. He may have had a herpes infection of the penis. He has been treated for hemorrhoids. He denies hepatitis. He drinks two six-packs of beer per week. He has never used intravenous drugs, but he does smoke marijuana occasionally. He has borrowed sleeping pills and alprazolam (Xanax) from a friend when he feels "stressed out." He tried "crack" once but felt his heart race and did not enjoy it. On further questioning, he admits to the use of "poppers."

FAMILY HISTORY. His father, a retired attorney, is in good health and is on no medications at age 77. His mother, age 67, works for an insurance company and is in good health. She had a hysterectomy 20 years ago for bleeding. His paternal grandfather died in World War I, and his paternal grandmother died in 1938 of tuberculosis. His maternal grandparents both died in their eighties from natural causes. Robert is an only child.

SOCIAL HISTORY. Robert divorced his wife 7 years ago after being married less than 1 year. They met while he was in law school. She lives in another state, and they had no children. He is currently involved in a monogamous relationship of 6 months' duration. He has had over 20 sexual partners, and he has performed both receptive and insertive anal intercourse. Although he and his current partner are practicing safe sex, neither is aware of their human immunodeficiency virus (HIV) antibody status.

His last heterosexual contact was with his wife 7 years ago. She was his only female sexual partner.

He just made partner in his law firm and earns in excess of $500,000 per year. His area of expertise is discrimination.

REVIEW OF SYSTEMS. Robert notes that two or three nights per week he has to change his bedding because of night sweats. In the afternoon he frequently has a low-grade fever. He denies headache, scotomata, cough, shortness of breath, dyspnea on exertion, nausea, vomiting, abdominal pain, dysuria, or paresthesias. He notes that his skin is drier and that he has had a scaling rash on his forehead, scalp, and chest for the last 9 months. He has two pet cats in good health. He travels overseas one to two times yearly. His most recent trip was to Thailand. He notes increasing insomnia, even though he is sleeping more hours per night. He has been having nightmares about death, and his friends have been teasing him about his memory lapses. He runs three to four times per week and he lifts weights at the gym 2 to 3 days per week. He enjoys swimming, racquetball, and tennis. Last year he ran a half-marathon.

Objective

PHYSICAL EXAMINATION. Robert is a muscular 195-lb man. His blood pressure is 105/60 mm Hg, pulse 58, respiratory rate 12, temperature 99.5°F. HEENT: pupils equally round and reactive to light (PERRL), extraocular movements intact (EOMI), cotton-wool spot O.S., and oral candidiasis. Lymphadenopathy: He has anterior and posterior chain cervical adenopathy. Thyroid: Normal. Lungs: Clear to auscultation. Cardiovascular: Sinus bradycardia without a murmur. Abdomen: Well-healed midline and McBurney incisions without hepatomegaly. Bowel sounds are present and normoactive. No guarding or rebound. No CVAT. Rectal: Decreased rectal tone with hemorrhoids. Guaiac negative. Genitourinary: Circumcised male with condyloma on the glans. Skin: Xerosis and seborrheic dermatitis of the face and scalp. Tinea cruris and pedis are present. Onychomycosis of the left hallux. Neurologic: Normal. No cognitive deficit noted on screening examination.

Assessment

DIFFERENTIAL DIAGNOSES

1. *Hyperthyroidism* is unlikely given the presence of bradycardia and a normal thyroid gland.

2. *Lipid storage disease* as an etiology of his lymph-adenopathy, such as Gaucher or Niemann-Pick disease, is unlikely secondary to the acute onset of symptoms and age presentation.

3. *Diabetes mellitus* could be considered. Robert's complaints of weight loss, voracious appetite, and dry mouth are consistent with hyperglycemia. His halitosis may represent ketosis. In fact, the diarrhea may have precipitated the clinical onset of diabetes mellitus. A serum glucose determination would be helpful.

4. An essential aspect of this patient's evaluation was obtaining the sexual history. This information has provided clues to various high-risk sexual and social behaviors. His clinical examination provides findings suggestive of *immunosuppression,* such as oral candidiasis, seborrheic dermatitis, and atypical lymphadenopathy. An infectious cause for his diarrhea and weight loss should be considered.

5. *Lymphoma* also must be considered and is consistent with weight loss, fatigue, night sweats, fever, and atypical lymphadenopathy. Lymphoma of the gastrointestinal tract also may cause protracted diarrhea. The types of lymphoma may include Hodgkin lymphoma and T- or B-cell lymphoma. The location of his lymphadenopathy provides an important clue to the differential diagnosis. In case of lymphadenopathy, it is important to assess the node location, patient's age, associated clinical symptoms, and physical characteristics of the lymph node (asymmetry, size, tenderness, texture, mobility). Under normal conditions in an adult patient, the inguinal nodes can range in size from 0.5 to 2.0 cm. Particular attention must be paid to anterior cervical, posterior cervical, occipital, axillary, and supraclavicular adenopathy.

In addition to a malignant cause of his lymph-adenopathy, infectious causes also must be considered. These can include (1) viral (hepatitis B virus [HBV], HIV, cytomegalovirus [CMV], and Epstein-Barr virus [EBV]); (2) bacterial (*Salmonella,* cat-scratch disease); (3) fungal (histoplasmosis, coccidioidomycosis); (4) mycobacterial (*Mycobacterium avium-intracellulare, Mycobacterium tuberculosis*); and (5) parasitic (toxoplasmosis) infections.

Not all lymph node enlargement is associated with local inflammation. However, Robert's clinical findings are not consistent with immunologic diseases such as rheumatoid arthritis, serum sickness, drug reactions, or systemic lupus erythematosus (although he does have a facial rash).

6. Based on his sexual and clinical history, *HIV infection* must be considered. All his clinical and physical findings are consistent with HIV infection.

In addition, he could have lymphoma in the presence of HIV infection, more specifically B- and T-cell lymphoma (versus Hodgkin lymphoma). Furthermore, although he does not have suggestive cutaneous or mucocutaneous findings, Kaposi sarcoma also may present as lymphadenopathy. In HIV infection, it is the presence of extrainguinal adenopathy that is considered clinically significant.

Plan

LABORATORY AND SPECIAL TESTS

1. During the initial patient visit, it is reasonable to obtain stool studies for ova and parasites, stool guaiac, and culture and sensitivites to look for a treatable cause of Robert's diarrhea.

2. A complete blood count, chemistry profile, and urinalysis would be helpful. Anemia may be present secondary to malabsorption, hemolysis, lymphoma, or HIV infection. In patients with advanced HIV infection or lymphoma, an absolute lymphocytopenia can be present. Eosinophilia can occur in parasitic infections or malignancies. The chemistry profile might reveal hyperglycemia, azotemia, hypokalemia, hypo- or hypernatremia, hyperuricemia, hypergammaglobulinemia, or liver enzyme elevation.

3. HIV antibody testing should be obtained in a confidential manner (Table 14–1). Before a serologic sample is drawn, Robert must be informed about the consequences of serologic testing and be assured of confidentiality. Pretest counseling includes a review of his risk behaviors, virus transmission, the incubation and latency period(s) of HIV infection, what positive and negative tests mean, reasons for false-positive and false-negative test results (Table 14–2), and how to reduce high-risk behaviors. At some testing sites, an informed consent and demographic form are completed. Finally, a follow-up appointment is made for the release of the test results.

If referral is needed for community services, this information can then be provided. At this time the patient may experience significant anxiety and a sense of fatality. Support services are essential. Risk assessment for potential suicide may be warranted.

DISPOSITION. Stool studies, a complete blood count, a chemistry profile, and HIV antibody test (enzyme-linked immunosorbent assay [ELISA] and Western blot) were obtained. The patient was scheduled for a follow-up visit within the week.

TABLE 14–1. Adult Human Immunodeficiency Virus (HIV) Serologic Testing: United States Recommendations

Pretest and Post-test Counseling

Pretest and post-test counseling must address the following issues: determination of individual potential risk status (past, current, future); implications of positive, negative, and indeterminate test results; pregnancy and contraception issues; behavior modification to reduce risk; low-risk sexual activities; and referral to appropriate agencies for follow-up.

Note: Pretest and post-test counseling provides an opportunity to tailor risk-reduction education. Health care providers may wish to consider the use of an informed consent form. Finally, a sample that is repetitively positive needs to be confirmed by an independent antibody assay.

Anonymous or Confidential Testing

A system must be implemented that has the ability to protect the anonymity and confidentiality of the test specimens and results. Preferably, results of testing are given in a face-to-face encounter.

Note: If testing is performed in a private office, the physician may wish to use numerically coded samples. If this is not feasible, use of alternative testing sites may be advisable.

Voluntary Versus Mandatory Testing

Although voluntary testing is preferable, in certain situations, mandatory testing is performed.

Mandatory testing: Testing of blood, plasma, sperm, and organ donation. Mandatory testing also occurs within the military and in specific legal interactions.

Voluntary testing: Previous or current high-risk behavior, pregnancy, prior blood transfusion, occupational exposure, new-onset tuberculosis, syphilis, and public health surveillance. Voluntary testing is also used to confirm a clinical diagnosis.

Interpretation of Results (Post-exposure)

A negative enzyme-linked immunosorbent assay screen and absence of antibody bands on the Western immunoblot test at 3, 6, 9, and 12 mo provide evidence that no immune response to HIV has occurred. Indeterminate test results require observation and repeat testing. HIV-1 RNA viral load testing may have a role in confirmation, or delineating primary infection.

Modified from Rakel RE. Textbook of Family Practice. Philadelphia, WB Saunders, 1995.

FIRST FOLLOW-UP VISIT

Subjective

Robert's diarrhea persisted. He was extremely anxious to know the test results and brought his significant other to the clinic to hear the findings.

Objective

Robert has lost an additional 2 lb. His stool studies revealed the presence of *Giardia lamblia*. His white

TABLE 14–2. Potential Sources of False-Positive or False-Negative Antibody Tests

False-positive	False-negative
Populations with low seroprevalence	Prior to host antibody response (i.e., "window period")
Passive transfer of antibody in immunoglobulin preparations	Late infection, resulting from deterioration of host antibody response
Cross-reactive antibodies secondary to multiple blood transfusions, serum proteins (cryoglobulins, rheumatoid factor), other retroviruses, or human leukocyte antigens (HLA class I and II)	Laboratory error*
Transplacental transfer of maternal antibody	
Laboratory error*	

* Laboratory error may include misinterpretation of weakly positive bands or the incorrect application of interpretive criteria.
Modified from Rakel RE. Textbook of Family Practice. Philadelphia, WB Saunders, 1995.

blood cell count (WBC) was 8200/mm³; hemoglobin (Hg) and hematocrit (Hct) were 11.7/34.1 respectively; platelet count was 94,000/mm³. Serum glucose was 104 mg/dl; potassium, 3.4 mEq/L; total protein, 9.1 g/dl; and cholesterol, 108 mg/dl. Both the ELISA and Western blot tests were positive.

Assessment

1. *G. lamblia* infection

2. Mild hypokalemia secondary to diarrhea

3. Decreased serum cholesterol

4. HIV infection with probable decreased CD4 lymphocyte counts and elevated HIV-1 RNA viral load

5. Elevated total protein probably secondary to B-cell activation as a result of HIV infection.

Plan

1. Metronidazole 500 mg orally three times daily for 7 to 10 days.

2. A chest radiograph to rule out occult tuberculosis and to serve as a baseline should future pulmonary symptoms develop.

3. Placement of a purified protein derivative (PPD) skin test and *Candida* control.

4. Assessment of his immunologic status. This can be achieved by obtaining CD4 lymphocyte subsets. A p24 antigen, β2-microglobulin, and CMV/EBV serology are not necessary at this time.

5. HIV-1 RNA viral load. Even with a normal CD4 lymphocyte count, patients with elevated viral loads are at increased risk of disease progression (Mellors et al., 1996).

6. Updating his immunization status. Tetanus toxoid, pneumovax, and annual influenza vaccines are considered standard. Hepatitis B vaccine may be considered if continued high-risk behavior is anticipated or if the patient is a health care worker. The HIB vaccine also should be administered. Live vaccines are generally avoided. Patients with low CD4 counts may not be able to mount an effective antibody response.

7. Toxoplasmosis IgG antibody. An HIV-infected person who is IgG seropositive has a 20 to 35 per cent chance of disease reactivation. Robert is at risk for exposure secondary to his travel and pet history.

8. A patient with positive serology for syphilis requires aggressive follow-up. Syphilis may be a co-factor for disease progression in HIV infection. In addition, syphilis is difficult to treat in the presence of immunosuppression and may more rapidly progress to the tertiary stage.

9. Female patients may require a pregnancy test and Pap smear. HIV infection is often overlooked in female patients and should be considered part of a differential diagnosis for sexually transmitted diseases (STDs), atypical Pap smears, unresolving gynecologic infections, pregnancy, atypical dermatologic problems, multiple sexual partners, history of blood transfusions (or spouse with a blood transfusion), rape, or substance abuse.

10. Safe-sex guidelines must be reviewed. HIV may be transmitted with oral sex. Contact tracing of known sexual partners (including his former wife) should be initiated.

11. Robert may need re-referral to community support groups. He also may wish to consider updating his will and power of attorney and obtaining a living will.

SECOND FOLLOW-UP VISIT

Subjective

Robert's diarrhea has resolved, although the metronidazole imparted a metallic taste to his food. His anxiety is diminished, but he still has not told his ex-wife about his serologic status.

His thrush is better. He noted mild fatigue, myalgias, and fever after receiving his vaccinations.

Objective

Chest x-ray study, rapid plasma reagin (RPR), *Toxoplasma* titer, and hepatitis B surface antigen/antibody were all negative. His total WBC was 8300/ mm^3 with a differential of 45 per cent polymorphonuclear lymphocytes (PMNs), 40 per cent lymphocytes, 0 per cent atypical lymphocytes, 3 per cent monocytes, 1 per cent eoosinophils, and 1 per cent basophils. His Hg/Hct were 11.4/34.6. His platelet count was 94,000/mm^3. His percentage CD4 lymphocyte count was 14 per cent and percentage CD8 lymphocyte count was 37 per cent. His PPD skin test was measured at 6-mm induration. His viral load was 100,000 copies per ml.

Assessment

1. The anemia and thrombocytopenia are probably related to Robert's HIV infection. The thrombocytopenia likely has an autoimmune etiology and is occurring in the presence of an asplenic patient. His WBC of 8300/mm^3 does not reflect acute infection, since his differential is normal and the count is relatively elevated for a patient with HIV infection. This "spuriously high" WBC is most likely secondary to asplenia. Therefore, his CD4 lymphocyte count of 465 cells/mm^3 is relatively high for the number of clinical symptoms he is having; hence his CD4 percentage is a better surrogate marker for the degree of immunosuppression. Any viral load greater than 10,000 copies/ml mandates aggressive therapy.

2. Robert is a candidate for antiretroviral therapy (Table 14–3). His CD4 lymphocyte count is between 200 and 500, and he is symptomatic for immunosuppression. His thrombocytopenia might improve with therapy.

3. In addition, Robert is also a candidate for *Pneumocystis carinii* pneumonia (PCP) prophylaxis (Table 14–4), since his CD4 percentage is less than 20 per cent. Since he is allergic to sulfa (e.g., Bactrim/Septra), Robert should receive dapsone (50 mg per day) or aerosolized pentamidine (300 mg every month). He should tolerate this fairly well, although his tobacco and marijuana use need to be curtailed, since these increase his risk of bronchospasm.

TABLE 14–3. Indications for Antiretroviral Therapy

Absolute	Probable
Prior opportunistic infection or AIDS-defining illness	Moderate-risk occupational exposure
Second- or third-trimester pregnancy in HIV-infected mother (Connor et al., 1994)	Viral load greater than 10,000 copies per ml (no matter the CD4 lymphocyte count)
Repeat pregnancy in HIV-infected mother	Primary infection (acute seroconversion)
An absolute CD4 lymphocyte count less than 200 cells/mm^3	High-risk sexual encounter with HIV-positive partner (rape, condom breakage)
An absolute CD4 lymphocyte count less than 500 cells/mm^3 (or a CD4+ percentage less than 25%)	
Symptomatic HIV disease (oral hairy leukoplakia, weight loss, recurrent fever, recurrent mucosal candidiasis)	
High-risk occupational exposure	

AIDS = Acquired immunodeficiency syndrome; HIV = human immunodeficiency virus.

4. Since his PPD skin test was less than 5-mm induration, isoniazid prophylaxis was not initiated.

DISPOSITION. Triple-combination antiretroviral therapy using two nucleoside analogues and a protease inhibitor was initiated. His viral load of 100,000 RNA copies per ml, symptomatic disease, and decreased CD4+ lymphocyte count places him at the highest risk of disease progression (Mellors et al., 1996).

The choice of initial therapy is based on severity of disease status, medication cross-resistance, baseline potential for resistance, concomitant medical conditions, side effects, and compliance. Monotherapy is a suboptimal regimen (Carpenter, 1996).

Robert was educated about potential side effects of the medications and what clinical symptoms warranted a return visit to the clinic. He also was edu-

TABLE 14–4. Indications for *Pneumocystis carinii* Pneumonia Prophylaxis

An absolute CD4 lymphocyte count less than 200 cells/mm^3 (CD4 percentage less than 20%)
Prior *Pneumocystis carinii* pneumonia
Unexplained or persistent fever or oropharyngeal candidiasis
Rapidly declining CD4 lymphocyte counts

Modified from Rakel RE. Essentials of Family Practice. Philadelphia, WB Saunders, 1993, p 246.

cated about local research study sites and potential future medications. Alternative treatment regimens were discussed. He was asked to keep a question diary of things he heard or read for future discussions. Arrangements were made for his ex-wife and current partner to receive serologic testing.

The preceding information was obtained (Table 14–5). A follow-up visit was scheduled in 1 week. Metronidazole and clotrimazole (Mycelex) troches were prescribed. Alcohol was prohibited. Reassurances and support were provided.

Discussion

HIV is a chronic, persistent viral infection. Before the effective initiation of antiretroviral therapy, the

TABLE 14–5. Suggested Protocol for Ambulatory Management of Human Immunodeficiency Virus (HIV) Infection

Establish an index of suspicion.
Evaluate past and current transmission risk.
Accurate assessment of HIV serology (e.g., sequential ELISA and Western blot testing).
Determine stage of infection.
Document baseline physical examination.
Record HIV-directed review of systems.
Update immunization status (dT, Pneumovax, annual influenza vaccine; consider HBV and HIB vaccines). *Note:* Prior BCG vaccination is not a contraindication to placement of a PPD. Review childhood infections and immunizations.
Laboratory evaluation:
  Baseline: Complete blood count, chemistry profile, chest radiograph, PPD with control, toxoplasmosis IgG antibody, rapid plasma reagin, absolute CD4 lymphocyte count and percentage, viral load.
  Other (based on clinical presentation): Hepatitis serology (A, B, C), cryptococcal antigen, stool for ova and parasites or cultures, sputum for AFB, Pap smear, pregnancy test, STD tests, drug screening, biopsy, blood culture for AFB.
Document drug allergies.
Consider antiretroviral and opportunistic infection prophylaxis therapy.
Safe-sex counseling.
Consider research protocols.
Document unconventional therapies.
Document living will and power of attorney status.
Obtain illicit drug history.
Refer to community resources.
Aggressive work-up of symptoms.
Assess compliance with current therapies.

AFB = acid-fast bacilli; BCG = bacille Calmette-Guérin; dT = diphtheria and tetanus toxoids, adult type; HBV = hepatitis B virus vaccine; HIB = haemophilus influenzae type B vaccine; O & P = ova and parasites; PPD = purified protein derivative of tuberculin; RPR = rapid plasma reagin; STD = sexually transmitted diseases.
Modified from Rakel RE. Essentials of Family Practice. Philadelphia, WB Saunders, 1993, p 246.

average length of time from infection to the onset of an AIDS-defining illness was approximately 10 years. Frequently, patients feel that HIV infection implies that they have AIDS and death is imminent. This fear of death supersedes the concept of HIV being a chronic illness and contributes to states of acute and severe anxiety. Fortunately new therapies developed within the last few years have significantly improved the long- and short-term prognosis of HIV infection.

The two most difficult decisions in the antiretroviral management of HIV infection are deciding when to initiate therapy and whether to change therapy. Although a complete understanding of HIV infection and pathogenesis is incomplete, the number of treatment alternatives have rapidly increased. Although there is no single treatment recommendation that can be prescribed for all HIV-infected individuals, the ability to prolong patients' lives has markedly improved with the availability of combination reverse transcriptase and protease inhibitor therapies.

HIV undergoes replication during all stages of disease in almost all patients; complete viral dormancy has been disproved (Ho et al., 1995). Even after the host generates cell-mediated and humoral antibody responses, only a partial reduction in viral load is observed. Significant numbers of virus continue to be produced, even if the host appears to be clinically asymptomatic. Viral load levels can be measured and exist in a "steady-state" representing an equilibrium between viral production, viral clearance, and host immune responses. The level of viral load is predictive of the rate of CD4 lymphocyte decline and time of progression to AIDS (Mellors et al., 1996). HIV-1 RNA levels reflect rates of active viral replication and CD4 lymphocyte destruction. Even in an advanced disease state, the host maximally reproduces CD4 lymphocytes. Unless antiretroviral therapy completely blocks HIV replication, CD4+ cells are subsequently destroyed. If antiretroviral therapy is discontinued, high-level viral replication resumes.

Historically the management of HIV infection involved the use of single chemotherapeutic agents, such as zidovudine monotherapy. Limiting factors of previous treatment regimens were the time-limited durability and sequential emergence of viral resistance (Havlir and Richmann, 1996).

In general, new recommendations suggest that a high viral load mandates the initiation of therapy regardless of the CD4 lymphocyte count. Therapy should be initiated for all patients with CD4 lymphocyte counts less than 500 cells/mm^3, and should probably be initiated for all patients with CD4 lymphocyte counts of greater than 500 cells/mm³ if they have an elevated HIV RNA viral load (i.e., viral load greater than 10,000 copies per ml) (Carpenter et al., 1996).

Aggressive initial therapy is currently defined as the use of a protease inhibitor in any treatment regimen. Because previous therapeutic recommendations did not prevent disease progression, patients were often reticent to consider therapy. New treatment alternatives using protease inhibitors are providing preliminary evidence that viral replication can be suppressed for substantially longer periods than that seen with previous monotherapy. These treated viral loads are below those seen in individuals who have historically remained clinically stable (i.e., long-term nonprogressors). Use of these combinations while the immune system is still functional may offer the best chance for long-term survival, especially in patients with impaired cellular and serologic responses to HIV.

Since the effectiveness of antiretroviral therapy is becoming more durable, a strong emphasis on patient education, patient autonomy, and patient responsibility regarding health is important. A medical treatment program may be divided into three components: (1) HIV infection, (2) opportunistic infections and malignancies, and (3) immune reconstitution. To date, antiretroviral therapy and op-portunistic infection management have had the most clinical success. Examples of available antiretroviral medications include reverse transcriptase inhibitors, protease inhibitors, and non-nucleoside reverse transcriptase inhibitors. Management of HIV-related opportunistic infections and malignancies include such medications as ganciclovir, foscarnet, cidofovir, fluconazole, itraconazole, valacyclovir, liposomal doxorubicin, intraocular implants, liposomal amphotericin B, atovaquone, clarithromycin, azithromycin, thalidomide, octreotide, paromomycin (to name a few). Immune reconstitution may be temporarily assisted with erythropoietin, granulocyte colony-stimulating factors, vaccinations, and interleukin-2.

Finally, management of substance abuse is essential. This includes not only the use of street drugs, but also the overprescribing of benzodiazepines and pain killers. These medications may cloud an individual's ability to think or modify behavior. The protease inhibitors increase the risk of medication toxicity and side effects when used in combination with prescribed medications. Referral to Alcoholics Anonymous or drug-treatment programs must be considered. It is extremely difficult to treat HIV infection in a person actively abusing drugs. Lack of compliance in this clinical situation increases the risk of resistance.

SUGGESTED READING

Carpenter CCJ, Fischl MA, Hammer SM, et al. Antiretroviral therapy for HIV infection in 1996: Recommendations of an international panel. JAMA 1996;276:146–154.

Connor EM, Sperling RS, Gelber R, et al. Reduction of maternal-infant transmission of human immunodeficiency virus type 1 with zidovudine treatment. N Engl J Med 1994;331:1173–1180.

Havlir DV, Richmann DD. Viral dynamics of HIV: Implications for drug development and therapeutic strategies. Ann Intern Med 1996;124:984–994.

Ho DD, Neumann AU, Perelson AS, et al. Rapid turnover of plasma virions and CD4 lymphocytes in HIV-1 infection. Nature 1995;373:123–126.

Mellors JW, Rinaldo CR Jr, Gupta P, et al. Prognosis in HIV-1 infection predicted by the quantity of virus in plasma. Science 1996;272:1167–1170.

Miller SM: Care of the adult HIV-1-infected patient. In Rakel RE (ed). Textbook of Family Practice, 5th ed. Philadelphia, WB Saunders Company, 1995, pp 292–410.

QUESTIONS

1. A false-positive HIV antibody test can occur under the following conditions:
   a. During the window period
   b. In patient populations with low seroprevalence
   c. Laboratory error
   d. Cross-reactive HLA antibodies

2. The following vaccinations are safe to give to HIV-infected adults:
   a. Measles

b. Hepatitis B
c. Influenza
d. Pneumococcal

3. Antiretroviral therapy should be initiated:
   a. During the first trimester of pregnancy
   b. When the viral load is greater than 100 copies per ml
   c. After any unprotected sexual intercourse
   d. When the CD4 lymphocyte count is less than 1000 cells/mm^3

e. All of the above
f. None of the above

4. Isoniazid prophylaxis is indicated when the PPD
   a. Induration is >15 mm
   b. Induration is >10 mm
   c. Induration is >5 mm
   d. Induration is >1 mm

Answers appear on **page 603**.

Chapter 15

Chronic Cough

Richard Neill, M.D.

CASE PRESENTATION

Subjective

Elaine R. is a 42-year-old woman who works as a schoolteacher and lives with her husband and two children. She presents to her family physician with a 6-month history of cough. A recent paroxysm of coughing prompted her to seek care.

She stated that the cough developed insidiously over the course of several months. There was no shortness of breath, wheezing, sputum production, fevers, sweats, weight loss, or sneezing. An antihistamine-decongestant combination had decreased the frequency of the cough only slightly. Over-the-counter cough preparations had no effect. The cough occurred throughout the day, with no predilection for morning, afternoon, or evening. She admitted having been awakened from sleep while coughing on several occasions over the preceding month. On these occasions she sometimes noted a sour taste in her mouth.

PAST MEDICAL HISTORY. Her past medical history revealed no chronic medical conditions. She had two uncomplicated pregnancies resulting in two healthy children by vaginal delivery in her twenties. After her second child she underwent semielective cholecystectomy for symptomatic cholelithiasis. A bilateral tubal ligation was performed at the same time. She denied any other surgery. She was on no medications and reported no drug or environmental allergies.

FAMILY HISTORY. All of her family were healthy throughout her illness. Neither she nor her husband smoke. She reported no recent travel outside her midwestern town.

Objective

PHYSICAL EXAMINATION. Her weight was 167 lb, height 5 feet 8 inches, blood pressure 118/77 mm Hg, pulse 65, and respirations 14.

Ear examination revealed normal external auditory canals and tympanic membranes. She had no sinus tenderness to percussion. Examination of the nose revealed normal-appearing mucosa and turbinates. The mouth and pharynx were unremarkable.

Neck examination revealed no thyromegaly, masses, or lymphadenopathy. Lung examination revealed no wheezing, rales, or rhonchi. The remainder of her examination was likewise unremarkable.

ASSESSMENT. Elaine was felt to have chronic cough due to gastroesophageal reflux disease (GERD). The absence of a smoking history combined with a "sour taste" in her mouth on history was felt to be sufficient evidence for a therapeutic trial before further evaluation.

PLAN. Elaine was informed of her probable diagnosis and educated regarding measures she should take to reduce the possibility of reflux. These included elevating the head of her bed by placing 4 inches of books under the legs of her bed frame near the head; eating smaller, more frequent meals; and avoiding meals for 2 hours before bedtime. She was also asked to begin taking ranitidine (Zantac), 75 mg by mouth, 2 hours before bedtime.

DIFFERENTIAL DIAGNOSIS. Because cough is a reflex triggered by cough receptors in well-defined locations throughout the body, understanding the location of cough receptors and the afferent limbs of the cough reflex arc can help guide the history and physical examination and in formulating the differential diagnosis. Cough receptors are located throughout the larynx, trachea, bronchi, ear canals, pleura, and stomach. All send afferent impulses via the vagus nerve to the cough centers located diffusely in the medulla. Receptors in the nose and sinuses send afferents via the trigeminal nerve, whereas receptors in the pharynx send afferents via the glossopharyngeal nerve. The pericardium and diaphragm also contain cough receptors that send afferent impulses via the phrenic nerve. The location of these receptors and reflex arcs makes the differential diagnosis of chronic cough easier to understand, and even predict.

Elaine certainly meets criteria for the diagnosis of chronic cough—undiagnosed cough persisting for 4 weeks or longer. Although this definition is somewhat arbitrary, it allows physicians to weed out the majority of causes of acute cough such as viral upper respiratory illness.

The most common causes for chronic cough differ according to the age and smoking status of the patient. For adult smokers, *chronic bronchitis* is the most common cause. This should be considered first in any smoker presenting with chronic cough. Chronic bronchitis generally produces moderate amounts of sputum, and is more prevalent on awakening from sleep. Bronchitic cough typically re-

solves within 1 month after smoking cessation. Elaine's lack of a smoking history and the pattern of her cough make this diagnosis less likely.

Postnasal drip syndrome (PNDS) is also a common cause of chronic cough in adult nonsmokers. These patients frequently report a "tickle" in their throat or frequent throat clearing, with little or no sputum production. Sinusitis and rhinitis due to colds and allergic conditions can each stimulate excess mucus production in the upper airways. This excess production can overwhelm the normal drainage mechanisms and cause stimulation of cough receptors in the sinuses, pharynx, larynx, and nose, resulting in persistent cough. PNDS can be confirmed by examination findings of cobblestoning and mucous drainage in the pharynx. Indolent or occult sinusitis can be detected by obtaining a three-slice screening computed tomographic (CT) image of the paranasal sinuses, which can often be performed at the same cost as plain x-ray films of the sinuses. Mucosal thickening with air-fluid levels is suggestive of chronic sinusitis. Treatment of either of these conditions can begin with topical decongestants. Sinusitis refractory to conservative management with mucolytics and decongestants may respond to surgical drainage. Elaine's normal physical examination results make this diagnosis less likely, although an occult chronic sinusitis should still be considered.

Angiotensin converting enzyme (ACE) inhibitors are the most common medication-related cause of chronic cough. This reaction can develop insidiously or abruptly anytime after beginning therapy and resolves with discontinuation of the medication. This idiosyncratic reaction cannot be predicted, and patients frequently fail to make the association between medication use and their symptoms. Losartan, an angiotensin II receptor blocker, does not cause cough to the same degree as traditional ACE inhibitors. Unfortunately, although losartan lowers blood pressure effectively, it does not appear to offer the benefits of traditional ACE inhibitors when used in diabetes mellitus or congestive heart failure. Elaine does not take ACE inhibitors, eliminating this possibility.

Cough variant asthma is another common cause of chronic cough in nonsmoking adults. These patients commonly have nonproductive paroxysms of cough precipitated by environmental stimuli such as changes in temperature, smoke, perfumes, or allergens. Unlike traditional asthma, however, these patients have no wheezing on physical examination. Pulmonary function testing may be normal or show a mild obstructive pattern that responds to bronchodilators. The diagnosis often requires demonstration of a 20 per cent decrease in the forced expiratory volume in 1 second (FEV$_1$) at lower than normal concentration thresholds on methacholine provocation testing. As with traditional asthma, treatment with inhaled steroids or β-agonists is the initial treatment of choice. An empirical diagnostic trial of these medications can often establish the diagnosis in the absence of more formal pulmonary testing. In children, the presence of cough variant asthma predicts eventual development of wheezing and full-blown asthma as adults. Certainly Elaine may have an element of cough variant asthma, but the lack of symptoms suggestive of allergic or environmental provocation makes this slightly less likely than GERD.

Along with GERD, these causes (chronic bronchitis, PNDS, ACE inhibitor use, and cough variant asthma) are felt to account for over 80 per cent of chronic cough in adults referred for evaluation, and over 90 per cent of adult cases presenting to primary care physicians. In children, *persistent or recurrent viral upper respiratory infection* is the most common cause. Often patients may have a combination of factors that contribute to their symptoms.

Less common causes of chronic cough in nonsmoking adults include interstitial pulmonary disease, cardiac causes such as congestive heart failure or pericarditis, foreign body impactions in upper or lower respiratory tracts, occult neoplasm, psychogenic cough, infectious causes such as tuberculosis or atypical pneumonia, aspiration syndrome in patients with swallowing difficulty due to neurologic or iatrogenic (e.g., nasogastric tube) causes, and in children, anatomic variations resulting in abnormal respiratory tract function. In the absence of findings suggestive of common causes as noted previously, many of these less common causes can be revealed by chest x-ray studies, tuberculin skin testing, radiographic imaging of swallowing function, or bronchoscopy with cultures, biopsy, or washings.

DISCUSSION

Elaine has few findings on physical examination, but her history is consistent with gastroesophageal reflux disease (GERD). GERD typically presents with symptoms of postprandial heartburn. Patients often report a sour taste in their mouth concurrent with their heartburn. The symptoms are usually exacerbated by recumbency or anything that increases intra-abdominal pressure. When considered as a cause of chronic cough, however, patients often are asymptomatic, with no abdominal or chest complaints. Indeed, in many patients the only symptom of their reflux is cough. In the absence of suggestive

symptoms on history, the diagnosis may be established by demonstrating reflux on radiographic swallowing examination or by documenting reflux on extended esophageal pH manometry. In the latter, correlation between decreasing esophageal pH and patient-recorded symptoms is suggestive. Some patients with GERD may develop intermittent reversible airway obstruction due to microaspiration of stomach acid into the bronchial tree with reflux. However, there are clearly patients with chronic cough that responds to GERD treatment who demonstrate no acid reflux into the lungs on radionuclide studies, and who respond normally to bronchial provocation testing. Presumably irritation of gastric or esophageal cough receptors plays a role in these patients. Treatment with antireflux precautions such as elevating the head of the patient's bed, smaller but more frequent meals, or treatment with antacids often reduces the patient's symptoms.

In Elaine's case, a barium swallow and upper gastrointestinal x-ray film demonstrated moderate reflux, and conservative treatment with antireflux precautions and nonsedating histamine (H$_2$) blockers eliminated her cough.

Other reasonable diagnostic measures in any patient with undiagnosed chronic cough include chest x-ray film, tuberculin (purified protein derivative, PPD) testing, and pulmonary function testing. Only rarely is bronchoscopy or nasopharyngoscopy necessary to establish the cause of chronic cough.

Cough Medications for Symptomatic Treatment

In general, the treatment of cough should be directed at the probable cause; however, symptomatic treatment is sometimes warranted. This treatment should generally be reserved for patients with self-limiting cough when other treatment is not available.

ANTITUSSIVES. *Codeine* and other opiates are the most effective antitussives; however, their abuse potential has limited their use for this indication. Codeine (40 to 160 mg every 24 hours in divided doses every 4 to 6 hours) is most practical and is available over the counter in some states. It can be used at bedtime in combination with other symptomatic treatments, as noted further on. Side effects include sedation, constipation, dry mouth, and histamine release causing bronchospasm. Sedation and bronchospasm limit the usefulness of opiates in patients with reversible obstructive airway disease.

Dextromethorphan has also been shown to be effective, but large doses are required (up to 180 mg per day) to obtain efficacy superior to placebo. Recent controlled-release forms (Delsym, Extend 12) and chewable (Mediquell) forms have made this the most popular over-the-counter cough remedy, accounting for 75 per cent of retail sales in this market. As with codeine, bronchospasm is a rare but notable side effect.

Mucolytics and Expectorants. The most common is *guaifenesin* (Robitussin), a relative of guaiacolate. It purportedly enhances output of secretions by reducing adhesiveness and surface tension of the mucus, making clearance by cough or cilia easier. However, at normal doses it can prolong the activated partial thromboplastin time and cause platelet dysfunction; higher doses can cause nausea and vomiting. Despite these side effects, it is a common ingredient in over-the-counter cough preparations.

Iodides (potassium iodide or iodinated glycerol) are used to increase sputum production and have been shown to be effective in animals and in humans, but the side effect profile is long, including rashes, metallic taste in the mouth, parotid swelling, and nodular enlargement of the thyroid. These complications prompt discontinuation of therapy in up to 14 per cent of those taking iodides.

N-Acetylcysteine (Mucomyst) is an effective mucolytic. However, its expense and the mode of delivery (inhalation of nebulized aerosol) limit its use to patients with particularly tenacious secretions, as in cystic fibrosis, or mucoid impactions, as in immotile cilia syndrome.

Other. Topical anesthetics such as *inhaled lidocaine* or *benzonatate* (Tessalon Perles) are effective at reducing cough in a variety of disorders. However, both drugs can reduce the gag reflex, putting patients at risk for aspiration. Use of inhaled lidocaine is generally limited to pulmonary procedures or experimental studies. Benzonatate is more commonly used in outpatient settings.

SUGGESTED READING

Corrao WM. Chronic persistent cough: Diagnosis and treatment update. Pediatr Ann 1996;25:162–168.

Ewig JM. Chronic cough. Pediatr Rev 1995;16:72–73.

Leung AK, Robson WL, Tay-Uyboco I. Chronic cough in children. Can Fam Physician 1994;40:531–537.

Mello CJ, Irwin RS, Curley FJ. Predictive values of the character, timing, and complications of chronic cough in diagnosing its cause. Arch Intern Med 1996;156:997–1003.

Patrick H, Patrick F. Chronic cough. Med Clin North Am 1995;79:361–372.

Pratter MR, Bartter T, Akers S, DuBois J. An algorithmic approach to chronic cough. Ann Intern Med 1993;119:977–983.

QUESTIONS

1. Which of the following medications has been implicated as a cause of chronic cough?
   a. Enalapril
   b. Benzonatate
   c. Losartan
   d. Digoxin
   e. Guaifenesin

2. Match the following causes of cough with the clinical findings in items (1) through (5).
   a. GERD
   b. Cough variant asthma
   c. Postnasal drip syndrome
   d. Chronic bronchitis
      (1) Frequent throat clearing.
      (2) Symptoms worse with recumbency or after large meals.
      (3) Productive cough worse in the morning.
      (4) Methacholine challenge testing may be useful in establishing diagnosis.
      (5) Usually attributable to smoking.

Answers appear on **page 603.**

Chapter 16

Fever and Chest Pain

John G. Prichard, M.D., M.H.S.

INITIAL VISIT

Subjective

PATIENT IDENTIFICATION. Joe is a 71-year-old retired engineer who provides his own history.

PRESENT ILLNESS. This active and intelligent man, who usually enjoys excellent health, was well until mid-June, 6 days before this visit, when he developed myalgia, fatigue, fever, and a minimally productive cough. Over the ensuing days the cough became persistent and severe with anterior midline chest pain and moderate to severe vertex headache occurring with each coughing episode. Fever reached a maximum of 102.5°F, unassociated with rigors. Fatigue persisted although the myalgia improved. On the third day of illness right ear pain without associated discharge occurred and persisted. Dyspnea was not present and hemoptysis had not occurred. Two weeks before the onset of illness he had traveled by car from southern to northern California for a music festival. He had stayed in a friend's home in which two teenagers had been ill with the "flu." He had no respiratory illness in the past and does not smoke.

PAST MEDICAL HISTORY. An appendectomy was performed at age 35. A cystoscopy was undertaken at age 65 following an episode of hematuria, the cause of which was never identified. He took no medicines other than an over-the-counter nonsteroidal anti-inflammatory agent (NSAID) for the present illness. No other serious illnesses have occurred.

FAMILY MEDICAL HISTORY. His mother and father died following a motor vehicle accident. He has two younger brothers who are in good health. He has no children.

HEALTH HABITS. He neither smokes nor drinks. He swims daily although he remains moderately overweight.

SOCIAL HISTORY. He lives with his wife of 40 years. Both are independent and active.

Objective

PHYSICAL EXAMINATION. He appears fatigued and moderately ill, although not dyspneic at rest. Paroxysms of cough occurred during which he complained of chest and head pain. His temperature is 100.9°F. Pulse is 90 per minute and regular. His blood pressure sitting was 155/90 mm Hg. The respiratory rate is 20 per minute and shallow. The pharynx, conjunctiva, and right tympanic membrane are injected. Rales are present over the left posterior lung fields without dullness on percussion. Mid- to end-expiratory wheezing is present throughout. Cardiac, abdominal, cutaneous, and neurologic examinations are unrevealing.

Assessment

Acute lower respiratory tract infection with bronchospasm.

Plan

DIAGNOSTIC. Obtain chest x-ray film. Attempt sputum induction for Gram stain and culture. Complete blood count.

THERAPEUTIC. Discontinue NSAIDs. Start inhaled bronchodilator and oral macrolide antibiotic.

PATIENT EDUCATION. Usual cautions regarding worsening and expected course. Instructions given regarding proper use of inhaler with spacer.

Discussion

This patient has symptoms and signs of pneumonia. At least 4 million episodes of pneumonia occur annually in the United States and account for about one-half million hospital admissions each year. During the winter months, as many as one in four office visits are prompted by symptoms similar to those described in this case vignette. The problem of community-acquired pneumonia continues to evolve in terms of cause, diagnostic methods, and treatment. From the perspective of ambulatory (as opposed to hospital) practice, however, certain fundamental issues remain as cornerstones of the approach to such patients. First, what is the *present* diagnosis? Fever, cough, wheezing, and chest discomfort may indicate bronchitis (usually not requiring antimicrobial therapy) or pneumonia or, indeed, noninfectious causes. Pneumonia may evolve from what was initially bronchitis (e.g., bacterial pneumonia complicating influenza) and may itself be self-limited or immensely complicated. In this instance, the finding of localized rales is suggestive of pneumonia.

An equally important issue is the degree of illness. This is most often a judgment made by the clinician during the course of the office visit, supplemented at times by impressions of family members. Does the patient require hospitalization or supplemental oxygen? Are blood cultures or arterial blood gases indicated? Is a chest x-ray film warranted? If the patient appears, at this juncture, to be a candidate for outpatient management, are there impediments to doing so? Are there underlying illnesses or conditions, such as chronic lung disease, diabetes, or an inability to mobilize secretions, that may limit the patient's ability to safely withstand some degree of worsening? Are conditions within the home conducive to support, adherence to a treatment regimen, as well as reasonable observation of the patient during the course of illness? Note that these issues are raised *before* the problems of cause and treatment are addressed. Indeed, most skilled office-based or emergency room clinicians answer these questions as a matter of course before considering diagnostic or therapeutic options.

Joe is thought to be moderately ill. He is, however, intelligent and has support within the home. Despite his age, he does not have known underlying diseases predisposing to pneumonia or conditions that may limit his respiratory reserve or otherwise interfere with his ability to cope with this illness. The clinician noted no dyspnea with rest and thus, at least at this point, was disinclined to order an oxygen saturation study or arterial blood gases. The x-ray study was ordered to confirm the impression of pneumonia, estimate its extent, and derive the clues implicating one cause as opposed to another.

The causes of community-acquired pneumonia have been defined by a number of studies over the past several decades (Sue, 1994; Bartlett and Mundy, 1995). *Streptococcus pneumoniae, Haemophilus influenzae, Chlamydia pneumoniae, Legionella* species, *Mycoplasma pneumoniae, Moraxella catarrhalis,* and viruses account for the majority of cases in which a precise cause is established. In numerous studies, defining the cause of community-acquired pneumonia was possible in only 40 to 60 percent of patients. This has remained true despite thorough use of invasive procedures and extensive laboratory testing. Accordingly, the cause of pneumonia in an ambulatory patient is unlikely to be established with certainty. The degree to which a diagnosis is sought, by the various methods available, depends on the severity of illness, extrapulmonary involvement, epidemiologic factors, or lack of response to empirical therapy.

The pathogens listed previously rarely produce clearly definable clinical syndromes; signs, symptoms, and clinical courses overlap to a considerable extent. Hence, one must use epidemiologic and laboratory data, along with clinical findings, in an attempt to narrow the spectrum of empirical therapy. In this instance, the history of Joe's travel through an endemic area for coccidioidomycosis may prompt serologic testing immediately or at a later time if his condition does not improve with initial antibiotic therapy. The patient's household contact with young adults having respiratory symptoms suggests *Chlamydia* or *Mycoplasma* could be a causative agent.

There are few instances of pneumonia in which chest x-ray findings are pathognomonic. Certain patterns on the radiograph may be suggestive, however. In the present case, a finding of hilar adenopathy ipsilateral to an infiltrate may provide stronger evidence for coccidioidomycosis, while interstitial infiltrates would favor *Mycoplasma* or *Chlamydia.* The complete blood count, although frequently performed, rarely sheds light either on the cause of pneumonia or the prognosis. The sputum Gram stain can be helpful in selecting initial therapy if a specimen can be produced. Sputum culture, performed in the usual manner, identifies some cases of streptococcal pneumonia and those caused by *Haemophilus* or *Moraxella,* although results are delayed a minimum of 24 hours.

With respect to empirical therapy, erythromycin was selected because of a clinical suspicion that *Mycoplasma* may have been the causative agent. Generally regarded as an infection of young adults, there is increasing evidence that *M. pneumoniae* may cause 15 percent of community-acquired pneumonia in older patients. Erythromycin has a reasonably broad spectrum, although a second-generation cephalosporin may be added if the patient has a complicating underlying illness such as chronic obstructive pulmonary disease or alcoholism.

Cough was a prominent symptom in this patient. The finding of wheezing indicates that the cough was, to some extent, induced by bronchospasm and may be relieved by an inhaled bronchodilator. NSAIDS were discontinued, as in some patients, they may aggravate bronchoconstriction.

FOLLOW-UP VISIT

The chest x-ray film showed patchy infiltrate in the posterior basal segment of the left lower lobe. Increased interstitial markings were present in the left and right lower lobes. No effusions or adenopathy were seen. The complete blood count gave normal results with the exception of a leukocytosis (13,400/mm^3, 78 per cent segmented forms). A sputum specimen could not be produced for stain or culture.

The patient's condition remained stable over the next 48 hours. An immediate decrease in cough was noted following use of the bronchodilator. Fever slowly resolved and fatigue lessened. When seen 5 days following the initial visit, the patient appeared improved. Antibiotics were continued for a total of 14 days. Bronchodilator use was according to need and soon discontinued. The illness resolved entirely within 2 weeks.

COMMENT

This case, a common circumstance encountered in ambulatory practice, illustrates several points. First, the precise cause of pneumonia is frequently never defined. Despite lacking a specific diagnosis, the vast majority of patients respond to empirical therapy in a satisfactory manner. Second, there are sociological as well as physiologic issues that determine the need for hospitalization, home visits, or evaluation (e.g., blood gases, serologies) beyond that usually obtained. Last, management of associated symptoms of pneumonia, such as pain or bronchospasm, is frequently necessary in addition to educating the patient and family on the use of medicines and expected course.

SUGGESTED READING

Bartlett, JG, Mundy LM. Community-acquired pneumonia. N Engl J Med 1995;333:1618–1924.

Casell GH. Severe mycoplasma disease—rare or underdiagnosed? West J Med 1995;162:172–175.

Farr BM, Sloman AJ, Fisch MI. Predicting death in patients hospitalized for community-acquired pneumonia. Ann Intern Med 1991;115:428–436.

Nelson HS. β-Adrenergic brochodilators. N Engl J Med 1995;333:499–506.

Rakel RE. Textbook of Family Practice, 5th ed. Philadelphia, WB Saunders, 1995, pp 419–424.

Sue DY. Community-acquired pneumonia in adults. West J Med 1994;161:383–389.

QUESTION

1. True or False: The etiology of community-acquired pneumonia may be definitively established by
   a. Clinical history
   b. Chest radiography
   c. Serology
   d. Blood cultures

Answer appears on **page 603.**

Chapter 17

Dyspnea

Amir Sweha, M.D.

INITIAL VISIT

Subjective

PRESENT ILLNESS. Mr. H.G. is a 59-year-old white man who presents with a 4-year history of an intermittent, productive morning cough and wheezing with gradually progressive dyspnea for the last 6 months. In the last 3 days he developed acute symptoms of upper respiratory congestion, fever of 101°F, worsening cough, and change of the sputum color from white to yellowish green. Currently, minimal activity precipitates dyspnea. He denies any chills, stridor, snoring, leg swelling, chest pain, hemoptysis, orthopnea, or paroxysmal nocturnal dyspnea. He also denies any abdominal pain or jaundice. He visited the emergency department three times in the last year for similar symptoms. He was never intubated or hospitalized for respiratory problems; however, he desires hospitalization and full resuscitation if needed. He has never used long-term oral steroid medication. His previous physician prescribed inhalers and pills. He stopped taking the pills because they caused insomnia and tremors, and he stopped using the inhaler, as it caused palpitations and "a rush" immediately after use. He had pulmonary function tests (PFT) performed 6 months ago, which showed decreased forced expiratory volume in 1 second (FEV_1) to 67 per cent of predicted, decreased FEV_1/forced vital capacity (FVC) ratio to 0.65, decreased peak expiratory flow rate (PEFR), increased residual volume (RV) to 110 per cent of predicted, normal total lung capacity (TLC), decreased diffusion capacity for carbon monoxide (D_{LCO}) to 79 per cent of predicted, and decreased D_{LCO}/alveolar volume (V_A) ratio.

HABITS. One pack of cigarettes per day for the last 38 years, and 12 cans of beer on weekends. He denies the use of recreational drugs.

PAST MEDICAL HISTORY. No history of pneumonia. Never received immunization for pneumonia or influenza. His tuberculin (purified protein derivative [PPD]) skin test was negative 2 years ago.

MEDICATIONS. Prescribed but not taking. Albuterol metered-dose inhaler (MDI) 2 puffs every 6 hours. Ipratropium bromide (Atrovent) MDI, 2 puffs every 8 hours. Theophylline 200 mg orally three times per day. He has a drug allergy to penicillin in the form of a severe allergic reaction and difficulty breathing.

SOCIAL HISTORY. Married and two children. He finished high school and 1 year of college education. No other family members smoke tobacco. His wife is an accountant. She is concerned and supportive. He is unable to perform his job requirements due to his limited functional capacity and easy fatigability. He worked in construction and the job is very physically demanding.

REVIEW OF SYSTEMS. Otherwise unremarkable.

Objective

PHYSICAL EXAMINATION. General: Weight 190 lb, not changed in last 6 months. Height 5 feet 5 inches. Blood pressure 130/84, respiratory rate 26, pulse 110, regular and no pulsus paradoxus. Temperature 99.8°F. H.G. is overweight. Mental status: Anxious and with good mentation. Decubitus: Sitting in moderate respiratory distress evidenced by use of the respiratory auxiliary muscles. He is able to finish short sentences without interruption; however, he is unable to blow out a match held 6 inches from his open mouth. HEENT: Nonicteric. Mucous membranes are moist and pink without cyanosis. Face is mildly plethoric with puffiness of the lower eyelids. Neck: No retraction of the supraclavicular fossa with inspiration. Jugular veins are mildly distended. Chest: Barrel-shaped with decreased chest wall movement. Hyper-resonant without dullness. Tactile vocal fremitus is slightly decreased all over. Decreased diaphragmatic excursion on percussion. Airflow is fair with a prolonged expiratory phase. Scattered expiratory wheezes and inspiratory rhonchi are present without basal crackles. Cardiac: Distant heart sounds, accentuated P_2, and no S_3 or S_4. Abdomen: Soft without tenderness or ascites. Liver is palpable 3 cm below the right costal margin with a normal span and a negative hepatojugular reflux. Extremities: Clubbing, grade I. No cyanosis or edema. Musculoskeletal: No kyphosis or scoliosis.

Diagnostic Tests

Pulse oximetry: Oxygen (O_2) saturation is 96 per cent on room air. Bedside peak flow meter (PFM) is 310 L/minute (55 per cent of predicted). Electrocardiogram (ECG): normal sinus rhythm rate 106/minute, right axial deviation, normal intervals (PR, QRS and QT), and normal P, QRS, and T morphologies. No evidence of ischemia or ventricular hypertrophy. Chest x-ray study showed hyperinflated lungs with depression and flattening of the diaphragm on a posteroanterior film, enlarged retrosternal space on the lateral film, and increased peribronchial and perivascular markings. No bullae, effusion, enlargement of the pulmonary artery, or infiltration. Blood count showed a hematocrit of 45 and a normal white blood cell count. A chemistry panel was normal.

Assessment

WORKING DIAGNOSIS

1. Chronic obstructive pulmonary disease (COPD); mixed type, uncomplicated, mild, secondary to cigarette smoking, with acute exacerbation, moderate, secondary to respiratory tract infection and possibly the patient's noncompliance. This is the most likely diagnosis due to the history of cigarette smoking, chronic cough, sputum production, dyspnea, and the presence of signs including rhonchi, distant breath sounds, and prolonged expiration on physical examination. The limitation of airflow on the PFM and PFT supports the diagnosis.

2. Tobacco use.

3. Candidate for immunization and health care maintenance.

DIFFERENTIAL DIAGNOSIS. Common causes of chronic dyspnea with acute exacerbation should be ruled out, as follows:

1. Cardiac causes including *congestive heart failure (CHF)* and mitral valve disease; dyspnea on exertion is usually associated with orthopnea and later on with paroxysmal nocturnal dyspnea. Basilar crackles and a third heart sound are specific signs for CHF. Also, the absence of apical murmurs argues against mitral valve disease.

2. Pulmonary causes.

   a. *Asthma.* Although characterized by episodes of chronic wheezing, dyspnea and cough, asthma is usually associated with complete or partial reversibility after bronchodilator therapy.

   b. *Bronchiectasis.* The physical findings are localized on chest examination. Features such as recurrent pneumonia, high grades of clubbing, copious production of purulent sputum, hemoptysis, and weight loss are sometimes helpful to differentiate bronchiectasis from COPD. Radiography may help to confirm the diagnosis.

   c. Parenchymal disease such as *interstitial lung disease.* In the majority of cases, no specific cause can be identified. In the remainder, exposure to drugs, inorganic and organic dust, gases and fumes, radiation, and infections should be identified. Usually interstitial lung disease presents with progressive dyspnea and dry cough. Physical examination is usually notable for the fine, diffuse, dry, and midexpiratory crackles. PFT indicate restrictive ventilatory defect and decreased D_{LCO}, however, with normal or slightly decreased D_{LCO}/V_A ratio due to the concomitant decrease in alveolar volume. Radiography may be normal in early stages, but later on diffuse ground-glass, nodular, reticular, or reticulonodular infiltrates that may progress to honeycomb appearance become evident. Lung biopsy may be used to confirm the diagnosis in early or difficult cases.

   d. *Primary (idiopathic) pulmonary hypertension.* Commonly occurs in middle-aged women and is diagnosed by exclusion.

   e. *Other ventilatory restrictive conditions* including kyphoscoliosis, massive obesity, ascites, and large pleural effusion were not evident.

   f. *Tracheal stenosis.* Dyspnea occurs in conjunction with stridor and inspiratory retraction of the supraclavicular fossa.

   g. *Cystic fibrosis.* Occurs in children and younger adults.

3. *Psychiatric causes.* Psychic dyspnea (anxiety) is a

common condition and usually takes the form of sighing respiration. The patient often reports chest tightness and cannot get enough air. Multiple bodily complaints, nervousness, and a normal physical examination are typical of such patients. Hyperventilation syndrome represents the acute exacerbation of the condition.

4. *Severe chronic anemia.* The underlying cause, e.g., gastrointestinal bleeding, may be evident. Pallor is usually noticeable on physical examination. Blood work-up is helpful to diagnose the type and severity of the condition.

Plan

OFFICE COURSE. A trial of albuterol inhaler resulted in improvement of dyspnea, respiratory rate and use of auxiliary muscles, air movement on auscultation, and the PFM reading to 340 L/minute (60 per cent of predicted). A nurse taught the patient the appropriate technique for the use of the MDI and PFM to monitor his condition at home.

DISPOSITION. The patient was sent home with the following:

1. Instructions for oral hydration and rest. Avoid alcohol and cigarette smoking.
2. Albuterol MDI, two puffs every 4 to 6 hours.
3. Prednisone 40 mg orally per day tapered in increments of 5 mg every 2 days over a 2-week period.
4. Trimethoprim-sulfamethoxazole (Bactrim DS) one tablet orally twice per day for 10 days.
5. Chest percussion and postural drainage as needed for copious sputum.
6. Follow-up in 10 days, with his wife, or sooner as needed.

FOLLOW-UP VISIT

The patient returned in 10 days accompanied by his wife. He feels much better. He is now able to walk three blocks without shortness of breath. His cough improved. Sputum is scant and white. He did not drink alcohol, but he continued to smoke half a pack of cigarettes per day. He denies side effects from the medications. On physical examination he appears comfortable. Respiratory rate is 16, neck veins are empty, and lung examination shows good air movement and no wheezing. Heart sounds are normal. His PFM reads 370 L/minute (65 per cent of predicted).

Plan

1. Thorough patient and family education regarding COPD. Discuss compliance with treatment.

2. Ipratropium bromide (Atrovent) MDI, two puffs every 6 hours.

3. Albuterol MDI, two puffs every 6 hours.

4. Triamcinolone acetonide (Azmacort) MDI, two puffs every 8 hours.

5. Pneumococcal vaccination today and influenza vaccination yearly.

6. Rehabilitation program and exercise training. Evaluate for vocational training. Start a smoking cessation program.

7. Avoid sedatives and alcohol.

8. Follow-up visit in 2 to 3 months or sooner as needed.

DISCUSSION

Chronic obstructive pulmonary disease (COPD) is a descriptive label often used to define chronic bronchitis and emphysema. Although they are two specific diseases, most patients have features of both conditions (mixed type) with one pathophysiology often predominating. More than 5 million Americans over the age of 55 have COPD, which directly causes or contributes to over 160,000 deaths per year. In evaluating a patient with COPD, the following areas need to be addressed.

TYPE OF COPD. The *chronic bronchitic type* is characterized by an onset after age 35, and with dyspnea that is intermittent mild to moderate. The cough is persistent, severe, and is associated with copious mucopurulent sputum production. The following features are commonly present: frequent respiratory infections, right-sided heart failure and edema, obesity, central cyanosis, plethora, and wheezing and rhonchi. Therefore, this type is sometimes called "blue bloaters'" type. Fever, increased expectoration, and particularly sputum purulence are indicators for the presence of bacterial infection. *Haemophilus influenzae, Streptococcus pneumoniae,* and *Moraxella catarrhalis* are the major pathogens; however, atypical bacteria such as *Chlamydia pneumoniae* may also play a role. Sputum Gram stain and culture may help in identifying the organism, particularly in a patient with an infiltrate seen on chest x-ray study; otherwise, their value may be limited because the organisms colonize most COPD patients. For treatment of the bacterial infection, the antibiotic should be at least active against the three major pathogens.

The chest x-ray results in the bronchitic type show increased peribronchial and perivascular markings. Blood count shows an increased hematocrit. Blood gases may show hypoxemia, hypercapnia, and respiratory acidosis in moderate to severe conditions. The PFT show decreased FEV_1, FEV_1/FVC, PEFR, and increased RV and TLC. In severe cases, the FVC is also decreased. The ECG may show evidence of cor pulmonale, a common complication of this type. Cor pulmonale usually presents with features of right-sided heart failure. Symptoms include leg swelling and right-sided abdominal pain. Signs include icterus, dilated neck veins, right upper quadrant tenderness and hepatomegaly, positive hepatojugular reflux, right ventricular sustained impulse and pansystolic murmur that increases with inspiration at the tricuspid area, accentuated second heart sound, and pedal edema. In cor pulmonale the ECG shows evidence of right axial deviation, "p pulmonale," and right ventricular hypertrophy (dominant R in V_1 and S in V_6, and T inversion in V_1 and V_2). On the ECG, right ventricular hypertrophy is more specific than right axial deviation to indicate the presence of cor pulmonale. The chest x-ray film shows evidence of pulmonary hypertension such as dilation of the main pulmonary artery and its proximal branches, right ventricular and right atrial enlargement, and in severe cases peripheral pulmonary oligemia.

The *emphysematous type* is characterized by a late onset after age 35. The dyspnea is progressive and severe. The cough and clear mucoid sputum production are mild or absent. In advanced disease, the patient is thin, wasted and tachypneic. Cyanosis and plethora are absent. Therefore, this type is sometimes called the "pink puffers'" type. The accessory respiratory muscles are usually hypertrophied and the chest has an increased anteroposterior diameter giving it a barrel shape. The lungs are hyper-resonant, the breath sounds are diminished, and the heart sounds are distant. The chest x-ray study may show parenchymal bullae, peripheral bleb, decreased peripheral lung markings, hyperinflation with flattening and lowering of the hemidiaphragms, enlargement of the retrosternal space, and reduction of the cardiac silhouette to a small vertical shadow. The arterial blood gas (ABG) analysis may show mild hypoxemia in advanced disease. The PFT show increase in TLC and decreased $DLCO$; however, the $DLCO/VA$ ratio is low due to the normal or increased alveolar volume. The ECG and blood count are usually normal. Cor pulmonale is uncommon.

SEVERITY AND EXACERBATION OF COPD. The severity of the disease can be determined by several factors related to COPD including the history of symptom progression, number of emergency department visits and hospitalizations for exacerbation, history of intubation for respiratory failure, chronic use of systemic corticosteriods, and the presence of complications including cor pulmonale. PFT may also help to determine the severity; an FEV_1/FVC ratio of greater than 0.70 indicates no, 0.61 to 0.69 mild, 0.45 to 0.60 moderate, and less than 0.45 severe, obstructive dysfunction. Similarly, a $DLCO$ less than 80 per cent of predicted suggests the presence of a diffusion defect. To determine the patient's baseline condition, it is generally recommended to perform PFT when the patient is clinically stable and at least 2 to 4 weeks after an exacerbation. PFM measures the PEFR and can be very helpful in the acute setting as well as for monitoring progression of the disease and the effectiveness of therapy. The PFM is portable and can easily be used in an office setting or lent to the patient for home use. It can be used for self-adjusting the time and dose of drug administration by the patient based on objective measurement of airway obstruction. The measurement of PEFR is converted to percentage of predicted value (for age, gender, and height), hence reflecting the severity of the obstruction. In the acute setting, a spirometer of PFM may be used to determine when to hospitalize the patient, for example, patients with an FEV_1 of 40 per cent or greater of predicted normal or no clinical evidence of respiratory distress after treatment may be safely discharged. Patients not meeting these criteria are at high risk for relapse and should either be admitted or have further aggressive therapy in the emergency department. Arterial blood gas (ABG) analysis is generally unnecessary unless hypoxemia or hypercapnia is suspected. It is helpful in determining the level of Po_2, Pco_2, and acidosis, and hence the severity of COPD. Chest x-ray study and ECG may show evidence of cor pulmonale. Several parameters have been used to predict a poor prognosis in COPD including an FEV_1 less than 40 per cent of predicted, especially when the absolute value is less than 1.0 L/minute, FVC less than 80 per cent of predicted, rate of decline of PEFR, arterial Po_2 less than 55 mm Hg, CO_2 retention, decreased diffusion capacity, heavy smoking, and the development of cor pulmonale. Discussing prognosis and advanced directives with the patient is usually helpful in the management.

RISK FACTORS FOR COPD AND PRECIPITATING FACTORS FOR EXACERBATION. Smoking, particularly cigarettes, is the most important cause. Other occupational and environmental pollutants are less common causes. Damp cold climate may enhance the pollutant's effect. Chronic upper respiratory tract infection, pulmonary embolism, pneumonia, and pulmonary congestion may worsen otherwise stable COPD. Deficiency of α1-antitrypsin due to an autosomal recessive trait may cause severe emphysema early in life. Upper respiratory infection and noncompliance with therapy are the most common causes for exacerbation of COPD. Early treatment of upper respiratory infection may prevent COPD exacerbation. Thorough patient and family education, addressing patients' concerns and identifying and minimizing undesirable medication side effects (e.g., teaching appropriate technique for using the MDI or use of a spacer device) usually improves patient compliance.

COMPLICATIONS. Pulmonary hypertension, cor pulmonale, arrhythmia, spontaneous pneumothorax, and chronic respiratory failure.

INVESTIGATIONS. Bedside spirometer or PFM. Blood count with differential. Chemistry panel. Sputum Gram stain and culture (if indicated). Theophylline level (if indicated). Pulse oximetry and ABG analysis (if indicated). ECG. Chest x-ray study. Others, e.g., echocardiogram if cor pulmonale is suspected.

PRINCIPLES OF TREATMENT

Treatment of an Exacerbation. The goal is to stabilize the patient and control bronchospasm. The objectives are:

1. Home treatment versus hospitalization according to the severity of the exacerbation.

2. Oxygen for hypoxemia; use cautiously and watch for respiratory depression.

3. Hydration; oral, parenteral, and topical (humidifier). Use cautiously in the presence of heart failure.

4. Bronchodilator; β-agonist (primarily), theophylline, others, as indicated.

5. Corticosteroid; for short-term use with taper versus long-term therapy according to the patient's baseline condition.

6. Antibiotic, if indicated.

7. Avoid sedatives, including alcohol.

8. Chest percussion and postural drainage for copious sputum.

9. Treat complications.

10. Smoking cessation.

Long-term Treatment. Goals over the long term are as follows:

1. To maximize lung function and improve the patient's functional status so that he or she can better carry out daily activities.

2. To eliminate or minimize precipitant and risk factors.

3. To minimize the frequency of exacerbations for better prognosis and cost-effectiveness.

4. To manage complications including hypoxemia and cor pulmonale.

The objectives are:

1. Thorough patient and family education regarding the disease process; the appropriate technique to use the MDI (effective for 60 per cent of patients and for the other 40 per cent add a spacer device to the MDI); the precipitating factors; compliance with the treatment plan; the patient's concerns including medication side effects, tolerance, and dependency; and the use of PFM for monitoring and deciding when to call or go to the emergency department.
   a. The appropriate technique for teaching the patient how to use the MDI is as follows: Assemble and shake the inhaler, hold the inhaler upside down; place the open end of the mouthpiece approximately 2 to 4 cm in front of the mouth, take a deep breath and blow out slowly through pursed lips, open the mouth as wide as possible, start slow inhalation through open mouth; while inhaling, press down firmly on cartridge to release medication; keep inhaling a full deep breath, hold breath for approximately 10 seconds, exhale slowly; rest 2 to 3 minutes, and repeat one or two more times.

2. Rehabilitation and exercise conditioning; physical therapy, occupational therapy, psychosocial counseling, vocational counseling and training, nutritional evaluation and counseling, and respiratory therapy.

3. Oxygen therapy; continuous, nocturnal (especially if there is concomitant sleep apnea), or with exercise according to the degree of hypoxemia. Oxygen therapy improves survival in a COPD hypoxemic patient.

4. Vaccination for influenza yearly and for pneumo-coccal pneumonia every 7 to 10 years. Monitor tuberculosis status particularly if steroids are used chronically.
5. Bronchodilator: ipratropium bromide (primarily), β-agonist, and theophylline.

6. Corticosteroid; inhaler and oral if needed.
7. Treat complications, e.g., heart failure.
8. Avoid sedatives and tranquilizers.
9. **Stop smoking;** smoking cessation program. Complete cessation of smoking slows progression of COPD more than any other form of therapy.

SUGGESTED READING

Bleecker E.R., Liu MC. Obstructive airways disease. In Baker LR, Burton JR, Ziefe PD (eds). Principles of Ambulatory Medicine, 5th ed. Baltimore, Williams & Wilkins, 1995, pp 604–637.

Goroll AH, May LA, Mulley AG Jr (eds). Primary Care Medicine: Evaluation of Chronic Dyspnea, 3rd ed. Philadelphia, JB Lippincott, 1995, pp 227–231.

Goroll AH, May LA, Mulley AG Jr (eds). Primary Care Medicine:

Management of Chronic Obstructive Pulmonary Disease (COPD), 3rd ed. Philadelphia, JB Lippincott, 1995, pp 252–261.

Katz D. The mini-Wright peak flow meter for evaluating airway obstruction in a family practice. J Fam Pract 1983;17:51–57.

Make B. COPD: Management and rehabilitation. Am Fam Physician 1991;43:1315–1323.

QUESTIONS

1. Which of the following indicates an emphysematous component in a patient with COPD?
   a. Persistent, severe, and productive cough
   b. Central cyanosis
   c. Decreased D_{LCO} with a normal D_{LCO}/V_A ratio.
   d. Hyperinflation with flattening and lowering of the hemidiaphragms on a chest x-ray film.
   e. Chronic anemia

2. The most common pathogen implicated in bacterial infection of the respiratory tract in COPD is?
   a. *Moraxella catarrhalis*
   b. *Escherichia coli*
   c. *Haemophilus influenzae*
   d. Anaerobes
   e. *Chlamydia pneumoniae*

3. Which of the following is *not* true regarding complications from COPD?
   a. Cor pulmonale is common in all types of COPD.
   b. Atrial fibrillation and multifocal atrial tachycardia are the most common arrhythmias associated with COPD.
   c. Spontaneous pneumothorax may result from rupture of peripheral bullae.
   d. Noncompliance with treatment results in increased cost for COPD management.

Answers appear on **page 604.**

Chapter 18

Acute Bronchitis

Kevin C. Oeffinger, M.D.

INITIAL VISIT

Subjective

PATIENT IDENTIFICATION. Mark C. is a 42-year-old married African American computer programmer, father of three, who presents with a cough.

PRESENT ILLNESS. Mark states that the cough began about 4 days ago. Initially, the cough was nonproductive, but for the past 2 days he notes that the sputum is thick and yellow. The cough is present throughout the day, but worsens at night. He had some low-grade fever on the first 2 days, but that has resolved. He denies any rhinorrhea, nasal congestion, earache, or sore throat. He notes no other new symptoms other than what he described. Mark missed work yesterday and today as a result of the cough, and is concerned because he will be flying to a conference in a week. Additionally, he exercises every other day, but has had to stop because the cough worsens with running. Mark denies previous episodes of cough or bronchitis in the past 1 to 2 years and did not experience any difficulty with breathing while running before this episode. His youngest son, age 4, had an upper respiratory infection about 9 days ago.

PAST MEDICAL HISTORY. Mark has been fairly healthy in the past. He has had no major medical illnesses, including asthma or recurrent bronchitis. He had a fractured radius at the age of 12 from a bicycle accident. He has not had any previous surgeries. He is currently on no medication other than occasional over-the-counter ibuprofen for muscle strains. He is allergic to penicillin; he thinks he had a rash, but was quite young at the time. He is up-to-date with his immunizations.

FAMILY HISTORY. Both of Mark's parents are alive and in reasonably good health. His mother has hy-

pertension and hypercholesterolemia. His father had a myocardial infarction at the age of 59, but has done well since. He also has hypertension and hypercholesterolemia. Mark is the oldest of the three siblings. His younger brother and sister are alive and well. Mark's paternal uncle died of a myocardial infarction at the age of 62. There is no history of asthma or atopic disease in the family.

HEALTH HABITS. Mark smokes a half to one pack of cigarettes a day, and is currently trying to cut down. He began smoking at the age of 21, while in college. He drinks about one to two glasses of wine a week and about a beer a month. He exercises consistently, running 2 to 3 miles every other day.

SOCIAL HISTORY. Mark has been happily married for 17 years. He works as a computer programmer and his wife is a first-grade teacher. They have three children.

REVIEW OF SYSTEMS. No other symptoms are elicited in the review of systems.

Objective

PHYSICAL EXAMINATION. Mark is a well-developed, well-nourished, physically fit individual in no apparent distress. Vital signs: height 6 feet, weight 161 lb, temperature 98.6°F, pulse 71, respiratory rate 18, and blood pressure 140/90 mm Hg in the right and left arm in the sitting position. HEENT: Scleras anicteric, conjunctiva without injection, pupils equal, round, and reactive to light and accommodation, extraocular muscles intact, fundi with sharp discs and normal vasculature, tympanic membranes clear with normal landmarks, nares are unremarkable, oropharynx is unremarkable. Percussion and transillumination of the frontal and maxillary sinuses are unremarkable. Neck: Supple without adenopathy or thyromegaly. No bruit audible. Lungs: Mild bilateral expiratory wheezes. No rales. Normal chest expansion with breathing. Cardiac: Regular rate and rhythm without murmur, S_3 or S_4. Abdomen: Soft, nondistended, no hepatosplenomegaly or palpable masses. Nontender to palpation. Extremities: No clubbing, cyanosis, or edema. Pulses are 2+ and symmetrical.

Assessment

WORKING DIAGNOSIS. The most likely diagnoses to explain Mark's findings are the following:

1. *Acute bronchitis.* The patient presents with an acute cough, described as productive and purulent, with bilateral wheezing noted on examination.

   Acute bronchitis is a clinical diagnosis, without a pathognomonic sign or symptom. The clinical diagnosis likely encompasses multiple diseases in a common pathophysiologic pathway. Infection, generally viral, is considered to trigger this process. An inflammatory response ensues, possibly complicated by secondary bacterial infection, bronchospasm, and/or overproduction of mucus. Cough is the primary complaint, often accompanied with a low-grade fever and chest discomfort. The cough can be productive or nonproductive, purulent or nonpurulent. The severity of the cough is generally mild to moderate. It frequently lasts for days before the patient presents for medical attention.

2. *Tobacco abuse or dependency.*

3. *Borderline elevated blood pressure.*

4. *Family history of early cardiac disease.*

Differential Diagnosis

1. *Upper respiratory infection.* Patients with a viral upper respiratory infection generally complain of significant nasal symptoms, such as rhinorrhea, sneezing, and congestion. The nasal symptoms are the primary problem with cough being a secondary complaint. Symptomatic treatment of the nasal symptoms usually results in improvement of the cough.

2. *Sinusitis.* Patients with acute sinusitis have purulent nasal discharge, often with facial or dental pain. The purulent discharge can be observed on examination with a nasal speculum. Transillumination of the frontal or maxillary sinuses often reveals abnormal findings. A patient may present with a concurrent sinusitis and bronchitis, and treatment should include an antibiotic such as amoxicillin or trimethoprim/sulfamethoxazole.

3. *Pneumonia.* Pneumonia caused by *Streptococcus pneumoniae* is not difficult to distinguish from acute bronchitis. Patients presenting with a pneumococcal pneumonia experience an abrupt onset of fever in the 102° to 104°F range, purulent cough (often of a rusty character), with associated chest pain. On examination, localized rales are heard. Patients with an atypical pneumonia, caused by *Mycoplasma pneumoniae* or *Chlamydia pneumoniae,* generally present with a persistent, harsh cough with minimally productive sputum. Careful auscultatory examination reveals rales, localized rhonchi, or bronchial breath sounds and dullness to percussion over the involved area of the lung. If the physician is unable to exclude pneumonia after the history and physical examination, a chest radiograph can be useful. The chest radiograph is generally normal in a patient with acute bronchitis, but may show peribronchial cuffing or overinflation of the lung fields. Findings consistent with pneumonia on a chest radiograph include patchy or consolidated infiltrates.

4. *Asthma.* Patients with asthma can present with an acute cough. However, a careful history of a patient with asthma reveals recurrent episodes of wheezing or coughing. An episode of acute bronchitis, particularly *Chlamydia pneumoniae,* can trigger adult-onset asthma.

Plan

DIAGNOSTIC. No diagnostic tests are appropriate at this time. Mark does not have any signs of acute sinusitis or pneumonia. Chest and sinus radiographs are generally not needed to distinguish between acute bronchitis and pneumonia or sinusitis. Sputum Gram stain and culture has not been found to be helpful in the management of a patient with acute bronchitis.

PATIENT EDUCATION. One primary and one secondary topic are addressed.

1. Treatment of bronchitis. Mark asks you to prescribe antibiotics for his bronchitis, so that he can get over it and get back to his daily routine. You use this opportunity to discuss the use, and potential overuse, of antibiotics. Erythromycin and trimethoprim-sulfamethoxazole have been shown to marginally improve symptoms. Albuterol, a β-2 agonist

bronchodilator, appears to be more effective in improving the cough. Antibiotic resistance is a growing problem that may limit our management of various illnesses in the future. Being a smoker, the patient has a higher likelihood of experiencing future respiratory infections, including pneumonia and sinusitis; having an effective antibiotic is important in his treatment. After discussing the pros and cons of treatment with albuterol, antibiotics, and cough suppressants, Mark is encouraged to select his therapy. He primarily wants symptom relief and to get back to his daily routine and decides to use the albuterol. It is important to make sure that the patient knows that he can discuss the matter with you again if he is not improving.

2. This can be a "teachable moment" in the care of Mark, an opportunity to discuss smoking, both for its role in this illness and the future health consequences. After briefly discussing smoking cessation, you encourage him to set a date to quit smoking.

THERAPEUTIC

1. Management of acute bronchitis. A prescription is written to use albuterol by metered-dose inhaler (MDI), two puffs four times a day for 7 to 10 days or until the cough resolves. After instructing Mark in the use of an inhaler, you observe his technique. You feel that he has good technique and will not need a spacer device. Mark is advised of the need for proper rest and hydration. He is instructed to call if there is any worsening of the cough, increase in fever, shortness of breath, or worsening in his sense of well-being.

2. Instruction concerning smoking cessation.

DISPOSITION. The patient is to return in 4 weeks for a recheck of his blood pressure and discussion of smoking cessation.

FIRST FOLLOW-UP VISIT

Subjective

Mark returns in good spirits. His cough improved within a few days on the albuterol MDI, and he stopped taking the medication after 1 week. He is back to running without difficulty. He denies any shortness of breath or coughing with exertion or at night. Additionally, he decided that during the episode of bronchitis, it was a good time to quit smoking. He decided to quit "cold turkey" and has not had a cigarette in nearly 4 weeks.

Objective

A focused examination is performed. Blood pressure is 130/85 in the right and left arms in the sitting position. His pulmonary and cardiac examinations are unremarkable.

Assessment

1. Resolved bronchitis.
2. Initial success in smoking cessation.
3. Improved blood pressure.
4. Family history of early cardiac disease.

Plan

DIAGNOSTIC. No diagnostic tests are indicated.

THERAPEUTIC PATIENT EDUCATION

1. Compliment the patient on smoking cessation and encourage follow-up. Discuss the role of smoking cessation in lowering Mark's risk of developing cardiac disease and recurrent pulmonary problems.

2. Compliment Mark on improvement in blood pressure. Briefly discuss hypertension and its manifestation as a silent disease. Emphasize that risk factors for early cardiac disease are lowered by smoking cessation and normalized blood pressure. Encourage Mark to continue exercising, being careful of his salt intake, and to have blood pressure checks periodically.

DISPOSITION. Schedule follow-up in 3 months to recheck patient's blood pressure and smoking status and to obtain a fasting lipid profile.

DISCUSSION

Acute bronchitis is a common problem encountered in primary care, ranking among the top 10 reasons for an office visit to the family physician. As noted earlier, the clinical diagnosis of acute bronchitis likely encompasses multiple disease in a common pathophysiologic pathway. The majority of episodes are viral in origin, including adenovirus, influenza

A and B, parainfluenza, rhinovirus, coronavirus, and coxsackievirus. *M. pneumoniae* and *C. pneumoniae*, two atypical respiratory pathogens, may cause 10 to 20 per cent of cases of acute bronchitis. The role of bacterial secondary infection is controversial. Bacterial pathogens include *S. pneumoniae*, *Haemophilus influenzae*, *Moraxella catarrhalis*, and *Bordetella pertussis*. Although the majority of episodes of acute bronchitis are self-limiting, many patients have a cough lasting longer than 10 to 14 days. Treatment is controversial; three methods that have been studied are discussed next.

The first option of treatment is to recognize that the illness is generally self-limiting and that either symptomatic relief or no treatment follows the precept of "First, do no harm." In the majority of patients treated with placebo in randomized clinical trials, the cough was still present 7 to 10 days after evaluation. The cough generally lasts around 2 weeks, often up to a month. It takes patients several days to note improvement in their symptoms, often with the patient missing 2 to 5 days of work. Patients generally do not return to their normal daily routine or a general sense of well-being for several days. Over-the-counter (OTC) symptomatic relief medications do not change the course of the illness. Dextromethorphan, a commonly used OTC cough suppressant, can help with the nighttime cough. Two findings from previous studies are worth noting. First, progression to pneumonia is a rare event in healthy patients with acute bronchitis treated with placebo. Patients treated with antibiotics have about the same chance of developing pneumonia. Secondly, the prolonged symptoms of acute bronchitis are very significant to patients and alter their daily routine enough to seek care.

The second option of treatment that has been studied is the use of antibiotics. Standard primary care texts recommend treatment with antibiotics only in severe cases, stating that symptomatic relief is preferred. In spite of these recommendations, antibiotics are often prescribed by the physician and expected by the patient. Erythromycin is used most often because of the theoretical advantage of treating potential pathogens such as *M. pneumoniae*, *C. pneumoniae*, and *B. pertussis*. To date, there are eight randomized, double-blinded trials of patients with acute bronchitis comparing the use of an antibiotic to placebo. Five trials, using dimethylchlortetracycline, doxycycline, or erythromycin, did not demonstrate statistically significant differences from placebo. The other three studies showed marginal improvement in symptom indicators with the use of trimethoprim-sulfamethoxazole or erythromycin. In one of the studies, patients with evidence of *Myco-plasma* infection were no more likely to respond to erythromycin than those without *Mycoplasma* infection. Two common reasons that patients are prescribed antibiotics are because the patient smokes or has a purulent, productive cough. In all of the randomized clinical trials, patients who smoked were no more likely to benefit from antibiotics than nonsmoking patients. Patients with a history of purulent sputum are able to produce a sputum sample less than half of the time. In patients with visibly purulent sputum, less than 25 per cent of the samples are abnormal on microscopic examination ($\geq$ 25 white blood cells per high-power field (HPF), $\leq$ 10 epithelial cells/HPF). Potential respiratory pathogens are cultured in only 20 to 25 per cent of microscopically abnormal sputum specimens. Thus in a patient with a history of a productive, purulent sputum, a bacterial pathogen can be isolated less than 5 per cent of the time. Patients with abnormal sputum samples do not respond to treatment with antibiotics differently than those with unremarkable sputum.

Because the symptoms of acute bronchitis are often prolonged and antibiotics have not been found to make a clinically significant impact on patients, investigators have begun to explore the possible role of bronchodilators. Bronchospasm plays an important role in many patients with bronchitis. Roughly one fourth to one third of patients with acute bronchitis have a history of wheezing with the episode or have audible wheezing on examination. Almost half of patients have bronchospasm demonstrable by spirometry. A double-blinded study comparing albuterol, a β-2 agonist bronchodilator, with erythromycin found that patients using albuterol were less likely to be coughing after 7 days of treatment. In a follow-up study, patients treated with albuterol were less likely to be coughing at 7 days compared with patients treated with placebo. In a Norwegian double-blinded study with a larger sample size, patients with acute bronchitis and objective findings of bronchial hyper-responsiveness experienced a significant reduction in cough on the second day when treated with fenoterol (β-2 agonist) compared with patients treated with placebo. There was no difference in patients without evidence of bronchial hyper-responsiveness.

To summarize, our understanding of the treatment of acute bronchitis in the healthy adult patient is slowly expanding, but an obviously clear-cut choice in treatment is lacking. Several points are important in considering treatment:

1. Symptoms of acute bronchitis usually last longer than a week and are significant enough to alter the patient's daily routine for several days.

2. Acute bronchitis rarely progresses to pneumonia, regardless of treatment.

3. A history of purulent sputum does not indicate a bacterial infection; less than 5 per cent of patients with a history of purulent sputum have a bacterial respiratory pathogen.

4. Nearly half of patients have demonstrable bronchospasm.

No treatment is an option that presents no harm. However, because of the lengthy duration of illness, patients and physicians are often not satisfied with this option. Treatment with erythromycin or trimethoprim-sulfamethoxazole can result in marginal improvement in patient symptoms. However, antibiotic resistance is a growing problem and careful consideration of the potential risks and benefits of antibiotic treatment is necessary. Bronchodilators, such as albuterol, have been shown to improve symptoms better than no treatment or erythromycin, especially in patients with a productive cough and wheezing on examination.

In the future, studies are needed to determine if specific clinical discriminators, such as productive versus nonproductive cough or abnormal versus normal spirometry, can be useful in predicting whether one treatment might be more useful than another. Further study of the β-2 agonist bronchodilators and similar medications is also needed.

SUGGESTED READING

Dunlay J, Reinhardt R, Roi LD. A placebo-controlled, double-blind trial of erythromycin in adults with acute bronchitis. J Fam Pract 1987;25:137–141.

Franks P, Gleiner JA. The treatment of acute bronchitis with trimethoprim and sulfamethoxazole. J Fam Pract 1984; 19:185–190.

Hueston WJ. A comparison of albuterol and erythromycin for the treatment of acute bronchitis. J Fam Pract 1991;33:476–480.

Hueston WJ. Albuterol delivered by metered-dose inhaler to treat acute bronchitis. J Fam Pract 1994;39:437–440.

King DE, Williams WC, Bishop L, Shechter A. Effectiveness of erythromycin in the treatment of acute bronchitis. J Fam Pract 1996;42:601–605.

Melbye H, Aasebø U, Straume B. Symptomatic effect of inhaled fenoterol in acute bronchitis: A placebo-controlled double-blind study. Fam Pract 1991;8:216–222.

QUESTION

1. True or false: Acute bronchitis in the otherwise healthy adult
   a. Frequently progresses to pneumonia if not treated with antibiotics
   b. Can be effectively managed with a β-2 agonist bronchodilator
   c. Is generally triggered by a viral infection
Answer appears on **page 604.**

Chapter 19

Blurring of Vision

Isaac Kleinman, M.D.

CASE 1

Subjective

PATIENT IDENTIFICATION. Rebecca is a 55-year-old white housewife, married with two children, both grown and living independently. She admits to some stresses in her marriage but otherwise has had no complaints, either physical or emotional.

PRESENTING PROBLEM. While lying awake in a darkened room Rebecca experienced abrupt onset of excruciating pain in the right eye associated with visual blurring and halos about lights, shortly followed by severe right-sided headache with nausea and vomiting. The patient described several prior transient episodes of blurred vision in the same eye associated with an aching pain that she related to periods of stress. She was unaware of any ameliorating, precipitating, or aggravating factors except that at times bright lights seem to help abort the attacks.

PAST HISTORY. Noncontributory; no known drug allergies, no history of ocular surgery or injury. She takes estrogen/progesterone, vitamin E 400 units, and a multivitamin daily, but no other medication.

FAMILY HISTORY. There is no history of eye diseases or blindness, no diabetes, hypertension, cardiovascular disease, or neurologic disorders. Both parents are living and well in their seventies. There are two younger siblings living and well.

HABITS. The patient does not smoke or use recreational drugs. She is an infrequent social drinker.

REVIEW OF SYSTEMS. Rebecca underwent an appendectomy at age 16 and has had no other surgery or hospitalization except for her obstetric admissions, both of which were uneventful. She went through an uneventful menopause.

Objective

Rebecca is a well-developed, well-nourished overweight white woman in severe discomfort. She is alert, coherent, and a good historian. Vital signs are normal. The general physical examination is negative except for the following findings: Visual acuity is 20/200 O.D. and 20/30 O.S. The affected eye appears congested and the cornea is slightly steamy making funduscopic examination difficult; the pupil is vertically oval, 5 mm in diameter and fixed; a relative afferent pupillary defect (RAPD)* is present. The anterior segment of the left eye is normal except for a shallow anterior chamber. The disc is somewhat pale with an increased cup-to-disc ratio. Digitally the right eyeball seems harder than the left. The carotids are full and bilaterally equal without bruits or abnormal pulsations. The extraocular movements are full without nystagmus or diplopia. There is no temporal artery tenderness on either side. The fundus of the unaffected eye reveals a disc that is somewhat pale with an increased cup-to-disc ratio.

LABORATORY TESTS. Blood count, urinalysis, chem 7 (serum glucose, K+, Na+, Cl−, BUN, creatinine), sedimentation rate are normal.

DIFFERENTIAL DIAGNOSIS AND ASSESSMENT. Acute angle-closure glaucoma, temporal arteritis, acute iritis, acute keratitis, ophthalmic migraine, central reti-

---

*To elicit RAPD have the patient look at a distant object and shine a light into the better eye. Constriction of the pupil should be seen and consensual constriction of the other pupil. Quickly move the light to the other eye. If the pupil dilates rather than remains constricted, a relative afferent pupillary defect is said to exist. Repeat several times. If RAPD is present it indicates optic nerve disease or severe retinal damage. RAPD is usually elicited in a patient with a lesion affecting the afferent pathway between the retina and the optic chiasm more severely on one side than the other.

nal artery occlusion, retrobulbar neuritis, vitreous hemorrhage, retinal vein thrombosis.

Discussion

Acute Loss of Vision Associated with Pain

1. *Acute angle-closure glaucoma.* We are directed to the diagnosis of acute angle-closure glaucoma, first by the history of onset while the patient was lying awake in a darkened room (this does not usually occur during sleep because a physiologic miosis occurs), then by unilaterality, halos around light, and associated symptoms of severe monocular pain and hemicrania. The presence of RAPD, intense conjunctival hyperemia, corneal edema, increased intraocular pressure (IOP), fixed dilated pupil, and shallow anterior chamber are physical findings that confirm the diagnosis. Because it is vision threatening it should be among the first diagnoses considered in a case of unilateral blurring with eye pain. The history of previous episodes aborted spontaneously suggests prior angle-closure attacks.

The other items in the differential diagnosis are sudden-onset painful ocular emergencies that must also be considered. Their differentiating characteristics are as follows:

2. *Temporal arteritis.* Pain is present but the eye itself is usually clear, and acuity is not affected. It tends to occur in patients over age 55, is usually associated with scalp or temporal artery tenderness, and the sedimentation rate is elevated. One sees a patient with profound decrease in vision, periocular pain, and a pale swollen disc with splinter hemorrhages. The anterior segment may be normal. Diagnosis is confirmed by temporal artery biopsy. Prompt treatment with high-dose systemic steroids is necessary usually at a starting dose of 80 mg daily. Vision loss occurs due to an ischemic optic neuropathy.

3. *Acute iritis.* Headache is common, but without nausea and vomiting. Pain is confined to the affected eye, which is reddened, and visual acuity may be decreased. The pupil is irregular or small. There is perilimbal or circumcorneal redness. Repeat attacks of acute iritis may lead to the formation of adhesions between pupil and cornea or lens which predisposes the patient to secondary glaucoma.

4. *Acute keratitis.* The affected eye is usually red and painful. There are usually halos, photophobia, and lacrimation. If there is loss of corneal transpar-

ency, vision may be decreased. There is a normal disc and fundus. The IOP is not increased. RAPD is absent.

5. *Ophthalmic migraine.* In the case of an acute ophthalmic migraine the anterior segment is normal and there is no increase in intraocular pressure. Retinal vessels may show some vasospasm but there are no other ophthalmoscopic findings and no RAPD.

Acute Loss of Vision Without Pain

1. *Central retinal artery occlusion.* It may be embolic (from the heart or carotids), vaso-obliterative (atheroma, gaint cell arteritis), vasospastic (ophthalmic migraine), or due to hyperviscosity states (polycythemia, sickle cell anemia, thrombocytosis, leukemia, multiple myeloma and Waldenström's macroglobulinemia). It is characterized by sudden monocular, painless loss of vision. There would be no significant eye congestion or edema of the cornea. A marked RAPD is present. There may well be a history of recurrent brief episodes of loss of vision (amaurosis fugax). Findings on ophthalmoscopy are characteristic and show an ischemic retina in which a cherry-red spot initially can be seen at the macula. Vessels are markedly narrowed. Treatment must be immediate. To promote vasodilatation the patient should rebreathe into a paper bag or inhale from a mixture of 5% to 10% carbon dioxide in oxygen. Acetazolamide (Diamox) should be given by mouth immediately and the eye massaged for 15 minutes to dislodge emboli, improve circulation, and decrease IOP. The patient must be referred immediately to an ophthalmologist for intravenous administration of acetazolamide; he or she may also perform a paracentesis of the eye to further decrease intraocular pressure. All patients with amaurosis fugax or central retinal artery occlusion must be worked up for carotid artery disease.

2. *Spontaneous vitreous hemorrhage.* The anterior segment of the eye is normal. The diagnosis should be suspected in diabetes or other causes of proliferative retinopathy (sickle cell, sarcoid), bleeding diatheses, or anticoagulant administration. Ophthalmoscopy should reveal an absent red reflex. Confirmation is made on slit lamp examination.

3. *Retrobulbar neuritis.* There are very few clinical findings. "The patient sees nothing and the examiner sees nothing." That is, the patient loses vision and the eye appears normal on examination. Pain

on movement of the globe and a positive RAPD may be the only signs. It is treated with systemic steroids.

4. *Retinal vein occlusion*. This is usually a posterior segment problem, with no eye congestion or corneal edema in the early stages. The retina should therefore be easily visualized and shows the classic red fundus with engorged, tortuous veins. The visual loss is painless. There may or may not be RAPD. In the late stages the anterior segment may become involved, with a painful congested eye and marked increase in IOP. Chronic open-angle glaucoma is a predisposing factor to central vein occlusion because of the compression of the retinal vasculature by the increased intraocular pressure.

CASE 2

Subjective

Lydia, a 65-year-old widow, is a retired office manager who lives alone. She has no children, and lives on Social Security and her late husband's pension.

PRESENTING PROBLEM. Lydia complains that for the past few months she has noticed a progressive blurring of vision in her right eye. She notes the blurring primarily with distance vision and has less trouble at near point. There is no diplopia. She also notes that for 2 years she has had increasing trouble driving at night because glare from bright lights bothers both eyes. Nothing she does makes it better or worse.

PAST MEDICAL HISTORY. The patient denies any significant past medical history. There is no history of surgery or hospitalization. The patient has rarely seen a doctor. She has never wanted to have her apparent infertility investigated and she's vague about the possibility of tubal disease in her youth. On review of systems, however, it is learned that she once had a diagnosis of hypothyroidism but that she no longer takes any thyroid replacement. The only medications she now takes are nortriptyline for insomnia and steroid eye drops that were given about 3 months ago for chronic eye irritation and dryness.

FAMILY HISTORY. Both parents are deceased. Her mother died of heart trouble in her eighties and her father of stroke in his sixties. Her father and paternal uncle were diabetic and the father may have had high blood pressure. She has six siblings,

all younger, and all well to the best of her knowledge.

HABITS. The patient is a nonsmoker and nondrinker and does not use drugs of any kind. She does not exercise regularly. Her main social activities are church related and she belongs to a quilting society that meets once a month. She enjoys watching TV and reading.

PHYSICAL EXAMINATION. This is well-developed, well-nourished white female in no acute distress. The neck is supple. There are no nodes. The carotids are full and equal, there are no bruits or abnormal pulses. There is no venous distention. The thyroid is small but palpable. It is firm and nontender. The pupils are round, regular and equal, and react to light and accommodation without RAPD. The extraocular movements are full without nystagmus. There is no inflammation or exudate. Visual acuity is 20/70 O.S. and 20/200 O.D. The cornea is clear and the conjunctivae are not injected. The red reflex is marked by patchy dark shadows. The right optic disc is not readily visualized but the left appears normal. Digitally both eyes are readily indented. The remainder of the physical examination is within normal limits.

LABORATORY. Blood glucose is 200 mg/dl; thyroid-stimulating hormone is 20 mU/L.

DIFFERENTIAL DIAGNOSIS. This is a case of blurred vision of gradual onset without associated symptoms and appears to be nonemergent. This occurs in cataract, refractive error (especially presbyopia), drugs, chronic glaucoma, early macular degeneration, and optic atrophy.

The scenario described best fits a cataract. The shadows cast on the red reflex by the opacities in the lens are characteristic. The pattern varies depending on whether the cataracts are nuclear or capsular. It may be unilateral or bilateral. In the present example there is no increase in intraocular pressure to support the diagnosis of glaucoma. Refractive error can be ruled out by the pinhole test which consists of having the patient view an illuminated Snellen chart through a pinhole in a dark piece of paper or cardboard. If refractive error is present, acuity improves using the pinhole. Diabetes and hyperthyroidism may be of concern as possible cofactors in the development of cataracts. Steroid eye drops are also associated with cataract formation but months of use on a regular basis are required. Difficulty with accommodation due to medications can produce unilateral blurring, but onset is more abrupt, there are usually no cataracts (in which case no shadows are seen on ophthalmoscopy), and the symptoms are relieved by discontinuation of the medications. In macular degeneration, central vision is affected and the patient complains that there is something blocking his or her central vision, pupils are usually normal and reactive, and ophthalmoscopy may show macular lesions (pigmentation, hemorrhage, cysts or holes in the retina). Further evaluation by a specialist is needed. If cataracts coexist it may be difficult to evaluate the retina. Optic atrophy occurs at an older age and is due to loss of optic nerve fibers. Onset is gradual. Loss of optic nerve fibers may parallel loss of brain fibers and thus be associated with dementia. Both near and far vision are affected.

DISCUSSION

These cases were chosen to illustrate as many of the usual history and physical findings as possible. History remains the most important feature in evaluation of blurred vision. In general it leads the physician close to the diagnosis even before any physical examination. The first questions to be asked are, Was the onset of blurring sudden or gradual? Is the eye painful? Is the blurring unilateral or bilateral? Is the "blurring" really diplopia? Is it episodic or constant? Are there associated symptoms, e.g., nausea, vomiting, fever, hemicrania, neurologic symptoms, history of trauma, and dementia (Table 19–1).

The first decision to make is whether the problem is life or vision threatening or relatively benign. Those that are sudden in onset are more likely to be vision threatening, e.g., acute angle-closure glaucoma, central retinal artery occlusion, cranial arteritis, central retinal vein occlusion, optic neuritis, papillitis, intraocular hemorrhage, hypertensive retinopathy, cerebral aneurysm, diabetic and sickle cell retinopathy, and retinal detachment. Central retinal artery occlusion may indicate carotid artery disease or aneurysm and as such may be life threatening. Other abrupt-onset causes include acute iritis, acute keratitis, endophthalmitis (uncommon), and acute keratoconus (uncommon).

Unilaterality suggests local rather than systemic disease. Bilateral disease suggests a systemic cause (e.g., hypertension and diabetes mellitus), a central process involving the optic chiasm or the occipital lobes (degenerative disease or vascular causes), or

topical instillation of mydriatic or cycloplegic eye drops.

Those disorders that tend to be painful are acute angle-closure glaucoma, acute iritis, acute keratitis, ophthalmic migraine, optic neuritis, retrobulbar neuritis, and certain cerebral aneurysms, particularly those involving the posterior communicating artery. Retinal detachment, retinal arterial or venous occlusion, hypertensive or diabetic retinopathy, macular degeneration, and spontaneous intraocular hemorrhage, on the other hand, tend to be painless.

The presence of a reflex afferent pupillary defect indicates optic nerve disease. Examination of the eye should proceed in an orderly manner from the most superficial to the deepest structures of the eye. The first examination must be a check of visual acuity with a Snellen chart. It is important to document visual acuity for legal as well as medical reasons before anything is done to the eye. If onset of blurring is gradual and the visual acuity is improved by use of the pinhole aperture, then the problem is probably due to refractive error. Begin with an evaluation of associated structures. Tenderness of scalp muscles or temporal arteries suggests temporal arteritis.

Examine the lids for retraction and symmetry. Unilateral complete ptosis with other signs of an isolated third cranial nerve involvement (dilated pupil, external ophthalmoplegia) suggests compression of the third cranial nerve from aneurysm, tumor, or uncal herniation. Diabetes may present with an isolated third nerve palsy. Parietal ptosis suggests Horner syndrome and intermittent ptosis suggests myasthenia gravis. Proptosis suggests thyroid disease, orbital tumor, or carotid-cavernous fistula, in which case a bruit may be heard over the congested pulsatile eyeball. Lid lag suggests thyroid disease.

Hyperemia of the conjunctivae may occur in acute angle-closure glaucoma, acute uveitis and keratitis, and carotid-cavernous fistula. It may appear in infection, inflammation, orbital cellulitis, or a venous obstruction. Tearing and photophobias, if associated with pain, suggest corneal disease, especially foreign body and ulceration.

Corneal haziness and edema occur in acute angle-closure glaucoma, prolonged contact lens wear, keratoconus, graft rejection, trauma, and infection.

Increase in intraocular pressure (greater than 21 mm Hg) by tonometry is the hallmark of glaucoma. Markedly decreased intraocular pressure (less than 10 mm Hg) suggests severe retinal detach-

TABLE 19–1. Summary of Clinical Characteristics in a Patient with Blurred Vision

	Sudden Onset?	Painful?	Unilateral?	Constant?	Eye Inflamed?	Near Vision Affected?	RAPD Present?	Comments
Central retinal artery occlusion	+	−	+	+	−	+	±	Pale fundus, vasospasm 5%, associated with cardiac or carotid disease, amaurosis fugax. Tx: inhale 5–10% CO_2 and massage eyeball through closed eyelid to decrease IOP
Central retinal vein occlusion	+	−	+	+	−	+	±	Hemorrhagic "bloody fundus" with engorged veins; associated with chronic glaucoma, coagulopathies and hyperviscosity states; may produce secondary glaucoma
Cranial arteritis	+	+	±	+	−	±	±	Pale disc with edema; associated hemicrania, myalgia, tender temporal artery; increased sed. rate. Tx: high-dose steroids
Optic neuritis	+	±	+	+	−	+	+	Disc edema, dilated retinal veins, exudates, ocular or periocular pain; may be secondary to inflammation; associated with degenerative disease, e.g., multiple sclerosis. Tx: steroids
Retinal detachment	+	−	−	+	−	±	±	Causes include tears or holes in retina; exudating: chronic renal failure, choroidal melanomas; tractional: diabetes, sickle cell disease; may also present with flashing lights and scotomas
Ophthalmic migraine	+	+	+	+	−	−	−	Periorbital pain with hemicrania, pale ischemic retina
Acute angle-closure glaucoma	+	+	+	+	+	+	−	Precipitated by darkness, mydriatics and stress, steamy cornea, hard eyeball, nonreactive pupil. Tx: 2% pilocarpine every 15 min for 1 hour; acetazolamide (Diamox) 250 mg
Macular degeneration	−	−	+	+	−	+	−	Disease of the elderly; problems with central vision; peripheral vision and color vision often spared. Needs fluorescein angiography
Spontaneous intraocular	+	−	+	+	−	+	−	Associated with bleeding diatheses, anticoagulant therapy

TABLE 19–1. Summary of Clinical Characteristics in a Patient with Blurred Vision *Continued*

	Sudden Onset?	Painful?	Unilateral?	Constant?	Eye Inflamed?	Near Vision Affected?	RAPD Present?	Comments
Acute uveitis	+	+	+	+	+	+	−	Turbidity in normally clear parts of the eye; conjunctival hyperemia; associated with systemic disease 40% of the time (e.g., ankylosing spondylitis, Reiter's syndrome)
Enophthalmitis	+	+	+	+	±	+	−	Uncommon; painful, cloudiness on ophthalmoscopic examination; usually associated with injury or eye surgery
Chronic glaucoma	−	−	−	+	−	+	+	Gradual onset, increased intra-ocular pressure and cup-to-disc ratio; suspect it in patients with halos or poor dark adaptation; five times more common in blacks
Cataract	−	−	±	+	−	−	−	Age related (other than congenital types); associated with diabetes, thyroid disease; can be drug induced (chronic use of steroids, phenothiazines)
Eye drops	+	−	±	−	−	+	−	Pupils fixed and dilated; loss of accommodation; no associated signs or mydriatics
Refractive error	−	−	−	+	−	±	−	Check with pinhole aperture test
Acute disc edema	+	+	+	+	−	−		Usually bilateral; vision may be normal early; no inflammatory cells in the vitreous; history of nausea, headache; also with hypertension and intracranial disease
Acute keratoconus	+	+	±	+	−	−	−	May be associated with acute glaucoma; chronic keratoconus is slowly progressive and characterized by frequent changes in eyeglasses
Acute conjunctivitis	+	+	±	+	+	−	−	Evident inflammation, mucoid or mucopurulent discharge
Acute keratitis	+	+	−	+	+	±	−	Eye red and painful; halos, photophora, lacrimation; normal disc and fundus

RAPID = Relative afferent pupillary defect; Tx = treatment; IOP = increased intraocular pressure; + = present; − = absent; ± = may or may not be present.

TABLE 19–2. Drugs Associated with Visual Blurring

Drugs Affecting Refraction
Cycloplegics: paralyzer of ciliary muscle; decreased reading
  ability while distance vision remains unchanged.
Anticholinergics: tricyclic antidepressants, antianxiety agents,
  barbiturates, antihistamines, atropine, scopolamine,
  chloroquine, phenothiazine
Drugs affecting glucose concentration in the lens: fluctuating
  visual acuity.
  Insulin, oral hypoglycemics
Myopics: vision blurred at a distance.
  Diuretics, carbonic anhydrase inhibitors, sulfonamides
Mydriatics: dilated pupil, photophobia, blurring due to glare.
  CNS stimulants: amphetamines, methylphenidate, cocaine
  Antihistamines: also affect accommodation
  Anticholinergics: affect accommodation
Miotics: constricted pupil; everything appears darker than
    usual; may appear to improve refractive errors; the
    pinhole camera effect
  Morphine, pilocarpine, codeine, heroin, anticholinesterases

Drugs Affecting Retina and Optic Nerve
Antimalariaes: patients on long-term therapy require
  ophthalmic monitoring.
Thioridazine
Ethambutol: monitor every 3 mo.
Chloramphenicol

Drugs Affecting the Lens Cataractogenic
Corticosteroids: topical or systemic. Patients on long-term
  steroids should be followed routinely.
Psoralens: require patients undergoing PUVA therapy to wear
  ultraviolet filter for 24 hours after each treatment.

Drugs Causing Dry Eyes (Decreased Tears)
Antihistamine, isotretinoin, anticholinergics, antiparkinsonian
  agents, β-blockers, phenothiazines, tricyclic antidepressants,
  monoamine oxidase inhibitors

PUVA = Psoralen plus ultraviolet A light therapy; CNS = central nervous system.

ment, severe intraocular inflammation, or ruptured globe.

The pupils may be constricted or dilated. If
dilation is an isolated finding it suggests cycloplegic
or mydriatic eye drops (Table 19–2). If there is
associated ptosis or extraocular muscle paralysis
look for oculomotor nerve involvement. If there is
contralateral hemiplegia and seventh cranial nerve
weakness, involvement of the corticospinal tract is
indicated. The presence of afferent pupillary reflex
defect (Marcus Gunn pupil) indicates optic nerve
disease or an extensive retinal lesion. The lens may
be opaque (cataract) or dislocated.

The vitreous may appear cloudy from posterior
uveitis, endophthalmitis, or possibly from retained
intraocular foreign body. In addition, vitreous hemorrhage may be seen in proliferative retinopathy

(diabetes mellitus, sickle cell disease, sarcoid),
bleeding diatheses, or anticoagulant therapy.

In retinal disease the patient may complain of
bright flashing retinal scotomas. A veil in the line
of vision suggests retinal detachment. Hemorrhages,
exudates, new vessel formation, and engorged veins
can be seen on ophthalmoscopy. The retina may be
elevated suggesting a detachment. Holes or tears
may be seen.

Examination of the optic nerve may show atrophy (e.g., papilledema), cupping (e.g., glaucoma),
disc edema (in optic nerve compression), or papilledema (in malignant hypertension). Extraocular
movements may be abnormal, causing strabismus.
This may be due to muscular (myopathies, thyroid
disease) or neurologic (palsy, paresis, diabetes, aneurysm) causes.

SUGGESTED READING

The Aging Eye and Low Vision. New York, The Lighthouse Inc.,
  1992 (800 2nd Ave., NY, NY 10017).
Bercow R (ed). The Merck Manual, 16th ed. Rahway, NJ,
  Merck & Company, 1992.
Dhillon B, Millar GT. The Child's Eye. New York, Oxford Univer-
  sity Press, 1994.

Kanski J. Clinical Ophthalmology, 2nd ed. Oxford, England,
  Butterworth, 1990.
Management of Cataracts. Ciba Symposia, Vol 42, No. 4. Summit,
  NJ, Ciba-Geigy Company, 1990.

1. Match the numbered disease with the appropriate letter.
   a. Acute angle-closure glaucoma
   b. Cranial arteritis
   c. Cataract
   d. Central retinal artery thrombosis
   e. Ophthalmic migraine
      (1) Periorbital pain and hemicrania; pale ischemic retina
      (2) Age greater than 55; tender temporal artery; hemicrania, pd sed imantation rate
      (3) Insidious onset; intolerance to glare; lens casts shadows on the red reflex
      (4) Steamy cornea; can be precipitated by mydriatics
      (5) Painless severe sudden vision loss; pale retina; carotid disease

2. Fixed dilated pupils without associated symptoms and signs suggest
   a. Acute angle-closure glaucoma
   b. Optic neuritis
   c. Use of mydriatic eye drops
   d. Acute keratoconus

Answers appear on **page 604**.

Chapter **20**

Ear Pain

John G. O'Handley, M.D.

INITIAL VISIT

Subjective

PATIENT IDENTIFICATION. Amy is a 5-year-old girl who lives with her biological parents and three older siblings. She completed preschool and is now enjoying the summer before beginning kindergarten. Her mother has taken time off work to bring Amy to the office.

PRESENTING PROBLEM. Fever of 102°F after a 1-week history of bilateral ear pain.

PRESENTING ILLNESS. Amy has been complaining of bilateral ear pain for 1 week, but the symptoms have improved each time acetaminophen (Tylenol) has been administered. She says the pain in the left ear is worse than in the right ear. She has had nasal drainage but no cough, and has been eating well. The previous night she had a fever of 102°F and her mother called this morning to make an appointment with her family physician.

PAST MEDICAL HISTORY. Amy was born after a term pregnancy. There were no perinatal complications. She was bottle-fed. Amy was hospitalized at age 9 months because of pneumonia. Reactive airways disease was diagnosed secondarily, and she has had intermittent wheezing since then treated with albuterol syrup and prednisolone syrup when necessary. At age 7 months she had her first episode of acute otitis media (AOM) in her right ear. AOM occurred in her left ear at age 15 months and recurred 6 weeks later. Three months before her present illness she was treated for left AOM. Her immunizations are current and were administered at the appropriate times.

FAMILY HISTORY. One older male sibling had a history of recurrent ear infections resulting in tympanostomy tube placement.

HEALTH HABITS. Amy is active with her friends and is involved in swimming lessons. Her appetite and sleep habits have been normal.

SOCIAL HISTORY. Both of Amy's parents work and she spends the day with a sitter who watches three to four other children. She enjoys swimming on the weekends in her family's backyard pool.

REVIEW OF SYMPTOMS. Essentially negative.

Objective

PHYSICAL EXAMINATION. Amy weighs 43 1/2 lb and is 43 inches tall (60th percentile by height, 80th percentile by weight). Her temperature is 97.3°F by ear thermometer (she had been given acetaminophen 2 hours before the appointment). Examination of the left ear reveals an erythematous tympanic membrane with poor landmarks but no bulging. Pneumatic otoscopy shows no movement of the eardrum. The right ear appears normal. There are some anterior jugulodigastric nodes present below the left ear. The lungs are clear. Purulent rhinorrhea is present.

LABORATORY TESTS. No laboratory tests were required.

Assessment

WORKING DIAGNOSIS. Based on the history of ear pain, AOM 3 months earlier, fever the previous night, and findings of an erythematous, immobile tympanic membrane, a diagnosis of AOM with effusion is made.

DIFFERENTIAL DIAGNOSIS. Although the clinical presentation in this case appears straightforward, a knowledge of the innervation of the ear is necessary in order to make a correct diagnosis whenever a normal physical examination follows the complaint of ear pain. A generous supply of sensory nerves innervate the ear. These are derived from four cranial nerves (trigeminal, facial, vagus, and glossopharyngeal) and two superior cervical nerves (lesser occipital and great auricular).

1. *Intrinsic causes* (Table 20–1). Otitis externa due

TABLE 20–1. Some Intrinsic Causes of Ear Pain

Otitis externa
Otitis media
Barotrauma
Foreign bodies
Infected cysts
Trauma
Carcinoma

to ear canal inflammation caused by pressure on the tragus or movement of the auricle exacerbates the pain and can differentiate it from otitis media. Barotrauma stretches the eardrum causing pain. Degrees of discomfort depend on the pressure change and can range from a "blocked" feeling to rupture of the eardrum. Foreign bodies in the ear can also be the source of pain, and the variety of small objects found in toddlers' ears attests to their ingenuity. Infected cysts result from plugged ceruminous glands and hair follicles in the ear canal and can be viewed with the otoscope. Trauma is another source of pain and can be diagnosed from the history and physical examination.

2. *Extrinsic causes* (Table 20–2). For patients younger than 10 years of age, referred ear pain is much less of a problem but should still be considered when intrinsic causes have not been found. Temporomandibular joint (TMJ) syndrome can be diagnosed by a history of pain with chewing and tenderness over the temporomandibular joint. One study (Uthman et al., 1986) documented that 78 per cent of patients with TMJ disorders had otalgia as a chief complaint. A recent history of dental work may also be a clue to the diagnosis. Cutting teeth and dental caries can cause ear pain and should be considered when no ear pathology is found.

TABLE 20–2. Some Extrinsic Causes of Ear Pain

TMJ syndrome
Cutting teeth
Dental caries
Pharyngitis and/or tonsillitis
Paranasal sinusitis
Eagle syndrome
Carotidynia
Cervical osteoarthritis
Cancer of oropharynx or larynx
Temporal arteritis
Acoustic neuroma

TMJ = Temporomandibular joint.

Pharyngitis and tonsillitis are frequent causes of otalgia; a history of ear pain with swallowing can lead the physician to look for these entities. Paranasal sinusitis can cause referred ear pain. Purulent rhinorrhea, facial or dental pain, and sinus tenderness point to the diagnosis. Ear pain brought on by swallowing, chewing, and/or yawning that is not associated with fever or upper respiratory congestion may be due to an elongated styloid process (Eagle syndrome). This is a rare syndrome that can be ruled out with a lateral neck radiograph. Another uncommon condition causing pain referred to the ear is carotidynia. It is more common in women than men and is associated with throat tenderness, specifically over the bifurcation of the carotid artery. An easily overlooked source of ear pain is cervical osteoarthritis. The two superior cervical nerves, the lesser occipital and the great auricular, can transmit pain from the neck to the external ear canal and the skin of the mastoid area.

Plan

DIAGNOSTIC. No other tests are necessary.

THERAPEUTIC. The patient was treated with cefaclor (Ceclor), 40 mg per kg in three divided doses effective against the common pathogens associated with otitis media as well as against β-lactamase–producing strains. There is also an option to give this dose of cefaclor every 12 hours. The duration of treatment was 10 days. Analgesic-containing glycerin otic drops were also prescribed for symptomatic treatment.

PATIENT EDUCATION. The proper administration of medications, possible complications, and signs of recurrent AOM were explained to Amy's mother. The possibility for placing tympanostomy tubes in the future was also discussed.

DISPOSITION. We scheduled a follow-up appointment for Amy in 3 weeks.

Discussion

DIAGNOSIS. Up to 80 per cent of pediatric visits involves symptoms referable to the ear. The majority of patients with ear pain presenting to a family practitioner's office have either AOM or otitis externa, especially in the younger age group. Practitioners are cautioned against making one of these diagnoses automatically when confronted by this symptom. Awareness of the ear's innervation and the various illnesses that are possible allows the physician the opportunity to include in the differential diagnosis the many causes of ear pain.

The intrinsic causes (see Table 20–1) are somewhat easier to diagnose because of history and visual inspection. The pneumatic otoscope should be available in every family physician's examination room. To make a diagnosis of otitis media without assessing the mobility of the tympanic membrane is akin to diagnosing kidney stones based on history and hematuria alone. Although the chances of making the correct diagnosis are good, it does allow room for error.

CLINICAL FEATURES. AOM is often associated with intense pain. Although older children can verbalize their discomfort, younger children may express their discomfort by ear pulling, irritability, and crying. However, studies have shown that up to 28 per cent of patients with AOM do not have ear pain (Hayden and Schwartz, 1985). Some of the associated findings in AOM include earache, rhinitis, fever, restless sleeping, cough, vertigo, tinnitus, otorrhea, and diminished hearing (Table 20–3). In children younger than 2 years, earache is present less often — although this fact may be related to their inability to communicate pain. Older children have earache with AOM the majority of the time.

Redness of the tympanic membrane by itself is not a reliable indicator of AOM unless accompanied by the other noted signs and symptoms. An immobile, bulging, red tympanic membrane confirms the diagnosis.

In the absence of upper respiratory symptoms, ear pulling does not indicate AOM. Along with upper respiratory infection symptoms, however, approximately 20 per cent of children pulling at their ears have AOM.

ETIOLOGY. The major mechanism in the pathogenesis of AOM is delayed innervation of the tensor veli

TABLE 20–3. Some Associated Symptoms in Acute Otitis Media in Order of Frequency

Greater Than 50% of Time	Less Than 50% of Time
Rhinitis	Vertigo
Cough	Tinnitus
Fever	Otorrhea
Restless sleeping	Diminished hearing
Earache	

palatini muscle. Swallowing causes this muscle to open the eustachian tube, thereby allowing drainage of accumulated fluid and equilibration of pressure. Children prone to AOM have delayed innervation of this muscle until age 6 or 7 years. Other factors that predispose to AOM are bottle feeding, especially in the supine position, male gender, ethnic factors (e.g., Inuit and Native Americans), exposure to upper respiratory tract infections, parental smoking, allergy, craniofacial abnormalities (e.g., cleft palate), Down syndrome, and previous history of AOM, especially in the previous 3 months.

TREATMENT. In order to treat AOM properly, a knowledge of the pathogens involved is necessary. Approximately two thirds of fluid samples from the middle ear in AOM grows bacteria, with the other samples growing viruses. In children less than 6 weeks old, 15 per cent of pathogens are *Escherichia coli* and *Klebsiella pneumoniae* and this must be taken into account to determine treatment. Depending on the geographic location 10 to 20 per cent of patients have β-lactamase–producing strains found in middle ear aspirates, principally from *Haemophilus influenzae* and *Moraxella catarrhalis*. *Streptococcus pneumoniae* is still the number one pathogen found in patients with AOM. Other bacteria are shown in Table 20–4.

The mainstay of treatment for AOM in the United States is still antimicrobial therapy. Amoxicillin (20 mg per kg per day in three divided doses for children weighing less than 20 kg; children weighing 20 kg or more should be given 250 mg every 8 hours) is the first-line antibiotic followed by a number of second-line antibiotics. Reasons for choosing alternative antibiotics are penicillin al-

TABLE 20–5. Drugs for Acute Otitis Media Effective Against β-Lactamase–Producing Strains

Amoxicillin–clavulanate (Augmentin)
Cefaclor (Ceclor)
Cefuroxime axetil (Ceftin)
Loracarbef (Lorabid)
Cefpodoxime proxetil (Vantin)
Cefprozil (Cefzil)
Cefixime (Suprax)
Erythromycin ethylsuccinate–sulfisoxazole (Pediazole)
Trimethoprim-sulfamethoxazole (Bactrim, Septra)
Azithromycin (Zithromax)
Clarithromycin (Biaxin)

lergy, a high incidence of resistant strains of bacteria in the community, treatment failure resulting in persistent infection after a full course of treatment, a recurrent episode of AOM within several weeks, persistent chronic effusion, or resistant bacterial strains identified on culture of middle ear fluid. Drugs effective against β-lactamase–producing strains are shown in Table 20–5. Trimethoprim-sulfamethoxazole (Bactrim, Septra) can be used against *S. pneumoniae* and *H. influenzae*, as well as the β-lactamase–producing organism, but is less effective against *Streptococcus pyogenes* (Group A, β-hemolytic *Streptococcus*). One must also weigh the potential side effects (renal tubular necrosis, Stevens-Johnson syndrome) against those of other antibiotics.

In addition to side effects, convenience of dosing is a consideration. A drug that is administered four times daily is much more difficult to complete than one given two or even three times daily. Cefixime (Suprax) is only given once a day, but is 10 per cent less effective against *S. pneumoniae* compared with other antibiotics in clinical trials and is only used as second-line therapy when there is persistent pain or fever beyond 72 hours.

Traditionally, the duration of therapy has been 10 days for AOM, but there is actually no proved rational basis for this. In England and several other European countries, a 5-day course is recommended for AOM, although French physicians commonly treat for 8 days. The advantages of a shorter course are fewer side effects, reduced cost, improved compliance, and less selecting-out of resistant organisms. One must consider bacteriologic as well as clinical cure. Studies of middle ear fluid obtained by tympanocentesis have shown that in most children greater than 2 years of age, the middle ear becomes sterile in 3 to 6 days (Cohen, 1996). For 5- and 10-day treatments of AOM with cefaclor 40 mg per kg per day, the percentages of treatment failures,

TABLE 20–4. Bacterial Pathogens Isolated from Middle Ear Fluid

	Percentage
Streptococcus pneumoniae	35
Haemophilus influenzae	23
Moraxella catarrhalis	14
Group A *Streptococcus*	3
α-*Streptococcus*	3
Staphylococcus aureus	1
Pseudomonas aeruginosa	1
Other bacteria	28

Totals are greater than 100% because of multiple pathogens.
From Bluestone CD. Current therapy for otitis media and criteria for evaluation of new antimicrobial agents. Clin Infect Dis 1992;14 (Suppl 2):S197–203.

relapses, recurrences, and otitis media with effusion are similar when the tympanic membrane is intact. When spontaneous perforation occurs, treatment failure is greater in the 5-day group compared with the 10-day group. In addition, 5- and 10-day courses of cefpodoxime proxetil (Vantin) in children with AOM show the only significant differences in favor of the 5-day regimen in terms of side effects, compliance, and acceptability (Cohen, 1996). The advantage of a 5-day course of antibiotics for children greater than 2 years of age with intact eardrums is hard to dispute; however, further studies may be necessary before this shorter course of therapy is generally accepted. Azithromycin (Zithromax) is currently the only antibiotic that has Federal Drug Administration approval for 5 days of treatment in AOM.

The natural history of effusions following AOM is resolution within 3 weeks in 75 per cent of cases and within 2 months in another 10 to 15 per cent. For those patients whose effusion persists beyond 2 months (formerly known as serous otitis media), there is still debate on the wisdom of prescribing a course of antibiotics. A meta-analysis in 1993 to examine the question (Williams et al., 1993) concluded that it was perhaps unreasonable to expect a brief course of antibiotics to produce a lasting benefit in this condition, given the continued role of eustachian tube dysfunction. Many factors play a role in the physician's decision-making regarding antibiotic use in otitis media with effusion (OME). These factors include infancy, concurrent hearing loss, vertigo, severe alterations of the tympanic membrane such as a deep retraction pocket, and ossicular involvement. The jury is still out, however, for run-of-the-mill OME. Antihistamines and decongestants have been shown to be ineffective in OME. Although there is some benefit in using systemic corticosteroids in OME, many clinicians believe the risks outweigh the possible benefits.

RECURRENT AOM. Recurrent AOM is defined as three episodes in 6 months, or four to five episodes in 12 months. Clinical trials have shown antimicrobial prophylaxis to be effective. Amoxicillin (20 mg per kg) given in one or two daily doses, or sulfisoxazole (50 mg per kg) once a day may be used. Trimethoprim-sulfamethoxazole (Bactrim, Septra) is contraindicated for prophylaxis. The *Physicians' Desk Reference* states that prophylactic or prolonged administration of this drug is not indicated at any age with otitis media. The duration of prophylaxis for recurrent AOM is 3 to 6 months depending on the season of the year and the response of the patient. While receiving prophylactic antibiotics, the patient needs to be examined every 1 to 2 months to check for effusion and hearing loss. Should either of these two conditions exist beyond 3 months or recurrent infections continue, surgical intervention with tympanostomy tubes should be considered.

COMPLICATIONS. Complications of otitis media are few in the antibiotic era but can occur. Hearing loss as the result of persistent effusion may lead to delays in language development in infants. The first 12 months of life are most critical for this skill, so middle ear effusions in this age group need to be treated aggressively. Other complications that can occur in order of frequency are perforation of the eardrum, cholesteatoma, mastoiditis, meningitis, epidural abscess, subdural empyema, and lateral venous sinus thrombosis.

SURGICAL PLACEMENT OF TYMPANOSTOMY TUBES. The two major indications for surgical intervention with tympanostomy tubes are chronic OME (3 months or greater) and persistent symptoms of vertigo. In some cases when extubation of the tympanostomy tube occurs, reinsertion may be indicated when antimicrobial treatment has failed and the effusion persists. This can happen several times to a young child, but usually by age 5 OME decreases. The average time that ventilation tubes remain in place is 10 to 12 months. Complications of the tubes can include tympanosclerosis (benign) or permanent perforation (less than 1 per cent of cases). In 15 to 20 per cent of patients with tubes in place, drainage from the middle ear can occur. This should be treated with appropriate oral antibiotics and/or ear drops containing an antibiotic–corticosteroid suspension. The treatment is based on culture and sensitivity of the middle ear fluid. The fluid in the ear canal is not satisfactory for culture because of contamination with *Pseudomonas* species and other flora in that area. The culture should ideally be obtained directly from the middle ear. If antibiotics fail to clear the otorrhea, re-evaluation for the presence of granuloma or chronic otomastoiditis may be indicated. Should a ventilation tube not be spontaneously extruded after 3 years, removal and myringoplasty can be performed.

CONCLUSION. The impact of otitis media can be felt not only by the patient but also by the entire family. Everyone who has experienced this illness can attest to the stress that an ill child crying in pain can bring to the parents. The economic impact alone has been estimated at $3.5 billion per year due to office visits, medication, and related surgeries. The frequency of medical visits and surgery for otitis media continue to increase. Although the reasons are not entirely clear, there could be a correlation with the increased use of day care facilities for infants and toddlers.

Children greater than 2 years of age who are prone to recurrent otitis media may benefit from pneumococcal vaccine, which has been shown to be effective in preventing infection from several different serotypes that cause otitis media. In children younger than 2 years, a poor immune response to the vaccine fails to make it useful in preventing otitis media.

Because of the frequency that patients with ear pain are seen by family physicians, it is incumbent on the practitioner to feel comfortable with the many diagnoses and treatments for this common problem.

SUGGESTED READING

Bluestone CD. Current therapy for otitis media and criteria for evaluation of new antimicrobial agents. Clin Infect Dis 1992;14 (Suppl 2):S197–203.

Cohen R. Shortened therapies in acute otitis media. Hosp Pract 1996;31 (Suppl 1):S5–10.

Eichenwald HE. Otitis media in the child. Hosp Pract 1985;20:51–61.

Hayden GF, Schwartz RH. Characteristic of earache among children with acute otitis media. Am J Dis Child 1985;139:721–723.

Heikkinen T, Runskanen O. Signs and symptoms predicting acute otitis media. Arch Pediatr Adolesc Med 1995;149:26–29.

Kligman EW. Treatment of otitis media. Am Fam Physician 1992;45:242–250.

Rakel RE. Saunders Manual of Medical Practice. Philadelphia, W.B. Saunders, 1996.

Thaller SR, DeSilva A. Otalgia with a normal ear. Am Fam Physician 1987;36;129–136.

Uthman AA, Sheth BJ, Gale EN. Prevalence of otological symptoms in a clinical setting. J Dent Res 1986;65 (Special Issue A):335.

Williams RL, Chalmers TC, Stange KC, et al. Use of antibiotics in preventing recurrent otitis media and in treating otitis media with effusion: A meta-analytic attempt to resolve the brouhaha. JAMA 1993;270:1344–1351.

QUESTIONS

1. Findings associated with acute otitis media greater than 50% of the time include:
   a. Cough
   b. Fever
   c. Pulling at the ears
   d. Vertigo
   e. Otorrhea

2. The major reason for acute otitis media is:
   a. Bottle feeding
   b. Delayed innervation of the tensor veli palatini
   c. Exposure to upper respiratory infections
   d. Allergy
   e. Parental smoking

3. All of the following antibiotics are effective against β-lactamase–producing strains of bacteria except:
   a. Trimethoprim-sulfamethoxazole
   b. Erythromycin ethylsuccinate–sulfisoxazole
   c. Cefpodoxime proxetil
   d. Cefixime
   e. Amoxicillin

Answers appear on **page 604**.

Chapter 21

Sinus Congestion

John W. Ely, M.D., M.S.P.H.

INITIAL VISIT

Subjective

PATIENT IDENTIFICATION. Susan J. is a 33-year-old married factory worker who presents with a 6-day history of nasal congestion and rhinorrhea.

PRESENT ILLNESS. Susan was well until 6 days ago when she developed nasal congestion, a nonproductive cough, and clear rhinorrhea. Her nasal discharge became greenish yellow on the day of her visit, and she now asks for antibiotics for what she believes is a sinus infection. She complains of a constant generalized headache and pain in her nose and cheeks when she bends forward. She admits to occasional chills and sweats but has not taken her temperature. She denies pain in her teeth and has obtained minimal relief from over-the-counter decongestants. She has no history of asthma or hay fever and no history of drug allergies. Her only long-term medication is an oral contraceptive, and she denies using decongestant nose sprays. She says she has at least one or two "sinus infections" every year, and she cannot seem to get over them unless she takes an antibiotic.

PAST MEDICAL HISTORY. Susan has had two vaginal deliveries but no other hospitalizations. She denies any history of serious illnesses or surgery.

FAMILY HISTORY. There is no history of hay fever or asthma in the family. Susan's father has a history of hypertension and elevated cholesterol. Her mother has a history of arthritis. Her only sibling, an older brother, is alive and well.

SOCIAL HISTORY. Susan is a nonsmoker and drinks alcohol occasionally. She is sexually active and monogamous, and she denies illicit drug use. She works on an electronics assembly line and helps her husband on the farm during the "busy season."

REVIEW OF SYSTEMS. Susan denies any history of heart or lung disease and her review of systems is otherwise unremarkable.

Objective

PHYSICAL EXAMINATION. Oral temperature 37.2°C, pulse 80, respiratory rate 20, blood pressure 110/75 mm Hg. General: Susan is alert and has obvious nasal congestion. Eyes: Pupils 3 mm bilaterally, regular and reactive to light. No conjunctival injection. Ears: Normal. Frontal and maxillary sinuses are nontender to palpation. Transillumination of the sinuses is normal. Nose: Swollen erythematous turbinates with no air movement on the left, clear mucus. Mouth and throat: No inflammation; mild posterior pharyngeal cobblestoning. Neck: Supple without lymph node enlargement. Lungs: Clear to percussion and auscultation. Heart: Regular rhythm, grade 1/6 systolic ejection murmur at the left sternal border. Abdomen: No organomegaly, no masses or tenderness.

LABORATORY TESTS. No laboratory tests were performed.

IMAGING STUDIES. No imaging studies were performed.

Assessment

WORKING DIAGNOSIS. Susan probably has a viral upper respiratory infection (URI). However, she may have a superimposed bacterial sinusitis. Factors in favor of sinusitis include her history of purulent nasal discharge and her failure to respond to decongestants.

DIFFERENTIAL DIAGNOSIS. Susan's symptoms may be secondary to other causes of nasal congestion such as

1. *Allergic rhinitis.* The absence of itching and paroxysms of sneezing makes allergic rhinitis ("hay fever") less likely. Also she has no history of atopic disease, and her symptoms are acute, not seasonal or chronic as would be expected with allergic rhinitis.
2. *Other rhinitis syndromes:*
   a. *Nonallergic rhinitis.* Patients with nonallergic rhinitis have symptoms similar to those with perennial allergic rhinitis, but their disease is not IgE-mediated and they have negative skin test findings. They may have large numbers of eosinophils in their nasal mucus. Susan's acute course argues against this diagnosis.
   b. *Vasomotor rhinitis.* This form of rhinitis is a chronic condition that may be aggravated by strong odors or changes in temperature or humidity. It has no allergic basis.
3. *Rhinitis medicamentosa.* Overuse of topical nasal decongestants can lead to tolerance and rebound nasal congestion when the medications are discontinued. Cocaine can also lead to nasal congestion.
4. *Endocrine causes.* Pregnancy and hypothyroidism can lead to nasal congestion.

Plan

LABORATORY AND SPECIAL TESTS. Imaging studies and laboratory tests are generally not indicated in the diagnosis of acute sinusitis and none were obtained in this case.

TREATMENT. Susan was started on an antihistamine-decongestant combination and a 3-day course of trimethoprim-sulfamethoxazole (Bactrim, Septra), one double-strength tablet twice a day. The decision to use antibiotics was based on her history of purulent nasal discharge and her failure to respond to decongestants. These clinical factors gave her a moderate likelihood of having bacterial sinusitis, as discussed later. There are no practical methods to reliably differentiate viral URIs from bacterial sinusitis in the primary care setting. In Susan's case, another option would have been to treat her symptomatically with close follow-up and later consideration of antibiotics depending on her course. She

was told she could use one of the over-the-counter decongestant nose sprays for the next 3 days.

PATIENT EDUCATION. Susan was instructed to return if she developed a fever or if her symptoms failed to improve within 2 or 3 days. She was warned about the adverse effects of prolonged topical decongestants and reminded not to use them for more than 3 days. She was also warned about the possibility of developing Stevens-Johnson syndrome and to stop the trimethoprim-sulfamethoxazole immediately if she developed a rash or oral mucosal lesions. Finally, she was told that her oral contraceptive may be less effective while taking the antibiotic.

DISPOSITION. Susan was asked to return in 1 week.

FIRST FOLLOW-UP VISIT

Susan returned as requested in 1 week, and she reported complete resolution of her symptoms. She had stopped all medications except for her oral contraceptive. She is a new patient and several health maintenance issues were discussed including Pap smears, diphtheria-tetanus immunization, and seat belts.

Objective

Vital signs were normal. Examination of her nose, ears, mouth, throat, and neck was normal.

Assessment

Acute maxillary sinusitis versus viral URI, resolved.

Plan

PATIENT EDUCATION. Susan was informed about symptoms that may help differentiate bacterial sinusitis from viral URIs, such as purulent nasal discharge and pain in the upper teeth. She was reminded about the importance of avoiding prolonged use of topical decongestants.

DISPOSITION. Susan was asked to return in 6 months for a complete physical examination and Pap smear.

DISCUSSION

Acute nasal congestion and rhinorrhea are among the most common complaints faced by family physicians. It is often challenging to differentiate sinusitis from a viral URI in patients with these symptoms. In the primary care setting, the differentiation necessarily rests on the history and physical examination rather than laboratory or radiologic studies. The dilemma is that the history and physical are often inadequate to distinguish between sinusitis and a viral URI. However, Williams and colleagues recently reported five clinical features that were found to improve the ability to predict sinusitis (Williams et al., 1992) (Table 21–1). If a patient has all five findings, the probability of sinusitis is 92 per cent, whereas if none of the findings are present, the probability of sinusitis is only 9 per cent. Most patients fall between these extremes. For these patients, the decision to use antibiotics depends on the physician's philosophy and his or her willingness to comply with patient requests.

Transillumination may help improve diagnostic accuracy in equivocal cases (Fig. 21–1). However, this procedure must take place in a completely dark room, and the physician must allow 2 to 3 minutes for visual adaptation to the dark before performing this test.

Laboratory tests are rarely indicated in patients with acute nasal congestion. However, in patients with underlying allergic rhinitis, a Hansel stain of the nasal mucus may reveal eosinophils. Nasal cultures are not helpful because they do not correlate with the causative organism in bacterial sinusitis. Cultures of the maxillary sinus, using antral puncture, are reserved for patients with resistant chronic sinusitis, immunocompromised patients, and patients with life-threatening complications.

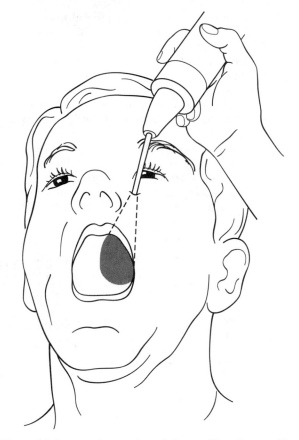

Figure 21–1. Transillumination of the maxillary sinuses. (From Williams JW, Simel DL. Does this patient have sinusitis? Diagnosing acute sinusitis by history and physical examination. JAMA 1993;270:1242–1246, with permission.)

TABLE 21–1.   Probability of Sinusitis

Number of Clinical Factors Present	Probability of Sinusitis (95% CI), %
0	9 (5–17)
1	21 (15–28)
2	40 (33–47)
3	63 (53–72)
4	81 (69–89)
5	92 (81–96)

Predictors of sinusitis:
1. Maxillary toothache
2. History of colored nasal discharge
3. Poor response to nasal decongestants
4. Abnormal transillumination
5. Purulent secretion on examination
(From Williams JW Jr, Simel DL, Roberts L, Samsa GP. Clinical evaluation for sinusitis: Making the diagnosis by history and physical examination. Ann Intern Med 1992;117:705–710. Used with permission.)

Radiographic studies are rarely ordered in the primary care setting, but they are occasionally helpful. For example, in patients with refractory symptoms despite multiple courses of antibiotics, a negative result from a sinus series may help avoid yet another course of antibiotics. Attention can then be turned to noninfectious causes of chronic nasal congestion and rhinorrhea. Computed tomography (CT) scans of the sinuses have high sensitivity but low specificity. In one study, 65 per cent of patients with viral URIs had abnormalities of their maxillary sinuses on CT scan (Gwaltney et al., 1994). Magnetic resonance images and ultrasound have little place in the diagnosis of sinusitis.

Acute sinusitis is most often caused by pneumococci, *Haemophilus influenzae*, and *Moraxella catarrhalis*. *Staphylococus aureus* is an unusual cause of acute sinusitis, but it is often present in chronic sinusitis. Anaerobes are also an important causative agent in chronic sinusitis.

Patients may derive symptomatic relief from

steam inhalations or nasal irrigations, although firm evidence of their efficacy is lacking. Topical decongestants (e.g., phenylephrine, oxymetazoline) and systemic decongestants (e.g., pseudoephedrine, phenylpropanolamine) may provide symptomatic relief and theoretically allow better sinus drainage. Patients should be warned not to use topical decongestants for longer than 3 days to avoid tachyphylaxis and rebound nasal congestion. However, these risks are minimal when the topical decongestants are used for 3 days or less. Antihistamines can be added if an allergic component is suspected.

Trimethoprim-sulfamethoxazole or amoxicillin is used to treat acute sinusitis. Although β-lactamase–producing strains of *H. influenzae* and *M. catarrhalis* can cause sinusitis, there is no good evidence to support the use of more expensive antibiotics for the initial treatment of acute sinusitis. A recent clinical trial found that a 3-day course of trimethoprim-sulfamethoxazole was just as effective as a 10-day course (Williams et al., 1995). If the patient fails to respond to the initial antibiotic, the spectrum can be broadened by changing to amoxicillin–clavulanate (Augmentin), or cefaclor (Ceclor), and 3- or 4-week courses may be required in such cases. Referral to an otolaryngologist is indicated if the patient's sinusitis fails to clear after these more intensive regimens.

SUGGESTED READING

Forstall GJ, Macknin ML, Yen-Lieberman BR, VanderBrug Medendorp S. Effect of inhaling heated vapor on symptoms of the common cold. JAMA 1994;271:1109–1111.

Gwaltney JM, Phillips CD, Miller RD, Riker DK. Computed tomographic study of the common cold. N Engl J Med 1994;330:25–30.

Williams JW, Hollerman DR, Samsa GP, Simel DL. Randomized controlled trial of 3 vs 10 days of trimethoprim/sulfamethoxazole for acute maxillary sinusitis. JAMA 1995;273:1015–1021.

Williams JW, Simel DL. Does this patient have sinusitis? Diagnosing acute sinusitis by history and physical examination. JAMA 1993;270:1242–1246.

Williams JW Jr, Simel DL, Roberts L, Samsa GP. Clinical evaluation for sinusitis: Making the diagnosis by history and physical examination. Ann Intern Med 1992;117:705–710.

QUESTIONS

1. Which organisms are most likely to cause acute sinusitis?
   a. *Haemophilus influenzae, Moraxella catarrhalis, Staphyloccus aureus*
   b. *Streptococcus pneumoniae, Haemophilus influenzae, Moraxella catarrhalis*
   c. *Haemophilus influenzae, Moraxella catarrhalis*, anaerobes
   d. Anaerobes, *Staphyloccus aureus, Haemophilus influenzae*
   e. *Moraxella catarrhalis, Streptococcus pneumoniae, Escherischia coli*

2. Which of the following imaging studies is most helpful and practical for differentiating sinusitis from rhinitis without sinus involvement?
   a. Magnetic resonance imaging
   b. Plain sinus radiographs
   c. Sinus ultrasound
   d. Isotope scanning
   e. Positron emission tomography

3. Which of the following clinical findings is least helpful in differentiating viral upper respiratory infections from bacterial sinusitis?
   a. Purulent nasal discharge
   b. Poor response to decongestants
   c. Pain in the maxillary teeth
   d. Abnormal transillumination
   e. Maxillary sinus tenderness

Answers appear on **page 604.**

Chapter 22

Dizziness

Jeanne M. Ferrante, M.D.

INITIAL VISITS

Subjectives

PATIENT IDENTIFICATION AND PRESENTING PROBLEM. Tom W. is a 41-year-old white man who presents for the first time with a complaint of dizziness.

PRESENT ILLNESS. Tom states that he began to feel ill 1 week ago with fatigue, slight sore throat, nasal congestion, and dry cough. This morning he awoke with severe dizziness, which he describes as "the room spinning" associated with nausea, vomiting, and generalized weakness. Any movement of his head makes his symptoms worse. He has been feeling dizzy and nauseated all day and has not been able to keep anything down. This is the first time he has experienced these symptoms. He denies recent head or neck trauma, barotrauma, headache, hearing loss, discharge from the ears, tinnitus, or fullness in his ears. There was no blurry vision, double vision, difficulty swallowing, changes in his speech, or weakness or numbness in his face, arms, or legs.

PAST MEDICAL HISTORY. Tom has had no major medical illnesses or surgery. He has no history of recurrent ear infections. He does not take any medications and has not been on antibiotics recently.

FAMILY HISTORY. Tom has no siblings. His parents are alive and well.

SOCIAL HISTORY. Tom is married and works as a mechanic. He has smoked one pack of cigarettes per day for 25 years. He drinks alcohol rarely on weekends. He denies illicit drug use.

REVIEW OF SYSTEMS. The patient denies headache, neck pain, shortness of breath, chest pains, palpitations, depression, anxiety, fainting, or falling.

Objectives

PHYSICAL EXAMINATION. Tom is a well-developed, well-nourished alert white male lying on the table in mild to moderate distress. Vital signs: Height 5 feet 10 inches tall, weight 165 lb, temperature 99.1° F, respiratory rate 20, blood pressure 138/88, pulse 90. There is no orthostatic change in blood pressure or pulse. Head, eyes, ears, nose, and throat: Head is without lesions or signs of trauma; external ear canals and tympanic membranes are clear bilaterally; hearing is intact by testing with tuning forks; conjunctiva pink; pupils equal, round and reactive to light and accommodation; extraocular muscles intact without nystagmus; nose clear; maxillary and frontal sinuses transilluminated and are nontender to percussion; mouth has poor dentition; oropharynx is clear. Neck: Supple, no bruits, no lymphadenopathy, normal thyroid. Lungs: Clear to auscultation. Heart: Normal sinus rhythm without murmurs, rubs, or gallops. Neurologic: Oriented to place, time, and person. He has a normal but slowed gait. Cranial nerves II to XII are intact. Deep tendon reflexes 2+ in upper and lower extremities bilaterally. Strength 5+ in all extremities. Sensorium is intact to light touch and pinprick. Cerebellar function is intact to finger-to-nose pointing and rapid alternating movements. Romberg test shows slight swaying toward the back. The Nylen-Barany test is positive on the left for nystagmus and vertigo after a latency of about 3 seconds. This lasted for less than 1 minute.

Assessment

WORKING DIAGNOSIS. The working diagnosis is peripheral vertigo caused by acute vestibular neuronitis or labyrinthitis. Vertigo can be caused by peripheral or central disorders. Peripheral causes of vertigo include lesions of the vestibular nerve, labyrinth, or both. Central vertigo is caused by disorders of the lower brain stem or cerebellum. Patients with brain stem disease have symptoms typical of vertebrobasilar insufficiency, such as diplopia, dysarthria, dysphagia, paresthesia, and changes in sensory and motor function. Patients with cerebellar disease may have truncal ataxia and difficulty with rapid alternating movements and finger-to-nose testing. Tom has none of the history or physical findings of central vertigo. The result of the Nylen-Barany maneuver also helps to point to a peripheral cause of the vertigo. The Nylen-Barany test (also referred to as the Dix-Hallpike maneuver) is a head hanging maneuver that helps to distinguish peripheral vertigo from central causes of vertigo. The Nylen-Barany test is performed with the patient initially sitting on the examination table. Quickly the patient is brought into the lying position by the examiner with the patient's head turned about 30 degrees to one side and slightly hyperextended over the end of the table (Fig. 22–1). The patient should be given clear instructions to keep the eyes open. The patient is then observed for symptoms of nausea and vertigo and signs of nystagmus. This maneuver is then repeated with the head turned to the opposite side. If the symptoms are reproduced and nystagmus occurs after a brief latency period (3 to 20 seconds) but resolves in less than 1 minute, then the dizziness is more likely to be a peripheral cause. If there are mild or no symptoms, and nystagmus is present immediately and persists for longer than 1 minute, then a central cause of vertigo should be suspected.

Vestibular neuronitis is thought to be due to a viral infection of the vestibular nerve. It is characterized by the acute onset of severe constant vertigo (made worse by head movement), nausea, and vomiting in the absence of hearing loss or tinnitus. Often, there is evidence of a recent or concurrent upper respiratory tract infection. Tom developed acute symptoms which have continued, and he had a recent upper respiratory tract infection. He has no hearing loss, tinnitus, or other signs of a central cause of the vertigo. Tom's history and physical findings make vestibular neuronitis a likely diagnosis.

DIFFERENTIAL DIAGNOSIS. Other causes of peripheral vertigo include several conditions.

1. *Benign paroxysmal positional vertigo.* This is the most common cause of vertigo. Patients usually have sudden intermittent episodes of vertigo on position change or head turning only. In most cases it is idiopathic and results from accumulation of organic debris in the posterior semicircular canal. A precipitating factor may be a recent middle ear infection, vestibular neuronitis, head trauma, or ear surgery.

2. *Meniere's disease.* Meniere's disease is defined by a classic triad of low-frequency sensorineural hearing loss, vertigo, and tinnitus. Ear fullness or pressure may also be present. Patients are usually

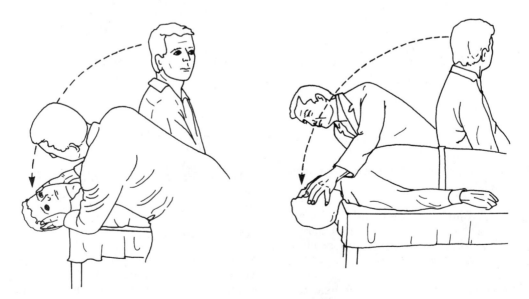

Figure 22–1. The Nylen-Barany maneuver. (From Reilly BM: Practical Strategies in Outpatient Medicine, 2nd ed. Philadelphia, W. B. Saunders Company, 1991.)

between the ages of 30 and 60 years at the onset. These patients have clusters of vertiginous exacerbations coinciding with increased hearing loss and intensity of tinnitus. During periods of remission, episodes of vestibular dysfunction and even hearing loss and tinnitus may significantly resolve for weeks or months.

3. *Recurrent vestibulopathy.* Patients with recurrent vestibulopathy usually have intermittent episodes of constant vertigo lasting for minutes or hours; there are no hearing deficits. The disease has a benign course and most patients have complete remission.

4. *Acoustic neuroma.* Acoustic neuroma is a benign tumor that usually causes progressive unilateral high-frequency hearing loss, tinnitus, and imbalance (particularly in the dark). Vertigo occurs in less than 20 per cent of patients because the neuromas grow slowly. The lesion is in the cerebellopontine angle and when advanced, affects other cranial nerves (i.e., fifth and seventh).

5. *Perilymphatic fistula.* A perilymphatic fistula allows leakage of inner ear fluids into the middle ear space resulting in hearing loss and vertigo. Patients with this rare clinical entity usually have a history of ambient pressure changes (diving, air flight), trauma, or congenital anomalies of the inner ear and temporal bone. Symptoms are typically worsened by straining.

6. *Cholesteatoma.* Cholesteatoma is a complication of chronic otitis media. It is caused by sacs of skin that arise from the tympanic membrane, collecting squamous debris as they enlarge. Eventually a fistula develops in the lateral semicircular canal. Patients have a history of chronic otitis media, conductive hearing loss, and drainage of the ear.

7. *Trauma and ototoxicity.* Temporal bone trauma can cause acute destruction of the inner ear leading to vertigo and hearing loss. Aminoglycoside antibiotics have a toxic effect on the vestibular labyrinth and can cause vertigo with or without hearing loss.

8. *Herpes zoster oticus (Ramsay Hunt syndrome).* Patients often have deafness, facial palsy, and vesicles in the ear canal.

Plan

DIAGNOSTIC. Since Tom does not have symptoms and signs of a more severe cause of vertigo, no tests are indicated at this time. If the symptoms do not resolve after 6 weeks or if hearing loss or tinnitus is present, then audiometry and vestibular assessment (including calorics with or without electronystagmography) may be indicated.

THERAPEUTIC. The patient is treated symptomatically with meclizine 25 mg three to four times a day.

PATIENT EDUCATION. The patient is educated on the benign course of vestibular neuronitis and that it gradually resolves over 2 days to 6 weeks. He is instructed to move slowly and to take the medication as needed for symptoms. He is also advised to stop smoking.

DISPOSITION. The patient is instructed to make a second appointment in 6 weeks or sooner if his symptoms are not relieved by the meclizine, or if he develops hearing loss, tinnitus, or other neurologic symptoms.

DISCUSSION

Dizziness is a common complaint in primary care, accounting for 2 per cent of all office visits (Sloane and coworkers, 1994). Dizziness can be caused by a disturbance in any of a number of balance control systems, including the visual pathways, the vestibular apparatus, the cardiovascular system, and the proprioceptive tracts of the central nervous system (CNS). Dizziness is a general and vague term that means different things to different people. History taking is most important to clarify what the patient means by dizziness. There is a broad spectrum of problems that can present with dizziness in a patient. These problems can be divided into four main categories: vertigo, impaired perfusion of the CNS or near-syncope, disequilibrium, and psychogenic causes. Vertigo is an illusion of movement, as if the patient or the room is spinning. Vertigo can be peripheral or central in origin (discussed previously). Central vertigo is caused by neoplastic, vascular, or neurologic disorders of the lower brain stem or cerebellum. In patients with posterior fossa tumors, vestibular dysfunction is usually slow in onset due to the slow growth of typical neoplasms. These patients usually have imbalance and coordination difficulties. Vascular diseases include vertebrobasilar transient ischemic attacks, cerebellar or brain stem strokes, and vertebrobasilar migraines. Neurologic disorders include complex partial seizures and multiple sclerosis. Complex partial seizures may present with an aura of dizziness, vertigo, or unsteadiness. In multiple sclerosis, vertigo can present initially in 5 per cent of patients and ultimately in up to 50 per cent of patients (Ruckenstein, 1995). Symptoms are usually episodic and associated with a wide variety of other neurologic symptoms.

In impaired perfusion or near-syncope, patients describe the feeling of lightheadedness or the world going gray and out of focus, especially when they stand. This can be caused by orthostatic hypotension due to decreased baroreceptor responsiveness, medications (antihypertensives, antidepressants), anemia, dehydration, metabolic diseases (i.e., diabetes mellitus, thyroid diseases), or cardiovascular disorders. Structural cardiac disease (i.e., aortic stenosis, mitral regurgitation, and hypertrophic cardiomyopathy), arrhythmias, and heart blocks may also cause dizziness associated with near-syncope or syncope.

Disequilibrium is a sensation of unsteadiness and imbalance when standing or walking. The patient feels a lack of coordination and a sense of an impending fall. This is commonly seen in the elderly. The cause is usually multifactorial including multiple sensory deficits (i.e., decreased visual acuity and peripheral neuropathy with impaired proprioception), medications affecting the CNS (i.e., anticonvulsants, benzodiazepines, neuroleptics, and antidepressants), or other neurologic disorders.

Psychogenic dizziness is consistently one of the most common diagnoses made for dizziness, especially in young adults less than 40 years of age. In one study at a military hospital, 40 per cent of patients with weakness and dizziness had an underlying psychiatric diagnosis (Kroenke et al., 1993). In psychogenic dizziness, symptoms are usually vague and may include sensations of lightheadedness, feeling apart or far away from the environment, fatigue, or tightness or fullness in the head. Patients may also complain of numbness or tingling around the mouth or in the hands. Common causes of psychogenic dizziness include depression, anxiety, panic attacks, somatization disorder, and substance abuse.

Once the character of the dizziness is determined, it is helpful to find out how long it has persisted, and whether or not it occurs in attacks. In addition, ask about what provokes or worsens the dizziness (standing up, head turning or rolling over in bed, coughing or straining, stress or emotional upset), and what was happening when the dizziness began (e.g., loud noise, blow to the head, flulike symptoms or a cold beforehand). Inquire about general health problems such as high blood pressure, diabetes, heart disease, thyroid disease, migraine headaches, seizure disorder, anxiety, or depression. Medications and drug use should always

be noted. A systems review is important to identify symptoms that are related to the dizziness including generalized weakness, loss of consciousness, headaches, nausea, vomiting, diplopia, blurry vision, dysarthria, dysphagia, hearing loss, discharge from the ears, tinnitus or a fullness in the ears, numbness or tingling in the face, around the mouth, or in the hands or feet, chest pain, or a pounding or rapid heartbeat.

The physical examination can help to narrow the differential diagnosis. Vital signs, especially postural changes in blood pressure, should be obtained to check for orthostatic hypotension. A head, eyes, ears, nose, and throat examination should focus on the ears, eyes, and sinuses. Spontaneous nystagmus can usually be observed in vertiginous patients. However, in peripheral vestibular disorders visual fixation can suppress spontaneous nystagmus. The neck examination includes checking for bruits and thyroid abnormalities. The cardiovascular examination is important to check for size of the heart, murmurs, and arrhythmias. The neurologic examination should focus on the cranial nerves, strength, sensory, and cerebellar functions. If the dizziness is described as vertigo, then the Nylen-Barany maneuver should be performed. If a psychogenic cause is suspected, a useful test is to have the patient hyperventilate for about 1 to 2 minutes. Exact reproduction of symptoms correlates strongly with psychogenic dizziness.

Laboratory tests are of little value in most patients complaining of dizziness. Patients who appear to have fatigue or metabolic abnormalities can be screened with a standard biochemical profile and complete blood count. Thyroid function tests may be indicated if thyroid disease is suspected. A rapid plasma reagin (RPR) or Venereal Disease Research Laboratories (VDRL) test may be useful in patients suspected of Meniere's disease because secondary or early tertiary syphilis may present with symptoms identical to those seen in Meniere's disease. An electrocardiogram can document cardiac abnormalities if they are suspected based on the history and physical examination. When the history, physical examination, and laboratory studies rule out organic disease, psychogenic factors should be addressed.

Advanced diagnostic tests are helpful if more severe causes of dizziness are suspected based on the history and physical examination. In patients with chronic peripheral vertigo or vertigo associated with hearing loss, audiometric testing and vestibular assessment by the audiologist are indicated. Patients with neurologic deficits should have imaging studies such as brain computed tomography or magnetic resonance imaging. Tests such as Holter monitoring and echocardiogram may be indicated in patients with underlying heart disease or an abnormal cardiac examination since these patients are more likely to have a cardiac cause for their dizziness.

Treatment of dizziness depends on the suspected underlying cause. Acute vertigo and associated vegetative symptoms can be treated symptomatically with the antihistamines meclizine or dimenhydrinate in doses of 25 to 50 mg three or four times a day. In severe cases diazepam, which decreases brain stem response to vestibular stimuli, in doses of 2.5 to 5.0 mg three times a day can be used. Benign paroxysmal positional vertigo can be cured by exercises that repeat the exact motion that leads to dizziness. The more serious causes of peripheral vertigo are best handled by otolaryngologic specialists. Corrective surgical procedures may sometimes be helpful. Patients with disequilibrium are usually managed supportively. Adjustment of medications may be necessary, and steps to improve function in the elderly (e.g., treatment of cataracts, use of walkers) can help to prevent secondary disability, isolation, depression, and falls. Cardiovascular and neurologic disorders are treated accordingly. Psychogenic dizziness can be managed by reassurance and addressing the specific psychogenic factors.

In summary, dizziness can be caused by a disturbance in any of a number of balance control systems. The history and physical examination are most important in the work-up for dizziness. Dizziness in primary care very rarely represents a life-threatening problem. Since the majority of cases are self-limited and benign, conservative management strategies, including observation and supportive treatment, are often appropriate.

SUGGESTED READING

Froehling DA, Silverstein, MD, Mohr DN, Beatty CW. Does this dizzy patient have a serious form of vertigo? JAMA 1994;271:385–388.

Kroenke K, Lucas CA, Rosenberg ML, Scherokman BJ. Psychiatric disorders and functional impairment in patients with persistent dizziness. J Gen Intern Med 1993;8:530–535.

Ruckenstein MJ. A practical approach to dizziness. Postgrad Med 1995;97:70–81.

Sloane P, Dallara J, Roach C, et al. Management of dizziness in primary care. J Am Board Fam Pract 1994;7:1–8.

Weinstein BE, Devons CAJ. The dizzy patient: Stepwise workup of a common complaint. Geriatrics 1995;50:42–50.

QUESTIONS

1. True or false: Vertigo associated with hearing loss is seen in:
   a. Acoustic neuroma
   b. Acute vestibular neuronitis
   c. Meniere's disease
   d. Perilymphatic fistula

2. True or false: Findings associated with peripheral vertigo include:
   a. Hearing loss
   b. Tinnitus
   c. Diplopia
   d. Nystagmus

3. True or false: Findings associated with central vertigo include:
   a. Nystagmus
   b. Ataxia
   c. Dysarthria
   d. Blurry vision

4. True or false: Management of patients with acute vestibular neuronitis include:
   a. Antihistamines
   b. Tricyclic antidepressants
   c. Benzodiazepines
   d. Antiepileptics

Answers appear on **page 604.**

Chapter 23

Sore Throat

Carlos A. Moreno, M.D., M.S.P.H.

INITIAL VISIT

Subjective

PATIENT IDENTIFICATION AND PRESENTING PROBLEMS. Ana is a 6-year-old girl who presents with fever, severe sore throat, and abdominal pain. She has decreased her eating complaining of some nausea but no vomiting or diarrhea. Her mother, Mrs. G., states that Ana was in good health until approximately 1 day before today's visit when she developed general malaise, headache, low-grade fever, and sore throat. She denies having any cough or nasal discharge. Her appetite has been slightly decreased. In addition, she states that her right ear has been "hurting a bit." Ana had one episode of culture-positive group A β-hemolytic streptococcus infection 6 months ago. Currently, the mother relates that a child in school has had similar symptoms and has been diagnosed with mononucleosis.

PAST MEDICAL HISTORY. Ana was the first child born when her mother was age 27, G3 P3 (gravida 3, para 3). Pregnancy and delivery were uneventful. Growth and development have been normal. Ana has had one episode of otitis media when she was 2 years old. Immunizations are up-to-date.

FAMILY HISTORY. Ana's parents are in good health. Her father is a professor and her mother is a law student. There is a positive family history on both the maternal and paternal sides of diabetes, hypertension, and hypercholesterolemia and coronary artery disease. Her four grandparents are all alive and well.

Objective

PHYSICAL EXAMINATION. Ana appears somewhat uncomfortable and fatigued. Vital signs: Temperature 102.2°F, respiratory rate 18, heart rate 92, weight 49 lb. Ana is alert and active. Her tympanic membranes are dull without erythema and with visible landmarks. Her nose has minimal clear rhinorrhea. Her throat is injected with bilateral tonsillar hypertrophy and with tonsillar exudate and small petechial lesions. Her neck is supple with bilateral tender anterior cervical adenopathy. There is no posterior cervical adenopathy. Lungs are clear. Examination of the heart is normal. Abdomen has minimal tenderness without any hepatosplenomegaly; no evidence of rebound tenderness. Neurologic examination is appropriate for her age. Skin is without rashes.

Assessment

WORKING DIAGNOSIS

1. Pharyngitis, probably streptococcal in origin
2. Viral pharyngitis
3. Abdominal pain
4. Mononucleosis

Plan

DIAGNOSTIC. A rapid streptococcal antigen test is conducted in the office. The results are negative. The nasopharyngeal swab is sent to the laboratory for culture. Because of the combination of fever and abdominal pain, a complete blood count (CBC) is sent to the laboratory. No x-ray films are obtained.

THERAPEUTIC

1. Because of her probable penicillin allergy, Ana is sent home on erythromycin estolate, 250 mg twice daily.

2. Acetaminophen, 320 mg, is prescribed every 4 hours.

PATIENT EDUCATION

1. Mrs. G. is advised that, although the rapid streptococcal antigen test is negative, there is a possibility that the culture will be positive. The child has been sent home on oral antibiotics. The office will call Mrs. G. in 48 hours to inform her whether to continue the antibiotics if the culture is positive or stop the antibiotics if the culture is negative. If Ana's course worsens, or if her temperature persists, she is to return to the clinic; otherwise, a follow-up appointment is scheduled in 2 weeks.

2. Because this is the child's third episode of pharyngitis for the current year, her mother is concerned about the need for tonsillectomy. You explain that three episodes of pharyngitis in 1 year is not sufficient for Ana to have a tonsillectomy.

3. Ana's mother is also advised that if any of the other children develop the following symptoms: sore throat and fever or other symptoms consistent with Ana's, she should call the office for advice and possible empirical treatment of these children.

FOLLOW-UP VISIT

Subjective

An office staff person calls Ana's mother in 48 hours to inquire how the child is doing, and she is informed that after 24 hours Ana became much improved with decreased sore throat and no recurrence of fever; the abdominal pain and ear pain have subsided, and the child's appetite is normal. Ana returned to school without any further complaints. She continues to be fatigued, however.

Objective

The nasopharyngeal culture tested positive for group A β-hemolytic streptococcus (GABHS). CBC showed a white blood cell count (WBC) of 11,300/mm³, a hemoglobin of 11 gm/dl, and a hematocrit of 35.

Assessment

1. Group A β-hemolytic streptococcal pharyngitis that is resolving.

2. Mild anemia.

Plan

DIAGNOSTIC. No tests are planned at this time. However, further testing of anemia and follow-up nasopharyngeal culture swab are planned in 2 weeks on Ana's return visit.

THERAPEUTIC

Patient is to continue oral antibiotics for 10 days.

PATIENT EDUCATION

1. Ana's mother is advised of the importance of finishing the course of oral antibiotics.

2. Because of the delay in coming to the physician, Ana's mother is advised of the possibility of a small risk for development of rheumatic heart disease and poststreptococcal glomerulonephritis.

DISPOSITION. Patient is to return for follow-up visit in 2 weeks.

DISCUSSION

Pharyngitis is the fourth most common reason for a visit to the family physician. Streptococcal pharyngitis is characterized by the abrupt onset of a sore throat, fever, tender anterior cervical adenopathy, malaise, and occasionally nausea or headache. Epidemiologically, streptococcal pharyngitis is more common in children. GABHS is the most common respiratory infection encountered in patients over 3 years of age. GABHS occurs primarily in January through May with a second peak incidence occurring with school exposure in September. Streptococcal pharyngitis frequently presents with sore throat, malaise, anorexia, and fever greater than 100°F.

Physical findings include erythema and edema of the tonsils and pharynx, with a pharyngeal exudate in some cases. Additional presenting signs include tender anterior cervical adenopathy. Coughing and rhinorrhea are generally suggestive of viral respiratory infection or other nonstreptococcal causes. Elevated WBC is seen more commonly in children than adults. Prior history of streptococcal infection or recent streptococcal exposure increases the probability of GABHS.

Pharyngitis generally is viral in origin, with rhinovirus, adenovirus, and coxsackievirus A being the common viral pathogens. Mononucleosis generally presents with pharyngitis accompanied by splenomegaly, atypical lymphocytosis, and a positive serologic test. In the unimmunized child, one must always consider diphtheria which generally presents with a grayish posterior pharyngeal pseudomembrane. Bacterial epiglottitis also presents with a sore throat but is characterized by odynophagia and difficulty in handling secretions. This diagnosis should be considered when the child's symptoms are disproportionate to findings on pharyngeal examination and must be treated urgently. Other less common causes of pharyngitis include herpangina, foot and mouth disease, and other systemic diseases. Treatment for viral pharyngitis is generally supportive therapy, with antibiotics not being indicated. On occasion, gargling or throat lozenges may be helpful to relieve symptoms.

The "gold standard" for diagnosis of GABHS is a throat culture on blood agar plate. This test requires 48 hours and can be performed by a commercial laboratory or in the office by trained office personnel.

The use of rapid streptococcal antigen testing allows one to start treating those with positive test results since commercially available preparations have a sensitivity from 85 to 90 per cent and a specificity from 98 to 99 per cent. Patients who have negative results on rapid streptococcal antigen testing should be cultured and treatment may be started immediately or after the results of the culture are available.

Patients presenting with symptoms consistent with high clinical suspicion, that is, sore throat, fever, difficulty swallowing, recent exposure, tender anterior cervical adenopathy, and absence of cough and rhinorrhea, may be treated empirically. A variety of algorithms to improve the decision analysis in the treatment of these patients has been developed for testing children.

Antibiotics are the treatment of choice for GABHS pharyngitis. Traditionally the use of a single-dose intramuscular injection of benzathine penicillin G is sufficient. Oral phenoxymethyl penicillin in divided doses for 10 days is also appropriate. An oral antibiotic for 10 days decreases compliance and has a greater number of treatment failures. The use of amoxicillin 20 to 40 mg per kg 3 times a day is also appropriate but may cause a maculopapular rash if the patient has mononucleosis instead of GABHS. Recently cephalosporins have also been used in a twice-a-day dose. Erythromycin is also an effective alternative.

The goal of therapy is to improve the clinical course, decrease the carrier state, and prevent complications including peritonsillar abscess as well as prevention of rheumatic fever. Surgical therapy for recurrent tonsillitis is indicated with the presence of a peritonsillar abscess, respiratory obstruction, or repeated episodes of tonsillitis.

Sequelae of untreated streptococcal pharyngitis include the development of acute rheumatic fever, which generally presents 2 weeks after the onset of pharyngitis and arthralgia.

SUGGESTED READING

Dajani A, Taubert K, Ferrieri, P. Treatment of acute streptococcal pharyngitis and prevention of rheumatic fever: A statement for health professionals. Pediatrics 1995;96:758–764.

Goldstein MN. Office evaluation and management of sore throat. Otolaryngol Clin North Am 1992;25:837–842.

Kline JA, Runge JW. Streptococcal pharyngitis: A review of pathophysiology, diagnosis and management. J Emerg Med 1994;12:665–680.

QUESTIONS

1. True or false: Treatment of group A β-hemolytic streptococcal pharyngitis can include the use of
   a. Intramuscular benzathine penicillin G
   b. Oral phenoxymethyl penicillin
   c. Oral amoxicillin
   d. Oral erythromycin

2. True or false: Causes of pharyngitis can include:
   a. Epstein-Barr virus (infectious mononucleosis)
   b. Rhinovirus
   c. Group A β-hemolytic streptococcus
   d. *Corynebacterium diphtheriae*
   e. *Entamoeba histolytica*

Answers appear on **page 604.**

Chapter 24

Oral Leukoplakia

Granvil L. Hays, D.D.S., M.S.

INITIAL VISIT

Subjective

PATIENT IDENTIFICATION. Margie R. is a 56-year-old white woman and homemaker. She was referred by her dentist for biopsy of a white, leukoplakic lesion in the floor of her mouth.

PRESENTING PROBLEM. During a recent dental examination a white, corrugated lesion was observed just to the right of midline in the floor of Margie's mouth. She is unaware of any problem and the dentist says the lesion was not present at last year's examination. Since Margie does not have dental insurance she asked to be referred to her health maintenance organization where the procedure can be done with little or no out-of-pocket cost to her.

PAST MEDICAL HISTORY. Margie is the mother of two sons who are in their early thirties. She has had no surgery or serious medical illnesses. After her second son left home she was treated approximately 1 year for mild depression. She currently takes no medication.

FAMILY HISTORY. Margie's father died at the age of 79 from the sequelae of prostate cancer. Her mother is in reasonably good health at age 82. She takes a diuretic for hypertension. Her brother is a certified public accountant and is in good health at age 52.

Both sons are reported to be in good health. There is no history of oral cancers.

HEALTH HABITS. Margie reports that she has smoked a pack of cigarettes each day for the last 30 years (30 pack years). She denies the use of chewing tobacco or the placement of a mint or candy in the area of concern. She reports that she and her husband have a cocktail or two when he arrives home from work, before dinner. They also usually drink a bottle of wine with their dinner.

Objective

PHYSICAL EXAMINATION. Margie's height is 5 feet 4 inches; she weights 110 lb; temperature is 98.2°F, blood pressure is 130/80 mm Hg. The examination is limited to the head and neck. No palpable nodes are found on examination of the neck. The teeth appear to be in good repair. The general color of the oral mucosa is somewhat inflamed and the patient's breath suggests that she had an alcoholic drink with her lunch. Examination of the floor of the mouth reveals an area of white plaque that measures 1 × 1.5 cm. The surface is corrugated and lies just to the right of midline. When the area is wiped with a sterile gauze the lesion remains. No other lesions are evident on the tongue, buccal mucosa, gingiva, palate, or tonsillar region.

Assessment

WORKING DIAGNOSIS. The fact that the lesion is still present would appear to rule out a chemical burn. Since the lesion does not wipe away and is localized, it is not candidiasis. Lichen planus is usually found bilaterally rather than localized. While there is a plaquelike variant of lichen planus, it usually appears with areas of striae on the periphery of the lesion or elsewhere in the mouth.

The location is critical in the diagnosis. The floor of the mouth is not the usual location for placement of tobacco or snuff; thus the lesion is most likely not caused by the chemical irritation of tobacco resting against the tissue. The patient wears no dental prosthesis that could irritate the area. The history of smoking and drinking of alcoholic beverages is of concern. Although the incidence of a solitary white lesion being a squamous cell carcinoma is not high, this lesion must be biopsied. Clinically one cannot distinguish a benign hyperkeratosis from a precancerous or cancerous lesion.

DIFFERENTIAL DIAGNOSIS. A number of conditions result in white plaques (leukoplakia) in the oral cavity. These include chemical burn, candidiasis, lichen planus, benign hyperkeratosis, leukoplakia or hyperkeratosis with dyskeratosis, carcinoma in situ, verrucous carcinoma, and squamous cell carcinoma.

1. *Chemical burn.* These white plaques may be caused by aspirin or other chemicals lying against oral mucosa. Cinnamic acid or cinnamon aldehydes found in cinnamon-flavored candies can cause chemical burns. Most chemical burns are of short duration and the burnt surface epithelium usually peels away.

2. *Candidiasis.* This is usually seen as multiple, curdlike patches. Fungal overgrowth can, however, take on a plaquelike variant and adhere to the oral tissues with tenacity. Most fungal lesions wipe off easily.

3. *Lichen planus.* In its classic pattern these are white, lacy lesions. The lesions can be found on almost any oral tissue and cannot be wiped off. This common dermatologic lesion has a plaquelike variant. A biopsy is required to differentiate the plaquelike variant of lichen planus from leukoplakia.

4. *Benign hyperkeratosis.* This white lesion may be flat or raised, fissured, rough or smooth. It usually is asymptomatic and can occur anywhere on the oral mucosa. This "callus" formed in response to a mechanical or chemical irritation cannot be wiped off.

5. *Leukoplakia.* As a clinical term leukoplakia is used to describe a white plaque. Histologically, this term is used to describe hyperkeratosis with dysplastic changes. Clinically, the lesions may appear the same as benign hyperkeratosis. The actual irritant may not be identifiable. The presence of red, erythroplakic changes within or at the periphery of the white plaque, would raise concerns of severe dysplastic changes.

6. *Carcinoma in situ.* The clinical appearance of carcinoma in situ may also be the same as hyperkeratosis. There may also be an erythematous component to these lesions, which increases the level of concern.

7. *Verrucous carcinoma.* This lesion resembles leukoplakia except for the papillary surface appearance. Histologically it is very similar to carcinoma in situ because the atypical cells are confined to epithelium.

8. *Squamous cell carcinoma.* About 5 per cent of oral squamous cell carcinomas present as white plaques. Concern increases when there is an associated ulcer. A mottled appearance of red and white would also increase the likelihood of cancer.

Plan

Margie should be advised that you concur with the referring dentist on a biopsy of the lesion if it is still present at the next appointment in 1 week. Margie should be encouraged to stop smoking and reduce alcohol consumption.

At her next visit the leukoplakic lesion is found to still be present. Lidocaine is infiltrated around the lesion. An area of the leukoplakic lesion including a margin of normal-appearing tissue is outlined with a 6-mm disposable, sterile dermatologic punch. After circumscribing the area to be removed and establishing the depth with the punch, the tissue is removed with tissue forceps and a No. 21 Bard-Parker blade. The tissue is placed in a 10 per cent formalin solution and submitted for microscopic examination. A single resorbable gut suture closes the wound.

FOLLOW-UP VISIT

Subjective

Margie reports that the site has healed without incident. She has tried but has little or no success in reducing smoking and states she will not give up her evening cocktails with her husband.

Objective

The area of the biopsy has healed. The leukoplakic plaque is smaller due to the removal of the tissue but is still present.

The results of the microscopic examination are given to the patient. The report reads—Leukoplakia, hyperkeratosis with moderate to severe dysplastic changes. The area of dysplastic change appears to be confined to the area under the plaque.

Assessment

Margie is advised that, although this is not cancer, it is a precancerous condition. The entire leukoplakic area must be removed and examined. A complete examination of the throat, pharynx, larynx, and lungs needs to be scheduled. Unless she is willing to give up smoking and drinking alcoholic beverages, this lesion will likely recur or another lesion develop elsewhere that could be cancerous. Untreated dysplastic leukoplakia of the floor of the mouth becomes invasive carcinoma up to 90 per cent of the time.

Plan

1. Referral to an oral surgeon for removal of the entire leukoplakic area with wide margins.

2. A complete examination of the entire upper aerodigestive tract must also be scheduled. This is to ensure that Margie has no other synchronous precancerous or cancerous lesion.

3. Margie must receive assistance to help her with smoking and alcohol cessation.

4. Margie must receive a complete oral cancer examination twice yearly.

5. Chemoprevention should be considered.

DISCUSSION

The term "leukoplakia" when used to describe a clinical lesion is descriptive of a white plaque. Before microscopic examination, any white plaque lesion in the oral cavity may be called leukoplakia. Pathologists may use the term leukoplakia to describe white lesions of the oral cavity in which dysplastic changes have occurred. Leukoplakia as a pathologic diagnostic term denotes premalignant changes in the tissue. The degree of atypia is usually ranked as minimal, moderate, or severe.

Patients with the diagnosis of moderate to severe dysplasia are at high risk for the development of oral cancer and must stop the use of tobacco and alcohol. Whereas smoking tobacco offers a more pronounced risk of oral cancer, combining alcohol and tobacco increases cancer incidence many times greater than the additive effect. This multiplying factor of alcohol and tobacco is called co-carcinogenesis. Approximately 75 per cent of all oral and pharyngeal cancers are caused by excessive smoking and heavy consumption of alcoholic beverages. Removal of the entire dysplastic area can result in a cure if the patient's social habits can be changed. The complete evaluation of the entire upper aerodigestive tract is imperative. When an oral cancer is found, there is approximately a one in four chance of finding a synchronous second primary cancer in the upper aerodigestive tract. This is because of field cancerization. The same carcinogens that caused the oral dysplastic lesion have irritated the entire upper aerodigestive tract.

Margie must quit smoking cigarettes and drinking alcoholic beverages. The erythematous appearance of her oral tissues suggests that she is underreporting the quantity of alcoholic beverages consumed. The actual mechanism for the synergistic effect of alcohol and tobacco use in the development of cancer is unclear. However, the present view is that alcohol promotes the effects of carcinogens found in tobacco. Theories advanced include:

Penetration of oral mucosa by nitrosamines and hydrocarbons found in tobacco is enhanced by the dehydrating effects of alcohol.

Alcohol affects liver function, increasing acetaldehyde content in tissues. This condition makes the oral tissues more susceptible to the carcinogens in tobacco.

Nutritional deficiencies as the result of alcohol interfering with the absorption of nutrients result in an immunocompromised state of health.

In addition to frequent oral examinations, you may wish to try a chemoprevention protocol. In the head and neck, systemic retinoids have shown promise in reversing oral premalignant lesions.

Franco EL, Kowalski LP, Kanda JL. Risk factors for second cancers of the upper respiratory and digestive system: A case-control study. J Clin Epidemiol 1991;44:615–625.

Hays GL, Lippman SM, Flaitz CM, et al. Co-carcinogenesis and field cancerization: Oral lesions offer first signs. J Am Dent Assoc 1995;126:47–51.

Lippman SM, Batsakis JG, Toth BB, et al. Comparison of low-dose isotretinoin with beta carotene to prevent oral carcinogenesis. N Engl J Med 1993;328:15–20.

Lippman SM, Hong WK. Retinoid chemoprevention of upper aerodigestive tract carcinogenesis. In Devita VT, Hellman S, Rosenbern SA (eds). Important Advances in Oncology. Philadelphia, JB Lippincott, 1992, pp 93–109.

Mashberg A, Boffetta P, Winkleman R, Garfinkel L. Tobacco smoking, alcohol drinking, and cancer of the oral cavity and oropharynx among U.S. veterans. Cancer 1993;72:1369–1375.

QUESTIONS

1. A pathologic report of leukoplakia indicates:
   a. Oral cancer
   b. A precancerous lesion
   c. A fungal overgrowth
   d. Lichen planus
   e. Erythroplasia

2. Alcohol and tobacco are estimated to be responsible for _____ per cent of all oral and pharyngeal cancers.
   a. 100
   b. 90
   c. 75
   d. 60
   e. 50

3. Which of the following lesions is most likely to be cancerous?
   a. A solid white plaque
   b. A white plaque with red areas interspersed
   c. A solid white plaque that wipes away
   d. A white lacy-appearing lesion
   e. A grayish white plaque

Answers appear on **page 604**.

Chapter 25

Nasal Congestion

Richard D. Clover, M.D.

INITIAL VISIT

Subjective

PATIENT IDENTIFICATION. Mary B. is a 30-year-old, married, white secretary, mother of two, who is being seen for the first time for facial pain, sinus congestion, and dental pain.

PRESENT ILLNESS. Mary has been experiencing pain on the right side of her face and right upper teeth for 48 hours. She has been suffering from "nasal and sinus" congestion for about 2 weeks, as she does every spring. She has noticed a greenish coloration to her nasal discharge over the last 2 days. She has felt mildly ill over the past 48 hours and has felt feverish, although she has not taken her temperature. She has had no chills or sweats. The pain in her face is on the right side over the cheekbone, and it is made worse by bending over. She also has noticed pain in the upper teeth on the right side of her mouth. She denies earache or sore throat. She has had a slight cough but has not been coughing up any phlegm. She has had no pain in her chest. She denies any neurologic symptoms.

PAST MEDICAL HISTORY. Mary has been generally healthy all her life. She has had no surgery, serious illnesses, or serious injuries. Her only hospitalizations have been for the birth of her two children, now ages 3 and 5, who were delivered vaginally. She has no known medication allergies. She takes no medications regularly, other than loratadine, which she takes as needed for "sinus problems" with good relief.

FAMILY HISTORY. Both of Mary's parents are in their late fifties and healthy. Her one younger sister is healthy. Both her father and sister also have "sinus problems." Mary's husband is healthy, and the children are basically healthy—both have had recurrent problems with otitis media, however.

HEALTH HABITS. Mary has smoked a pack of cigarettes daily for 10 years. She denies alcohol consumption or use of illicit drugs. She wears seat belts when she drives or rides in a car. She participates in "jazzercise" at a local health club for 30 minutes three times a week. She tries to eat "healthy."

SOCIAL HISTORY. Mary has been married for 8 years and states that she has a happy, stable, monogamous sexual relationship with her husband. They use barrier contraception. Her husband is a certified public accountant, and she works as a secretary for a local oil and gas firm. She identifies no unusual stressors in her life and notes that she and her husband are involved in a local church and have a number of close friends.

REVIEW OF SYSTEMS. Mary denies ear problems, recurring sore throats, or history of asthma or bronchitis.

Objective

PHYSICAL EXAMINATION. Blood pressure is 120/80 mm Hg, normal heart rate of 80, respiration rate 16, temperature 98.6°F. Head: Right maxillary sinus is tender to palpation and percussion. Ears: Tympanic membranes are clear and mobile bilaterally. Nose: The nasal mucosa is somewhat inflamed and edematous. Speculum examination shows a purulent discharge exuding from the middle meatus on the right. Mouth and throat: Teeth are in good repair, and there is no periodontal disease. The throat is not inflamed. There is some cobblestoning of the posterior oropharynx. Neck: Without adenopathy. Lungs: Resonant to percussion, clear to auscultation. Transillumination of the sinuses is performed and reveals opacification of the right maxillary sinus.

LABORATORY TESTS. No laboratory tests were performed.

Assessment

WORKING DIAGNOSIS. Two likely diagnoses best explain Mary's symptoms and findings:

1. *Seasonal allergic rhinitis* would explain the recurring symptoms of nasal congestion, responsive to antihistamines, occurring each spring and the cobblestoned appearance of the posterior oropharynx.

2. *Acute right maxillary sinusitis* is suggested by the constellation of the patient's symptoms and physical findings. Acute sinusitis is a common complication of allergic rhinitis.

DIFFERENTIAL DIAGNOSIS. Mary's symptoms and findings suggest a few other possibilities, which include:

1. *Allergic rhinitis/sinusitis.* The presence of facial and dental pain, purulent nasal discharge, and sinus tenderness and the decreased transillumination suggest that this is more than allergic rhinitis/sinusitis and that there is a complicating bacterial sinusitis.

2. *Viral upper respiratory infection.* Although a viral upper respiratory infection can cause nasal and sinus congestion and, occasionally, purulent rhinorrhea, the presence of the facial and dental pain as well as the decreased transillumination suggest a bacterial sinus infection.

Plan

LABORATORY AND SPECIAL TESTS. The symptoms and physical findings are highly suggestive of a diagnosis of acute right maxillary sinusitis. The physician does not need additional diagnostic confirmation before instituting treatment for this problem.

TREATMENT

1. Amoxicillin 500 mg every 8 hours for 14 days is prescribed.

2. The patient is advised to use oxymetazoline 0.05% (Afrin), an over-the-counter nasal spray, in the following manner: Spray each nostril twice, 5 minutes apart, every 12 hours for 3 days. If, at the end of this time, nasal and sinus congestion is still a problem, begin taking pseudoephedrine (Sudafed), 60 mg orally every 6 hours, until symptoms of congestion have subsided.

3. The patient is advised that she might want to perform steam inhalations two or three times daily to help liquefy the nasal secretions.

4. The patient is advised to take acetaminophen orally as needed for pain relief.

PATIENT EDUCATION

1. The patient is educated about the pathophysiology of acute sinusitis and the importance of taking all the antibiotics as prescribed. She also is educated about the importance of decongestants and the importance of not using topical decongestant nasal spray for more than 3 days at a time. She is told that her seasonal allergic rhinitis may have precipitated the acute sinusitis and that a treatment plan for this more chronic problem will be discussed at the next visit.

2. The patient is advised that smoking is not only dangerous to her general health but also might be a contributing factor to the cause of her sinus infections. She is encouraged to stop smoking and told that whenever she desires to do so, she may be counseled on effective smoking cessation methods.

DISPOSITION. The patient is asked to return for follow-up in 3 weeks' time.

FIRST FOLLOW-UP VISIT

Mary returned 3 weeks after her initial visit as scheduled. She has completed her course of antibiotics as prescribed. Her facial and dental pain and purulent nasal discharge have resolved after 5 days of prescribed therapy. She is now feeling well, although she is still having some intermittent nasal stuffiness and clear nasal discharge, along with intermittent sneezing, as is usual for this time of year. She is still smoking and expresses no desire to quit.

Objective

Vital signs are normal. Nose: Nasal mucosa is somewhat violaceous and boggy. Clear rhinorrhea. Throat: Cobblestoning of the posterior oropharynx.

Assessment

1. Persistent seasonal allergic rhinitis.

2. Acute maxillary sinusitis resolved.

Plan

DIAGNOSTIC. A nasal smear was submitted for Wright's stain and showed multiple eosinophils per microscopic high-power field.

THERAPEUTIC. Mary is started on topical nasal beclomethasone spray, one puff in each nostril three times daily, to be used during the months of the year when she usually has allergic rhinitis symptoms.

PATIENT EDUCATION. Mary is advised that it will take 2 to 3 weeks before she notes an improvement in her allergic rhinitis symptoms from the topical beclomethasone spray. She is advised that she should use this three times daily every day during the months of the year when she is prone to allergic rhinitis symptoms. She is again reminded of the adverse effects of smoking on her health.

DISPOSITION. Mary is asked to return in 6 weeks for follow-up of her allergic rhinitis symptoms.

DISCUSSION

Seasonal allergic rhinitis is a common affliction, caused by respiratory allergens, that is manifested by nasal congestion, sneezing, and clear rhinorrhea, which occur on a seasonal basis. Common physical findings include nasal mucosa that is edematous and violaceous in appearance and a cobblestone appearance to the posterior oropharynx. Nasal smears usually show many eosinophils. Symptomatic treatment includes antihistamines. Prophylactic treatment can include topical nasal steroids or topical nasal cromolyn sodium (Nasalcrom). Patients who do not respond to these therapies are candidates for allergic desensitization therapy.

Acute sinusitis is a common problem in primary medical practice. Acute sinusitis is usually preceded by a viral upper respiratory infection or an exacerbation of allergic rhinitis. The pathophysiology of acute sinusitis involves obstruction of the osteomeatal complex. The most common infecting organisms include *Streptococcus pneumoniae, Haemophilus influenzae,* and *Moraxella catarrhalis.* There is not one single symptom or sign that is pathognomonic for acute sinusitis. Common findings include a history of sinus pain, purulent nasal discharge, poor response to nasal decongestants, and generalized malaise in the presence of preceding acute upper respiratory infection or allergic rhinitis symptoms. One symptom, maxillary toothache, is highly specific (93 per cent), but occurs in only 11 per cent of patients with acute sinusitis. Tenderness over the frontal and/or maxillary sinuses and decreased transillumination of the involved sinuses may be present. Although plain x-ray films of the sinuses may be helpful as diagnostic aids in equivocal situations, they are neither very sensitive nor very specific tests. Limited computed tomography (CT) and nuclear magnetic resonance (NMR) imaging studies are more sensitive tests than radiography, but they probably have no place in the primary-care management of the patient with sinusitis. Therapy is aimed at treating the bacterial infection with appropriate antibiotics, relieving obstruction through the use of topical and systemic decongestants, and providing adjunctive symptomatic measures of relief.

Suboptimal management of acute sinusitis can lead to the development of chronic sinusitis. Patients who either have suffered more than three bouts of acute sinusitis in a year or have developed chronic sinusitis should be referred to an otorhinolaryngologist for further evaluation and treatment.

The most likely explanation for the failure of the current therapeutic regimen would be infection with a β-lactamase–producing organism such as *H. influenzae* or *M. catarrhalis.* This would be an indication for broadening the spectrum of antibiotic coverage by using something like amoxicillin with clavulanate (Augmentin), cefuroxime axetil (Ceftin), or a newer macrolide (clarithromycin [Biaxin] or azithromycin [Zithromax]). Changing the antibiotic to Augmentin would achieve this goal.

Acute sinusitis frequently involves more than one sinus. However, the classic symptoms may be helpful in localizing the involved sinus. Ethmoid and sphenoid sinusitis are more difficult to diagnose clinically than maxillary and frontal sinusitis. Limited CT images may be necessary to confirm these diagnoses.

SUGGESTED READING

Rakel RE. Textbook of Family Practice, 4th ed. Philadelphia, W.B. Saunders, 1990, pp 552–554.

Williams JW, Simel DL. Does this patient have sinusitis? JAMA 1993;270:1242–1246.

Williams JW, Simel DL, Roberts L, Samsa GP. Clinical evaluation for sinusitis: Making the diagnosis by history and physical examination. Ann Intern Med 1992;117:705–710.

Winther B, Gwaltney JM. Therapeutic approach to sinusitis: Anti-infectious therapy as the baseline of management. Otolaryngol Head Neck Surg 1990;103:876.

QUESTIONS

1. Match each of the following types of sinusitis with the typical clinical presentation.
   a. Frontal sinusitis
   b. Maxillary sinusitis
   c. Ethmoid sinusitis
   d. Sphenoid sinusitis
      (1) Retro-orbital pain, occipital headache
      (2) Pain over the bridge of the nose and behind the eye
      (3) Pain radiating to the teeth
      (4) Causes generalized headache, may progress rapidly

Answers appear on **page 604.**

Chapter 26

Wheezing

Greg L. Ledgerwood, M.D.

INITIAL VISIT

Subjective

PATIENT IDENTIFICATION. Amy K. is a 26-year-old white woman who presents with problems of increasing respiratory distress.

PRESENTING PROBLEM. Amy has had problems of "allergies" since childhood. In infancy, she had recurrent otitis media, resulting in tympanostomy tube placement four different times, difficulty with atopic dermatitis, and asthma. At age 10, while playing soccer, she became so short of breath that she had to watch the rest of the game from the sidelines. Shortly thereafter, Amy was taken to an allergist where skin tests were found positive to pollen, environmental pollutants, and dust. She was placed on immunotherapy for an extended period of time. "Shots" were eventually discontinued because she was not convinced that it was helping her allergic condition and, more specifically, she wasn't convinced that her asthma was any better. She stated that she had had allergic rhinitis for as long as she could remember, resulting in severe nasal obstruction.

At age 21, after almost a continuous year of "sinus infections," an ear, nose and throat surgeon performed some type of surgery, improving her nasal airway and removing the "blockage" from her sinuses. Since the surgery she feels that there has been an improvement as far as the number of infections she has experienced. She states that since her senior year in high school she has had more difficulty with her asthma. She feels that perhaps it is worse in the fall, but her asthma symptoms are present throughout the year. Over the past month, before this evaluation, Amy has been awakening once a night with difficulty breathing. She has been using a metered-dose inhaler more frequently, about one canister every 2 weeks. Her other medications include a slow-release theophylline preparation, 300 mg twice a day. She notices that her asthma is exacerbated by emotional upset, such as crying or laughing. She continues to have a great deal of difficulty with exertional wheezing, particularly in cold air. At age 22, during her first pregnancy, she developed a severe "head cold" with marked increase in respiratory difficulty resulting in a hospitalization during her first trimester.

Amy does not smoke cigarettes. Her husband is a smoker, but he smokes outside the house. In childhood, her father was also a smoker and she remembers distinctly having a great deal of difficulty being around him because it created problems with her breathing.

She currently operates a day care center and is exposed to frequent upper respiratory infections from the children and states that she has had a "cold" ever since the fall began.

Amy lives in a mobile home that was built in the mid-1970s and has done so for the past 3 years. The home is constructed over an unfinished basement. Urea formaldehyde may have been used in the wall construction, but Amy is unaware of any odors in her home at this time. She does notice, however, that whenever she is in the basement, the musty smell seems to "choke her up." She and her husband have no pets. She is aware, however, that the previous owners did have cats and apparently they were kept indoors. The carpet in her home is old and she is planning to replace it soon. Electric forced-air heat is used, with a wall-unit "swamp cooler." She believes this cooling unit is as old as the home itself.

Shortly after her first pregnancy, complicated by blood pressure elevations, she was started on a long-acting propranolol preparation, with the resultant effect of causing a marked increase in her wheezing and shortness of breath. This was subsequently replaced with an angiotensin converting enzyme inhibitor, which she currently takes without difficulty. She is able to use aspirin and aspirin-containing products without any exacerbation of her symptoms.

PAST MEDICAL HISTORY. Other than her chronic respiratory problems and high blood pressure, Amy has otherwise been in good health. She currently is on birth control pills in addition to the medications already mentioned. She denies any medicine allergies.

FAMILY HISTORY. Amy has one child, age 4, who has had problems with recurrent otitis media since age 1. She has one older brother, age 27, who has been diagnosed with "mild asthma." Her father, who is in his late fifties, has "chronic bronchitis." Her mother, also in her late fifties, has no known medical problems. Amy has a maternal grandmother with adult-onset diabetes.

SOCIAL HISTORY. Amy works in a day care center 5 days a week, and on weekends she enjoys outdoor activities including gardening and, during the winter months, skiing. She states that her outdoor activities have been limited recently because of increased wheezing and shortness of breath, particularly when the wind blows, or she overexerts herself. She has found that perfumes and hair sprays create respiratory difficulties, so she avoids using them. She has been happily married for the past 6 years and five of those years have been spent working outside the home. She describes her marital life as excellent and denies any current stressful situations, other than those related to her illness. She admits that she has frequently been discouraged about her health. She does not feel better, and often cannot participate with her family in some of their outdoor activities.

REVIEW OF SYSTEMS. Amy has noticed no change in her appetite or weight, but she does note that her energy level seems to have dropped off over the past several years and relates this to her respiratory problems. She denies any headaches or change in vision. She states that she frequently experiences "rawness" in her throat on awakening in the morning. She has significant dyspnea on exertion with any vigorous activity, including swimming and bicycling. Other than high blood pressure, she denies any cardiovascular problems. Gastrointestinal: She denies any problems. Musculoskeletal: Other than being "out of shape" she denies problems. Neurologic: Noncontributory. Endocrinologic: Noncontributory. Mental: She does admit to being de-

pressed at times related to her general overall health.

Objective

PHYSICAL EXAMINATION. Amy is a pleasant, healthy-appearing, white woman who is alert and cooperative and gives a good medical history. Her blood pressure is 138/88 mm Hg in the left arm sitting. She weighs 133 lb, pulse 78 and regular, respiratory rate 20 and slightly labored. She does describe frequently during the history and physical the frustration of having to use the inhaler and not wanting to "live like this."

Her physical examination is significant for the following: Skin: She has a dry, lichenified area over the flexor surfaces of her forearms with an erythematous base. ENT: The examination is unremarkable with the exception of a clear to gray rhinorrhea, with good nasal patency. Her throat shows erythematous streaking in the lateral walls of the pharynx. Neck: There is no cervical or supraclavicular adenopathy, no thyroid enlargement. Chest: Expands symmetrically with respirations. There is a certain coarseness to her breath sounds, but no rales, rhonchi, or rubs are heard. Wheezing and a prolonged expiratory phase at rest are present in both lung fields. Cardiac: The rhythm is regular at a rate of 90. There are no murmurs, rubs, or gallops.

The rest of her examination is normal.

LABORATORY TESTS. A complete blood count shows 8200/mm^3 white blood cells with a differential showing 13 per cent eosinophils; otherwise, it is normal. Pulse oximetry done at rest is 90 per cent on room air. Spirometry examination is significant showing a decrease in the forced expiratory volume in 1 second (FEV_1) of 78 per cent of predicted and a forced expiratory flow, midexpiratory phase ($FEF_{25\%-75\%}$) of 46 per cent of predicted. These both returned to greater than 80 per cent of predicted after using albuterol with an inhaler. A chest x-ray study is interpreted as within normal limits. Nasal cytology is negative for eosinophils, but does show 2+ neutrophils. Sputum cytology is positive for 2+ eosinophils.

Assessment

WORKING DIAGNOSES

1. *Reactive airway disease/asthma.* This is the primary diagnosis, established not only by her long-standing history, but confirmed by her abnormal

function tests, returning to normal after bronchodilator therapy, and a normal chest x-ray study.

2. *Allergic nasal disease.* Her previous allergy tests, showing a positive reaction to pollen and dust, and her history confirm this diagnosis.

3. *Chronic sinusitis/nasal obstruction.* Her history of recurrent sinusitis, otitis media, and nasal obstruction support this diagnosis.

4. *Essential hypertension.* Although not mentioned here, a previous negative hypertensive work-up and a family history of hypertension support this diagnosis.

DIFFERENTIAL DIAGNOSIS

1. *Hyperventilation syndrome.* This is generally associated with anxiety and nonpulmonary symptoms and relieved through relaxation with reassurance, often differentiating it from "asthma."

2. *Pulmonary emboli.* In older patients this can be differentiated by a history of predisposing factors (thrombophlebitis, cardiac failure, oral contraceptive use, prolonged bed rest, recent surgery, or malignancy).

3. *"Cardiac" asthma.* History of cardiac disease, moist rales in the chest, and a third heart sound distinguish cardiac asthma from extrinsic asthma. Cardiac asthma usually manifests in a patient with underlying, long-standing obstructive lung disease who develops left-sided heart failure.

4. *Chronic bronchitis.* Although patients with this condition do have wheezing and coughing as part of their symptoms, purulent sputum production, particularly in the morning, is the hallmark of this disease.

5. *Allergic bronchopulmonary aspergillosis.* See later discussion.

Plan

THERAPEUTIC

1. Discussion with Amy of etiology and expectations of her disease.

2. Demonstrate to Amy the proper use of a metered-dose inhaler with a spacer device. Many patients are given metered-dose inhalers without proper instruction and frequently are not getting the prescribed dose. Using a spacer device eliminates the problems of "timing with breathing" associated with metered-dose inhalers.

3. Start patient on an inhalable anti-inflammatory agent, such as inhaled corticosteroids, sodium cromolyn (Intal), or nedocromil (Tilade). Regular daily use of a β2-agonist as first-line therapy for chronic asthma is contraindicated. A rule of thumb would suggest that if a patient uses a β2-agonist more than once a day to control asthma, the severity of the disease dictates adding an anti-inflammatory agent, as previously mentioned.

4. Continue the use of long-acting theophylline and/or consider switching or adding a long-acting inhaled β2-agonist such as salmeteral.

5. Consider a computed tomography (CT) scan of the sinuses. Standard radiographs of the sinus cavities are of limited value after nasal surgery because of the scarring associated with the procedure. Untreated infections, particularly sinusitis, are a frequent, often-missed diagnosis in all patients with the diagnosis of asthma. A neural-mediated reflex can occur when any infection is present, resulting in bronchospasm. The exact mechanisms of these reflexes are unknown. If this problem, however, is not addressed, control of asthma will continue to be very difficult.

PATIENT EDUCATION

1. Develop a patient treatment plan for severe exacerbations. Infections should receive prompt attention. Both steroid- and nonsteroid-dependent asthmatic patients should be instructed on the addition of oral corticosteroids for moderate or severe exacerbations.

2. Counsel the patient on the need for a yearly influenza vaccine shot and a pneumococcal vaccine immunization.

3. Instruct the patient on the avoidance of areas of high pollution and on dust and dander control.

4. Encourage the patient to become an "active" participant in treating his or her disease.

DISPOSITION. CT scan of Amy's sinuses did demonstrate an air-fluid level present in her right maxillary sinus cavity. She is started on amoxicillin 500 mg three times daily for 14 days, begun on inhalable beclomethasone (Beclovent, Vanceril), two inhalations four times a day, paired with her short-acting bronchodilator, and started on a pulse dose of prednisone 40 mg tapering off over a 10-day period. She is instructed to return for follow-up in 2 weeks.

FIRST FOLLOW-UP VISIT

Subjective

Amy returned for her 2-week visit, noticing not only an improvement in her respiratory state, but also a decrease in the amount of nocturnal shortness of breath. She states that she finds it difficult using the medications on a regular basis, as prescribed, and admits to having missed some of the doses during the day. She does relate, however, that she seems to be able to do more without developing shortness of breath and that she is pleased with how she is feeling at this time.

Objective

PHYSICAL EXAMINATION. This visit reveals a normal examination. Repeat spirometry without bronchodilator therapy shows normal FEV, and $FEF_{25\%-75\%}$, compared with her first visit.

Assessment

The patient has appeared to stabilize.

Plan

1. Continue patient education about the importance of regular use of her metered-dose beclomethasone.

2. Reinforce the importance of early intervention with infections.

3. Consider other medications if treatment failure occurs including additions of sodium cromolyn, ipratropium (Atrovent), or nedocromil (Tilade).

4. Consider adding a long-acting β-agonist, salmeterol (Serevent).

5. Re-examine the possibility of instituting immunotherapy.

DISCUSSION

Asthma is a reversible obstructive disorder of the tracheobronchial tree characterized by paroxysmal episodes of respiratory distress often interspersed with periods of apparent well-being. Asthma can begin at any age, but it most often appears in childhood, commonly with a familial disposition. When the onset is early, prognosis is excellent, and most patients improve at puberty. Until puberty, asthma is twice as common among boys as among girls. This distribution reverses between puberty and early adulthood, so that among adults with asthma, women are affected more frequently than men. Asthma can be conveniently divided by causative factors into two main groups, as seen in Table 26–1. In intrinsic asthma, most commonly seen in adults, symptoms are provoked and worsened by infection, exertion, emotion, and nonspecific environmental factors, and are not related to allergy exposure. The majority of extrinsic asthma patients are atopic with symptoms related to environmental allergens. Over

TABLE 26–1. Clinical Features of Extrinsic and Intrinsic Asthma

| | Extrinsic Asthma | | Intrinsic Asthma (Idiopathic) |
	Atopic	Nonatopic	
Age of onset	Usually childhood	Adult	Usually after age 25
Symptoms	Variable with environment and season	Usually occupation related	Unpredictable fluctuation, often chronic
Associated conditions	Allergic rhinitis, atopic dermatitis	None	Bronchitis, sinusitis, nasal polyps
Family history of atopic disease	Strong	Minor	Asthma only (?)
Skin tests (wheal-erythema)	Several positive, related to history	Negative, or one reaction only	Usually negative
Total IgE	High	Usually normal	Normal
Eosinophilia	High during allergen exposure	Sometimes high during allergen exposure	High
Prognosis	Good, especially with allergen avoidance	Good, especially with allergen avoidance	Fair, remissions uncommon

the past several years, re-examination of the prevalence of extrinsic/allergic asthma has suggested that it is much more common than once was thought. The characteristic physiologic change in asthma is airway obstruction due to bronchial smooth muscle spasm, mucous plugging, edema, and inflammation of the bronchial wall. As a result of such airway narrowing, inspiration and expiration are impeded. Obstruction of airflow results in air trapping and hyperinflation of the lungs. Smooth muscle spasm can occur in large, medium, or small airways. When large airways are involved, wheezing predominates. When small airways are involved, the predominant symptoms are dyspnea and cough, rather than wheeze. It is well understood that asthma has both an immediate (bronchospastic) and a late (inflammatory) phase in response to inhaled allergens and certain other provoking agents. The occurrence of this dual asthmatic response has important therapeutic implications.

The history often provides a diagnosis. Asthma should be suspected in any person with unexplained episodes of dyspnea, cough, repeated chest colds, or bronchitis, particularly in children. Even cough by itself may be a symptom of asthma. In evaluation of the acute attack, severity is related to frequency, duration, intensity, and response to previous medications and their side effects, as well as symptom-free intervals. When symptoms are chronic or continuous, the condition may be confused with irreversible chronic obstructive pulmonary disease (COPD). A family history may be positive for asthma, or atopy, and a search for provocative environmental factors, including occupational exposure, smoking, stress, infection, exercise, and medication (aspirin, propranolol, angiotensin converting enzyme [ACE] inhibitors), may yield important information. A familial triad of aspirin sensitivity, nasal polyp formation, and severe asthma should always be excluded.

Propranolol and β blockers, including topical β blockers used in the treatment of glaucoma, should be avoided. Many cases of sudden, severe, life-threatening asthma have occurred with the inadvertent addition of these agents in patients with an established diagnosis of asthma. When considering therapy for associated diseases, such as hypertension and glaucoma, one must always keep this in mind. ACE inhibitors, also used for the treatment of hypertension, can have an associated idiopathic cough that might be mistaken for a symptom of asthma. In assessing the patient physically, recording blood pressure is important, since steroids, adrenergic agents, and theophylline may elevate blood pressure. Monitoring oxygen saturations has become an important tool in assessing the severity of asthma.

During an asthmatic episode, the patient presents with difficulty in respiration with an increased respiratory rate, using accessory muscles and suprasternal retraction, pursed-lip expiration, and flaring of the nostrils. Expiration is prolonged, with intercostal retraction. Cardiac dullness may be present, and the liver edge may be palpable owing to a lower diaphragm from pulmonary hyperexpansion.

To supplement the history and physical examination, the response to a bronchodilator may be used to establish the presence of reversible obstructive lung disease. Measurements of FEV_1 and $FEF_{25\%-75\%}$ are often extremely helpful before and after bronchodilation. Sputum analysis is also helpful in assessing in general terms the potential for developing obstructive lung disease. Care should be taken to note the type of cells, whether lymphocytic, neutrophilic, or eosinophilic. Worsening of asthma symptoms is usually accompanied by an increase in the total blood eosinophil and sputum eosinophil counts. Both are decreased when glucocorticoid therapy is instituted.

A chest x-ray study is often not helpful in evaluating the noncomplicated asthmatic patient, since it is usually normal. However, it does provide a baseline for future comparisons. A majority of asthmatic patients show hyperinflation with increased bronchial markings and flattening of the diaphragm during the acute episode.

The total serum IgE level is not particularly useful information for the management of asthma. It is normal in intrinsic asthma, but not always elevated in extrinsic asthma. Its main significance is an aid in diagnosing bronchopulmonary aspergillosis, which commonly has marked elevated serum IgE levels and this is a treatable cause of "asthma." Baseline pulmonary function studies are extremely helpful, not only in defining the type of lung disease that is present, but also in serving as a reference source for future episodes and as a way of measuring medication efficacy. In patients who do not have abnormal pulmonary function studies when examined, but complain of symptoms occurring at other times that suggest asthma, a bronchial challenge with histamine or methacholine may be useful. These procedures, however, should be done with properly trained personnel because of their potential danger in initiating a life-threatening asthma attack. Portable peak flow meters, now easily available to all patients, serve as an important guide to disease management in patients with moderate or severe asthma. Monitoring peak flow rates daily in patients with moderate or severe disease heralds the onset of respiratory difficulty and allows the patient to initiate a treatment plan that has been previously outlined.

The aim of management is to keep the patient as symptom free as possible with minimal medication. It is essential that the patient understand the disease and its precipitating and aggravating factors and recognize its early manifestations so that an acute episode can be treated early in order to prevent hospitalization. Recognition of the impact of emotional factors on asthma from a personal, family, and work standpoint can facilitate an acceptance of the limitations of the disease without over-reaction and frustration. Patients can be taught to practice relaxed breathing to help prevent the panic that is often associated with the onset of acute symptoms.

In children it is important to differentiate asthma from bronchiolitis in infancy, bronchitis, croup, epiglottitis, and aspiration of foreign body. An inspiratory stridor differentiates hypertrophic tonsils, laryngeal disease, subglottic stenosis, or a foreign body from asthma. Among chronic conditions, childhood cystic fibrosis is distinguished by malabsorption and failure to thrive and a sweat chloride concentration of greater than 16 mEq/L. In both children and adults, nocturnal respiratory distress has been associated with sleep apnea related to upper airway obstruction and should always be considered in the differential diagnosis.

The concept of preventive therapy in the treatment of asthma is the rule. In 1991 an expert panel was convened under the sponsorship of the National Heart, Lung, and Blood Institute, affiliated with the National Institutes of Health in Bethesda, Maryland. Their report with its treatment recommendations has become the foundation for current medical management of asthma and serves as an excellent resource for all clinicians treating this disease (International Consensus Report, 1992).

Preventive therapy encompasses the use of specific pharmacologic agents capable not only of ablating the immediate phase of the asthmatic reaction, but also suppressing the ensuing late-phase inflammatory component. Guidelines established by the NIH expert panel using both a step-up and step-down approach to the asthmatic patient should be followed (Table 26–2).

For a patient with mild paroxysmal asthma, a β2-adrenergic bronchodilator, such as albuterol, administered by a metered-dose inhaler with a spacer usually provides relief for at least 6 hours. Should repeated use of β2-adrenergic agents become necessary to control symptoms, inhalable anti-inflammatory agents, such as glucocorticoid steroids, nedocromil sodium, or sodium cromolyn must be added. "Nocturnal" breakthrough is one of the more annoying symptoms associated with asthma. Aminophylline, once the foundation of therapy for the treatment of asthma in the United States, still has a therapeutic role, particularly in the sustained-release forms, when given at bedtime to control nocturnal breakthrough symptoms. With the recent release in the United States of salmeterol, a long-acting β2 agonist, the addition of this medication likewise has provided nocturnal relief. It must be recognized, however, that this particular drug has a slow onset of action and should never be used for "rescue" therapy. Recent information in the literature suggests the possibility that both short- and long-acting β2 agonists have been associated with increasing morbidity and mortality (Busse, 1996). At this time, however, there is no scientific support that these agents are directly associated with increased morbidity and mortality. An oral β2-adrenergic drug may provide some additional benefit, but usually has no advantage over, and more side effects than, the same drug given by inhalation.

Status asthmaticus must be treated aggressively in order to promote rapid reversibility. Continuous oxygen, nebulized β2-adrenergic agents, subcutaneous β2 agonists, and systemic corticosteroids may all be necessary to promote rapid reversibility (Table 26–2).

The management of chronic asthma presents a different challenge, again with the goal being to maintain the patient as symptom free as possible. Inhaled anti-inflammatory agents, paired with an inhaled β2-adrenergic agent, delivered with a spacer device, is the accepted form of therapy at this time. The patient should be counseled on rinsing the mouth after the use of inhalable steroids to decrease the risk of oral pharyngeal candidiasis. If continuous oral glucocorticoid therapy is necessary, using the lowest dosage possible and administering it on alternate days minimizes the side effects. Unfortunately, most patients who require oral steroid therapy often find that they have a flare of bronchospasm during their "off" day. Ipratropium bromide, an anticholinergic bronchodilator, has proved effective as an additive agent in patients with chronic disease, particularly that associated with chronic bronchitis and COPD. Its effectiveness in asthmatic patients is variable; generally, it is less effective than β2-adrenergic agents, and it has no effect on the late-phase asthmatic response.

Environment control by reducing exposure to common indoor allergens (house dust mite, cockroach, animal dander, and molds) is also extremely important. "Swamp" coolers often allow significant amounts of mold spores to circulate within a home and should not be used. Dust mite and animal dander can be reduced using a high efficiency air filter (HEPA) in the heating/cooling system of the

TABLE 26–2. Management of Chronic Asthma*

Step-up:	Progression to the next higher step is indicated when control cannot be achieved at the current step and there is assurance that medication is used correctly. If PEFR ≤ 60% predicted or personal best, consider a burst of oral corticosteroids and then proceed.
Step-down:	Reduction in therapy is considered when the outcome for therapy has been achieved and sustained for several weeks or even months at the current step. Reduction in therapy is also needed to identify the minimum therapy required to maintain control.

Outcome: Control of Asthma
- Minimal (ideally no) chronic symptoms, including nocturnal symptoms
- Minimal (infrequent) episodes
- No emergency visits
- Minimal need for p.r.n. beta$_2$-agonist
- No limitations on activities, including exercise
- PEF circadian variation <20%
- (Near) normal PEF
- Minimal (or no) adverse effects from medicine

Outcome: Best Possible Results
- Least symptoms
- Least need for p.r.n. beta$_2$-agonist
- Least limitation of activity
- Least PEFR circadian variation
- Best PEFR
- Least adverse effects from medicine

Step-down
- Once control is reached at any step, and sustained, a step-down—reduction in therapy—may be carefully considered and is needed to identify the minimum therapy required to maintain control.
- Advise patients of signs of worsening asthma and actions to control it.

STEP 1: MILD

Therapy†
- Short-acting inhaled beta$_2$-agonist p.r.n. not more than 3 times a week
- Short-acting inhaled beta$_2$-agonist or cromolyn before exercise or exposure to antigen
- Leukotriene inhibitor

Clinical Features Pretreatment*‡
- Intermittent, brief symptoms <1–2 times a week
- Nocturnal asthma symptoms <1–2 times a month
- Asymptomatic between exacerbations
- PEFR or FEV:
  —>80% predicted
  —variability <20%

STEP 2: MODERATE

Therapy†
- Inhaled anti-inflammatory daily
  —Initially: inhaled corticosteroid 200–500 μg or cromolyn or nedocromil (Children begin with a trial of cromolyn)
  —If necessary: inhaled corticosteroid 400–750 μg (Alternatively, particularly for nocturnal symptoms, proceed to Step 3 with additional long-acting bronchodilator)
  and
- Short-acting inhaled beta$_2$-agonist p.r.n., not to exceed 3–4 times a day

Clinical Features Pretreatment*‡
- Exacerbations >1–2 times a week
- Exacerbations may affect activity and sleep
- Nocturnal asthma symptoms >2 times a month
- Chronic symptoms requiring short-acting beta$_2$-agonist almost daily
- PEFR or FEV:
  —60–80% predicted
  —variability 20–30%

STEP 3: MODERATE

Therapy†
- Inhaled corticosteroids 800–1000 μg daily (>1000 μg under specialist's supervision)
  and
- Sustained-release theophylline, oral beta$_2$-agonist, or long-acting inhaled beta$_2$-agonist, especially for nocturnal symptoms; may consider inhaled anticholinergics
  and
- Short-acting inhaled beta$_2$-agonist p.r.n., not to exceed 3–4 times a day

STEP 4: SEVERE

Therapy†
- Inhaled corticosteroid 800–1000 μg daily (>1000 μg under specialist's supervision)
  and
- Sustained-release theophylline and/or oral beta$_2$-agonist, or long-acting inhaled beta$_2$-agonist, especially for nocturnal symptoms with or without
- Short-acting inhaled beta$_2$-agonist once a day; may consider inhaled anticholinergic
  and
- Oral corticosteroids (alternate-day or single daily dose)
  and
- Short-acting inhaled beta$_2$-agonist p.r.n., up to 3–4 times a day

Clinical Features Pretreatment*‡
- Frequent exacerbations
- Continuous symptoms
- Frequent nocturnal asthma symptoms
- Physical activities limited by asthma
- PEFR or FEV:
  —<60% predicted
  —variability >30%

*PEFR, peak expiratory flow rate; PEF, peak expiratory flow; FEV, forced expiratory volume.

†All therapy must include patient education about prevention (including environmental control where appropriate) as well as control of symptoms.

‡One or more features may be present to be assigned a grade of severity; an individual should usually be assigned to the most severe grade in which any feature occurs.

From International Consensus Report on Diagnosis and Management of Asthma (Publication No. NIH-92-3091). Bethesda, MD, U.S. Department of Health and Human Services, 1992, p 34.

home. Commercial agents (Aearoson, benzoate powder, tannic acid) also help reduce the number of dust mites. If at all possible, all animals should be removed from the home, certainly the bedroom, and tobacco smoke totally avoided.

Asthma following exercise (exercise-induced asthma [EIA]) is common in children and young adults (Rakel, 1995). Some patients have asthma only with exercise. Premedicating patients immediately before exercise with a β2 agonist, or cromolyn sodium generally prevents an asthmatic attack. Salmeterol, a long-acting β2 agonist, can be used in the morning for school-age children, protecting them during school-sponsored physical activities. Zafirlukast (Accolate), a leukotriene inhibitor, is also very effective in blocking EIA. Its counterpart zileuton (Zyflo) may

also be effective but has more side effects and probably should be reserved for patients with aspirin triad (nasal polyps, aspirin allergy, and asthma).

Other medications that have been used to treat chronic asthma include troleandomycin, methotrexate, and gold salts. Their use is beyond the scope of this discussion.

With identification of the mediators of the late-phase response, including platelet activating factor, various leukotrienes and cytokines, a whole new line of medications is now on the horizon. Soon to be released in the United States will be a medication that blocks one of the leukotrienes that participates in the late-phase response and offers a whole new therapeutic modality in the treatment of this chronic disease state.

SUGGESTED READING

Busse WW. Long- and short-acting beta 2-adrenergic agonists. Effects on airway function in patients with asthma. Arch Intern Med 1996;156:1514–1520.
deShazo RD, Smith DL. Primer on Allergic and Immunologic Disease, 2nd ed. Chicago, American Medical Association, 1987.
International Consensus Report on Diagnosis and Management of Asthma. Publication No. NIH-92-3091. Bethesda, MD, U.S. Department of Health and Human Services, 1992.
Rakel RE. Textbook of Family Practice, 5th ed. Philadelphia, W. B. Saunders, 1995.
Szefler SJ, Chambers CV. Diagnosis and Management of Asthma, Vol 2. American Family Physician Monograph. New York, Health Science Communications, 1995.

QUESTIONS

1. Patients with a diagnosis of asthma and hypertension should never use which of the following drugs?
   a. ACE inhibitors
   b. Diuretics
   c. β blockers
   d. Calcium channel blockers

2. Answer true (T) or false (F) to the following statements:
   a. Asthma frequently occurs only *after* puberty.
   b. Infections play a significant role in asthma.
   c. Oral steroids should only be used as a *last* resort in an acute asthma attack.

3. Metered-dose inhalers (MDIs) containing β2 agonists should:
   a. Be used 4 to 6 times a day as the only treatment for asthma.
   b. Used with a spacer device to assist in delivery of the medication.
   c. Never be used with inhaled steroids.

Answers appear on **page 604.**

Chapter 27

Diarrhea

Jerry E. Jones, M.D., M.S.

INITIAL VISIT

Subjective

Melva H. is a 32-year-old white woman, mother of two active boys. Her visit is for a problem with diarrhea.

PRESENTING PROBLEM. Melva comes to your office complaining of watery stools of 3 days' duration.

PRESENT ILLNESS. She states she was in her usual state of good health prior to this time. The onset of diarrhea was sudden and associated with slight abdominal cramping and some nausea but no vomiting. She has felt generalized malaise and denies fever, chills, or night sweats. She denies seeing blood or mucus in the stools. She states that the number of stools has been as high as six to eight per 24-hour period, with the last stool being some 2 hours before her office visit. She has been able to tolerate her usual diet but states that she has not felt hungry.

PAST MEDICAL HISTORY. Melva has had no surgeries, accidents, or serious injuries. She had to be hospitalized for one episode of renal stones 6 years before but has been on no recent medications for this. She has no known medication allergies.

FAMILY HISTORY. Both of the patient's parents are living and reported to be in good health. There is a history of diabetes mellitus in a grandmother and a history of hypertension in both grandfathers. Her only sister is alive and well. No one else in the family has been ill.

HEALTH HABITS. The patient does not smoke or drink alcohol. She does not actively exercise, but states that keeping up with two small children gives her plenty to do.

SOCIAL HISTORY. Melva is married to a third-year dental student. She has two children ages 2 and 5 years. She works outside the home part time as a visiting nurse. She denies a recent travel history. She denies known exposures to hepatitis. She lives in a community of 2500 and drinks city water.

REVIEW OF SYSTEMS. She reports a decrease in appetite over the last several days. She has had an occasional headache. She has noted some increase in "gas." She has had difficulty sleeping owing to the bouts of diarrhea. She denies rashes.

Objective

PHYSICAL EXAMINATION. The patient appears comfortable, with blood pressure 118/72 mm Hg, heart rate 88, temperature 99°F, weight 142 lb, and height 5 feet 8 inches. Her mucous membranes appear moist. Her physical examination was notable for active bowel sounds, slight upper abdominal and left lower quadrant abdominal tenderness, and a somewhat flushed appearance. Her rectal vault was empty.

LABORAORY TESTS. A stool test for blood is negative. A microscopic examination of the stool shows no red blood cells and only a few white blood cells. The urinalysis is negative for ketones. The white blood cell count and liver enzyme studies are normal. No parasitic ova or cysts were identified in stool obtained during the digital rectal examination.

Assessment

WORKING DIAGNOSIS. A diagnosis of viral gastroenteritis is most likely in this case (rotavirus or Norwalk agent). Additional considerations could be early vital hepatitis, which may present with diarrhea

TABLE 27–1. Common Infectious Agents Causing Diarrhea in Various Age Groups Seen by Family Physicians

Agent	Age Group					
	Neonate	*Infant*	*Child*	*Adolescent*	*Adult*	*Elderly*
Viruses						
Rotavirus group A	−	+ + + +	+ + +	−	+ +	+ +
Enteric adenovirus	−	+ + + +	+ + +	−	−	−
Norwalk	−	−	+ +	+ +	+ +	+ +
Calicivirus	−	+ + + +	+ + +	−	−	−
Astrovirus	−	+ + + +	+ + +	−	−	−
Bacteria						
Escherichia coli						
Enterotoxigenic	+ + + +	+ + +	+ +	+ +	+ +	+ +
Enteropathogenic	−	+ + + +	−	−	+ +	−
Enteroinvasive	−	−	+ +	+ +	−	−
Strain O157:H7	−	+ +	+ +	+ +	+ +	+ +
Salmonella spp	−	+ +	+ +	+ +	+ +	+ +
Shigella spp	−	+ + + +	+ + +	+ +	+ +	+ +
Vibrio spp	−	+ +	+ +	+ +	+ +	+ +
Campylobacter spp	−	+ + + +	+ +	+ + +	+ + +	+ +
Yersinia spp	−	+ + +	+ + + +	+ +	+ +	−
Clostridium difficile	−	−	+ +	+ +	+ +	+ +
Protozoa						
Giardia lamblia	−	+ + +	+ + + +	+ +	+ +	−
Entamoeba histolytica	−	+ +	+ +	+ +	+ +	−
Cryptosporidium spp	−	+ +	+ + +	+ +	+ +	−

+ + + + = Most common; + + + = frequent; + + = outbreaks; − = data unclear.

before onset of liver involvement, and a protozoal infection with *Giardia lamblia.*

DIFFERENTIAL DIAGNOSIS. Table 27–1 outlines the most common infectious agents responsible for diarrhea in the human host. Certain agents may predominate within age groups. For adults, outbreaks due to viral, bacterial, and protozoal causes are possible. Even under the best of circumstances, an identifiable infectious agent is identified in less than 50 per cent of the cases.

With the stool negative for red and white blood cells, a bacterial cause would be less likely.

If there is a negative exposure history, drug- or toxin-induced diarrhea would be unlikely.

No one else has been ill in the immediate family, so food poisoning would be unlikely. Food poisoning with *Staphylococcus* and mushrooms is associated with vomiting as well.

Protozoan infections with *Entamoeba histolytica* present with blood and mucus in the stools.

Plan

CLINICAL MANAGEMENT. The key issues in the clinical management of a patient with diarrhea associated with nausea and/or vomiting are (1) severity of illness and its duration; (2) the travel history; and (3) special considerations of high-risk groups.

The physical examination should include consideration of fluid status (dehydration?), high fever, weight loss, and blood in the stools. If the diarrhea has lasted longer than 24 to 48 hours, there may be a need to proceed with a more extensive work-up. In a patient with a recent travel history (within 2 to 4 weeks), parasitic infections may be more likely. The possibility of high-risk behaviors for human immunodeficiency virus infection necessitates special stool tests such as acid-fast staining.

THERAPEUTIC TREATMENT PLAN. The patient has continued to tolerate her usual diet. A discussion of replacing fluids orally is helpful along with symptomatic treatment of the diarrhea. Effective replacement of lost fluid and electrolytes is the cornerstone of treatment. Oral rehydration fluid can be obtained commercially or produced from common food items. Table 27–2 outlines a simple formula for making a rehydration solution at home. Nonprescription oral rehydration solutions include Rehydralyte, Ricelyte, and Pedialyte. A simple rule of thumb is to give 5 ml (1 teaspoon) every 1 to 5

TABLE 27–2. Oral Rehydration Fluid Using Common Household Ingredients

1 Quart of clean water
(1.05 L)
1 Teaspoon of baking soda
(2.5 g of sodium bicarbonate)
1 Cup of orange juice*
(1.5 g of potassium chloride)
4 Tablespoons of sugar
(20 g of glucose)
3/4 Teaspoon of table salt
(3.5 g of sodium chloride)

*May substitute two bananas.
Modified from Guerrant RL, Bobak DA. Bacterial and protozoal gastroenteritis. N Engl J Med 1991;325:327–340.

minutes in a child and 15 ml (1 tablespoon) every 1 to 5 minutes in an adult.

Therapeutic use of bismuth subsalicylate (Pepto-Bismol) in volunteers with gastroenteritis caused by Norwalk virus has produced some reduction in abdominal cramps without affecting the rate of viral excretion.

PATIENT EDUCATION. A review of the most likely causes is helpful in educating the patient regarding "viral gastroenteritis." It is important to discuss the fact that antibiotics are not indicated in a viral illness. Careful hand washing is indicated. A decision on oral rehydration fluids needs to be made and directions provided on how to use or give these fluids.

DISPOSITION. The patient is told to return for re-evaluation if the number and frequency of stools do not diminish. Otherwise, the natural course of the illness would be that of gradual improvement and the return to normal function.

FIRST FOLLOW-UP VISIT

Subjective

The patient returned in 2 weeks stating that the initial bout of diarrhea seemed to clear. However, 2 days before this visit there was a second bout of foul-smelling diarrhea associated with epigastric discomfort and increased gas. The patient noted increasing nausea without vomiting and experienced a 10-lb weight loss over the past 2 weeks. There was generalized fatigue. She stated that her oldest son had also started having loose stools.

Objective

The patient appears fatigued. Blood pressure is 110/68 mm Hg, pulse 90, respiration rate 20, and temperature 98.8°F. Her weight is 136 lb. Abdominal examination reveals slight epigastric tenderness and diffuse active bowel sounds. A digital rectal examination revealed soft stool in the ampulla and was again negative for occult blood. A microscopic examination of the stool revealed cysts of *G. lamblia*.

Assessment

A diagnosis of giardiasis was made.

Plan

1. The patient is started on metronidazole (Flagyl) 250 mg orally three times a day for 7 days.

2. Stool examinations were obtained on the remaining family members. In both children, stool samples were positive for cysts of *Giardia*.

3. On further investigation, it was found that the patient's community water supply had recently experienced problems with a breakdown in water treatment. The community at large had experienced bouts of diarrhea, and local health officials were notified of the clustering of these cases. The patient was instructed to use bottled water for drinking and cooking until the community water supply problem could be corrected.

4. The children were treated with furazolidone (Furoxone) suspension. The recommended dose for children is 5 mg per kg in four equally divided doses during a 24-hour period for 7 days.

5. Repeat stool examinations are requested for all family members in 4 weeks.

DISCUSSION

Giardiasis is the human infection caused by the flagellated protozoan *Giardia lamblia*. It occurs in all age groups and can present to the physician with a range of symptoms. In the acute phase, the patient presents with diarrhea, abdominal pain, bloating, and flatulence. As in this case, it may initially be manifested as the "garden variety" gastroenteritis. The cyst passage is variable, with high numbers being passed initially during the acute phase. Stool samples for ova and parasites are helpful but frequently are overlooked during the acute episodes. Even without treatment, its natural course is to spontaneously improve.

Following the initial bout, the host may either recover without further problems or become a chronic carrier with intermittent episodes of recurrent diarrhea. This "chronic" phase may be prolonged and last several years after the first contact with this organism. This phase of giardiasis presents with flatulence, upper abdominal pain, epigastric gnawing, nervousness, and weight loss. Diagnosis is at times difficult.

Digital rectal examination is one way to obtain samples for microscopic examination in the office setting. This also provides a method to examine for red and white blood cells in the stool.

It is helpful to place the presenting signs and symptoms into an "acute" or a "chronic" episode. If it appears that the symptoms represent a chronic infection (duration of recurrent symptoms greater than 3 months), it may be necessary to use the "string test" to obtain duodenal samples for diagnosis. In this test, the trophozoite phase is identified. This procedure can be used in the office setting and provides a fairly simple method for upper intestinal sampling. An additional laboratory procedure for the detection of the giardial antigen is available, GSA 65 (ProSpecT Giardia, Alexon Inc., Sunnyvale, CA). It is based on a solid-phase immunoassay and can be obtained using fecal specimens with the stool kit methods described later. Figure 27–1 outlines a diagnostic approach to giardiasis.

Since any intestinal protozoan infection indicates that the patient has experienced fecal contamination, it is important to explore the possible sources of this contamination. Melva has several possible sources including her young children (giardiasis is a major cause of day care epidemics), her part-time job (working as a home health care nurse places her in situations of chronic care), and the breakdown of her community water supply. In this

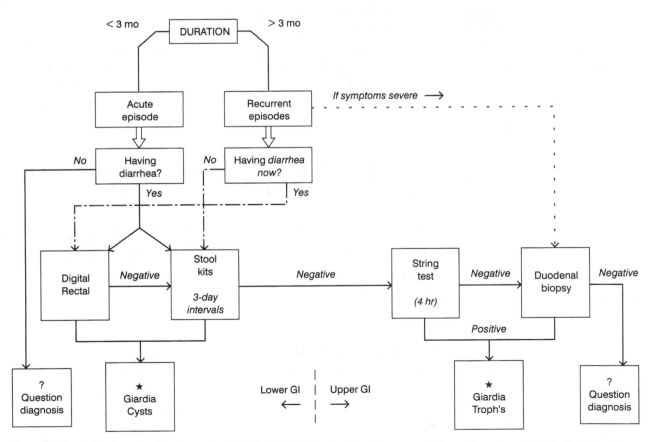

Figure 27–1. A flowchart for the diagnosis of *Giardia lamblia* infection. Troph's = trophozites. (From Jones JE. Giardiasis. In Balows A, Hausler WJ, Lennette EH (eds). Laboratory Diagnosis of Infectious Diseases: Principles and Practice, vol. 1. New York, Springer-Verlag, 1988, with permission.)

situation, the local health department identified problems that were helpful in correcting a community outbreak.

Collecting fecal specimens is often embarrassing and frequently difficult to accomplish in the office setting. Stool collection kits are available and helpful in improving compliance. It is important to check other family members for possible infections since many infections may be asymptomatic and provide a source for reinfection. Careful instructions on how to collect a stool sample at home are necessary. The use of plastic kitchen wrap under the toilet seat is a helpful way to instruct individuals in the collection of a stool specimen. By placing this wrap beneath the toilet seat, one can obtain a sample of stool without having to dip into the toilet bowl or try to pass stool into a container. The sample is placed into a prepared kit containing two vials: polyvinyl alcohol (PVA) and buffered formalin. These kits are available commercially (Meridian Diagnostics, Inc., Cincinnati, Ohio).

Morphologic characteristics that distinguish the cyst are its shape, size, and intracytoplasmic structures. The cyst is approximately the size of a white cell and has a distinctive oval shape. On wet preparation, a refractile body called the axostyle is seen obliquely within the cytoplasm. One to two of the four nuclei are usually seen in any one field of focus. Dilute iodine dropped on the edge of the coverslip helps outline the nuclear characteristics of the cysts.

TABLE 27–3.   Drug Treatment of Giardiasis

Adults	
Quinacrine HCl (Atabrine)	100 mg tid for 5 days
Metronidazole (Flagyl)	250 mg tid for 5 days
Furazolidone (Furoxone)	100 mg qid for 7–10 days
Paromomycin (Humatin)*	25–30 mg/kg in three divided doses for 7–10 days
Children	
Quinacrine HCl	2 mg/kg tid for 5 days (maximum, 300 mg/day)
Metronidazole	5 mg/kg tid for 5 days
Furazolidone	1.25 mg/kg qid for 7 days

*For first trimester of pregnancy if treatment is deemed necessary.

Trophozoites are easily recognized on wet preparation by their irregular motion and activity. The trophozoite is pear-shaped, and on special stains the two large nuclei give it its characteristic "monkey face" appearance.

Treatment with metronidazole is generally effective, although some treatment failures have been reported. Quinacrine is equally effective. Table 27–3 outlines the available drugs for the treatment of giardiasis. Special consideration is needed for the pregnant patient since metronidazole is contraindicated during the first trimester.

SUGGESTED READING

Blacklow NR, Greenberg HB. Viral gastroenterits. N Engl J Med 1991;325:252–264.

Goepp JG, Katz SA. Oral rehydation therapy. Am Fam Physician 1993;47:843–848.

Gracey M (ed). Diarrhea. Boca Raton, FL, CRC Press, 1990.

Guerrant RL, Bobak DA. Bacterial and protozoal gastroenteritis. N Engl J Med 1991;325:327–340.

Jones JE. Giardiasis. Prim Care 1991;18:43–52.

Jones JE. Giardiasis. In Balows A, Hausler WJ, Lennette EN (eds). Laboratory Diagnosis of Infectious Disease: Principles and Practice, Vol I. New York, Springer-Verlag, 1988, pp 872–882.

QUESTIONS

1. The *cornerstone* of treatment for diarrhea associated with nausea and/or vomiting is:
   a. The clear identification of a causative agent at the first office visit
   b. Treatment of the nausea
   c. Effective replacement of lost fluid and electrolytes
   d. Treatment of diarrhea with antibiotics

2. The acute phase of giardiasis is characterized by
   a. Constipation
   b. Fever
   c. Vomiting

d. Diarrhea
e. Blood in stools

3. The chronic phase of giardiasis is characterized by
   a. Vomiting

b. Flatulence
c. Blood in stools
d. Mucus in stools
e. Fever

Answers appear on **page 604**.

Chapter **28**

Pregnancy

Randy Wertheimer, M.D.

INITIAL VISIT

Subjective

Rachel is a 23-year-old G2 P0 (gravida 2, para 0) ab1 woman who presents with a 4-week history of fatigue, nausea, and breast tenderness. She had a positive pregnancy test 2 weeks ago, and she is experiencing symptoms similar to those she had 5 years ago when she was pregnant for the first time. Rachel stopped her birth control pill 3 months ago with the hope of becoming pregnant within the next year. She had a normal withdrawal menses at that time, and had a few days of spotting around 8 weeks ago. She is unsure of the exact date of her last menstrual period, as the spotting episode was not typical of her menses. She expressed concern about becoming pregnant so soon after using the contraceptive pill.

Rachel has been on a multivitamin preparation with folic acid as prescribed by her family physician when she went off the birth control pill with plans to become pregnant. She has been immunized against hepatitis B with the full triple vaccine within the last 5 years. We know from her previous pregnancy that she is immune to rubella and that her blood type is B−. She remembers having chickenpox as a child. Her last Pap smear 6 months ago was within normal limits, and she has had normal Pap smears yearly since age 18.

Ben, Rachel's husband of 3 years, is excited about this pregnancy according to Rachel. Although they have no family close by, they have been living in the area since college and have a community of close friends. Rachel plans to work part-time as a computer programmer after the baby is born and her husband will continue to work full-time in his job as an electrical engineer.

PAST MEDICAL HISTORY. Menarche at age 13. Menstrual cycle 31 days, 5 days' flow. Oral contraceptives used 1990 to 1996. Pregnancy 1990—Elective first-trimester termination. No complications. Rh immune globulin (RhIG) given after procedure. Hospitalizations: None. Allergies: None.

FAMILY HISTORY. Maternal mother (Rachel's mother) has hypertension and hypercholesterolemia. Paternal father (Ben's father) has type II diabetes. No family history of congenital defects or genetic disorders.

SOCIAL HISTORY. Rachel is a computer programmer. Her husband is an electrical engineer. They are both excited about starting a family.

HEALTH HABITS. Alcohol intake of one glass of wine a few times per week was stopped 3 months ago. Past history of occasional marijuana use. No cocaine or other substance use. No smoking.

REVIEW OF SYSTEMS. History of occasional headaches. Urinary tract infection twice in the past 10 years. No history of pyelonephritis.

Objective

Rachel is a well-appearing, mildly overweight young woman. Blood pressure 110/70 mm Hg, pulse 76, regular. Height 5 feet 3 inches, weight 140 lb. Skin: No rashes. HEENT: Normal. Neck: Supple. No adenopathy. Thyroid normal size. Lungs: Clear. Cardiovascular: S_1 normal, S_2 normal. No murmur. Breasts: No masses, inverted nipples bilaterally. Abdomen: Bowel sounds normoactive. No hepatosplenomegaly. No fetal heart tones audible by Doppler. Pelvic: External genitalia normal, vaginal vault has scant discharge. Cervix shows bluish discoloration. *Chlamydia* culture taken. Uterus is anterior, enlarged, 8 weeks in size (size of large orange). Ovaries not palpated. No adnexal masses palpated. Diagonal conjugate (distance between sacral promontory and inferior aspect of symphysis) 13 cm, distance between ischial spines 12 cm, pelvic side walls concave. Extremities: No edema.

LABORATORY TESTS. Urine dipstick test negative for albumin and glucose.

Assessment

Intrauterine pregnancy. History, physical examination, and laboratory data all point to an early intrauterine pregnancy. Establishing the due date is the first order of business. In addition, the physician needs to identify screening tests to diagnose and treat prenatal disease. Last, he or she wants to promote a healthy pregnancy by assessing the woman's home and work environment and by promoting a healthy lifestyle.

DISCUSSION

1. *Establishing the due date.* The diagnosis of pregnancy in this case is relatively straightforward. Rachel has had unprotected sex, is amenorrheic, and is exhibiting many of the frequent symptoms of early pregnancy, i.e., fatigue, breast swelling and tenderness, nausea.

Her physical examination reveals changes in the cervix and the uterus which are also consistent with early pregnancy. Her cervix has a bluish hue, known as the Chadwick sign. She has an enlarged uterus,

about the size of a large orange, corresponding to 8 weeks' gestation. The physician does not hear a fetal heart beat by Doppler. Fetal heart tones may be audible by Doppler as early as 9 weeks' gestation, depending in part on the position of the uterus and the body habitus of the woman. By 12 weeks' gestation, fetal heart tones are audible by Doppler in most pregnant women.

Rachel did not need a urine pregnancy test done in the office, because she had a positive test that she had done at home, and physical examination confirmed an intrauterine pregnancy. The commonly performed urine test measures the presence of an elevated level of human chorionic gonadotropin (hCG). Normally nonpregnant women have low circulating levels, .02 to .08 IU of hCG. With early pregnancy, levels double every 1.3 to 2.3 days and peak at 7 to 10 weeks (100,000 IU). Elevated hCG levels are generally detected in the urine by 7 to 10 days after conception. By the time menses is missed, 98 per cent of pregnant women have a positive test.

The most commonly used method to ascertain a pregnant woman's due date is the last menstrual period (LMP). When a woman can recall with clarity the first day of her last menstrual period, can define it as a normal period with regard to regularity and duration, and there has not been a recent use of birth control pills, then the LMP is a remarkably accurate predictor of the due date. However, in this case, Rachel's last normal menses was attached to her last cycle of oral contraceptives. The few days of spotting 4 weeks later may represent the LMP, but it is difficult to determine with accuracy by this history. Women may not ovulate regularly the first few months after stopping the pill. Her physical examination, however, with a uterus the size for an 8-week fetus, suggests that this spotting was in fact the LMP.

If the LMP was believed to be more accurate, one could estimate the due date by using a pregnancy wheel or by applying the Nägele rule. One begins with the first day of the LMP, adds 1 year plus 7 days and subtracts 3 months. The length of human gestation is estimated at 280 days, or 40 weeks counting from the first day of the LMP. This assumes a 28-day cycle and that the time from ovulation to menses was 14 days. In women with a longer cycle, as is true with Rachel who has a 31-day cycle, one should add a few days to the expected due date.

Because we are not able to estimate a due date with certainty by history and physical examination at this point, it is reasonable to order an ultrasound as an additional tool to help establish accurate dating. First-trimester scans can identify the gestational age of a pregnancy within 3 to 5 days using the crown-rump length. This method of measurement is not used after 12 weeks' gestation because of fetal spine flexion. Transvaginal scanning uses a higher frequency transducer, and structures may be seen earlier than in transabdominal screening. Fetal poles can be seen as early as 6 weeks transvaginally and 7 to 8 weeks transabdominally. It is important to note that the use of ultrasound is not recommended as a routine screening test in pregnancy. Neither early, late, or serial ultrasounds have demonstrated an improved perinatal morbidity or mortality (U.S. Preventive Services Task Force, 1996). However, it is an appropriate tool to use for gestational age assessment in cases of uncertain dates.

2. *Diagnose and treat prenatal disease.* Rachel did have adequate preconception care within the year before pregnancy. During this time, risk assessment, health promotion, and medical and psychosocial intervention were addressed by her family physician. We know that the greatest sensitivity to the environment for the developing fetus occurs during the 17 to 56 days after conception, yet as many as one fourth of pregnant women fail to initiate care until after the first trimester. Because healthy women are more likely to have healthier babies, the time to treat illness or change unhealthy behavior is before pregnancy.

A number of screening tests must now be ordered as part of the initial prenatal visit. Many of the tests ordered in the preconception period need not be repeated. Table 28–1 lists recommended screening laboratory tests during pregnancy.

First the hemoglobin–hematocrit level should be determined. During pregnancy, the increase in plasma volume is disproportionately greater than the red blood cell mass, causing physiologic dilution and a normal drop in hematocrit by 3 to 5 per cent. Therefore the definition of anemia in pregnancy is different from that in the nonpregnant adult woman. For women living at sea level, a hemoglobin of 11 gm/dl in the first and third trimester, and 10.5 gm/dl in the second trimester is acceptable. Although hemoglobin values well below 10 per cent have been associated with an increased risk of low birth weight, preterm delivery, and perinatal mortality in numerous longitudinal cross-sectional studies, most of these studies did not control for other factors such as smoking and maternal malnutrition. Whereas a large body of data suggests that iron supplements improve hematologic indices in hemoglobin levels above 10 gm/dl, there is no consistent evidence that iron supplementation actually improves clinical outcomes. Therefore there is no medical reason to recommend routine iron supple-

TABLE 28–1. Prenatal Screening Tests

Initial Prenatal Visit

Blood pressure
Hemoglobin or hematocrit
Antibody screen
Rapid plasma reagin (RPR)
HBsAg (if status unknown)
Blood group and Rh factor (if status unknown)
Rubella titer (if status unknown)
Varicella titer (if status unknown)
Urine culture (12–16 wk)
Chlamydia (if woman <25 yr of age or high risk)
Gonococcal culture (if high risk)
Pap smear (if not done within past 6–12 months)
Hemoglobin electrophoresis (if status unknown in at-risk racial groups)
HIV screen (counsel and offer to all)

16–18 wk
α-Fetoprotein

24–28 wk
Glucose (Glucola) screen
Antibody (if Rh-negative)
RPR (if high risk)

HBsAg = Hepatitis B surface antigen; HIV = human immunodeficiency virus.

mentation in pregnant women with hemoglobin values greater than 10 gm/dl.

Testing for antibodies is done also during this first prenatal visit. One needs to know blood type (ABO/Rh) and antibodies for each pregnancy. Because Rachel was pregnant previously, we already know that she is B−, and blood type testing need not be repeated. Antibodies must be checked with each pregnancy, however. The most prevalent antibody of concern during pregnancy is the anti-Rh(D) antibody. Rh incompatibility occurs when an Rh-negative woman is pregnant with an Rh-positive fetus. This occurs in 9 to 10 per cent of pregnancies. Consequences for the fetus include hemolytic anemia, hyperbilirubinemia, kernicterus, or intrauterine death due to hydrops fetalis. Without preventive measures, 0.7 to 1.8 per cent of Rh negative women become isoimmunized antenatally, and develop Rh(D) antibody through exposure to fetal blood, 8 to 15 per cent become isoimmunized at birth, 3 to 5 per cent become isoimmunized after spontaneous or therapeutic abortion, and 2.1 to 3.4 per cent become isoimmunized after amniocentesis (U.S. Preventive Services Task Force, 1996).

All pregnant women need to be screened for syphilis with a rapid plasma reagin (RPR) titer, even if they have been tested within the past year. The incidence of congenital syphilis has increased over the past 15 years. The neurologic sequelae for the surviving newborn are devastating, and there is a 40 per cent fetal or perinatal death rate in pregnancies compromised by congenital syphilis. Penicillin is an inexpensive, easily available treatment.

Rachel's rubella status (immune) is already known and she also has a positive hepatitis B surface antigen (HbsAg) documented on her chart. It is unnecessary to repeat these. If these results were not known as part of her medical history, they would have to be checked at the first prenatal visit. Similarly there is no need to repeat a normal Pap smear that was done within the past 6 months in a patient with no other known risk factors and with documented yearly normal Pap smears.

Rachel is not at high risk for sexually transmitted diseases (STDs). Gonorrhea is more prevalent in specific high-risk groups, namely in prostitutes, in women less than 25 years of age with two or more sexual partners within the past year, or with recurrent episodes of STDs. Routine screening for women at high risk is recommended. At this first prenatal visit, Rachel is screened for *Chlamydia*, however. Patient characteristics associated with a higher prevalence of infection include a history of a prior sexually transmitted disease, new or multiple sexual partners, inconsistent use of barrier contraceptives, cervical ectopy, and age under 25. Rachel is only 23 years old and thus fits into one of the high-risk categories.

Rachel is advised to have human immunodeficiency virus (HIV) testing, as the overall prevalence in her community of seropositive newborns has increased to greater than 0.1 per cent. The U.S. Preventive Services Task Force recommends that all pregnant women from communities in which prevalence of seropositive newborns has increased be offered testing as soon as the woman is known to be pregnant. The probability of vertical transmission varies from 13 to 35 per cent, increasing with the severity of disease in the mother. Recent randomized controlled trials have shown that zidovudine therapy, begun between 14 and 34 weeks' gestation and continued through delivery reduces infant perinatal HIV infection (8.3 per cent versus 25.5 per cent) in seropositive mothers (Connor et al., 1994). Other benefits of early detection include *Pneumocystis carinii* pneumonia prophylaxis, prevention of vertical transmission associated with breast feeding, early treatment of the infant, and early accessing of social service support.

Rachel does not need hemoglobin electrophoresis, as she is not a member of one of the ethnic groups at high risk for a hemoglobinopathy, namely, women of Caribbean, Latin American, Mediterranean, Southeast Asian, or African descent.

3. *Promote a healthy pregnancy.* Rachel needs to be counseled on a healthy lifestyle. She is advised to eat a diet high in calcium (1200 to 1500 mg daily) with generous amounts of protein, fruit, and vegetables. She is advised to continue her folic acid. Ninety to ninety-five per cent of pregnancies complicated by neural tube defects occur in the absence of a positive history. It is recommended that all women planning a pregnancy take a multivitamin containing folic acid at a dose of 0.4 mg, beginning at least 1 month before conception and continuing through the first trimester to reduce the risks of neural tube defects. Rachel had been started on folic acid when she discontinued her birth control pill 3 months ago. Adequate studies have not been completed to evaluate whether adequate dietary intake without vitamin supplementation could achieve the same results.

Rachel stopped drinking her usual one glass of wine a few times a week when she stopped the birth control pill. Her physician supports that decision, although there is no proven association between occasional light drinking and birth problems. There is a known association between problem drinking (two or more drinks per day or binge drinking) and fetal alcohol syndrome. According to the U.S. Preventive Services Task Force, there is insufficient evidence to prove or disprove harm from occasional light drinking during pregnancy.

Fortunately, Rachel does not smoke cigarettes. Tobacco use contributes to low birth weight, placenta previa, congenital anomalies, and spontaneous abortion.

Rachel is encouraged to exercise regularly, at the same level that she was exercising before her pregnancy, providing she feels up to it. She should not work to increase her exercise stamina at this time.

Sexual activity needs to be addressed by the physician early in pregnancy. If the patient does not ask about it, the physician must feel comfortable initiating the topic. There is no contraindication to sexual intercourse in a normal healthy woman during her pregnancy.

We perform a screening interview to elicit any history of domestic violence, an underdiagnosed problem. Rachel was asked if she had ever been emotionally or physically abused by her partner, and if she had been hit, slapped, kicked, or otherwise physically hurt by someone within the past year. She was surprised by the questions and responded with a clearly negative answer. Surveys from women in urban clinics state that 7 to 18 per cent of women report physical abuse or forced sex during pregnancy (Norton et al., 1995). One well-controlled study suggests that detection rates improve when more than one question pertaining to violence is asked in a single interview, and with repeated questions on subsequent visits. However, there is insufficient data to recommend for or against use of specific screening instruments, as methods have not been adequately evaluated to change behaviors once the problem is identified.

Rachel's workplace is a computer room at a college campus. No occupational hazards were discovered in review of her work site.

Plan

1. Ultrasound for dating.

2. Hematocrit, antibodies, *Chlamydia*, RPR, HIV.

3. Continue multivitamins with folic acid.

4. Diet, exercise, sexual activity discussed.

5. Follow-up in 1 month.

FIRST FOLLOW-UP VISIT

Subjective

Rachel and her husband return 4 weeks later. Ben is looking forward to hearing the fetal heartbeat today. Rachel's nausea and fatigue have passed. She has gained weight and is enjoying her pregnancy. She plans to keep working as long as possible.

Ultrasound done 4 weeks ago confirmed an 8-week-old fetus, making her 12 weeks pregnant today. She is concerned about her 5-lb weight gain over the past month. She continues to take her multivitamins with folate.

Her normal laboratory studies are reviewed. Her hematocrit is 35. Antibodies, *Chlamydia*, and HIV testing are all negative.

Objective

Well-appearing gravid woman. Blood pressure 115/70 mm Hg, weight 145 lb. Fundus palpated just above the symphysis pubis. Fetal heart audible by Doppler at 150 beats per minute.

Urine is negative for glucose and albumin.

Assessment

Normal pregnancy. Rachel's due date has been confirmed by ultrasound and she is growing well.

Discussion

A 5-lb weight gain over the past month is acceptable. Rachel has gained around 10 lb from her pregravid weight, and a total pregnancy weight gain of 25 to 35 lb, or 11 to 16 kg, is desirable in a woman of normal weight. Low pre-pregnant weight and inadequate weight gain are both contributors to intrauterine growth retardation. Conversely, in obese women, perinatal morbidity begins to increase with a weight gain of greater than 15 lb (ACOG Technical Bulletin No. 179, 1993). Extreme obesity increases the risk of gestational diabetes, hypertension, macrosomia, shoulder dystocia, and prolonged dysfunctional labor.

At 12 weeks' gestation, Rachel may now be screened for occult bacteriuria. All pregnant women need to be screened for occult bacteriuria. The occurrence of this condition in pregnancy varies in studies between 2 and 7 per cent. If untreated, pregnant women are at increased risk for pyelonephritis, with subsequent preterm delivery and a low-birth-weight infant. The timing of a urine culture may vary, although most cases of asymptomatic bacteriuria are detected if the specimen is taken between 12 and 16 weeks' gestation. Urine dipstick testing for leukocyte esterase is not an acceptable alternative screening test in the pregnant woman. Sensitivity for dipstick testing of urine is only 50 per cent.

Plan

1. Urine culture today.

2. Follow-up in 1 month.

SUBSEQUENT FOLLOW-UP VISITS

Rachel is seen monthly over the next 24 weeks. Her uterine growth, blood pressure, and weight gain continue to be normal.

Specific objectives, e.g., screening tests, physical findings, or anticipatory guidance issues, are highlighted at subsequent visits.

1. *At 16 weeks.* Rachel is screened for potential neural tube defects with a maternal serum α-feto-

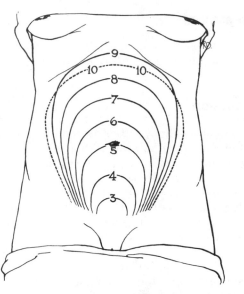

Figure 28–1. Relative height of the fundus at the various months of human pregnancy. (From Hellman LM, Pritchard JA. Williams Obstetrics, 14th ed. New York, Appleton-Century-Crofts, 1971, with permission.)

protein test (MSAFP). This is recommended for all women at 16 to 18 weeks' gestation. False-positive results can occur with multiple gestations, fetal demise, or incorrect gestational age. A test is considered abnormal if it is 2 to 2.5 times above the median value for gestational age. A very low AFP is suggestive of Down syndrome. Rachel's results are normal.

2. *At 20 weeks.* Rachel is now at the midpoint of her pregnancy. Her physician asks her if she has begun to feel movement. "Quickening," as it is commonly called, occurs at 18 to 20 weeks' gestation in a primipara. It is subtle at first, and Rachel describes fleeting, faint movements over the last few days. On physical examination, the fundus is at the umbilicus and measures 20 cm above the upper rim of the symphysis pubis. Over the next 12 to 16 weeks, her growth corresponds to a centimeter per week (Fig. 28–1).

3. *At 24 weeks.* Rachel expected to be screened for gestational diabetes at this visit. At 24 to 28 weeks, the goal is to identify women with glucose intolerance and treat them with diet or insulin as needed. This should reduce associated perinatal morbidity, specifically fetal macrosomia, and neonatal hypoglycemia. A 50 gm glucose drink is given, and the blood sugar is checked 1 hour later. A normal reading is below 140 ng/dl. Glycosuria is

not an accurate predictor of diabetes in the pregnant woman because the renal threshold for glucose is lowered.

New 1997 guidelines from the American Diabetes Association were published during Rachel's pregnancy, and she was delighted to hear that she did not fit into the newly specified high-risk groups. Individuals now recommended for screening include those who are obese, are age 25 or older, have a positive family history of diabetes, or are members of ethnic groups with a high prevalence of diabetes, namely African Americans, Asians, Native Americans, and Hispanics.

4. *At 28 weeks.* Antibodies are repeated at this visit because Rachel is Rh-negative. She has negative results and thus is given an intramuscular injection of 300 mg of Rh immune globulin (RhIG), which should prevent any isoimmunization over the third trimester.

5. *At 30 weeks and later.* Beginning at 30 weeks, the uterus is examined at each visit using Leopold maneuvers (Fig. 28–2; Table 28–2) to detect the baby's position. Rachel is seen weekly by her physician after 36 weeks' gestation.

Health education and risk assessment continue at each visit throughout the second and third trimesters. During the second trimester signs of labor are discussed and Rachel is encouraged to attend prenatal classes. In the third trimester, signs of labor are reviewed, birth plans are discussed including specifics of anesthesia, labor support, and episiotomy. Rachel's wishes for a natural childbirth are supported and documented on her prenatal form. Breast feeding, circumcision, and postpartum contraception are also addressed, as are Ben and Rachel's plans for help with the newborn.

TABLE 28–2. Leopold Maneuvers

Maneuver	Action	Question
First	Examine the fundus	What fetal part is in the fundus?
Second	Palpate the lateral abdomen	Where is the fetal back?
Third	Palpate the suprapubic area	Is the presenting part engaged?
Fourth (vertex only)	Find the cephalic prominence	Is the head flexed?

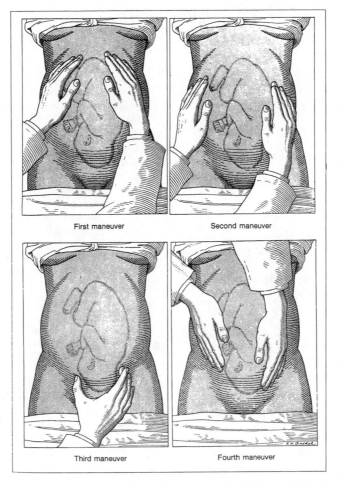

Figure 28–2. Palpation in left occiput anterior position. (From Cunningham FG, MacDonald PC, Gant NF [eds]. Williams Obstetrics, 18th ed. East Norwalk, CT, Appleton & Lange, 1989, with permission.)

SUGGESTED READING

ACOG Technical Bulletin No. 179: Nutrition during Pregnancy. Washington, DC, American College of Obstetricians and Gynecologists, 1993.

Caring for our Future: The Content of Prenatal Care. Washington, DC, U.S. Public Health Service, 1989.

Connor EM, Sperling RS, Gelber R, et al. Reduction of maternal-infant transmission of HIV-1 with zidovudine treatment. N Engl J Med 1994;331:1173–1180.

Norton LB, Peipert JF, Zierler S, et al. Battering in pregnancy: An assessment of two screening methods. Obstet Gynecol 1995;85:321–325.

Rakel, Robert E. Textbook of Family Practice, 5th ed. Philadelphia, W.B. Saunders, 1996, pp 528–567.

U.S. Preventive Services Task Force. Guide to Clinical Preventive Services. Baltimore, Williams & Wilkins, 1996.

1. Establishing the accurate due date in pregnancy is an essential component of good prenatal care. The physician relies on the following clues in diagnosis (true or false):
   a. By 8 weeks' gestation, fetal heartbeats are audible by Doppler.
   b. The LMP, if recalled with clarity by the woman and defined as normal with regard to its regularity and duration, is a very accurate predictor of the due date.
   c. Recent use of the birth control pill does not affect ovulation history.
   d. A screening first-trimester ultrasound is recommended for all women to confirm the estimated gestational age.
   e. The length of gestation estimated at 40 weeks assumes a 28-day cycle and a 14-day window from ovulation to menses.

2. Which one of the following statements about neural tube defects and their prevention is true?
   a. Ninety to 95 per cent of neural tube defects in pregnancy occur in women with a positive family or personal history.
   b. It is recommended that all women planning a pregnancy begin taking a multivitamin preparation with at least 0.4 mg folic acid daily.
   c. Studies confirm that adequate dietary intake of folic acid is as effective as vitamin supplementation in preventing neural tube defects.

   d. Folic acid supplementation need only be taken during the early part of the first trimester.
   e. If one takes folic acid as recommended, a screening AFP blood test can be avoided.

3. All pregnant women are screened for bacteriuria. Which of the following statements about this condition are true?
   a. Bacteriuria in pregnancy occurs in 15 per cent of all pregnancies.
   b. If untreated, women are at risk for pyelonephritis and subsequent preterm delivery.
   c. Urine dipstick testing for leukocyte esterase is an acceptable screening test in the pregnant woman.
   d. Most cases of asymptomatic bacteriuria are detected if the specimen is taken between 12 and 16 weeks' gestation.

4. Which of the following statements about screening tests in the pregnant woman are true?
   a. Risk factors for *Chlamydia* include age less than 25 independent of other variables, multiple sexual partners, other STDs.
   b. All pregnant women should be screened for gonorrhea, regardless of risk factors.
   c. A Pap smear should be done at the first prenatal visit regardless of the most recent Pap smear result or Pap smear history.
   d. Varicella titer need not be drawn if the patient remembers having chickenpox as a child.

Answers appear on **page 604.**

Chapter **29**

Newborn Care

Rebecca H. Gladu, M.D.

INITIAL VISIT

Subjective

Patient Identification and Presenting Problem

Baby Randall is a 1800-gm male infant born at 37 weeks via vacuum-assisted vaginal delivery to a 17-year-old G1 P0 Ab0 Caucasian female. His mother's pregnancy was complicated by scant prenatal care; she was seen in the Family Practice Center only twice, at 20 and 28 weeks. Growth of the baby was appropriate for gestational age at these two visits, but dating was never confirmed because the mother was unsure of her last period and missed her ultrasound appointment. Prenatal laboratory results were normal (Pap smear, hepatitis B surface antigen, human immunodeficiency virus [HIV], gonococcus and chlamydia screen, urine culture, hematocrit and hemoglobin).

Randall's mother, Natalie, had a difficult labor and delivery. She presented to the triage area in intense pain with bounding contractions. Her 18-year-old boyfriend, Paul, explained that she had been having contractions for several hours now, but it took them a while to get a ride to the hospital from their friend who had a car. Her bag of water broke early that morning, about 12 hours ago. He went on to tell the hospital staff that Natalie had been feeling ill for several days, but didn't want to go to the doctor. Paul then left, explaining that he couldn't handle watching a birth with "all that blood."

In the triage area, the nurse assessed Natalie's vital signs and placed her on the fetal monitor. She was found to be hypertensive and febrile with a blood pressure of 174/98 and a temperature of 101.5°F. The fetal monitor strip showed variable decelerations with each contraction from a baseline of 120 to 90. Her contractions were 2 minutes apart.

A urine dip stick test showed 3+ proteinuria. The physician was called.

Natalie's physical examination by the physician on call for the family practice group showed a very agitated teen in severe pain. Her uterine fundus measured 32 cm, and the baby's presentation was cephalic. The cervix was 6 cm dilated and completely effaced, and the baby's head was at −1 station. Thick meconium and blood stained the examining glove. Contractions were nonindentable, but the uterus was not tender to palpation between contractions.

Natalie was immediately admitted to a labor bed with the diagnosis of active labor, pregnancy-induced hypertension, and possible chorioamnionitis. Internal monitors were placed and she was given an infusion of magnesium sulfate to prevent seizures. Cultures of the cervix were taken and intravenous antibiotics given. Epidural anesthesia was administered, which immediately calmed her pain. Over the next 2 hours, Natalie's cervix completely dilated and she pushed. She became exhausted, and thus her physician performed a vacuum extraction to deliver baby Randall.

After delivery and before Randall could cry, Natalie's doctor suctioned baby Randall's nasopharynx with a DeLee catheter to remove meconium and prevent aspiration. She then cut the cord and quickly handed Randall to the physician who would resuscitate Randall. A foul-smelling placenta was delivered and sent to the pathology laboratory. Natalie's episiotomy was then repaired. Natalie had minimal blood loss (250 ml). After delivery, her blood pressure decreased to 140/90, and her temperature was 100.5°F.

Randall was taken to the warmer, and his larynx examined with direct laryngoscopy to determine if indeed any meconium had been aspirated below the vocal cords. Such aspiration can cause a severe pneumonia in a newborn. Randall's examination showed he was clear of any meconium below the

TABLE 29–1. Apgar Scoring

Score	Heart Rate	Respiratory Effort	Muscle Tone	Reflex Irritability	Color
0	Absent	Absent	Limp	No response	Blue or pale
1	Less than 100	Slow, irregular	Some flexion	Grimace	Body pink, extremities blue
2	Over 100	Good	Good motion	Cough or sneeze	Pink

cords, and he was routinely resuscitated with stimulation and nasal and oral suctioning. An Apgar score of 7 (-1 for tone, color, and respirations) and 9 (-1 for color) was assigned at 1 and 5 minutes (Table 29–1). His fingerprints and footprints were taken, identification bands were placed, and he was swaddled in receiving blankets. The nurse gave him to his mother to hold, but she refused and began to cry.

Natalie's mother arrived but did not greet her daughter verbally. She held the baby for a few moments, then left the room. The tension between Natalie and her mother was palpable.

Objective

In the Transitional Nursery

Baby Randall arrived to be evaluated in the transitional nursery. His rectal temperature was 100.0°F, with mildly labored respirations at 18 per minute and pulse of 160. A complete physical examination was performed, which revealed the following:

General: 1800-gm (<10th percentile) small for gestational age (SGA) infant of 36 weeks' maturity by examination scoring (Fig. 29–1). Length: 42.5 cm (15th percentile). Head circumference: 29 cm (10th percentile) Normal tone, color, and cry

Skin: No jaundice. Moderate diffuse erythematous papules and pustules on trunk, face, and legs

HEENT: Mild cephalohematoma and molding. Anterior fontanel flat. Positive red reflex bilaterally. Normal palate, lips, and gums. No grunting or nasal flaring

Cardiovascular: Heart regular rate and rhythm without murmur, rub, or gallop. Femoral, jugular, brachial, pedal, and radial pulses 2+ throughout

Chest: Clear to auscultation and percussion. Mild intercostal retractions

Abdomen: Soft without masses. Three-vessel cord

Genitalia: Testes descended bilaterally, normal male genitalia. Patient urinated during the examination

Anus: Patent, passing meconium

Trunk and spine: Normal without skeletal abnormalities. Straight spine. Hair noted over the sacrum

Extremities: Normal clavicles, no hip click, normal feet, no clubbing or deformities

Reflexes: Moro, grasp, suck, and swallow intact

Because Baby Randall's mother had a temperature elevation during her labor, the physician went to the labor and delivery suite to discuss plans for Randall's treatment with his mother and father. He found Natalie crying in her bed with her boyfriend Paul at her side. Paul explained that she was upset because she hadn't seen her mother in 6 months and that seeing her after the delivery was difficult. He explained that Natalie and he had been living together since the pregnancy was discovered and that her mother had "disowned" her.

The physician acknowledged their difficult situation and then discussed a rule-out sepsis workup for Randall with the parents. They consented without questions. Natalie said nothing, nodded, and did not make eye contact. Paul signed the consent form.

Assessment

1. Possible bacteremia resulting from maternal chorioamnionitis. Begin intravenous antibiotics and rule-out sepsis protocol

2. Tachypnea. Blow-by oxygen. Chest radiograph. Close observation

2. Prematurity—unsure dates and 36 weeks by examination

3. SGA infant—low birth weight most likely due to mother's pregnancy-induced hypertension

NEWBORN MATURITY RATING & CLASSIFICATION

ESTIMATION OF GESTATIONAL AGE BY MATURITY RATING
Symbols: X - 1st Exam   O - 2nd Exam

Gestation by Dates_____wks

Birth Date_____ Hour_____am/pm

APGAR_____1 min_____5 min

NEUROMUSCULAR MATURITY

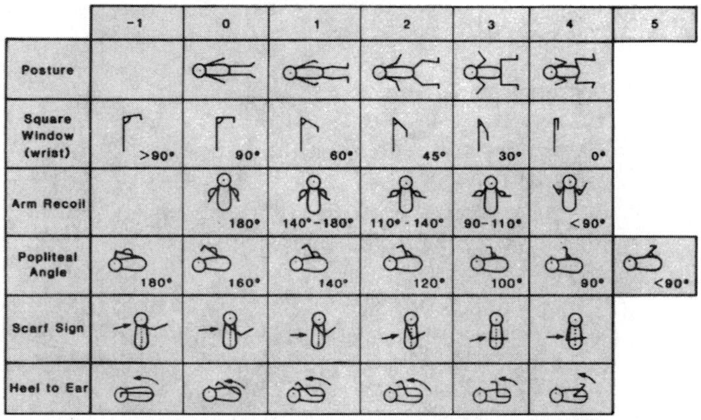

	-1	0	1	2	3	4	5
Posture							
Square Window (wrist)	>90°	90°	60°	45°	30°	0°	
Arm Recoil		180°	140°-180°	110°-140°	90°-110°	<90°	
Popliteal Angle	180°	160°	140°	120°	100°	90°	<90°
Scarf Sign							
Heel to Ear							

PHYSICAL MATURITY

Skin	sticky friable transparent	gelatinous red, translucent	smooth pink, visible veins	superficial peeling &/or rash, few veins	cracking pale areas rare veins	parchment deep cracking no vessels	leathery cracked wrinkled
Lanugo	none	sparse	abundant	thinning	bald areas	mostly bald	
Plantar Surface	heel-toe 40-50mm:-1 <40mm:-2	>50mm no crease	faint red marks	anterior transverse crease only	creases ant. 2/3	creases over entire sole	
Breast	imperceptible	barely perceptible	flat areola no bud	stippled areola 1-2mm bud	raised areola 3-4mm bud	full areola 5-10mm bud	
Eye/Ear	lids fused loosely:-1 tightly:-2	lids open pinna flat stays folded	sl. curved pinna; soft; slow recoil	well-curved pinna; soft but ready recoil	formed &firm instant recoil	thick cartilage ear stiff	
Genitals male	scrotum flat, smooth	scrotum empty faint rugae	testes in upper canal rare rugae	testes descending few rugae	testes down good rugae	testes pendulous deep rugae	
Genitals female	clitoris prominent labia flat	prominent clitoris small labia minora	prominent clitoris enlarging minora	majora & minora equally prominent	majora large minora small	majora cover clitoris & minora	

Scoring system: Ballard JL, Khoury JC, Wedig K, Wang L, Eilers-Walsman BL, Lipp R. New Ballard Score, expanded to include extremely premature infants. *J Pediatr.* 1991;119:417-423.

MATURITY RATING

score	weeks
-10	20
-5	22
0	24
5	26
10	28
15	30
20	32
25	34
30	36
35	38
40	40
45	42
50	44

SCORING SECTION

	1st Exam=X	2nd Exam=O
Estimating Gest Age by Maturity Rating	_____Weeks	_____Weeks
Time of Exam	Date_____ Hour_____am/pm	Date_____ Hour_____am/pm
Age at Exam	_____Hours	_____Hours
Signature of Examiner	_____ M.D./R.N.	_____ M.D./R.N.

Figure 29–1. Newborn maturity rating and classification. (From Ballard JL, Khoury JC, et al. New Ballard Score, expanded to include extremely premature infants. J Pediatr 1991;119:417–423.)

3. Teen parents—poor prenatal education. Begin parenting education

4. Family conflict—high risk for family disruption and dysfunction. Discuss social situation with family. Consider social work or psychology consultation

5. Erythema toxicum

Plan

Orders were written as follows:

1. Admit to low-risk nursery, Family Practice service

2. Diagnosis: Rule out sepsis, prematurity, tachypnea

3. Vitals q 8 hours

4. Allergies NKDA

5. IV D10W at 10 ml/hr

6. Begin IV antibiotics: Ampicillin 45 mg IV (100 mg/kg/day divided q 6 hr) and gentamicin 5.4 mg IV per day (3 mg/kg/24 hr)

7. CBC with differential and platelets

8. Chest radiographs—PA and lateral

9. Cerebrospinal fluid (CSF) for culture, cell count, differential, Gram stain, glucose, and protein

10. Blood cultures ×2

11. Urine latex agglutination test for *Escherichia coli* and group B streptococci.

12. AquaMEPHYTON 1.0 IM stat

13. Credé ointment: erythromycin SO$_4$ Ophthalmic Ointment 0.5% OU

14. Cord blood: (a) rapid plasma reagin test; (b) type, group, and direct Coombs

15. Dextrostix prior to feeds × 24 hours

16. Feed q 3 hours with formula, hospital stock (20 cal/oz). If mother decides to breast feed, feed as soon as mother's condition permits and every 2 to 3 hours thereafter

17. Report any Dextrostix value <35 to physician.

18. Bathe if axillary temperature is >97.6°, HR and RR are stable. If infant is unstable for any reason, hold bath

19. Triple dye to cord and 1-inch abdominal perimeter after bath

20. Trim nails prn. Lubriderm prn dry skin

21. Newborn screening test at 24 hours of age

22. Recombivax 0.25 ml IM × 1 (10 mEq/ml). If mother tests HbsAg-positive, give another dose (0.25 ml) so it totals 0.50 ml. Then give in a different site hepatitis B immune globulin (HBIG) 0.5 ml IM and notify physician

Discussion

Diagnosis of Neonatal Sepsis

Bacterial sepsis and meningitis continue to be serious causes of illness in newborns, with an incidence of one to eight cases per 1000 live births. Infants at high risk for neonatal bacterial sepsis or meningitis include those with low birth weight, respiratory distress, temperature instability, feeding intolerance, hepatosplenomegaly, jaundice, lethargy, irritability, or apnea. Maternal risk factors are chorioamnionitis, prolonged rupture of membranes, fever during labor, maternal peripartum infection, excessive bleeding, and premature rupture of membranes. In Randall's case, his low birth weight and his mother's prolonged rupture of membranes, fever during labor, and probable chorioamnionitis made him a high-risk case.

The differential diagnosis of sepsis in a neonate can include respiratory distress syndrome, pneumonia, amniotic fluid aspiration syndrome, persistent fetal circulation, meningitis, osteomyelitis, septic arthritis, sepsis from other infections (*Listeria monocytogenes*, *Haemophilus influenzae*, *Streptococcus pneumoniae*, and *Neisseria meningitidis*), and metabolic derangements.

Infants with sepsis can present clinically with poor feeding, cyanosis, apnea, tachypnea, grunting, nasal flaring and retractions, seizures, lethargy, a bulging fontanel, and rapid onset and deterioration.

Cultures of the blood or CSF or both are definitive for diagnosis; antigen identification tests may have a false-positive rate of up to 8 per cent, but they are helpful because results are rapidly available.

SGA Infant

Small for gestational age is defined as a birth weight and weight:length ratio falling two SD or more below the mean (Fig. 29–2). The majority of cases of growth retardation occur late in gestation and are

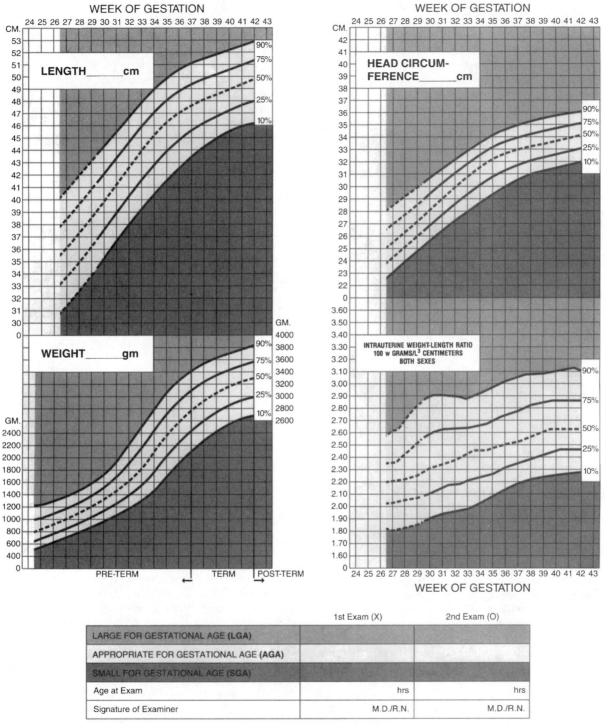

CLASSIFICATION OF NEWBORNS –
BASED ON MATURITY AND INTRAUTERINE GROWTH
Symbols: X-1st Exam   O-2nd Exam

	1st Exam (X)	2nd Exam (O)
LARGE FOR GESTATIONAL AGE (LGA)		
APPROPRIATE FOR GESTATIONAL AGE (AGA)		
SMALL FOR GESTATIONAL AGE (SGA)		
Age at Exam	hrs	hrs
Signature of Examiner	M.D./R.N.	M.D./R.N.

Adapted from Lubchenco LO, Hansman C, and Boyd E: Pediatr. 1966; 37:403; Battaglia FC, and Lubchenco LO: J Pediatr. 1967; 71:159.

Figure 29–2. Classification of newborns—based on maturity and intrauterine growth. (Adapted from Lubchenco LO, Hansman C, Boyd E: Intrauterine growth in length and head circumference as estimated from live births at gestational ages from 26 to 42 weeks. Pediatrics 1966;37:403; Battaglia FC, Lubchenco LO: A practical classification of newborn infants by height and gestational age. J Pediatr 1967;71:159.)

mild in degree. The retardation is usually in birth weight alone, with normal height and head circumference. Such cases may be found on ultrasound examination, showing sluggish growth of the biparietal diameter of the fetal head, shortened femurs, or a discrepancy of the trunk:head ratio. Causes of such growth retardation may include viral infections, maternal pregnancy-induced hypertension, twinning, drug and alcohol addiction, and primary placental abnormalities. More severe cases may have been caused earlier in gestation by trisomies, congenital viral diseases, radiation exposure, or early drug or alcohol exposure.

SGA neonates are particularly susceptible to cold stress and hypoglycemia from deficient fat stores. Because of the low availability of nutrients and oxygen, the stress of labor is particularly difficult for these infants, often leading to fetal distress noted on the fetal monitor.

Erythema Toxicum

Lesions are described as firm, yellow-white 1- to 2-mm papules or pustules with a surrounding erythematous base. Lesions are clustered in several sites. These lesions develop in the first 1 to 2 days of life. The cause is unknown, although microscopic examination reveals eosinophilia. The differential diagnosis includes pyoderma, candidiasis, herpes simplex infection, transient neonatal pustular melanosis, and miliaria. No treatment is required because the course is self-limited.

FIRST FOLLOW-UP EXAMINATION

The following morning, Baby Randall was examined and found to be doing well. The baby was afebrile with normal vital signs. The lungs were clear. He was breathing normally on room air. An intravenous (IV) needle was in his hand for his antibiotics and IV fluids. He was taking formula feeds well and was stooling and urinating well. His mother and father were visiting during the examination and had multiple questions about the baby. Natalie was more animated and talkative and held her baby for the first time. She asked about breast feeding, admitting that although she was scared, she was willing to try. She then asked if a circumcision could be performed on Randall. When asked about the situation with her mother, Natalie admitted she and Paul needed help with the baby and advice from her mother. She hoped that the new baby would help bring her and her mother closer and help her mother accept her relationship with Paul.

Laboratory studies showed a white blood cell count of 25 with 10 bands. Cultures of the blood showed no growth so far. Randall's blood type was O positive. Cord blood gases were normal. CSF result was normal; cell count showed 7 WBCs, no RBCs, glucose of 80, protein of 90 mg per dl, cultures still pending. Latex testing of the urine was positive for group B streptococcal organisms, and negative for *E. coli*. Chest radiograph was normal. Natalie's laboratory values were also checked. Her placental Gram stain was positive for streptococcal species. Her blood type was also O positive.

Assessment and Plan

1. Group B streptococcal sepsis. Continue antibiotics for a full course of 10 days.

2. Elective circumcision. Will schedule elective circumcision within the first month of life, after full course of antibiotics given for sepsis.

3. Breast feeding. Plan to institute immediately. Discuss breast feeding in detail with mother and assist as needed. Notify nurses of change in feeding plans.

Discussion

Group B Streptococcal Sepsis Treatment

When the etiology of sepsis is confirmed by culture to be group B streptococci, the antibiotic regimen can be changed from broad coverage to penicillin G intravenously. Because the early latex test can give a false-positive result, however, the present antibiotics are continued until the definitive identification of the organism is known by culture, usually by day 3.

Group B streptococcus may present as an early-onset and late-onset disease. Early-onset disease occurs shortly after birth. Late-onset disease may occur during the second week of life. The mortality rate of early-onset disease ranges from 10 to 40 per cent; mortality is highest in very low birth weight infants and in those with a low neutrophil count, low Apgar scores, hypotension, apnea, or a delay in starting antimicrobial therapy.

Breast Feeding

Breast feeding imparts numerous benefits to the infant. Among them, the early administration of maternal colostrum, the protein excreted initially before the milk comes in, gives babies a source of maternal antibody directly to the gut. This antibody can protect the gut from viruses and can decrease the incidence of gastroenteritis and its diarrhea. Breast-fed infants also have a lower incidence of upper respiratory infections. Especially for the first 2 months of life, when the baby is most vulnerable to infection, the maternal antibodies play a major role in the baby's immune status.

Bonding between mother and infant is enhanced. Breast feeding imparts a natural closeness and requires a frequency of feedings about every 2 hours. This frequency is necessarily higher than for formula-fed babies because breast milk is thin and watery with natural proteins that the baby can easily digest. Formula is thicker and more difficult for the baby to digest, and thus it stays in the stomach longer.

Breast milk is the most natural and efficient food for the baby to take. Most interesting is how the composition of breast milk changes as the baby grows. It meets the nutritional needs of the baby at different stages of development. Breast milk nutrient analysis when the baby is 6 months of age is completely different from nutrient analysis at birth.

For the mother, breast feeding is very convenient. Middle-of-the-night feedings do not require getting up to warm bottles. Should the mother and infant need to be separated, the mother can prepare bottles of breast milk ahead of time. Otherwise, no bottles need be prepared for outings with the baby. Another benefit for parents is that stools of breast milk–fed infants do not have an odor.

Circumcision

The decision to perform a circumcision on a male infant is entirely elective. Usually it depends on the parents' preference or the cultural norm. Studies have shown that circumcision can in fact have health benefits for the child. Such infants have a lower incidence of urinary tract infection. Circumcision is contraindicated in infants demonstrating hypospadias because the foreskin is needed for the urologic repair.

The main risks of circumcision are bleeding and infection. Bleeding can be controlled by observing the circumcision for up to 2 hours after the procedure. If bleeding occurs, it can be controlled with pressure, lidocaine with epinephrine drops, silver nitrate, or sutures placed at the bleeding site. Infection is very infrequent if the circumcision is cared for with petrolatum jelly application to the surgical site and if the wound is kept clean. Occasional local infection is easily controlled with topical Bactroban ointment or oral antibiotics that cover dermal streptococcal and staphylococcal infections. Less likely complications from neonatal circumcisions are sepsis, meatal ulceration, and poor cosmetic results.

There are three types of clamps used for circumcision: Plastibell, Gomco, and Mogen. Each has its benefits and downfalls. The Plastibell is placed over the glans and the foreskin is essentially ligated with a string. The majority of the foreskin is cut above the ligature. The baby is sent home and over the next few days the remaining foreskin necroses. Because the circumcision is done during the same time that the umbilical cord is necrosing, parents generally are accepting of this phenomenon. The great benefit of the Plastibell is that the risk of bleeding with the procedure is virtually zero.

The Gomco clamp is definitely the most difficult to use because it is cumbersome and requires some practice to use with ease. The major benefit is the excellent cosmetic result it gives. Its major drawback is that there is a higher rate of bleeding after its use than with the other two devices. The bell and the base must fit perfectly to ensure complete hemostasis of the foreskin. After many uses, nicks in the steel bell or base may leave a space in the foreskin that was not adequately crimped, so that excision over that part of the foreskin begets bleeding.

By far the easiest instrument for circumcision is the Mogen clamp. Very few complications are associated with the use of this clamp, and its ease of use makes it a favorite for many physicians.

SECOND FOLLOW-UP VISIT

On day 2 of life, Randall was examined again. He was afebrile with normal vital signs. His weight had decreased to 1780 g. He was noted to be visibly jaundiced. His mother began to breast feed him yesterday, but no true milk had yet been expressed. Randall continued to receive IV fluids because of his risk for hypoglycemia of low birth weight. Natalie asked about the jaundice and wondered if it was dangerous. Her mother had come by yesterday and was discussing this with her. She told her that in the old days when Natalie was born, infants had to be placed under lights because jaundice was so dangerous for them. The physician explored this subject further with Natalie. Natalie expressed how good she felt that her mother was coming to visit and was interested in the health of the baby. Her mother held the baby for a while and even helped Natalie with the positioning of the baby for breast feeding. Psychologically, Natalie was doing very well compared with the night of her delivery. The physician congratulated her on her success with her mother and encouraged her to continue to work on the relationship. She invited Natalie, Paul, and Natalie's mother to come to the office together for family therapy later to work on issues that might be causing stress between them so that the baby could grow up in a positive, loving environment.

Laboratory results were checked. Group B streptococcal culture of the cervix was positive for beta-hemolytic streptococci (such as Group B), and more importantly, Randall's blood culture result was positive for group B streptococci. His CSF culture still had no bacterial growth.

Assessment and Plan

1. Group B streptococcal sepsis confirmed. Discontinue ampicillin and gentamicin; start penicillin G 250,000 U/kg/day in three divided doses for 150,000 U IV q 8 hr. Continue for a total of 10 days of antibiotics (8 more days).

2. Jaundice. Check bilirubin, total and direct fractions.

Discussion

Jaundice

The issues surrounding the subject of the jaundiced newborn and hyperbilirubinemia are widely debated. High levels of bilirubin can cause yellow staining of the brain known as kernicterus in the globus pallidus, putamen, basal ganglia, and caudate nucleii. Necrosis, neuronal loss, and replacement of neurons by glial cells may occur. Kernicterus can appear subtly as a poor Moro reflex, decreased tone, lethargy, poor feeding, or more dramatically with seizures, fever, rigidity, paralysis of upward gaze, and spasticity. Late sequelae may be catastrophic and may include athetosis, deafness, mental retardation, and paralysis of upward gaze. Because of these serious possible sequelae, much research has been done to identify risk factors and practice guidelines for practitioners to use when dealing with a jaundiced newborn.

Hyperbilirubinemia, the cause of jaundice, must be understood as *physiologic* or *nonphysiologic*. The clinical pattern of physiologic jaundice usually manifests as an indirect bilirubin level that rises and falls in the first 3 days of life in a normal term neonate, to a level of about 6 to 8 mg per dl by 3 days of life, and may peak at about 12 mg per dl. Preterm infants may have a peak of about 10 to 12 mg per dl on the 5th day of life, with a peak of about 15 mg per dl. This physiologic hyperbilirubinemia is caused by an increased bilirubin load presented to the liver cells with decreased clearing of the bilirubin by the plasma and poor excretion of the bilirubin. These are merely immature processing systems in the infant. It is most common in breast-feeding infants (because they may have a decreased fluid intake compared with formula-fed infants), infants of maternal diabetics, Asian or Greek infants, and infants with poor caloric intake.

Nonphysiologic hyperbilirubinemia may not be easy to distinguish from physiologic hyperbilirubinemia. It may be caused by blood group incompatibility with hemolysis, infection, or metabolic derangements. Clues that may signal that jaundice is due to nonphysiologic unconjugated (indirect) hyperbilirubinemia may be prematurity, SGA, and presence of microcephaly, pallor, petechiae, or hepatosplenomegaly. The following findings suggest nonphysiologic hyperbilirubinemia and require investigation.

1. Clinical jaundice before 36 hours of age

2. Serum bilirubin concentrations increasing by more than 5 mg per dl per day

3. Total serum bilirubin level greater than 15 mg per dl in a formula-fed term infant

4. Total serum bilirubin level greater than 17 mg per dl in a breast-fed term infant

5. Clinical jaundice lasting longer than 8 days in a term infant or 14 days in a premature infant

It is important to differentiate direct hyperbilirubinemia from the indirect or unconjugated hyperbilirubinemia described earlier. Direct-reacting bilirubin is *not* neurotoxic to the infant (i.e., it does not cause kernicterus). It signifies a serious underlying disorder, however, and must be investigated. Underlying disorders may be perinatal congenital infections (the TORCH infections), inspissated bile from prolonged hemolysis, neonatal hepatitis, sepsis, cytomegalovirus infection, cholestasis, and biliary atresia.

Indirect hyperbilirubinemia can be treated with phototherapy, which reduces the serum bilirubin concentration by a series of photochemical reactions. Because of the confusion among physicians treating this common problem, and because there is no specific bilirubin level that is definitely safe or toxic for all infants, guidelines for treatment have been developed to incorporate risk factors and weight of the infants at risk:

1. Infants under 1500 gm: phototherapy if the bilirubin level is over 5 mg per dl

2. Infants between 1500 and 2000 gm: phototherapy at bilirubin levels of 8 to 12 mg per dl

3. Infants between 2 and 2.5 kg: phototherapy at bilirubin levels of 13 to 15 mg per dl

4. Term formula-fed healthy infants: consider phototherapy when the bilirubin level is between 15 and 20 mg per dl

5. Term breast-fed healthy infant with frequent nursing: (a) if bilirubin >15, be certain that there is adequate fluid intake; (b) if bilirubin is >18, consider stopping nursing for 48 hours; (c) if the bilirubin level is approaching 20, phototherapy.

All of these treatments must be adjusted according to the age of the baby at the time of the bilirubin level.

In our example, Randall was a premature infant with low birth weight and sepsis. He clearly was ill and at risk for nonphysiologic jaundice. With a bilirubin level of 12 at day 2 of life, his risk of kernicterus was high. Therefore, phototherapy, as well as aggressive hydration, will be instituted.

Phototherapy is not without risk. Phototherapy causes insensible water loss and watery diarrhea, and thus the infants must be aggressively hydrated during therapy. Because retinal damage can occur from the fluorescent lamps, eye shields must be placed. The scrotum should also be shielded during phototherapy because cell damage can occur.

The main problem with phototherapy is that it interrupts the normal maternal-infant bonding interactions and can cause significant stress for the mother and the baby. In several studies, mothers of previously jaundiced infants were unwilling to leave their babies, were more likely to regard other illness in their infants as serious, and were much more likely to have stopped breast feeding. Mothers found phototherapy upsetting, and 70 per cent thought its use implied their child was moderately to seriously ill. For this reason, the institution of phototherapy must be a well-thought-out process.

THIRD FOLLOW-UP VISIT

Baby Randall underwent phototherapy. In the course of 24 hours his bilirubin level decreased from 12 mg per dl to 8 mg per dl. His mother stayed close to him during the therapy, determined not to stop breast feeding. She understood that his jaundice was due to his infection and his small size, not to her breast milk. His weight increased by 40 g to 1820 g with hydration and breast feeding.

Randall's condition was very stable clinically. He would require phototherapy until his bilirubin levels decreased consistently for at least two consecutive bilirubin tests and would require 7 more days of IV antibiotics to complete his course. His weight should be checked daily to ensure progressive weight gain before discharge home.

SUGGESTED READING

Behrman RE, Kliegman RE. Nelson Essentials of Pediatrics. Philadelphia, W.B. Saunders, 1994, pp 163–213.
Burns, CE, Barber N, Brady MA, et al. Pediatric Primary Care. Philadelphia, W.B. Saunders, 1996, pp 809–825.
Cloherty JP, Stark AR. Manul of Neonatal Care. Boston, Little, Brown, 1991.
Holman JR, Lewis EL, Ringler RL. Neonatal circumcision techniques. Am Fam Physician 1995;52:511–518.
Ziai M. Pediatrics. Boston, Little, Brown, 1990, pp 125–161.

QUESTIONS

1. Phototherapy is indicated
   a. Whenever the bilirubin level rises above 15 mg per dl
   b. In every jaundiced infant
   c. In a term infant with a bilirubin level of 5 mg per dl at day of life 7
   d. In all breast-feeding jaundiced infants
   e. In an 1800-gm preterm infant with a bilirubin level of 10 mg per dl on day 1 of life

2. Mortality from group B streptococcal sepsis is highest in infants with

a. Low Apgar scores
b. High neutrophil count
c. Jaundice
d. Hypotension
e. Early empiric antibiotic therapy

3. Which of the following are parameters assessed in determining the Apgar score?

a. Respiratory effort
b. Heart rate
c. Color
d. Muscle tone
e. Reflex irritability

Answers appear on **page 604.**

Chapter **30**

Hyperactivity

Lawrence H. Miller, M.D.

INITIAL VISIT—SUBJECTIVE

PATIENT IDENTIFICATION. Kevin M. is a 7-year-old white male elementary school student.

PRESENTING PROBLEM. Mrs. M. brings Kevin to the office at the request of his teacher with concerns that he has difficulty obeying school rules, he is easily distracted and inattentive, he is hyperactive, and he turns in incomplete school work.

PRESENT ILLNESS. Kevin is a second-grade, special-education student with developmental disabilities including borderline IQ and poor gross motor function. He has been in speech therapy classes since the age of 4 years. The distractibility, hyperactivity, and incomplete work problems have become more noticeable over the past 6 to 8 months.

PAST MEDICAL HISTORY. Kevin is the product of a 39-week gestation pregnancy, with an uneventful labor and spontaneous vaginal delivery. Apgar scores were 9–10–10. Developmentally he was quite slow, however. His first words were spoken at age 2½ years, he spoon-fed himself at 4 years, toilet trained at 4 years, and walked unassisted at 4½ years.

FAMILY HISTORY. Kevin is the younger of two boys. His 9-year-old brother has attention-deficit/hyperactivity disorder (ADHD), which was diagnosed at the age of 6 years. His mother is 28 years old. She is obese and has an eighth-grade formal education. She works as a waitress part-time. His father is 33 years old and works as an auto mechanic. He is in generally good health but has "trouble holding down a steady job;" he has a high school education.

SOCIAL HISTORY. Kevin is a student. He is taking no medications. He neither smokes nor consumes alcohol. He sleeps 9 to 10 hours a day. His diet is average for age for breakfast and lunch, but he prefers to play outside rather than eat dinner. Discipline at home is "a challenge" but not a problem. Kevin and his parents deny emotional or physical abuse. He relates appropriately to his peer group.

REVIEW OF SYSTEMS. Except as noted earlier, this is noncontributory.

OBJECTIVE

Physical Examination

Kevin is a shy but active young man who relates to others in a normal age-appropriate manner. Height is 52¼ inches, weight 61 lb, blood pressure 96/50, pulse 84 and regular, respirations 20 and regular, temperature 98.4°F. His physical examination was completely unremarkable except for the neurologic component. Cranial nerves II to XII were intact. Deep tendon reflexes were symmetric at 2+. No tremors were present. Sensory examination was normal. Balance, heel-to-toe walking, eye-hand coordination, and spatial perception were abnormal.

Laboratory Tests

CBC and urinalysis were completely normal. Serum lead screening was negative.

ASSESSMENT

Working Diagnoses

1. ADHD (Table 30–1). The DSM-IV Criteria for ADHD shows that Kevin fulfills the criteria for ADHD, combined type.

2. Learning disabilities. This refers to a generic inclusion of all types of specific learning disability (e.g., dyslexia—reading, dyscalculia—math, dysgraphia—writing). Although Kevin has required speech therapy, there is insufficient evidence to identify or confirm specific learning disabilities.

Differential Diagnoses

1. Cerebral palsy. Typically there are severe motor control difficulties associated with birth trauma, hypoxia, or labor and delivery abnormalities. No such history is present in this case, although there is considerable developmental delay in motor functions.

2. Affective illness (mania, depression, bipolar). This is manifest by a disturbed sleep-wake cycle, somatic complaints, lowered energy, agitation, hostility, and even rages of anger. Kevin does not display these attributes.

3. Primary disorder of vigilance. A system complex of poor attention, poor concentration, distractibility, daydreaming, fidgeting, talking, yawning, stretching when sitting still, or falling asleep when prevented from being active. This case does not fulfill the boredom to the point-of-sleep qualities of hypovigilance.

4. Conduct disorder. People with this disorder

TABLE 30–1. DSM-IV Criteria for Attention-Deficit/Hyperactivity Disorder*

1. Inattention: At least six of the following symptoms of inattention have persisted for at least 6 months to a degree that is maladaptive and inconsistent with developmental level:
   a. Often fails to give close attention to details or makes careless mistakes in schoolwork, work, or other activities
   b. Often has difficulty sustaining attention in tasks or play activities
   c. Often does not seem to listen when spoken to directly
   d. Often does not follow through on instructions and fails to finish schoolwork, chores, or duties in the workplace (not due to oppositional behavior or failure to understand instructions)
   e. Often has difficulties
   f. Often avoids, dislikes, or is reluctant to engage in tasks that require sustained mental effort (such as schoolwork or homework)
   g. Often loses things necessary for tasks or activities (e.g., toys, school assignments, pencils, books, or tools)
   h. Is often easily distracted by extraneous stimuli
   i. Is often forgetful in daily activities
2. Hyperactivity-impulsivity: at least six of the following symptoms of hyperactivity-impulsivity have persisted for at least 6 months to a degree that is maladaptive and inconsistent with developmental level:
   Hyperactivity
   a. Often fidgets with hands or feet or squirms in seat
   b. Often leaves seat in classroom or in other situations in which remaining seated is expected
   c. Often runs about or climbs excessively in situations in which it is inappropriate (in adolescents or adults, may be limited to subjective feelings of restlessness)
   d. Often has difficulty playing or engaging in leisure activities quietly
   e. Is often "on the go" or often acts as if "driven by a motor"
   f. Often talks excessively
   Impulsivity
   g. Often blurts out answers before questions have been completed
   h. Often has difficulty awaiting turn
   i. Often interrupts or intrudes on others (e.g., butts into conversations or games)

*Attention deficit hyperactivity disorder, combined type, is diagnosed if both criteria 1 and 2 are met. Attention deficit hyperactivity disorder, predominantly inattentive type, is diagnosed if criterion 1 is met but not criterion 2. Attention deficit hyperactivity disorder, predominantly hyperactive-impulsive type, is diagnosed if criterion 2 is met but not criterion 1.
Reprinted with permission from the Diagnostic and Statistical Manual of Mental Disorders, 4th ed. Copyright 1994, American Psychiatric Association.

display a pattern of consistent violation of social rules and rights of others, including aggression toward other people and animals, property destruction, deceitfulness, theft, and other serious rule violations. Kevin does not display these qualities.

5. Oppositional defiant disorder is a pattern of

negativistic, angry behavior consistently present for at least 6 months. In adult interactions, these children are defiant and argumentative without identifiable cause.

Laboratory and Special Tests

No laboratory tests are specific in the diagnosis of ADHD. Complete thyroid function and serum lead screening should be done to rule out the rare cases of familial ADHD due to peripheral resistance to the actions of thyroid hormone (RTH) and lead toxicity, which is at least partially reversible. The diagnosis of ADHD should be based on a complete history plus the use of the Conner questionnaire, a 28-query teacher version and a 48-query parent version.

Treatment

Treatment must be tailored to the needs of each patient and family. It is usually multifaceted and may include:

1. Stimulant medication tends to reduce impulsivity, distractibility, and inattention. Amphetamines 5–40 mg, methylphenidate (Ritalin) 10–60 mg, and Pemoline 37–75 mg (Cylert) used in children result in a 70 per cent favorable response.

2. Antidepressants have been an adjunct in some cases of stimulant failure or in combination with stimulants. Tricyclics 1–3 mg/kg, monoamine oxidase inhibitors (MAOIs) 10–15 mg, antipsychotics, and benzodiazepines have all been used with success.

3. Antihypertensives have been found to be helpful, especially in cases with marked hyperactivity. Clonidine 0.05 tid, beta blockers, and SSRIs (selective serotonin reuptake inhibitors) have all been used with success.

4. Dietary manipulation. Some anecdotal reports exist of elimination diets (concentrated sweets, chocolate,) resulting in improved symptomatology in some ADHD cases.

5. Psychosocial interventions. Cognitive therapy, family therapy, behavioral management, biofeedback, individual counseling, and psychoeducational couseling have all been employed with varying results.

6. Prostheses, such as laptop computers, electronic notebooks, white noise generators, private study carrels, test isolation, and curricular modifications have also proven to be therapeutic in some cases.

Patient Education

Educating the patient, parents, and teachers is important to the understanding of this handicap and the recognition of the impact this disability has on all concerned. The variety of treatment options suggests its multimodal origins, and all parties must work in concert to effect improvement in the affected child.

Disposition

Kevin was started on methylphenidate 5 mg morning and noon with promptly noted improvement in daily behavior and school attentiveness. His case was so recently diagnosed that other therapeutic interventions have not yet been instituted.

DISCUSSION

ADHD is a multimodal behavioral disorder diagnosed by specific criteria (see Table 30–1) with onset before age 7 years and signs present for at least 6 months. The prevalence in school-age children is estimated to be 3 to 5 per cent. ADHD is not simply a contrived disorder designed to put children in chemical straightjackets for the sake of orderly classrooms. Untreated children with ADHD are 20 times more likely to develop delinquent behaviors as adolescents. Even if treated, up to one third of ADHD children develop a major psychiatric illness as adults (adult ADHD, alcoholism, somatization, or personality disorders).

No matter what combination of therapeutic interventions is used, it is important that a cooperative informed approach be shared among the child, parents, teachers, and health care professionals.

It is not unusual for children with ADHD to experience failure or to do poorly in school. The child has resultant low self-esteem, has difficulty in making and getting along with friends, and becomes involved with drugs and alcohol. ADHD children have more physical problems, accidents, and sleep disturbances than non-ADHD children. Twenty to thirty per cent of children with ADHD have specific learning disabilities and may test 7 to 15 points below average on standardized IQ tests.

There are a number of commonsense parental

interventions that may be of benefit even before a diagnosis of ADHD is made:

1. Accept the child's limitations

2. Provide an outlet for the release of excess energy

3. Keep your home well organized

4. Try not to let your child become fatigued

5. Avoid taking your child to formal gatherings

6. Maintain firm discipline

7. Enforce rules with nonphysical punishment

8. Stretch your child's attention span

9. Buffer your child against overreaction by neighbors

10. Get away from it all occasionally

11. Use special programs at school

SUGGESTED READING

Elia J. Drug treatment for hyperactive children. J Am Acad Child Adolesc Psychiatry N Y 1995;34:987–1000.

Faigel HC. Attention Deficit Disorders during Adolescence. Society for Adolescent Medicine. New York, Elsevier Science, 1995, pp 174–184.

McAnarey ER. Textbook of Adolescent Medicine. Philadelphia, Harcourt Brace Jovanovich, 1992, pp 1018–1028.

Safer DJ. Major Treatment Considerations for Attention Deficit Hyperactivity Disorder. Current Problems in Pediatrics. New York, Mosby–Year Book, 1995, pp 137–143.

Weinberg WA. The myth of attention deficit hyperactivity disorder. J Child Neurol 1992;7:431–458.

QUESTIONS

1. True or false. ADHD is a disorder characterized by
   a. Excessively talking
   b. Difficulty organizing tasks
   c. Nodding off in boring situations
   d. Easily distracted by extraneous stimuli
   e. Forgetfulness in daily activities

2. True or false. Long-term management of ADHD may include
   a. Elimination diets
   b. ECT
   c. Behavioral management
   d. Family therapy
   e. Barbiturates

3. True or false.
   a. Excessive exposure to lead in infancy may cause ADHD
   b. ADHD is a childhood diagnosis, not affecting adults
   c. Untreated ADHD is associated with increased rates of delinquet behaviors in teens
   d. A child with ADHD does not respond to firm discipline

Answers appear on **page 604**.

Chapter **31**

Short Child

Sanford R. Kimmel, M.D.

INITIAL VISIT—SUBJECTIVE

PATIENT IDENTIFICATION. Johnny J. is a 5-year-old Caucasian boy seen for a prekindergarten "well-child" physical examination.

PRESENTING PROBLEM. Johnny's mother notes that he is smaller than other boys his age. His 3-year-old sister is almost as tall as he is.

PRESENT ILLNESS. Johnny's only recent illness has been a cold, which was treated with an over-the-counter antihistamine-decongestant medicine. His appetite and physical activity are normal. He is a picky eater who generally has cold cereal and milk for breakfast, macaroni and cheese for lunch, and hamburger or pizza for supper. He likes apples, bananas, and corn but few green or yellow vegetables. He plays and keeps up with other boys his age.

PAST MEDICAL HISTORY. Johnny was the product of a full-term, uncomplicated pregnancy. His birth weight was 7 lb 8 oz (3.4 kg), and his length was 20 in (51 cm). A chart of his growth is presented in Figure 31–1.

His developmental milestones include the following: he smiled at 2 months, sat without support at 6 months, said "dada" specifically at 11 months, walked alone at 13 months, and now dresses himself without supervision. He speaks in understandable sentences.

Immunizations include diphtheria, tetanus, and pertussis (DTP) and *Haemophilus influenzae* B (HIB) vaccines at 2, 4, 6, and 15 months of age; oral polio vaccine (OPV) at 2, 4, and 18 months of age; and a measles, mumps, rubella vaccine (MMR) at 15 months of age.

Johnny has had four to five upper respiratory infections per year and three lifetime episodes of otitis media. He has not had varicella; he has not been hospitalized and has not required major surgery.

FAMILY HISTORY. Johnny's mother is 26 years old and in good health. She is 5 ft 4 in tall and weighs 132 lb. His 30-year-old father is 5 ft 8 in tall and weighs 150 lb. Johnny's father recalls being smaller than his peers as a child and being a "late bloomer." Johnny's 57-year-old paternal grandfather had a heart attack 2 years ago. His other grandparents are in their fifties and in good health. Johnny's 3-year-old sister is 37 in tall and weighs 33 lb.

HEALTH HABITS. Johnny wears his seatbelt when traveling in the car. His parents limit television viewing to 2 hours per day. He is learning to ride a bicycle.

SOCIAL HISTORY. Johnny is currently in nursery school but will be starting kindergarten next year. His mother, who is a teacher, reports that he interacts well with other children his age. She and her executive husband are concerned that his small size may place him at a disadvantage in school.

REVIEW OF SYSTEMS. Other than slight rhinorrhea, the review of systems is unremarkable.

Objective

PHYSICAL EXAMINATION. Johnny's height is 38 1/2 in; weight is 33 lb; blood pressure is 94/58; and pulse is 76 and regular. He appears normally proportioned and has no detectable deformities. Examination of the head, neck, eyes, ears, nose, and throat is normal. The cardiorespiratory and abdominal examinations are also normal. His genitalia are prepubertal (Tanner stage I). He follows directions and can balance on one foot for 6 seconds, catch a bounced ball, and draw a man with a head, eyes, ears, nose, mouth, body, arms, and legs.

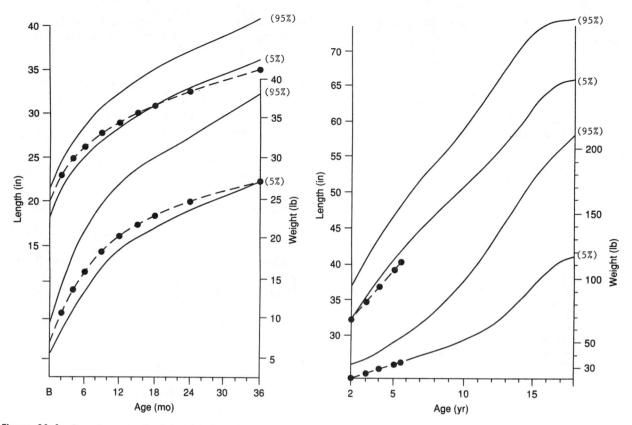

Figure 31-1. Growth curves for Johnny J. for length/height *(top curve)* and weight *(lower curve)*. The 95th and 5th percentiles for each parameter are also outlined.

LABORATORY TESTS. An office hemoglobin level was 12.5 g per dl. Urinalysis demonstrates a specific gravity of 1.022, pH 6.0, with negative results on dipstick and microscopic examination.

Assessment

WORKING DIAGNOSIS. The most likely diagnosis is *constitutional growth delay* in an otherwise well child. Although Johnny's height is below the 5th percentile and his weight is at the 5th percentile, his rate of growth parallels the growth curve. His deceleration in growth occurred before age 2 years with crossing of percentile lines. Since age 2 years, his linear growth has averaged 4 to 5 cm per year. Johnny's family history of delayed physical development also supports this diagnosis.

DIFFERENTIAL DIAGNOSES. Almost any serious chronic illness can have an adverse impact on a child's growth in addition to genetic and environmental causes. Common causes of short stature are listed in Table 31-1 and discussed later in this chapter (see Discussion).

Plan

Diagnostic

1. Proper evaluation of the growth curve is the most important consideration. A normal rate of linear growth excludes most organic causes of short stature. Children younger than 36 months of age should have their length measured in the supine position. Children 3 or more years old should have their shoeless standing height measured with a right angle held at their head. Children should be wearing minimal clothing when they are weighed at each visit, preferably on the same scale. Height and weight are then plotted on a growth chart developed by the National Center for Health Statistics. *Height age* is the age at which the child's height intersects the 50th percentile curve on this chart.

2. A *bone-age* radiograph of the left hand and

TABLE 31–1. Common Causes of Short Stature in Children

Familial
Constitutional growth delay
Familial short stature
Congenital
Down syndrome
Skeletal dysplasias (dwarfism)
Turner syndrome
Systemic Illnesses
Endocrine disorders
    Congenital adrenal hyperplasia (short adult)
    Cushing syndrome
    Diabetes mellitus (poorly controlled)
    Growth hormone deficiency—congenital or acquired
    Hypopituitarism
    Hypothyroidism
Heart disease
    Chronic heart failure
    Congenital heart disease
Gastrointestinal disease
    Celiac disease
    Chronic liver disease
    Crohn disease
    Malabsorption syndromes
Pulmonary diseases
    Asthma (poorly controlled)
    Cystic fibrosis
Renal disease
    Chronic renal failure
    Renal tubular acidosis
Environmental
Malnutrition
Psychosocial deprivation
Toxin or drug exposure

wrist is compared with published age-specific standards. Children must be at least 2 years of age for clinicians to reliably identify epiphyseal ossification centers. Bone-age films help differentiate familial short stature from constitutional growth delay and various endocrinologic disorders (Table 31–2).

3. The upper segment:lower segment ratio for the child is determined by measuring the distance from the top of the symphysis pubis to the floor for the lower segment. The distance subtracted from the total height then equals the upper segment. This ratio decreases from 1.7 at birth to 1.3 at 3 years of age and 1.0 after 7 years of age.

4. In the underweight child, a complete blood count (CBC) with differential may reveal anemia or malignancy, whereas an erythrocyte sedimentation rate (ESR) may detect nonspecific inflammatory disorders such as inflammatory bowel disease or collagen vascular disease.

5. Serum thyroxine (T_4) and thyroid-stimulating hormone (TSH) determinations should be considered, because hypothyroidism is easily detected and treated.

6. Renal and liver function tests, blood glucose, cholesterol, calcium, phosphorus, and electrolyte determinations are also available in the chemistry panel. Because a panel typically costs less than individual tests, it is useful in ruling out renal or hepatic disease, diabetes, or hyperlipidemia. The cholesterol level is important in this case because the family history is suspicious for early cardiac disease.

Therapeutic

The appropriate preschool immunizations should be given, including a booster DTaP (DT with acellular pertussis vaccine), OPV, and MMR. Varicella vaccine should also be given separately at a different site or 1 month later. In some states, the second MMR is not required until admission to middle school or junior high school and may be deferred until then.

Patient (Parent) Education

1. The parent's concerns were acknowledged. Johnny's satisfactory rate of growth despite his small absolute size was then demonstrated on the growth curve. The parents were told that although some children constituted the lower percentiles of the normal population, the family history suggested that Johnny may be a "late bloomer" like his father.

2. Anticipatory guidance should include injury prevention issues such as locking up poisons, medicines, dangerous tools, or firearms; teaching children to follow the proper rules of the road when bicycling, wearing a helmet when bicycling or rollerblading, and modeling this behavior. Children should be taught to swim; they should be constantly supervised when in or near the water. The child should know his or her name, address, and telephone number and to say "no" to strangers. Age-appropriate chores should be encouraged at home, as should quality family time. Appropriate and consistent limit setting should balance the child's need for autonomy. Playing well with other children, taking turns, following simple directions, and dressing one's self indicate skills appropriate for school entry.

Disposition

Johnny is scheduled to return in 6 months for a follow-up of his growth parameters. Laboratory re-

TABLE 31–2. Causes of Short Stature and Relationship to Bone Age and Growth Rate

Growth Rate	Bone Age < Chronological Age	Bone Age = Chronological Age	Bone Age > Chronological Age
Initially increased (Short adult)			Congenital adrenal hyperplasia Exogenous androgenic steroids Sexual precocity
Normal or slightly decreased	Constitutional growth delay	Familial short stature Skeletal dysplasias Rickets	

Decreased	Endocrine disorders
	  Cushing syndrome
	  Growth hormone deficiency
	  Hypothyroidism
	  Sex hormone deficiency
	Chronic systemic disease
	  Crohn disease
	  Heart failure
	  Renal failure
	Severe malnutrition
	Severe psychosocial deprivation
		Chromosomal disorders
		  Down syndrome
		  Turner syndrome	

sults and any subsequent necessary action will be communicated by telephone.

FIRST FOLLOW-UP VISIT

Subjective

Johnny returned 6 months later accompanied by his mother. He has been in kindergarten several months and is adjusting well.

Objective

Johnny's height is now 39 ¾ in, and his weight is 35 lb. His bone-age film of the wrists done shortly after his first visit approximated 3 years and 6 months. His chemistry panel demonstrated normal levels of electrolytes, calcium, phosphorus, total protein, and albumin. His creatinine level was normal at 0.6 mg per dl (53 μmol/L), as was his BUN level at 7 mg per dl (2.50 mMol/L). His alkaline phosphatase level was elevated above the normal adult value at 172 U per L. Other liver enzymes were normal. Serum T_4 level was normal at 8.2 μg per dl (105 nMol/L), and the TSH level was 3.5 μ U per L. The ESR value was normal at 4 mm per h. Serum cholesterol level is 156 mg per dl (4.04 mMol/L).

Assessment

1. The diagnosis of constitutional growth delay is supported by the delayed bone age consistent with height age and a normal growth velocity.

2. An alkaline phosphatase level elevated two or three times the adult normal is appropriate for a child with active skeletal growth.

Plan

Diagnostic

1. Continued monitoring of Johnny's growth at yearly intervals is essential.

2. No further diagnostic testing is necessary at this time. The serum cholesterol determination may be repeated in 5 years.

Therapeutic

At this time, Johnny does not seem to be suffering any adverse psychologic effects such as poor self image or social isolation. Continued reassurance is sufficient. If a child is sustaining deleterious psychological effects, referral to a pediatric endocrinologist to consider a trial of human growth hormone therapy may be in order.

Patient Education

Johnny's mother is reassured that his delayed bone age indicates that he has additional time to "catch up" in growth. His family can expect that he will enter puberty later and be a "late bloomer" like his father.

DISCUSSION OF DIFFERENTIAL DIAGNOSIS

Parents (and grandparents) are greatly interested in their child's growth. They are especially concerned about children smaller than their peers. A careful history should include prenatal factors such as nutrition, smoking, and drug use; problems in the perinatal period; and the child's subsequent growth and development. A family history to detect short stature, delayed maturation, genetic abnormalities, and chronic diseases is also necessary. Accurate measurements of the child's height, weight, and head circumference should be made. Arm span and upper segment:lower segment ratio should also be measured if indicated, and a careful physical examination should be performed including assessment for dysmorphic features. After age 2 years, normal children grow linearly at a rate of 5 cm or more per year and gain approximately 5 lb per year until the adolescent growth spurt (Table 31–3). Growth occurs in spurts rather than continuously.

Constitutional Growth Delay

Constitutional growth delay is a variant of normal growth that occurs more frequently in boys who enter puberty and develop later than their peers.

Their bone age is correspondingly delayed by 2 to 4 years and is approximately equal to their height age. Review of the growth chart demonstrates an average birth size with deceleration in the growth rate during the first 2 years of life. The growth rate subsequently returns to normal, but the child now follows a lower percentile on the growth curve. The pubertal growth spurt and adolescent development will also be correspondingly delayed. A family history of delayed growth and development in either parent is obtained in about 50 per cent of these children.

Familial Short Stature

Familial short stature (FSS) is less likely because Johnny was a normal size at birth. Children with FSS generally have below-average birth weights. In addition, their parents or close relatives are short. Johnny's parents are of average height. Children with FSS have a bone age that is approximately equal to their chronological age but less than their height age. Their growth curve is below the 5th percentile but parallels the normal curve, indicating a normal growth velocity. Children with FSS will have a below-normal adult height.

Constitutional growth delay and familial short stature are both characterized by a normal growth rate. The *mean predicted adult height* for a boy can be calculated as

[father's height + (mother's height + 5 inches)] ÷ 2

If the child is a girl, the mean predicted adult height is

[(father's height − 5 inches) + mother's height] ÷ 2

TABLE 31–3. Rules of Thumb: Growth Guidelines for Children

Age	Length or Height	Weight
Newborn	50 cm (20 in) average	3.4 kg (7½ lb) average
NB–3 months		1 kg/month (½ –1 oz/day)
4–5 months		Doubles birth weight
6 months		0.5 kg/month
12 months	Increases by 50%	Triples birth weight
12–24 months		0.25 kg/month
>2 years	>5 cm (2 in)/year until adolescent growth spurt	2.3 kg (5 lb) per year until adolescent growth spurt
4 years	Doubles (40 in approximately)	40 lb approximately

Adapted from Keefer CH. Normal growth and development: An overview. In Dershewitz RA (ed.). Ambulatory Pediatric Care. Philadelphia, J.B. Lippincott, 1988, p 24.

Ninety-five per cent of the population attains an adult height within 3 to 4 inches above or below their predicted height. If the child is growing at a rate that will enable him to achieve his predicted adult height, careful observation of growth parameters is appropriate. If the child's growth rate is declining, further investigation is warranted.

Malnutrition and Psychosocial Deprivation

Adverse nutritional or socioeconomic factors should always be considered in the evaluation of a child's growth. The diagnosis of psychosocial deprivation should not be made, however, until an appropriate nutritional assessment and trial have been conducted and organic causes excluded. Some chronic illnesses that can result in poor growth are listed in Table 31–1.

Chronic Systemic Illness

Chronic systemic illness usually has an adverse effect on body mass (weight) before linear growth. Failure to grow is sometimes the only manifestation of inflammatory bowel disease or renal disease. A CBC, ESR, and electrolyte and other blood chemistry tests may be required if these conditions are suspected. A normal result on urinalysis with a specific gravity greater than 1.020 assists in ruling out diabetes insipidus whereas a negative result on dipstick test for glucose rules out diabetes mellitus. Poor growth due to malnutrition may be caused by malabsorption syndromes characterized by loose or foul-smelling stools and diminished caloric intake.

Endocrinologic Causes and Hypothyroidism

Endocrinologic causes of short stature are less common but treatable diseases that must be considered. Most children with endocrine causes of poor linear growth have a normal weight for height-age. Despite prenatal screening, *hypothyroidism* may appear later in childhood, either as an acquired condition or as a diagnosis missed in earlier testing. Clinical features include constipation, slow pulse, dry skin, thinning hair, cold intolerance, sluggishness, and developmental delay. Bone age is also delayed. The TSH level is elevated in primary hypothyroidism, whereas low T_4 and low TSH levels suggest pituitary or hypothalamic defects. Thyroid hormone is necessary for normal growth hormone synthesis, and levels must be assayed before growth hormone (GH) studies are done.

Cushing Syndrome

Cushing syndrome is usually caused by the administration of pharmacologic doses of glucocorticoids but may rarely be due to an adrenocortical tumor or excess adrenocorticotropic hormone (ACTH). It is characterized by truncal obesity, "moon" facies, "buffalo hump," violet striae, easy bruisability, glucose intolerance, hypertension, and osteoporosis or cataracts. The linear growth rate (height velocity) is decreased and bone age is delayed in children with Cushing syndrome.

Congenital Adrenal Hyperplasia

Undetected and untreated congenital adrenal hyperplasia ultimately leads to short stature as an adult, although the initial signs are ambiguous genitalia and virilization. Initial growth is accelerated and bone age is advanced, leading to premature closure of the epiphyses.

Growth Hormone Deficiency

Congenital or acquired GH deficiency causes severe retardation of skeletal growth that may be accompanied by central adiposity and immature facies. A history of neonatal hypoglycemia may accompany the poor growth that is usually apparent by 6 to 12 months of age in the congenital form of this disorder. Boys with micropenises (stretched length less than 2.8 cm [1.1 in] in a term infant) may have luteinizing hormone deficiency from panhypopituitarism. Specific causes of GH deficiency include congenital abnormalities such as septo-optic dysplasia, trauma, tumors such as craniopharyngiomas, and central nervous system infections or irradiation.

Children with classic GH deficiency fail to release normal amounts of GH in response to standardized drug stimuli. Emotional deprivation can produce functional hypopituitarism with inadequate response of GH to provocative stimuli. Any coexisting hypothyroidism must be corrected before GH testing or the response to stimuli may be blunted. Children with GH neurosecretory dysfunction may exhibit a normal GH response to the usual provocative tests but demonstrate a marked deficiency of pulsatile secretion of GH over a 24-hour period. Because of the variation in testing, referral to a pediatric endocrinologist is in order when GH deficiency is suspected.

Chromosomal Disorders

Children with chromosomal disorders usually have apparent dysmorphic features. *Turner syndrome* should always be considered in short girls, especially if there is no family history of short stature. Characteristic features include low birth weight, webbing of the neck, low posterior hairline, broad chest with widely spaced nipples (shieldlike chest), cubitus valgus, and lymphedema of the hands and feet. If mosaicism is present, short stature may be the only manifestation. Consequently, short girls with subnormal growth rates should have banded karyotyping performed, because Turner syndrome may be as common as GH deficiency. Special growth charts are available for girls with Turner syndrome as well as children with Down syndrome.

Skeletal Dysplasias

Skeletal dysplasias or osteochondrodysplasias are usually inherited; they cause disproportionate short stature. The term *dwarfism* is frequently used to refer to this group of disorders, although there are more than 200 varieties. Skeletal dysplasias are frequently characterized by a greater than normal upper segment:lower segment ratio. In contrast, children with hypogonadism have longer extremities and a less-than-normal ratio caused by failure of the epiphyses to close. Complete skeletal radiographs may be required in addition to determination of serum calcium, phosphorus, protein, and alkaline phosphatase levels to rule out hypophosphatasia and vitamin D–resistant and vitamin D–dependent rickets. Urine screening for metabolic and storage disorders should also be considered.

GH Treatment

Most children with constitutional growth delay will reach their predicted midparental height. Some may remain several inches below their target height. Children with familial short stature will grow up to be short adults, a fact that some families may not accept. In the United States, taller college graduates earn more money, and most presidents have been the taller candidate. Consequently, there has been greater pressure to give human growth hormone (hGH) to children who do not have classic GH deficiency. Although the administration of hGH may initially accelerate linear growth in these children, it also may accelerate the rate of epiphyseal closure. Studies demonstrate conflicting results, and it remains unclear whether such therapy produces a greater-than-predicted adult height. Therapy is costly and rarely is accompanied by such adverse effects as allergy, impaired glucose tolerance, pseudotumor cerebri, slipped capital femoral epiphysis, and possibly leukemia. The child must also tolerate daily or thrice weekly injections.

SUGGESTED READING

Bercu BB. The growing conundrum: Growth hormone treatment of the non-growth hormone deficient child. JAMA 1996;276:567–568.

Denniston CR. Assessing normal and abnormal patterns of growth. Primary Care 1994;21:637–654.

Duck SC. Identification and assessment of the slowly growing child. Am Fam Physician 1996;53:2305–2312.

Kimmel SR, Fay L. Growth and development. In Rakel RE (ed). Textbook of Family Practice, 5th ed. Philadelphia, W.B. Saunders, 1995, pp 610–633.

Plotnik LP. Growth, growth hormone, and pituitary disorders. In Oski FA, et al (eds). Principles and Practice of Pediatrics, 2nd ed. Philadelphia, J. B. Lippincott, 1994, pp 1973–1980.

1. Which developmental milestone is not appropriate for a 5-year-old child?
   a. Can balance on one foot for 5 seconds
   b. Able to put on clothing without help
   c. One-half of speech is understandable
   d. Can draw a person with 6 body parts

2. All except which one of the following are characteristics of familial short stature?
   a. Below average size at birth
   b. Normal or slightly subnormal growth rate
   c. A family history of delayed maturation (i.e., "late bloomer")
   d. An ultimate adult height that is below normal

3. Match the following diseases to their respective clinical characteristics. Each answer may be used once, more than once, or not at all.
   a. Cushing syndrome
   b. Hypothyroidism
   c. Growth hormone deficiency
      (1) Micropenis
      (2) Moon facies
      (3) Cold intolerance
      (4) Developmental delay

Answers appear on **page 604.**

Chapter 32

Preschool Physical Examination

Bruce T. Vanderhoff, M.D.

INITIAL VISIT

Subjective

PATIENT IDENTIFICATION. Patrick O. is a 4-year-old boy brought to the office by his mother for a preschool physical examination.

PRESENTING PROBLEM. Because Patrick will not be 5 years old until late September his mother is concerned about his readiness to begin kindergarten this fall. Patrick's mother also wants to know if he might have "attention deficit." Her sister's son, who is 6 months older than Patrick, was recently diagnosed with attention deficit hyperactivity disorder (ADHD). Patrick's mother has noticed that Patrick sometimes seems "hyper" and "does not always do what he is told," although he is generally "a good boy."

PRESENT ILLNESS. Patrick's mother indicates that although Patrick seems to her to be better behaved than his cousin, there are episodes when he seems "hyper" at play. These episodes typically occur when he is playing with his cousins and sometimes when playing alone with his dinosaurs. She also notes that she must sometimes repeat some instructions to him several times before he complies, especially when she wants him to turn off his computer for bed.

Despite these behaviors, Patrick's mother

admits that he is able to play quietly by himself for extended periods, such as when she is paying bills. He is relatively well behaved in the pew at church, he helps her with household chores, and he is good about remembering safety instructions such as looking both ways before crossing the street and always wearing his bicycle helmet. Moreover, his preschool teachers report that he is well behaved, displays above-average academic performance, and interacts well with the other children.

PAST MEDICAL HISTORY. Patrick was the product of an uneventful term pregnancy; his weight was 7 lb, 14 oz. During the pregnancy his mother did not smoke, did not consume alcohol or drugs, and had no transmittable diseases. Patrick had a single episode of otitis media at 14 months and chickenpox at age 3 years. He has been otherwise healthy with only occasional "coughs and colds." The office chart documents that he has always received his immunizations in a timely fashion. Immunizations received to date include: diphtheria, tetanus, pertussis (DTP), and *Haemophilus influenzae* type B (Hib) vaccines at 2, 4, and 6 months; diphtheria, acellular pertussis (DTaP) at 18 months; oral polio vaccine (OPV) at 2, 4, and 18 months; measles, mumps, rubella (MMR), and Hib at 15 months. Patrick had a normal screening hematocrit level at 6 months of age. Lead screening, however, was deferred by his parents. Patrick had his first dental visit at age 3 years.

FAMILY HISTORY. Patrick's family history, with the exception of his cousin's recent diagnosis of attention deficit hyperactivity disorder, lacks any report of significant childhood illnesses, learning disabilities, or behavioral problems. Patrick's father is "a bit overweight" and takes antihypertensive medication. Patrick's paternal grandfather had a heart attack at age 64 years, and his maternal grandmother is diabetic.

HEALTH HABITS. Patrick's mother describes a fairly sedentary lifestyle for a preschool child. Patrick spends much of his time at home watching television, playing computer games, or playing with his toys. He seldom plays outside because there are no children his age nearby. None of the members of Patrick's family, including his grandparents, smoke at this time.

SOCIAL HISTORY. Patrick's parents were divorced when he was 2 years old. He lives with his mother in a condominium complex and visits his father on alternate weekends. Patrick attends a daycare/

preschool center during the week. Patrick has no siblings but has several cousins close to his age whom he sees frequently. Patrick has a cat named Max.

REVIEW OF SYSTEMS. Patrick seems well to his mother. She denies any additional problems or concerns.

DEVELOPMENTAL MILESTONES. Patrick has achieved all the screening milestones normally expected of a 5-year-old (gross motor: skips, alternating feet, and jumps over low obstacles; fine motor: ties his own shoes and can spread with a knife; language: prints his first name and asks what a word means; social: plays competitive games and abides by the rules, and likes to help around the house).

Objective

Physical Examination

Patrick's general appearance is that of an alert and cooperative boy. Vital signs reveal a temperature of 98°F, respiratory rate 22, pulse 90, blood pressure 104/60, weight 46 lb, and height 43 in (yielding a stature-weight ratio around the 90th percentile). His skin is normal in color and without rashes. His HEENT examination demonstrates: a head of normal shape; eyes with normal conjunctivae, corneas, pupils, and extraoccular movements; normal cover testing; ears with normal pinnae, canals, and tympanic membranes; a nose with normal turbinates and nares; and a mouth with normal teeth, oral mucosa, tonsils, and pharynx. His neck is supple with no thyromegaly and only some age-appropriate shoddy anterior cervical adenopathy. Lymph node examination demonstrates no other significant adenopathy.

His chest is clear to auscultation throughout. His heart examination demonstrates regular rate and rhythm without murmurs, rubs, or gallops.

His abdomen is soft and nontender, with normal active bowel sounds. No mass or organomegaly is appreciated. Patrick's back is without scoliosis or sacral defects. Genitourinary examination reveals normal Tanner stage I male genitalia with bilaterally descended testicles and no inguinal hernias.

His extremities are without limitations of range of motion, tenderness, clubbing, edema, or perfusion abnormalities. Patrick's gait is normal, and his neurologic examination is nonfocal with normal deep tendon reflexes.

Tests

Screening audiometry demonstrates normal hearing bilaterally. Visual acuity is 20/20 left eye (OS), 20/15 right eye (OD), and 20/20 both eyes (OU).

Assessment

Working Diagnosis

Patrick is a healthy but overweight 4 11/12-year-old boy who appears ready for school entry. He needs to receive immunizations today to remain in compliance with the recommended immunization schedule for children.

Differential Diagnosis

1. Kindergarten readiness. The information that has been elicited at this visit strongly suggests that Patrick is ready to enter kindergarten. He is at low risk for medical problems; his family appears to be able to meet his needs; he has demonstrated adequate developmental progress in the preschool years; and he appears to have adequate social skills as assessed by the screening developmental milestones.

2. Attention deficit hyperactivity disorder seems an unlikely diagnosis for Patrick based on the information currently available. Patrick has not demonstrated a pattern of behavior that is typical of this diagnosis and, based on today's interview, it seems unlikely that he meets the diagnostic criteria for this condition.

3. A behavioral disorder also seems an unlikely diagnosis. Patrick's mother describes him as typically "a very good boy." His ignoring her instructions to discontinue enjoyable activities to go to bed is not adequate evidence of a pervasive behavioral disorder, particularly in a child who is not routinely defiant.

Plan

Diagnostic

1. Because of maternal concerns about school readiness and attention deficit/hyperactivity disorder (ADHD), administer a Denver Developmental Screening Test (Fig. 32–1).

2. Provide mother with a parental rating scale for ADHD, such as the Conners Parent Rating Scales. Ask her to complete this and return it to you when Patrick returns for his Denver Developmental Screening Test. Request that his teachers also complete rating scales.

3. Recommend lead screening, which has never been performed. The Centers for Disease Control and Prevention (CDC) considers nearly all children in the United States to be at risk for lead poisoning. Even low-level long-term exposure to lead can result in adverse neurodevelopmental effects.

Therapeutic

Today Patrick will receive the DTaP, OPV, and MMR immunizations. Patrick's mother is reminded that he will be due to receive a tetanus, diphtheria toxoids (Td) vaccination when he returns at 11 years of age for his junior high school examination. The mother also is advised that Patrick should receive the hepatitis B vaccination series. Patrick's mother, however, continues to decline hepatitis immunization for Patrick.

Parental Education

1. Suggest or provide appropriate reading materials about ADHD to Patrick's mother.

2. Provide Patrick's mother with reading material or a video about parenting children of Patrick's age.

3. Discuss Patrick's weight with his mother. Encourage a shift in family activities away from sedentary pursuits, especially television viewing, toward active pursuits. Review Patrick's diet with his mother and suggest appropriate reductions in caloric intake, especially in snacking. Provide the mother with reading materials outlining appropriate dietary recommendations for Patrick, and offer consultation with a qualified nutritionist.

4. Provide Patrick's mother with reading materials about the hepatitis B immunization series.

Disposition

Patrick is scheduled to have a Denver Developmental Screening Test in the office later this week and, provided that this reveals age-appropriate development, for a follow-up visit in 6 weeks.

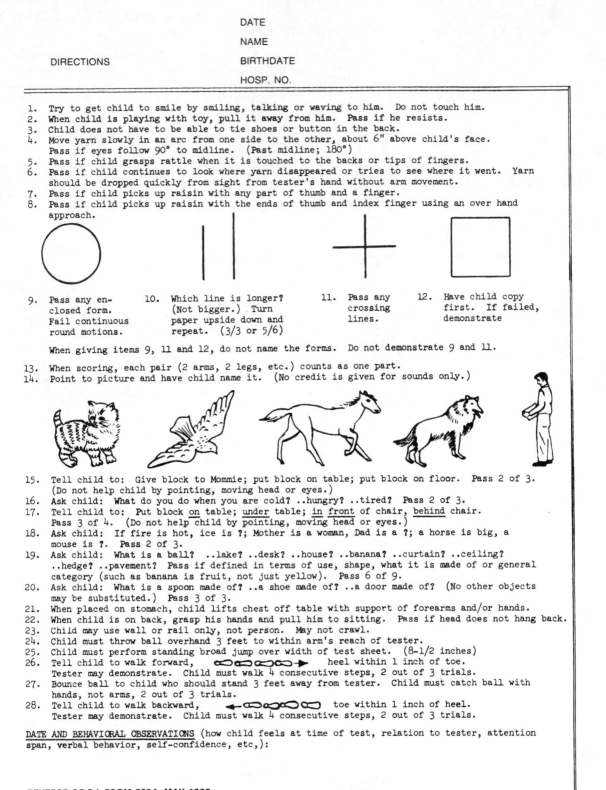

1. Try to get child to smile by smiling, talking or waving to him. Do not touch him.
2. When child is playing with toy, pull it away from him. Pass if he resists.
3. Child does not have to be able to tie shoes or button in the back.
4. Move yarn slowly in an arc from one side to the other, about 6" above child's face. Pass if eyes follow 90° to midline. (Past midline; 180°)
5. Pass if child grasps rattle when it is touched to the backs or tips of fingers.
6. Pass if child continues to look where yarn disappeared or tries to see where it went. Yarn should be dropped quickly from sight from tester's hand without arm movement.
7. Pass if child picks up raisin with any part of thumb and a finger.
8. Pass if child picks up raisin with the ends of thumb and index finger using an over hand approach.

9. Pass any enclosed form. Fail continuous round motions.
10. Which line is longer? (Not bigger.) Turn paper upside down and repeat. (3/3 or 5/6)
11. Pass any crossing lines.
12. Have child copy first. If failed, demonstrate

When giving items 9, 11 and 12, do not name the forms. Do not demonstrate 9 and 11.

13. When scoring, each pair (2 arms, 2 legs, etc.) counts as one part.
14. Point to picture and have child name it. (No credit is given for sounds only.)

15. Tell child to: Give block to Mommie; put block on table; put block on floor. Pass 2 of 3. (Do not help child by pointing, moving head or eyes.)
16. Ask child: What do you do when you are cold? ..hungry? ..tired? Pass 2 of 3.
17. Tell child to: Put block on table; under table; in front of chair, behind chair. Pass 3 of 4. (Do not help child by pointing, moving head or eyes.)
18. Ask child: If fire is hot, ice is ?; Mother is a woman, Dad is a ?; a horse is big, a mouse is ?. Pass 2 of 3.
19. Ask child: What is a ball? ..lake? ..desk? ..house? ..banana? ..curtain? ..ceiling? ..hedge? ..pavement? Pass if defined in terms of use, shape, what it is made of or general category (such as banana is fruit, not just yellow). Pass 6 of 9.
20. Ask child: What is a spoon made of? ..a shoe made of? ..a door made of? (No other objects may be substituted.) Pass 3 of 3.
21. When placed on stomach, child lifts chest off table with support of forearms and/or hands.
22. When child is on back, grasp his hands and pull him to sitting. Pass if head does not hang back.
23. Child may use wall or rail only, not person. May not crawl.
24. Child must throw ball overhand 3 feet to within arm's reach of tester.
25. Child must perform standing broad jump over width of test sheet. (8-1/2 inches)
26. Tell child to walk forward, ⟳⟳⟳⟳→ heel within 1 inch of toe. Tester may demonstrate. Child must walk 4 consecutive steps, 2 out of 3 trials.
27. Bounce ball to child who should stand 3 feet away from tester. Child must catch ball with hands, not arms, 2 out of 3 trials.
28. Tell child to walk backward, ←⟳⟳⟳⟳ toe within 1 inch of heel. Tester may demonstrate. Child must walk 4 consecutive steps, 2 out of 3 trials.

DATE AND BEHAVIORAL OBSERVATIONS (how child feels at time of test, relation to tester, attention span, verbal behavior, self-confidence, etc,):

REVERSE OF DA FORM 5694, MAY 1988

Figure 32–1. The revised Denver Developmental Screening Test (DDST-R) screens developmental skills in children up to 6 years of age. Delays identified by the test require repeat or more definitive testing, since the test itself is not diagnostic. (From Frankenburg, W. K. Ladoca Publishing Foundation, Denver, Colorado, 1978.)

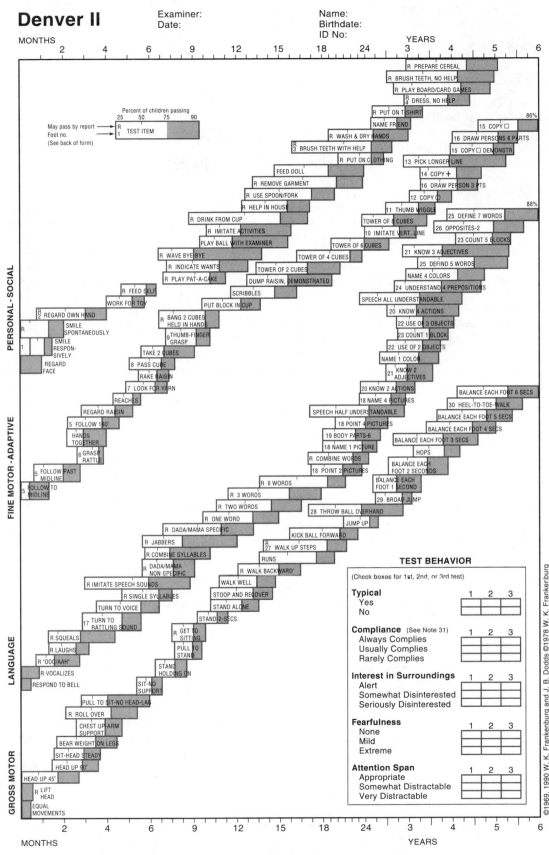

Figure 32–1 *Continued*

FOLLOW-UP VISIT

Subjective

Patrick is very happy in kindergarten and his teachers report that he is well behaved and interacting appropriately with the other children. The family has substantially reduced the amount of time they spend watching television and playing computer games, and they now schedule regular outings. Patrick's mother, aunt, and grandparents are sharing responsibility for taking him to the park to play regularly. Patrick's father has incorporated similar changes in activity into their weekends together. Patrick's mother did meet with a nutritionist and has made changes in their diet. After watching the parenting video on 4- to 5-year-olds that Patrick's mother borrowed from the office library, there has been less conflict over going to bed.

Both Patrick's mother and his new kindergarten teacher have completed behavior rating scales. The findings are not those expected for a child with ADHD.

Objective

With the exception of his weight, which has decreased 1 lb, to 45 lb, Patrick's vital signs are essentially unchanged. His general appearance, HEENT, cardiopulmonary, abdominal and extremity examinations are unchanged and unremarkable. The Denver Developmental Screening Test, performed since his last visit, demonstrated age-appropriate development in all four areas assessed (personal-social, fine motor, language, and gross motor). Patrick's lead screen resulted in a level of 2 µg/dl, which is within normal limits.

Assessment

Patrick is doing well with the transition to kindergarten and does not appear to have ADHD like his cousin. The family has made an excellent start toward improving his weight.

Plan

Reassure Patrick's mother that he does not appear to have ADHD; however, remind her to contact the physician if he develops any behaviors that concern her or his teachers. Applaud the family's behavioral modifications and encourage continued efforts to modify Patrick's weight.

Disposition

Schedule Patrick for a follow-up visit in 6 months to reassess his weight.

DISCUSSION

School Readiness

At the time of the preschool examination it is not uncommon for parents to seek the assistance of their family doctor in assessing whether their child is ready to enter school. All schools set cutoff dates, typically ranging from September 1 to October 1, by which children must reach their fifth birthday to enter kindergarten. Parents whose children have birthdays close to the cutoff date are often particularly concerned about the preparedness of their relatively younger child to successfully participate in formal schooling.

For a child to be ready to successfully participate in formal schooling, that child must have the physical, developmental, and behavioral skills typical of the child's peers entering school. The child must also have adequate physical health, emotional maturity, general knowledge, and social and emotional development.

Certain groups of children are at increased risk for grade retention or failure. These children are thus less likely than their peers to be ready for school entry. Younger kindergartners, such as Patrick, generally do have achievement levels that are lower than those of their peers. These differences in achievement, however, tend to be small, and they diminish during the elementary years. Nevertheless, a birthday close to the cutoff date for entry into school may increase a child's risk of retention or failure, particularly when age is added to other risk factors.

Children with certain clinical histories are among those more likely to have difficulty performing adequately in school. Such children include those of low birth weight; those born preterm; those exposed to substances of abuse, such as cigarettes, alcohol, and cocaine, during pregnancy; and those who are malnourished as infants and toddlers. Moreover, children of low birth weight are not only at risk for school failure but are also at risk for learning and language disabilities, impairments of vision and hearing, and behavioral problems.

The family physician's assessment of a child's readiness for school begins with the medical history. Pertinent features of this record include a history of low birth weight, prematurity, or small-for-gestational-age status; a maternal history of substance abuse, including tobacco; and a maternal history of transmittable diseases during pregnancy. Past childhood conditions that can affect a child's ability to perform effectively in the classroom, such as lead poisoning, chronic or recurrent otitis media with associated hearing loss, cerebral injury, or iron deficiency anemia, should be noted. The family physician should remember that chronic active diseases such as diabetes mellitus, seizure disorders, and asthma can impede a child's school performance because of medication effects, absenteeism, and their impact on self-esteem.

A complete physical examination should be performed on all children before school entry. Abnormalities of growth parameters, such as microcephally, may provide clues to conditions associated with developmental disability. Physical anomalies can provide clues to the presence of syndromes associated with developmental and/or learning disabilities, such as Down syndrome and Turner syndrome. Possibly the most important components of the preschool physical examination, however, are the screens of vision and hearing. Uncorrected deficits of vision or hearing can impede a child's ability to achieve his or her potential in the classroom.

The family physician should consider the child's family environment, preschool experience, and development. The quality of a child's family environment is one of the best predictors of school achievement. Children who receive adequate support and stimulation from their families are much more likely to succeed in school than those who do not. Information from preschool teachers can be very useful, because these teachers are often very aware of whether a child has the self esteem and social skills necessary for school entry. Developmental screening tests, such as the Denver Developmental Screening Test, allow the family physician to assess whether a child has age-appropriate gross motor, fine motor, language, and social skills. Abnormal scores on the Denver Developmental Screening Test should prompt reconsideration of a child's readiness for school.

Although young age confers an initial slight disadvantage, this disadvantage disappears within a few years. Holding a child out of school solely to eliminate this disadvantage is generally not recommended; some work suggests that such an approach may negatively affect social development and self esteem without conferring any academic benefits.

Childhood Obesity

Patrick is at risk for developing childhood obesity. He is currently very close to the 95th percentile of weight for height, which represents the screening threshold for childhood obesity. Although heredity plays a role in the development of obesity, environment clearly plays a major role as well. Thus, the fact that Patrick's father is "overweight" does not dictate that Patrick must share that feature on a genetic basis. Some of the most important risk factors for the development of obesity are related to the family environment. Such environmental risk factors include higher socioeconomic class; higher levels of parental education; small family size; and parental inactivity, because children whose parents are active are leaner than those whose parents are inactive.

Another important environmental influence on the development of childhood obesity is television viewing. Television viewing is a sedentary activity that displaces active recreation and increases consumption of foods advertised on television. Thus, there is a direct association between duration of television viewing and childhood obesity. Region of residence, season of the year, and degree of urbanization represent other environmental risk factors associated with childhood obesity. In the United States, obesity is most prevalent in the Northeast and least prevalent in the West. Obesity is more prevalent in winter and spring than in summer and fall, and more prevalent in major metropolitan areas than in sparsely settled areas.

Although parents often speculate that their child's obesity can be "a gland problem," less than 1 per cent of childhood obesity is the result of an underlying medical condition. Medical disorders that can contribute to obesity include conditions such as hypothyroidism, growth hormone deficiency, Turner syndrome, and Cushing syndrome. Such disorders are, however, usually associated with abnormalities of growth and development that may be evident after a complete history and physical examination.

Because obesity is the result of an imbalance of energy intake and expenditure, the prevention and treatment of obesity must focus on both decreasing caloric intake and increasing physical activity. Decreasing the amount of time spent watching television can be an important first step toward increasing a child's activity level while decreasing television's food-promoting effects. A family-wide pattern of increased physical activity and proper caloric intake should be promoted. Moreover, children should receive immediate, frequent, and consistent positive reinforcement. This positive reinforcement may take the form of reward stickers, positive verbal support and praise, and contractual agreements. Successful modification of a child's obesity or risk for obesity depends upon the family's commitment to changing those factors that promote the development of this condition.

Attention Deficit/Hyperactivity Disorder

ADHD is among the most common chronic behavioral disorders in children. It is more common in boys than in girls. Although symptoms may persist into adulthood, they must begin before age 7 years. Hyperactivity, impulsivity, distractibility and short attention span, emotional lability, and low tolerance for frustration are characteristic symptoms of this disorder. The criteria outlined by the American Psychiatric Association in the *Diagnostic and Statistical Manual of Mental Disorders* are among the most widely accepted for making this diagnosis (Table 32–1).

Children who are reported to have the cardinal

TABLE 32–1. Characteristics of Attention Deficit/ Hyperactivity Disorder

Inattention

- Often fails to give close attention to details or makes mistakes in schoolwork or other activities
- Often has difficulty sustaining attention
- Often does not seem to listen when spoken to directly
- Often does not follow through on instructions and fails to finish schoolwork or chores not due to oppositional behavior or failure to understand instructions
- Often has difficulty organizing tasks and activities
- Often avoids or dislikes tasks that require sustained mental effort
- Often loses things necessary for tasks or activities
- Often easily distracted by extraneous stimuli
- Often forgetful in daily activities

Hyperactivity-impulsivity

- Often fidgets with hands/feet or squirms in seat
- Often leaves seat in classroom or in other situations in which remaining seated is expected
- Often runs about or climbs excessively in situations in which it is inappropriate
- Often has difficulty playing or engaging in leisure activities quietly
- Often "on the go" or often acts as if "driven by a motor"
- Often has difficulty awaiting turn
- Often interrupts or intrudes on others

Onset before age 7 years
Some impairment from symptoms in two or more settings
Symptoms are not result of a pervasive developmental disorder or another mental disorder

Modified from American Psychiatric Association: Diagnostic and Statistical Manual of Mental Disorders, 4th ed. Washington, DC, American Psychiatric Association, 1994, pp. 83–85.

features of ADHD should be evaluated in a thorough and systematic fashion by the family physician. A complete history and physical examination should be performed including screens of vision and hearing; developmental assessment; and consideration of the child's emotional, environmental, and familial situation. Evaluation of the child's attention and behavior in the home as well as at school should be pursued. Various parent and teacher rating scales are available to assist with this evaluation. All children suspected to have this diagnosis should have a complete evaluation of their cognitive capacities, speech and language abilities, academic functioning, and psychological condition. This final assessment can often be accomplished with assistance from the school, using a multidisciplinary team to perform cognitive, psychological, achievement, and speech/language testing.

In Patrick's case, the office evaluation, coupled with evaluations from the home and preschool environments, failed to identify the cardinal features of ADHD. The family physician elected, after discussion with Patrick's mother, not to pursue further evaluation for ADHD before school entry, but to continue to closely monitor Patrick's behavior in and out of the classroom. Had Patrick manifested behaviors suggestive of ADHD, however, it would have been appropriate to work with his school to conduct a multidisciplinary evaluation as outlined earlier.

Lead Poisoning in Children

Although surveys in this country have reported that 14 to 67 per cent of preschool children have blood lead levels exceeding 10 µg/dl, the level considered unsafe by the CDC, Patrick has not been screened for lead poisoning to date. Children may be exposed to lead from chips or dust from lead-based paint, contamination of soil and dust, air contamination from nearby smelters or battery manufacturing plants, and less commonly, from tap water. Unfortunately, although lead has only a 10 per cent bioavailability in adults, it has a 40 per cent bioavailability in children and more readily enters their central nervous systems, particularly before age 3 years. Most children with elevated blood lead levels are asymptomatic. Nevertheless, long-term low-level exposure to lead is associated with irreversible developmental effects including decreased IQ, and higher levels can lead to a variety of symptoms including hyperactivity. Fortunately, lead toxicity is both preventable and, when identified, treatable. Thus, screening Patrick for lead toxicity, which the

CDC advises for all children, will be performed by his family physician.

Immunizations

The immunizations administered to Patrick at this visit were chosen based on the Recommended Childhood Immunization Schedule, United States, which has been approved by the Advisory Committee on Immunization Practices of the American Academy of Pediatrics and the American Academy of Family Physicians (Fig. 32–2). This schedule recommends ages for administration of the hepatitis B (Hep B); DTP; Hib; OPV; MMR; and varicella-zoster (Var) vaccinations.

Patrick never received the hepatitis B vaccination series. It is recommended that all children in the United States complete this three-shot vaccination series within the first 18 months of life. The series usually begins with the first vaccination in the newborn nursery or at the 1- to 2-month visits. The second vaccination is then administered at 1 to 4 months of age. At least 1 month, however, should be allowed between the first and second hepatitis B vaccination. The third and final hepatitis B vaccination should be administered between 6 and 18 months of age. An interval of at least 4 months after the first vaccination and 2 months after the second vaccination should be allowed. For children such as Patrick who have not received three doses of hepatitis B vaccine, the series can be started at any age.

The DTP and Hib vaccinations are administered at 2, 4, and 6 months. They are now often administered as a conjugate vaccination, which reduces the number of required injections. A fourth DTP dose should be given once at 12 to 18 months of age and a fifth DTP dose should be given at 4 to 6 years of age. The DTaP (diphtheria and tetanus toxoids and acellular pertussis) vaccine is now preferred to the whole-cell DTP vaccine for all doses in this series. The DTaP vaccine contains an acellular pertussis vaccine that causes fever less frequently than the whole-cell pertussis vaccine. A fourth Hib vaccine should be given at 12 to 15 months of age. Patrick had received DTP vaccinations at 2, 4, and 6 months; a DTaP at 18 months; and Hib vaccinations at 2, 4, 6, and 15 months. Hence, he received a DTaP vaccination at this visit.

In September 1996, the Advisory Committee on Immunization Practices (ACIP), which advises the Centers for Disease Control and Prevention regarding the most appropriate use of vaccines in the United States, recommended a change in the polio vaccination schedule. The ACIP recommended that IVP be administered at 2 and 4 months, followed by two doses of oral polio vaccine (OPV) at 12 to 18 months and 4 to 6 years. The ACIP noted that the only cases of indigenously acquired polio in the United States in the last 17 years have been vaccine related. None of the cases were due to wild poliovirus. The risk of recipients acquiring paralytic poliomyelitis from the first OPV is about 1 in 1.4 million, while the risk for contacts is about 1 in 2.2 million. After later doses, this risk declines markedly. Thus,

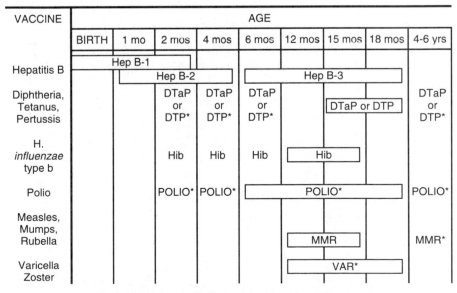

Figure 32–2. Recommended childhood immunization schedule, United States, January–December 1997, to age 6 years. (Adapted from Recommended Childhood Immunization Schedule United States, January–December 1997. Contemp Pediatr 1997;14(1):24–25.)

VACCINE	AGE								
	BIRTH	1 mo	2 mos	4 mos	6 mos	12 mos	15 mos	18 mos	4-6 yrs
Hepatitis B	Hep B-1								
		Hep B-2			Hep B-3				
Diphtheria, Tetanus, Pertussis			DTaP or DTP*	DTaP or DTP*	DTaP or DTP*		DTaP or DTP		DTaP or DTP*
H. influenzae type b			Hib	Hib	Hib	Hib			
Polio			POLIO*	POLIO*		POLIO*			POLIO*
Measles, Mumps, Rubella						MMR			MMR*
Varicella Zoster						VAR*			

*See text regarding schedule options for this vaccination.

this change in the polio vaccination schedule was recommended to reduce the already small risk of vaccine-associated paralytic polio in recipients and their contacts in an area of the world where the wild virus has been eliminated. Patrick had no contraindication to receiving live oral poliovirus vaccine and, hence, he received a fourth OPV at this visit.

Patrick had received an initial MMR vaccination, as recommended, at 12 to 15 months of age. A second MMR vaccine is routinely recommended at 4 to 6 years of age or 11 to 12 years of age. Patrick's family physician elected to provide the second vaccination at this time.

The varicella vaccination can also be administered to susceptible children at any time after 12 months of age, and unvaccinated children who lack a reliable history of chickenpox should be vaccinated at the 11- to 12-year-old visit. Patrick, however, had a reliable history of chickenpox at age 3 years and is not a candidate for vaccination at this time.

SUGGESTED READING

Casey PH, Evans LD: School readiness: An overview for pediatricians. Pediatr Rev 1993;14(1):4–10.

Chao J, Kikano GE: Lead poisoning in children. Am Fam Physician 1993;47(1):113–120.

Dietz WH, Robinson TN: Assessment and treatment of childhood obesity. Pediatr Rev 1993;14:337–343.

Kelly DP, Aylward GP: Attention deficits in school-aged children and adolescents. Current issues and practice. Pediatr Clin North Am 1992;39:487–512.

Levy HB, Harper CR, Weinberg WA: A practical approach to children failing in school. Pediatr Clin North Am 1992;39:895–928.

Reiff MI, Banez GA, Culbert TP: Children who have attentional disorders: Diagnosis and evaluation. Pediatr Rev 1993;14:455–464.

Shefflin Zal AJ: Attention deficit disorders: A family physician perspective. Fam Practice Recert 1994;16(8):21–32.

Tucker ME: Academy may not endorse CDC polio recommendation. Fam Practice News 1996;26(14):1–2.

QUESTIONS

1. True or false: In order to successfully participate in kindergarten, a preschool child must have
   a. Adequate physical health
   b. His or her 5th birthday at least 1 month before school entry
   c. Developmental skills typical of his or her peers
   d. The ability to read simple sentences

2. True or false: Groups of children more likely to have difficulty performing adequately in school include
   a. Children with low birth weight
   b. Children whose mothers smoked during pregnancy
   c. Preterm infants
   d. Children exposed to alcohol during pregnancy

3. True or false: The typical preschool child is a candidate for the following vaccinations:
   a. DTaP
   b. Hib
   c. MMR
   d. OPV

Answers appear on **page 605**.

Chapter 33

Abdominal Pain

Daniel T. Earl, D.O.

SUBJECTIVE

Eugene is a 19-year-old Caucasian male college student who has come to the emergency room with complaints of abdominal pain and vomiting. He had been well before this malady, noting that he had developed this pain rather suddenly about 12 hours ago.

Present Illness

Eugene noted that he has not had any unusual dietary patterns or precedent illness. He had no constipation, diarrhea, or fever. No other family members are or have been ill. He describes the abdominal pain as beginning in the midepigastrium, not relieved with position. The origin of the pain has gradually migrated to the right lower quadrant.

Past Medical History

Eugene had some exertional asthma when he was a child, which was relieved with the periodic use of an inhaled beta agonist. He has not seen a physician in the past 3 years, his last physical examination having been just before beginning college. He does not recall his last tetanus immunization, but did receive the hepatitis B vaccine. He denies any use of alcohol or tobacco products. He denies any other drug use. He has never been sexually active.

Family History

Eugene's father, an archeologist, is 53 years old and has well-controlled hypertension. His mother is 52 years old and is a professor at the local college. She has no significant medical problems. She takes estrogen and progestins daily for replacement therapy. Eugene's paternal grandparents are both deceased. His paternal grandfather died in World War II and his paternal grandmother died at age 75 years from complications following a cerebrovascular accident. His maternal grandfather is dead as well, succumbing to a myocardial infarction at age 70. His maternal grandmother is 85 years old and has well-controlled hypertension and non–insulin-dependent diabetes, for which she is taking an oral hypoglycemic twice a day. Eugene has one sibling, a sister, who is 24 years old and in excellent health.

Social History

Eugene is in his second year at a local college, where he is studying computer science. He is an excellent student. He has a part-time job at a local ice cream store, where he works mainly on the weekends. He lives in a dormitory on campus. He eats mostly at the cafeteria on campus, but goes home on most weekends where he eats with his parents. He has not noted any particular unique stressors in his life.

Review of Systems

Eugene notes no significant changes in his bowel habits, and he tends to have a bowel movement on a daily basis. He denies any fluctuations in his weight, and he has never had this kind of abdominal pain before. He denies any symptoms of reflux. His travel history is unremarkable.

OBJECTIVE

Physical Examination

Eugene is a young man of normal build, weighing 150 lb. Notably, he appears on examination to be in significant pain, unable to find a comfortable position. Vital signs include a blood pressure of 130/85 mm Hg, a pulse of 118, a respiratory rate of 22, and a temperature of 100.4°F.

Skin: no jaundice
HEENT: PERRL, EOMI, throat normal
Lungs: clear to auscultation
CV: tachycardic rate, but no gallops
Abdomen: The examination was done with the patient in supine position. He was wriggling and writhing in discomfort throughout, seemingly unable to find a comfortable position. His abdomen was scaphoid and without any scars. Bowel sounds were hypoactive. He was noticeably tender on palpation of the right lower quadrant, and muscle guarding was noted. Rebound pain was noted as well. A significant grimace was elicited with striking the heels.
Rectal: normal tone, guaiac negative, but nonspecific tenderness was elicited anteriorly.
GU: circumcised male phallus, Tanner stage V, testicles nontender, no hernia

Laboratory examinations revealed a white blood cell count of 15,500 per mm³, with 70 per cent segmented neutrophils and 30 per cent lymphocytes. Serum electrolyte levels were normal, as was a serum amylase level. A urinalysis revealed three to five white blood cells per high power field in an otherwise unremarkable sample. Radiographs of the abdomen (acute abdominal series) revealed no free air under the hemidiaphragm, and a nonspecific bowel gas pattern was noted. No fecolith or appendicolith was noted.

ASSESSMENT

Working Diagnosis

The most likely diagnosis is appendicitis with right lower quadrant pain, guarding, rebound tenderness, and leukocytosis.

Differential Diagnosis

1. Gastroenteritis. Gastroenteritis caused by a variety of agents, including *Campylobacter, Salmonella,* and *Shigella,* can produce severe abdominal pain, often with low-grade fever. In the absence of diarrhea or vomiting and with the duration of the severe pain (12 hours), however, gastroenteritis becomes less likely.

2. Mesenteric adenitis is inflammation of the lymph nodes surrounding the intestine. It is often diagnosed surgically when appendicitis is suspected. Its presentation can be very similar to that of appendicitis, but it is often preceded by an illness such as a viral infection. Adenitis usually resolves spontaneously.

3. Meckel diverticulum, classically described as "left-sided appendix." The inflammation of a Meckel diverticulum may cause symptoms similar to those of appendicitis. Meckel diverticulum problems usually occur in younger patients (those under 3 years old).

4. Hepatitis. Abdominal pain and anorexia can denote the beginning of hepatitis. The abdominal pain of acute hepatitis is usually not severe, however, and nausea and jaundice are usually associated.

5. Genitourinary disorder. Kidney stones, pyelonephritis, and other genitourinary problems can be associated with severe abdominal pain.

6. The differential diagnosis of acute abdominal pain in females is significantly more extensive than that in males. Gynecologic sources for pain are multiple, including infectious causes like pelvic inflammatory disease (PID), tubo-ovarian abscess (TOA), and salpingitis. Other causes include dysmenorrhea, which may range in intensity from mild to severe. Mittelschmerz is common but usually insignificant, except in rare cases when it produces enough bleeding to necessitate laparotomy. Anatomic causes may include endometriosis, ovarian cysts, ovarian torsion, and rarely an intrauterine device (IUD) that has migrated into the peritoneal cavity, producing peritonitis. One of the most feared conditions is ectopic pregnancy alone or ruptured ectopic pregnancy; therefore, ruling out pregnancy in women of childbearing status is critical.

7. Other phenomena may produce acute abdominal pain, including sickle cell crisis, withdrawal from drugs (particularly heroin), herpes zoster outbreak, pneumonia, inflammatory bowel disease, and typhoid fever. In acute myocardial infarction, abdominal pain may be the presenting complaint.

DIAGNOSIS

Abdominal pain is a common complaint, accounting for between 5 and 40 per cent of all emergency department visits. Almost half of the persons with abdominal pain are released without a definitive cause for their pain. Deciding which patients have a serious etiology for their pain can be frustrating.

Although many diseases can produce abdominal pain, acute and severe pain nearly always is a symptom of intra-abdominal pathology. It may be the sole guide to the need for an emergency or elective operation or determination whether the treatment should be nonsurgical.

Textbook descriptions of abdominal pain have significant limitations, because each individual reacts differently. Infants and children may be unable to localize their discomfort, and they have many diseases not seen in adults. Obese or elderly patients tend to tolerate pain better than others but may find it difficult to localize the pain. In contrast, some overwrought patients tend to exaggerate symptoms.

The challenge is in making the decision as to whether the patient has a "surgical abdomen," that is, one that has pathology necessitating surgical intervention. Abdominal pain can be acute, in which the question of urgent surgery always arises, or it can be chronic, in which case therapy (at least for a time) is medical.

The diagnosis of abdominal pain can be confusing, because there are myriad potential causes. The cause is established by a history, physical examination, and a carefully selected group of laboratory tests; however, of these, the history and physical examination are the most important.

The history, whenever possible, must be detailed, and in many cases it is sufficient to make the diagnosis. Remembering that "common things occur commonly," the clinician must direct the questions to the patient to clarify certain areas. Certain questions are always important (Table 33–1).

In Eugene's case, a surgical consultation was requested and surgery was performed. An inflamed appendix was removed, and Eugene had an uneventful hospital course, being discharged home 3 days after surgery.

DISCUSSION

Appendicitis is usually diagnosed with the combination of physical signs and symptoms, including sudden onset of epigastric or periumbilical pain followed by nausea and vomiting and, after a few hours, movement of pain to the right lower quadrant (RLQ). Right lower quadrant pain, rebound tenderness (pain in the RLQ with pressure on the left lower quadrant), low-grade fever (100–101°F) and leukocytosis (12,000 to 15,000/μL) characterize appendicitis.

The RLQ tenderness is classically located at McBurney's point (junction of the middle and outer

TABLE 33–1. Key Points in the History of Persons with Abdominal Pain

Pertinent Questions	Significance of Answers
Pain acute/chronic?	Chronic pain often is functional; however, a perforated duodenal ulcer or diverticulum can present with chronic pain
Onset sudden/gradual?	Sudden pain may reflect perforation of a viscus, ruptured ectopic pregnancy
Duration of the pain?	Colicky (on/off) pain may be biliary or renal in origin
Severity of pain?	Difficult to assess in some patients, particularly hysterical patients. Severe pain may reflect more serious intra-abdominal pathology (e.g., ruptured aneurysm)
Location of pain?	May directly reflect origin (e.g., renal pain over flank, radiating to testicle) or as referral of pain to particular areas (e.g., shoulder pain referred from gallbladder)
Character of the pain?	Is it ripping or tearing (aneurysm dissection) or knife-like, episodic (colicky?) or an ache (pyelonephritis)?
Associated symptoms?	Diarrhea? (gastroenteritis?) Vomiting? (appendicitis, gastroenteritis, or abdominal obstruction?)
Medication history?	Potassium tablets, tetracycline, and prednisone can all precipitate esophagitis, abdominal pain

thirds of the line joining the umbilicus to the anterior superior iliac spine). Rovsing's sign (pain felt in the RLQ resulting from palpation in the left lower quadrant) suggests peritoneal irritation. The psoas sign (worsening of pain with extension of the right hip joint, stretching the iliopsoas muscle) or adductor pain (produced by internal rotation of the flexed thigh) may suggest irritation of the appendix and surrounding peritoneum.

Bowel sounds are very important. Active peristalsis of normal pitch suggests a nonsurgical disease (e.g., gastroenteritis). High-pitched peristalsis or borborygmi in rushes suggest intestinal obstruction. Severe pain combined with a silent abdomen is an indication of intestinal paralysis and warrants surgical exploration. The pathophysiology usually is impaction of an appendicolith, with subsequent obstruction of the outflow of the appendix and inflammation of the intestinal wall. Obstruction of lumen by lymphoid hyperplasia (60%), fecolith (33%), foreign body (4%), stricture, tumor, parasitic infestation, and Crohn's stricture are also causes.

Atypical presentations of appendicitis are relatively common, particularly among children and elderly and obese patients. A high index of suspicion should be maintained for those patients, and additional tests to rule out appendicitis may be necessary. The presence of a few red blood cells (RBCs) in the urine may occur in appendicitis because of irritation of a ureter.

Other diagnostic tools that can be used include radiographic techniques. Plain radiographs of the abdomen (kidney, ureter, bladder—KUB) are helpful only in patients in whom bowel obstruction is considered or in whom an appendicolith is noted. An appendicolith is noted in about 15 per cent of surgically proven cases of appendicitis, and if visualized, it has a positive predictive value of greater than 95 per cent. Computed tomography (CT) of the abdomen is helpful in cases of abscess or perforation, but it is relatively ineffective in diagnosis of uncomplicated appendicitis. Barium enema used to be popular, but it has a fairly high false-positive rate. Ultrasonography (US) of the abdomen in the diagnosis of appendicitis is the subject of several studies and, with certain restrictions, is helpful. Sensitivity of US for diagnosis is about 80 per cent and specificity about 95 per cent. Positive predictive value is about 90 per cent. Those cases in which US is of less value include obese patients, in whom scanning is difficult. A reasonable algorithm for US may be that in typical cases of appendicitis, no scanning is necessary. Atypical cases, particularly in female patients, should be scanned by US. Patients with positive results on scans go to surgery; those with negative results either are watched or undergo further testing.

SUGGESTED READING

Catto JA. Acute appendicitis. In Tintinalli J, Ruiz E, Krome RL (eds). Emergency Medicine: A Comprehensive Study Guide, 4th ed. New York, McGraw-Hill, 1996, pp 461–463.

Rice PE, Abdominal pain: Predicting who will need an operation. Emerg Med 1996; April:14–25.

Silen W: Abdominal pain. In Isselbacher KJ, et al (eds): Harrison's Principles of Internal Medicine, 13th ed. New York, McGraw-Hill, 1994, pp 61–64.

Silen W. Cope's Early Diagnosis of the Acute Abdomen, 18th ed. New York, Oxford University Press, 1991.

Trott AT, Trunkey DD, Wilson SR. Acute abdominal pain: A guide to crisis management. Patient Care 1995; August 15:104–133.

QUESTIONS

1. Classic presentation of acute appendicitis occurs about what percentage of the time?
   a. 5%
   b. 20%
   c. 40%
   d. 75%
   e. 95%

2. Which of the following statements is *true* regarding the role of imaging in the diagnosis of acute appendicitis?
   a. CT scanning of the abdomen is a very effective method for diagnosing uncomplicated, unperforated appendicitis
   b. Radiographic imaging is unnecessary in most typical cases of uncomplicated appendicitis
   c. Routine plain radiographs of the abdomen are usually sensitive and specific in the diagnosis of acute appendicitis
   d. Ultrasonography of the abdomen is most helpful in diagnosis of acute appendicitis when the patient is obese

Answers appear on **page 605**.

Chapter 34

Breast Lump

Colleen Conry, M.D.

Breast cancer is the most common cause of cancer in women and the second leading cause of death from cancer, second only to lung cancer. In 1996, approximately 184,300 new cases of invasive breast cancer are expected to be diagnosed, and 44,300 women are expected to die from this disease (American Cancer Society, 1996). Evaluation of breast lumps is a common problem that demands that the family physician be alert for breast cancer and identify the etiology of the lump without delay. Fortunately, in combination with a good history and physical examination, various techniques are available to evaluate the breast in a step-wise logical manner.

Breast cancer survival is dependent on early detection; in general, more advanced stages at diagnosis have a lower survival rate. Five-year survival rates are estimated at 96 per cent when cancer is confined to the breast (local stage). Only 58 per cent of breast cancer is diagnosed at this early stage, however. Regional stages (cancer with spread to surrounding tissue) have a 75 per cent 5-year survival rate, and distant stages (cancer with metastases) have a 20 per cent 5-year survival rate (American Cancer Society, 1996). In addition to effective screening programs, efficient identification and evaluation of breast masses can help lower morbidity and mortality from breast cancer.

CASE EXAMPLE 1

Mrs. L.B. is a 46-year-old who presents with a 1-month history of a right breast lump. She has never had a lump before and does regular self-breast examination. The lump is nontender, and she has noted no nipple discharge. She has never had a mammogram. Her past medical history is significant for the birth of two children; the older is now 12. There is no family history of cancer; she is premenopausal, on no medications, does not smoke, and is 20 pounds overweight. The lump has seemed to increase in size over the past month; she expects her period to start any day.

On examination, the breasts are moderately dense with a 1×1-cm smooth, round mass in the upper outer quadrant of the right breast. The mass is somewhat mobile and nontender. There are no skin abnormalities. The remainder of the breast is normal.

CASE EXAMPLE 2

Ms. S.K. is a 62-year-old who presents with a 2-month history of a nontender breast lump. She is postmenopausal, on both estrogen and progestin hormone replacement. She smokes one pack of cigarettes per day. Her mother died at age 72 of breast cancer. She breast fed her six children. She has never had a mammogram and her last clinical breast examination was 5 years ago. On examination, the breasts are easy to examine with a 1×1-cm mass in the right upper outer quadrant. The mass is fixed to the underlying tissue and has irregular borders. The remainder of the breast is normal; no axillary nodes and no skin retractions are identified.

HISTORY

The initial step in the evaluation of a breast lump is a careful history about the lump itself. Duration of the mass, changes in the mass with time, associated pain, associated trauma, nipple discharge, and previous breast surgery are important factors. For premenopausal women the date of last menstrual period, length and regularity of cycles, and use of oral contraceptives should be elicited. Changes with the menses should be noted as well. Time since the onset of menopause and the use of estrogen replacement therapy are part of the history for postmenopausal women. The majority of breast complaints are breast masses; approximately 10 per cent of women presenting with breast complaints have breast pain and no mass, and nipple discharge accounts for approximately 3 to 10 per cent of breast complaints (Haagensen, 1986).

An assessment of the woman's risk factors for breast cancer should be included in the history.

Primary risk factors are female gender, increasing age, and family history. Although breast cancer is uncommon in men, about 1400 cases occur annually and should be considered in masses of the chest wall. The incidence of breast cancer in women rises rapidly in the fifth decade, and about 77 per cent of breast cancers occur in women over 50 years of age (American Cancer Society, 1996). The clinician must be aware, however, that 63 to 80 per cent of women who sued physicians for a delay in the diagnosis of breast cancer were younger than 50 years of age (Physicians Insurers Association of America, 1990).

Family history is a significant risk factor for breast cancer; the risk for women who have a first-degree relative (mother, sister, daughter) with breast cancer is 1.4 to 2.8 times higher than the risk for women with no family history of this cancer (National Cancer Institute, 1987; Harris and colleagues, 1992) (Table 34–1). New research has identified at least two genes located on chromosomes 17 and 13, BRCA1 and BRCA2, respectively, in patients in whom mutations are related to the development of breast cancer. An estimated 8 per cent of women have a genetic basis for inheriting breast cancer and up to 85 per cent of women with one of the abnormal breast cancer genes develop breast cancer (Szabo and King, 1995). Additionally, these abnormal genes have been linked to ovarian, colon, and prostate cancer. A careful family history can elicit

those women who are likely to have a genetic component to their cancer. Technology is available commercially to identify these genetic carriers, although the family physician must carefully counsel women on the implications of genetic testing.

Prior history of breast abnormalities is important in the initial evaluation of breast masses. Clinicians must be careful to ask for specific biopsy results, not just assurance that the results were benign. A biopsy-confirmed diagnosis of benign breast disease is associated with an increased risk of breast cancer, although several studies have suggested this increased risk is attributable to the pathologic diagnosis atypical hyperplasia (RR 2.2–5.0) (National Cancer Institute, 1987; Harris and colleagues, 1992).

Hormonal factors such as early age at menarche, late age at menopause, late age at first live birth, and exogenous hormones such as oral contraceptives and estrogen replacement therapy may increase a woman's risk of developing breast cancer (National Cancer Institute, 1987; Harris and colleagues, 1992). Hormones may promote cell division in breast tissue and increase the risk of mutation. Of five meta-analyses of postmenopausal hormones and breast cancer risk, two concluded that there was no increased risk, and three found only a small associated risk with long-term use (Colditz and colleagues, 1995). The addition of progestins to the estrogen therapy does not seem to increase the risk (Colditz and colleagues, 1995).

A summary of risk factors for breast cancer is outlined in Table 34–1. Care must be taken in interpretation of risk factors, because only 25 per cent of women with breast cancer have identifiable risk factors other than age and gender.

PHYSICAL EXAMINATION

Once a careful history has been obtained, a clinical breast examination (CBE) can be done. Ideally, the examination can be accomplished when ovarian hormones exert the least influence. For premenopausal women and women on cyclical postmenopausal estrogen replacement therapy, this date is 3 to 10 days after the onset of menstruation. Findings must be carefully documented in the patient record. Figure 34–1 demonstrates a sample documentation form. Excellent written descriptions and videotapes can be obtained to learn CBE (see Suggested Reading).

Many women's breasts are not identical, and small differences in size are of no concern. Changes in breast shape such as bulges of the breast contour

TABLE 34–1. Risk Factors for Breast Cancer

Risk Factor	Relative Risk
Family history of breast cancer (1st degree)	
One	1.4–2.8
Two	4.2–6.8
Nulliparity	1.5–1.9
First child born after age 30 years	1.9
First menstrual period before age 12 years	1.2–1.3
Last menstrual period after age 55 years	1.5–2.0
Atypical hyperplasia on previous biopsy	2.2–5.0
Obesity	1.2
Current oral contraceptive use	1.5
Past oral contraceptive use	1.0
Postmenopausal estrogen-replacement therapy	1.2–2.1
Alcohol use	
1 drink/day	1.4
2 drinks/day	1.7
3 drinks/day	2.0

Adapted from Harris JR, Lippman ME, Veronesi U, Willett W. Breast cancer. I. N Engl J Med 1992;327:319–328 and Dawson DA. Breast cancer risk factors and screening. DHHS publication number (PHS) 90–1500. Hyattsville, MD, U.S. Department of Health and Human Services, 1990.

Patient Name _____

Date _____

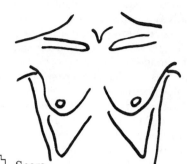

Comments:

✛ Scars

☆ Palpable Mass

// Dimpling

Right:
__ Normal
__ Abnormal, no change from previous visit
__ Abnormal, new changes but not suspicious
__ Abnormal, new changes suspicious for malignancy
Left:
__ Normal
__ Abnormal, no change from previous visit
__ Abnormal, new changes but not suspicious
__ Abnormal, new changes suspicious for malignancy

Figure 34–1. Breast physical examination.

or retractions can indicate a malignancy. Superficial tumors may cause skin retraction due to direct extension of tumor or fibrosis; deep tumors that involve the Cooper ligaments may also cause retraction. Edema of the skin of the breast (peau d'orange) is found most often in the inferior aspect of the breast and periareolar area. Edema usually occurs from obstruction of the dermal lymphatics with tumor cells, but the condition may also be caused by metastatic tumors of the axillary lymphatics. Erythema may be due to cellulitis or abscess in the breast, but a diagnosis of inflammatory carcinoma should always be considered. The new onset of nipple inversion should be regarded with a high index of suspicion, except when it occurs immediately after cessation of breast feeding. Ulceration and eczematous changes of the nipple may be the first signs of Paget disease.

Many premenopausal women have normal nodular irregularities of the breast tissue, particularly in the upper outer quadrants of the breast. Generalized lumpiness is not a pathologic finding. Many benign lesions have symmetrical examinations in both breasts, helping the examiner decide on further evaluation. A dominant breast mass has a density that differs from that of the adjacent breast tissue. The overall risk that a mass detected by either the patient or the physician will be cancer is 20 per

cent, unless there are indications that the mass is benign. Benign masses tend to feel soft or cystic, to have regular borders, and to be mobile. Even with these characteristics, however, a mass has a 10 per cent chance of being malignant (Mushlin, 1985). When a breast mass is associated with enlarged axillary lymph nodes, the chance of cancer is high.

Evaluation of the Breast Mass

An approach to the evaluation of a breast mass is shown in Figure 34–2. Initial management consists

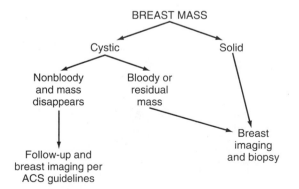

Figure 34–2. Breast mass evaluation. ACS = American Cancer Society.

of determination of whether the mass is cystic or solid. This determination may be accomplished by either cyst aspiration or ultrasound examination.

Cyst aspiration is both diagnostic and therapeutic and may be done in the office. The mass is stabilized with the nondominant hand, and a 22-gauge needle on a small syringe is placed directly into the mass. Thereafter, the plunger of the syringe is withdrawn. Local anesthesia is usually unnecessary, and its use may obscure the breast landmarks. It is important to document the exact location of the cyst before aspiration so that if an excisional biopsy is necessary it will include the involved area and the needle track.

Few complications arise from fine-needle aspiration. Ecchymosis and formation of a clinically apparent hematoma can occur, but they are rare. If a hematoma does occur, however, it can result in a false-positive mammogram reading. This risk should not deter aspiration, but the radiologist should be informed of the procedure. If the mass is not suspicious the mammogram should be delayed for 2 weeks. Other rare complications include infection and pneumothorax. There is a theoretical risk of spread of tumor along the needle track, although this has never been reported and it is felt to be a smaller risk with small-bore needles.

If the aspirate does not contain blood and the mass disappears completely, the patient should return for a follow-up visit in 1 to 2 months. In general, cytologic examination of the aspirated fluid is not performed because of low yield. Breast imaging to screen for other occult abnormalities should also be performed following the screening guidelines of the American Cancer Society (Table 34–2).

If aspiration of the mass is nonproductive, ultrasound can accurately distinguish between cystic and solid masses, and it may be used to guide cyst aspiration. Ultrasound is less accurate in differentiating between benign and malignant solid masses and should not be used in this manner.

TABLE 34–2. American Cancer Society Screening Guidelines for Breast Cancer

---

Breast self-exam
   Monthly for women age 20 years and older
Clinical breast exam
   Every 3 years for women age 20–40 years
   Every year for women over age 40 years
Screening mammography
   Every 1–2 years for women age 40–49 years
   Every year for women age 50 years and
   older

Diagnostic mammography and biopsy should be performed on cysts that contain bloody fluid or do not resolve with aspiration, and on masses from which no fluid can be removed. Because mammography has a sensitivity of only 75 to 90 per cent in distinguishing between benign and malignant disease, biopsy should also be performed on mammographically normal masses.

All masses must be resolved—they should disappear on aspiration or a tissue diagnosis should be made. When a mass is palpable, a biopsy always should be considered. Mammography before biopsy can confirm the presence of a malignant mass and can detect occult, nonpalpable malignant masses in either breast but does not rule out cancer in the palpable abnormality.

Biopsy

Fine-needle biopsy is becoming a popular procedure, because it can be done under local anesthesia in the office or radiology suite, it is minimally traumatic to the patient, and results can be obtained relatively quickly. The sensitivity of fine-needle biopsy is reported to be between 65 and 98 per cent, depending on the skills of the physician and pathologist (Kline, 1995). For optimal sensitivity the physician must be skilled in performing the procedure and must work closely with the pathologist to ensure that the slides are processed appropriately. Combining the procedure with ultrasound to confirm needle placement has improved the sensitivity. With fine-needle biopsy false-positive results are rare, but false-negative rates may be as high as 35 per cent (Layfield and colleagues, 1989). Common reasons for false-negative readings include inadequate sampling, usually due to inexperience; insufficient cells; tumors less than 1 cm, for which the target has presumably has been missed by the aspirating needle; tumors containing a large degree of fibrosis, large tumors with necrosis of the center or edema at the periphery; and interpretive errors, especially in cases of well differentiated tumors (Harris and colleagues, 1996). A positive test result provides information for appropriate treatment. If the result of fine-needle biopsy is negative and it is unclear if the biopsy was from the proper site, however, open biopsy is required.

Fine-needle biopsy is performed using a 22- to 25-gauge needle that is attached to a 10- to 20-ml syringe. When the needle enters the mass, suction is applied by retracting the plunger of the syringe. With suction maintained, the needle is advanced. To obtain sufficient tissue, the needle is directed to different areas of the mass, maintaining suction on the syringe at all times. This procedure allows cells to be drawn into the hub of the needle.

The suction should be slowly released before the needle is withdrawn from the mass. This technique prevents sudden aspiration of the contents into the barrel of the syringe, which makes collection of the specimen difficult. The needle contents are discharged onto one or more glass slides. A smear is made, and the material is prepared for staining. Alternatively, a fixative solution may be mixed with the cells; this step is followed by centrifugation and staining.

The other primary modality of biopsy is an open surgical biopsy, either excisional or incisional. Today, most biopsies are performed in the outpatient setting. This approach is more cost-effective; and if the biopsy sample is positive for malignancy, treatment options can be discussed with the patient before further intervention.

The decision of whether to refer the patient to a surgeon depends on the family physician's degree of comfort in managing breast complaints, his or her skills in performing cyst aspiration, and availability of fine-needle biopsy, surgical biopsy, and radiologic procedures.

DIFFERENTIAL DIAGNOSES

Possible results of biopsy include normal breast tissue, fibroademona, fibrocystic masses, breast cysts, and malignancy. The relative distribution is dependent on the woman's age. Fibroadenomas are most likely to occur in young women; it is uncommon to have a palpable fibroadenoma in a woman over the age of 40 years. Benign breast disease, also known as fibrocystic changes, can occur in any age group, but again is more common in women under the age of 40 years. Breast cysts are commonly found in women of age 40 to 55 years and are likely due to the hormonal fluctuations common in this perimenopausal age group. Carcinomas are found with increasing frequency as women age.

FOLLOW-UP

A critical element in the management of any breast abnormality is appropriate follow-up of the patient. All women with a benign breast mass should be seen within 1 to 2 months after diagnosis to confirm either resolution or absence of other problems. At this visit the family physician should confirm that appropriate mammographic screening has been completed and the result is normal, and that no new abnormalities have arisen. The psychological impact the evaluation of the breast mass has had on the woman and her current breast self-examination practice should be elicited. Because of the high incidence of breast cancer and widespread knowledge about the disease, simply being evaluated for a mass can have significant impact on a woman, even with a benign outcome. Some women may cease regular screening practices because of fear, reluctance to repeat the experience, or a false belief that they are now protected from further problems.

CASE DISCUSSIONS

CASE 1

Mrs. L.B.'s history is significant for a new breast lump that is increasing in size. She has not completed a menstrual cycle since noting the lump, thus its changes with the cycle are unknown. The lump is nontender and not associated with any other signs of malignancy. Her only risk factor for breast cancer is mild obesity. Mrs. L.B. is younger than 50 years of age; however, 20 per cent of breast cancers occur in women younger than 50 years. On examination, the mass has benign characteristics of smoothness and roundness, yet she still has a 10 per cent risk of this mass being malignant.

The initial step in managing Mrs. L.B.'s breast mass is needle aspiration of the mass. An alternative is careful documentation of the size and location of the mass and observation through one menstrual cycle. If the mass resolves, it can be assumed to be a cyst. Screening mammography should also be completed because she has never undergone mammography.

On needle aspiration, clear, straw-colored fluid was obtained and the mass disappeared. Screening mammography was normal. She returned for follow-up in 1 month and was noted to have no recurrence of the mass. Her final diagnosis was breast cyst, a common diagnosis particularly as women near menopause. Mrs. L.B. has a normal risk of developing breast cancer in the future and should receive annual clinical breast examinations and annual mammography beginning at age 50 years.

CASE 2

Mrs. S.K. presents with a worrisome breast mass and significant risk factors for breast cancer. She is older than 50 years and has a family history of breast cancer. No note is made of family members other than her mother who may have had breast cancer or other malignancies; this information should be obtained to evaluate for genetic carrier states. She is postmenopausal and is taking estrogen replacement therapy, which may slightly increase her risk. Studies do not suggest that smoking increases the risk of breast cancer. Older women's breasts are often easy to examine because much of the breast stroma has been replaced with fat. The irregular borders and fixed nature of the mass are very suggestive of malignancy.

Initial evaluation of this breast abnormality included

needle aspiration, which was negative for fluid. Ultrasound examination showed a solid mass, and fine-needle biopsy confirmed a breast carcinoma. Mrs. S.K. was referred to a surgeon for definitive therapy, and a modified radical mastectomy was done, with lymph nodes testing positive for metastasis at the time of surgery.

This case highlights the need for early screening for all women. All women should have yearly clinical breast examinations beginning at age 20 years and annual mammography testing after the age of 50 years. Although mammographic screening between the ages of 40 and 50 years is somewhat controversial, all organizations recommend annual screening for those older than 50 years. It is likely that Mrs. S.K.'s cancer could have been identified much earlier had she presented for regular screenings.

SUMMARY

A palpable breast mass must be carefully evaluated by history, physical examination, and mammography. The initial objective is to differentiate between a solid and cystic mass. All masses must either resolve or undergo tissue diagnosis. Mammography is an important adjunct to physical examination and cyst aspirations, but a negative mammography reading must never be substituted for pursuing a mass to a final diagnosis.

REFERENCES

American Cancer Society, Rosary CL, Ries LAG, Miller BA, et al: SEER Cancer Statistics Review, No. 95-2789. Bethesda, MD, 1995.

American Cancer Society: Cancer Facts and Figures—1996. Atlanta, American Cancer Society, 1996.

Colditz GA, Egan KM, Stampfer JM. Hormone replacement therapy and risk of breast cancer: Results from epidemiologic studies. Am J Obstet Gynecol 1993;168:1473–1480.

Colditz GA, Hankinson SE, Hunter DJ, et al. The use of estrogens and progestins and the risk of breast cancer in post-menopausal women. N Engl J Med 1995;332:1589–1593.

Dawson DA. Breast cancer risk factors and screening: United States, 1987. DHHS publication number (PHS) 90-1500. Hyattsville, MD, U.S. Department of Health and Human Services, 1990.

Haagensen CD. Diseases of the Breast, 3d ed. Philadelphia, W.B. Saunders, 1986, pp 501–533.

Harris JR, Lippman ME, Morrow M, Hellman S. Diseases of the Breast. Philadelphia, Lippincott-Raven, 1996.

Harris JR, Lippman ME, Veronesi U, Willett W. Breast cancer. I. N Engl J Med 1992;327:319–328.

Kline TS. Fine-needle aspiration biopsy of the breast. Am Fam Physician 1995;52:2121–2125.

Layfield LJ, Glasgow BJ, Cramer H. Fine-needle aspiration in the management of breast masses. Pathol Annu 1989;24:23.

Mushlin AI. Diagnostic tests in breast cancer. Clinical strategies based on diagnostic probabilities. Ann Intern Med 1985;103:79–85.

Physician Insurers Association of America. Breast cancer study. Lawrenceville, NJ, Physicians Insurers Association of America, 1990. National Cancer Institute. 1973–1992: Tables and Graphs. NIH Publication.

Szabo CI, King MC. Inherited breast and ovarian cancer. Hum Mol Genet 1995;4:1811–1817.

SUGGESTED READING

Clinical Breast Examination: Proficiency Criteria and Guidelines. American Cancer Society, California Division, 1989.

Haagensen CD. Diseases of the Breast, 3d ed. Philadelphia, W.B. Saunders, 1986.

Harris JR. Lippman ME, Morrow M, Hellman S. Diseases of the Breast. Philadelphia, Lippincott-Raven, 1996.

Love SL, Lindsey K. Dr. Susan Love's Breast Book. Reading, MA, Addison-Wesley, 1990.

QUESTIONS

Circle all the correct answers.

1. Which of the following increase a woman's risk for developing breast cancer?
   a. Age
   b. Gender
   c. Smoking
   d. Family history of breast cancer
   e. Family history of uterine cancer
   f. Atypical hyperplasia on breast biopsy
   g. Fibroadenoma on breast biopsy

2. Current American Cancer Society recommendations for screening include

a. Baseline mammogram at age 35 years
b. Biannual to annual mammogram beginning at 40 years, followed by annual mammogram from age 50 years
c. Annual mammogram beginning at age 50 years
d. Biannual mammogram from age 50 years
e. Mammography only in symptomatic women

3. Which of the following statements about patient follow-up are true?
   a. A patient with a cyst aspirate that is not bloody may be followed up at the next regular well-woman examination.

b. A 46-year-old patient with a mobile, smooth-walled mass on examination may be watched for one menstrual cycle prior to further evaluation.
c. A 58-year-old patient with a normal mammogram and solid mass by ultrasound should have a biopsy performed.
d. A 52-year-old patient has a cyst with a bloody aspirate. She should be re-evaluated in 3 months. If the cyst has recurred, the mass should be biopsied.

Answers appear on **page 605**.

Chapter **35**

Laceration Repair

Louis A. Kazal, Jr., M.D.

INITIAL VISIT—SUBJECTIVE

PRESENTING PROBLEM. Gus is a 32-year-old Caucasian male rancher who drove himself to the emergency room for evaluation of a 4-hour-old lacerated arm injured while he was hunting.

HISTORY OF PRESENTING ILLNESS. Gus had "dressed out" a five-point bull elk, and as he hoisted one of the hindquarters onto the bed of his truck, the broken end of the elk's femur lacerated the inside of his left arm. He applied pressure over the wound with a clean folded bandana, which stopped the bleeding. On arriving home 3 hours later, Gus was not going to seek medical attention, but his wife insisted that he see their family physician.

In the emergency room, his only concern was to ensure that stitches would not be necessary. There was no associated numbness or weakness.

PAST MEDICAL HISTORY. Gus has no history of a bleeding disorder or other medical illness. He has

been immunized against tetanus; his last tetanus booster was 12 years ago; there were no known allergies to, or current use of, any medications.

FAMILY HISTORY. Gus's father died of a myocardial infarction at age 48 years, as did his paternal grandfather at age 55 years. Gus's mother and two sisters are in good health.

HABITS. Gus does not use a seatbelt when driving. He has smoked two packs of cigarettes per day for 15 years. He rarely drinks alcohol.

SOCIAL HISTORY. Gus is a high school graduate who is currently a successful rancher in western Wyoming. He and his wife of 8 years have two healthy children.

REVIEW OF SYSTEMS. Gus last saw a physician 12 years ago after stepping on a rusty nail. His cholesterol level has never been checked. He coughs up yellow-

303

ish phlegm every morning. There is no history of hemoptysis.

Objective

Physical Examination

Gus was alert, cooperative and in no apparent distress. Alcohol was not detected on his breath. His vital signs were blood pressure 140/92, pulse 80, respirations 20, and temperature 98.6°F. He weighed 188 lb and stood 5 ft 10 in tall. A pack of cigarettes was noticed in his shirt pocket.

Examination of his left arm revealed a 2.5-cm laceration of the midforearm on the flexor surface. Small portions of the wound edges were jagged. Some dried blood covered the wound. He had no weakness with resistance to flexion of the left hand at the wrist or to pronation of the forearm. His biceps and brachioradialis reflexes were normal. The distal sensation and circulation in that extremity were intact.

Laboratory

No tests were ordered.

Assessment

1. Gus was diagnosed with what appeared to be an uncomplicated 2.5-cm laceration of the left forearm. (The full extent of the injury cannot be determined until it is explored.)

2. Gus does not use a seatbelt, which places him at increased risk for traumatic injury or death if he is involved in a motor vehicle accident. (Motor vehicle injuries are the number one cause of years of potential life lost before age 65 years. It is estimated that crash mortality can be reduced 40 to 50 percent with the use of lap and shoulder belts.)

3. Gus has a 30-pack-year history of smoking cigarettes (15 years × 2 packs per day). (Cigarettes are the leading preventable cause of death in the United States.)

4. Gus has an elevated blood pressure reading. (He is not labeled as hypertensive based on one measurement. This diagnosis typically requires two or more blood pressures recorded at separate times, and then the measurements, including the initial one, are averaged.)

5. Gus is mildly obese. (His body mass index [weight in kilograms divided by height in meters squared] is 27. A body mass index of 27 or greater is associated with an increased risk for obesity-related diseases.)

Plan

1. These findings were reviewed with Gus, and he gave verbal permission to assess and repair his injury. (Lacerations of the body and extremity should not be closed if older than 6 hours because they are prone to infection. An exception is sometimes made for those of the head and neck, which have excellent blood supply and may be repaired up to 12 hours after injury.)

2. Tetanus toxoid was given in his nondominant arm. (Tetanus prophylaxis is a priority in laceration care. If the patient has not been immunized against tetanus, 0.5 ml toxoid is given, repeated in 6 weeks, and again in 6 to 12 months. If the wound is tetanus-prone, 250 units of human tetanus antitoxin also is given at the initial visit. If the patient has been immunized and the wound is tetanus-prone, a booster is recommended when more than 5 years have lapsed since the last dose. For the immunized patient with a clean wound, a tetanus booster is not necessary unless it has been more than 10 years since the last dose.)

3. Gus's poor health maintenance record will be addressed during the laceration repair.

Procedure

1. Two milliliters of 1% lidocaine HCl (1% Xylocaine) without epinephrine were injected with a sterile 1.5-in 27-gauge needle through the open wound, infiltrating the surrounding tissue in a fanlike fashion.

   a. 1% Xylocaine is the drug of choice as a local anesthetic in laceration repair. Approximately 1 ml is required for each 2 cm of wound. The maximum adult dose with epinephrine is 7 mg per kg, and without epinephrine it is 4.5 mg per kg. *Note:* Each milliliter of 1% Xylocaine contains 10 ≧ of lidocaine HCl.

   b. Aqueous epinephrine combined with lidocaine is useful in closing lacerations of the scalp and other vascular areas. In tissues with less blood supply or in dirty wounds, routine use of lidocaine with epinephrine is discouraged because it decreases blood supply, leading to delayed healing and possible infection. Its use is contraindicated in the fingers, toes, penis, nose, and earlobes.

c. Anesthetic solutions should not be injected into rigid fascial compartments (tamponades neurovascular bundles). Regional blocks are preferred in these circumstances *after* evaluation of sensation and function.

d. Important cosmetic landmarks should be marked before injecting, and the least amount of local anesthetic should be used so as not to cause distortion and malalignment of the wound edges.

e. Pain can be minimized by injecting (1) slowly to avoid rapid distention of the tissue (using a 27-gauge needle assists in this goal); (2) through the opening of the wound in a fan-like fashion rather than repeatedly through the skin; and (3) with a longer needle (1.5 in), reducing the number of "sticks."

f. Local anesthetic should be infiltrated 1 cm into the wound margins. (Subcutaneous fat does not need to be anesthetized.)

g. Nonsterile gloves may be worn while administering the local anesthetic and sterile gloves used during the repair.

h. Small (1- to 2-cm) superficial lacerations requiring only a couple of sutures or staples (scalp) may be closed without an anesthetic.

2. After adequate local anesthesia was obtained, the wound was irrigated copiously with sterile saline, and the skin surrounding the wound was scrubbed with Hibiclens antiseptic. The field was then draped in a sterile fashion and illuminated.

a. Commonly used surgical preps are chlorhexidine gluconate (Hibiclens), povidone-iodine (Betadine), and hydrogen peroxide. Debate exists about which is the best solution because each has cytotoxic properties that interfere with wound healing and local immune response. Regardless, antiseptics should be kept from entering open wounds.

b. Irrigation is best accomplished using a large syringe (10–50 ml) with an 18-gauge Angiocath, providing jet-stream turbulence.

c. The practice of shaving hair about the wound should be avoided because it increases the rate of infection.

3. There was some oozing of blood easily controlled with sterile 4 × 4s and pressure.

4. The wound edges were slightly ragged. The laceration extended through the subcutaneous tis-

sue and fascia without injury to the underlying musculature. No debris was seen. Digital examination using a sterile gloved finger revealed no foreign body or disruption of the underlying structures.

5. Ample skin was present to permit débridement of the wound without resulting in excessive tension with closure. The damaged wound edges were trimmed with tissue scissors to produce symmetrical, freshly "squared off" edges with intact blood supply (Fig. 35–1).

a. Depending on the region of the body (i.e., how thick the skin is), it may be necessary to use a No. 15 blade scalpel instead of tissue scissors.

b. Débridement of devitalized tissue is essential whenever possible, except when it will compromise function or result in greater cosmetic deformity than expected if the crushed edges were closed.

c. If large areas of the wound margins are devitalized, or the edges are too jagged, the revision may need to be more extensive. When feasible, the tension lines or wrinkles in the skin are followed when revising a wound to

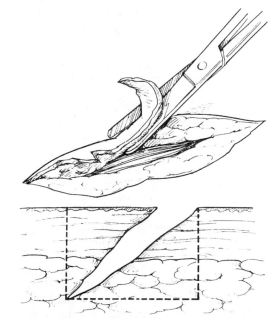

Figure 35–1. Wound revision. Jagged wound edges should be trimmed with tissue scissors or a No. 15 blade scalpel to produce a wound with even and vertical edges. Tangential wound edges, either left as such or made during revision, create a wider, more depressed scar due to retraction. (From Zuber TJ: Procedure: Wound management. In Rakel RE [ed]: Saunders Manual of Medical Practice. Philadelphia, W.B. Saunders, 1996, p 1008.)

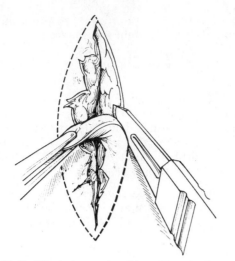

Figure 35–2. Elliptical wound revision. Wound edges with significant traumatic injury need to be revised, location permitting, by making an elliptical (ratio of length to width 3:1) excision of the wound with a No. 15 blade scalpel. (From Zuber TJ: Procedure: Wound management. In Rakel RE [ed]: Saunders Manual of Medical Practice. Philadelphia, W.B. Saunders, 1996, p 1008.)

minimize the retractive forces on the wound. An ellipse is made with a No. 15 blade scalpel parallel to the lines of tension (Fig. 35–2). It requires a length:width ratio of approximately 3:1 to avoid an uneven closure.

6. The new wound edges were bluntly undermined with tissue scissors.

   a. Most wounds require some degree of undermining, especially if there has been loss of tissue.
   b. Undermining the edges 4 to 5 mm reduces tension on the wound by disrupting the elastic fibers that cause inversion of the skin edges.
   c. The safest level at which to undermine is just below the dermal-fat junction. Such a precaution helps avoid injury to deeper blood vessels and nerves. In some lacerations of the trunk and extremities, it may be necessary to undermine at the fat-fascial level.
   d. The ends of slightly opened tissue scissors can be entered between the dermis and fat and the tissue spread apart by gently opening the scissors. The edge of a scalpel blade can also be used to tease open this tissue plane.

7. The wound was reirrigated with sterile saline.

8. Hemostasis was achieved with steady compression of the wound with a sterile 4 × 4 for 5 minutes. Health maintenance issues were discussed during this time.

   a. Hemostasis usually can be attained in 5 to 10 minutes with compression.
   b. Prevention of hematoma formation is critical for proper wound healing. Hematomas cause wider scars by increasing wound tension and by separating the skin edges. Wound edges also may necrose when capillary ingrowth to the skin is prevented by hematoma formation. Additionally, hematomas promote infection by providing a source of culture medium for bacteria.

9. The revised laceration was closed in layers, the *deep* layer first, with interrupted simple sutures of 4–0 Vicryl with inverted knots (Fig. 35–3).

   a. Closing all "dead space" is essential. Closing the space reduces tension on the healing skin edges and decreases the chance of hematoma formation.
   b. The size of suture is dependent on the location of the laceration and degree of tension. The smaller the number, the thicker and stronger the suture. For the deep layer, a 2–0 or 3–0 absorbable suture is used in the extremities, and a 4–0 or 5–0 size is used in the face.
   c. Absorbable sutures such as polyglactic acid (Vicryl), polyglycolic acid (Dexon), or chromic catgut swedged on a curved cutting needle are typically used to close the deep and subcutaneous layers.
   d. Knots should be inverted (buried), with the ends of the suture closely cut.
   e. The deeper layers should be approximated so that the skin edges come together evenly

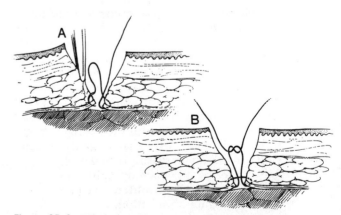

Figure 35–3. The inverted knot. Deep sutures should be tied so that the knots are buried below the layer being closed. This prevents the knots from interfering with the approximation of wound edges and minimizes tissue reaction to suture near the skin's surface. *(A)* Start under one edge, and *(B)* end underneath on the opposite side.

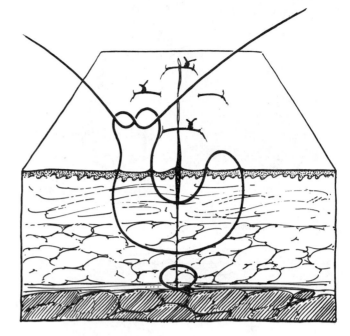

Figure 35–4. Alternating simple and vertical mattress sutures. The vertical mattress suture is an excellent technique to evert wound edges. The increased width of the deep portion of this double-layered suture also provides added wound support.

with little tension. These layers include the dermal-fat and fat-fascial junctions, depending on the depth of the laceration. In this case, the skin on the inside of the forearm was thin, and, therefore, the dermal-fat layer was able to be approximated with the skin closure, as described later.

10. The skin was closed with a combination of alternating vertical mattress and simple sutures using 4–0 Ethilon (Fig. 35–4).

   a. A major goal in laceration repair is the gentle approximation of everted skin edges, which allows for the matching of the regenerating basal layer of skin to produce a thinner scar that heals flatly without a ridge.

   b. Simple sutures evert the wound edges if (1) the needle enters and exits the skin at identical distances from each edge; (2) they are deeper than they are wide; and (3) the "base" of the loop incorporates more tissue than its epidermal counterpart (Fig. 35–5).

   c. In areas of thin skin or increased tension, a vertical mattress suture effectively everts the wound edges. A mattress suture is stronger than the simple suture and is often used on extremities. Alternating vertical mattress and simple sutures is a common practice. This takes some of the remaining tension off the larger vertical mattress sutures, decreasing stitch scarring.

   d. Use the smallest suture possible: 6–0 on the face, 5–0 or 4–0 on the trunk and extremities, and 4–0 on the back or other thick-skinned areas.

   e. Stitch marks occur when sutures are (1) too heavy a gauge; (2) too long (distance from entrance to exit sites); (3) too tight; (4) left in too long; or (5) when they incorporate too much tissue.

   f. The skin layer is usually closed with nonabsorbable monofilament suture, either nylon (Ethilon or Dermalon) or polypropylene (Prolene or Surgilene) on a curved needle.

   g. Start the closure at one corner of the wound and work toward the other (unless an anatomic landmark is present, which is then approximated first). The needle should enter and exit the skin at a distance from the edge equal to the skin's thickness, usually about 3 to 4 mm. Sutures should be placed at a distance from each other equal to their length.

   h. The skin needs to be handled as atraumatically as possible by using skin hooks or by gently grasping the fat-dermal junction with tissue forceps held parallel to the plane of the skin.

   i. Knots are tied with the needle holder by a technique known as the "instrument tie." A surgeon's knot is made, followed by a second knot that is not squared and is incompletely tightened, leaving a tiny loop. The third and

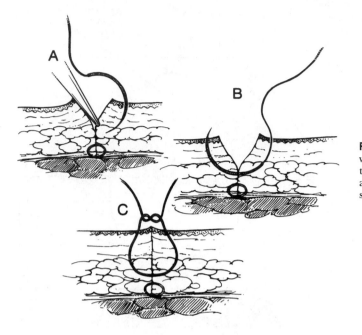

Figure 35–5. The simple suture. This basic suture everts wound edges when placed correctly. *(A)* Begin by piercing the skin with the needle at a right angle or greater. *(B)* Take a bite of tissue that is deeper than it is wide. *(C)* Exit the skin symmetrically on the opposite side of the wound.

fourth knots are squared. The clinician must remember to approximate, not strangulate, the tissue when tying knots.

11. The laceration repair was cleansed and dried. Benzoin was applied with a cotton swab to the skin on both sides of the closed laceration. Steri-Strips were placed across the wound, and the drapes were removed.

  a. Repairs are cleansed with either normal saline or hydrogen peroxide.
  b. Steri-Strips are sterile microporous tape of various widths that add support to the repair, thus taking some tension off the sutures. They are applied on one side of the laceration up to the skin edge, drawn across the repair, and then pressed down on the other side.
  c. Tincture of benzoin is a liquid that makes the skin more adhesive after it dries, allowing the Steri-Strips to be more effective and help them remain in place longer.

Disposition

1. Gus was asked to keep the wound clean and dry and to rest and elevate his arm over the next 24 hours.

2. Signs of infection (i.e., fever, redness, tenderness, increased local warmth, or purulent discharge) were explained, for which he would need to return earlier than the scheduled follow-up in 2 days.

3. The dressing was to be changed after 24 hours, and any dry blood removed from the sutures with hydrogen peroxide.

4. Gus was educated about the need to use a seatbelt when driving and advised to stop smoking.

5. Gus's blood pressure will be rechecked at the time of follow-up and again when his sutures are removed. Because of his risk factors for coronary artery disease (cigarette smoking, male sex, positive family history, and obesity), a fasting lipid profile instead of a random screening cholesterol will be ordered.

6. Gus was encouraged to give consideration to a diet and exercise program.

FIRST FOLLOW-UP VISIT—SUBJECTIVE

Gus returned for follow-up and had no concerns about his arm. He was not aware of any fever and had no pain or paresthesias. He was happy to report that he stopped smoking cigarettes and has already started to "watch" what he eats. His wife says he wore his seatbelt today.

Objective

Gus had no fever, and his blood pressure was 118/78, with a pulse of 70. There were no cigarettes in his pocket. The dressing was dry, and no distal edema was noted. His circulation, sensation, and function remained normal. The dressing was removed. The wound was clean and dry without signs of infection. There was no necrosis of the skin edges or hematoma formation. The wound edges were slightly everted and well approximated.

Assessment

1. The revised layered repair of Gus's 2.5-cm laceration of the left forearm was healing well without signs of infection.

2. Gus's blood pressure was within normal limits today.

3. Gus has discontinued his cigarette habit.

Plan

1. Gus will return in 7 days for suture removal.

2. Gus will continue to keep the wound clean and protect it with an adhesive bandage.

3. Gus was congratulated on his cessation of smoking, use of a seatbelt, and attention to diet.

4. Gus's blood pressure will be recorded by a friend (nurse) each week for 3 weeks, and he is to return to the office with these readings.

5. Blood for the lipid profile was drawn, and the results will be discussed with him at his next visit. At that time, an appropriate diet and exercise plan also will be outlined.

DISCUSSION

The schedule for suture removal is approximately 3 to 5 days for the face, 5 to 7 days for the scalp, 7 to 10 days for the trunk and extremities, and 10 to 14 days for the back, hands, and feet. If a patient returns for suture removal and has a slow-healing wound with areas that may separate, partial suture removal should be considered as an option to minimize stitch scarring. Steri-Strips are applied in places where sutures were removed, and the remaining sutures are taken out as soon as possible.

Scars require 2 years to fully mature, during which time they become less erythematous and hypertrophic. Progressive collagen turnover results in retraction and produces a softer scar. Any revision should be delayed until this process of remodeling is complete.

Scarring in areas of cosmetic significance may be minimized by daily massage and protection from the sun. Massaging is started approximately 2 weeks after laceration repair and a regimen of 5 minutes twice daily for about 3 months is recommended. Sunblock and shading are used to limit sun exposure until the scar is mature. This after-laceration care may produce a softer, flatter, and less noticeable scar.

SUGGESTED READING

Breitenbach KL, Bergera JJ. Principles and techniques of primary wound closure. In Snell GF (ed.). Office Surgery. Primary Care Clin Office Pract 1986;13:(3):411–431.

Dushoff IM. A stitch in time. Emerg Med 1973;5:21–43.

Moy RL, Lee A, Zalka A. Commonly used suturing techniques in skin surgery. Am Fam Physician 1991;44:1625–1634.

Zuber TJ. Wound management. In Rakel RE (ed.). Saunders Manual of Medical Practice. Philadelphia, W.B. Saunders, 1996, pp 1007–1008.

QUESTIONS

1. An 18-year-old female whose immunizations are up-to-date presents on Sunday afternoon with a 1-cm laceration of the lower leg caused by a piece of rusted barbed wire. The injury occurred the previous morning. Her last tetanus booster was 2 years ago. Appropriate intervention(s) is/are

   a. Immunoglobulin
   b. Cleansing of the wound
   c. Tetanus booster
   d. Steri-Strip closure of the laceration
   e. Suture repair of the laceration

2. Scarring from skin sutures is a problem when they

remain in place longer than required. Match the ideal time of suture removal with the appropriate wound location.

a. 3 to 5 days
b. 7 days
c. 10 to 14 days

d. 21 days
   (1) A 3-cm elliptical excision of a 1-cm melanocytic nevus on the back.
   (2) A superficial 1.5-cm laceration of the forehead.
   (3) A 2-cm laceration of the scalp over the external occipital protuberance.

Answers appear on **page 605.**

C h a p t e r   36

Vaginal Discharge

Karl E. Miller, M.D.

Subjective

Sandra, a 23-year-old woman, presents to the office with a 2-week history of vaginal discharge. She describes the discharge as being white and thin with a fishy odor. She states that she has never had this type of discharge in the past. She has noticed that the odor and discharge are worse after she has intercourse. She denies any itching with the discharge. She also denies any swelling or pain in the genital area. She denies any dyspareunia, abdominal pain, nausea, vomiting, fevers, chills, or sweats. She is currently sexually active and is using an intrauterine device (IUD) as her contraceptive method. For the last 6 months she has been in a monogamous relationship and her partner is having no symptoms. She does state that age of first intercourse was 16 and that she has had six partners. She does have a past history of a chlamydial infection 1 year ago that was treated with oral antibiotics. Her last menstrual period was 3 weeks ago and was normal. She denies any chronic medical problems and is on no routine medications. She also denies any recent antibiotic therapy.

Objective

PHYSICAL EXAMINATION. The patient is afebrile with normal vital signs. General appearance shows no acute distress. Abdominal examination demonstrates no tenderness, rebound, or guarding. No liver edge tenderness is noted. Genital examination reveals a small amount of thin white, homogeneous discharge around the introitus with no erythema, lesions, or swelling around the labia. The cervix is normal in appearance and no discharge is noted in the os. The IUD string is in place. Copious amounts of a thin homogeneous white discharge that has a fishy odor is noted in the vaginal vault and part of the discharge is adherent to the vaginal wall. *Chlamydia* and gonorrhea specimens are obtained from the os. Wet preparation/potassium hydroxide sample is obtained from the vaginal vault. The uterus is normal size, nontender with cervical manipulation, and nontender on palpation. The adnexa is negative for any tenderness, and the ovaries are normal in size.

LABORATORY TESTS. The pH on the discharge is 5.5 and clue cells are noted on the wet preparation. The "sniff" test, adding potassium hydroxide to the discharge, is positive with a fishy odor. The *Chlamydia* and gonorrhea tests are negative (results were available later).

Assessment

Vaginal discharge—bacterial vaginosis.

Plan

The patient is treated with metronidazole (Flagyl) 500 mg twice daily for 7 days. She is advised to avoid alcohol consumption while taking the metronidazole.

DIFFERENTIAL DIAGNOSIS

1. *Bacterial vaginosis.* This is the most likely diagnosis because the patient meets the following criteria: (1) an off-white, adherent vaginal discharge; (2) vaginal pH greater than 4.5; (3) clue cells present microscopically; and (4) a positive sniff test. Patients must have at least three out of four of these criteria present in order to make a diagnosis of bacterial vaginosis.

2. *Vulvovaginal candidiasis.* The presenting symptom with this diagnosis is a thick whitish, almost cottage cheese–like discharge that has no odor and the patient complains of significant pruritus on both external and internal genitalia. On physical examination, the vulvovaginal area can be edematous with erythema. The discharge has a vaginal pH between 4.0 and 5.0. Microscopically, there is budding yeast and hyphae after applying potassium hydroxide.

3. *Trichomoniasis.* The discharge from this infectious process is a thin, frothy, green-yellow or gray malodorous discharge. Women can present with vaginal soreness or dyspareunia. On physical examination, the cervix can have a "strawberry" red appearance or there may be erythema on the vagina or external genitalia. The vaginal secretions have a pH greater than 5.0 and more than 10 white blood cells (WBCs) per high-power field. Using a wet mount preparation, the diagnosis can be confirmed by identifying mobile trichomonad.

4. Chlamydia *Infection and Gonorrhea.* These two infections need to be considered anytime a female patient presents with a vaginal discharge. The main risk factors for these infections are patient under age 25, history of multiple sexual partners, previous history of sexually transmitted diseases (STDs), and nonbarrier contraception. The patient in this case meets all the risk factors for these two STDs. The presentation of a vaginal discharge is the most common presenting complaint with these two infections, but the majority of women are asymptomatic. The cultures are negative for both STDs.

5. *Pelvic inflammatory disease (PID).* In any female patient who presents with a vaginal discharge, this diagnosis needs to be considered in the differential diagnosis. Any patient who is at risk for *Chlamydia* or gonorrhea infection should have cultures performed to evaluate for these two organisms. However, the patient does not meet the criteria to establish this as the appropriate diagnosis.

DISCUSSION

Bacterial Vaginosis

Bacterial vaginosis is the most common vaginal infection seen in the ambulatory setting. This infection develops when there is a change in the normal vaginal flora allowing the growth of multiple organisms that are responsible for the symptoms associated with this infection. The cause of this change is unclear at the present time, but there are certain factors that place the patient at risk for this infection including menstruation, concomitant vaginal infection, sexual activity, multiple sexual partners, hygiene, contraceptive use, and abnormal uterine bleeding.

The presenting symptoms in bacterial vaginosis range from asymptomatic infections found on various routine screening examinations to symptoms consistent with pelvic inflammatory disease. The majority of women are asymptomatic. If they do present with a discharge it is usually a malodorous white, homogeneous vaginal discharge with no associated pruritus.

Establishing an accurate diagnosis of bacterial vaginosis is sometimes difficult. There are four criteria developed to assist in improving the accuracy of the diagnosis, and at least three of the following four criteria must be met: (1) off-white, creamy adherent vaginal discharge; (2) vaginal pH greater than 4.5; (3) clue cells present microscopically; and (4) a positive sniff test. Clue cells are squamous epithelial cells coated with bacteria that are observed using normal saline preparation to create a microscopic slide. The sniff test is performed by applying potassium hydroxide to the secretions. The addition of this chemical releases a "fishy" odor. Vaginal cultures do not assist in making the diagnosis because of the polymicrobial nature of this infection.

Treatment options for bacterial vaginosis include oral and topical vaginal preparations. The oral options are metronidazole (Flagyl) 500 mg twice daily for 7 days or 2 gm twice daily for 1 day, and clindamycin 300 mg twice daily for 7 days. The topical vaginal creams include metronidazole vaginal gel (MetroGel) 5 gm daily for 5 days and clindamycin vaginal cream 5 gm vaginally for 7 days. There are no advantages to any of these regimens with regard to cure rates and post-treatment vulvovaginal candidiasis; however, patients report more satisfaction with the vaginal preparations.

Chlamydia Infection

Chlamydia infection is one of the most common STDs in the United States. In women the reported infection rate may be lower than what it actually should be because the majority of infected women are asymptomatic. Another important fact is that the majority of *Chlamydia* infections in women cannot be accurately assessed by physicians based on patients' risk assessments and physical findings. These two factors make it difficult to detect and treat chlamydia infections in the early stages.

The most common presenting complaint, if any are present, of women with *Chlamydia* infections is a vaginal discharge. Other possible symptoms include vaginal bleeding or spotting, particularly after intercourse, lower abdominal pain, and irregular or heavy menses. Pleuritic right upper quadrant abdominal pain with or without pelvic pain can be a rare presentation of *Chlamydia* infection. The pelvic examination findings include a mucopurulent discharge coming from the cervical os and a friable and edematous-appearing cervix. Other possible physical findings include uterine and/or cervical motion tenderness from endometritis or PID, and adnexal masses or tenderness related to salpingitis or abscesses. The presenting complex of right upper quadrant pain with a fever and tenderness in the right upper quadrant (with or without pelvic tenderness) is indicative of perihepatitis (Fitz-Hugh–Curtis syndrome) related to *Chlamydia* infections.

Because there are a large number of asymptomatic patients with *Chlamydia* infections, the following criteria were developed to determine which patients should be screened: (1) sexually active adolescents; (2) women who do not use barrier contraceptive devices and have had more than one sexual partner in the last 3 months; (3) women who are pregnant; (4) women who are undergoing an abortion; (5) women with a mucopurulent cervical discharge; and (6) women with rectal pain, tenesmus, bleeding, or discharge.

The "gold standard" for establishing the diagnosis of *Chlamydia* infections is culturing the discharge. In order to collect an adequate sample for these cultures, a Dacron swab must be used, placed in the cervix for at least 30 seconds, and then placed in the appropriate culture media. The disadvantage to using cultures is that they are expensive and take 3 to 7 days before test results can be finalized.

Nonculture techniques are available that are less expensive and test results are much quicker. These tests are specific but have a higher false-negative rate than the culture method. If these nonculture tests are negative, this needs to be confirmed by the culture technique.

If the patient has a significant number of signs and symptoms suggesting PID or salpingitis, a WBC count with a differential should be performed. Also, a serum pregnancy test and a pelvic ultrasound may be required in patients with salpingitis to rule out ectopic pregnancy.

The recommended treatment for *Chlamydia* infections is doxycycline 100 mg orally twice a day for 7 days. This agent is inexpensive in its generic form and is very effective against *Chlamydia* infections. Azithromycin (Zithromax) in a single 1-gm dose orally is an alternative regimen. The advantage to this regimen is that it can enhance compliance with the disadvantage being that this medication is more expensive than doxycycline. Doxycycline remains the drug of choice unless there are concerns about patients' compliance. Potential side effects from doxycycline and azithromycin include nausea, diarrhea, vomiting, and stomach pain. If patients cannot tolerate either of these two drugs, ofloxacin (Floxin) and erythromycin are possible alternatives. Pregnant patients with *Chlamydia* infections need to be treated with an erythromycin base 500 mg four times per day for 7 days. In patients unable to tolerate erythromycin, amoxicillin 500 mg three times per day for 7 to 10 days is a less effective, but better tolerated regimen.

In patients requiring hospitalization because of the severity of the illness or because of inadequate response to outpatient treatment, the PID treatment should be used (see discussion later in the chapter).

Gonorrhea

One of the most commonly reported STDs is gonorrhea. There has been an overall decline in the total number of reported gonorrhea cases except in the adolescent and inner-city populations. The incubation time tends to be 3 to 5 days after exposure and women are at greater risk for contracting this infection.

The most common site of gonorrhea infection is the endocervix, but it can involve the urethra, Bartholin glands, or anus. Women with this infection can exhibit symptoms such as vaginal discharge, dysuria, abnormal vaginal bleeding, and pelvic pain. Similar to *Chlamydia* infections, the majority of women with gonococcal infections are asymptomatic. On physical examination, the cervix can appear normal or can be inflamed with mucopurulent exudate.

There are nongenital gonococcal infections that can develop from direct or contiguous spread or by dissemination through the blood stream. The nongenital infections include the following: PID, anorectal gonorrhea, perihepatitis (Fitz-Hugh–Curtis syndrome), conjunctivitis, and pharyngitis. One common nongenital form is anorectal gonorrhea, which can occur from either direct sexual contact or by extension of the vaginal infection. The presenting symptoms in patients with anorectal infections can range from no symptoms, to mild pruritus and mucoid discharge, to severe proctitis. Gonococcal pharyngitis usually presents with no symptoms but when patients are symptomatic they usually present with a mild sore throat and an erythematous pharynx. An exudative tonsillitis or oral ulcer lesion can also occur with this infection. Gonococcal conjunctivitis occurs after a direct-contact exposure and patients present with extensive inflammation and copious amounts of purulent secretions.

Gonorrhea can develop into disseminated infections, which occurs in two stages. The bacteremic stage is first and is distinguished by fevers, chills, and typical skin lesions. The skin lesions appear initially as small vesicles, then develop into pustules with a hemorrhagic base and central necrosis. These skin lesions usually occur on the volar aspect of the hands and digits. Other symptoms in this stage consist of joint stiffness and pain. In the second, or septic arthritis, stage a purulent synovial effusion occurs more commonly in the knees, ankles, and wrists.

In order to establish the diagnosis of gonococcal infections in women the isolation of the organism by cultures is required. Appropriate sampling and handling techniques are vital to assure an accurate diagnosis. The specimen samples are taken from the endocervical canal or the suspected area in nongenital infections using a cotton-tipped applicator. The sample is then plated out on Thayer-Martin medium, and placed in a carbon dioxide–rich environment.

The classic treatment of gonorrhea was penicillin. However, there has been a significant increase in gonococcal strains that are resistant to penicillin. Because of these resistant strains, the treatment recommendation is ceftriaxone (Rocephin) 125 mg intramuscularly. Alternative therapies are ciprofloxacin (Cipro) 500 mg, or ofloxacin (Floxin) 400 mg, in one single oral dose. These two options are less than ideal because there has been an increase in the number of gonococcal strains that are resistant to the fluoroquinolones. Therefore, ceftriaxone continues to be first-line therapy. Because of the high number of concomitant *Chlamydia* infections in patients suspected of having a gonococcal infection, treatment for both gonorrhea and *Chlamydia* is recommended. In the case of disseminated gonorrhea infections, intravenous ceftriaxone for 1 week is the recommended treatment.

Pelvic Inflammatory Disease

Pelvic inflammatory disease (PID) includes a broad spectrum of ascending infections that involve the upper reproductive tract in women. The diagnosis of PID includes any combination of endometritis, salpingitis, tubo-ovarian abscess, and pelvic peritonitis. The infection has a significant impact on women during their reproductive years with approximately 1 in 10 in this age group developing PID. Not only is PID prevalent, it can also cause a significant morbidity in infected women including infertility, ectopic pregnancy, and chronic pelvic pain.

The difficulty in diagnosing acute PID is that patients can present with a wide variety of symptoms. The presenting symptoms are directly correlated to the severity of the infection. The most common presenting complaint is lower abdominal pain. However, in some patients with PID, this symptom may be absent. The abdominal pain is usually exacerbated by coitus or Valsalva maneuvers. The other symptoms associated with PID include vaginal discharge or bleeding, gastrointestinal upset, and urinary tract symptoms.

Lower abdominal tenderness, adnexal tenderness, and cervical motion tenderness are some of the physical examination findings in patients with PID. Other findings that can be present include fever, and abnormal cervical or vaginal discharge.

In evaluation of patients with PID a sedimentation rate or a C-reactive protein level can assist in establishing the diagnosis and evaluating the severity of the infection. These two tests are nonspecific and can be elevated in any inflammatory condition, or they can be normal in patients with known PID. Nonculture *Chlamydia* testing can be performed and if negative, followed with cultures in order to reduce the number of false-negative results. The other culture that must be performed is for gonorrhea. Because PID is a polymicrobial process, negative tests for *Chlamydia* and gonorrhea do not rule out PID. One important point to consider is that cultures need to be obtained before initiation of any antibiotic therapy. Because of the similarity between PID and ectopic pregnancy, a serum pregnancy test should be performed on all patients suspected of PID.

Two other evaluative methods that can be used in patients suspected of PID include the pelvic ultrasound with a vaginal probe and laparoscopy. The ultrasound can help evaluate the pelvic structures if the physical examination suggests abdominal tenderness or if obesity makes the pelvic examination difficult to assess. The ultrasound can also assist in evaluating any suspected tubo-ovarian abscesses or assessing the adnexa for ectopic pregnancy. The best method for establishing the diagnosis of PID is laparoscopy. Because there are risks associated with this procedure, laparoscopy is reserved for those patients who are hospitalized and are not responding to appropriate antibiotic therapy. It can also be used when an adnexal mass is discovered to evaluate for tubo-ovarian abscesses.

The accurate diagnosis of PID is difficult to establish in patients because of the spectrum of presentations. In order to reduce the number of unrecognized PID cases, diagnostic criteria were developed by the Centers for Disease Control and Prevention (CDC). The minimal criteria that all patients must have is lower abdominal pain, adnexal tenderness, and cervical motion tenderness. Additional criteria include an elevated temperature, abnormal cervical or vaginal discharge, an elevated sedimentation rate or C-reactive protein levels, or a positive screen or culture for *Chlamydia* or gonorrhea. One important factor to consider is that in any suspected case of PID, it is critical to initiate therapy before confirming the diagnosis. It is preferable to treat presumptively than to wait until a definitive diagnosis has been established.

The majority of time patients with PID can be treated as outpatients. When determining if the patient is a candidate for inpatient therapy, there are established criteria developed by the CDC to assist in making this decision. The criteria for inpatient therapy includes uncertain diagnosis; presence of pelvic abscess; pregnant patients; patients at high risk for poor compliance; patients with human immunodeficiency virus (HIV), severe illness, or nausea and vomiting; patients unable to tolerate outpatient therapy; or patients who fail to respond clinically or cannot be followed up in 72 hours. Inpatient therapy with parental antibiotics is indicated in patients who meet any of these criteria.

The recommended outpatient treatment of PID is ceftriaxone (Rocephin) 250 mg intramuscularly, (or other parental third-generation cephalosporin) plus doxycycline 100 mg orally twice a day for 14 days. An alternative regimen is ofloxacin (Floxin) 400 mg twice a day for 14 days plus clindamycin 450

mg four times per day or metronidazole (Flagyl) 500 mg two times per day for 14 days. If outpatient PID therapy is used, it is vital to reassess patients in 72 hours to determine their response to the therapy.

In patients who require inpatient therapy, there are two treatment options. The first option is cefoxitin (Mefoxin) 2 gm intravenously (IV) every 6 hours or cefotetan (Cefotan) 2 gm IV every 12 hours plus doxycycline 100 mg IV every 12 hours. The second option is clindamycin 900 mg every 8 hours plus gentamicin IV in a loading dose followed by maintenance therapy. Both regimens need to be maintained for at least 48 hours or until the patient has a clinical response. In order to complete the treatment regimen after stopping the IV therapy, doxycycline 100 mg orally for 14 days is the recommended regimen. Because doxycycline is contraindicated in pregnancy, inpatient therapy consists of either clindamycin or erythromycin and gentamicin until the patient is afebrile for 24 to 48 hours. To complete the treatment course, the patient is switched to oral erythromycin base for 14 days.

Patients who have PID need to be aware of potential complications and long-term sequelae. These include the potential for recurrence of PID, the development of tubo-ovarian abscess, chronic abdominal pain, infertility, and the increased risk for ectopic pregnancy. It is important to inform patients of these potential problems and advise them on the appropriate follow-up for each of these complications.

Vulvovaginal Candidiasis

Vulvovaginitis is among one of the most common reasons women present to primary care physicians' offices. One of the major types of vulvovaginitis is caused by an overgrowth of candidiasis from *Candida albicans, C. tropicalis,* or *C. glabrata.* The first pathogen is the more common, with the latter two being more responsible for resistant infections. Intense pruritus on both the external and internal genitalia is the most common presenting complaint for vulvovaginal candidiasis. The vaginal discharge that patients complain about is an odorless, thick cottage cheese–like discharge. Certain factors can predispose patients to vulvovaginal candidiasis including recent antibiotic use, oral contraceptive use, pregnancy, tight-fitting clothing, partner with candidiasis, or diabetes mellitus.

In order to establish the diagnosis of vulvovaginal candidiasis physicians must use clinical impression and basic laboratory evaluation. On physical examination, the vulvovaginal area is edematous with erythema. On examination of the vaginal vault, there is a cottage cheese–like discharge present with a pH of 4.0 to 5.0. Microscopically, there are budding yeast or hyphae present after applying potassium hydroxide. Fungal cultures are not necessary to confirm the diagnosis, but they are indicated if the infection recurs or is unresponsive to treatment.

The treatment regimens available for patients with vulvovaginal candidiasis are varied and include over-the-counter preparations. There is little difference in cure rates among these regimens. In certain cases in which there is resistance to treatment, or an increased risk for treatment failure, terconazole (Terazol) may provide a better cure rate. This antifungal is available in a 3- or 7-day intravaginal regimen. Recently, fluconazole (Diflucan) 150 mg, one dose given orally, has been approved as an alternative to the vaginal preparations. This oral preparation is as effective as the vaginal preparations in curing vulvovaginal candidiasis.

Recurrent vulvovaginitis presents a dilemma in a significant number of women. When recurrences respond to standard therapy and occur at intervals that are greater than every 4 months, no further evaluation needs to be performed. If recurrences are developing at shorter intervals, then fungal cultures need to be performed. In recurrent cases of vulvovaginal candidiasis, the fungal infections may mask other underlying pathogens. In resistant cases, patients need to be assessed for HIV infection.

Trichomoniasis

Trichomoniasis is caused by the pathogen *Trichomonas vaginalis* and is classified as a sexually transmitted disease. The incubation period is 3 to 21 days after exposure. There are certain factors that predispose women to this infection including multiple sexual partners, sexual activity, pregnancy, and menopause.

The presenting complaint with trichomoniasis is copious amounts of a thin, frothy green-yellow or gray malodorous vaginal discharge. Other complaints can include vaginal soreness or dyspareunia. Women are at increased risk for this infection around or during their menses because blood raises the pH of the vagina creating an ideal environment for trichomonad reproduction. Because of this fact, patients' symptoms may start during or immediately after menses, or they may be exacerbated during this time period. However, similar to other STDs in women, the majority infected with trichomoniasis are asymptomatic.

In order to establish the diagnosis of trichomoniasis, there are physical examination and laboratory findings unique to this infection. During the physical examination there are noted copious amounts of a malodorous vaginal discharge that is yellow-green or gray and occasionally is frothy in appearance. In some cases the cervix has a "strawberry" appearance (red and inflamed with punctations), or redness of the vagina or perineum is present. The vaginal discharge has a pH greater than 5.0 and more than 10 WBCs per high-power field on the wet mount preparation. Also, motile trichomonads can be discovered microscopically using the wet mount preparation. However, the microscopic examination cannot be used as the definitive test because there are a significant number of false-negative results. Cultures may be necessary in cases in which the definitive diagnosis cannot be established by using clinical impression and laboratory evaluation.

The recommended treatment for trichomoniasis is oral metronidazole (Flagyl), 2 gm in a single dose for both the woman and her sexual partner. Other treatment options include metronidazole 500 mg twice per day, or 250 mg three times per day, for 7 days. If patients develop persistent or recurrent infections, it is vital to assess for other STDs and other sexual contacts. The suggested treatment for persistent or recurrent infections is metronidazole, 500 mg orally twice a day for 14 days or 2 gm orally for 3 days. In order to ensure better cure rates in women for this STD, it is critical to treat their partners.

SUMMARY

When providing care for female patients with vaginal discharge it is also important to screen for those patients at risk for exposure to human immunodeficiency virus. In many cases the behaviors that place patients at risk for the aforementioned infections also place them at risk for HIV exposure. While evaluating and assessing patients with vaginal discharge, risk assessment, counseling about risk reduction, and offering HIV screening in appropriate patients is vital in an attempt to reduce the impact this virus has on patients.

Using the information discussed, and following the recommendations for evaluation and treatment of female patients who present with vaginal discharge, physicians can reduce the number of inaccurate diagnoses and inappropriate treatment regimens for this presenting problem. These strategies provide physicians with the best opportunity to re- solve one of the more common presenting complaints in the ambulatory environment.

SUGGESTED READING

Centers for Disease Control and Prevention. 1993 sexually transmitted diseases treatment guidelines. MMWR Morb Mortal Wkly Rep 1993;42 (RR-14):266:75.

Centers for Disease Control and Prevention. Recommendations for the prevention and management of *Chlamydia trachomatis* infections, 1993. MMWR Morb Mortal Wkly Rep 1993;42 (RR-12):1–39.

Heath CB, Heath JM. *Chlamydia trachomatis* infection update. Am Fam Phys 1995;52:1455–1461.

Kassler WJ, Cates W Jr. The epidemiology and prevention of sexually transmitted diseases. Urol Clin North Am 1992;19:1–12.

Kent HL. Epidemiology of vaginitis. Am J Obstet Gynecol 1991;165:1168–1176.

Newkirk GR. Pelvic inflammatory disease: A contemporary approach. Am Fam Physician 1996;53:1127–1135.

Reed BD, Eyler A. Vaginal infections: Diagnosis and management. Am Fam Physician 1993;47:1805–1815.

QUESTIONS

1. To establish the diagnosis of bacterial vaginosis, there are four criteria developed to improve the accuracy of this diagnosis. Which of the following is *not* one of those criteria?
   a. Off-white, creamy adherent vaginal discharge
   b. Greater than 10 WBCs per high-power microscopic field
   c. Vaginal pH greater than 4.5
   d. Clue cells present microscopically
   e. Positive sniff test

2. A patient returns to the office for treatment of a positive *Chlamydia* culture. She is pregnant and at 14 weeks' gestation. Which of the following is the appropriate antibiotic regimen in this patient?

   a. Azithromycin (Zithromax) 1 gm orally for one dose
   b. Doxycycline 100 mg bid for 7 days
   c. Ofloxacin (Floxin) 400 mg bid for 7 days
   d. Erythromycin base 500 mg qid for 7 days
   e. Ceftriaxone (Rocephin) 250 mg IM for one dose

3. Certain factors can predispose female patients to vulvovaginal candidiasis. Which of the following is *not* one of these factors?
   a. Menopause
   b. Diabetes mellitus
   c. Recent antibiotic use
   d. Oral contraceptive use
   e. Pregnancy

Answers appear on **page 605**.

Chapter 37

Amenorrhea

Carol A. Baase, M.D.

INITIAL VISIT

Subjective

Lori is a 26-year-old white woman who presents with the complaint of not having her menstrual period for the last 8 months. She reports that she had been on the birth control pill for contraception until about 1 year ago when she and her husband decided to start their family. While on the birth control pill, her menstrual cycles had been regular with light flow. She reports that menarche was at age 14. Lori's menstrual cycle was initially irregular, with heavy flow. She was started on oral contraceptive pills at the age of 17 to "regulate her periods" and has been on them continuously until she stopped 1 year ago. She has had a total of three sexual partners. She has never been pregnant.

Her health is otherwise good. She takes no medications. She does not smoke or use alcohol. She normally runs 3 miles a day 5 days a week and has done this for the last 4 to 5 years. She reports that recently she has been training for a marathon. She has lost about 10 lb since she intensified her training. Lori has been married for 14 months. She works as a secretary in what she describes as a "stressful environment." She also states that she has been under more stress recently because of having purchased a new home, being expected to work longer hours at work, and her grandfather's having suffered a heart attack.

Her parents are both alive and in good health. Her mother did have a hysterectomy at the age of 48 because of "heavy bleeding." She has no siblings. Other than her grandfather, she is not aware of any other health problems in the family.

Objective

PHYSICAL EXAMINATION. Lori's general appearance is a thin woman with no obvious abnormalities. Her height is 5 feet 4 inches, weight is 104 lb; vital signs are normal. There is no hirsutism or acne noted. There is normal breast development and no galactorrhea noted. There is normal distribution of axillary and pubic hair. Her pelvic examination is unremarkable except for a decrease in cervical mucus. The remainder of her physical examination is normal.

LABORATORY TESTS. A urine pregnancy test is negative.

Assessment

Lori presents with secondary amenorrhea, which is defined as the absence of menstrual bleeding for greater than 6 months in a woman in whom normal menstruation had been established. The most common reason for secondary amenorrhea is pregnancy, which must be ruled out before further diagnostic evaluation is performed. This diagnosis is unlikely given the negative pregnancy test.

DIFFERENTIAL DIAGNOSIS. The differential diagnosis for amenorrhea can be categorized according to the level of organ or endocrine function that is disrupted. In Lori's case the most likely diagnosis is *hypothalamic amenorrhea*. This is caused by a disruption in the hypothalamic-pituitary-ovarian axis. Hypothalamic amenorrhea can be caused by emotional stress, concurrent illness, sudden or extreme weight loss (as in anorexia nervosa), or strenuous exercise. It is important to remember that this is a diagnosis of exclusion; therefore, a full evaluation is required to rule out other possibilities in the differential. Her recent training for a marathon and recent emotional stressors are likely causes for her amenorrhea.

Another cause for amenorrhea that must be considered is a *disorder of the pituitary*, specifically a prolactin-secreting pituitary adenoma. Up to 20 per cent of cases of secondary amenorrhea are caused by hyperprolactinemia. Only about one third of women with high prolactin levels have galactorrhea. An unusual disorder of the pituitary is Sheehan syndrome. This is caused by ischemia and infarction of the pituitary and usually occurs in the setting of an obstetric hemorrhage. Certain medications, including phenothiazines, thioxanthines, and other dopamine antagonists, can induce hyperprolactinemia.

Hyperandrogenic chronic anovulation must also be considered in the differential diagnosis of secondary amenorrhea. This disorder is characterized by hyperandrogenism and hyperestrogenism. Causes of this condition include obesity, polycystic ovary syndrome, Cushing syndrome, thyroid disease, adrenal hyperplasia, and androgen-producing tumors. The "typical" patient with this syndrome may be noted to have truncal obesity, hirsutism, and acne (signs of androgen excess). Lori does not demonstrate these characteristics.

Also to be considered in the differential diagnosis are *disorders of the ovary*, specifically premature ovarian failure. If the person is less than age 30, karyotyping must be done to rule out the presence of a Y chromosome (as in Turner mosaicism). If the patient is older than age 30, one can assume that the chromosomes are normal, although an autoimmune disorder may be a cause for the premature ovarian failure.

Disorders of the uterus and outflow tract can also cause amenorrhea. Congenital absence of the uterus or vagina or an imperforate hymen presents as primary amenorrhea (no menses by the age of 16). Asherman syndrome is usually the result of overly vigorous curettage that results in intrauterine scarring with destruction of the endometrium.

Plan

DIAGNOSTIC. Since Lori's pregnancy test is negative further testing must be done to determine the cause of amenorrhea. Since hypothyroidism and hyperprolactinemia are both fairly common causes of amenorrhea, a thyroid-stimulating hormone (TSH) and prolactin level should be drawn. If the prolactin level is elevated, a computed tomographic (CT) scan or magnetic resonance image (MRI) of the sella turcica is warranted. If the TSH is elevated, the patient should be started on levothyroxine.

After these initial screens, the next step is to determine the relative estrogen status in the patient if she is not pregnant. This is done by administering a progestin challenge test. This test is performed by administering medroxyprogesterone acetate, 10 mg by mouth for 5 to 10 days. Any uterine bleeding within 2 to 7 days after stopping the medication is considered a positive test. If the patient bleeds, the test has confirmed adequate endogenous estrogen and that the amenorrhea is caused by anovulation (hyperandrogenic chronic anovulation). If the prolactin level is normal, further evaluation is not needed.

If the progestin challenge test is negative, then Lori should be given 2.5 mg of conjugated estrogen daily for 21 days. Medroxyprogesterone acetate 5 to 10 mg is added for the last 5 days of the 21-day cycle. Presence of a responsive endometrium and an intact outflow tract is confirmed if withdrawal bleeding occurs within 2 to 7 days after the last dose of progesterone.

If Lori is found to have hypoestrogenic amenorrhea, then a follicle-stimulating hormone (FSH) level should be drawn. If the FSH level is elevated (greater than 50 mIU per ml), then the diagnosis of premature ovarian failure has been made. A work-up for autoimmune disease is in order since 20 to 40 per cent of cases of premature ovarian failure are associated with autoimmune disorders.

An FSH level that is normal or low and a low estrogen level indicate pituitary or hypothalamic dysfunction. An MRI should be done to rule out a pituitary tumor. If the MRI scan is normal, then a diagnosis of hypothalamic amenorrhea can be made.

THERAPEUTIC. The decision for type of therapy depends on the cause for the amenorrhea as determined by the diagnostic evaluation, as well as Lori's desire to start her family at this time. If Lori is found to be anovulatory, she will require regular progestin withdrawal (10 mg of medroxyprogesterone acetate every day for 10 days each month) to prevent hyperplasia of the endometrium which can occur with chronic unopposed estrogen stimulation. Birth control pills can also be used if she desires contraception. If Lori does wish to become pregnant, clomiphene can be used to induce ovulation.

If the amenorrhea is found to be secondary to hyperprolactinemia, treatment is usually with bromocriptine 2.5 mg daily to reduce the prolactin level. Surgery is indicated if a large macroadenoma is found.

If the diagnosis of ovarian failure is made, Lori needs to be started on estrogen replacement therapy to prevent osteoporosis and to decrease the cardiovascular risks that occur with hypoestrogenic states. If she desires to start a family, she needs to be told that it is unlikely for her to be able to get pregnant on her own, although she may be a candidate for some of the assisted reproductive technologies.

If hypothalamic dysfunction is the cause of Lori's amenorrhea, she again will need estrogen replacement to prevent osteoporosis. This can be done with the use of birth control pills or restarting the menstrual cycle with conjugated estrogen and medroxyprogesterone acetate. The appropriate dose of hormone supplementation for hypoestrogenic premenopausal women has not been established. Lori is a candidate for pregnancy induction when she decides to start her family. This does not include clomiphene since it depends on a functioning pituitary axis.

PATIENT EDUCATION. Lori needs to be instructed in the importance of a complete evaluation for amenorrhea to determine the cause and to tailor therapy accordingly. At the present time hypothalamic amenorrhea is the most likely cause of her complaint because of her family stressors and her recent undertaking of marathon training. Hypothalamic amenorrhea can resolve spontaneously when some of the underlying causes are treated or modified. She should be encouraged to modify her exercise regimen and to eat a well-balanced, nutritious diet.

She also needs to know that if the cause for the amenorrhea is found to be secondary to chronic anovulation, ovulation can still sporadically occur. Therefore, she will need to use a method of contraception if she decides to postpone pregnancy.

DISPOSITION. Lori is given a prescription for medroxyprogesterone acetate (Provera) 10 mg to be taken by mouth for the next 5 days. If she fails to have a withdrawal bleed, she then needs to call the office so that she can be started on 2.5 mg of conjugated estrogen on days 1 through 21. She should again take 10 mg of medroxyprogesterone acetate with the estrogen for the last 5 days of her menstrual cycle. Bleeding should occur within 7 days of completing the regimen. She then needs to have an FSH level drawn and an MRI of the sella turcica scheduled. She is scheduled for a return visit after the completion of all the tests.

FIRST FOLLOW-UP VISIT

Subjective

Lori returns after completion of both tests. She had called the office when she failed to have a withdrawal bleed after completing the progesterone

challenge. She was then given the cyclic estrogen and progesterone, after which she had a normal period. She also reports that she has completed her marathon race and has now returned to running only 2 to 3 miles, 4 days a week. She states that her grandfather is doing much better, and that she generally feels better. After a long discussion, she and her husband have decided to postpone having children for a while longer.

Objective

Lori's weight is up 8 lb (to 112 lb). Her prolactin level is 5 ng/ml (normal). Her TSH is 2.6 μU/ml (normal). Her FSH is normal, as is the MRI of the pituitary.

Assessment

After a complete investigation it has been determined that the cause of Lori's amenorrhea is hypothalamic dysfunction. This is a diagnosis of exclusion and is likely secondary to Lori's life stressors and recent exercise intensity and weight loss.

Plan

Because Lori is in a hypoestrogenic state, she needs to be given supplemental hormonal therapy to prevent osteoporosis. She should also be instructed in the importance of an adequate calcium intake in preventing osteoporosis. Since she has decided to postpone starting her family, she can be given birth control pills which will provide her with both estrogen and contraception.

She needs to be counseled that when she stops the birth control pills again her menses may resume normally since she has cut down on her running and has gained some weight. If her periods do not resume normally, she will continue to need estrogen therapy to prevent osteoporosis. She also needs to be told that if the amenorrhea does not resolve and she desires pregnancy, then she will need ovulation induction.

DISCUSSION

Hypothalamic amenorrhea is a disruption in the hypothalamic-pituitary-ovarian axis caused by psychological stress, depression, anorexia nervosa, severe weight loss, or strenuous exercise. Generally the disruption causes inadequate gonadotropin-releasing hormone (GnRH) stimulation to the pituitary gland, which leads to inadequate release of FSH and luteinizing hormone with resultant low estrogen levels. It has not been determined what the physiologic link is between exercise, stress, or weight loss and GnRH release.

Nutritional factors and psychological stress contribute to the amenorrhea that develops with anorexia nervosa, but their contribution is inconsistent in the amenorrhea seen in the woman athlete. Energy expenditure (stress) and level of body fat both have critical roles contributing to amenorrhea in the woman athlete. Rapid increases in training intensity cause luteal phase shortening and anovulation.

Exercise-related amenorrhea is found to be reversible within a few months of decreased training intensity. Amenorrhea can persist in the anorexic patient despite weight gain. There is no evidence that fertility is compromised after the return of normal menstruation.

Osteoporosis is a major problem for hypoestrogenic, amenorrheic women. They have been found to have a 10 to 20 per cent decrease in lumbar bone density when compared with age-matched controls. Even if they resume menses, they continue to have lower bone mass than women who have not had amenorrhea. Estrogen deficiency is a strong stimulation for bone resorption that cannot be totally overcome by increased calcium intake or weight-bearing exercise.

There is also concern that the hypoestrogenic state at such a young age can increase a woman's risk for cardiovascular disease, although this has not yet been specifically studied. Because of these risks, hormonal replacement should be strongly recommended for all young women who are found to have hypothalamic amenorrhea with estrogen deficiency.

SUGGESTED READING

Kiningham RB, Apgar BS, Schwenk TL. Evaluation of amenorrhea. Am Fam Physician 1996;53:1185–1194.

Lobo RA. The syndrome of hyperandrogenic chronic anovulation. In Mishell DR Jr, Davajan V, Lobo RA (eds). Infertility, Contraception and Reproductive Endocrinology. Boston, Blackwell Scientific, 1991, pp 447–487.

Marshall LA. Clinical evaluation of amenorrhea in active and athletic women. Clin Sports Med 1994;13:371–377.

Skolnick AA. "Female athlete triad" risk for women. JAMA 1993;270:921–923.

Speroff L, Glass RH, Kase NG. Clinical Gynecologic Endocrinology and Infertility, 5th ed. Baltimore, Williams & Wilkins, 1994, pp 401–456.

QUESTIONS

1. During evaluation for amenorrhea, a patient experiences a withdrawal bleed after being given the progestin challenge. This is consistent with a diagnosis of
   a. Hypothalamic amenorrhea
   b. Hyperandrogenic chronic anovulation
   c. Pituitary failure
   d. Ovarian failure
   e. Pituitary adenoma

2. The patient in question 1 should be counseled about
   a. Her potential for osteoporosis
   b. Her need to pursue adoption if she desires children
   c. Regular progesterone challenge to provide effective contraception
   d. Her need for hormonal replacement
   e. Her risk for endometrial hyperplasia

3. A 17-year-old woman has a negative progestin challenge test, but responds to progestin and estrogen. Her prolactin and TSH levels are normal, and MRI scan is negative. Her FSH level is elevated. These test results are consistent with
   a. Turner syndrome
   b. Sheehan syndrome
   c. Asherman syndrome
   d. Polycystic ovary syndrome

Answers appear on **page 605**.

Chapter 38

Postmenopausal Vaginal Bleeding

Angela J. Shepherd, M.D.

INITIAL VISIT

PATIENT IDENTIFICATION AND PRESENT ILLNESS. Mrs. Joanna B. is a 65-year-old black woman who presents to the clinic reporting vaginal bleeding. She had an uneventful menopause at 51 years of age, and has experienced no menstrual flow for more than a decade until approximately 8 months ago, when another physician recommended and prescribed continuous conjugated estrogens (Premarin) and medroxyprogesterone acetate (Provera) as hormone replacement. Seven months after beginning hormone replacement therapy, she began to experience vaginal bleeding. The bleeding was painless and moderate, requiring three pads per day and it stopped 4 days before the appointment. As the interview proceeds, the patient reveals that she took only the Premarin and never filled the Provera prescription.

PAST MEDICAL HISTORY. Mrs. B. reported menarche at age 13. Her first pregnancy occurred at age 22, and was followed by three more. Three ended in term vaginal deliveries, one ended in a first-trimester spontaneous abortion. Her menstrual history was otherwise unremarkable. She did not breast feed or take oral contraceptives. Surgical history included an open cholecystectomy at age 44. She has hypertension diagnosed 5 years ago, treated with hydrochlorothiazide 25 mg and lisinopril 20 mg.

FAMILY HISTORY. Mrs. B.'s parents are both deceased. Her father died in his early forties in an industrial accident; her mother died at the age of 78, after suffering several strokes. She has three sisters and two brothers; two siblings have hypertension. There is no history of cancer of the breast, reproductive organs, or colon in her family. Her children are healthy.

HEALTH HABITS. Mrs. B. started smoking in her teens, and reports smoking two packs of cigarettes per day for 30 years, then quitting at the age of 60. She drinks rarely. She walks 1 to 2 miles several times a week.

SOCIAL HISTORY. Mrs. B. lives with her husband, one daughter, and two grandchildren. She is a member of the Southcentral Baptist Church and sings in the choir. She enjoys gardening.

REVIEW OF SYSTEMS. Mrs. B. reports that she has some dizziness if she "starts out too quickly," and mild vaginal dryness. She denies bleeding from her gums or rectum, weight loss, and abdominal bloating or pain.

Objective

PHYSICAL EXAMINATION. Mrs. B. is a talkative woman who looks younger than her stated age. Blood pressure is 148/92 mm Hg, pulse 78 and regular, weight 190 lb, height 5 feet 4 inches. Gynecologic examination reveals normal external genitalia, slightly rugated vaginal wall, and a 2-cm erythematous polyp protruding from the cervical os. A scant amount of old blood is present in the vaginal vault. Her uterus is anteverted and normal size, nontender, without nodularity. Adnexal examination is unremarkable, and rectal examination is normal with a stool occult blood test negative. A Pap smear is done and sent to the reference laboratory.

TABLE 38–1. Differential Diagnosis of Postmenopausal Vaginal Bleeding

Source	Anatomic Cause
Uterus	Atrophy
	Hyperplasia
	Adenocarcinoma
	Leiomyoma (fibroids)
	Polyps
	Foreign body (IUD)
	Sarcoma and other cancers
Ovary	Thecal cell tumors (very rare)
Cervix	Cervicitis
	Endocervical polyps
	Cervical ulcers
	Cervical carcinoma
Vagina	Atrophy
	Vaginitis
	Postcoital (traumatic)
Nongynecologic	Hypothyroidism
	Cirrhosis
	Bleeding dyscrasias
	Perirectal and periurethral sources

IUD = Intrauterine device.

Assessment

WORKING DIAGNOSIS. Postmenopausal vaginal bleeding, most likely from a cervical and/or uterine source.

DIFFERENTIAL DIAGNOSIS (see Table 38–1). *Postmenopausal bleeding* is defined as any vaginal bleeding after 6 months of amenorrhea. In the setting of hormone replacement therapy, irregular bleeding (or a change in the bleeding pattern) after 6 months of a consistent dose of hormone replacement is also abnormal. Many women on simultaneous estrogen and progesterone experience spotting during the first 6 months of hormone therapy. Bleeding during this time does not require sampling, but can be observed or treated by adjusting hormone dosages. Likewise, there is no recommendation for endometrial sampling before initiation of combination replacement hormones in asymptomatic women.

Uterine cancer (adenocarcinoma of the endometrium) is the most worrisome of the potential causes of postmenopausal bleeding, so much so that all postmenopausal bleeding should be considered "cancer until proved otherwise." Only 8.2 to 20 per cent of those women presenting with bleeding after menopause are diagnosed with endometrial cancer,

but because stage I disease has a 5-year survival rate of 93 per cent, early diagnosis is most important. Bleeding is the presenting symptom in 85 per cent of women with endometrial carcinoma. It is important to note that studies have shown that the complaint of "spotting" is as likely as "heavy bleeding" to be the first sign of the disease.

Endometrial cancer is usually a disease of older women. Only 5 per cent of the diagnosed endometrial cancer occurs in women before age 50, with a steady rise in disease occurrence until a peak is reached in women ages 60 to 65. It is more often diagnosed in white women than black women. Endometrial hyperplasia is most prevalent in women ages 45 to 55, who may also present with abnormal bleeding.

The nomenclature of *endometrial hyperplasia* is still confusing and in progress. For clinical purposes, the hyperplasias can be classified into two groups: those with atypia and those without. Hyperplasia with atypia should be considered as a premalignant lesion. Without any specific treatment, at least 30 per cent of hyperplasia with atypia progresses to carcinoma within 4 years and 15 to 25 per cent is associated with well-differentiated carcinoma already present in the uterus.

Hyperplasia without atypia should be considered a risk for progression to carcinoma, but a 14-day regimen of oral progesterone induces a regression in many cases within 2 to 6 months. More importantly, an appropriate dose of progesterone for 12 or more days per month reduces the incidence of new cases of hyperplasia to almost zero.

Uterine *polyps* or *leiomyoma (fibroids)* are benign uterine sources of vaginal bleeding after menopause, although both are more likely to be causes of bleeding in pre- and perimenopausal women. Both conditions can coexist with hyperplasia and cancer; therefore, the presence of either a uterine polyp or leiomyoma should not be considered the definitive cause of abnormal bleeding without a thorough evaluation of the endometrium.

In asymptomatic women over age 30, leiomyomas are found in 50 per cent of blacks and in 20 per cent of white women. After menopause, a leiomyoma usually becomes inactive, but in the hormonal surges of the perimenopausal period, it may be stimulated or degenerate, causing excessive bleeding. Less likely possibilities of uterine sources of bleeding include foreign body–induced bleeding from an intrauterine device, and rarely sarcoma.

Cervicitis and *endocervical polyps* are the common causes of vaginal bleeding, followed rarely by syphilis, tuberculosis, and malignancy. Polyps appear beefy red on examination, and are usually amenable to twisting as a means of removal. Endocervical polyps are associated with a higher than expected incidence of endometrial hyperplasia, and necessitate endometrial sampling when discovered in the postmenopausal woman. In the cervix that appears inflamed, properly collected samples for infectious organisms should be taken, with appropriate therapy instituted based on the results. Ulceration of the cervix (especially in the setting of prolapse) can also cause vaginal bleeding.

Vaginal sources of bleeding include *atrophic vaginitis*, *postcoital bleeding*, and *vaginal infections*. Infections should be sampled for causative agent and treated appropriately, and atrophy is easily discernible by physical examination, with pallor, loss of rugae, dryness, and friability. Inspection of the perineum should also include the urethra (for caruncles), rectum (for inflamed hemorrhoids), and vulva (for atrophy, malignancy, or trauma).

Ovarian tumors are very rare causes of vaginal bleeding and typically occur in younger women, but thecal cell tumors do occur in older women. Abdominal ultrasound is usually the initial step in the work-up.

Nongynecologic causes of bleeding, also rare, include bleeding dyscrasias such as idiopathic thrombocytopenic purpura, leukemia, and iatrogenic prolongation of the bleeding time with heparin or warfarin (Coumadin); disorders of the adrenal, thyroid, or pituitary; and liver disease. History and physical examination usually tip the clinician toward these diagnoses.

Plan

DIAGNOSTIC. The recommended procedure for removing an endocervical polyp and endometrial biopsy is discussed with the patient. After obtaining informed consent, the vaginal canal and cervix are swabbed with povidone-iodine (Betadine). The endocervical polyp was twisted from its stalk with ring forceps. A tenaculum was placed in the anterior lip of the cervix and a 4-mm Pipelle endometrial sampler was inserted into the cervical os. The uterus sounded to 7 cm, and a 4-mm core sample of endometrial tissue 4 cm long was aspirated. The patient tolerated the procedure well.

THERAPEUTIC. A progesterone challenge test is prescribed. It consists of medroxyprogesterone acetate (Provera) tablets, 10 mg, to be taken once daily for 2 weeks.

PATIENT EDUCATION. The physician and nurse educator have discussed treatment with the patient, explaining that she might experience withdrawal bleeding after finishing the 14-day course, and instruct her to call if the bleeding becomes excessive.

FOLLOW-UP VISIT

Subjective

Mrs. B. returned for her follow-up visit 3 weeks later. She reports that she had spotting only for 1 day after her biopsy and polyp removal. She reports compliance with the Provera, and did not experience any bleeding in the 2 weeks after finishing the dose.

Objective

Her blood pressure is 138/88 mm Hg, pulse 72 and regular. Pelvic examination is done and reveals a normal-appearing cervix with no blood in the vaginal vault. Her uterus is nontender.

LABORATORY TESTS. Her Pap smear is reported as "no evidence of dysplasia." The polyp is reported as "endocervical cells without atypia," and the endometrial biopsy report indicates "mildly proliferative endometrium with no signs of hyperplasia." Thyroid-stimulating hormone is 1.2 μIU/ml (normal 0.35 to 5.50 μIU/ml); her blood count, including platelet count, is normal.

Assessment

Vaginal bleeding most likely due to inflamed endocervical polyp and several months of unopposed estrogen stimulation. Lack of bleeding after progesterone challenge test ruled out hyperplasia.

Plan

Hormone therapy is discussed with the patient. She declined another try at any form of hormone therapy, but did agree to take the pamphlets home and discuss it with her sister and daughter, who are both registered nurses. A follow-up visit for routine blood pressure check is set for 4 months.

DISCUSSION

The in-office endometrial biopsy is the standard of outpatient evaluation in postmenopausal bleeding

TABLE 38–2. Indications for In-Office Endometrial Sampling* in Postmenopausal Women

Strongly Recommended	Bleeding 6 months after ceasing menstruation
	Irregular bleeding after 6 months of HRT†
	Any endometrial cells seen on a Pap smear report
	Continued withdrawal bleeding after 4 months of PCT‡
	Endometrial thickness over 5 mm by vaginal ultrasound
Suggested	1. Conditions with history of prolonged endogenous estrogen excess
	a. History of infertility
	b. Obesity (especially with upper body fat pattern)
	c. History of failure to ovulate (Stein-Leventhal syndrome)
	2. Conditions with current exogenous estrogen excess
	a. Estrogen alone therapy (every 2 yr after initial evaluation)
	b. Tamoxifen therapy

*Same indications can be used for vaginal or abdominal ultrasound to measure endometrial thickness.

†Hormone replacement therapy (estrogen and progesterone).

‡Progesterone challenge test (10 mg progesterone every day × 14 days).

OF SPECIAL NOTE

The Pap Smear in Postmenopausal Bleeding. Detecting endometrial cancer on a Pap smear is almost fortuitous. The Pap smear, widely accepted as the screening modality for cervical cancer and its precursors, is only 25 to 60 per cent accurate in the detection of endometrial cancer. The false-negative rate ranges from 50 to 80 per cent. Although it cannot be used to rule out uterine cancer, the reported presence of *any* endometrial cells (normal or abnormal) on the Pap smear of a postmenopausal woman should prompt further investigation with endometrial sampling.

Tamoxifen's Effects on the Uterus. Tamoxifen is a nonsteroidal synthetic antiestrogen used in the treatment of some breast cancers. Tamoxifen replaces estradiol on its receptors and, contrary to its effect on the breast, in the uterus, the tamoxifen-receptor complexes are suspected to exert a persistent low-grade estrogenic environment. This is the theory for the increased risk of endometrial cancer found in women on tamoxifen therapy for breast cancer. Tamoxifen-related cancers tend to be poorly differentiated and more aggressive than those developing in women on estrogen replacement therapy. All women taking tamoxifen should be considered for endometrial sampling every 2 years, regardless of symptoms.

(Table 38–2). Endometrial sampling with a plastic suction device, such as the Pipelle endometrial sampler, can be done with or without lidocaine as local anesthesia. Potential adverse outcomes such as perforation of the uterus and infection are rare. Rarely, women not on estrogen replacement (and who have significant atrophy) may have cervical stenosis and be unable to tolerate insertion of the endometrial sampler. Once the endometrial biopsy results are known, they should direct treatment (see Table 38–3).

The newest technique for evaluating the endometrium, not yet available in most family practice offices, is vaginal ultrasound. A probe inserted into the vagina can be used to accurately measure endometrial thickness. Several studies have shown that an endometrial thickness of 5 mm or less is not associated with atypical hyperplasia or carcinoma. A thickness of 8 mm or more is definitely abnormal, and a thickness of 5 to 8 mm is questionable. An endometrial biopsy should be done for an endometrial thickness over 5 mm.

TABLE 38–3. Endometrial Biopsy Results and Actions

Tissue Report	Therapy
Atrophic	Consider individual patient—hormone replacement therapy or nothing
Proliferative	Progesterone (14 days)*
Hyperplasia without atypia	Progesterone (14 days)*
	Follow-up biopsy or ultrasound in 4 mo
Hyperplasia with atypia	Hysteroscopy and full surgical D&C
Cancer	Referral for staging and treatment

* If bleeding persists after 4 mo on progesterone, hysteroscopy and full surgical dilation and curettage (D&C) is recommended, for presumed hyperplasia.

SUGGESTED READING

de Lignieres B, Moyer DL. Influence of Sex Hormones on Hyperplasia/Carcinoma Risks. In Lobo RA (ed). Treatment of the Postmenopausal Woman. New York, Raven Press, 1994, pp 373–384.

Lorrain J, Ravnikar VA, Charest N. Peri- and postmenopausal abnormal bleeding. In Lorrain J (ed). Comprehensive Management of Menopause. New York, Springer-Verlag, 1994, pp 229–245.

Parsons AK. Detection and surveillance of endometrial hyperplasia/carcinoma. In Lobo RA (ed). Treatment of the Postmenopausal Woman. New York, Raven Press, 1994, pp 385–395.

Stubblefield PG. Abnormal uterine bleeding. In Branch WT Jr (ed). Office Practice of Medicine. Philadelphia, W.B. Saunders, 1994, pp 469–474.

Sutton GP, Stehman FB, Look KY. Endometrial cancer and uterine sarcomas. In Kase NG, Weingold AB (eds). Principles and Practice of Clinical Gynecology, 2nd ed. New York, Churchill-Livingstone, 1990, pp 921–943.

Weingold AB. Abnormal bleeding. In Kase NG, Weingold AB (eds). Principles and Practice of Clinical Gynecology, 2nd ed. New York, Churchill-Livingstone, 1990, pp 511–543.

QUESTIONS

1. Match each of the following statements with the single best answer. (Use each answer once.)
   a. Hyperplasia with atypia
   b. Hyperplasia without atypia
   c. Both
      (1) Will regress with discontinuation of exogenous estrogen
      (2) Should be considered definitely premalignant
      (3) Will likely normalize with progesterone therapy

2. Adequate evaluation of the endometrium is possible with all the following tests, *except*:
   a. Pipelle endometrial biopsy
   b. Dilation and curettage
   c. Pap smear
   d. Vaginal ultrasound

3. Endometrial biopsy is indicated in all the following situations, *except*:
   a. In an asymptomatic woman before beginning combined estrogen and progesterone therapy
   b. In a postmenopausal woman who reports spotting after 6 months of amenorrhea
   c. In a woman who reports an irregular bleeding pattern after 2 years on hormonal therapy
   d. In a woman who has been on 1.25 mg of Premarin without progesterone for 6 years

Answers appear on **page 605**.

Chapter 39

Contraception

Louisa C. Coutts–van Dijk, M.D.

INITIAL VISIT

Subjective

PATIENT IDENTIFICATION AND PRESENTING PROBLEM. Patricia V. is a 36-year-old part-time librarian and single mother of two boys. She attends the Family Practice Center (FPC) on Monday with a request for contraceptive advice. She is using condoms but is concerned about becoming pregnant using this method alone. She has been sexually active with her fiancé for about a year. She is not sure if she will like to have any more children, but is very sure that a pregnancy this early on during their relationship would be unwelcome.

PRESENT ILLNESS. Her menstrual periods are regular, lasting 4 to 5 days and occurring every 29 to 30 days. Her last menstrual period started 8 days ago, at the normal time and is not heavier or lighter than usual. She usually has some premenstrual bloating and cramping during the first few days of her menses. She reports the amount of bleeding as fairly light with no clots. She has not had any vaginal bleeding between periods or after intercourse. There is no vaginal discharge or itching. She has no history of sexually transmitted diseases, but has had occasional candidal vaginosis (confirmed by wet mount preparation) in the past. She describes her current relationship as stable and mutually monogamous.

Patricia is g3p2; she had one first-trimester miscarriage followed by two normal spontaneous vaginal deliveries. Her children, both boys, are 7 and 9 years old. Before she started her family she used the combined oral contraceptive pill (COC) for 6 years. She recalls having had difficulty remembering to take the pill each day. In addition she fears that taking the pill for many years may increase her chances of getting breast cancer. She has had cervical (Pap) smears every 2 years and these have all

been normal. Her last Pap smear was 18 months ago.

PAST MEDICAL HISTORY AND MEDICATION HISTORY. Patricia's past surgical history consists of an appendectomy at age 11. Her past medical history includes seasonal allergic rhinitis and conjunctivitis which started when she was a child. She has recently been attending the FPC for monitoring of her blood pressure. It has been elevated above 140/90 mm Hg on three occasions. She is currently trying nonmedication treatment for her hypertension, under her family physician's supervision. This involves diet, limitation of alcohol, weight loss, and exercise. Patricia uses over-the-counter acetaminophen (Tylenol) for tension headaches, antihistamines for allergies, and occasional over-the-counter vaginal antifungal preparations. She has no known drug allergies.

FAMILY HISTORY. Patricia is of African American heritage. Her mother had a myocardial infarction at age 63, and has been doing well following an angioplasty. Her father is currently age 64, and has hypertension. Patricia's sister, who is 44 years old, was diagnosed with breast cancer 2 years ago and has completed treatment. Her brothers, ages 32 and 39, are healthy.

HEALTH HABITS. Patricia smokes a half pack of cigarettes a day and drinks approximately three to six alcoholic beverages a week. Smoking cessation has been discussed on several occasions but Patricia says she is not ready to quit. She tells you she has difficulty controlling her weight and is worried that this could get worse if she stops smoking. She exercises one to two times a week; this usually consists of 30 minutes of cycling or swimming.

SOCIAL HISTORY. Patricia has been divorced for 2.5 years. She lives with her two children in a three-bedroom house. Her two boys, ages 7 and 9, attend the local elementary school. She works part-time as a librarian and finds it difficult to make ends meet. Her ex-husband does not see the children as frequently as she would like. Her fiancé gets along well with the two boys but is not ready to have children of his own. Patricia and her fiancé are planning a wedding later this year.

REVIEW OF SYSTEMS. Other than an occasional dry and unproductive cough, the review of systems is unremarkable. She has not had any nausea, vomiting, or breast tenderness.

Objective

PHYSICAL EXAMINATION. Patricia is a healthy-looking, mildly obese 34-year-old African American woman. She looks tired but is in no apparent distress. Her pulse is 76 and regular, blood pressure 135/96 mm Hg, and she is afebrile. Her blood pressure is repeated after 5 minutes rest and is 132/93 mm Hg. Heart sounds are normal, with regular rate and rhythm. Chest is clear to auscultation bilaterally with good air entry. Breast examination reveals no masses, abnormal skin dimpling or discharge, and there are no lymph nodes palpated in the axillae and supraclavicular areas. The abdomen is nontender, and no uterine or other masses are palpated. Vaginal speculum examination shows no vaginal or cervical discharge. The cervix appears normal. On bimanual pelvic examination a normal-sized uterus is palpated which is anteverted, mobile, and nontender; ovaries are not enlarged. No cervical or adnexal tenderness is noted.

LABORATORY TESTS. Patricia had her cholesterol checked last year and it was normal. Microscopic examination of vaginal saline and potassium hydroxide preparations (wet mounts) are negative for vaginosis. Vaginal swabs are sent for gonorrhea and *Chlamydia* testing. In low-risk patients with no history of abnormal Pap smears the time interval between Pap smears may be extended from the 1-year interval after three consecutive normal Pap smears have been obtained. They should, however, still be performed at least once every 3 years. Patricia has had normal Pap smears done at 2-year intervals. Her last one was 18 months ago. Therefore, no Pap smear is indicated today.

Assessment

WORKING DIAGNOSIS. Patricia V. is a single mother of two, who is currently in a stable monogamous relationship and in need of effective contraception. On history and physical examination there is no indication of pregnancy, vaginosis, or pelvic inflammatory disease. The risk factors that need to be taken into account while considering her contraceptive options include her tobacco use, elevated blood pressure, and a family history of breast cancer, hypertension, and coronary artery disease.

Discussing Contraception with Patients. When giving contraceptive advice the family physician's task is to guide the patient (and her partner if appropriate) through a decision-making process that is both personal and private. Patients and their partners come to the encounter with their family physician with personal experiences and moral and religious beliefs that shape their own views on the acceptability of particular methods. These must be taken into account. The physician should also be aware of his or her own personal views and be careful not to impose these on the patient. Receiving information concerning the advantages, disadvantages, risks, and benefits of the many methods available will enable Patricia to make an informed decision. A physician–patient relationship based on trust, sensitivity, mutual respect, and strict confidentiality is essential to this process. The questions that need clarification are listed in Table 39–1.

Contraceptive Options. There are many options available. Each method has its own failure rate, ease of compliance, reversibility, side effects (both positive and negative), and contraindications. Failure rates are user dependent, varying by patient age and patient lifestyle characteristics. Averages are listed in Table 39–2. Contraceptive methods that are relatively compliance independent are sterilization, intrauterine devices (IUDs), and progestin implants or injectables. However, such methods make women

TABLE 39–1. Contraceptive Questionnaire

How high a contraceptive failure rate is acceptable to this patient?
Is she at risk from sexually transmitted diseases?
Does she intend having children, and if so how soon?
Is compliance likely to be difficult with certain methods?
Does she or her partner find it distracting or embarrassing to use contraceptive methods at the time of intercourse?
Are there methods she has had bad experiences with, or that she fears to use?
Does she have any religious or cultural beliefs affecting her choice of contraceptive method?
How much can she afford to spend on contraceptives?

TABLE 39–2. Per Cent of Women with Accidental Pregnancy in the First Year of Use of Common Contraceptive Methods

Method	Percentage Accidental Pregnancy	
	Typical Use	Perfect Use
Chance	85	85
Spermicides	21	6
Periodic abstinence	20	1–9*
Withdrawal	19	4
Cap (with spermicide)		
Parous	36	26
Nulliparous	18	9
Sponge		
Parous	36	20
Nulliparous	18	9
Diaphragm (with spermicide)	18	6
Condom (without spermicide)		
Male	12	3
Female (Reality)	21	5
Oral contraceptives		
Combined	3	0.1
Progestin only	3	0.5
Intrauterine device		
TCu 380A	0.8	0.6
Progesterone T	2.0	1.5
Depo-Provera	0.3	0.3
Norplant	0.09	0.09
Female sterilization	0.4	0.4
Male sterilization	0.15	0.1

* Varies with type of method used. Lowest rates with postovulation method.
From Hatcher RA, Trussell J, Stewart F, et al. Contraceptive Technology. New York, Irvington Publishers, 1994. Adapted with the permission of Contraceptive Technology Communications, Inc.

more dependent on their physician for certain procedures. Oral contraceptives are examples of continuous compliance–dependent methods. Hormonal contraceptive methods may consist of progestin alone or a combination of estrogen and progestin. Episodic methods such as barrier methods include spermicide, condoms, sponges, diaphragms, and cervical caps. Another example of an episodic method is the rhythm method. These methods are easily reversible but may interfere with intercourse. Many contraceptive methods have noncontraceptive benefits. In addition, the family physician must always consider the risk of sexually transmitted diseases (STDs) including human immunodeficiency virus infection (HIV). Using a combination of two different contraceptive methods, which includes a

barrier method, may be necessary to reduce this risk.

Combined Oral Contraceptives (COCs). COCs consist of estrogen and progestin, are highly effective at preventing pregnancy, and are easily reversible. Commonly used estrogens are ethinyl estradiol and mestranol. Progestins used in COCs include norethindrone, norgestrel, norgestimate, levonorgestrel, ethynodiol diacetate, or desogestrel. The main mechanism of action of the COC is inhibition of ovulation. They are taken for 21 days followed by 7 days with no pill or with a placebo pill. Side effects are mild, often transient, and consist of breast tenderness, nausea, and breakthrough spotting or bleeding. Contraindications to COCs are listed in Table 39–3. The COC has many noncontraceptive benefits, which are listed in Table 39–4. This

TABLE 39–3. Contraindications to Use of Oral Contraceptives (OCs)

Contraindications
Thromboembolism
Cerebrovascular disease
Coronary artery disease
Breast cancer, known or suspected
Estrogen-dependent malignancy, known or suspected
Pregnancy, known or suspected
Undiagnosed abnormal vaginal bleeding
Liver neoplasm, benign or malignant
Active liver disease
Cholestatic jaundice of pregnancy, or jaundice with prior use

Other Conditions That May Make OC Use Less Desirable
Hypertension
Diabetes mellitus
Hyperlipidemia
Smoker over 35 years old
Gallbladder disease
Migraine headaches
Seizure disorder
History of serious depression
Chloasma (melasma)
Morbid obesity
Vasomotor rhinitis
Congenital or rheumatic heart disease
Inflammatory bowel disease
Neurofibromatosis
Hereditary hemorrhagic telangiectasia
Psoriasis
Systemic lupus erythematosus
Renal disease
Porphyria
Lactation (controversial)
Sickle hemoglobinopathies (controversial)
Elective surgery (controversial)

TABLE 39–4. Noncontraceptive Benefits: Conditions for Which Oral Contraceptive Use Offers Protection

Ovarian carcinoma
Endometrial carcinoma
Ectopic pregnancy
Pelvic inflammatory disease
Functional ovarian cysts
Menstrual irregularities
Dysmenorrhea
Iron deficiency anemia
Benign breast disease
Premenstrual syndrome

method has the advantage of being familiar to Patricia, but her previous problems with compliance may decrease its effectiveness. Patricia also has a concern about breast cancer risk. There are many studies and intense surveillance on the issue of oral contraceptives and breast cancer. Many studies show no increased risk, but some have shown a slightly increased risk in women on COCs. It is not clear if this is due to increased detection (women taking COCs see their physician more often) or an actual increased incidence. Patricia has several risk factors for cardiovascular disease. Hypertension and smoking over the age of 35 are both relative contraindications to COCs. The newer progestins (desogestrel, gestodene) are expected to have less adverse effects on lipids than the older progestins, but they have recently raised concerns about increased risk of thromboembolic events.

Progestin-Only Contraceptives. These are available in different forms: pill, injection, implant, or IUD. These methods offer highly effective contraception. They may be used in breast-feeding women or in women with contraindications to COCs. Mechanism of action includes inhibition of ovulation, thickening of cervical mucus, and a thin, atrophic endometrium. The minipill consists of a low-dose progestin-only pill which is taken continuously with no pill-free break, as with COCs. This progestin-only pill needs to be taken at the same time each day, and compliance is more demanding than with COCs. Because Patricia already has had trouble remembering to take her COC at regular times, this method will not be very effective in her case. Progestin injectables, implants, and progestin are useful for patients for whom compliance is a problem. Side effects may include irregular periods, amenorrhea, weight gain, and headaches. Osteoporosis may also be a long-term concern. Pregnancy needs to be ruled out before use of a progestin-only contraceptive. This is especially important as some of these methods are not immediately reversible. Injectable progestin is given by deep intramuscular injection every 12 weeks but may last several weeks longer. The progestin implant consists of six silicone tubes that are surgically inserted under the skin on the inside of the arm. Its effects last for 5 years, but removal may prove difficult and it is relatively expensive if used for shorter periods of time. Delayed return of fertility may be seen after long-term use of the injectables. Patricia has a strong preference not to use this method because of her concerns about weight gain.

Intrauterine Devices (IUDs). IUDs are available in two forms. The copper T IUD may remain in place for up to 10 years, the progestin T IUD needs to be replaced annually. They are suitable for parous women who are at low risk for pelvic inflammatory disease. Contraindications are listed in Table 39–5. Side effects may include heavier menstrual periods and dysmenorrhea. Bleeding is less with the progestin IUD. Risks are infection, perforation, and spontaneous expulsion. These risks are greatest at, and immediately after, insertion. IUDs do not cause increased rates of ectopic pregnancy. However, because IUDs prevent intrauterine pregnancy more than extrauterine pregnancy, women who become

TABLE 39–5. Contraindications to Use of Intrauterine Devices (IUDs)

Known or suspected pregnancy
Undiagnosed abnormal genital bleeding
Known or suspected uterine or cervical malignancy,
    including unresolved abnormal Pap smear
Active genital infection
    Pelvic inflammatory disease (PID)
    Acute cervicitis
    Vaginitis
    Genital actinomycosis
    Postpartum or postabortal endometritis within the last
        3 months
Uterine abnormality resulting in a distorted uterine
    cavity
High risk of STDs
    Patient or her partner has multiple sexual partners
    History of PID
Decreased resistance to infection (e.g., acquired
    immunodeficiency syndrome, chronic steroid therapy)
Presence of a previously inserted IUD
For copper-bearing IUDs
    Wilson disease
    Allergy to copper
History of ectopic pregnancy (controversial)

STDs = Sexually transmitted diseases.

pregnant with an IUD in place have a higher possibility of this pregnancy being ectopic than women who do not have IUDs. Because Patricia is at low risk for STDs this method is a definite possibility for her.

Barrier Methods. Barrier methods are episodic contraceptive methods used at the time of intercourse. They prevent sperm penetration and are often used together with spermicides containing nonoxynol-9. Examples of barrier methods are the diaphragm, cervical cap, sponges, and condoms. They are less effective than hormonal methods of contraception (see Table 39–2). These methods reduce risks of STDs, including HIV and papillomavirus (HPV). This is why women using these methods may have a lower incidence of cervical neoplasia. Women need to have diaphragms measured to fit snugly between the posterior fornix and the back of the symphysis. The diaphragm is inserted before intercourse and left in place for at least 6 hours after intercourse, but no longer than 24 hours. Side effects include increased incidence of urinary tract infections (UTIs) in some women, and rarely toxic shock syndrome. Cervical caps are smaller and also need to be fitted. They are kept in place by suction and may be left in place longer. Cervical caps are more effective in nulliparous women (women who have not had children). The female condom consists of a pouch with two rings, one of which is inserted into the vagina. It is less effective than the male condom (see Table 39–2). Latex used in barrier methods may cause allergy and may be damaged by lubricants that are oil or petroleum based. For lubrication, petroleum jelly (K-Y jelly), water, or spermicidal jelly or foam may be used. These are appropriate methods for Patricia. However, she prefers to use a method that is more effective and that does not interfere with the spontaneity of intercourse.

Sterilization. Sterilization of either the man or woman is highly effective but should be considered permanent. Vasectomy is a safe and simple office procedure done under local anesthetic. Following a small scrotal incision, a segment of each vas deferens is excised. Female sterilization requires laparoscopy and is associated with slightly higher rates of complications. During this procedure patency of the fallopian tubes is interrupted by banding, clipping, or coagulation. Because Patricia may want to have more children in the future this method is not appropriate for her.

Rhythm Methods. Rhythm methods involve periodic abstinence during the fertile phase of a woman's cycle. These methods require a mutually cooperative relationship. The fertile phase of the cycle is identified by the calendar method, cervical mucous changes, or basal body temperature change. The postovulation method is the most effective. These methods are attractive to many women because they do not involve the use of chemicals or hormones and because of their low cost. Patricia, however, would like a more effective method at this time.

Withdrawal or Coitus Interruptus. Coitus interruptus is the withdrawal of the penis from the vagina before ejaculation. Together with condoms it is one of the few contraceptive options men are able to use. The main disadvantage is the amount of self-control required. Its effectiveness is comparable to that of the diaphragm.

Lactational Amenorrhea Method (LAM). LAM is an unreliable method of contraception because the postpartum return of ovulation is difficult to predict. Ovulation may precede menstruation. Daily, frequent stimulation of the breast, of adequate duration is required to suppress ovulation. Its effectiveness as a contraceptive method decreases with time since delivery.

Abstinence. Abstinence should be included in the list of contraceptive options, as it is a common and acceptable choice for many people at different times in their lives. Withstanding peer or partner pressure is not often easy, especially for teenagers. Providing education about contraceptive options can be coupled with teaching techniques for saying "no." Educating teenagers on how to avoid high-risk situations by staying sober and in the company of reliable friends, may also be appropriate. The possibility of sexual abuse needs to be kept in mind.

Emergency (Postcoital) Contraception. It is estimated that almost one half of all pregnancies in the United States are unintended. This does not necessarily mean that all of these are also unwanted. Many elective terminations of pregnancy can be prevented if more patients and their physicians are aware of the methods available for emergency contraception. Physicians need to be aware that some people may have moral or religious objections to the use of emergency contraception. The main methods of postcoital contraception are as follows:

1. The combined oral contraceptive may be used for emergency contraception up to 72 hours after unprotected intercourse has taken place. Effectiveness depends on how soon after unprotected inter-

course the tablets are taken. The failure rate per event of unprotected intercourse is 3 per cent. Two tablets of an oral contraceptive containing ethinyl estradiol 50 μg and norgestrel 0.5 mg (Ovral) are given immediately together with an antiemetic. A further two tablets of Ovral and an antiemetic are taken 12 hours after the first dose. Mechanism of action is believed to be a combination of interference with implantation and cervical mucus and tubal mobility changes.

2. A copper IUD may be used up to 5 days after unprotected intercourse for emergency contraception. It has a 0.1% failure rate and is highly effective. Its mechanism of action is believed to be prevention of implantation and possible interference of tubal function. If left in place it also provides long-term contraception.

3. Mifepristone (RU 486). This newer method of postcoital contraception appears to be more effective than the other methods currently available.

Plan

DIAGNOSTIC. The presence of vaginosis is excluded by examination of the wet mount preparation. Swabs are sent to the laboratory to test for gonorrhea and *Chlamydia*.

THERAPEUTIC. Patricia's options for long-term contraception are reviewed. Her views and feelings about continuation of a pregnancy, if contraception failed, are also discussed. Because of her previous problems with compliance and the presence of two relative contraindications, a combined oral contraceptive is not considered to be a first choice. Her close experience with breast cancer in her immediate family also makes this a method that will cause her unnecessary anxiety. Patricia prefers not to continue with barrier methods because of their lower effectiveness and because of what she perceives as interference with sexual spontaneity. She will, however, use condoms in addition to other methods if she needs protection from STDs in the future. Patricia also prefers a method that is immediately reversible if she decides to have more children. She chooses to have an IUD fitted because it provides effective and compliance-free contraception without interfering with intercourse.

PATIENT EDUCATION. Patricia is told that common side effects of IUDs include spotting, increased menstrual flow, menstrual cramps, and increased mucous discharge. Complications include infection and, rarely, perforation of the uterus on insertion.

She is informed that pelvic infections can manifest as fever, vaginal discharge, abnormal bleeding, painful intercourse, or abdominal pain. The IUD can remain in place for up to 10 years, and removal requires a return visit. If pregnancy occurs while using this method a pelvic ultrasound scan is indicated to determine fetal location. Patricia is told to expect some cramping and spotting the first few days following insertion of the IUD. She is told that the highest risk of expulsion and infection are immediately after insertion and during the first few menstrual periods. She is asked to repeat important information to ensure it has been properly understood.

DISPOSITION. Patricia is instructed to return to the clinic to have an IUD fitted. She is instructed to take one dose of an antibiotic and one dose of a nonsteroidal anti-inflammatory drug (NSAID) 1 hour before the procedure and another dose of antibiotic 12 hours later.

PROCEDURE. Patricia completes a procedure consent form. She agrees that she is well informed about potential complications and side effects of this method. Uterine position, shape, and size is determined by bimanual examination. Following cleansing of the cervix with antiseptic solution the cervix is stabilized with a tenaculum. Using sterile technique a sound is inserted to measure the uterine cavity. The IUD applicator is adjusted to the correct size and the IUD inserted into the uterine cavity. Following removal of the applicator the IUD strings protruding from the cervical os are trimmed.

PATIENT EDUCATION. Patricia is instructed to contact her physician if there is any unexpected bleeding, expulsion of the IUD, vaginal discharge, fever, excessive cramping, or abdominal pain. She is instructed when to take the second dose of antibiotic and to use the NSAID for any pain or cramping. Patricia is informed that she can continue to use condoms until her next visit to reduce further any risk of infection or unwanted pregnancy should the IUD be expelled. Patricia is instructed in the proper use of condoms. To be effective the penis must be removed from the vagina before loss of erection. The rim of the condom needs to be held at the base of the penis during removal. She is aware that women in mutually faithful relationships have little increased risk for infection.

DISPOSITION. Patricia is scheduled for an appointment following her next menstrual period to have the IUD checked. If her period is late she is advised to keep the appointment to have pregnancy testing.

Her blood pressure also needs to be checked again at the next visit.

FIRST FOLLOW-UP VISIT

Subjective

Patricia reports that she experienced mild spotting and cramping for a few days following insertion of the IUD. She has not had any fever, vaginal discharge, or abdominal pain. Her menstrual period started on time and has been slightly heavier than usual. She did not find this problematic. It lasted for 5 days and stopped yesterday. She is satisfied with this contraceptive method so far.

Objective

Patricia's blood pressure is 135/90 mm Hg. She is apyrexial. Abdomen on examination is nontender. On speculum examination the cervix is closed and the IUD threads are visible protruding from the cervical os. There is no abnormal vaginal or cervical discharge present. On bimanual examination the uterus is normal in size, mobile, and nontender. Adnexa are nontender and not enlarged. The laboratory tests for gonorrhea and *Chlamydia* have both returned negative.

Assessment

Patricia appears to tolerate this form of contraception well. There are no apparent complications, such as infection or heavy bleeding. The IUD is correctly placed and no expulsion has occurred.

Plan

Patricia is taught how to identify the threads in the vagina herself so that she can be sure the IUD remains in place. If the threads cannot be palpated, ultrasound can be used to determine location of the IUD. She is to return to the clinic if there are signs of infection or problems with heavy, irregular, or painful bleeding. Her next Pap smear is due in approximately 6 months, at which time the IUD will also be checked. She is encouraged to come in sooner to discuss smoking, exercise, and diet and to monitor her blood pressure. She is also cautioned about drug interactions. She is advised not to use over-the-counter antihistamines and antifungal preparations simultaneously, without consulting a physician, because of a potential risk for cardiac arrhythmias.

SUGGESTED READING

Hatcher RA, Trussell J, Stewart F, et al. Contraceptive Technology, 16th ed. New York, Irvington Publishers, 1994.

Heath CB. Helping patients choose appropriate contraception. Am Fam Physician 1993;48:1115–1124.

Johnson CA, Johnson BE, Murray JL, et al. Women's Health Care Handbook. Philadelphia, Hanley and Belfus, Inc., 1996.

Rakel RE. Textbook of Family Practice, 5th ed. Philadelphia, W.B. Saunders, 1996, pp 715–728.

Rakel RE. Conn's Current Therapy 1996. Philadelphia, W.B. Saunders, 1996, pp 1087–1091.

QUESTIONS

1. Of the following, the most effective method of contraception is
   a. Male condom
   b. Diaphragm with spermicide
   c. Periodic abstinence
   e. Female condom

2. True or false: The following are absolute contraindications to use of the combined oral contraceptive pill
   a. Breast cancer
   b. Pelvic inflammatory disease
   c. Hepatitis
   d. Age over 35

3. True or false: Contraceptive methods that are suitable for patients for whom compliance is difficult include
   a. Progestin-only pill
   b. Intrauterine device
   c. Injectable progestin (Depo-Provera)
   d. Diaphragm

Answers appear on **page 605**.

Chapter **40**

The Abnormal Pap Smear

Mark M. Bajorek, M.D.

Subjective

Susan M., a 46-year-old woman, presents to the clinic to follow up an abnormal Pap smear. She reported good general health. Menarche began at age 12 and she began having intercourse at age 18. She denies a history of severe menstrual cramps. Her periods are every 28 days with a 4- to 5-day flow. Her last period ended about 1 week ago.

Susan's obstetric history includes three pregnancies, with the first ending in a miscarriage at 8 weeks and the two subsequent pregnancies going to term without sequelae.

After the birth of her second child, Susan used an intrauterine device (IUD) for 5 years. Shortly after the IUD was removed the patient had a tubal ligation. This patient is sexually active and reports no pain with, or spotting after, sexual intercourse.

Susan denies any vaginal discharge but has noted some skin tags in the vulvar area. There is no history of herpes, gonorrhea, syphilis, or *Trichomonas* infection. She had asymptomatic candidal infections in the past. She reports two male sexual partners, neither with overt genital warts or a history of promiscuity. She recounts no risk factors for human immunodeficiency virus (HIV) disease. Vaginal cultures at the time of her last pelvic examination were normal.

Susan's mother did not use diethylstilbestrol. The patient denies any history of smoking.

The patient reports having been diagnosed with inflammation on a Pap smear 10 years ago and used oral antibiotics. The remainder of her Pap smears had been unremarkable until 6 months ago when one showed atypical squamous cells of undetermined significance (see Discussion further on).

Objective

On physical examination, the patient has labial skin tags, and small external warts. No perianal warts are noted. The introitus, vagina, and cervix have normal mucosa. No leukoplakia, pigmented lesions, or friable tissue are noted. The external cervical os is slightly open. No endocervical polyps or IUD strings are noted. Pap smear is repeated and wet mount preparation is negative for *Candida, Trichomonas,* and bacterial vaginosis. The bimanual examination is not repeated.

Assessment

Atypical cells of undetermined significance in a 46-year-old woman with a remote history of a prior abnormal Pap smear and external evidence of human papillomavirus (HPV). The patient has no current signs or symptoms of vaginitis.

Plan

Susan is educated about HPV and its association with cervical dysplasia. Future management will be based on the results of the Pap smear. If the Pap smear is normal, the patient will be scheduled for Pap smear follow-up in 6 to 12 months. If the Pap smear shows more atypical cells, signs of HPV, or squamous intraepithelial lesions then colposcopy is indicated.

DISCUSSION

Pap smears are the mainstay for detecting precancerous changes of the uterine cervix. Women who are sexually active or over age 18 are advised to have regular Pap smears. A representative Pap smear may be obtained at any time in a woman's cycle except menses. During menses the red blood cells obscure the appearance of sloughed epithelial cells. Ideally Pap smears should be obtained 6 to 8 weeks after treatment of vaginitis or cervicitis to avoid the diagnosis of inflammatory changes.

In addition to timing, collection method is important to quality of the specimen. Obtain the Pap smear before the bimanual examination to avoid lubricant artifact. After the speculum is placed, remove excess cervical mucus with a cotton swab. Collect the squamous cells of the cervix with an Ayre spatula applied to the cervix in a circular motion, then spread the cells across the slide with a single, even stroke. Collect the endocervical cells with a cytobrush in the external os. A quarter of a turn gathers enough cells to roll onto a slide. Spray the slide with a cell fixative immediately to prevent drying artifact. A slide with squamous cells and endocervical columnar epithelium is more likely to represent the zone of metaplasia, that is, the squamocolumnar junction, which is the area most vulnerable to squamous cell cancer of the cervix. Metaplasia on Pap smear is a normal finding and generally means a good cell sample.

At least 20 per cent of patients with normal Pap smears have undiagnosed cervical pathology. Precancerous lesions may not shed enough cells for recognition or scar tissue may overlie abnormal cells. Cells might not be collected from dysplastic sites. Inflammation or atypical cells also make cervical screening difficult. In 1988 pathologists began using the Bethesda system, a four-part Pap smear description, to aid clinicians in clinical decision making thorough, detailed cytologic descriptions. The first component of the Bethesda system is a statement of adequacy of the specimen. Three categories are available: satisfactory for evaluation, satisfactory for evaluation but limited, or unsatisfactory. Interpretation may be obscured by drying artifact, blood, inflammation, or vaginal lubricant. The second component of the Bethesda system is a summary of the slide's cytologic findings into one of three classifications: within normal limits, benign cellular changes, or epithelial cell abnormalities. The third component is the detailed descriptive diagnosis of the smear: benign cellular changes, infection reactive changes, and epithelial cell abnormalities. Low-grade squamous intraepithelial lesions (LGSIL) describe cell findings consistent with mild dysplasia. The diagnosis of high-grade squamous intraepithelial lesions (HGSIL) represents moderate and severe dysplasia as well as carcinoma in situ.

The fourth component of the Bethesda classification describes the cell findings in terms of hormonal changes: compatible with age and history, incompatible with age and history, or not able to specify. Clinicians can use this information to identify women who need further evaluation or routine follow-up.

Occasionally, the cells on Pap smear appear atypical without specific diagnosis. Pathologists describe these smears as atypical cells of undetermined significance (ASCUS). Pathologists should classify less than 5 per cent of all Pap smears in this indeterminate category. Women determined as having ASCUS on their Pap smears are encouraged to have a repeat Pap smear in 3 to 6 months depending on their risk factors for cervical cancer. Some researchers have found high-grade dysplasia in up to 20 per cent of women who have been in the ASCUS category on a prior Pap smear. If a repeat Pap smear also is described as ASCUS, colposcopy is recommended.

The colposcope is a magnification instrument paired with a light source and filters. Colposcopes resemble a tall microscope. Power magnification of 3 to 15× is used to view the cervical surface for vascular changes and color changes after application of acetic acid and iodine. Cervical biopsies are directed at the most abnormal areas. Colposcopy is indicated in women with persistent inflammation, ASCUS category on two successive Pap smears, and for women in categories LGSIL and HGSIL on their Pap smears. Women with these changes need to be examined to locate the source of the dysplasic cells. Biopsies directed at suspicious sites are sent for diagnosis and staging.

Atypical glandular cells of undetermined significance, AGUS, is a Pap smear diagnosis category that encompasses proliferative benign reactive changes through endocervical adenocarcinoma in situ. Pathologists often describe the endocervical glandular cells as favoring either a benign process or a neoplastic process. Management of this Pap smear finding depends on the patient's history and risk factors. For low-risk patients with AGUS of an endocervical origin, a repeat sample of endocervical cells with the cytobrush is appropriate. Other women may need endocervical curettage. Patients with persistent changes may require a cone biopsy.

Part of delivering the most appropriate patient care in light of the Pap smear result is also to consider the patient's risk factors for cervical cancer. In the United States 600,000 women yearly are diagnosed with premalignant cervical cytologic findings. Patients most likely to have cervical cancer include women with a history of onset of intercourse at

16 or younger, sexually transmitted disease, HPV infection, active or passive exposure to cigarette smoke, multiple sexual partners, prior genital tract cancer, and immunosupression.

Susan reports being sexually active at age 18. She denies a history of herpes, gonorrhea, syphilis, or *Trichomonas* infection. She is a nonsmoker. Candidal infections are not a risk factor for cervical cancer. Condyloma on physical examination, however, puts her in a higher risk group. HPV, the cause of condyloma, is associated with cervical cancer. Researchers have identified subtypes of HPV that are associated with more aggressive dysplasia. Currently, viral probes to identify these subtypes have had limited clinical value but may be helpful in the future.

Leukoplakia, friable tissue, or a nodular cervical surface are often signs of squamous cell cancer of the cervix. Patients with these findings require aggressive evaluation, often needing colposcopy and biopsy. Susan had a history of a prior inflammatory Pap smear. Cervical polyps and foreign bodies, such as IUD strings, may cause inflammatory changes. IUDs are associated with *Actinomyces* infection and are best treated with penicillin. If Susan has inflammatory changes on her current Pap smear, management should include physical examination for a foreign body irritant, wet mount preparation for *Trichomonas* infection, candidal infection, bacterial vaginosis, and cultures for gonorrhea and *Chlamydia*. Patients with persistent inflammation and negative cultures benefit from colposcopy. Empirical antibiotics, oral or topical, do not appear to have a significant effect.

Susan is having regular menses, but postmenopausal women without estrogen supplementation have atrophic genital tracts. In these women, squamous cells may cover the entire cervix and the Pap smear lacks the endocervical component, the columnar epithelial cells. Five days of oral estrogen supplementation before the Pap smear improves the quality of the Pap smear.

Many authors have created flowsheets for the management of these patients depending on the Pap smear diagnosis (see Suggested Reading). The astute clinician will devise a plan for the patient considering the recommendations based on cell diagnosis with attention to the patient's risk factors, mental state, and history of compliance.

SUGGESTED READING

Cannistra SA, Niloff JM. Cancer of the uterine cervix. N Engl J Med 1996;334:1030–1038.

Kurman RJ, Henson DE, Herbes AL, et al. Interim guidelines for management of abnormal cervical cytology. JAMA 1995;271:1866–1869.

Lonky NM, Navarre GL, Saunders S, et al. Low-grade Papanicolaou smears and the Bethesda system: A prospective cytopathologic analysis. Obstet Gynecol 1995;85:716–720.

McIntyre-Seltman K. The abnormal Papanicolaou smear. Med Clin North Am 1995;79:1427–1442.

Nuovo J, Melnikow J, Paliescheskey M. Management of patients with atypical and low-grade Pap smear abnormalities. Am Fam Physician 1995;52:2243–2250.

Roland PY, Naumann RW, Alvarez RD, et al. A decision analysis of practice patterns used in evaluating and treating abnormal Pap smears. Gynecol Oncol 1995;59:75–80.

QUESTIONS

1. The diagnosis of metaplasia on Pap smear is indicative of
   a. A normal squamocolumnar junction
   b. Inflammatory changes
   c. Low-grade squamous intraepithelial lesion
   d. High-grade squamous intraepithelial lesion
   e. Carcinoma in situ

2. If a patient has atypical cells of undetermined significance (ASCUS) on two successive Pap smears, the next appropriate step is
   a. Colposcopy
   b. DNA probe for human papillomavirus
   c. Electrosurgical loop biopsy
   d. Two months of cyclic estrogen and progesterone
   e. Dilation and curettage

3. Initial evaluation of women with atypical glandular cells of undetermined significance (AGUS) without a history of a prior abnormal Pap smear is to
   a. Perform colposcopy with directed biopsies
   b. Obtain a DNA probe for human papillomavirus
   c. Repeat the Pap smear in 4 to 6 months
   d. Perform hysteroscopy
   e. Schedule dilation and curettage

Answers appear on **page 605**.

Chapter 41

Menopause

Jon C. Calvert, M.D., Ph.D.

SUBJECTIVE

M.K., a 46-year-old white female gravida 3 para 2 (2 term deliveries, 0 preterm deliveries, 1 miscarriage, 2 living children), presents with the complaint of persistent back pain for several weeks. In good health since her last physical 10 months ago, she noted the onset of pain 4 weeks ago after working in her flower beds. Sudden in onset and sharp in nature, the pain is located in the mid to lower back. It radiates bilaterally to the flanks and has been relatively constant although somewhat less apparent at rest than with activity. Some relief is obtained by lying on her side with knees and hips flexed, moving as little as possible. For several days after the pain began she was constipated and noted that bearing down to have a bowel movement aggravated the pain, as did sitting straight up in bed. Having lessened over the past 2 weeks, pain continues to be present. No change in gait or weakness in the lower extremities has been observed and loss of sensation has not been noted. There are no symptoms of urinary tract infection.

Review of clinic records reveals a hysterectomy and bilateral oophorectomy 8 years ago. She had a normal screening examination with a Pap smear at the vaginal cuff and a mammogram 7 months ago. Cholesterol and stool examination results for occult blood were normal at that time. A review of systems is negative. M.K. continues to smoke two packs of cigarettes per day. More directed questioning reveals that she has not been taking her continuous estrogen replacement therapy since her hysterectomy, even though she continues to have periodic hot flushes, difficulty getting a complete night's sleep, and dyspareunia. She continues in her job as an administrative secretary and except for gardening leads a relatively sedentary lifestyle. Other than the extra-strength acetaminophen for the pain and aluminum-based liquid antacids, she takes no medications.

Past medical history is positive for seasonal allergies, peptic ulcer disease, and anemia following the delivery of her youngest child. Past surgical history includes the above-mentioned hysterectomy with bilateral oophorectomy and cesarean section for her second child.

Family history reveals a father, paternal uncle, and paternal grandmother with insulin-dependent diabetes mellitus. Her mother died last year in a nursing home of pneumonia following a fall and hip fracture.

OBJECTIVE

The patient data is the following: blood pressure 132/80; pulse 90; respiratory rate 16; temperature 98.6°F; height 5'2": weight 102 lb. There is absence of ocular prominence with slight pallor of conjunctiva. Thyroid is not palpable. Chest is unremarkable except for tenderness to palpation over the spinous processes of the tenth thoracic vertebra. Breast examination is negative except for a fine nodularity, unchanged since last examination less than a year ago. Cardiac and abdominal examination are unremarkable. Examination of the back reveals absence of tenderness or spasm of the paraspinous muscles. There is full range of motion of the thoracolumbar spine with no localized pain in the muscle groups or their attachments. Pelvic examination reveals pallor and dryness of the vaginal mucosa with loss of rugation. Neurologic examination of the lower extremities is normal.

A complete blood count revealed a mild normochromic normocytic anemia with a hemoglobin of 11.7 g/dl. Urinalysis and chemistry panel results were within normal limits, as was a sedimentation rate. Thoracolumbar spine radiographs revealed a compression fracture of the body of the tenth vertebra with evidence of marked osteopenia for age.

Assessment

The patient is assessed for the presence of (1) hypo-estrogenemia; (2) osteoporosis; (3) compression fracture, thoracic vertebrae; and (4) anemia.

Plan

The plan of management includes (1) Pain management for fracture; (2) estrogen replacement therapy; (3) densitometry study; (4) patient education regarding osteoporosis; (5) stop aluminum-based antacid use; (6) begin calcium therapy; (7) encourage smoking cessation; (8) additional studies: thyroid function studies, serum alkaline phosphatase; (9) consider bisphosphonate therapy; (10) characterize anemia with further studies.

DIFFERENTIAL DIAGNOSIS

In addition to osteoporosis, the differential diagnosis includes those secondary causes of osteoporosis listed in Table 41–1. Other considerations include thoracolumbar strain/sprain, and metastatic disease to the bone. Given this patient's presentation and findings, the differential diagnosis most likely includes multiple myeloma, thoracolumbar sprain/strain, osteomalacia, and hyperparathyroid disease.

TABLE 41–1.   Causes of Secondary Osteoporosis

Systemic	Bone marrow disorders
Connective tissue	Lymphoma
Marfan syndrome	Multiple myeloma
Ehler-Danlos syndrome	Carcinoma, disseminated
Endocrine	Leukemia
Hypogonadism	Ectopic
Hyperadrenocortisolism	adrenocorticotropic
Hyperthyroidism	hormone (ACTH)
Hyperparathyroidism	syndrome
Diabetes mellitus	Gastrointestinal system
Drugs	Obstructive jaundice,
Alcohol	chronic
Aluminum antacids	Malnutrition, severe
Anticonvulsants	Malabsorption syndromes
(phenytoin)	Miscellaneous
Cyclosporin	Immobility
Glucocorticoids	Radiation therapy
Gonadotropin-	Rheumatoid arthritis
releasing hormones	Osteogenesis imperfecta
Heparin	Chronic renal failure
Isoniazid	Chronic obstructive
Lithium	pulmonary disease
Methotrexate	
Phenothiazines	

Multiple Myeloma

Presenting primarily in women with average age around 50, multiple myeloma should be near the top of the list of possible causes of back pain for this patient. The back pain can be chronic in its presentation and can be associated with vertebral compression fractures. Other localized bone pain may be present. Physical examination reveals an anemia and focal pain with compression of spinous processes over vertebrae involved or other areas of bony involvement. Radiograph of the spine may reveal an associated osteoporosis with vertebral body compression fractures. Survey of the skeleton may reveal multiple, widespread lytic lesions. Laboratory studies can be helpful. Urinalysis may reveal the presence of Bence Jones protein and a 24-hour urine electrophoresis result will be positive for kappa or lambda light chain proteins. Blood studies may demonstrate a mild anemia, elevated sedimentation rate, and rouleaux formation on peripheral smear. Less commonly, hypercalcemia is present. Serum immunoelectrophoresis reveals a characteristic monoclonal gammopathy. Aspiration studies of the bone marrow are necessary to confirm the diagnosis.

Thoracolumbar Sprain and Strain

Given the onset of back pain related to activity, muscle strain is in the differential. The constancy of the pain and the physical examination that cannot identify evidence of muscle tenderness or spasm does not support the diagnosis of back sprain and strain. Compression over bony structures (spinous process of the vertebrae) elicits pain and suggests skeletal involvement rather than muscle involvement.

Osteomalacia

In some cases it may be difficult to distinguish osteomalacia from osteoporosis based on clinical and/or radiologic criteria. The aching in bones, tenderness over bones of the proximal extremities, and pelvic girdle muscle tenderness are present in adult osteomalacia. Absent in this patient's presentation is a history of renal disease or renal failure. Not present also is a low serum phosphate level and elevated serum calcium, alkaline phosphatase, and parathyroid hormone levels.

Hyperparathyroid Disease

In hyperparathyroid disease, the hypercalciuria and hypercalcemia commonly result in urinary system calculi and occasionally generalized bone pain due to osteitis fibrosa cystica. Rarely there may be bone fractures at the site of these bone cysts. Physical findings are usually absent. Serum calcium and alkaline phosphatase levels tend to be high and serum phosphate level low. Relative to the level of serum calcium, the parathyroid hormone is elevated. Unlike osteoporosis, cortical bone rather than trabecular bone is more commonly affected.

DISCUSSION

Background

It is estimated that 10 to 15 million people in the United States, primarily women, have osteoporosis. Osteoporosis is the most common cause of fracture in the postmenopausal woman. Fifty per cent of women over the age of 70 years are below the fracture threshold and therefore highly susceptible to fracture. By age 60 years, 25 per cent of Caucasian and Asian women have evidence of spinal compression fractures resulting from osteoporosis. It is estimated that only 7 per cent of all those with osteoporosis receive therapy. Only 20 per cent of those diagnosed with osteoporosis receive therapy.

Significant clinical consequences of osteoporosis and its sequalae are observed. These include increased mortality, acute and chronic pain, deformity, and loss of independence. Ten to twenty per cent of elderly persons who have a hip fracture die within 6 months and 15 to 25 per cent have an abrupt change in lifestyle. Each year, 60,000 elderly persons move into nursing homes following osteoporosis-related hip fractures. Annual costs related to osteoporosis have been estimated to be as high as $7 to $10 billion. With the number of elderly persons continuing to increase, it is expected that osteoporosis and its sequelae will be of increasing medical concern.

Definitions

Osteoporosis is defined as a deterioration of bone microarchitecture with decreased bone mass, increased bone fragility, and increased incidence of fracture. Two types of osteoporosis are identified—primary and secondary. Primary osteoporosis has no identifiable cause and makes up about 80 per cent of all types of osteoporosis. Secondary osteoporosis (see Table 41–1) is represented by bone loss consequent to an identifiable cause (e.g., disease, drugs, immobility from any cause). Twenty per cent of females with osteoporosis have the secondary type, whereas 40 per cent of males with osteoporosis have the secondary type.

Pathophysiology

Bone is a metabolically active organ undergoing continual turnover. It is composed of an outer shell of cortical (compact, laminar) bone making up 75 per cent of bone mass and central trabecular (cancellous) bone making up the remaining 25 per cent. The metabolism of bone is divided into two competing but interdependent functions. The first continually destroys bone in a process of bone breakdown termed *resorption*. The second competing function is the continual building up of bone, which is termed *formation*. The primary cell type involved in bone resorption is the osteoclast and in bone formation is the osteoblast. Resorption and formation are interdependent, and when osteoclast activity is relatively greater than osteoblast activity, osteoporosis results over time. A biochemical marker for the level of osteoclast activity is urine deoxypyridinoline. Markers for osteoblast activity are serum osteocalcin and alkaline phosphatase.

Sex steroids play an important role in bone metabolism. They block the action of parathyroid hormone on bone, preventing bone resorption. Specifically, estrogen raises calcitonin levels, which act on the osteoclast to prevent bone resorption and increase calcium absorption in the gastrointestinal tract. Thus, in menopause-related osteoporosis there is excessive bone resorption by osteoclasts. By contrast, in age-related osteoporosis (primary osteoporosis), there is reduction in bone formation due to decreased osteoblast activity.

Peak bone mass plays an important role in the prevention of osteoporosis. Peak bone mass is reached around the age of 35 years and is 80 per cent greater in men than in women. In women factors that increase or improve peak bone mass include exercise, calcium in the diet, and the presence of estrogen. Because the postmenopausal loss of calcium from bone follows a known rate, the greater the peak bone mass, the longer it takes to lose enough calcium to reach the fracture threshold. Postmenopausal bone mass loss is 1 to 2 per cent per year, primarily in trabecular bone. This loss, which is the result of resorption exceeding bone formation, can be slowed by exercise, calcium intake, and estrogen supplementation. Postmenopausal bone loss can be accentuated by the absence of weight-bearing exercise, lack of calcium, and lack of estrogen supplementation. During the first 3 to 7 years following the onset of menopause, there is an accelerated bone loss that is independent of the age at which menopause begins and independent of whether the menopause is physiologic or surgically induced. This same accelerated bone loss can also be seen if postmenopausal estrogen replacement therapy is stopped.

Other factors that affect peak bone mass include genetics, race, calcium intake, nutrition, hormone levels, and lifestyle. Some evidence exists that female children and female relatives of women with osteoporotic fractures have lower peak bone mass and increased susceptibility to fracture. Genetic determinants of body size and build (ectomorphic body habitus) affect peak bone mass as they predispose to lower peak bone mass. Osteoporosis is less common in African Americans than in Caucasians or Asians.

Calcium nutrition plays a significant role in the level of peak bone mass. The three periods in life during which calcium intake is most important are childhood, adolescence, and old age. Children receiving calcium-rich diets have a higher hip bone density as adults. Malnutrition, for example, anorexia nervosa, is associated with decreased bone mass. Inadequate calcium intake during pregnancy results in mobilization of calcium to the baby with resultant loss from the maternal bone. In the elderly, increased calcium intake is necessary to overcome less efficient gastrointestinal absorption of calcium.

Hormones associated with bone metabolism are parathyroid hormone, calcitonin, growth hormone, insulin, and sex hormones (estrogen, progesterone, testosterone). In the female with low estrogen levels, there is increased osteoclast activity with increased bone resorption relative to formation. Hypogonadism in the male decreases peak bone mass and increases the rate of age-related bone loss. Some believe insulin-dependent diabetes mellitus predisposes to osteoporosis.

The three primary lifestyle factors that alter bone metabolism are physical activity, cigarette smoking, and alcohol consumption. Physical activity acts to increase bone formation before and during puberty. After puberty, weight-bearing exercise helps to maintain bone mass. Prolonged immobilization of any cause results in a decrease in bone mass and predisposes to fractures. Smokers have a 1.5 to 2.0 times higher incidence of vertebral (men) and hip (women) fractures. In women, cigarette smoking increases estrogen metabolism in the liver and lowers circulating estrogen levels. Alcohol consumption of 7 oz or more per week has been demonstrated to decrease bone mass, increase bone loss, and increase the incidence of fractures.

Because the best approach to osteoporosis management is prevention, modifiable risk factors should be addressed by the physician. In addition to the above three factors, attention must be paid to the environment in which an osteoporosis-prone person lives. This environment should be made safe so that falls are prevented.

Several medical problems that contribute to bone loss or depressed bone formation are modifiable through medical management. Examples of these include hyperthyroidism, pregnancy, diabetes, non–pregnancy-related amenorrhea, oligomenorrhea, hypoestrogenic states such as gonadal dysgenesis (Turner syndrome), and early menopause (see Table 41–1). Proper management of these conditions can help to maintain bone mass and prevent or slow the onset of osteoporosis.

Diagnosis

Many times the diagnosis of osteoporosis is discovered as an incidental finding during evaluation for another medical concern. Some aspects of the history and physical examination identify those with osteoporosis or those at risk for developing osteoporosis. A common historical finding is back pain related to vertebral compression fracture. Other findings are a history of fractures; significant prolonged oligomenorrhea or amenorrhea, early menopause (either physiologic or medical); hyperparathyroidism, hyperthyroidism; Turner syndrome; family history of osteoporosis or fractures at a relatively early age; alcohol use; sedentary lifestyle; and smoking. Medications associated with osteoporosis include long-term heparin use, discontinuation of estrogen replacement therapy, high-dose fluoride use, and high-dose or long-term corticosteroid use (see also Table 41–1. Physical findings associated with osteoporosis include short stature, small body frame, decrease in height when compared with maximal height, dowager's hump, kyphoscoliosis, hepatomegaly, spider angioma, palmar erythema, and moon facies of Cushing disease.

Biochemical tests can be used in addition to static indicators to complement the historical screening for those at risk. Indicators of increased bone resorption include a fasting urine calcium level corrected by creatinine excretion, which is an inexpensive test but it lacks sensitivity. Markers for increased bone formation include alkaline phosphatase (lacks sensitivity and specificity) and osteocalcin. Osteocalcin has been identified as a marker for bone fragility associated with hip fractures.

Currently, the most accurate method available to selectively screen for those at risk for developing osteoporosis and/or fractures is bone densitometry. As a screening procedure bone densitometry should be limited to those who, based on history and physical finding, demonstrate multiple risks for the development of osteoporosis (Table 41–2). Vertebral abnormalities on radiographs or suspicious fractures, asymptomatic primary hyperparathyroidism, chronic alcoholism, or long-term glucocorticoid use are some examples. Bone densitometry can also be used to follow the progress of patients who are being treated with the goal of arresting the progress of osteoporosis. Procedures available for assessment of bone density or mass include conventional radiography, single-photon and x-ray absorptiometry, dual-photon absorptiometry, radiographic absorptiometry, quantitative computed tomography, and ultrasonography. Of these, dual-energy x-ray absorptiometry (DXA) is currently believed by many to be the most precise.

The World Health Organization cutoff values for low bone density and for osteoporosis are: low bone density is a bone mineral density (BMD) 1 to 2.5 standard deviations (SD) below the reference group mean; osteoporosis is BMD greater than 2.5 SD below the mean. A decrease in 1 SD in bone mineral density increases the fracture incidence 50 to 100 per cent. Evaluation of the spine and hip are more important than evaluation of peripheral bone (e.g., radius). Universal bone densitometry screening has not been demonstrated to be cost-effective.

Management

The approach to management can in general be divided into two parts. The first is prevention. The second is management after osteoporosis and/or fracture has been identified. Preventing or delaying bone loss is just as efficacious as treatment after diagnosis. Therapy should be selected based on underlying pathophysiology, increased bone resorption, or decreased bone formation. In menopausal patients, management should be directed toward decreasing bone resorption. In age-related osteoporosis, management may be directed at increasing bone formation. When osteoporosis is the consequence of a specific medical problem or medication, management of the medical problem or use of another medication should be addressed.

Antiresorptive drugs such as estrogen and bisphosphonates act to decrease excess osteoclast activity and have a greater effect on trabecular bone, stabilizing structural integrity but not necessarily improving or reversing the process. Bone formation–enhancing drugs such as sodium fluoride, parathyroid hormone, and anabolic steroids serve to activate the number of bone-forming units and increase the activity of individual osteoblasts. The integrity of the new bone is not always optimal. For example, it has been noted that with sodium fluoride use, although there is measurably more bone formed, there is also an increase in the number of fractures.

Estrogens should be begun at the time of menopause to prevent the early, rapid phase of bone loss. Even if this early phase is past before estrogen is started, estrogen should be started to prevent further bone loss. In postmenopausal osteoporosis, estrogen has been demonstrated to decrease the rate of fracture by 50 per cent. The minimal effective dose of estrogen is 0.625 mg of conjugated equine estrogen (Premarin), or 1.0 mg of estradiol (Estrace). If the patient has a uterus, a progestin must be given to decrease the chance of developing endometrial hyperplasia or endometrial cancer. It can be given in either a cyclic or a continuous fashion. No evidence exists that progestins used with estrogen inhibit bone formation.

Bisphosphonates act to inhibit osteoclast activity for very long periods of time (years) and must be given cyclically with long rest periods. The bone

TABLE 41–2. Risk Factors for Osteoporosis

Age: elderly
Race: Caucasian, Oriental
Reduced weight for height (ectomorphic body habitus)
Early menopause (spontaneous or surgical)
Family history of osteoporosis
Diet: deficient calcium or vitamin D, excessive caffeine or alcohol
Medications: heparin, corticosteroids, GnRH antagonists
Cigarette smoking
Calcium deficiency
Sedentary lifestyle/immobilization
Endocrine disorders
  Diabetes mellitus
  Hyperparathyroid
  Turner syndrome
  Oligomenorrhea
  Hyperthyroid
  Cushing disease
  Precocious menopause
  Amenorrhea

TABLE 41-3.   Optimal Calcium Requirements

Age Group	Optimal Daily Intake of Calcium (mg)
Birth–6 months	400
6 months–1 year	600
1–5 years	800
6–10 years	800–1200
11–24 years	1200–1500
Men, 25–65 years	1000
Men, over 65 years	1500
Women, 25–50 years	1000
Pregnant or nursing	1200–1500
Postmenopausal, estrogen	1000
Postmenopausal, no estrogen	1500
Women over 65 years	1500

formed with this treatment has been demonstrated to be biochemically and histologically normal. Their use has been demonstrated not only to decrease fractures but to a modest degree increase bone mass in the vertebral bodies. Alendronate (Fosamax) is well tolerated and has a low side effect profile, primarily gastrointestinal. Newer bisphosphonates are being developed. Bisphosphonates are useful in the woman who is not able to take estrogen (e.g., one with breast cancer, endometrial cancer) or who is at high risk for fracture or recurrent fracture.

When given by itself in postmenopausal women, calcium has demonstrated a decrease in bone loss. This benefit is lost after 5 years of use. Adequate calcium is essential throughout a woman's life and the requirement varies with age (Table 41–3). Only elemental calcium is absorbed. Table 41–4 lists the amount of elemental calcium available in various products. A side effect of calcium intake in high doses is renal calculi. Vitamin D–fortified foods should be eaten along with calcium because vitamin D facilitates positive calcium metabolism.

Calcitonin inhibits bone resorption and is useful in high turnover osteoporosis. It has been shown to increase bone mass in postmenopausal women taking estrogen. It also reduced the incidence of fractures of the hip, vertebrae, and forearm. Interestingly, calcitonin also has an analgesic effect for 50 per cent of those with pain from osteoporosis-related fracture. Calcitonin use particularly favors cortical (cancellous) bone. The drug is available in an intranasal dosage route. It is expensive. Side effects include nausea with or without vomiting, site-of-injection reactions, and flushing of face or hands.

Infrequently used, there are three drugs that stimulate bone formation—sodium fluoride, androgens, and parathyroid hormone. Fluorides increase bone mass, but the bone formed is more fragile and there is an increase in fracture rate with its use. Therefore, fluorides have a narrow margin of safety. Androgens increase bone mass. In women, however, they also lead to acne, hirsutism, hoarseness, and mild increase in facial hair. Other side effects include risk of hepatotoxicity and lowering of high-density lipoprotein (HDL). Parathyroid hormone stimulates bone growth in low doses or when given in intermittent doses. Parathyroid hormone, however, stimulates bone resorption in higher doses.

Nonpharmacologic therapies include increased use of weight-bearing exercises. In all ages the benefit persists only while exercising continues. Women who exercise excessively (e.g., female Olympians) may become amenorrheic (hypoestrogenemic). The positive effect of exercise on bone mass is lost owing to the adverse effect of exercise-induced hypogonadotrophic hypogonadism. Exercises that appear to be beneficial are those in which there is direct weight bearing such as walking, hiking, stair climbing, jogging, dancing, tennis. Further efforts should be made to decrease environmental hazards that increase the risk of falling and to improve health conditions that may contribute to the risk of falling (e.g., avoid medications that may lead to falls, avoid polypharmacy).

TABLE 41-4.   Relative Amounts of Elemental Calcium

Source	Elemental Calcium (mg)
Calcium carbonate (1000 mg)	400
Tribasic calcium phosphate (1000 mg)	390
Yogurt (8 oz)	300
Orange juice (Ca fortified, 8 oz)	300
Cheese (1.5 oz)	300
Milk (8 oz)	300
Calcium citrate* (1000 mg)	240
Calcium lactate* (1000 mg)	130
Calcium gluconate* (1000 mg)	90
Calcium glubionate (1000 mg)	65

*Solubility is pH-dependent.

Association of Professors of Gynecology and Obstetrics. Osteoporosis; Diagnosis, Treatment, Monitoring. APGO Educational Series on Women's Health Issues. Washington, D.C., 1996.

Gamble CL. Osteoporosis: Making the diagnosis in patients at risk for fracture. Geriatrics 1995;50:24–33.

Gamble CL. Osteoporosis: Drug and nondrug therapies for the patient at risk. Geriatrics 1995;50:39–43.

Lufkin EG, Zilkoski M. Diagnosis and Management of Osteoporosis. American Family Physician Monograph No. 1, 1996.

Nightingale SL. From the Food and Drug Administration: Alendronate approved for bone disorders. JAMA 1995;274:1578.

NIH Consensus Conference. Optimal calcium intake. JAMA 1994;272:1942–1948.

Stanford JL, Weiss NS, Voigt LF, et al. Combined estrogen and progestin hormone replacement therapy. I: Relation to risk of breast cancer in middle-aged women. JAMA 1995;274:137–142.

QUESTIONS

1. Peak bone mass is reached at the age of
   a. 30 years
   b. 35 years
   c. 40 years
   d. 45 years
   e. 50 years

2. In the postmenopausal woman, which of the following would *not* accelerate the development of osteoporosis?
   a. Hypothyroidism
   b. Alcohol abuse
   c. Smoking
   d. Early menopause
   e. History of fractures

3. The recommended daily amount of calcium for a postmenopausal woman not on estrogen replacement therapy is
   a. 500 mg
   b. 1000 mg
   c. 1500 mg
   d. 2000 mg
   e. None of the above

Answers appear on **page 605**.

Chapter **42**

Chest Pain

Jane E. Corboy, M.D.

SUBJECTIVE

Presenting Problem

Jim W. is a 61-year-old white male accountant who has had chest pains for the past month.

Present Illness

Jim first noticed the pains when he was cleaning the apartment of his younger sister, who had committed suicide the previous week by jumping from the window of her third floor apartment. Jim and his oldest daughter drove 700 miles to his sister's home the day after learning of the suicide. They started packing and cleaning the apartment the following day. Jim noticed an aching tightness in his throat and mid-chest while carrying boxes up and down stairs, scrubbing and vacuuming floors. The pain did not radiate or change location. He had no nausea, diaphoresis, or shortness of breath with the pain. The discomfort lasted for 2 to 5 minutes after he reached the top of the stairs. He took Tums without relief or prevention of the pain.

Since he returned home, Jim has noticed the pains less frequently. He has had one or two episodes a week that have occurred with the moderate exertion of lifting and unpacking boxes. He had not had similar pain in the past, but admits that his activity level had been quite low for several years. None of the episodes has lasted more than 30 minutes.

Past Medical History

Jim has had a hiatal hernia and reflux esophagitis for several years. He regularly takes an antacid/antigas medication after meals and at bedtime. He has no history of hypertension, diabetes, previously known heart disease, asthma, or psychiatric disease.

Family History

Jim's father died at the age of 32 years from peritonitis due to appendicitis. His father's two brothers died suddenly in their sixties of uncertain causes. His mother is 89 years old and has hypertension and osteoarthritis. Jim had no other brothers or sisters. No family history exists of premature heart disease, diabetes, hyperlipidemia, or stroke.

Social History

Jim is the plant accountant for the local factory of a national manufacturing company. He has worked for the same company since his teens with time off for military service during World War II. He describes his work as stressful because of his management responsibilities. Jim completed high school and some college. He has been married for 35 years. He and his wife have three daughters, ages 19, 28, and 29 years, all living away from home. Since his sister's death, his mother has moved in with Jim and his wife.

Health Habits

Jim has never smoked. His alcohol intake is less than one drink per week. Jim usually eats three meals a day with moderately high fat intake, and enjoys a late-night snack of ice cream or cheese and crackers. He drinks one or two cups of coffee daily. Jim occasionally plays tennis or golf, but has no regular exercise routine.

Review of Systems

Positive results are observed only as in the history of present illness. His esophageal reflux symptoms had been somewhat worse over the past several months and are associated with increased weight.

OBJECTIVE

Physical Examination

Jim is a moderately obese white man in no acute distress. His vital signs are: height 5'8"; weight 180 pounds; blood pressure 160/102; pulse 82. Significant physical findings involving the cardiovascular system include mild arteriovenous narrowing on funduscopic examination, no carotid bruits, cardiac examination normal except for distant heart sounds, peripheral pulses mildly decreased in the lower extremities. Abdominal examination showed slight epigastric tenderness. The remainder of the examination, including the neurologic system, is normal. Jim does not want to discuss his feelings about his sister's death.

Laboratory

A fasting multitest chemistry panel was notable for a total cholesterol level of 266. His high-density lipoprotein (HDL) cholesterol level was 42, triglycerides level 175, and the calculated low-density lipoprotein (LDL) cholesterol level was 189.

ASSESSMENT

Working Diagnoses

The most likely diagnoses to explain Jim's symptoms are as follows.

Angina Pectoris. Jim gives a classic description of chest tightness or pain brought on by exertion and emotional stress and relieved by rest. In a man with cardiovascular risk factors of hypertension, sedentary lifestyle, and elevated cholesterol, angina pectoris is the most likely, as well as the most critical, diagnosis to consider.

Grief Reaction, Unresolved. Jim's unwillingness to discuss his feelings about his sister's recent unexpected violent death may be due to his immediate concerns about his own health. It would be useful to know if he had discussed his reactions to the event with his family or church pastor, because unresolved grief may negatively affect his physical well being.

Hypercholesterolemia. With a total cholesterol level over 240, LDL cholesterol level over 160, and a total to HDL cholesterol ratio of 6.4, Jim's cholesterol profile places him in high risk for atherosclerotic heart disease.

Differential Diagnosis

Costochondritis or Musculoskeletal Chest Pain. Chest pain arising from the chest wall, ribs and costochondral joints is usually sharp in nature. The pain lasts seconds rather than minutes. It may worsen with moving the arms or a severe cough. Physical examination shows tenderness on palpation of the chest wall. Movement of the arms often reproduces the patient's pain. With Jim's history of lifting heavy boxes at the time the pain started, this diagnosis is possible. Without the chest wall tenderness, it must be a diagnosis of exclusion.

Esophageal Disease. Esophageal pain may be from reflux or spasm. Reflux pain is classically burning in nature and occurs shortly after meals. It may worsen with activities that increase reflux, such as reclining or straining, thereby increasing intra-abdominal pressure. Antacids usually provide rapid relief of the pain of reflux. Esophageal spasm causes a substernal pressure-type pain, which may last 2 to 5 minutes, similar to that in angina. It usually radiates to the back rather than the arms. The pain is more likely to occur after meals, and usually it is not associated with exertion. Antacids provide variable relief of the pain of esophageal spasm. Jim's history of hiatal hernia makes esophageal disease a reasonable inclusion in the differential diagnosis.

Pericarditis or Pleuritis. Chest pain from inflammation of the pleura or pericardium is sharp, worsened by a deep breath or cough. It is usually associated with other symptoms reflecting the primary disease or condition, such as fever and cough with pneumonia, dyspnea with a pulmonary embolism, positional pain and fever with pericarditis. Physical examination reveals friction rubs over the inflamed pleura or pericardium. Jim's history and physical findings are not consistent with this diagnosis.

Anxiety. Either situational anxiety or a primary anxiety disorder may cause chest pain, discomfort, or palpitations. Usually, situational anxiety occurs in association with stressful life events, and the symptoms are transitory. With generalized anxiety disorder, the patient may have unrealistic worries about several life events. Physical symptoms reflect muscle tension, autonomic hyperactivity, and excessive central nervous system arousal. Panic attacks may cause intense discomfort and multiple symptoms including dyspnea, dizziness, trembling, sweating, nausea, chills, fear of dying or of losing control, along with chest pain or palpitations. Jim certainly has undergone a stressful event and may have worries and concerns, but his symptoms are not consistent with a true anxiety disorder.

PLAN

Diagnostic

The goal of the diagnostic plan for angina is to establish the significance of the patient's symptoms. The specific objectives are:

Evaluate Risk Factors for Accelerated Atherosclerosis. The history reveals smoking, poor exercise habits, and family history of heart disease. Physical examination may reveal hypertension, xanthomata or xanthalasmata. Abnormal levels of cholesterol, creatinine, or glucose may suggest hyperlipoproteinemia, renal insufficiency, or diabetes. Jim has two major cardiac risk factors, hypertension and hypercholesterolemia. His family history is unclear, but it is suggestive of heart disease.

Identify Conditions That May Exacerbate or Trigger Angina Symptoms. Conditions that increase myocardial oxygen demand, such as thyrotoxicosis or fever, are detectable on history and physical examination. The history and physical may suggest certain conditions that decrease oxygen supply, such as anemia and hypoxemia. Laboratory tests including hemoglobin or hematocrit and arterial blood gases provide confirmation.

Determine the Presence and Extent of Coronary Artery Disease. Jim's *resting electrocardiogram* was normal, and he did not have pain during the office visit. An *exercise electrocardiogram* (ECG) or treadmill stress test may elicit ECG changes with exercise. Jim's physician scheduled him for an exercise ECG to be done before his next visit in 1 week.

Coronary angiography to define the coronary artery anatomy and left ventricular function is important in determining the patient's prognosis. The risks and indications for angiography are discussed later.

Education

The goal of patient education in angina is to enable the patient to reduce his morbidity and mortality from cardiovascular disease. The specific objectives are as follows.

Inform the Patient of the Meaning of His Chest Pain Symptoms. Jim's physician advised him that his chest discomfort is likely to represent an imbalance of the heart muscle's oxygen supply and demand. It therefore signifies a threat to the health of the heart. He and his physician discussed that he should stop and rest immediately at the onset of pain to avoid prolonging the precarious situation.

Recommend Lifestyle Modifications to Reduce Further Cardiovascular Risk. Jim and his physician discussed a low-fat, low-cholesterol, reduced-caffeine diet. Because of the mild hypertension, he also received instructions on reducing his salt intake.

Educate the Patient on Basic Pathophysiology of Angina, Rationale for Therapy, and Treatment Options Available. Jim received information on basic coronary artery anatomy. He learned that treatment aims to increase blood flow to the heart, either with medications or by mechanical means. He received nitroglycerin sublingual tablets (0.4 mg) with instructions to carry them with him at work and home. He understood that he should use one under his tongue at the onset of pain and a second tablet if his pain does not disappear after about 5 minutes. He and his physician also briefly discussed the treatment plan of medical versus surgical management, depending on the outcome of his treadmill test.

Therapeutic

The goal of therapy of angina is to reduce mortality from coronary artery disease.

The specific objectives are

1. Reduction of cardiovascular risk factors, as discussed earlier

2. Treatment of coexisting conditions that aggravate angina

3. Amelioration of the fundamental disparity between myocardial oxygen supply and demand

The methods include pharmacologic (medical) therapy and "invasive" therapy, which are discussed at greater length in the Discussion section, later. Jim's physician prescribed propranolol, 40 mg four times daily.

RETURN VISIT—SUBJECTIVE

Jim had only one episode of chest pain in the preceding week. The pain occurred while he was climbing stairs at work and was promptly relieved with the nitroglycerin. He and his family have sorted his sister's belongings and have given away or discarded most of the household goods and clothing. He reports that he read some of her letters and diaries in an attempt to understand her suicide. He has begun to discuss the event with his wife.

OBJECTIVE

Jim has no significant changes in his physical examination, including vital signs. His exercise ECG showed downsloping ST segment depression in leads I, II, aVF, and V3 to V6, which occurred 5 minutes into the exercise portion of the test at a heart rate of 120 (75 per cent of predicted maximal heart rate). Jim reported chest tightness at the time of the ECG changes, and the examination was stopped. No fall in blood pressure occurred, and the ECG changes and pain resolved approximately 5 minutes after stopping exercise.

ASSESSMENT

Coronary Artery Disease. With Jim's symptoms, cardiac risk factors and a positive stress test, the diagnosis of atherosclerotic cardiovascular disease is almost certain. The diffuse ST segment depression indicates that a large portion of the myocardium is at risk.

Grief Reaction. Jim has begun to address his questions and come to terms with his sister's death.

PLAN

Jim was referred to a cardiologist for a coronary angiogram and left ventriculogram. The angiogram showed 90 per cent occlusion of the left main coronary artery, 95 per cent occlusion of the left anterior descending artery proximal to the obtuse marginal branch, and 95 per cent blockage of a dominant right coronary artery in its mid-portion. Left ventricular function was good with a 60 per cent ejection fraction and no discrete areas of hypokinesis. Jim was referred to a cardiovascular surgeon for coronary artery bypass surgery.

DISCUSSION

Angina pectoris is one of the four cardinal manifestations of ischemic heart disease. The other three are myocardial infarction, congestive heart failure, and arrhythmia. The major determinants of myocardial oxygen consumption are listed in Table 42–1. Because angina usually represents a *transient* imbalance in myocardial oxygen supply and demand, patients may present with angina before the myocardium is permanently damaged. Because patients with angina pectoris have a better prognosis than those with silent ischemia or prolonged ischemia, the physician must recognize classic angina symptoms and diagnose and treat the condition accurately and promptly.

Diagnosis

The resting ECG may show an old myocardial infarction, but it may be completely normal if the

TABLE 42–1. Determinants of Myocardial Oxygen Consumption

I. Determinants of oxygen demand
  A. Heart rate
  B. Wall tension
    1. Blood pressure
    2. Ventricular size
    3. Ventricular wall tension
  C. Contractility
  D. Metabolic rate
II. Determinants of oxygen supply
  A. Coronary artery patency
    1. Spasm
    2. Fixed obstruction
    3. Platelet aggregation
  B. Blood oxygen carrying capacity
    1. Hemoglobin content
    2. Oxygen saturation

TABLE 42–2. Correlation Among ECG Changes, Location of Ischemia, and Coronary Artery Involved

ECG Leads with ST Segment Depression	Area of Ischemic Myocardium	Coronary Artery
II, III, aVF	Inferior	Right coronary artery
V1, V2 (elevation)	Posterior	Right coronary artery
V2–V4	Anteroseptal	Left anterior descending branch
V3–V5	Anterior	Left anterior descending branch
I, aVL	High lateral	Circumflex or diagonal branch
V5, V6	Apical	Left anterior descending branch, or posterior descending of right CA

Adapted from Ischemic heart disease: Angina pectoris. Sci Am Med 1994;1–20.

patient does not have pain. An ECG done while the patient has pain may show transient ST segment depression or T wave inversion in the leads that correlate with the location of the ischemic segment (see Table 42–2). This finding helps to predict the coronary artery obstruction, as well as establish that the pain is indeed angina.

Patients who have classic angina and numerous risk factors for heart disease may not need an exercise ECG, because the outcome of this test should not dissuade the physician from suspecting heart disease in those patients. If the diagnosis is uncertain, however, an exercise ECG may assist the diagnosis. Exercise-induced ECG changes associated with typical anginal pain, fatigue, or a fall in blood pressure are strongly predictive of the presence of coronary artery disease. The exercise ECG is also useful in detecting exercise-induced ECG changes or arrhythmias that have not caused angina pain. These changes represent "silent ischemia." Table 42–3 lists the criteria for ECG changes that most reliably indicate the presence of myocardial ischemia. False-negative test results (a negative result in a person with coronary artery disease) occur about one third of the time, and false-positive results occur in about 10 per cent of people who do not have coronary artery disease. Because of the imperfect sensitivity and specificity of the test, the physician should consider the likelihood of the disease before performing the test. A negative test result does not

TABLE 42–3. Exercise ECG Criteria for Ischemia

ST segment depression that:
   Is over 1 mm in amplitude
   Is a horizontal or downsloping contour
   Occurs early in exercise
   Persists for a few minutes after exercise

rule out angina in a person with numerous risk factors and a high likelihood of disease.

Other noninvasive diagnostic studies include the thallium or sestamibi stress test, which combines electrocardiographic measurements with a radioisotope uptake scan. It provides increased sensitivity and specificity over the standard exercise ECG, but it is a more expensive test. Other imaging techniques are available, including gated wall motion studies of left ventricular function, magnetic resonance imaging of the heart, and others.

Coronary angiography provides the most accurate information about the status of the coronary arteries and left ventricular function. Because of its invasive nature it also has greater risks than the previously discussed examinations. These risks include myocardial infarction, stroke, and death. The physician must balance these risks against the value of the information gained by the procedure and recommend the procedure only for those patients for whom the benefits outweigh the risks. These patients include:

1. Young or vigorous patients who have a large area of cardiac muscle at risk

2. Patients who are incapacitated by atypical chest pain, to exclude the diagnosis of coronary artery disease

3. Patients undergoing cardiac surgery for valvular heart disease, to assess the presence or extent of coronary artery disease

4. Patients on maximal medical therapy who continue to have incapacitating angina

Treatment

The rationale for medical therapy is to reduce the discrepancy between myocardial oxygen demand and oxygen supply to the heart. Oxygen demand is reduced by lowering heart rate at rest and with exercise, decreasing blood pressure, lowering left ventricular volume, and decreasing contractility. The oxygen supply may be enhanced by increasing

coronary artery patency by preventing spasm, dilating fixed obstructions, or preventing platelet clumping. Each of the major categories of antianginal medications acts on one or more of these mechanisms. Some classes of drugs are complementary or synergistic with others. Some target different mechanisms; others interfere with the compensatory responses that limit the effectiveness of the other agent. Table 42–4 is a summary of the three categories of antianginal drugs.

Beta blockers act on the demand side of the myocardial oxygen equation by reducing heart rate, blood pressure, and myocardial contractility. Beta blockers are effective in the treatment of angina. They may reduce the risk of myocardial infarction and ischemia-related arrhythmia. Side effects include worsening or provocation of congestive heart failure or asthma. Other adverse effects include impotence, decreased exercise tolerance, and lethargy. They may block the hypoglycemic symptoms in patients with insulin-dependent diabetes mellitus. Beta blockers are classified as nonselective or cardioselective. Those that are cardioselective have less risk of inducing bronchospasm at standard therapeutic doses. Other characteristics that distinguish the different beta blockers include duration of action, degree of lipid solubility, and presence of intrinsic sympathomimetic activity. Each of these characteristics affects the agent's side effect profile or dosing frequency. These qualities may affect the patient's acceptance of and adherence to therapy.

Nitrates primarily affect ventricular volume by reducing left ventricular filling pressure. The mechanism of action is venous dilation and some arteriolar dilation. A secondary effect of nitrates is to dilate coronary arteries, relieve coronary artery spasm, and improve collateral flow. Side effects of nitrates are related to their vasodilating effects. Reflex tachycardia results from the decreased blood pressure. Headache and flushing resulting from vasodilation may discourage the patient from using these effective drugs. Beta blockers counter the tachycardia of nitrates and may also decrease the headache. Nitrates may be taken sublingually, as nitroglycerin, with rapid onset and short duration. Other dosing routes for angina are oral and transdermal. Patients on maintenance nitrates develop tolerance and loss of efficacy if the drugs are used continually. The patient should omit the bedtime dose of oral nitrates or remove the nitroglycerin patch at bedtime to prevent tolerance to the drug.

The *calcium antagonists* each have different effects on the myocardial oxygen demand/supply ratio. Verapamil decreases heart rate, blood pressure, and contractility. Its effects are similar to those of

TABLE 42–4. Drugs Commonly Used for Stable Angina Pectoris

Beta Blockers

Name	Cardiac Effects	CNS Effects (Lipid Solubility)	Dosage (mg/day)	Frequency (times/day)
Atenolol (Tenormin)	Cardioselective	Low	25–100	1
Metoprolol (Lopressor)	Cardioselective		50–200	2
Metoprolol (extended release) (Lopressor X-R)	Cardioselective		50–200	1
Nadolol (Corgard)		Low	20–240	1
Propranolol (Inderal)	Membrane stabilization		40–240	2
Propranolol (long-acting) (Inderal-LA)	Membrane stabilization		60–240	1

Calcium Channel Blockers

Name	Anti-arrhythmic Effect	Myocardial Depressant	Vasodilator		
			Systemic	Coronory	Cerebral
Verapamil	+ + +	+ +	+	+	+
Diltiazem	+ +	+	+ +	+ +	+ +
Nifedipine	−	+	+ + +	+ + +	+ + +
Felodipine	−	−	+ + +	+ + +	+ + +
Amlodipine	−	−	+ + +	+ + +	+ + +
Isradipine	−	−	+ + +	+ + +	+ + +
Nicardipine	−	−	+ + +	+ + +	+ + +

Nitrates

Name	Category	Route of Administration	Dosage (mg/dose)	Frequency (times/day)
Nitroglycerin	Immediate release	Sublingual	0.3–0.6	prn angina
Nitroglycerin	Immediate release	Topical	1″–2″	3–4 (12/hr/day)
Nitroglycerin	Sustained release	Transdermal	1 patch	12–14 hr/day
Nitroglycerin	Extended release	Oral	2.5–6.5	2–4
Isosorbide dinitrate	Immediate release	Sublingual	2.5–10	6–8
Isosorbide dinitrate	Immediate release	Oral	20–30	2–3
Isosorbide dinitrate	Sustained release	Oral	40–80	1–3
Isosorbide-5-mononitrate	Immediate release	Oral	20	2 (7 hr apart)
Isosorbide-5-mononitrate	Extended release	Oral	60–120	1

the beta blockers, but it does not precipitate asthma. Nifedipine, nicardipine, and israpidine have a greater effect on peripheral and coronary dilation. In this way, they behave similarly to the nitrates. Diltiazem's effects are between those of the other two groups. The different calcium antagonists have different side effects as well. The most common side effects with verapamil are constipation, bradycardia, and fatigue. Nifedipine most commonly causes headache, dizziness, and flushing.

Calcium antagonists are useful additions to the standard beta blocker and nitrate combination in patients who have not responded to maximal therapy. Another use is in patients who cannot tolerate beta blockers because of lung disease, diabetes, or other conditions.

Other components of medical management include treating hypertension, congestive heart failure, and other underlying medical conditions. In addition, aspirin 325 mg daily has been shown to prevent myocardial infarction by reducing platelet aggregation.

Surgical therapy or angioplasty is recommended for patients who have certain conditions.

Each of these groups has a large amount of myocardium at risk from myocardial infarction.

1. Those with left main coronary artery disease have better survival with surgery than with medical therapy.

2. Patients with three-vessel disease and decreased left ventricular function also have improved survival rates with surgery.

3. Two-vessel disease is also an indication for surgery, if one of the vessels is the proximal left anterior descending artery.

4. Those with intractable angina or silent ischemia on maximal medical management may benefit from surgery.

The indications for percutaneous transluminal coronary angioplasty (PTCA) are similar to those for coronary artery bypass grafting. Because the procedure is less invasive, however, it may be appropriate to use angioplasty on single-vessel lesions, as well.

SUGGESTED READING

Aspirin for prevention of myocardial infarction. Med Lett Drugs Ther 1995;37:14–16.

Drugs for stable angina pectoris. Med Lett Drugs Ther 1994;36:111–114.

Hjemdahl P, Eriksson SV, Held C, Rehnqvist N. Prognosis of patients with stable angina pectoris on antianginal drug therapy. Am J Cardiol 1996;77:6D–15D.

Nishiyama S, Iwase T, Ishiwata S, et al. Comparison of long-term efficacy of medical treatment versus coronary artery bypass grafting (CABG) in multivessel coronary artery disease. Jpn Heart J 1995;36:709–717.

Rakel RE. Textbook of Family Practice. 5th ed. Philadelphia, W.B. Saunders, 1995, pp 712–720.

Ischemic heart disease: Angina pectoris. Sci Am Med 1994:1–21.

Varnauskas E, The European Coronary Surgery Study Group. Twelve year follow-up of survival in the randomized European Coronary Surgery Study. N Engl J Med 1988;319:332–338.

QUESTIONS

1. Match each of the following antianginal drug classes with mechanism of action or side effects in items (1)–(4).
   a. Venous pooling, decreased ventricular filling pressure, coronary artery dilation, tachycardia
   b. Reduction of arrhythmia, fatigue, exacerbation of congestive heart failure, bradycardia
   c. Decreased myocardial contractility, constipation, fatigue
   d. Antiprostaglandin, gastrointestinal irritation, exacerbation of asthma
      (1) beta blockers
      (2) calcium antagonists
      (3) platelet inhibitors
      (4) nitrates

Answers appear on **page 605.**

Chapter 43

Shortness of Breath

Stephanie Wiman Wells, M.D.

SUBJECTIVE

PATIENT IDENTIFICATION AND PRESENTING PROBLEM. Janet O. is a 57-year-old mother of three children. She and her husband have owned and operated a reasonably successful bar and grill for the past 30 years. Janet works as the primary bartender. She presents to the doctor because of increased difficulty working her late-night shifts. Except for prenatal care during her teens and twenties, Janet has not made regular visits to her physician.

PRESENT ILLNESS. Janet states that she has always been "healthy as a horse" until approximately 6 months ago when she began to experience difficulty catching her breath. She is fine when she is working behind the bar, but when she carries cases of beer up the stairs from the basement storage she has to stop midway to catch her breath. This symptom has worsened to the point where she has to stop after two or three steps. She feels excessively tired just a few hours into her shift, and her customers are noticing that she is starting to slow down. She wonders if she is just getting "too old" for this kind of work.

Janet is also having problems sleeping. She has never had a problem with sleep because, she says, "I'm on my feet from 8 A.M. to 2 A.M. the next morning." Lately, though, she cannot sleep through the night because she constantly wakes up feeling as though she is choking. She gets a slightly better night's sleep if she sleeps in her husband's La-z-Boy downstairs; however, she still has to get up to go to the bathroom three to four times each night.

Janet states that her ankles have been staying swollen all day long. They have always tended to swell up by the end of the day, but the swelling no longer disappears throughout the night. Janet also jokes that the "rest of my body must be swelling" since her jeans seem to be getting "tighter and tighter."

PAST MEDICAL HISTORY. Janet had three normal vaginal deliveries during her late teens and twenties. She states that her doctor was worried about her blood pressure during her last pregnancy, but she never followed up after her delivery. Janet had her cholesterol level checked at a county fair several years ago and was told that it was high. Her children wanted her to see her doctor, but she was too busy. She has never had any surgeries. She takes no regular medicines except Maalox every once in a while for heartburn. She stopped having her periods about 6 or 7 years ago.

FMILY HISTORY. Janet's mother is 88 years old and has mild high blood pressure. She has never had a heart attack or stroke. Janet's father was a heavy drinker and died from a "bleeding ulcer" in his fifties. Janet is an only child and states that her grandparents died of "old age."

HEALTH HABITS. Janet used to drink heavily, but 20 years ago she cut back to two beers per night. Unfortunately, she replaced heavy drinking with heavy smoking. She has been smoking one and one-half packs of cigarettes for the past 20 years. She does not use illicit drugs. She gets no regular exercise beyond "running around the bar and grill all day" and has never lost the weight that she gained during her third pregnancy. Her diet consists primarily of "grill food" with very little fruits and vegetables. She "usually" wears her seatbelt.

SOCIAL HISTORY. Janet and her husband have been happily married since their teens. They were high school sweethearts and, for the most part, have enjoyed developing their business together. Janet admits that the bar is very stressful to operate and that she and her husband do not have a chance to properly care for themselves. Her three adult children are very supportive and are "constantly nagging" her to take better care of herself.

REVIEW OF SYSTEMS. No cough, chest pain, palpitations, visual changes, polydipsia, polyphagia, or dysuria. No gastrointestinal symptoms.

OBJECTIVE

PHYSICAL EXAMINATION. Blood pressure is 164/104; pulse 90; respiratory rate 12; oxygen saturation on room air 100%; height 5'4"; weight 160 lb. Pertinent findings include normal funduscopic examination, nonpalpable thyroid, normal neck veins, hyperdynamic apical impulse, S_4 on cardiac auscultation, clear lungs, obese abdomen, and 2+ pitting edema at the ankles.

LABORATORY TESTS. Blood chemistry panel revealed normal glucose and electrolyte levels, normal renal function and liver enzyme levels. Random cholesterol level was elevated at 260. Complete blood count (CBC) and urinalysis results were normal. Thyroid function tests were normal. ECG showed left ventricular hypertrophy (LVH) with no evidence of past or acute ischemic injury. Chest radiograph was normal.

ASSESSMENT

DIFFERENTIAL DIAGNOSES. The following are the most likely working diagnoses.

Congestive Heart Failure (CHF) as a Consequence of Untreated Hypertension. This is the most likely diagnosis based on the history alone. Janet relates some of the common presenting symptoms of CHF, namely dyspnea on exertion and fatigue (symptoms of left heart failure). Associated also with left heart failure are Janet's symptoms of paroxysmal nocturnal dyspnea (PND) and orthopnea. PND is often described as a sensation of choking or suffocating that causes awaking and causes patients to gasp for air. Orthopnea is shortness of breath that occurs in a recumbent position. These symptoms are due to the redistribution of fluid from the lower extremities to the thorax, which occurs when sleeping in the prone or supine position. Patients often try to ameliorate these symptoms by using several pillows (i.e., "four-pillow orthopnea") or by sleeping in a recliner or chair. Janet also relates symptoms of right heart failure and volume overload including nocturia, persistent lower extremity edema, and, possibly, increasing abdominal girth. Janet has functional class II disease according to the New York Heart Association classification of heart disease (Table 43-1).

TABLE 43-1. New York Heart Association Functional Classification of Heart Disease

Class I: No limitation of physical activity; no dyspnea, fatigue, or palpitations
Class II: Slight limitation of physical activity, dyspnea with ordinary physical activity, no dyspnea at rest
Class III: Marked limitation of physical activity, symptoms during mild exercise, no dyspnea at rest
Class IV: Severe limitation of physical activity, dyspnea at rest

Adapted from Yakubov SJ, Bope ET. Cardiovascular disease and arrhythmias. In Rakel RE (ed). Textbook of Family Practice, 5th ed. Philadelphia, W.B. Saunders, 1995, p 791.

Signs on Janet's physical examination consistent with the diagnosis of CHF are pitting edema of the lower extremities, left ventricular heave, and a fourth heart sound. The latter two findings combined with her elevated blood pressure and LVH on ECG make hypertension the likely etiology of her heart failure. Other signs of CHF that were not found include distended neck veins, lung rales and/or wheezing, third heart sound, tachycardia, hepatomegaly, and ascites.

Pulmonary Disease Consequent to Smoking. Janet's long history of smoking brings chronic obstructive pulmonary disease (COPD) and possibly asthma into consideration as causes of her dyspnea on exertion and fatigue. Pulmonary disease by itself does not explain all of her symptoms, especially her lower extremity edema and nocturia. These symptoms can be explained only by long-standing pulmonary disease leading to right heart failure (i.e., cor pulmonalc). If this were the case, Janet should be expected to have some abnormalities on lung examination, perhaps with some tachypnea and low oxygen saturation levels. Thus pulmonary disease may contribute to Janet's symptoms, but it is not likely to be the primary etiology.

Less Likely Diagnoses. Janet's physician likely considered a host of possible diagnoses as Janet listed her symptoms. For example, her dyspnea can be explained by CHF, exertional asthma, COPD, anemia, lung cancer, and anxiety with hyperventilation. Her extremity edema brings many diagnoses to mind: CHF, diabetes, nephrotic syndrome, venous stasis or obstruction, anemia, and hypothyroidism. The challenge to her physician is to come up with one diagnosis that can explain most, if not all, of Janet's symptoms and signs.

PLAN

DIAGNOSTIC. Because CHF has a high morbidity and mortality, the physician's first task is to look for a reversible cause such as hyperthyroidism, anemia, valvular abnormalities, or hypertension (Table 43–2). The search begins with a baseline laboratory evaluation, chest radiograph, and ECG.

Patients with CHF may have abnormal blood chemistry values including elevated blood urea nitrogen from decreased renal perfusion and elevated liver function tests from hepatic congestion. The chest radiograph often shows cardiomegaly from dilated heart chambers and evidence of pulmonary congestion such as cephalization (prominence of upper lobe pulmonary veins), Kerley's B lines (interstitial edema at the base of the lungs), and sometimes pleural effusions. The ECG may be normal or may show evidence of chamber enlargement, hypertrophy, or ischemia.

Janet has very few laboratory abnormalities, which is not uncommon in early CHF. Her LVH on ECG is a result of her long-standing hypertension, and the malfunction with her heart is likely to be diastolic rather then systolic dysfunction. Diastolic dysfunction is relatively common and occurs in approximately 40 per cent of people with CHF (Opie,

TABLE 43–2. Etiologies of Congestive Heart Failure

Left-sided
Primary myocardial failure (idiopathic, myocarditis)
Structural abnormalities
  Valvular regurgitation (aortic insufficiency, mitral regurgitation)
  Congenital heart disease
  Pericardial disease
  Ischemic heart disease
Secondary etiologies
  Viral
  Hypertension
  High-output failure (e.g., thyrotoxicosis)
  Toxins (e.g., cobalt, lead)
  Cardiac depressants (e.g., disopyramide)
  Drugs (e.g., Adriamycin)
Right-sided
Primary pulmonary hypertension
Cor pulmonale
Congenital heart disease
Collagen vascular diseases (e.g., systemic lupus erythematosus, scleroderma)
Tricuspid regurgitation or stenosis
Right ventricular infarction
Secondary to left ventricular failure

From Yakubov SJ, Bope ET: Cardiovascular disease and arrhythmias. *In* Rakel RE (ed). Textbook of Family Practice, 5th ed. Philadelphia, W.B. Saunders, 1995, p 790.

1995). An echocardiogram helps to confirm this (by documenting a normal systolic ejection fraction) and evaluates any valvular or regional wall motion abnormalities. Once Janet's symptoms are improved, she should be evaluated for ischemic heart disease using noninvasive testing first (stress test, nuclear imaging) and invasive cardiac catheterization if indicated. The possibility of ischemic heart disease is high, especially given Janet's numerous risk factors (smoking, hypertension, obesity, postmenopausal state without estrogen replacement and possible hypercholesterolemia).

THERAPEUTIC

1. The diagnoses of CHF and hypertension were discussed with Janet. The various treatment strategies and the need to quit smoking, reduce weight, and improve her diet were discussed as well. She was reassured about the continued support of her physician during these changes.

2. Hydrochlorothiazide 25 mg/day was started to alleviate Janet's leg edema as well as treat her hypertension. She was instructed to keep a record of her daily weight to monitor the effectiveness of diuretic treatment.

3. Instructions on a reduced-sodium (3–4 g/day) diet as well as low-fat diet were given.

4. Instruction to avoid activities that cause symptoms (i.e., climbing stairs) were given.

5. Janet was asked to return to the office in 1 week.

First Follow-Up Visit

SUBJECTIVE. One week later Janet states that her legs feel less swollen and that she has been able to move back into the bed to sleep. Her shortness of breath while climbing stairs has improved somewhat. Her husband and children are very worried about her health and are pressuring her to hire some extra help around the bar.

OBJECTIVE. Her blood pressure is 150/98. Janet appears somewhat depressed. Lungs are clear. S4 persists on cardiac examination. Extremities appear to have trace edema at the ankles. Fasting total cholesterol level is 240, LDL 148, HDL 47, and triglyceride level 225.

ASSESSMENT

1. Congestive heart failure—improving
2. Hypertension—moderately controlled
3. Hypercholesterolemia—mild

PLAN

1. Add lisinopril 5 mg/day po
2. Further instructions on fat/cholesterol reduction diet. Janet stated that she and her husband are considering changing the menu at their bar and grill.
3. Further counseling and support
4. Referral for echocardiogram
5. Follow-up appointment in 1 to 2 weeks to assess progress and for further counseling

DISCUSSION

CHF is a complex syndrome that occurs when the heart cannot meet the demands of the body or when the heart muscle cannot relax appropriately. It is an extremely common condition that affects approximately 3 million patients in the United States and occurs in approximately 400,000 patients each year (Yakubov, 1995). It is a leading cause of hospital admissions in all age groups and especially in people older than 65 years. CHF is associated with high morbidity and mortality. Despite numerous treatment modalities, approximately 40 per cent of patients with CHF die within 4 years of therapy (Yakubov, 1995).

Management begins with a search for a precipitating, and possibly reversible, cause of CHF. If such a cause is found, the primary treatment involves trying to reverse the underlying etiology (e.g., reversing hyperthyroidism or revascularizing an ischemic heart). General treatment measures independent of the etiology of the CHF include dietary salt restriction, exercise rehabilitation and weight loss, and psychological support. Pharmacologic treatment usually begins with diuretics and angiotensin converting enzyme (ACE) inhibitors and may progress to inotropic agents (e.g., digoxin), vasodilators (e.g., nitroglycerin), and fluid restriction in severe cases.

SUGGESTED READING

DeGowin RL. DeGowin and DeGowin's Diagnostic Examination, 6th ed. New York, McGraw-Hill, 1994, pp 327–333.

Elkayam U. Congestive heart failure. In Rakel RE (ed). Conn's Current Therapy. Philadelphia, W.B. Saunders Company, 1997, pp 288–294.

Opie LH. Drugs for the Heart, 4th ed. Philadelphia, W.B. Saunders Company, 1995, pp 112–114 and 323–325.

Yakubov SJ, Bope ET. Cardiovascular disease (congestive heart failure). In Rakel RE (ed). Textbook of Family Practice, 5th ed. Philadelphia, W.B. Saunders Company, 1995, pp 789–794.

QUESTIONS

1. True or False: Etiologies of congestive heart failure include
   a. Aortic stenosis
   b. Myocardial infarction
   c. Antidepressants
   d. Hypertension

2. True or false: The chest radiograph in patients with congestive heart failure may reveal
   a. Kerley's B lines
   b. Cardiomegaly
   c. Hilar adenopathy
   d. Pleural effusions

Answers appear on **page 605.**

Chapter 44

Hypertension

David E. Burtner, M.D.

SUBJECTIVE

Bill P. is a 44-year-old white male who presents as a work-in patient. Earlier today he had tried to give blood but was turned away because of having a blood pressure of 170/107 mm Hg. After a quick evaluation, he is found to be asymptomatic. He specifically denies any headaches, changes in mentation, chest pain, shortness of breath, or lack of urination. He is instructed to come in for two blood pressure checks weekly and schedule a thorough evaluation in 3 weeks.

Blood pressure measurements are 167/102 mm Hg and 181/106 on the two weekly visits; thus, the diagnosis of hypertension is established. A complete evaluation is begun with a thorough history. Bill had only one previous elevated blood pressure on an insurance physical 8 years ago. He has no history of renal problems. There has been no change in weight. He has not experienced heat, cold intolerance, or flushing episodes. He is on no medications. His job does not involve chemical or toxin exposures.

PAST MEDICAL HISTORY

Bill had a normal childhood other than some early asthma. He had the usual childhood illnesses. He was hospitalized once for a compound fracture of his left leg from an auto accident at age 25 years. He was treated as an outpatient 4 years ago for pneumonia without sequelae. He has mild allergic rhinitis. He is on no long-term medications but does take clemastine (Tavist), intermittently. His allergies are the seasonal environmental type only. His immunizations are up to date including a diphtheria and tetanus shot 6 years ago and an influenza shot last fall.

Review of Systems

No problems are noted other than muscle tension–type headaches about once monthly. He requires corrective lenses for distant vision.

Social History

Bill works as an insurance adjuster. He is married a second time, with two children, ages 13 and 11 years from the previous marriage, and a 5-year-old from this marriage of 6 years. He hunts and fishes as a hobby but gets little aerobic exercise. He has smoked one-half pack of cigarettes per day since age 20 years. He drinks an average of one beer a day.

Family History

A maternal uncle had early-onset hypertension and died from a myocardial infarction at age 59 years. Parents are both alive and well. He has a sister who is now 39 and a survivor of thyroid cancer at age 24 years. No other family members have premature myocardial infarctions or cerebrovascular accidents.

OBJECTIVE

Height 69″ Weight 190 lbs
 Temperature 97.8
 Pulse 86 and regular
 Respiratory rate 16
 Blood pressure
  168/102 right arm sitting
  172/100 left arm sitting
  178/106 left arm standing
  165/100 left arm recumbent
 General Impression: Mildly obese white male in no distress and appearing stated age.

Skin: Multiple café-au-lait spots noted.

HEENT: Normocephalic. TMs and canals normal with grossly normal hearing.

PERRLA: Conjunctiva and sclera normal. Fundoscopic examination showed sharp discs. A:V ratio was 1:2 with some early crossing changes. Nose and throat are normal.

Neck: No masses or bruits noted. Normal thyroid to palpation.

Chest: Clear to percussion and auscultation.

Heart: Regular rhythm with physiologically split S_2 and tambor quality to S_2 in aortic area. PMI is in the midclavicular line, fourth intercostal space. Pulses are all 2+ and equal bilaterally. Radial and femoral pulses are simultaneous. There are no abdominal, flank, or femoral bruits.

Abdomen: Normal bowel sounds. Nontender without masses.

Genitalia: Normal circumcised male with testes descended bilaterally and no evidence of hernia.

Rectal: No masses. Normal prostate. Occult blood negative.

Extremities: Normal

Neurologic: Normal

Laboratory examinations:

   CBC: normal

   U/A: trace protein

   Chem 18: Cholesterol 287 mg/dl

      HDL: 28

      Glucose, potassium, calcium, uric acid, protein, BUN, and creatinine are all normal

ECG: mild LVH by voltage criteria only

24-hour urine for metanephrines and VMA: normal

ASSESSMENT

Findings are consistent with essential hypertension.

PLAN

The patient is strongly advised on the importance of smoking cessation. He had already been restricting salt intake. He is also advised to continue to limit his alcohol to 1 ounce per day. He agrees to attempt a diet reduced in calories, saturated fats, and cholesterol.

Antihypertensive therapy is begun with atenolol, although plans are to watch closely its effect on the patient's lipid profile. Follow-up in 4 to 6 weeks is planned.

DISCUSSION

Diagnosis

Establishing the diagnosis of hypertension clearly begins with the documentation of elevated blood pressures. The blood pressures must be measured with the proper cuff in a quiet room after rest. The American Heart Association recommends the use of a cuff that is at least 40 per cent the upper arm's circumference in width and 80 per cent in length. If one arm measures higher, it is used as the estimate of central blood pressure. The obese arm and the calcified atherosclerotic vessel in many elderly can introduce measurement error. *White coat hypertension* is a term used when blood pressures are consistently high only in the doctor's office. Blood pressures often run lower at home, but studies documenting the morbidity of hypertension and the benefits of therapy are primarily based on office determinations. Ambulatory blood pressure measurement is technologically available but not clear in its application to date.

Normally, blood pressures vary greatly throughout our changing emotional and activity levels. The first step in diagnosis is to document that the level being used for diagnosis is based on three different measurements taken at rest. A specific diagnosis of emergency hypertension (malignant or accelerated hypertension) must be ruled out before taking the time to document elevated blood pressure on at least two different occasions. For this reason, physicians screen for acute brain, heart, and renal symptoms. Malignant hypertension is defined by the presence of papilledema. The patient in our case study denied headaches, change in mentation, chest pain, shortness of breath, or lack of urination. Therefore his physician felt comfortable in documenting the blood pressures measured over time.

What level then defined the diagnosis of hypertension? The American Heart Association has long recommended the 90 mm Hg diastolic and the 140 mm Hg systolic pressures as criterion levels. The Joint National Committee on Detection, Evaluation, and Treatment of High Blood Pressure (JNC) has outlined a series of categories stressing the concept that cardiovascular risk increases over the entire range of normally occurring blood pressures (Table 44–1). In fact, data from the Framingham study show dramatically (Fig. 44–1) that risk of cardiovascular disease increases almost logarithmically over the range of blood pressures commonly seen. Note the dramatically different plots for men versus women.

Hypertension must be viewed more as a risk factor than a disease. It is common, affecting at least 15 per cent of the adult population of the United States and 65 per cent of those older than 65 years. The outcomes to be avoided are stroke and myocardial infarction. Heart failure and renal disease are also of concern, but the value of medical therapy in their prevention is not as clearly established. The

TABLE 44–1. Classification of Blood Pressure for Adults Aged 18 Years and Older*

Category	Systolic (mm Hg)	Diastolic (mm Hg)
Normal†	<130	<85
High normal	130–139	85–89
Hypertension‡		
Stage 1 (mild)	140–159	90–99
Stage 2 (moderate)	160–179	100–109
Stage 3 (severe)	180–209	110–119
Stage 4 (very severe)	≥210	≥120

* Not taking antihypertensive drugs and not acutely ill. When systolic and diastolic pressures fall into different categories, the higher category should be selected to classify the individual's blood pressure status. For instance, 160/92 mm Hg should be classified as stage 2, and 180/120 mm Hg should be classified as stage 4. Isolated systolic hypertension is defined as a systolic blood pressure of 140 mm Hg or more and a diastolic blood pressure of less than 90 mm Hg and staged appropriately (e.g., 170/85 mm Hg is defined as stage 2 isolated systolic hypertension).

In addition to classifying stages of hypertension on the basis of average blood pressure levels, the clinician should specify presence or absence of target-organ disease and additional risk factors. For example, a patient with diabetes and a blood pressure of 142/94 mm Hg, plus left ventricular hypertrophy, should be classified as having "stage 1 hypertension with target-organ disease (left ventricular hypertrophy) and with another major risk factor (diabetes)." This specificity is important for risk classification and management.

† Optimal blood pressure with respect to cardiovascular risk is less than 120 mm Hg systolic and less than 80 mm Hg diastolic. However, unusually low readings should be evaluated for clinical significance.

‡ Based on the average of two or more readings taken at each of two or more visits after an initial screening.

From the fifth report of the Joint National Committee on Detection, Evaluation and Treatment of High Blood Pressure. Arch Intern Med 1993;153:154.

level at which an operational diagnosis of hypertension is made is related to concomitant risk factors (Fig. 44–2) clearly shows the impact of concomitant risk factors on cardiovascular sequelae. For this reason, the history has to evaluate all cardiovascular risk factors including family history, tobacco use, cholesterol level, diabetes, and lack of exercise.

Having established the diagnosis, the work-up of hypertension addresses four areas:

1. Identify all risk factors for cardiovascular disease.

2. Identify and rule out secondary causes of hypertension.

3. Identify concomitant diseases that may modify therapy.

4. Establish a baseline of target end-organ damage.

The risk factors for heart attack and stroke are

family history, tobacco use, hypercholesterolemia, diabetes, obesity, and lack of exercise. A thorough history plus a fasting blood glucose and cholesterol level can identify these factors.

The secondary causes of hypertension can be divided into four categories (Table 44–2). Almost all (90–99 per cent) diagnosed hypertension is the idiopathic or essential type. Initial evaluation should consider potentially reversible causes. This evaluation is predominantly based on a well-directed history and physical. In this case, secondary hypertension should be more suspected because of the age of onset. Primary hypertension is familial, with onset often in the 20s and 30s. The skin finding of multiple café-au-lait spots suggests the *possibility* of pheochromocytoma because they are both of neural crest origin. The patient denied flushing, tachycardia, and sweating, which are symptoms of pheochromocytoma. The urinary vanillylmandelic acid (VMA) level and metanephrines were ordered because of the physical findings, but they should not be done routinely. The basic principle when considering secondary hypertension is to order only those tests that are indicated by the history and physical.

Renal disease is screened for using a routine urinalysis and serum blood urea nitrogen (BUN) or creatinine level. Renal vascular hypertension is considered by listening over the epigastrium, flanks, and back for bruits. Coarctation is actually screened in all newborns when their femoral pulses are checked. Collateral circulation develops by adult age and then the femoral pulse may be near normal. If the coarctation is between the brachioce-

TABLE 44–2. Secondary Causes of Hypertension

   I. Renal
      Renal parenchymal
      Polycystic kidney disease
  II. Renal vascular
      Coarctation of the aorta
      Renal artery stenosis
 III. Endocrine
      Pheochromocytoma
      Primary hyperaldosteronism
      Cushing syndrome
      Hyperthyroidism
 IV. Environmental
      Medications
        Oral contraceptives
        Antidepressants
        Decongestants
        Steroids
        Others
      Toxic chemicals

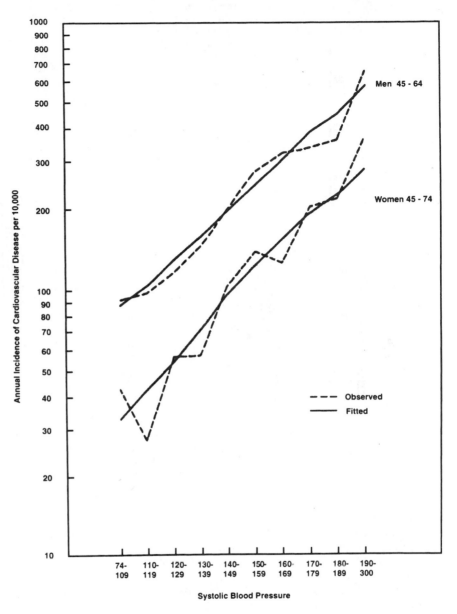

Figure 44-1. Annual incidence of cardiovascular disease by systolic blood pressure at entry, observed *(dotted line)*, and fitted *(solid line)* in the Framingham cohort over an 18-year follow-up. (From Kannel WB, Sorlie P. Hypertension in Framingham. In Paul O [ed]: Epidemiology and Control of Hypertension. Miami, Symposia Specialists, 1975, p 566.)

phalic and subclavian arteries, there is a large differential between pressures in the arms. Radial and femoral pulses should occur simultaneously. In coarctation, the femoral artery pulse can be delayed. Leg pressures can be taken with the proper size cuff while listening over the popliteal region. They can be normal or low in coarctation. Chest radiographs can show rib notching from the collateral circulation and sometimes may demonstrate the coarctation.

Endocrine diseases are largely screened via the history, considering flushing, sweating, weight loss, heat intolerance, and skin changes. Hyperaldo-steronism should be suspected if the serum potassium level is low.

A number of medications can cause hypertension. Oral contraceptives particularly must be questioned in female patients. Antidepressants can also be a factor Decongestants can potentially cause hypertension. Corticosteroids and many other less commonly used medications such as cyclosporine and erythropoetin are causes of hypertension. Lead intake can cause hypertension. A thorough medication and toxin history is clearly required in the evaluation of elevated blood pressures.

Antihypertensive medications can affect other

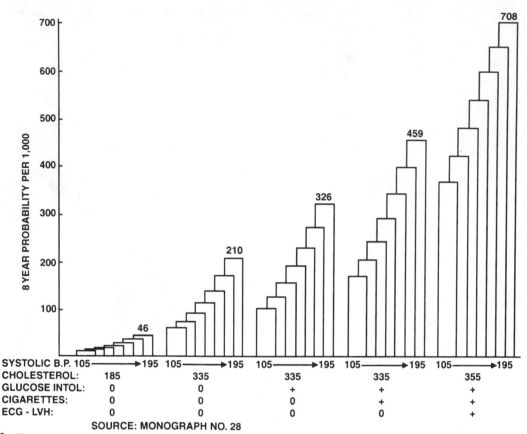

SOURCE: MONOGRAPH NO. 28

Figure 44-2. The 8-year risk of cardiovascular disease for 40-year-old men in Framingham according to progressively higher systolic blood pressure at specified level of other risk factors. (From Kannel WB. An overview of the risk factors for cardiovascular disease. In Kaplan NM, Stamler J [eds]. Prevention of Coronary Heart Disease. Philadelphia, W.B. Saunders, 1983.)

diseases both positively and negatively (see Table 44–3). Angiotensin converting enzyme (ACE) inhibitors can benefit heart failure and diabetes. Calcium channel blockers can benefit migraine and asthma. Ischemic heart disease can benefit from ACE inhibitors and beta blockers. Beta blockers can also help migraine but are contraindicated in asthma, diabe-tes, and heart failure. Alpha blockers can benefit patients with prostatic hypertrophy. Both thiazides and beta blockers can have negative effects on lipid profiles. ACE inhibitors can aggravate or cause chronic urticaria.

The use of evaluation to establish baseline dam-age is mainly of prognostic significance. An ECG

TABLE 44-3. Antihypertensive Effects on Concomitant Diseases

Medication	Beneficial Effect	Negative Effect
Thiazides	Edema	Diabetes, hyperlipidemia, gout
Beta blockers	Migraine, ischemic heart disease, anxiety, essential tremor, hyperthyroidism	Hyperlipidemia, heart failure, asthma, chronic obstructive pulmonary disease, diabetes, peripheral vascular disease
Calcium blockers	Migraine, asthma, cardiac dysrhythmias	Heart failure, heart block
ACE inhibitors	Heart failure, diabetic nephropathy, ischemic heart disease	Urticaria, renovascular hypertension

can demonstrate LVH. Retinal examination can indicate vascular changes. As arteriolar walls thicken the arteriolar venous (A:V) ratio decreases from the normal of 2:3. The arteries can make a greater indentation on veins as they cross them, giving rise to A:V nicking. The BUN or creatinine level can indicate the level of existing renal damage A chest radiograph can indicate severe LVH and findings of heart failure.

In summary the evaluation of hypertension should focus on a comprehensive history and physical examination with special attention to the retina, blood vessels, heart, lungs, and renal system. Routine laboratory examination includes a CBC, urinalysis, potassium, calcium, uric acid, cholesterol, fasting blood sugar, and BUN or creatinine levels. ECG and chest radiography should be considered. Further tests are done if they are indicated by the above evaluation. In this case there was suggestion of a need to rule out a pheochromocytoma. Other findings can lead to more specialized testing.

Therapy

Initially, nondrug therapy can be attempted. Some patients are sensitive to salt and can be managed by dietary salt reduction. More than one ounce of ethanol intake daily can raise blood pressure. Relaxation and biofeedback therapy can reduce blood pressure in the motivated patient.

Weight reduction can also reduce blood pressure. Weight reduction is also a part of the general cardiovascular risk reduction. An aerobic exercise program should be introduced. Smoking cessation as an independent risk variable probably has more impact than blood pressure control.

The lowering of blood pressure by the use of medications has been demonstrated to reduce the incidence of stroke and possibly myocardial infarction. Elevated blood pressure itself is asymptomatic except in the extreme. The goal is to maintain blood pressure control without inducing symptoms from the therapy. Many choices of agents for the lowering of blood pressure are now available (see Table 44–4). The JNC has recommended favoring beta blockers and thiazides because these are currently the only agents that have clearly demonstrated benefits in long-term large controlled studies. The concomitant conditions are also weighed in the choice of therapy (see Table 44–3).

Thiazides are the most well-established medications for the treatment of hypertension. They are inexpensive and can be given once daily. These characteristics are important in patient compliance.

Seventy per cent of African Americans and 50 per cent of Caucasians are controlled on thiazides as single agents. Concern exists that negative effects counteract some of the beneficial impact of thiazides. Some studies even suggest increased mortality in patients on thiazides with milder hypertension.

Beta blockers are the other clearly proven antihypertensive agents. In choosing the agent for any patient, there are many options. Contraindications narrow the choices some. Concomitant diseases then can give specific direction. For example, diabetic and heart failure patients receive additional benefits from ACE inhibitors. Cost is another consideration. Medication costs can be anywhere from $5 to $100 a month for a single agent. Additional laboratory requirements such as monitoring potassium levels can add to the cost of medications. The choice of agents can be a joint decision with the patient, actively indicating how his or her values should be factored.

Sometimes single-drug therapy is inadequate to reach the therapeutic target blood pressure. The choice is either to switch to or add another drug. Any additional drug should come from a different class. Diuretics are particularly complementary to most antihypertensive agents. Minimizing the number of drugs can increase compliance, but sometimes a smaller dose of two agents can have a better side effect profile than pushing a single agent closer to maximal dose. Combination medications are often available with a diuretic, but this vehicle restricts flexibility in dosage adjustment.

The management of hypertension and other cardiovascular risks is a lifetime partnership with the patient. If a patient fails to respond to usual therapy the clinician should reconsider secondary hypertension as well as noncompliance. Renal function should be monitored during therapy, as should electrolyte levels if diuretics are used. Patients should be educated regarding side effects to report relative to adverse medication results. Sexual dysfunction is a common side effect of antihypertensive therapy. Patients should know that there are many choices in antihypertensives and that erectile dysfunction and other sexual difficulties should not just be accepted as a normal part of aging. Although the myriad antihypertensive agents available can seem overwhelming to the practitioner, the multiple alternatives allow most patients effective treatment with few to no side effects. With all the new agents available and expected, the student of medicine should review this area frequently. Large studies currently underway promise to give better guidance for the optimal choice of treatment in the future.

TABLE 44–4. Selected Antihypertensive Medications

Class	Examples	Comments	
		Positive	*Negative*
Diuretics			
	Hydrochlorothiazide	Inexpensive, well proven, once daily, effective	Can raise glucose, uric acid, triglycerides; lowers potassium
	Furosemide	Well proven	Not effective as antihypertensive except in cases of high volume
Beta blockers			See concomitant diseases
	Propranolol		
	Atenolol	Once daily, more water soluble	Peripheral edema, headache, constipation, negative inotropic, conduction blockade
Calcium channel blockers			
	Nifedipine	Dihydropyridine family—less negative inotropic effects	
	Verapamil		
ACE inhibitors		Prolongs survival for congestive heart failure, postmyocardial infarction patient; positive effects on diabetic proteinuria	Can cause angioneurotic edema, cough, hyperkalemia, renal failure
	Captopril		
	Enalapril		
Alpha inhibitors		Favorable lipid effects, improves prostate obstructive symptoms	Orthostatic hypotension
	Prazosin		
	Terazosin		
Central adrenergic blockers			
	Clonidine	Available in a transdermal patch	
	Methyldopa		Fatigue, drowsiness, sexual dysfunction
Vasodilators			
	Hydralazine	Combines well with beta blockers	Tachycardia, positive ANA titer
	Minoxidil	Potent antihypertensive	Hirsutism

SUGGESTED READING

Bennett JC, Plum F. Cecil's Textbook of Medicine, 20th ed. Philadelphia, W.B. Saunders, 1996.

Joint National Committee on Detection, Evaluation and Treatment of High Blood Pressure, 5th ed. Arch Intern Med 1993;153:154.

Kaplan NM. Clinical Hypertension, 6th ed. Baltimore, Williams & Wilkins, 1994.

Perloff D, Grim C, Flack J, et al. Human Blood Pressure Determination by Sphygmomanometry. Dallas, American Heart Association, 1994.

Rakel RE (ed). Textbook of Family Practice, 5th ed. Philadelphia, W.B. Saunders, 1995.

QUESTIONS

1. The American Heart Association recommends the cuff size for blood pressure measurement be
   a. 80 per cent of the arm circumference in length and 40 per cent in width
   b. Twice the width of the forearm in length
   c. Four finger-breadths overlapping
   d. At least 12 inches in length
   e. At least 6 inches in width

2. Which of the following suggests secondary hypertension?
   a. Onset late in life
   b. Onset early in life
   c. Failure to respond to usual therapy

d. Low serum potassium level
e. All of the above

3. Which of the following is *not* a cardiovascular risk factor?
   a. Hypertension

b. Diabetes
c. Tobacco use
d. Family history of hypertension
e. Asthma

Answers appear on **page 605.**

Chapter 45

Hypercholesterolemia

Michael A. Crouch, M.D., M.S.P.H.

SUBJECTIVE—INITIAL VISIT

Patient Identification

Gary A. is a 24-year-old Caucasian freshman medical student being seen for a preschool physical examination.

Presenting Problems

Although his general health has been quite good in the past, Gary has been experiencing abdominal pain, loose bowel movements, chest discomfort, and palpitations intermittently for about 2 weeks.

Present Illness

Gary began experiencing cramping periumbilical pain and loose bowel movements following a farewell weekend with college friends, just before moving to University City to begin medical school. The abdominal pain originally began while he was packing his belongings in his car. The most severe episode occurred midway through the first day of orientation week and was quite uncomfortable (8 on a scale of 10). Each episode has lasted from 30 to 45 minutes. The pain has occurred at all different times of the day but has not awakened him from sleep. The pain is unrelated to mealtime or physical activity. Neither antacids nor bismuth subsalicylate (PeptoBismol) has produced prompt pain relief, but a dose of bismuth subsalicylate seemed to normalize his bowel movements for about 12 hours. His bowel movements have been a normal brown color, with a quite loose, but not liquid consistency. The stool has contained small amounts of mucus at times, without visible blood.

Gary began experiencing bilateral chest discomfort and palpitations sometime after the onset of the abdominal pain. He has had episodes lasting 5 to 10 minutes, occurring two to three times a week, associated with unusually forceful and rapid heartbeat. The episodes typically occurred at rest, after he had been experiencing abdominal pain for an hour or more. The symptoms were relieved by his getting up and moving around restlessly.

Past Medical History

Gary has had no surgery, accidents, or serious injuries and has never been hospitalized. He has no known medication allergies. He takes no medications on a regular basis and denies using cathartic laxatives or stool softeners.

Family History

Gary's father, a dairy farmer, died suddenly at age 48, presumably from a heart attack. His mother is in good health at age 58 years. His only brother has hypercholesterolemia. His only sister has had no serious health problems. His paternal grandfather died from colon cancer at age 75 years. His other three grandparents died from unknown causes past the age of 80 years. He admits to worrying quite a bit about the possibility of his having inherited a predisposition to heart disease from his father. He is also worried about getting colon cancer like his grandfather did.

Health Habits

Gary does not smoke. He drinks small amounts of alcohol on rare occasions and denies using any illicit drugs. He always wears seatbelts when driving his car. For the past 5 years he has always used latex condoms when having intercourse. He exercises regularly, usually running about three to four miles at least three times a week. He has avoided eating red meat, pork, and whole milk dairy products for 2 years, after reading that they could increase the risk of heart disease and cancer.

Social History

Gary is single. He has been seeing one girlfriend regularly for 2 years and is sexually active exclusively with her. They are planning to marry following his second year in medical school. He describes his relationships with his girlfriend, mother, and siblings as close and supportive. He is unsure that he will be able to compete well academically in medical school and is concerned about how he will handle the heavy academic load and mental stress he has heard about. He made excellent grades in college while being active in intramural sports and social life with friends.

Review of Systems

Gary has had no change in his appetite, weight, energy, or general mood. He has experienced no nausea or vomiting. He has felt somewhat jittery and restless while sitting in lectures for the past few days. He has also had uncharacteristic difficulty getting to sleep recently. He denies having thoughts of imminent life-threatening illness or death.

OBJECTIVE

Physical Examination

Vital signs were all within normal limits, including blood pressure of 110/70, heart rate of 92, weight of 160 pounds, and height of 70 inches. Affect was normal except for appearing mildly nervous. The physical examination was notable only for cool clammy hands, moist axillae, mild diffuse tenderness of the abdomen, and questionably diminished deep tendon reflexes and slow recovery. The thyroid gland and Achilles tendons were normal on inspection and palpation. Peripheral pulses were all normal.

Laboratory Tests

A multitest "executive profile" drawn 2 days before Gary's office visit was notable only for a total cholesterol level of 300 mg/dl (7.7 mMol/L). The panel did not include cholesterol subfractions or triglyceride levels, but it did include normal liver and renal function test results.

ASSESSMENT

Working Diagnoses

Two likely diagnoses best explain the patient's symptoms and findings.

1. Adjustment disorder with anxious mood, expressed as situational anxiety, mild sleep disorder, symptoms of autonomic overactivity, and irritable bowel syndrome.

2. Familial heterozygous hypercholesterolemia (type IIa in the Frederickson classification), based on the suggestive family history and the very high total cholesterol value despite a "heart-healthy" lifestyle. This inherited condition is the most common cause of severe hypercholesterolemia. Although unlikely, secondary causes of hypercholesterolemia should be kept in mind.

Differential Diagnosis

Gary's symptoms and findings suggest several other plausible possibilities.

1. Hypertriglyceridemia is a distinct possibility that can produce a fasting triglyceride level above 200 mg/dl and carries a lesser degree of risk for

heart disease than low-density lipoprotein (LDL) cholesterol elevation.

2. Hypothyroidism is unlikely because of the mild tachycardia, but it is a cause of secondary hypercholesterolemia worth keeping in mind. Patients with hypothyroidism usually present with fatigue and lethargy in younger people but some can be completely asymptomatic, especially elderly people.

3. Generalized anxiety disorder is not an appropriate diagnosis at this point because of the short duration of symptoms.

4. Somatization disorder is not an appropriate diagnosis at this point because of the relatively limited scope and duration of somatic symptoms. If this episode is not handled well, however, the patient may gradually become more preoccupied with somatic symptoms.

5. Panic disorder is unlikely because of the lack of intense acute fear of imminent personal catastrophe. If the patient were biologically predisposed to panic disorder (despite a lack of suggestive family history in this case), sustained or severely heightened concerns can eventually be expressed as panic attacks.

6. Hypochondriasis with cardiac and cancer neuroses should be kept in mind as a plausible possibility, given the patient's family history and current symptoms. If he does not already have this disorder, he may well be vulnerable to developing an exaggerated fear of heart disease as he approaches the age at which his father died. A certain amount of fear is actually rational, given his lipid disorder and family history.

Even less likely diagnoses include the following:

1. Acute pancreatitis, resulting from severe hypertriglyceridemia is unlikely because of the relatively brief duration and mild severity of the pain episodes, and the patient's slenderness, regular aerobic exercise, low alcohol intake, and nondiabetic status.

2. Hyperalphalipoproteinemia is unlikely, especially in a male. Patients with this condition have a very high level of high-density lipoprotein (HDL) cholesterol (above 70 mg/dl, and as high as 125 mg/dl). High levels of HDL cholesterol are usually associated with low risk for atherosclerosis. In rare cases, however, the HDL cholesterol does not function normally in transporting peripheral cholesterol to the liver, and the patient can be at risk for coronary disease despite having a high HDL cholesterol level.

3. Angina pectoris caused by atherosclerotic coronary artery disease is highly unlikely in such a young adult. Patients with *homozygous* familial hypercholesterolemia develop heart disease early in life, but if he had the homozygous form, he would have already experienced severe atherosclerotic consequences (stroke or myocardial infarction).

4. Coronary vasospasm causing atypical angina is rare in this age group and is less likely in men than in women.

PLAN

Diagnostic Laboratory and Special Tests

1. Fasting lipoprotein analysis (lipid profile) is the most appropriate initial test. Measurement of total cholesterol, HDL cholesterol, and triglyceride levels, and a calculated estimate of LDL cholesterol allow verification and categorization of common lipid disorders.

2. Thyroid stimulating hormone (TSH) level is the most cost-effective test for excluding hypothyroidism, a treatable secondary cause of high cholesterol level.

3. Electrocardiogram (ECG), although very unlikely to show abnormalities, may provide useful reassurance to the patient if the reading is normal. Neither the patient nor the physician thought an ECG was necessary at this point.

Therapeutic Treatment Plan

1. Diet low in saturated fat and cholesterol—recommended to follow step II American Heart Association (AHA) dietary guidelines by avoiding whole milk dairy products and fatty cuts of beef and pork. Given the level of total cholesterol, a step I AHA diet would be ineffective for significantly lowering what is likely to be a severe LDL cholesterol elevation. Also recommended is a regular high intake of water-soluble fiber (e.g., oat bran).

2. Aerobic exercise. Gary was advised to continue his current routine throughout medical school and residency training, as much as possible. Regular aerobic exercise sometimes lowers LDL and total cholesterol modestly, usually raises HDL cholesterol by 5 to 15 mg/dl, and often dramatically lowers elevated triglyceride levels. Exercise also has an acute

relaxation effect that can reduce the patient's level of chronic anxiety, and it can have a moderately effective lowering effect on elevated blood glucose level.

3. Lipid altering medication—probably advisable if lipid profile results show the anticipated severe LDL cholesterol elevation. A discussion of pros and cons and specific alternatives was deferred until the second visit.

4. Relaxation techniques. Gary was introduced to options of deep breathing, progressive muscle relaxation, and visual imagery to help reduce effects of stress and deal with acute and chronic anxiety by taking his mind off the many demands being made on his time.

Patient Education

1. The cholesterol elevation was provisionally characterized as severe, pending two repeat measurements to confirm persistence and severity of the elevation, and to establish a pre-treatment baseline.

2. The strong role of cholesterol level elevation as a risk factor for heart disease was explained. The physician gave the patient a pamphlet with answers to common questions about cholesterol to read and discuss during the return visit.

3. The importance of rechecking the cholesterol level and obtaining a fractionated fasting lipid profile to look at LDL and HDL cholesterol levels was stressed.

4. The patient was urged to encourage his sister and fiancée to have their cholesterol levels checked if they had not already done so.

5. He was asked to keep a 3-day food diary, recording everything he ate and drank for 72 hours, noting serving sizes and method of preparation.

6. His anxiety as an entering medical student was deemed normal, and a likely good adjustment was predicted. Anxiety was reconnoted as a useful signal of stress and as an energy mobilizing catalyst.

Disposition

The patient was asked to return in 1 week for follow-up of his cholesterol level and anxiety problems. Referral was not thought to be indicated for either problem at this point.

SUBJECTIVE—FIRST FOLLOW-UP VISIT

Gary returned for follow-up 1 week after his initial visit. He was feeling much better. He attributed his improvement mainly to relief from worry about his symptoms indicating some serious underlying illness such as heart disease or cancer. His abdominal pain, chest discomfort, and palpitations had resolved. He was still having occasional loose bowel movements but was not bothered by them. Gary was anxious to discuss his lipid profile results. In the intervening week he had discovered that a paternal aunt and a paternal uncle both developed heart disease in their 50s, and that both had high cholesterol levels. He had already encouraged his sister and fiancée to undergo cholesterol screening. He expressed curiosity about the wisdom of taking fish oil capsules.

OBJECTIVE

The patient looked less nervous than on the first visit. His heart rate was 72 (compared with 90 the previous week). His 3-day food diary showed a very low intake of foods high in saturated fat and cholesterol, congruent with the step II American Heart Association dietary guidelines. He had increased his intake of water-soluble fiber, with oatmeal for breakfast and oat bran muffins for lunches.

The fasting lipoprotein analysis showed a total cholesterol level of 310 mg/dl (8.0 mMol/L), HDL cholesterol of 40 mg/dl (1.0 mMol/L), triglycerides of 100, and an estimated LDL cholesterol level of 250 mg/dl (6.5 mMol/L). The TSH result was 2.0—within normal limits.

ASSESSMENT

1. Familial heterozygous hypercholesterolemia (FHC) with:
   a. Severely elevated total and LDL cholesterol levels (Figs. 45–1 and 45–2).
   b. Below average HDL cholesterol level. The average for males is 45 mg/dl (1.15 mMol/L), and for females the average is 55 mg/dl (1.42 mMol/L).
2. Adjustment disorder with anxious mood of mild severity, responding well to reassurance and education about stress-coping strategies.

PLAN

Diagnostic Laboratory and Special Tests

1. Repeat fasting lipid profile. It is advisable to examine short-term variation and establish pretreat-

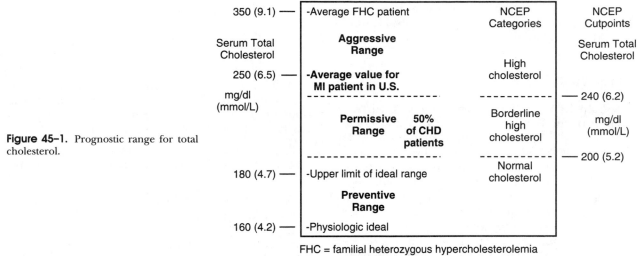

Figure 45–1. Prognostic range for total cholesterol.

FHC = familial heterozygous hypercholesterolemia
NCEP = National Cholesterol Education Program
MI = myocardial infarction

ment baseline values for LDL cholesterol level. This repeat analysis should be done several weeks later. Once treatment is started, a lipid profile should be repeated about 4 weeks after each change in the regimen is made. Once a regimen has achieved satisfactory results, a lipid profile should be repeated every 6 to 12 months to monitor the ongoing response.

2. Soft tissue radiographs of the Achilles tendons. Xanthomas show up as tendon thickening. Remeasurement after a year of treatment can be used as an index of therapeutic response to lipid-

altering medications in the patient with long-standing dyslipidemia. Although measurement is not done routinely in clinical practice, it is reasonable to provide tangible evidence of benefit for selected patients. It is unlikely to be beneficial for this patient.

3. Apolipoprotein B level. Although elevation indicates higher risk for atherosclerosis, this measurement would add little or nothing to this patient's risk assessment.

4. Lp(a) level elevation indicates higher risk for

Figure 45–2. Prognostic range for LDL cholesterol.

FHC = familial heterozygous hypercholesterolemia
NCEP = National Cholesterol Education Program
MI = myocardial infarction

atherosclerosis. This test may be useful in a patient with marginally high risk for heart disease. It would not add to this patient's risk assessment.

Therapeutic Treatment Plan

1. Step II AHA diet. Recommended further restriction of foods high in saturated fat and cholesterol, to be continued lifelong to help reduce LDL cholesterol level elevation. The physician recommended use of nonhydrogenated corn, safflower, soybean, and olive oil in cooking, and avoidance of oils high in saturated fat, including coconut and palm oils. Gary was encouraged to bring his fiancée along to the next visit for a more detailed discussion of food selection and preparation and was offered a referral to a dietitian for an even more detailed dietary consultation.

2. Lipid altering medication. Aggressive medical treatment was recommended to lower LDL cholesterol level to less than 130 mg/dl (3.4 mMol/L) and keep it in an atherosclerosis-preventive range lifelong. Pros and cons of lipid medications in general and specific drugs were discussed. Atorvastatin (a HMG CoA reductase inhibitor) was recommended as the medication most likely to produce good results with monotherapy because of its superior efficacy (50% to 60% reduction of LDL cholesterol, compared with 30% to 45% with the other "statins"). The proven benefit of pravastatin for preventing heart disease was presented as a potential advantage of that medication, which may be more applicable to the patient with established coronary artery disease than to younger men with a low likelihood of advanced atherosclerosis.

Psyllium hydrophilic mucilloid and niacin were presented as inexpensive over-the-counter choices for adjunctive treatment. Sustained-release niacin alone gives good results at 1 to 2 g per day, but the possibility of liver toxicity should be observed during the first few months by monitoring liver enzymes periodically.

Cholestyramine was presented as a costly adjunctive treatment for use at a low to medium dose to avoid the constipation caused by a high dose.

Plans were made to initiate drug therapy after obtaining the results of a second lipid profile.

3. Relaxation techniques. The physician explained deep breathing, progressive muscle relaxation, and visual imagery in more detail, encouraged trying them, and loaned Gary an audiotape with relaxation instructions.

Patient Education

1. The physician discussed the general pros and cons of the over-the-counter and prescription medications for lowering LDL cholesterol levels.

2. The genetic inheritance pattern of familial hypercholesterolemia and the reproductive implications of the patient's marrying someone who also has familial hypercholesterolemia were discussed.

3. The heart disease risk factor pamphlet was discussed and the patient's questions were answered.

4. The physician told the patient that although one or two capsules of fish oil high in eicosapentaenoic acid (EPA) would not be harmful, the preparation probably is not helpful either. Higher doses affect blood lipids but deliver high amounts of fat-soluble vitamins that could be toxic, as well as a substantial caloric intake. Intake of fish high in EPA (e.g., halibut, sardines) was encouraged.

Disposition

The patient was asked to return in 4 weeks for a repeat fasting lipid profile. An office visit was scheduled in 5 weeks to discuss the lipid level results and tentatively to initiate lipid altering medical treatment with atorvastatin or pravastatin.

DISCUSSION

Gary's symptoms are quite common expressions of anxiety related to difficulty coping with stress at home, school, or work. Most patients in this situation respond well to simple reassurance, normalization, and empathic support, coupled with developing an effective repertoire of strategies for preventing and coping with stress and anxiety. This patient's anxiety appears to stem partly from irrational fear about acute heart disease and a more rational fear of eventually having heart disease. Discussing and treating his major risk factor for heart disease can greatly reduce his anxiety, if the treatment is successful and well tolerated. If treatment does not go well, however, his anxiety can escalate.

This particular form of severe hypercholesterolemia is asymptomatic until atherosclerotic lesions progress to a critical extent, or until a plaque ruptures and triggers formation of a coronary thrombus. This scenario usually occurs after the age of 30. The average age of developing clinical heart disease is 42 for men and 52 for women with this disorder. Although the likelihood of Gary's having symptomatic coronary artery disease now is quite low, he most likely already has some degree of coronary atherosclerosis. His concern about developing early heart disease in his 30s or 40s is well founded. The severity of cholesterol elevation may be exacerbated by the stress of beginning medical school and ambivalence about his ability to succeed academically and cope well with the demands of his chosen profession. It is important to clarify that his long-term LDL cholesterol range is the important determinant of prognosis, not any particular LDL cholesterol level.

Familial heterozygous (type IIa) hypercholesterolemia is not uncommon, with a prevalence of about one in 400 in the general population. Mild and moderate hypercholesterolemia are extremely common. Over 50 per cent of American adults have levels of LDL cholesterol high enough to promote coronary atherosclerosis, especially in the presence of other identified risk factors. Over one half of patients who experience myocardial infarctions have total cholesterol values between 200 and 239 mg/dl (5.2-6.1 mMol/L) and LDL cholesterol levels below the NCEP cutpoint for defining elevated LDL cholesterol—160 mg/dl (4.1 mMol/L). Individuals with diabetes, hypertension, or tobacco abuse (cigarette smokers and users of oral tobacco) are at especially high risk if their LDL cholesterol levels are even mildly elevated and/or their HDL cholesterol levels are below average. After menopause, women rapidly catch up to men with respect to their risk for heart disease unless they receive estrogen replacement therapy.

When starting a program of dietary change to lower LDL cholesterol, it can be very helpful to ask patients to bring in their spouse, children, and other key family members for a conference to discuss the rationale and details of a heart-healthy diet. Teaching patients and spouses how to interpret the information on food labels is an important component of patient education. Figuring out ways to deal with ethnic food preferences and customs is an important need for some families.

The main dietary changes for lowering elevated LDL cholesterol entail reducing the intake of foods high in saturated fat—fatty cuts of beef and pork, and whole milk dairy products. Healthier replacements for these foods include chicken, fish, low- or nonfat dairy products or substitutes (not those with coconut or palm oil), and complex carbohydrates (starches such as rice, breads, and potatoes, and water-soluble fiber such as oat bran). The best oils for cooking include monounsaturated olive oil and polyunsaturated corn, safflower, and soybean oils. Olive oil has recently gained favor because it lowers

LDL cholesterol as much as polyunsaturated oils, and it does not have the HDL cholesterol–lowering effect seen with the polyunsaturated oils.

Patients who have an average American intake of saturated fat and cholesterol usually respond to dietary modification by lowering their total and LDL cholesterol levels by about 10 to 15 per cent of the baseline value. Patients who already have a low intake of saturated fat seldom respond well to dietary modification because they have so little room for change. Increased intake of water-soluble fiber often lowers LDL cholesterol levels by 5 to 15 per cent. Cholesterol-lowering medication usually lowers the LDL cholesterol an additional 20 to 60 per cent below the level achieved by dietary modification, depending on the medication.

Although the cost effectiveness of treating patients with "borderline high" LDL cholesterol level is controversial, several large prospective studies have established that lowering the elevated LDL cholesterol level with medication reduces the risk of coronary heart disease events (myocarcial infarction and CHD death) greatly during the ensuing 5 to 10 years in men. Although patients with severe LDL elevation and/or very low HDL cholesterol level are most likely to benefit from treatment, pravastatin has also shown primary prevention benefit in asymptomatic individuals with moderate LDL elevation (130 to 159 mg/dl).

Some experts advocate withholding medical treatment until three lipid profiles have been obtained over a several month period, to observe variation over a longer time interval. Many patients prefer to delay starting lipid-lowering medication until persistently elevated values on several lipid profiles convince them that they cannot obtain satisfactory results with dietary and exercise measures alone.

Guidelines are also available for the diagnosis and management of hypercholesterolemia in children. Dietary prevention should ideally begin relatively early in life to minimize or postpone the development of atherosclerosis in adulthood. Although most clinicians are reluctant to use lipid-altering drugs in children, medication should be considered if a child's severely elevated LDL cholesterol level does not respond well to dietary modification.

The benefit of lipid-lowering medication has not been adequately studied in females. Limited information suggests that women probably benefit about as much as men with similarly elevated LDL cholesterol and comparable risk factors. Postmenopausal estrogen replacement may have more powerful preventive potential than LDL-lowering medications, especially for women with low HDL cholesterol levels.

Treatment of high LDL cholesterol in the elderly is even more controversial. The estimated potential benefit of treatment (enhanced quality of life for more of the remaining life span) must be weighed carefully against the expense and possible adverse effects of medications being considered for each elderly patient.

The importance of triglyceride elevation as a heart disease risk factor continues to be controversial. Severe elevation above 400 mg/dl appears to increase the risk for heart disease in female patients, especially those with diabetes, and should be treated with niacin, gemfibrozil, or an HMG CoA reductase inhibitor. It is unclear whether lesser elevations of triglycerides should be treated medically if weight loss, exercise, alcohol abstinence, and improved control of diabetes do not satisfactorily lower the fasting level of triglycerides.

A low HDL cholesterol level is a powerful independent risk factor, even if LDL cholesterol is only mildly elevated (130 to 159 mg/dl) or in the high range of normal (100 to 129 mg/dl). Although the latest NCEP guidelines do not recommend medical management for low HDL cholesterol in particular, the results of the Helsinki Study suggest that treating low HDL cholesterol level is at least as beneficial as lowering an elevated LDL cholesterol level. Hygienic approaches, including regular aerobic exercise, weight loss, and smoking cessation, tend to raise HDL cholesterol by 5 to 15 mg/dl, as does treatment with niacin or gemfibrozil. HMG CoA reductase inhibitors and cholestyramine sometimes elevate HDL cholesterol slightly.

The prognosis for patients with lipid problems can be greatly improved by lasting lifestyle changes, long-term lipid-altering medication, and diligent follow-up care.

REFERENCES

Rakel RE. Textbook of Family Practice, 5th ed. Philadelphia, W.B. Saunders, 1995, pp 640–641, 769–770, 1087, 1149–1153, 1581–1582.

Sacks FM, Pfeffer MA, Moye LA, et al. The effect of pravastatin on coronary events after myocardial infarction in patients with average cholesterol levels. N Engl J Med 1996;335:1001–1009.

Scandinavian Simvastatin Survival Study Group. Randomized trial of cholesterol lowering in 4444 patients with coronary heart disease: The Scandinavian Simvastatin Survival Study (4S). Lancet 1994;344:1838–1839.

Shepherd J, Cobbe SM, Ford I, et al. Prevention of coronary heart disease with pravastatin in men with hypercholesterolemia. N Engl J Med 1995;333:1301–1307.

Summary of the second report of the National Cholesterol Education Program (NCEP) expert panel on detection, evaluation, and treatment of high blood cholesterol in adults (Adult Treatment Panel II). JAMA 1993;269:3015–3023.

QUESTIONS

1. Which of the following is not a risk factor for hypertriglyceridemia?
   a. High intake of dietary cholesterol
   b. High intake of alcohol
   c. Diabetes mellitus
   d. Obesity
   e. Sedentary lifestyle

2. Which of the following is most consistently and favorably affected by regular aerobic exercise?
   a. Elevated LDL cholesterol level
   b. Low HDL cholesterol level
   c. Elevated total cholesterol level
   d. Elevated blood sugar level
   e. Elevated triglycerides level

3. Which medication lowers elevated LDL cholesterol the most effectively?

   a. Cholestyramine
   b. Simvastatin
   c. Pravastatin
   d. Atorvastatin
   e. Niacin

4. Which of the following foods contain the *least* saturated fat and cholesterol when eaten in average serving amounts?
   a. Eggs and liver
   b. Beef and pork
   c. Olive and safflower oil
   d. Whole milk and butter
   e. Coconut oil and palm oil

Answers appear on **page 606.**

Chapter 46

Atrial Fibrillation

Daniel J. David, M.D.

INITIAL VISIT—SUBJECTIVE

Patient Identification and Presenting Problem

Paul M., a 52-year-old university professor, was seen for evaluation of an episode of shortness of breath and lightheadedness while attending the county fair. He was evaluated by emergency medical technicians (EMTs) who found his blood pressure to be "normal," pulse "irregular." He declined to be taken to the hospital because he had "experienced this before" and agreed to follow up with his family physician. He reports experiencing a "fluttering" sensation in his chest once or twice a year over the past 2 years. Two months ago, just before moving to the area, he went to a walk-in clinic with one of these episodes where he had an electrocardiogram (ECG) and was told he was in atrial fibrillation, but the rhythm returned to normal before the ECG was disconnected.

Past Medical History

Paul has no history of cardiac disease, rheumatic fever, drug use, or any other significant medical problems.

Family History

Both parents are living. His father has a history of hypertension and had a myocardial infarction a year ago at age 70 years.

Health Habits

Paul is a nonsmoker and has an alcoholic drink once or twice a month. He eats a low-fat diet and runs regularly, having completed three marathons since college.

Social History

Paul has been married 25 years, has three children, and has taught economics at the college level for 20 years. He recently relocated to the area but reports no significant life stresses.

Review of Systems

General health is good. He has never experienced any chest pain. He occasionally has musculoskeletal aches and pains related to running.

OBJECTIVE

Physical Examination

Paul's blood pressure is 126/74, heart rate is 60 and regular, height is 73 inches, and weight is 175 pounds. He appears to be in excellent health, younger than his stated age. Skin is warm and dry. Thyroid is palpably normal. No carotid bruits are heard. Cardiac examination reveals a regular rate and rhythm with no murmers or gallops. Peripheral pulses are full and equal bilaterally. Abdominal examination reveals no abnormalities.

Laboratory Tests

An ECG reveals a sinus bradycardia and is otherwise normal.

ASSESSMENT

Paul has palpitations. By history, his symptoms are paroxysmal in nature and possibly are the result of atrial fibrillation. History and physical examination are negative for apparent cardiac disease otherwise.

PLAN

Diagnostic

A complete blood count (CBC), chemistry panel, thyroid studies, an echocardiogram, and an exercise treadmill test were ordered.

Therapeutic

Paul was advised to abstain from dietary and over-the-counter stimulants, e.g., caffeine, decongestants.

FIRST FOLLOW-UP VISIT—SUBJECTIVE

Paul returned for his 2-week follow-up visit having experienced no further symptoms.

OBJECTIVE

Physical examination was unchanged. Results of laboratory studies were all within normal limits. The echocardiogram revealed no chamber enlargement or valvular abnormalities, and left ventricular function was normal. The exercise tolerance test was negative for symptoms or ECG changes. Records from the walk-in clinic revealed only an ECG and rhythm strip showing atrial fibrillation initially, which abruptly converted to a sinus rhythm.

DISCUSSION

Historically, atrial fibrillation may have been first described by a Chinese emperor and physician around 2000 B.C. William Harvey described it in annuals in 1628. Despite a variety of clinical reports and descriptions through the 1800s and early 1900s, the mechanism and importance of atrial fibrillation were not appreciated until the 1970s. The epidemiologic importance of atrial fibrillation was not known until the Framingham study data in the early 1980s, which identified the cerebrovascular implications.

Atrial fibrillation seems to be one of the most commonly encountered arrhythmias. Its prevalence, clinical manifestations and significance, long-term implications, and management can be quite variable based on the clinical circumstances in which it occurs.

From Framingham and other epidemiologic data there are several generally accepted premises regarding atrial fibrillation. An estimated 1.5 to 2.2 million Americans have atrial fibrillation; patients have a median age of 75 years. Prevalence increases with age from less than 1 per cent in young adults, to 1 to 5 per cent from ages 40 to 65 years, and 6 to 10 per cent over age 65 years. The latter group accounts for approximately 70 per cent of all cases of atrial fibrillation. The condition seems to be slightly more common among men.

The prevalence at any age is significantly affected by other factors. Framingham data identified diabetes, hypertension, congestive heart failure, and valvular heart disease as significant risk factors for atrial fibrillation in both sexes. Valvular heart disease was associated with a greater risk for women and myocardial infarction with a greater risk for men.

Other studies have reported various other cardiac processes that have been associated with atrial fibrillation: myocarditis, pericarditis, conduction system disease (e.g., Wolff-Parkinson-White syndrome), hypertrophic cardiomyopathy, and congenital heart disease (e.g., atrial septal defect and patent ductus arteriosus). Noncardiac causes that have been reported are thyrotoxicosis, alcohol use, severe infections, and pulmonary pathology (cancer, infection, embolism, and chronic lung disease).

The epidemiologic finding of greatest significance is the well-documented association of increased risk for thromboembolism and stroke among patients with atrial fibrillation. The general risk is 5 to 6 per cent among patients without rheumatic heart disease. In patients with rheumatic heart disease, the risk of systemic embolism has been reported as approximately 18 per cent. The presence of other cardiac risk factors noted earlier seems to increase the relative risk. Other risk factors for thromboembolism with atrial fibrillation include dilated cardiomyopathy, dilated left atrium, recent onset, and/or a history of prior embolism, transient ischemic attack (TIA), or stroke. Several major clinical trials have proven significant reduction of stroke risk with anticoagulation (Atrial Fibrillation Investigators, 1994).

Atrial fibrillation begins in one of the atria as a result of sinus node dysfunction or disruption of the atrial conduction system as a result of ischemia, degeneration, or anatomic factors (distention, scarring, others). As a result of the short-circuiting of sinoatrial (SA) node impulses or the generation of non-SA node impulses, which are thought to be rerouted over and over (re-entry phenomenon) through atrial tissue but never reaching the AV node, atrial fibrillation results.

The clinical manifestations of atrial fibrillation can be quite variable as a result of the influence of the coexisting factors described earlier. Symptoms may range from none or an awareness of otherwise asymptomatic palpitations to general fatigue or lethargy, angina, limited exercise tolerance, dyspnea, overt congestive heart failure, or syncope, TIA, or cerebrovascular accident (CVA).

Physical examination of the patient may reveal signs consistent with any of the above symptoms. Specific findings that may point toward atrial fibrillation include: (1) absent or variable amplitude of the a-wave of the jugular venous pulsations; (2) irregular pulse of variable intensity; and (3) irregularly irregular rate and rhythm on auscultation with variable intensity of the first heart sound. These findings are related to the role that coordinated atrial function plays in the cardiac cycle. These cardiovascular manifestations may be clinically more difficult to discern if the heart rate is slow or fast.

Electrocardiographically, atrial fibrillation is well characterized by the classic terminology "irregularly irregular" referring to both the ventricular rate and rhythm. There are no discrete, identifiable p-waves. Atrial electrical activity can usually be seen as small, variable amplitude, irregular undulations of the baseline. These are referred to as *f-waves* and are best seen in lead V_1 but are usually evident also in leads II, III, and aVF. In the absence of any visible atrial electrical activity, a grossly irregular ventricular rhythm is suggestive of atrial fibrillation. Other arrhythmias that may be considered based on clinical findings, although they are usually distinguishable on ECG, include a sinus rhythm with frequent extrasystole, sinus tachycardia, atrial flutter, and junctional tachycardia.

Evaluation of the patient with atrial fibrillation includes a thorough assessment of the clinical status in an effort to identify predisposing factors and hemodynamic status. An ECG is necessary to confirm the diagnosis. If the atrial fibrillation is not persistent, a 24-hour Holter monitor recording may be indicated. Basic laboratory studies (CBC, chemistries, thyroid functions) are indicated. An echocardiogram assesses valvular anatomy and function and chamber size, with left atrial enlargement being an additive risk for thromboembolic disease. An

exercise treadmill test can be helpful in assessing the presence of coronary artery disease.

No universal consensus exists on all aspects of the management of atrial fibrillation, but there are some well-founded principles on which to guide treatment. The urgency to control the ventricular response rate and/or attempt to convert the atrial fibrillation to a sinus rhythm depends primarily on the hemodynamic stability of the patient. The probability of converting to a sinus rhythm is inversely related to the duration of the atrial fibrillation, patient's age, underlying disease, and left atrial diameter. Of note, approximately 50 per cent of recent-onset (less than 48 to 72 hours) atrial fibrillation episodes revert spontaneously to a sinus rhythm. The general objectives of treating atrial fibrillation are to relieve symptoms, improve cardiac performance, minimize the risk of thromboembolism, and ultimately reduce mortality. Research has suggested that the approach to treatment may be subcategorized based on the duration (and associated comorbidity) of the atrial fibrillation (i.e., paroxysmal, persistent [typically more than 48 to 72 hours], and chronic atrial fibrillation).

Patients with hemodynamically unstable conditions (hypotension, angina, CHF, syncope, other) are the primary candidates for immediate direct-current (DC) cardioversion. Elective DC cardioversion is typically reserved for those patients who cannot be converted to a sinus rhythm medically and who are likely to benefit significantly from a hemodynamic standpoint. Cardioversion should be done in a monitored hospital setting with full resuscitation capabilities. Cardioversion also requires sedation to reduce the discomfort of the DC shock. Because of the increased risk of thromboembolism with conversion of atrial fibrillation of greater than 72 hours' duration, it is generally accepted that patients be anticoagulated before and for 3 to 4 weeks afterward. Overall cardioversion has an 80 per cent success rate. DC cardioversion can, however, produce adverse effects—embolic events and cardiac arrhythmias.

A broad range of medications has been used for ventricular rate control. Digoxin has probably been the most commonly used drug to control the ventricular rate in atrial fibrillation. Typically, a loading dose of 0.25 to 0.5 mg is given orally or IV followed by 0.25 mg every 6 hours to a total of 1.0 to 1.5 mg. An average maintenance dose is 0.125 to 0.375; the dose needs to be adjusted downward in the presence of impaired renal function or certain concomitant medications (antacids, cholestyramine, erythromycin, tetracycline, quinidine, amiodarone, or verapamil). Drug levels should be obtained after three to four half-lives and periodically thereafter, based on clinical response and/or suspicion of toxicity. Digoxin toxicity, however, correlates poorly with serum level.

Digoxin slows the ventricular rate by enhancing vagal effects on the AV node. One of its advantages is its positive inotropic effect for patients with impaired left ventricular function. It does not control ventricular rate well in response to exercise or in conditions with a high sympathetic drive, however. It has been commonly held to play a role in conversion of atrial fibrillation to a sinus rhythm; however, there is no evidence to support this. There seems to be a trend away from the use of digoxin in atrial fibrillation for rate control in favor of other agents—calcium channel blockers and beta blockers.

Verapamil and diltiazem have been used for rate control with a fair degree of success. Calcium channel blockers provide some degree of rate control even in response to exercise but variably may adversely affect left ventricular function. Diltiazem is relatively mild in this regard. An initial bolus of 20 to 25 mg can be given intravenously over 2 minutes and repeated in 15 minutes if the ventricular rate remains greater than 120. After reduction in heart rate, an infusion of 10 to 15 mg per hour can be given for up to 24 hours. Oral diltiazem can then be used to maintain rate control.

Beta blockers are effective in slowing the ventricular rate in atrial fibrillation, including in response to exercise. They also have negative inotropic effects and must be used with caution in CHF. Propranolol may be given IV in a dose of 1 to 3 mg not to exceed 1 mg per minute. The patient should be monitored closely and sufficient time allowed for the drug to act. A second dose may be given after 2 minutes but subsequent doses should not be given for 4 hours. The oral maintenance dose is 10 to 30 mg tid or qid.

Esmolol may also be used but is available only IV. The drug is very short-acting. A loading infusion of 0.5 mg per kg per minute is given. Ventricular rate can be controlled by an additional loading dose and/or increase in the rate of infusion.

Other beta blockers available for oral maintenance include metoprolol, atenolol, nadolol, acebutolol, timolol, and pindolol.

As for rate control, there are several options for medical conversion of atrial fibrillation. Antiarrhythmics typically used are from class IA, IC, and III drugs. It is important to have a general understanding of these options, their indications, and potential side effects. The maintenance of sinus rhythm after electrical cardioversion is enhanced by oral antiarrhythmic therapy. In patients not requiring cardioversion, antiarrhythmic therapy converts atrial fibrillation to a sinus rhythm in 30 to 80 per cent of patients. Side effects may occur with the same frequency, however.

Quinidine is a prototype class IA drug. It depresses automaticity and slows depolarization, repolarization, and action potential amplitude. Quinidine sulfate is given orally in a dose of 300 to 600 mg every 6 hours. Quinidine gluconate, an extended-release formulation may be given as one to two (324-mg tablets) every 8 to 12 hours. It is effective in converting and/or maintaining sinus rhythm in approximately 50 per cent of patients. Side effects, primarily gastrointestinal, are not uncommon (25 to 40 per cent) and not infrequently result in discontinuation of therapy. Of concern also is the reported two- to three-fold increase in overall mortality among patients treated with quinidine.

Procainamide can be administered intravenously and orally. In the acute stage, 100 mg by slow IV push until conversion or 500 mg has been given. With cardioversion, a maintenance infusion of 2 to 6 mg per minute is started. If the arrhythmia recurs, a bolus is repeated and the infusion rate increased. Procainamide is about 50 per cent effective in converting atrial fibrillation to a sinus rhythm. It has a side effect frequency of 25 to 50 per cent, primarily a lupus-like syndrome, which resolves with discontinuation.

Disopyramide also converts and prevents atrial fibrillation with an efficacy reportedly comparable to that of quinidine. It is available only in oral form. For rapid control, an initial bolus of 300 mg (immediate release) can be given, followed by a maintenance regimen of 100 to 200 mg every 6 hours (immediate-release form) or 100 to 300 mg every 12 hours (extended-release form). Disopyramide is a myocardial depressant, and it can precipitate CHF, particularly if there is a prior history. Its anticholinergic activity requires that it be avoided if possible in patients with glaucoma, myasthenia gravis, and urinary retention.

Class IC agents include flecainide and propafenone, which have been found to be 80 to 90 per cent effective in converting atrial fibrillation to sinus rhythm. A recommended starting dose for flecainide is 50 mg bid, increasing by 50 mg bid every 4 days to a maximal dose of 300 mg per day. One study reported a 91 per cent conversion rate within 8 hours and 95 per cent in 24 hours after a single 300-mg dose. Sixty-five per cent of patients in another study remained in a sinus rhythm after 9 months on an average daily dose of 200 mg with infrequent side effects. Flecainide, however, has pro-arrhythmic and negative inotropic effects and should be avoided or used with caution in patients with a history of ischemic heart disease or CHF. Propafenone is a relatively new antiarrhythmic class IC drug with an efficacy similar to flecainide with similar negative inotropic potential. The usual dosage (oral) is 150 to 300 mg tid.

Amiodarone is a class III agent with alpha and beta adrenergic and calcium channel blocking properties. It has been proven to be very effective (40 to 85 per cent) in converting to and maintaining a sinus rhythm even in patients in whom other drugs have failed. It is slow in onset. Full antiarrhythmic effects may not be seen for up to 10 weeks. Loading dose recommendations vary from 400 mg per day to 600 to 800 mg per day for 1 to 4 weeks. When cardioversion is achieved (or prominent side effects occur) the dosage should be reduced gradually to a maintenance dose of 200 mg per day (or less). Patients must be monitored closely for side effects, which may include pulmonary fibrosis, thyroid dysfunction, and corneal microdeposits. Hepatic transaminase levels transiently increase but dosage reduction or discontinuation is not indicated unless the increase exceeds three times the normal level. Asymptomatic bradycardia and prolonged AV conduction are frequently seen. Amiodarone also potentiates warfarin effect and increases flecainide and digoxin levels. Maintenance doses over 400 mg per day are more frequently associated with side effects.

Sotalol, another class III drug, also prolongs the duration of the action potential and has some class II (beta blocking) properties as well. It has less organ toxicity than amiodarone, is well tolerated, and may be useful in patients unresponsive to other medications. With its class II properties it may be valuable as monotherapy (i.e., rate control and cardioversion potential). Initial dosage is 80 mg bid, which may be increased as needed to 240 to 320 mg per day in divided doses, bid to tid. Dosage should not exceed 480 mg per day. Patients should be monitored for class III adverse effects, especially QT prolongation and torsades de pointes.

Some patients who fail electrical and pharmacologic cardioversion may be candidates for dual-chamber pacing. Techniques using radiofrequency catheter ablation or surgical interruption of intra-atrial conduction fibers or the AV node may provide other therapeutic options in the future.

The role of anticoagulation therapy in atrial fibrillation was outlined earlier. The data regarding thromboembolic risk is irrefutable. Mitral stenosis is the primary valvular lesion associated with embolism. In conjunction with atrial fibrillation, the risk increases seven-fold. Patients with valvular disease and atrial fibrillation benefit significantly from anticoagulation with a recommended INR range of 2.0 to 3.0. INR recommendations with prosthetic valves are 2.0 to 3.0 (tissue valves) and 2.5 to 3.5 (mechanical valves). A review (Atrial Fibrillation Investigators, 1994) of five major multicenter randomized trials provides guidance for anticoagulation management in nonvalvular atrial fibrillation:

1. Patients with lone atrial fibrillation (no underlying systemic or cardiac disease) under age 60 years do not need anticoagulation. Their risk of embolism is low (0.5 per cent per year or less) increasing to about 2.0 per cent per year over age 70 years. Management of such patients (over age 60 years) remains less definitive and ranges from no treatment to aspirin 325 mg per day to oral anticoagulation. The benefits of aspirin are less clear. Combined data from two studies indicate a modest (30 per cent risk reduction) but not statistically significant benefit for stroke with persistent deficit. There was, however, significant benefit (28 per cent reduction) for combined outcomes (stroke, systemic embolism, or death).

2. Patients under age 75 years with atrial fibrillation and one risk factor for stroke benefit from anticoagulation to an INR of 2.0 to 3.0. Studies have shown warfarin therapy reduces the frequency of all strokes by 68 per cent and deaths by 33 per cent.

3. Patients over age 75 years, even those without other risk factors, benefit from anticoagulation because of the increased risk with advancing age. This age group is thought to be at higher risk for bleeding complications with anticoagulation therapy. The annual frequency of major bleeding events was 1.0 per cent in control groups, 1.3 per cent with anticoagulation, and 1.0 per cent with aspirin. Intracranial bleeding was associated with higher blood pressures and an INR greater than 3.0.

Atrial Fibrillation Investigators. Risk factors for stroke and efficacy of antithrombotic therapy in atrial fibrillation: Analysis of pooled data from five randomized controlled trials. Arch Intern Med 1994;154:1449–1457.

Benjamin EJ, Levy D, Vaziui SM, et al. Independent risk factors for atrial fibrillation in a population-based cohort. JAMA 1994;271:840–844.

Fineberg WM, Blackshear J, Lanpacis A, et al. Prevalence, age distribution, and gender in patients with atrial fibrillation: Analysis and implications. Arch Intern Med 1995;155:469–473.

Lip GYH, Beevers DG: History, epidemiology, and importance of atrial fibrillation. Br Med J 1995;311:1361–1363.

QUESTIONS

1. True or False. The following medications are effective in converting atrial fibrillation to a sinus rhythm.
   a. Digoxin
   b. Quinidine
   c. Flecainide
   d. Sotalol
   e. Propranolol

Answers appear on **page 606.**

Chapter 47

Knee Injury

Jon Divine, M.D.
Steven C. Van Noord, M.D.
John Lombardo, M.D.

SUBJECTIVE

A 22-year-old male collegiate volleyball player presented to the training room with recurrent anterior knee pain. He localized the pain to the infrapatellar region of the right knee. The pain began during the last few volleyball practices and became more painful with jumping. This incident was not a new source of knee pain, because he had experienced the same pain in the same location for "many years," beginning in adolescence. In years past, the pain recurred during the early phase of training and became more tolerable as the competitive season progressed. He could not recall a single isolated event resulting in immediate pain, instability, or swelling during any episode. He had no sensation of locking, catching, or grinding when bending or straightening the knee. Pain symptoms generally occurred only during practice; however, he did have mild pain going up and down stairs. He also reported occasional stiffness after long periods of sitting. Review of records demonstrated a consistent history of similar knee pain during the preseason. In the past, his symptoms were relieved with post-activity icing, nonsteroidal anti-inflammatory drugs (NSAIDs), and phonophoresis. On two previous episodes his pain could not be relieved with medications or pain-relief modalities and he was rested for 1 to 2 weeks, which temporarily lessened his symptoms. He had no history of additional knee problems and had no pain in the left knee. Generally, he was healthy without significant medical problems.

In this episode he felt the knee pain was adversely affecting his performance and he asked to be rested for at least 1 week to resolve the pain. He also believed that the knee pain was adversely affecting his regular training habits, resulting in the sensation of being "tired, overweight, and out of shape." Teammates and coaches also noticed that the athlete appeared to "wear down" and appeared at times to be apathetic early in practice sessions. He was a very popular member on the volleyball team and was being looked upon as a team leader in the upcoming season. Outside of vigorous preseason volleyball training, his school work was going very well; he had little difficulty maintaining a high grade point average. His relationships with family, friends, and teammates were very good. He was in a steady, monogamous relationship with a girlfriend for several months. He drank alcohol occasionally but reported no episodes of binge drinking. He used no other recreational drugs or dietary supplements. He described a diet that was well balanced, but he had been eating an increasing amount of "junk food." His sleeping habits were described as "staying awake until late at night" studying, or socializing, yet he continued to awaken in time for early morning classes. Although he was discouraged about his recurrent knee pain, he felt no extraordinary anxiety or sadness. His interests in most activities had not decreased; however, he did admit to having less interest in preseason training.

OBJECTIVE

On physical examination, this was a healthy, pleasant Hispanic male, 73 inches tall and 180 lb, with a very good general appearance. Because of the feelings of "being tired," a complete general examination was done. Special attention was given to the lower extremities. Mini-mental status examination was completely normal, and the athlete's affect, rate and content of speech, and appearance were all

unremarkable. HEENT was normal; there were no signs of conjuctival pallor or scleral icterus and no evidence of upper respiratory infection. The neck was supple without adenopathy. Chest was clear with symmetrical air movement. Cardiovascular examination was also normal with a regular heart rate and rhythm, without murmur, rub, gallop, or click. The abdomen was also normal; there was no hepatosplenomegaly or inguinal adenopathy.

On examination of the extremities, there was focal tenderness to light palpation of the right tibial tubercle and distal patellar tendon. The pain increased slightly with full flexion but was unaffected by extension. The tibial tubercles were prominent but not grossly enlarged. The player had visible genu varus of both knees and bilateral foot pronation. The Q angle was roughly 15 degrees. There were no signs of knee swelling, effusion, or ecchymosis. Results of ligamentous testing including Lachman test, anterior and posterior drawer tests, collateral and posterior-lateral stability test were all normal. No joint line pain occurred with flexion, and none occurred with either internal or external tibial circumduction. Mild superior-medial patellofemoral tenderness was noted. No visible patella tracking defect or palpable enlargement of the retinaculum was seen. Patella apprehension testing was negative. Quadriceps muscle tone, especially the vastus medialis oblique (VMO) portion, was excellent. The remainder of the extremity examination, including that of the left knee, was normal.

Radiographs of the right knee revealed an increased radiodensity of the distal patellar tendon extending from the tibial tubercle. The proximal tibial epiphysis was closed, and no defect was detected along its course. There was an 8-degree genu varus. No evidence of patella alta, osteochondral defect, or loose body was noted. No joint space abnormality appeared on AP, lateral, or notch views. On the sunrise view, the patellofemoral joint space was well preserved without significant abnormality.

Because of fatigue, a screening complete blood count (CBC), thyroid stimulating hormone (TSH) and serum glucose levels, and monospot tests were done, and results were well within normal limits.

ASSESSMENT

Given the location of pain, radiographic findings, and chronic, recurrent nature of anterior knee pain the most likely diagnosis is adult complications of Osgood-Schlatter disease. Although the patient is well past the period of epiphysis closure, many adults continue to have anterior knee pain with activities as a result of previous Osgood-Schlatter disease during adolescence. The presence of a distal patellar tendon calcification, although not often seen, is an adult remnant of Osgood-Schlatter disease and can contribute to recurrent anterior knee pain.

"Being tired" is a common complaint in athletes during strenuous preseason training, and the complaint can have multiple potential causes. Following a normal physical examination and screening laboratory tests, the cause of "tiredness" or subjective fatigue should focus on volume of training, and psychosocial and potential lifestyle causes. Although fatigue, change in sleep habits, and disinterest in activities are signs of clinical depression, they are also early signs of overtraining, a condition in athletes that is difficult to differentiate from depression. In addition to the recurrence of a chronic injury adversely affecting his performance on the court, this athlete was also having difficulty adjusting to his perception of an "ideal" team leader. At this point, it was believed that this athlete was overtraining and was having an acute adjustment reaction to his recurrent injury; however, he was going to be followed closely for signs of clinical depression.

PLAN

The athlete was started on quadriceps and hamstring flexibility training, naproxen (Naprosyn) 500 mg bid, and postactivity icing. Phonophoresis (ultrasound directed application of anti-inflammatory medications to subsurface tissue) with dexamethasone was added 2 weeks later after initial measures to control pain symptoms failed. The athlete believed that the phonophoresis was actually causing more pain, which is a common complaint when ultrasound is used over an area of bony injury, and treatments were discontinued after the second dose. The athlete was then rested from jumping and weight training activities for 2 weeks. During this time he was seen by a physician in his home town and was injected with dexamethasone around the insertion of the patella tendon. He was rested completely for 5 days following the injection. During the subsequent active rest period he was permitted to jog, ride a stationary cycle, and continue with upper body weight training activities; however, he did no jumping or squatting activities. He also continued an aggressive quadriceps and hamstrings flexibility program. Following the active rest period he was allowed to progressively increase his jumping activity during training drills. He reported having

some pain, but pain was not as severe as before the rest period. His energy level during training sessions also improved. Before returning to full play he was instructed to always wear protective knee padding, which he had worn on a limited basis throughout his volleyball career. Surgery to remove the ossicle in the tendon was presented as an option to control chronic pain following the competitive season.

DIFFERENTIAL DIAGNOSIS

Anterior knee pain is a common complaint in athletes, especially jumping athletes. The differential diagnosis for chronic anterior knee is extensive. The initial evaluation of an athlete with anterior knee pain must include a thorough history and physical examination. It is essential to determine if the knee pain first occurred with an acute activity or event. The onset of acute pain following a specific event often indicates a more serious injury, rather than a chronic case of anterior knee pain. Acute injuries include damage to the major ligaments: medial collateral (MCL), lateral collateral (LCL), anterior cruciate (ACL), and posterior cruciate (PCL). Other acute traumatic knee injuries include tears to the medial and lateral meniscus, osteochondral or growth plate fractures, and patellar dislocation. These types of injuries are also generally associated with some degree of swelling and joint effusion, and they are often associated with instability. Nonacute injuries are those that do not have a specific inciting event but rather evolve insidiously over time. Nonacute injuries include Osgood-Schlatter disease, as in this case, patellofemoral dysfunction, and patellar tendinitis.

The most common cause of chronic anterior knee pain is pain at the patellofemoral joint.

Patellofemoral syndrome is a generalized term used to describe anterior knee pain involving several factors affecting the patellofemoral joint, including malalignment, trauma, overuse, and plica disorders. Tendinitis, bursitis, and osteochondritis dissecans are specific causes of pain; however, they have been lumped incorrectly into the category of patellofemoral syndrome. Patellofemoral dysfunction is characterized by insidious onset of pain in the anterior aspect of the knee. Discomfort is present during activities that stress the joint between the patella and the femur, classically walking up stairs or hills, or sitting with a bent knee for a prolonged period of time. The onset of pain can rarely be associated with an isolated event. Many explanations are given for this syndrome, but usually it is the result of maltracking of the patella in the femoral groove.

This can adversely alter cartilage on the undersurface of the patella. The patella tracking problem can be associated with malalignment of the entire lower extremity, which increases stresses at multiple sites including the patellofemoral joint. The term "miserable malalignment," a condition seen more often in females, refers to increased anteversion of the femoral head with forward placement of the femoral head in relation to the shaft and increased internal rotation of the femur to allow satisfactory coverage of the femoral head in the pelvis. There is also a widened Q angle, often giving a "knock-knee" appearance. The Q angle is the angle formed by a line drawn from the anterior superior iliac spine through the mid-patella and a line drawn from the tibial tubercle extending through the patella.

Lower extremity malalignment is further complicated by the presence of external tibial rotation and foot pronation. Decreased flexibility of the lateral retinaculum, iliotibial band, or hamstrings also contributes to adverse stresses at the patellofemoral joint. Weak VMO muscles can also contribute to recurrent patellofemoral problems including lateral subluxation and symptomatic irritation of the medial and lateral patella retinaculum. Diagnosis is made by history and peripatellar pain. Retropatellar pain and even crepitation are reproduced by compression of the patella against the femur while contracting the quadriceps. Treatment includes avoiding aggravating activities; giving ice and NSAIDs; and improving the flexibility and strength of the hamstrings and quadriceps, particularly strengthening the VMO. Clinicians should regularly monitor the balance between quadriceps and hamstring flexibility and strength; ideally, quadriceps:hamstring strength ratios should be 1.6:1 or less.

Acute trauma resulting in patella contusion, fracture, subluxation, or dislocation also results in patellofemoral joint pain. Delayed effects of acute trauma, or chronic microtrauma, can further result in degenerative changes in the patellofemoral chondral cartilage (chondromalacia patellae), osteoarthritis, or retinacular fibrosis.

A synovial *plica* is a symptomatic fold in the synovial lining of the joint, usually located along the medial border of the patellofemoral joint, that can become also inflamed as a result of trauma and overuse. All of these entities have been lumped along with malalignment into the patellofemoral syndrome diagnosis "basket." Although all are similar causes of anterior knee pain, each should be recognized as a separate potential problem and appropriately treated.

Another cause of chronic anterior knee pain is *Osgood-Schlatter disease (OSd)*, the most common of the growth-related causes of knee pain in skeletally immature athletes. OSd is characterized by gradual onset of pain and swelling on the tibial tubercle, typically without a traumatic event. Symptoms develop during a growth spurt, usually between the ages of 11 and 15 years; it is seen more frequently in boys and is bilateral in one third of the cases. Pain increases with eccentric quadriceps work or weight bearing on a flexed knee. Common provoking activities include running, jumping, squatting, and occasionally kneeling. It often occurs in those who are active in more than one sport. Athletes with OSd present with anterior knee pain localized over the tibial tubercle or distal patella tendon. They may have localized heat, tenderness, and enlargement of bony tissue at the tubercle. Tenderness is elicited on the tubercle and extends proximally on the tendon. There may be restricted passive flexion, and tight hamstrings are usually present. OSd is generally believed to be caused by repetitive traction on the tibial tuberosity apophysis, at the insertion of the patella tendon. Excessive traction on the apophysis at the tibial tubercle by the patellar tendon creates the well-recognized apophysitis, or enlarged tender tibial tubercle. Radiographs may be normal or may reveal fragmentation of the tibial tuberosity. Patella alta is a common finding.

Treatment focuses on pain relief, balance between quadriceps and hamstring flexibility and strength, and reduction of exercise or activity below the soreness threshold (active rest) in severe cases. Symptoms often resolve completely when skeletal maturity is reached. Occasionally, pain persists into adulthood after apophyseal closure. After skeletal maturity has been reached, the apophysis may fragment, which results in an ossicle forming in the distal patellar tendon, resulting in chronic irritation and pain. The enlarged tubercle area continues to be tender and may require surgical excision for relief of recurrent pain. In severe cases, traumatic avulsion of the patella tendon at the apophysis can occur in those who have OSd, often necessitating immediate surgical repair.

Bursitis of the knee is another common diagnosis in the presence of anterior knee pain. Inflammation of one of many bursae surrounding the knee can cause anterior pain and stiffness. Bursae commonly causing anterior knee pain include the large prepatellar bursa, located between the patella and skin; the superficial infrapatellar bursa, located between the proximal patella tendon and the skin; and the deep infrapatellar bursa, located between the distal patella tendon and the proximal tibia.

Prepatellar bursitis, also known as *carpet layer's* or *housemaid's knee*, is generally caused by frictional stress directly over the bursae resulting from repetitive kneeling or direct trauma. Penetrating injuries to this bursae can also result in pyogenic or infectious bursitis. *Superficial infrapatellar bursitis* is also caused by repetitive microtrauma and friction and usually arises from repetitive kneeling in the upright position—hence the name *vicar's knee*. Patients present with pain, obvious swelling, and tenderness surrounding the patella, which may also cause limited range of motion due to discomfort.

Deep infrapatellar bursitis is more likely to result from a direct blow or fall on the knee than are injuries of the other two bursae. Chronic overuse injuries involving the deep infrapatellar bursae can result in anterior knee pain felt deep to the distal patellar tendon; the condition is difficult to distinguish from other causes of infrapatellar area pain. Patients present with vague tenderness over the mid-distal portion of the patella tendon and are unable to fully flex and extend the knee. The onset of symptoms usually follows isolated or repetitive blows on the knee, such as incurred by a volleyball player diving to pass a ball. Symptoms can also be due to overuse. Often, there are very few signs of swelling. These symptoms cause difficulty in distinguishing this condition from other common causes of anterior knee pain including patellar tendinitis, hemorrhage into the retropatellar fat pad, and OSd. A partial tear in the patella tendon can also present in a similar vague fashion, without significant weakness in leg extension. In general, bursitis and fat pad pain are felt deep to the tendon, whereas pain caused by inflammation of the tendon is felt more superficially. Ossification of the tendon at either pole on plain films may also help in determining the diagnosis. Diagnosis can be more confusing when bursitis and one or more of these conditions coexist. For persistent symptoms a magnetic resonance imaging (MRI) examination may be necessary to accurately make the diagnosis.

Patellar tendinitis is a very common cause of chronic anterior knee pain, and it can be confused with deep infrapatellar bursitis and OSd. Anterior knee pain made worse with jumping has been labeled *jumper's knee*, often due to patellar tendinitis. *Jumper's knee*, however, may also refer to pain at the quadriceps tendon insertion or stress reactions involving the proximal or distal poles of the patella. Repetitive, explosive forces generated by athletic activities, especially jumping, place a tremendous axial load, more than 10 times body weight, on the tendon. Athletes generally present with chronic pain at the inferior pole of the patella but can have pain along the entire length of the tendon. The onset of pain is gradual, and there is rarely a single event that results in pain. Because of the superficial location of the tendon, tenderness can be elicited by light palpation of the tendon. Pain due to bursitis often requires more pressure with direct palpation. Most athletes with patellar tendinitis have normal radiographs; however, findings on films may include osseous changes at the inferior patellar pole, intratendinous calcifications, and patella alta. Treatment for tendinitis focuses on pain relief, relative rest from explosive (jumping) activities, and working toward balance in flexibility between the quadriceps and hamstrings, along with improving heel cord flexibility. In addition, quadriceps and eccentric ankle dorsiflexion-strengthening exercises have also been found to be beneficial.

Therapeutic modalities such as ice, heat, ultrasound, phonophoresis, and iontophoresis (low-volume electrical current used to direct the medication to deep tissues) have been helpful in inflammation reduction and pain control. The use of an infrapatellar strap to reduce pain has had variable results. Several investigators report having more consistent success with the McConnell patellofemoral taping technique than with the various brands of straps. Pain management of less severe cases of patella tendinitis (short duration of pain following activity) includes the regular use of NSAIDs, taping or strap use during activities, and ice following activities. Pain during activities may require periods of active rest from pain-provoking activities. Prolonged pain after athletic activities, pain with activities of daily living, or prolonged rest pain adversely affects performance, and prolonged rest is necessary. In the past, direct injection of corticosteroids into the patella tendon has been used in patients with severe tendinitis. Although no information from controlled studies is available, data from animal studies indicate a temporary, 3- to 4-week reduction in the tensile strength of the tendon following corticosteroid injection. Because of the potential for tendon rupture, direct injection of corticosteroids into the tendon has no place in the successful management of acute or chronic patellar tendinitis.

Patients with severe pain not responding to at least 6 months of conservative therapy may have *angiofibroblastic tendonosis* of the patella tendon. This chronic cause of anterior knee pain is characterized by proximal-medial tendon thickening along with an increased signal intensity on MRI. Grossly, the affected portion of the tendon is thickened and has a loss of normal longitudinal fiber orientation. Histologically, the affected tissue has hyaline degeneration, collagen fiber disorganization, and inefficient angiogenesis. When this chronic condition is suspected, the athlete should be referred to an orthopedist, because surgery may be an option to correct chronic pain and allow the athlete to return to training and competition.

The MCL and LCL are injured by an acute trauma. The MCL, which runs from the medial femoral condyle to the proximal medial tibia, is more commonly injured. The history includes a valgus stress to the knee and pain in the medial aspect of the knee. The diagnosis is confirmed by medial knee pain on the femoral condyle or the proximal tibia. A valgus stress to the knee reproduces the medial joint pain and may also widen the medial joint line. This injury generally heals well without surgery. The LCL runs from the lateral femoral condyle to the head of the fibula. It is injured by a varus stress to the knee. The patient feels tenderness on the lateral femoral condyle or near the head of the fibula. Diagnosis is confirmed by applying varus stress and reproducing the lateral joint pain. This may be accompanied by widening of the lateral joint line. The injury often does not occur alone; therefore, a high index of suspicion for associated injuries must be present. Special attention should be given to skeletally immature athletes with collateral ligament sprains because avulsion epiphysis injuries can occur.

The *medial and lateral menisci* are crescent-shaped "shock absorbers" that are located between the tibia and femur. They are cartilaginous structures that cover one to two thirds of the articular surface of the tibial plateau. They are damaged as a result of a rotation or twisting of the knee. The knee typically is mildly swollen, with pain in the medial or lateral joint line, and the patient may complain of a knee that locks or gives way. The physical examination is that of a knee that may or may not have an effusion and pain along the joint line. Positive meniscal tests such as McMurray's test, along with reproducing locking or catching of the knee, can be present. The medial meniscus is much less mobile than the lateral and consequently is injured more often. As one ages, the menisci can lose moisture, become more friable, degenerate, and tear with much less force than when one was younger. Occasionally, the diagnosis is not clear-cut, and an MRI is needed if the patient continues to have symptoms and the examination is equivocal. Treatment consists of arthroscopic surgery, which can often have a patient back to the sport or hobby in a few weeks. Those older patients with degenerative tears and minimal functional disability may benefit from a trial of nonoperative rehabilitation.

The most impressive acute knee injury is that due to a tear of the ACL. The ACL is a major ligament within the knee that supplies significant rotational stability to the knee and prevents anterior translation of the tibia on the femur. The history is that of a single event that may or may not involve contact. A blow may occur to the lower leg, or the patient may be making a cut resulting in rupture of the ACL. An audible pop is often heard, with immediate swelling and inability to bear weight. The knee may feel unstable. The examination confirms the diagnosis by a positive Lachman's or anterior drawer test with the knee flexed 30 degrees. Associated injuries to the other ligaments or meniscus may be present. The ACL is a very poor healer; therefore, a torn ACL should be surgically repaired. A knee can function without an ACL; however, this requires a decrease in demanding activities such as quick starts, stops, cutting, and jumping. Having an ACL-deficient knee can lead to instability, and chronic instability can result in premature degenerative changes. Therefore, the younger and more active a patient is, the more likely that an ACL reconstruction is required.

The PCL also is an intrinsic stabilizer of the knee that prevents posterior translation of the tibia on the femur. It is injured less frequently than the ACL. The mechanism involves a traumatic blow to the anterior tibia, as with a motor vehicle accident in which the tibia strikes the dashboard. If the injury is isolated the patient may have minimal pain, swelling, and dysfunction. The injury is confirmed by a positive posterior drawer sign and/or a positive tibial sag sign. The treatment is usually nonoperative, involving rehabilitation that focuses on quadriceps strengthening. This treatment strategy may be changing somewhat in the future because more is being learned about this injury.

Patellar subluxation or *dislocation* is an acute event in which the patella is displaced laterally. By definition, subluxation is a spontaneous dislocation and relocation of the patella, whereas dislocation requires the patella to be manipulated back into the normal position. Both can occur as a result of a valgus stress to the knee, by external rotation of the tibia, or as the result of a direct blow to the patella. Significant pain and moderate effusion often develop. Physical findings following a subluxation include effusion, pain medial to the patella, and significant apprehension in the patient when the patella is manually pushed laterally. Treatment includes immobilization of the knee followed by rehabilitation. Those who have had a dislocated patella are at an increased risk for future dislocations. If the patient is a recurrent "dislocator," surgical treatment is an option.

DISCUSSION

Deciding on the cause of anterior knee pain is difficult. Multiple anterior knee structures are affected by extensive mechanical forces even with routine activities. Active people can have even greater mechanical forces affecting the knee, which may lead to overuse type injuries or may worsen pre-existing problems. After examining the volleyball player presented here, the location and chronic recurrent nature of anterior knee pain is most likely adult complications from OSd. Being 22 years old and well past adolescence, other possible causes were initially considered to be more likely sources of pain. In "jumping athletes" the most likely cause of chronic anterior knee pain is patellar tendinitis, followed by symptomatic plica, patellofemoral syndrome, or complications following an acute injury. Although some argue that a plica can be diagnosed only by arthroscopy, a plica causing significant symptoms is generally palpable on examination and was not found in this athlete. The location of point tenderness at the tibial tubercle, more common with deep infrapatellar bursitis or symptomatic OSd, is less common with patellar tendinitis, which usually causes pain and tenderness at the inferior pole of the patella or proximal patella tendon. This athlete's tenderness was elicited by light palpation at the tibial tubercle, and little discomfort was present on flexion and extension. Inflammation of the bursa causing tenderness with light palpation also produces considerable pain on active and passive leg extension and flexion. Radiographic findings helped to rule out significant bony abnormalities and confirmed the strongly suspected, postadolescent closure of the tibial epiphysis. Many adults continue to have anterior knee pain with activities well past the period of epiphysis closure. The calcification seen in the distal patellar tendon can very well be the result of chronic patellar tendinitis; however, given the athlete's history of adolescent knee pain, the most likely cause is a fragmented apophysis with ossicle formation within the patellar tendon as a consequence of OSd. The presence of distal patellar tendon calcification is a cause of recurrent pain and stiffness, especially with acute or repetitive blunt trauma over the ossicle. Thus, not only was repetitive jumping a cause for knee irritation, but also the repetitive direct trauma to the knee with diving on the floor during volleyball training also played a contributing role in worsening knee pain.

The athlete failed to respond to conservative therapy, which included naproxen (Naprosyn) 500 mg bid and phonophoresis with dexamethasone. Rest from jumping and weight training activities was then implemented. After the localized injection of corticosteroids, the athlete did no athletic activities for 5 days. During the next 10 days, he was permitted to jog, ride a stationary cycle, and continue with upper-body weight training activities all below the threshold of knee pain. He also started an aggressive quadriceps and hamstring flexibility program. Following the 10-day active rest period he was allowed to progressively increase his jumping activity during training drills. He reported having some pain but not as severe as before the rest period. His energy level during training sessions also improved. Before returning to full play he was instructed to always wear protective knee padding, which he had worn on a very limited basis throughout his volleyball career.

Injection with dexamethasone around the insertion of the patellar tendon during the rest period by the athlete's primary care physician probably assisted in reduction of inflammation and pain. It is important to remember, however, that injections in this area should be done with caution, and the athlete should be required to rest for at least 1 to 2 weeks following the injection to reduce the risk of patellar tendon rupture. Injections should never be made directly into the patellar tendon. Surgery to remove the ossicle in the tendon is a last resort following conservative therapy but it does not guarantee complete resolution of pain.

It is important to remember that athletic injuries also have significant psychological and emotional impact on the athlete. As in this case, the athlete's psychological and emotional state may have contributed to the risk of injury as well. Fatigue and "being tired" are common complaints from athletes during strenuous preseason training. Multiple exercise and non–exercise-related causes of fatigue, too numerous to describe in any detail within this chapter, exist. In well-trained athletes, consideration should be given to the possibility of overtraining as a cause of fatigue. Although fatigue, change in sleep habits, and apathy are signs of clinical depression, they are also early signs of overtraining. Overtrained athletes may also have an inability to concentrate, mood instability, and a feeling of heaviness or staleness. Athletes with an acute musculotendinous injury or a recurrence of a chronic injury also should be evaluated for overtraining. Oddly enough, injured athletes are also predisposed to developing signs and symptoms of clinical depression. Thus, a vicious circle of overtraining and depression may develop. Initially, a review of training volume is essential to help differentiate clinical depression from overtraining, because there are no reliable clinical or laboratory markers that consistently correlate with overtraining. Symptoms due to depression generally do not improve and may worsen with inactivity. Symptoms associated with overtraining usually respond quickly to a substantial decrease in the volume of training, as they did in this athlete. In retrospect, his perception of a "team leader" as one who works hard and performs well led to significantly increasing his training volume. When his performance expectations on the court were not met, his training volume increased, his chronic knee pain recurred, and the vegetative symptoms of depression appeared. The active rest period allowed the injury to heal and decreased the athlete's depression symptoms. It is possible that relative overtraining played a significant role not only in the athlete's knee pain but also in his sensation of "being tired."

SUGGESTED READING

Blazina ME, Kerlan RK, Jobe FW, et al: Jumper's knee. Orthop Clin North Am 1973;4(3):665–678.

Brukner P, Khan K. The tired athlete. In Clinical Sports Medicine. Sydney, McGraw-Hill, 1993, pp 618–626.

Richmond C. The knee. In Sports Medicine for Primary Care. Cambridge, MA, Blackwell Scientific, 1996, pp 387–444.

Roland GC, Beagley MJ, Cawley PW. Conservative treatment of inflamed knee bursae. Physician Sports Med 1992;20(2):67–78.

Stanitski, CL. Patellofemoral mechanism. In Stanitski CL, DeLee JC, Drez D (eds). Pediatric and Adolescent Sports Medicine. Philadelphia, W.B. Saunders, 1994, pp 294–370.

Yu JS, Popp JE, Kaeding CC, Lucas J. Correlation of MR imaging and pathologic findings in athletes undergoing surgery for chronic patellar tendinitis. Am J Radiology 1995;165:115–118.

QUESTIONS

1. Patellar tendinitis
   a. Typically occurs with an acute event
   b. Should not be treated with injectable corticosteroids
   c. Surgery should be considered early in the course of the injury
   d. a and b
   e. None of the above

2. Which statements are false?
   a. Osgood-Schlatter disease is more common in boys
   b. OSd usually peaks after the growth plates have closed
   c. OSd is an apophysitis
   d. OSd involves the distal pole of the patella
   e. a and d
   f. b and d

3. Deep infrapatellar bursitis
   a. Causes tenderness on examination at the proximal patellar tendon.
   b. Tenderness is difficult to distinguish from that caused by OSd.
   c. Is commonly referred to as "carpet layer's knee."
   d. Is associated with an enlarged tibial tubercle.

Answers appear on **page 606**.

Chapter 48

Neck Pain

Jon Divine, M.D.

SUBJECTIVE

Patient Identification and Presenting Problem

A 45-year-old female courtroom reporter presented with a 2- to 3-week history of neck pain. She could not recall a specific traumatic event, previous history of neck injury, or chronic neck pain. She denied working longer than her accustomed 6- to 8-hour work day; however, she had recently been working during a "stressful" trial that had attracted increased local media attention. She did not have a regular exercise schedule but had been doing "some weight training" 3 months before presentation. The volume of her household activities had not changed before the onset of neck pain. Her pain was localized to the posterior portion of the neck, mainly in the "middle and left side" and was described as "dull and fairly constant." The patient stated that her neck "felt stiff"; the stiffness was more noticeable throughout the day with turning her head to the left and when looking down—a frequent position in her job. She had no early morning stiffness. There was no change in the quality of pain with movement, although the pain increased while she was lying on her left side. The pain seemed to be lessened in the morning and increased throughout the day until she could "rest" at night, when there would be "some" improvement. Over the 3-week period she did notice an increase in pain radiating to the lower scapula and shoulder without any numbness, weakness, or sensation of pain in the upper extremities. She had been taking up to 1 g of over-the-counter (OTC) ibuprofen three times a day with little improvement in pain symptoms.

The patient was being treated for depression with paroxetine (Paxil) and had no other current medical problems. She was not taking any other medications (besides OTC ibuprofen and Paxil) and had allergies to "codeine." She had had back surgery for a "protruding disk" in the lumbar area 10 years ago and breast augmentation surgery roughly 15 years ago. Her family history was remarkable for degenerative arthritis (mother, still living) and cerebral vascular accident resulting in death (father). Socially, she had been happily married to an attorney for 15 years, with no children. She had been working for the same court for approximately 10 years, was a nonsmoker, and had fewer than three drinks per week. No symptoms of fever, weight loss, night sweats, respiratory difficulties, chest or abdominal discomfort, or incontinence were reported.

OBJECTIVE

Examination and Laboratory Findings

On examination, this was a very pleasant woman who appeared younger than her stated age, sitting with her head slightly flexed and bent toward the left. No other postural abnormality or neck deformity was observed. No visible muscle spasm, swelling, neck mass, or skin discoloration was seen. Localized tenderness was noted in the midposterior cervical region on the left, and mild tenderness at the inferior poles of the scapula on both the right and the left; no palpable muscle cord or mass was found at tender sites. Active range of motion was slow and progressively painful with both flexion and extension. Rotation and bending to the right was "stiff" but not painful. Rotation to the left was also stiff and became painful at the midpoint of rotation. She could not bend to the left because of pain. Resisted range of motion caused mild pain in all directions but was worse on bending to the left. Cervical compression was not painful. No anterior neck tenderness, spasm, masses, or adenopathy were present. Neurologic examination was remarkable for decreased left side tricep deep tendon reflex (DTR 1/4 versus 2/4 on the right), without any other abnormal neurologic findings. The thyroid, heart, lung, and abdominal examinations were normal. A midline surgical scar was noted on the lower lumbar area of the back, and there was "stiffness" with active range of motion on the remainder of the spinal examination, with no other abnormality. Pulses in the upper extremity were strong and symmetrical and did not change with abduction of the arm. Radiographs of the neck were remarkable for a loss of normal cervical lordosis and degenerative changes at the C5 to C7 areas without foramen obstruction at any level.

Laboratory tests within normal limits included complete blood count (CBC), chemistry profile, Westergren erythrocyte sedimentation rate (ESR), and antinuclear antibody (ANA). Rheumatoid factor and HLA-B27 antibody tests were negative. The patient was initially treated conservatively with nonsteroidal anti-inflammatory drugs (NSAIDs), muscle relaxers, and supervised physical therapy. Her symptoms did not improve over 4 weeks, and she began having radicular pain on the left side, from the neck to the middle finger. On repeat examination, in addition to an asymmetrical tricep DTR, there was a subtle loss of arm extension strength on the left compared with the right and a diminished ability to distinguish light touch on the dorsal aspect of the midportion of the left hand. No other abnormality with strength, sensation, or reflexes was present.

ASSESSMENT

This case describes a middle-aged female courtroom reporter with worsening symptoms of apparently chronic neck pain and new significant neurologic findings involving her left arm. She described her pain as "dull and constant" and improving with rest. The current onset of pain was associated with increased job stresses and an increased amount of postural stress. She has a family history of osteoarthritis as well as previous back surgery for a herniated lumbar disk, indicating a predisposition toward degenerative changes. She had no other symptoms to suggest rheumatologic disease as a cause of premature spinal degeneration. On examination there was tenderness over the trapezius muscle, without a specific trigger point site, and pain with flexion and rotation of the head. Perhaps most important are the neurologic findings involving the left arm, indicating a disease process causing impingement or compression of the nerve root, specifically of C7

(Fig. 48–1). In a 45-year-old female without rheumatic disease, the most likely cause of neck pain with neurologic symptoms is degenerative disk disease, with compression of the nerve root caused by a herniated disk. The reason for the early onset of significant disease is unknown; however, her familial and occupational predisposition seems to be the only identifiable cause. It appears that the degenerative cervical spine disease was already present and the increased psychological and position stresses may have aggravated the condition to the point of provoking neurologic symptoms.

PLAN

The initial management of this patient began with efforts to control pain, make an accurate diagnosis, help her regain function, and prevent worsening of a chronic degenerative process. She was initially treated conservatively with NSAIDs and muscle relaxers. Radiographs of the neck were obtained along with baseline rheumatologic laboratory tests, including CBC, chemistry profile, ESR, ANA, rheumatoid factor, and HLA-B27 antibody. She was started on a program of supervised physical therapy, which included range-of-motion exercises and basic postural exercises and training. When her symptoms

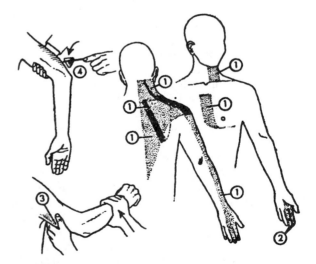

Figure 48–1. Should the disk cause entrapment of the 7th cervical nerve root, pain will radiate into the neck, trapezius region, vertebral border of the scapula, anterior chest wall, outer aspects of the arm, and index and middle finger *(1)*. The patient will experience paresthesias of the index and middle fingers particularly *(2)*. There will be diminished muscle power evident, particularly in the triceps *(3)*. The triceps reflex tends to be diminished *(4)*. (From Connolly JF, Jardan OM. Orthopedics. In Rakel RE [ed]. Textbook of Family Practice, 4th ed. Philadelphia, W.B. Saunders, 1990, p 1072.)

did not improve over 4 weeks and she began having radicular pain on the left side, from the neck to the middle finger, she was given a tapering dose of oral steroids and a trial of cervical traction. She was referred to a neurosurgeon. A magnetic resonance imaging (MRI) examination of the neck demonstrated the nerve root obstruction at the C7 level by a herniated disk. Because of chronic pain and progressive worsening neurologic symptoms, surgery was performed to relieve the compression.

Since the surgery, the patient has had alleviation of pain and complete resolution of neurologic symptoms. She continues to use Paxil and has been instructed in progressive relaxation techniques for stress management. To prevent future problems she has also been instructed in proper posture and ideal work ergonomics. She was advised to limit long periods of excessive neck flexion and extension, and avoid sleeping on multiple pillows and in the prone position.

DIFFERENTIAL DIAGNOSIS

The key to an accurate diagnosis and appropriate management is obtaining important information during the history and physical examination. Important points to know in the history of all patients and those that should raise the red flag when present include traumatic injury, especially that associated with a head injury; pain not relieved by rest; pain associated with severe headache and/or change in mental status; and pain radiating to the extremities in a dermatomal fashion. Other important information is history regarding the patient's lifestyle, including sleep habits and posture; exercise and activity habits; and regular and recent irregular physical and psychological demands.

Listening to how the story is told may provide the initial clue to an acute or ongoing process. Patients with traumatic or acute injuries usually start their explanation in a chronological fashion: "I had a car wreck" . . . "slept on it funny" . . . "heard something pop," and so forth, "and the pain followed." Their injuries often represent muscle strain, ligamentous sprain, or vertebral fracture. These patients should expand upon the details of their acute, painful event because details shed light on the anatomy involved. In contrast, patients with a chronic pain history usually start their explanation with the location of pain, because they are unable to recall a specific painful onset. A history of chronic neck pain is more likely to indicate myofascial, degenerative, or neoplastic disease. In these

patients the anatomic site of pain is less predictive of the anatomic site involved in the disease process.

Regardless of presentation, any previous neck injury or pain before presentation is an important portion of the history and may represent a recurrent or worsened injury. All patients with neck pain should have a thorough examination, paying particular attention to focal areas of increased tenderness, especially midline pain; active, passive, and resisted range of neck motion, noting immobility or painful areas; and a thorough neurologic examination, focusing on the upper and lower extremities. Radiographic imaging studies are not required for all patients with neck pain. Whenever there is a question concerning the integrity of the cervical skeleton, neurologic findings, or pain following trauma, baseline films of the cervical spine should be obtained to assist in the diagnosis (Table 48–1).

The axiom that "common things happen commonly" is one to keep in mind while formulating an accurate diagnosis from a broad and varying differential diagnosis for neck pain (Table 48–2). Neck pain is a common complaint; it is estimated that 35 per cent of all persons will have neck pain in their lifetime for which they will seek medical attention. The vast majority of neck pain is of a nonserious nature: 70 per cent of patients with neck pain have complete resolution of symptoms in less than 1 month. Because several important structures in the neck are required to function well for the patient in future occupational and leisure activities, it is also important to rule out less common but more debilitating disease processes such as cervical instability, infection, neoplastic disease, or referred pain from the chest.

To formulate a thorough and accurate diagnosis, a consistent thought process should be used with each patient. An organized method of grouping pathologic processes together to rule out disease is used to discuss this patient. A helpful way to orga-

TABLE 48–1. How to Read a Cervical Radiograph

1. Count the vertebrae
2. Check vertebrae position
3. Check vertebral alignment
4. Assess bony integrity
5. Measure sagittal and transverse spinal canal space
6. Examine the intervertebral disk spaces
7. Examine the facet joints
8. Check the spinous processes
9. Assess the atlanto-occipital relationship
10. Inspect the odontoid
11. Examine the prevertebral soft tissues

TABLE 48–2.   Differential Diagnosis for Neck Pain

Postural causes
Myofascial pain
  Trapezius muscle trigger points
  Autochthonous muscles of the back (postural cervical spine
    pain syndrome)
  Semispinalis capitis
  Splenius capitis
  Longissimus (capitis portion)
  Sternocleidomastoid
  Scalenus
Torticollis (acquired)
Fibrositis (transient stiff neck)
Coracoid pressure syndrome
Teres muscle syndrome
Cervical nerve root compression

Osteoarthritis
Cervical osteoarthritis
Multiple or single joint involvement
Degenerative disk disease (see Table 48–3 for specific findings)
Mass effects caused by degenerative changes
  Cervical myelopathy
  Esophageal compression
  Cervical spondylitis

Inflammatory/Infectious
Viral myalgia
Rheumatoid arthritis
Ankylosing spondylitis
Osteomyelitis or Pott's disease
Meningitis
Cervical spine bursitis
Neurogenic pain
  Post-herpetic neuralgia
  Occipital neuralgia
  Glossopharyngeal neuralgia (often with syncope)

Trauma
Neck sprain
  Acceleration-extension sprain
    Normal cervical spine
    Diseased spine
  Acceleration-flexion sprain
    Normal cervical spine
    Children
    Diseased spines
    Lateral flexion with rotation
Bilateral facet dislocation below C3
Vertebral fractures
C1–C2 dislocation
Posterior cervical sympathetic syndrome
Atlanto-occipital flexion/extension injury
Vertebral artery injury

Congenital
Basilar invagination
Occipitalization of atlas to occiput
Klippel-Feil syndrome
Arnold-Chiari malformation
Anomalies of atlantoaxial vertebrae
Congenital cervical spine stenosis
C-spine anomalies associated with other total body syndromes

Vascular/Compression
Anatomic compression syndrome causes
  Cervical rib
  Scalenus anterior muscle
  Costoclavicular
  Thoracic outlet
  Pectoralis minor hyperabduction
Vascular causes
  Vertebrobasilar insufficiency
  Migraine headaches

Endocrine/Metabolic
Tophaceous gout
Acute suppurative thyroiditis
Thyroglossal duct abscess
Diffuse idiopathic skeletal hyperostosis syndrome
Calcification of ligamenta flava

Neoplastic
Primary and metastatic tumors of spinal vertebrae
Primary intraspinal and extramedullary tumors
Foramen magnum tumor
Horner syndrome
  Third neuron of cervical sympathetic system
    Hyperfunction
    Hypofunction
    Deranged function
      Idiopathic hemifascial hyperhidrosis
      Hemifascial anhidrosis

Referred pain to the neck
Sinus infection
Temporomandibular (TMJ) inflammation
Upper extremity inflammation
  Acromial-clavicular (AC) joint trauma/arthritis (C4)
  Rotator cuff muscles/subacromial bursa (C4–C5)
  Lateral epicondyle of elbow (C5–C6)
  Carpal tunnel syndrome (C5–C7)
Myocardial ischemia (C3–C6)
Superior sulcus (Pancoast) tumor of lung (C3–C5)
Aortic dissection (C5–C7)
Irritation of the surface of the diaphragm (C3–C5)
Distal esophagus, or inferior pulmonary tumors, hepatic/
  gallbladder inflammation, or tumor (C4–C6)

Idiopathic
Fibromyalgia
Torticollis
  Congenital
  Acquired
    Musculoskeletal injury
    Soft tissue contracture
    Functional
Hyoid bone syndrome
Neck-tongue syndrome with sudden head movement
Calcific retropharyngeal tendinitis
Functional syndromes with osteoarthritis

nize the differential diagnosis thought process is to consider symptoms and examination findings and to answer three important clinical questions: (1) Is the neck pain due to an acute or chronic problem(s)? (2) Is there neurologic involvement? (3) What is the prevalence of the potential problems? If all three questions can be answered, an accurate assessment of the cause of neck pain can be made.

Perhaps the most common causes of neck pain are *posture* problems. Typically, the patient's occupation requires the neck to be flexed for prolonged periods, resulting in chronic tension on portions of the muscle, causing, over time, imbalances in muscle strength and flexibility. Chronic *psychological stress* can also produce a "hyperalert" (anxious, neck extended) or "pensive" (depressed, neck flexed) state that typically results in similar chronic postural stresses. Most patients in the early stages of disease find relief with position changes and rest; however, the process may slowly progress to the point of continued, unrelenting pain and stiffness. An acute episode of strain from rapid unaccustomed lifting or movement may result in a localized muscle spasm that may persist for some time, causing chronic pain. Typically, the muscles of the upper and lower trapezius, the cervical spine extensors, splenius capitis, or cervical erector muscle groups are affected, resulting in posterior and posterolateral neck pain, inflexibility, and posterior headaches. Owing to relative inactivity, the anterior flexor groups contribute to the problem because of progressive weakness. Neurologic symptoms are rare, the exception being the patient who has a prolonged history of chronic, repeated hyperextension of the cervical spine resulting in vertebral compression of the cervical spinal roots. Radiographic findings associated with postural disorders are usually nonspecific, often showing a loss of cervical lordosis or early degenerative osteoarthritic changes.

Treatment involves pain reduction with medications (NSAIDs and muscle relaxers) and pain control modalities, including alternating ice and heat, and ultrasound. The bulk of treatment is directed at improving balance in flexor/extensor muscle strength and flexibility. Efforts to improve workplace ergonomics by promoting work-related activities that require the head and neck to function in the neutral position are essential to recovery and prevention of future problems.

A common cause of debilitating chronic neck pain is *cervical arthritis*. Whether from inflammatory, infectious, or degenerative causes, arthritic changes in the cervical spine can result in chronic, progressive neck pain and a variety of peripheral neurologic symptoms. Cervical spinal osteoarthritis is virtually universal after the age of 50 years, and it affects the cervical spine at multiple levels, resulting in symptoms and signs specific to the level of involvement. The intervertebral disks, vertebral body and arch, and apophyseal joints are all variably affected. Localized joint involvement may in turn affect nearby soft tissue structures such as muscles and ligaments; cervical spine nerve roots; the intervertebral and transverse foramina; the spinal cord esophagus; and the vertebral vasculature supply, including the vertebral artery. Symptoms in patients with cervical arthritis are variable and include stiffness; limited movement; crepitus; and pain that may be general, localized, or referred to other areas in the neck or upper extremities. Significant examination findings vary by the site of involvement and include point tenderness, muscle spasm, and limited range of motion. If neurologic or vascular structures are involved, examination findings are varied (Table 48–3). Radiologic findings that define degenerative disease include four key points: (1) narrowing of the intervertebral disk space; (2) osteophyte formation on the anterior and posterior vertebral bodies adjacent to the neurocentral lip and at the apophyseal joints; (3) vertebral body end-plate sclerosis; and (4) narrowing of the sagittal diameter of the spinal canal.

Because the degree of degenerative changes is highly variable and not entirely age specific, it is important to differentiate osteoarthritis specifically affecting the cervical intervertebral disk from arthritis affecting the remainder of the cervical spine. Disk disease is more likely to cause significant episodes of nonspecific atraumatic neck pain, frequently with a variety of neurologic symptoms, and can produce clinically recognizable symptoms well before the age of 50 years. A progressive sequence of events indicative of *intervertebral disk disease* can occur early in life. Persons in their teens and 20s may experience sudden, atraumatic episodes of sharp neck pain and unilateral neck spasms, generally referred to as torticollis. These signs last for 24 to 72 hours, resolve spontaneously, and are indicative of a sudden displacement of the cartilaginous portion of the intervertebral disk with a spontaneous return to near-normal position. Usually there is an annual recurrence of torticollis symptoms. As the disease progresses, persons in their 20s to 30s experience unilateral episodes of scapular pain lasting 3 to 4 weeks before resolution. This scenario also represents a sudden displacement and return to position of the disk. As the degeneration progresses, the previous spontaneous return of the displaced disk is less likely to occur, resulting in more

TABLE 48–3.   Common Findings at Cervical Nerve Root Levels

Nerve Root	Disk Level	History	Sensory Loss	Reflex Loss	Weakness
C3	C2–C3	Pain into the back of the neck and around the mastoid process	Neck and posterior scalp		Neck flexion/extension Shoulder shrugging, inspiration
C4	C3–C4	Pain into the posterior neck, scapula, and high thoracic spine	Clavicle and tip of shoulder		Head and neck flexion, rotation Inspiration (phrenic nerve)
C5	C4–C5	Pain into side of neck, the superior lateral shoulder, and arm. Numbness from shoulder to lateral arm/forearm	Lateral shoulder, upper arm, and forearm	Biceps	Arm abduction, external rotation Forearm flexion, inspiration
C6	C5–C6	Pain to the lateral aspects of the arm and forearm into the thumb and index finger with numbness of thumb and dorsum of hand	Radial forearm, thumb, and index fingers	Brachioradialis	Forearm flexion, wrist extension Forearm pronation/supination Thumb flexion/abduction
C7	C6–C7	Pain below elbow, into the mid-forearm, to the second and third fingers	Dorsal forearm and hands palmar second and third fingers	Triceps	Forearm extension, hand flexion, and second and third finger flexion
C8	C7–T1	Pain to the medial aspect of the forearm into the ring and small fingers with numbness of fourth and fifth fingers	Ulnar forearm, fourth and fifth fingers	Fingers	Ulnar deviation wrist Thumb extension and adduction Finger extension

frequent episodes or constant scapular pain. If the disk protrudes posterolaterally resulting in impingement on a cervical nerve root, radicular pain can occur. Radicular pain (radiculopathy) refers to pain felt distal to the site of nerve root impingement, generally in a dermatomal fashion. The pain is often worse at night, and it is associated with a sensation of "pins and needles." Site-specific muscle weakness is also common, and it can result in muscle atrophy after a relatively short period of continuous impingement. The most common cluster of symptoms involves disease at the C7 level (see Fig. 48–1). Ultimately, as the disease progresses, especially in elderly patients, compression on the spinal cord can result from disk protrusion into the posterior longitudinal ligament, causing constant pain from the occipital area to the scapula, bilateral paresthesias, weakness, and eventually paralysis.

Degenerative disease of the cervical spine also occurs in patients with rheumatic diseases. *Rheumatoid arthritis* can affect the apophyseal joints and the synovium, as well as the soft tissues surrounding these joints. Unlike osteoarthritic degeneration, parts of the upper cervical spine area are more commonly affected than lower cervical areas. Intervertebral disks may become involved when granula-

tion tissue forms on the vertebral bodies, causing compression of the disk. Clinical symptoms are similar for patients with rheumatic cervical disease and osteoarthritis of the cervical spine with regard to pain, neck stiffness, radiculopathy, and neurologic signs. Symptoms are rarely caused by osteophyte formation, a radiographic finding that often distinguishes the two disease processes. It is important to consider *ankylosing spondylosis* in young patients (25–40 years) who present with painless "neck and back stiffness" or a gradual onset of marked limited range of motion. Clinical suspicion should prompt radiographic examination of the neck as well as testing for HLA-B27 antibody, which is present in 95 per cent of patients. Ankylosing spondylosis as a cause of neck pain and/or stiffness should be considered in patients with chronic iritis, uveitis, or inflammatory bowel disease. Incidental radiographic findings of sacroiliac erosion or "squaring off" of lumbar vertebrae should also prompt clinical suspicion.

Common secondary problems with rheumatic causes of cervical degeneration include atlantoaxial subluxation and mental status changes associated with vertebrobasilar artery compression; in advanced stages of apophyseal erosion the odontoid may migrate through the foramen magnum, producing basilar invagination symptoms. Effective management begins with early recognition of symptoms associated with radiographic evidence of early bony atrophy, apophyseal joint erosions, and narrowed upper cervical disks.

A less common but related cause of neck pain is a mass effect on localized cervical soft tissues that can produce various symptoms. Typically, these patients have a known history of degenerative cervical disease. Isolated neck pain, pain with central neurologic symptoms, and post-traumatic injury can become worse, owing to mass effect. Neurologic symptoms can also result from compression of vascular or neurologic structures by the mass effect of soft tissue or bony external compression. The most common is *vertebrobasilar insufficiency*, manifesting as paroxysmal symptoms of pain, or central neurologic symptoms occurring with head movement. Most patients are elderly, with degenerative changes near the apophyseal joints resulting in encroachment on the vertebral artery. In addition to external compression, the vertebral artery itself may have evidence of arteriosclerosis or aneurysm that may complicate external compressive defects. Similar central nervous symptoms may be present in younger as well as elderly patients following traumatic neck injuries. Compression at the suboccipital triangle as a result of cervical instability, bony external compression, or localized muscle spasm causes similar central nervous symptoms and requires urgent attention. Treatment may include thrombolytic agents if thrombosis is present, in addition to cervical traction, pain relief, and/or vasodilator therapy.

Pain and peripheral neurologic defects are also commonly seen in patients with *cervical* or *thoracic outlet compressive conditions*. Patients generally are athletic or have strenuous occupational demands. Pain radiating from the lower portion of the neck to the arm and hand, usually increasing with activity and often associated with dermatomal sensory changes or paresthesias in the ulnar distribution, is the most frequent presenting complaint. Compression can be the result of anatomic causes, such as a cervical rib, or pathophysiologic causes, such as a blood clot or localized inflammation creating a transient external compression. On examination, the pain increases with the arm flexed overhead, resulting in lost pulses at the wrist (positive Addison sign), indicating a vascular compression most commonly due to a congenital cervical rib. Sensory changes observed in this position may also be due to a hypertrophied anterior scalene muscle compressing a portion of the trunk of the brachial plexus. Thrombotic compression can result in pain,

weakness, paresthesias, and sensory loss. Treatment is directed at the specific cause of compression. Surgery may be required to locally decompress the point of compression due to anatomic causes. Thrombolytic agents are used if arteriogram-documented thrombotic obstruction is present.

Other causes of neck pain may be the result of irritation, injury, or *disease outside the neck*. Visceral structures having cervical nerve root innervation cause referred pain to the neck. Patients may or may not have symptoms outside the neck to indicate the origin of the problem. Pain may be described as burning, irritating, or stabbing and may be associated with nausea and vomiting. On examination, if the source of pain is outside the neck, there is no site in the neck with localized tenderness or spasm. An *infectious* cause of neck pain may be the result of bony infection (Pott's disease, osteomyelitis), or soft tissue infection. Neck pain due to meningitis should be suspected in all ill-appearing patients with fever and neck pain that worsens with flexion of the spine. *Primary* and *metastatic tumors in the neck* cause pain and symptoms by either mass effect or tissue erosion. Bony tumors are extremely painful, and pain is not often relieved with rest.

An idiopathic yet very frequent cause of neck pain is trigger point tenderness associated with *fibromyalgia*. Patients with this common syndrome present with various symptoms including chronic pain; fatigue; unexplainable, atypical neurologic symptoms (frequently numbness and tingling in a nonspecific anatomic pattern); multiple "allergies" or hypersensitivities; mitral valve prolapse; irritable bowel syndrome; dysmenorrhea in females, or prostadynia in males; and affective disorders. A family history of similar or "undiagnosed" chronic problems is usually revealed. Neck pain in these patients is related to specific trigger point or localized sites of muscle spasm and tenderness with direct palpation. Patients often complain of neck site–specific morning stiffness, loss of range of motion, "knots" in the neck, and increased nonlocalizing pain that can be precipitated by a variety of external factors including poor posture, increased activity, loss of sleep, weather changes, and increased mental or emotional stress. The pain may be anywhere; however, the American College of Rheumatology has identified 18 common trigger point sites, including three bilateral areas in the posterior neck at the suboccipital muscle insertion site, the anterior aspect of intertransverse spaces at C5–C7, and the midpoint of the upper trapezius border. Pain in at least 11 of the 18 trigger point sites as well as a history of widespread chronic (more than 3 months) pain in the axial skeleton and all four body quadrants is diagnostic. Neurologic symptoms or findings on physical examination are rare. Although fibromyalgia is a common problem, it is a diagnosis of exclusion, and other causes of neck pain should be prudently ruled out, usually by repeated thorough body examination and baseline laboratory tests (CBC, routine chemistries, thyroid function screen, and plain film neck radiographs).

Treatment of fibromyalgia includes educating the patient regarding the frustrating and fluctuating nature of the clusters of seemingly unrelated symptoms. Therapy is directed at minimizing emotional stress through diet, regular exercise and sleep habits, and stress management techniques, such as progressive muscle relaxation. Many patients' symptoms are relieved with massage. Because etiologic theory indicates that these patients have low levels of serotonin, the serotonin reuptake inhibitors fluoxetine (Prozac), sertraline (Zoloft), and venlafaxine (Effexor) have been found to be beneficial. Bedtime doses of amitriptyline (Elavil) and cyclobenzaprine (Flexeril) have also been helpful. During acute periods of trigger point pain, injection with localized anesthetic, alone or in combination with corticosteroids, may temporarily relieve symptoms. It is questionable whether the medication is the actual therapeutic agent, because some patients report similar trigger point pain reduction with localized acupuncture. Fibromyalgia is a chronic problem for patients and their primary care providers. Early identification of the pattern of symptoms; a directed, prudent work-up; and regular follow-up improve the patient's medical management and quality of life.

Although most tend to think of congenital causes as disease first occurring in children, it is important to remember that several congenital causes of neck pain initially manifest in adult life. Conditions vary from an uncomplicated asymptomatic fusion of two vertebrae (usually found incidentally) to a more complicated cluster of problems involving other body systems. For example, the incidence of congenital heart trouble in persons with congenital cervical spine problems is higher than in the general population. Presenting complaints and symptoms are diverse and variable. Congenital defects may be asymptomatic until the fourth or fifth decade, and they may become evident only following the onset of symptoms associated with cervical osteoarthritis, rheumatoid arthritis, or trauma. Important points in the history include unexplainable, intermittent, debilitating neck stiffness; recurrent pain in the occipital area; headaches and neck pain associated with true vertigo; or ataxia.

The most common anomaly is *basilar impression (invagination)* affecting the atlanto-occipital region

that results in an upward bulging of the margins of the foramen magnum with subsequent decrease in the volume of the posterior cranial fossa. There may or may not be an associated fusion of the anterior arch of the atlas to the skull, *occipitalization of the atlas,* the second most common congenital defect of the cervical spine.

The third most common anomaly, *Klippel-Feil syndrome,* or congenital vertebral fusion, is possible at all levels of the cervical spine and usually presents as a painless loss of cervical range of motion; however, the majority of diagnoses are by an incidental finding on radiographs.

Other less common but clinically significant congenital anomalies include cervical spinal stenosis, os odontoid, and cervical ribs. All are almost always present without symptoms and are found incidentally during the evaluation of an acute or chronic neck pain or an upper extremity problem. These anomalies are clinically important because congenital malformations commonly lead to significant degenerative changes early in life. Neurologic symptoms associated purely with congenital anomalies are rare; however, basilar invagination and occipitalization of the atlas can occur with neurologic symptoms, in particular, *Arnold-Chiari (A-C) syndrome.* This syndrome refers to the prolapse of central nervous structures, usually the cerebellar tonsils caudally through the foramen magnum. The childhood form of A-C syndrome, because of a common association with hydrocephalus, is more severe than the adult form. Symptoms are variable, often mimicking those associated with cervical osteoarthritis or multiple sclerosis. These include neck pain, headaches as a result of obstructed flow of cerebrospinal fluid (CSF); limb paresthesias, weakness, and muscle atrophy. Symptoms of vertigo or ataxia may also be present. The diagnosis is often made clinically and may be confirmed by MRI abnormalities in the craniocervical border area. Patients with no neurologic symptoms can be managed conservatively with pain control modalities and medications. Exercises may be used to improve range of motion. Patients with increasing pain or onset of neurologic symptoms require neurosurgical consultation.

Another common cause of neck pain is injury due to *trauma.* The effects of traumatic injury to the neck can range from minor to catastrophic. The vast majority of pain associated with neck injury responds to conservative therapy within 1 month of onset. Because of the potentially debilitating injuries that can mimic minor injuries, neck pain due to trauma deserves very close attention in obtaining an accurate diagnosis. As for the majority of pathophysiologic causes of neck pain, consideration should be given to the potential for spinal cord compression; sympathetic nervous system compression or traction; nerve root compression; vascular insufficiency; and superimposed diseases present at the time of injury, such as degenerative changes, infection, or malignancy worsening the condition. The work-up begins with the patient's recall of the events causing the injury.

Jeffreys (1980) groups mechanisms for neck injury into three major categories based on mechanisms of injury: the acceleration extension sprain (whiplash mechanism); the acceleration flexion sprain (head-on collisions); and the lateral flexion with rotation sprains (side impact, landing on shoulder/neck, and so forth). The mechanism classes are then subdivided based upon the level of inherent spinal disease and age (adult or child). Important points in the history include the presence of other severe injuries; altered mental status, especially loss of consciousness; immediate pain radiating to the back, shoulders, or extremities; upper extremity paresthesias; and continued neck pain present for 6 months following the initial injury. The examination should focus on palpating the entire cervical vertebral area, noting areas of tenderness and severity of tenderness and muscle spasm. An ominous physical sign is visible soft tissue swelling or bruising shortly after an injury. If the patient is not immobilized, postural changes in the neck and back should be noted. A focused neurologic examination done initially and repeated regularly is essential. In patients who present immobilized, with localized neck tenderness, swelling, or spasm, radiographs should be completed immediately to assist in ruling out vertebral fractures, cervical instability or spinal canal narrowing, or compression. The use of radiographic studies in nonimmobilized, post-traumatic patients is prudent but not necessary in all cases. Because of the potential for serious injuries to be missed, it is better to be conservative when considering patients for radiographs. All patients with a known history of degenerative cervical disease should have radiographs, especially flexion/extension views, because of the increased potential for cervical instability occurring after trauma.

The most common cause of neck pain following trauma is an uncomplicated ligamentous neck sprain. Injury to tendons, ligaments, muscles, and multiple joints of the spine can occur by the mechanisms described earlier. Patients may often present days after an acute episode of trauma, with daily worsening of neck pain, occipital headache, poor range of motion, upper extremity pain, and transient paresthesias. Findings on examination may in-clude localized tenderness and muscle spasms. Tenderness may be found along the midline if the ligaments or bursae joining the spinous processes were involved. Following traumatic injury, most patients have tender points lateral to the midline within the bulk of the trapezius muscle or deeper. Active and passive movement of the neck through full range of motion usually helps in locating the areas of injury. Patients may have reproducible occipital headache symptoms with direct palpation on the atlanto-occipital border. The presence of reproducible paresthesias into the occipital area indicates localized swelling caused by intrinsic muscle injury, locally compressing the superficial occipital sensory nerves. Anterior post-traumatic neck pain is localized to tenderness and spasm over the sternocleidomastoid muscles following acceleration extension injuries. Other soft tissues in the neck must also be considered to be damaged, including major blood vessels, hyoid bone, trachea, and esophagus. These structures generally require considerable trauma to be damaged and are rarely harmed in routine injuries.

DISCUSSION

Numerous important points are illustrated in the history and examination of the patient presented. Her initial complaint was, "The back of my neck hurts on the left side"—rather than seeking medical attention after an isolated pain-causing event—was indicative of a chronic process. Her age at presentation indicates that she is more likely to have early symptoms of arthritic changes, or disk disease. Patients in this age group are less likely than elderly ones to present with cervical osteodegenerative disease and are also less likely to have the first onset of neck pain associated with fibromyalgia after age 30 years.

The location and description of the pain were fairly nonspecific but did rule out other anatomic processes involving the anterior portion of the neck. This woman had no history of anterior neck pain and had no anterior adenopathy or thyroid masses or enlargement. She did not experience tenderness over the sternocleidomastoid muscle or trachea. Referred pain to the neck from a disease process in the chest almost always involves nonspecific pain in the anterior, rather than posterior, neck. The nonspecific location of neck tenderness over the trapezius muscle, without a specific trigger point site, also helps eliminate fibromyalgia as a potential source of pain. A muscle strain of the deeper muscles in closer proximity to the spine cannot be ruled out, however. The subjective description of the pain as "dull and constant" is somewhat helpful.

Emotional factors caused by increased job stresses certainly may have played a role in the exacerbation of neck pain. A history of depression and the chronic posture associated with depression (contemplative posture) also can contribute to the overall pain and degenerative process. The increased amount of postural stress, brought on by a coupling of increased anxiety (tight muscles) with increased head flexion may have contributed to the increased subjective symptoms of neck pain and stiffness. In addition, if cervical spine disease was already present, the psychological and position stress may have aggravated a previous condition.

"Dull," "deep," or "constant" usually describes bone, disk, or ligamentous pain, whereas muscle pain is frequently described as "cramping" and "stiff." In contrast, pain associated with fractures is described as "sharp," "severe," and often "intolerable." The fact that the pain increased with movement is of little help; most neck pain worsens with movement and improves with rest. Any pain that does not improve with rest or is worse at night indicates a neoplastic process such as metastatic disease or a primary bone disease such as Paget's disease or osteoid osteoma. Cervical osteomyelitis or cervical Pott's disease also is associated with increased pain at rest. The patient's pain seemed to improve with rest, which made a neoplastic growth less likely.

Significant findings on the physical examination, including pain with flexion and rotation as well as neurologic findings involving the left arm, indicate a disease process causing impingement or compression of the nerve root, specifically C7 (see Fig. 48–1). The early onset of degenerative changes producing neurologic findings is not common: It is important to rule out other causes of early degenerative disk disease. The fact that there had been no traumatic onset of symptoms lessens the likelihood of cervical instability as a cause. Likewise, there was no obvious congenital anomaly seen on initial radiographs that would have contributed to an early degenerative process. The patient had no other rheumatologic symptoms, and laboratory test results were all negative for rheumatic causes for degeneration. Her family history of osteoarthritis as well as a previous back surgery for a herniated lumbar disk indicates a predisposition toward degenerative changes, especially degenerative disk disease, as being a primary cause of her neck pain and symptoms. Her occupation as a courtroom recorder requires a great deal of concentration and requires her to sit for prolonged periods with the neck flexed, predis-

posing her to an increased risk of early bony and disk degenerative changes. In a 45-year-old female without rheumatic disease, the most likely cause of neck pain with neurologic symptoms is degenerative disk disease, with compression of the nerve root caused by a herniated disk. The reason for the early onset of significant disease is unknown; however, her familial and occupational predisposition appears to be the only identifiable cause.

Management of degenerative disk problems should begin early in order to prevent future problems. Torticollis in young patients should raise suspicion for future degenerative neck problems. They should be advised on proper posture and ideal work ergonomics, limiting long periods of excessive neck flexion and extension. They should avoid sleeping on multiple pillows and in the prone position. Although no direct evidence has linked regular exercise with decreased incidence of degenerative disease, regular neck strengthening and flexibility exercises should be encouraged. In symptomatic patients, early pain control combined with appropriate rehabilitation is crucial to regain normal function and return to normal activities. In the initial phase of neck pain, patients should be advised to rest and avoid potentially aggravating activities, use NSAIDs, and apply ice to painful areas. Muscle relaxers and narcotics are used, with variable results, for pain management. Cervical collars may alleviate pain from muscle spasm by actively resting the supporting vertebral musculature following an acute episode of pain. Patients should be encouraged, however, to perform range-of-motion exercises as soon as possible following the acute onset of pain. Other methods for control of acute or chronic localized neck pain include vapocoolant spray application to the tender site, followed by stretching (spray and stretch) and localized injections of topical anesthetics alone or in combination with corticosteroids. Manipulation therapy, in the capable hands of an expert in cervical spine manipulation, is an acceptable form of pain management and can more rapidly improve range of motion following an acutely displaced disk. Persons with chronic neck pain benefit from localized heat application before activities followed by ice afterward. These persons should strongly consider lifestyle or activity modifications to avoid activities that provoke recurrent pain.

Patients with radicular symptoms are a diagnostic and management puzzle. The majority of patients respond to conservative pain control and return to normal range of motion and activities. In addition to the above-named modalities, these patients may respond to cervical traction, which serves to relocate the displaced disk and reduce muscle spasm. A short, tapering dosage of corticosteroids may also benefit the patient with radicular symptoms.

The majority of patients with intervertebral disk disease without significant neurologic findings can be adequately managed without surgery. Neurosurgical or orthopedic consultation should be obtained in all patients who have documented upper extremity weakness, muscle atrophy, and sensory loss, as well as in patients with unrelenting pain who respond poorly to conservative therapy.

SUGGESTED READING

Aptaker, RL. Neck pain. Part 1: Narrowing the differential. Physical and Sports Med 1996;24(10):37–46.

Aptaker, RL. Neck pain. Part 2: Optimizing treatment and rehabilitation. Physical and Sports Med 1996;24(11):54–61.

Bland JH. Congenital anomalies. Differential diagnosis and specific treatment. In Bland JH (ed). Disorders of the Cervical Spine: Diagnosis and Medical Management, 2nd ed. Philadelphia, W.B. Saunders, 1994.

Clauw DJ. Fibromyalgia: More than just a musculoskeletal disease. Am Fam Physician 1995;52(3):843–851.

Connolly JF, Jardan OM. Orthopedics. In Rakel RE (ed). Textbook of Family Practice, 4th ed. Philadelphia, W.B. Saunders, 1990.

Jeffreys E. Soft tissue injuries of the cervical spine. In Jeffreys E (ed). Disorders of the Cervical Spine. London, Butterworth, 1980.

Sheon RP. Soft tissue cervical spine syndromes. In Bland JH (ed). Disorders of the Cervical Spine: Diagnosis and Medical Management, 2nd ed. Philadelphia, W.B. Saunders, 1994.

Watkins RG. Cervical spine injuries. In Watkins RG (ed). The Spine in Sports. St. Louis, Mosby–Year Book, 1996.

QUESTIONS

1. Which of the following is true?
   a. Less than 20 per cent of individuals have neck pain in their lifetime.
   b. Radiographic studies are required in all patients who present with neck pain.
   c. 70 per cent of persons with neck pain have a complete resolution of symptoms in less than 1 month.

2. All of the following are true regarding fibromyalgia *except*
   a. It is a common cause of neck pain.
   b. It is often associated with multiple allergies.
   c. Morning stiffness and "knots" in the neck are a common complaint.
   d. No other testing is necessary when fibromyalgia is clinically suspected.

3. All of the following indicate possible involvement of the C7 nerve root *except*
   a. Pain radiating from the neck to below the elbow
   b. Loss of the triceps reflex
   c. Loss of the biceps reflex
   d. Sensory loss involving the dorsal hand

Answers appear on **page 606**.

Chapter 49

Shoulder Pain in a Recreational Athlete

James E. Dunlap, M.D.

SUBJECTIVE

A 30-year-old female presents with a 1-month history of right shoulder pain. She is an avid recreational athlete who enjoys tennis three to four times per week and swims 1 mile per day. She has pain lifting her arm and occasionally feels "pins and needles" going down her arm when she serves or hits hard forehands. This pain also radiates into her neck. She had to quit swimming because her arm "goes dead" after about 200 yards. The shoulder pain awakens her at night when she lies on it. She has tried ice and ibuprofen once in a while but found them not helpful. She denies a history of early morning stiffness, other joint problems, and previous neck problems. Her past medical history is significant for a previous right shoulder dislocation a few years ago that she was able to put back in place on her own and that has not given her any further trouble. She also had "tennis elbow" recently.

Her current medications include an oral contraceptive.

A review of systems is remarkable only for mitral valve prolapse, which has been asymptomatic. An echocardiogram showed no significant regurgitation or abnormalities of the aorta.

OBJECTIVE

She is 5 feet 11 inches tall and weighs 140 lb. Her other vital signs are normal. Inspection reveals a slightly drooped right shoulder but no significant muscle atrophy. Shoulder and neck range of motion were full, but pain was felt at 90 degrees of passive forward flexion and abduction. She was tender to palpation 1 to 2 inches lateral and slightly inferior to the coracoid process. She was tender over the trapezius, the levator scapulae, the midsubstance of the deltoid, and the posterior aspect of the shoulder.

Assessment of strength revealed 5/5 resisted shoulder abduction, extension, and internal rotation; 3 to 4/5 resisted external rotation because of pain; 3/5 resisted shoulder flexion with the arm at 90 degrees of flexion and 45 degrees of horizontal abduction with the thumbs facing down (empty can test) because of pain and weakness.

On neurologic examination she had mildly diminished sensation over her biceps and forearm down to the wrist. Biceps, triceps, and brachioradialis reflexes were equal bilaterally. She had pain with the apprehension test (the shoulder is placed at 90 degrees' abduction with the elbow bent at 90 degrees and forced into external rotation—the position of a pitcher's arm before release of the ball). This pain diminished when a hand was placed over the anterior shoulder during the same maneuver (relocation test). She also had the impingement sign—the shoulder is at 90 degrees' abduction and internally rotated with the elbow flexed at 90 degrees (like a chicken wing). She had a positive sulcus sign (a dimple develops above the deltoid with downward traction of the humerus). She also had increased anteroposterior translation of the humeral head on the right compared with the left side. Adson maneuver (Fig. 49–1), the drop arm test (inability to hold an abducted arm up against mild resistance—supraspinatus tear), and Spurling maneuver results were negative.

DIFFERENTIAL DIAGNOSIS

Thoracic outlet syndrome

Cervical spine pathology

Biceps tendinitis

Rotator cuff tendinitis

Bursitis

Multidirectional instability

Shoulder subluxation

Thoracic Outlet Syndrome

In a patient who presents with vague shoulder pain, "a dead arm" sensation, and "pins and needles" type of pain, thoracic outlet syndrome and cervical spine pathology must be considered. Thoracic outlet syndrome is a catch-all term to describe neurovascular compression within the thoracic outlet where the subclavian vessels and brachial plexus pass through the scalene triangle over the first cervical rib and into the axilla. Frequently, the pain is difficult to reproduce and poorly localizable. In our

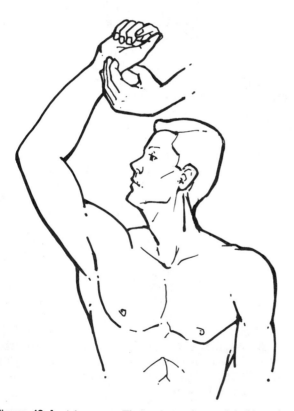

Figure 49–1. Adson test. The patient takes and holds a deep breath, the arm is adducted, the neck is extended, and the chin is turned to the side being tested. (From Bennett JB, Mehlhoff TL: Thoracic outlet syndrome. In DeLee JC, Drez D Jr [eds]: Orthopaedic Sports Medicine: Principles and Practice, volume 1. Philadelphia, WB Saunders Company, 1994.)

case, the plethora of physical findings around the shoulder joint and a negative Adson test result (no pulse diminution with the arm abducted, extended, and externally rotated behind her) safely excluded this diagnosis.

Cervical Spine Pathology

The history may also suggest cervical spine pathology, especially with a neurologic examination that shows diminished sensation over the biceps and lateral forearm and pain in the trapezius and levator scapulae. The patient does not describe any neck trauma or a past medical history of neck pain, however, and there are enough other physical findings to lead in a different direction.

Tendinitis, Bursitis

Rotator cuff and biceps tendinitis appear to be the most likely diagnoses given a positive empty can test result, painful external rotation, positive impingement sign, and tenderness over areas of the anterior and posterior shoulder. If she had felt tenderness just beneath the lateral tip of the acromion and had few other physical findings, subacromial bursitis may have been the diagnosis. Usually tendinitis and bursitis overlap, and the treatments are similar. Occasionally, the impingement test, in which a local anesthetic is injected into the subacromial space, is performed when the diagnosis is difficult to make (Fig. 49–2). Patients with supraspinatus and biceps long head tendinitis and bursitis experience relief. If our patient had been given the appropriate treatment for tendinitis (ice, NSAIDs, modified activity), the pain probably is reduced for a while.

Multidirectional Instability

Unfortunately, other clues from the physical examination suggest that the patient will have continued pain unless other symptoms are addressed. Positive apprehension and relocation test results indicate anterior shoulder subluxation and dislocation. With a sulcus sign that suggests inferior laxity and instability and increased anteroposterior (AP) translation of the humeral head, a diagnosis of multidirectional instability was made. A comparison between the shoulders should be made because overhead athletes (e.g., in swimming, baseball, tennis, and volleyball) frequently have shoulder laxity without instability. The search for pathologic etiologies of

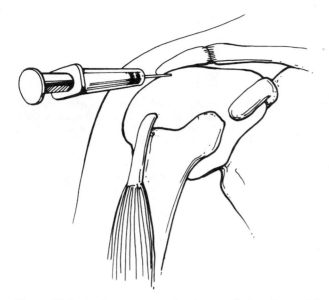

Figure 49–2. Impingement test showing needle in subacromial region. (From Hawkins RJ, Mohtadi N: Rotator cuff problems in athletes. In DeLee JC, Drez D Jr [eds]: Orthopaedic Sports Medicine: Principles and Practice, volume 1. Philadelphia, WB Saunders, 1994.)

multidirectional instability such as connective tissue diseases and Marfan syndrome should also be conducted.

Shoulder Subluxation

To distinguish between subluxation and dislocation, the current history and the past episode of the shoulder coming out and relocating must be reviewed. In the patient's case, the shoulder spontaneously came out without trauma and she returned to her activities within a week. Usually, a first-time dislocation occurs because of trauma. The pain and inflammation take a few weeks to subside before the patient can return to play or work, but 90 per cent of these individuals, if younger than 30 years, have redislocations despite immobilization and physical therapy. In first-time shoulder dislocations in young, active individuals, the standard of care is now surgical stabilization.

After obtaining plain radiographs of the shoulder to exclude any other shoulder pathology, a diagnosis of multidirectional instability with recurrent anterior subluxation leading to biceps and rotator cuff tendinitis was made. The patient was given a modified exercise prescription, a 2-week course of an anti-inflammatory drug, a twice-weekly physical therapy prescription for 3 weeks, and instructions

to follow-up in 3 weeks. After several more weeks of home exercises and progressive return to activity, she did quite well.

DISCUSSION

Recurrent subluxation and multidirectional instability represent diagnoses that are not frequently observed in the general population. Nevertheless, these two problems can be used to demonstrate the need for a comprehensive understanding of shoulder anatomy and biomechanics and physical examination techniques. The shoulder joint actually has four articulations: the glenohumeral, acromioclavicular, sternoclavicular, and scapulothoracic joints. The glenohumeral joint is said to be a ball and socket joint but really is more of a glide and roll joint (like a bowling ball skidding down an alley before it begins to roll). Static and dynamic stabilizers help to checkrein the glide mechanism, allowing the head to roll efficiently. Glide (i.e., translation) is an ineffective means for force generation, and, in excess, it leads to injury.

Of the static constraints, the inferior glenohumeral ligament (a conspicuous thickening of the glenohumeral capsule) is the most important stabilizer, especially with the arm in the throwing position (Fig. 49–3). The dynamic stabilizers include the large shoulder girdle muscles (e.g., trapezius, deltoid, latissimus dorsi, serratus anterior, rhomboids) and the biceps and rotator cuff. With capsular laxity or loss of protection of the inferior glenohumeral ligament (IGHL), there is too much translation. The rotator cuff muscles and the long head of the biceps compensate but eventually fail with repetitive overload. Tendinitis occurs. If the instability is particularly severe, the humeral head can shear off a piece of the bony glenoid or the cartilaginous glenoid labrum. Occasionally, the tendon insertions of the biceps and supraspinatus into the glenoid labrum may tear, necessitating surgical repair.

Radiographs should be obtained in anyone who has a history of shoulder dislocation or subluxation. Radiographs should always include an AP view parallel to the plane of the glenohumeral joint, a transscapular Y lateral view, and the axillary view. The latter is valuable for assessing the position of the humeral head relative to the glenoid and reveals humeral head impression fractures. The AP view can be performed with internal and external rotation to search for a fracture of the glenoid, humeral head, or greater tuberosity. The AP view also demonstrates signs of arthritis-like sclerosis, cystic

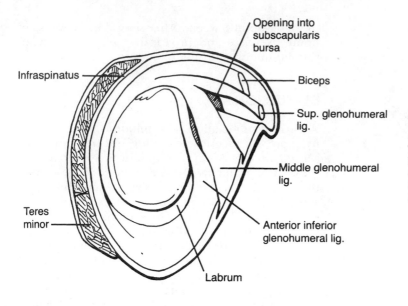

Figure 49–3. The static stabilizers of the ligamentous labral complex as well as the dynamic stabilizers of the rotator cuff are demonstrated. (From Tibone JT, Patek R, Jobe FW, et al. The shoulder: Functional anatomy, biomechanics, and kinesiology. In DeLee JC, Drez D Jr [eds]: Orthopaedic Sports Medicine: Principles and Practice, volume 1. Philadelphia, WB Saunders, 1994.)

changes, and osteophyte formation. The lateral (or outlet) view shows the shape of the acromion and the position of the humeral head. If a large spur is seen or if the acromion is severely hooked, rotator cuff tendinitis and impingement should be considered. The humeral head should sit in the intersection of the arms of the scapular Y. If the position is abnormal, dislocation should be considered.

Once a diagnosis of instability or subluxation has been made, a progressive treatment plan must be implemented. In addition to using ice, nonsteroidal anti-inflammatory drugs (NSAIDs) if needed and stretches to regain full range of motion, the rehabilitation program must include exercises to strengthen the scapular rotators. Examples include shoulder shrugs, horizontal adduction maneuvers, pull-downs, chin-ups, and push-ups with the hands close together and apart. Rotator cuff exercises progress through resistances, i.e., various thicknesses of rubber tubing or Theraband to dumbbell exercises or Nautilus or isokinetic (Cybex) machines. Four exercises have been identified through electromyographic data that specifically strengthen the glenohumeral muscles and do not require any expensive equipment to master.

1. Elevation of the arm in the scapular plane with the arm internally rotated and the thumbs down (supraspinatus)

2. Elevation of the arm in the sagittal plane (deltoid)

3. Horizontal adduction from the prone position with the arm externally rotated (deltoid and inferior cuff muscles)

4. The press-up exercise. In a seated position, the hands are placed upon the seat, and the body is lifted from the chair by extending the upper extremities.

If rotator cuff inflammation is present, the first of these exercises should be avoided.

Once strength is normal, return to sport is allowed and progressive advances in distance, intensity, duration, and frequency of the specific sport activities are encouraged.

SUGGESTED READING

DeLee JC, Drez D Jr. Orthopaedic Sports Medicine: Principles and Practice. Philadelphia, W.B. Saunders, 1994.

Hoppenfeld S. Physical Examination of the Spine and Extremities. East Norwalk, CT, Appleton-Century-Crofts, 1976.

Jobe FW, Bradley JP. Rotator cuff injuries in baseball: Prevention and rehabilitation. Sports Med 1988;6:378–387.

Rowe CR. The Shoulder. New York, Churchill Livingstone, 1988, pp 103–155.

Townsend H, Jobe FW, Pink M, Perry J. Electromyographic analysis of glenohumeral muscles during a baseball rehabilitation program. Am J Sports Med 1991;19:264–272.

1. True or false: When a diagnosis of multidirectional instability has been made, careful attention should be given to which of the following areas during the physical examination?
   a. Heart examination
   b. Vital signs
   c. Thyroid examination
   d. Musculoskeletal examination
   e. Eye examination

2. An athlete dislocates his shoulder and complains of numbness over the lateral shoulder and inability to abduct the arm. Which nerve has been injured?
   a. Musculocutaneous
   b. Ulnar
   c. Median
   d. Axillary
   e. C6 nerve root

3. True or false. Appropriate initial diagnostic tests for shoulder pain, a dead arm, and weakness include
   a. Cervical spine radiographs
   b. MRI of the shoulder
   c. Electromyography (EMG)
   d. Impingement test
   e. Shoulder radiographs

Answers appear on **page 606.**

Chapter **50**

Elbow Pain

Allan V. Abbott, M.D.

SUBJECTIVE

Patient Identification

John N. is a 48-year-old right-handed white male, who works as a college English professor.

Presenting Problem

John complains of pain in his right elbow for the past month and thinks he has "tennis elbow." He feels no pain most of the time, but the pain is brought on by certain activities. The pain came on gradually, but was especially bad the last few days when he was picking up books and boxes while he was moving his office. He also notices the pain when he grips and carries his briefcase and when he plays tennis. The pain usually resolves completely within seconds or minutes after resting, but it recurs immediately with any heavy use of the right hand.

Past Medical History

John has had an unremarkable medical history with no previous major illness or hospitalizations. He has had a few episodes of minor low back pain for which he has never sought medical attention.

Family History

John is an only child. His mother is living and well and is under treatment for high blood pressure. His father died 2 years ago of a myocardial infarction at the age of 75 years. His father was overweight and sedentary. John has a wife and two children who are in good health.

Health Habits

John prides himself on his good health. He has never smoked and drinks "a glass of wine" occasionally. He follows a low-fat diet and has tried to stay thin. He jogs three mornings each week for about 3 miles and takes long hikes most weekends. He started playing tennis with a friend about 2 months ago. He takes no medications.

OBJECTIVE

Physical Examination

Vital signs include weight 156 lb, height 69 inches, blood pressure 120/70, pulse 60 and regular, temperature 99°F orally.

John is pleasant and well nourished and appears physically fit. As he describes his elbow pain, he cups and holds his right elbow with his left hand. Both upper extremities appear muscular and symmetrical and there is no apparent deformity, swelling, or inflammation of either elbow. Passive and active range of motion of both hands, wrists, elbows, and shoulders is normal. Mild tenderness to palpation occurs over and immediately distal to the lateral epicondyle of the right elbow. Otherwise, there is no other palpable warmth, tenderness, or deformity.

John demonstrates that it hurts his elbow most when he makes a fist and extends his right wrist. Indeed, extension of his wrist against resistance causes pain near the lateral epicondyle, especially when the forearm is pronated.

Laboratory Tests

Radiographs of the elbow are normal.

ASSESSMENT

Working Diagnosis

The most likely diagnosis is lateral epicondylitis or tennis elbow. The onset and association of the pain with lifting and with playing tennis, as well as the tenderness over the lateral epicondyle, are typical.

Differential Diagnosis

In racquet sports, the differential diagnosis includes lateral and medial epicondylitis, medial collateral injury, bony articular injuries, and ulnar neuropathy (Table 50–1).

Medial epicondylitis, or medial tennis elbow (sometimes also called golfer's elbow), occurs much less often than lateral epicondylitis, but the symptoms are similar. The pain is localized to the medial epicondyle at the site of the flexor pronator tendon origins. Pain results from resisted wrist flexion and pronation. Management is similar to that for lateral epicondylitis. This patient had no medial elbow pain or tenderness.

Medial collateral ligament injury causes medial elbow pain and can overlap with other injuries such as medial epicondylitis. The medial collateral ligament receives valgus stress in tennis serves and overhead strokes. A tennis player may report medial elbow pain during vigorous overhead serves. Tenderness may be elicited over the medial collateral ligament, or instability or pain may be produced when the examiner applies valgus stress to the elbow in 30 degrees of flexion.

TABLE 50–1. Differential Diagnosis of Tennis Elbow

Conditions commonly associated with racquet sports
   Lateral epicondylitis (most common)
   Medial epicondylitis
   Medial collateral ligament injury
   Bony articular injuries
   Ulnar neuropathy
Other conditions
   Trauma
      Radial neck fractures
      Distal humerus fractures
   Neuropathy
      Radial tunnel syndrome
      Entrapment
         Of posterior interosseous nerve
         Of musculocutaneous nerve
         Of median nerve
   Inflammation
      Arthritis
      Synovitis
      Gouty arthritis
      Joint infection
   Referred pain
      Cervical radiculopathy
      Shoulder arthritis
      Carpal tunnel syndrome
      Angina pectoris
   Other
      Tumor
      Bone cyst

Bony articular injuries can result from excessive articular compression during vigorous and repeated use of the elbow in racquet sports. This injury can lead to degenerative changes, osteophytes, and loose body formation, especially in older adults. Poorly localized pain, stiffness, and limitation of motion are the most common findings. This patient had well-localized pain and no limitation of motion, as well as normal radiographs.

Ulnar neuropathy can result from traction or compression of the nerve, direct trauma, and subluxation. Medial elbow joint instability, degenerative arthritis, and soft tissue scarring can lead to ulnar nerve compression. Numbness and tingling in the fourth and fifth fingers are common symptoms and are often associated with medial elbow pain that radiates into the forearm. Careful palpation of the ulnar nerve where it crosses the elbow and observation of the nerve in its groove as the elbow moves through its full range of motion help rule out entrapment. This patient had no neurologic abnormal findings.

The differential diagnosis includes also the following.

Radial tunnel syndrome can closely simulate lateral epicondylitis. The radial nerve becomes compressed in the radial tunnel as it passes laterally around the posterior surface of the humerus and pierces the lateral muscular septum. Pain may be referred to the lateral epicondyle, and paresthesias may occur along the course of the superficial radial nerve. Most commonly, pain is elicited when the forearm is forcefully supinated. A Tinel sign (a distal tingling sensation in an extremity when a nerve is percussed) may be elicited over the radial head, and tenderness may be palpated in the extensor muscles more distally than 1 or 2 cm from the lateral epicondyle (as in lateral epicondylitis). Tenderness over the lateral epicondyle, as in this patient, is not expected.

Entrapment of the posterior interosseous, musculocutaneous, or median nerves can lead to elbow pain. Entrapment of the posterior interosseus nerve by the supinator muscle can cause elbow pain and weakness of extension of the fifth finger, mimicking the radial tunnel syndrome. Musculocutaneous nerve entrapment can result in anterolateral elbow pain and decreased sensation in the anterior (volar) forearm. Compression of the median nerve can produce pain in the volar forearm that is worse with repeated use (pronator syndrome). Pain may be produced by resisting flexion at the third finger proximal interphalangeal joint or by resisting forearm pronation. The patient had none of these findings.

Fractures of the radial neck or distal humerus can be suspected if the patient has had a fall or another acute trauma. The elbow is swollen and movement is painful. The diagnosis is confirmed radiographically.

Inflammation associated with arthritis or synovitis can be suspected in cases of a swollen painful elbow, especially in individuals with inflammation in other joints. Joint infection should be suspected if the joint is swollen, erythematous, or warm or if the patient is febrile.

Referred pain from cervical radiculopathy, shoulder arthritis, carpal tunnel syndrome, or angina pectoris can be ruled out through examination of the neck, shoulder, and wrist, with careful history-taking. When results of the history and physical examination are inconclusive, radiographic examination can rule out rare bone tumors or cysts.

PLAN

Diagnostic

The diagnosis of lateral epicondylitis is based entirely upon the history and physical examination results. Radiographs of the elbow are normal in lateral epicondylitis but should be performed to rule out other causes of pain.

Therapeutic

Treatment of lateral epicondylitis begins with patient education. The patient must avoid or reduce activities that produce extensor stress on the lateral epicondyle. Racquet sports should be avoided initially. Lifting of heavy objects should also be avoided; when lifting is necessary, the weight should be lifted close to the body with the elbow extended and the forearm supinated.

Tennis-elbow bands are helpful for some patients. These bands wrap around the forearm, placing pressure over the epicondyle and forearm and reducing discomfort.

Repeated application of ice several times daily directly to the painful area may provide the most effective local anti-inflammatory treatment. Various other physical therapies including heat, ultrasound, whirlpool, massage, and electrical stimulation may be helpful. Gentle active and passive full range-of-motion exercises are begun with the initial visit, and performing them should be painless.

A nonsteroidal anti-inflammatory drug (NSAID) may be helpful in most cases and may be continued for several weeks. Corticosteroid injections should be reserved only for those patients in whom the pain is disabling, and more conservative treatments are not satisfactory. Injection should be in the most tender area and into the subaponeurotic space with approximately 10 to 30 mg of methylprednisolone and lidocaine. Superficial subcutaneous injection, and injection into the tendon, should be avoided. No more than three injections should be performed within 1 year, and repeat injections should be avoided in athletes who continue to engage in activities that aggravate the condition. Surgery is rarely indicated but may be considered if all else fails under the following conditions: severe pain in the epicondylar area for more than 6 months, or no response to 2 or 3 weeks of immobilization and two injections of steroids.

In more severe cases, a splint can be placed on the wrist with the wrist in mild (20- to 30-degree) extension. Splinting shortens the extensor musculature and reduces the tension on the origin of the extensor brevis muscle at the lateral epicondyle. The splint should be maintained for several days to 2 weeks.

Rehabilitation is essential to avoid recurrences. After the pain has resolved, passive stretching of the extensor forearm muscles should be performed. A strengthening exercise program for the forearm beginning with light (1-lb) weights should progressively prepare the patient for returning to normal activities. After strength and endurance have returned to normal, a regular strengthening regimen should continue to avoid recurrence.

For an athlete or person who must participate in the activity that caused the lateral epicondylitis, a more formal rehabilitation and physical and occupational therapy program may be necessary. A tennis professional may be consulted to correct the backhand technique and to select the correct racquet with larger head size, reduced string tension, and soft or loose grip.

DISCUSSION

Tennis elbow has been used to describe pain at or near the origin of the extensor carpi radialis brevis since 1882. It occurs most commonly in white middle-aged males, and nearly always in the dominant hand (Fig. 50–1). The majority of cases of lateral epicondylitis do not occur as the result of racquet sports, but they result from repetitive movements in certain occupations. Tennis elbow affects about 50 per cent of recreational tennis players and is related

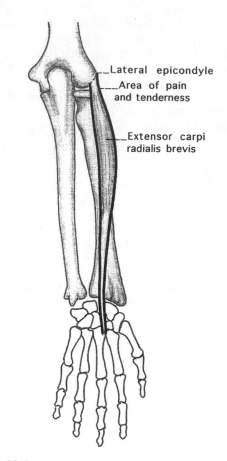

Figure 50–1. Posterior view of the right forearm showing the extensor carpi radialis brevis and the area of pain and tenderness in tennis elbow.

to overuse and poor technique, especially during the backhand stroke.

The exact etiology is unknown, but repeated stress on or near the lateral epicondyle by the action of the wrist extensor muscles, especially the extensor carpi radialis brevis, and the carpi radialis longus, extensor carpi ulnaris, and brachioradialis, results in recurrent microtrauma and inflammation of the periosteum with the formation of granulation tissue and adhesions. Lateral epicondylitis rarely results from direct local trauma or systemic connective tissue disease.

Lateral epicondylitis is a clinical diagnosis and, as in this patient, most patients present with typical signs and symptoms. This patient typically had pain relieved by rest, but he notices pain while gripping objects with the involved hand, especially with the right wrist extended. The pain developed gradually, but it was exacerbated with heavy repetitive use of his hand and arms. Morning stiffness and achiness throughout the day are common symptoms.

On physical examination, tenderness over and just distal to the lateral epicondyle, and pain on extension of the pronated wrist, is usually diagnostic. If the patient with tennis elbow is asked to hold a 5-lb object such as a book in the affected hand with the elbow flexed at 90 degrees, there is usually little pain with the hand supinated but marked pain and associated weakness when the hand is pronated. Grip strength is usually decreased. There is usually no visible swelling. The presence of swelling should alert the examiner to the possibility of another etiology.

PREVENTION

The racquet sports player who fails to follow a comprehensive conditioning program or who uses poor technique is more likely to develop lateral epicondylitis. Strengthening exercises should be done routinely using progressive resistance. Forearm extensor muscle stretching should be done consistently during the playing season and immediately before sports participation. Proper technique and equipment are also important.

SUGGESTED READING

Field LD, Altchek DW. Elbow injuries. Clin Sports Med 1995;14:59–78.

Foley AE. Tennis elbow. Am Fam Physician 1993;48:281–288.

Geoffroy P, Yaffe MJ, Rohan I. Diagnosing and treating lateral epicondylitis. Can Fam Physician 1994;40:73–78.

Noteboom T, Cruver R, Keller J, et al. Tennis elbow: A review. J Orthop Sports Phys Ther 1994;19:357–366.

Roetert EP, Brody H, Dillman CJ, Groppel JL. The biomechanics of tennis elbow. An integrated approach. Clin Sports Med 1995;14:47–57.

QUESTIONS

1. Match each of the following disorders that is included in the differential diagnosis of lateral epicondylitis with the clinical manifestations in items (1) to (4).
   a. Radial tunnel syndrome
   b. Elbow bony articular injury
   c. Medial epicondylitis
   d. Ulnar neuropathy
      (1) Pain with resisted wrist flexion and pronation, and tenderness over the medial epicondyle
      (2) Pain of the lateral elbow with forced supination of the forearm, and tenderness of the extensor muscles 4 to 8 cm distal to the lateral epicondyle
      (3) Numbness of the 4th and 5th fingers and medial elbow pain
      (4) Poorly localized elbow pain, elbow stiffness, and limitation of range of motion

Answers appear on **page 606.**

Chapter 51

Wrist and Hand Pain

Thomas R. Terrell, M.D., M.Phil.

SUBJECTIVE

Chief Complaint

Sue M. is a 53-year-old factory worker who has had right wrist and hand pain for 6 months.

History of Present Illness

Sue's complaints involve numbness of "all her fingers" and pain in her right wrist, which is exacerbated by pinching movements. The pain has been getting worse over the past 5 months and is much worse at night. Occasionally, the pain shoots up into her forearm and hurts at the outside of her right elbow. Her hand often "falls asleep" and this improves by "getting it moving." She also reports mild weakness in pinch grip, but she has not been dropping objects. She is having difficulty performing some tasks at work due to her discomfort. She reports no evidence of blanching or discoloration of the fingertips. There is no history of wrist or hand trauma, shoulder pain, or worsening of symptoms with overhead activities. In addition, she has had some neck pain for 2 months that occasionally radiates into her right shoulder. This pain is not exacerbated by neck positioning, coughing, or sneezing.

Past Medical History

Right tennis elbow 2 years ago resolved with activity modification and counterforce bracing. Sue has no previous neck injury and no history of hospitalizations. She is taking no medications.

I would like to thank Michael Andary, M.D., and Mike Woods, M.D., for their help with this chapter.

Family History

Her mother had mild type II diabetes mellitus.

Social History

She has no detrimental habits. She is married with two children.

Review of Systems

Systems review is essentially negative, with no history of bilateral joint pain, morning stiffness, or rheumatoid arthritis. No history of symptoms of diabetes, anemia, or hypothyroidism is noted. She denies numbness or tingling in the legs, leg weakness, gait disturbance, visual problems, dizziness, or diplopia (symptoms of multiple sclerosis).

OBJECTIVE

Physical Examination

Vital signs are normal. HEENT exam is normal with normal thyroid.

Right Wrist and Hand Examination

The right wrist skin color is normal with no trophic skin changes. No atrophy of the abductor pollicis brevis or thenar eminence muscles is present. No medial or lateral epicondyle tenderness is noted. The right wrist has full range of motion with palmar flexion reproducing some wrist paresthesias. Radial and ulnar pulses are equal. Result of the Allen test, which evaluates collateral blood flow through the ulnar and radial arteries, is normal.

Sensory examination reveals reduced light touch sensation in the right thumb and index, middle, and ring fingers. Two-point discrimination is abnormal in the same distribution. Motor examination reveals muscle bulk (abductor pollicis brevis) and strength equal in both hands and arms. Reflexes were 1+ and equal bilaterally at the biceps, brachioradialis triceps, patellar, and Achilles tendons. Plantar reflexes are flexor.

Provocative testing of resisted wrist extension, which often reproduces lateral epicondyle pain, showed a negative result. Testing of resisted wrist flexion, supination, and pronation were pain-free and of normal strength. The carpal compression test result was negative. It involves placing direct pressure over the carpal canal to elicit pain in the area and reproduce paresthesias in the median nerve sensory distribution to the thumb and index, middle, and radial side of the ring finger. This test did not elicit pain or paresthesias within 5 seconds. Tinel test at the wrist at the carpal canal over the median nerve gave a positive result. Tinel test involves lightly tapping over a nerve with resulting paresthesias or electric shock sensations in a given distribution being indicative of regenerating axons of an injured nerve. In a positive test result over the carpal canal, which may indicate median nerve regeneration, paresthesias radiate along the median nerve sensory distribution. Tinel test result over the ulnar nerve was negative. The result of the Phalen test was positive. Phalen test at the wrist involves bilateral palmar wrist flexion for 1 minute with reproduction of paresthesias in the fingers due to constriction of structures within the carpal tunnel. Resisted middle finger extension test for radial tunnel syndrome is slightly weak and causes vague pain.

Neck Examination

Neck examination shows full range of motion with no palpable tenderness. The result of the Spurling maneuver is normal. In the Spurling maneuver, the patient's neck is extended, rotated toward the involved arm, and compressed. A positive test result reproduces the pain or symptoms, particularly in patients with intervertebral foraminal narrowing, which can produce nerve root compression. If cervical spinal nerves are compressed by cervical disk herniation or facet hypertrophy, for instance, radiating pain from the cervical spine down the shoulder in a dermatomal distribution occurs with the Spurling maneuver. Valsalva maneuver does not reproduce neck pain. Plain radiographs, including ante-roposterior, oblique, and lateral views of the right wrist were normal.

DIAGNOSTIC DECISION MAKING AND INITIAL PLAN

This patient may be diagnosed with mild carpal tunnel syndrome (CTS) with strong clinical certainty. CTS is a clinical diagnosis supported by nerve conduction studies and electromyogram (NCS/EMG). When a diagnosis of CTS is uncertain or when one must exclude or confirm other associated disease or alternative diagnoses, NCS/EMG should be obtained. Because of loss of job function and the possibility of radiculopathy, the decision was made to obtain confirmatory NCS/EMG. NCS/EMG revealed mildly prolonged median sensory and motor latencies across the wrist when compared with the ulnar latencies. Amplitudes were normal. The primary problem was demyelination and not axonal loss. The ulnar nerve study results were normal. EMG results revealed no evidence of abnormal findings in eight muscles studied in the right arm or cervical paraspinals, which would be consistent with cervical radiculopathy or a "double crush" phenomenon (simultaneous compressive injury to the median nerve both distally and proximally in the neck). The normal NCS makes other problems such as radiculopathy much less likely. If the patient prefers nonoperative treatment, there is no permanent nerve damage while pursuing conservative treatment. If the NCS result had been negative, other problems should be seriously considered (e.g., degenerative joint disease or idiopathic arm pain).

Initial Treatment

The treatment of right CTS was initially managed conservatively with a nonsteroidal anti-inflammatory medicine and a right wrist splint to wear at night to hold the wrist in neutral position. The patient's work activities were modified to reduce wrist flexion and repetitive hand motion.

Follow-up Visit

After 2 months of treatment, her symptoms had improved slightly, but she still had night pain in her right wrist and numbness in her fingers, particularly at work. The repeat physical examination was unchanged. Because of her persistent pain with conservative treatment, she was offered an injection or surgery. She chose an injection of lidocaine and a long-acting corticosteroid preparation into the carpal canal, which was performed by a family physician very experienced in this technique. She continued to wear the night splint and take nonsteroidal drugs.

Second Follow-up Visit

Her pain subsided for 2 months following the injection, but then symptoms returned including increasing difficulty performing her job functions. Physical examination was unchanged. She was referred to an orthopedic surgeon for consideration of surgical carpal tunnel release. This procedure involved open division of the transverse carpal ligament and adjacent palmar aponeurosis. After surgery, the patient's symptoms resolved and she enjoyed a full return to work and recreational activities.

ASSESSMENT

Working Diagnosis

The working diagnosis is CTS of the right hand involving an entrapment neuropathy of the median nerve. Entrapment neuropathies may occur from the hand to the shoulder and involve a peripheral nerve being compressed by an anatomic structure such as fibrous tissue (a tendon) or by a bony structure. Nocturnal wrist pain, paresthesias in the fingertips, weakness of hand grip, and a sensation that one must "shake one's hands to relieve numbness" are all classic symptoms of CTS. The positive results to Tinel and Phalen signs and a positive result in NCS support the diagnosis. A number of different causes of CTS that should be considered have been described in the literature (Table 51–1).

Differential Diagnoses

Hand and wrist pain is a frequent presenting complaint with a broad differential diagnosis. The sources of pathology may involve peripheral nerves, muscles and tendons, vascular structures, or bony anatomy of the wrist, hand, and elbow. Other potential diagnoses are as follows.

Cervical Radiculopathy

A history of neck pain with paresthesias raises the question of a cervical radiculopathy, the most com-

TABLE 51–1. Physical Examination for Carpal Tunnel Syndrome

Examine thenar eminence for wasting
Tinel sign—tapping over the carpal tunnel causes pain, numbness, and dysesthesias in a median distribution
Phalen test—flexing the wrist 90 degrees for one minute causes numbness and dysesthesias in a median distribution
Carpal compression test—symptoms are elicited when examiner presses his or her thumbs over the patient's carpal tunnel for 30 seconds
Flick test—when patient is asked "What do you actually do with your hand(s) when symptoms are at their worst?" the patient exhibits a movement similar to shaking down a thermometer

From Katz RT. Carpal tunnel syndrome: A practical review. Am Fam Physician 1994;49:1371–1379.

mon cause of upper extremity pains, weakness, and sensory deficits. Cervical radiculopathy may occur through compression and inflammation of cervical nerve roots at or near the neuroforamen through which they exit the spinal column. This condition may occur as a result of cervical disk herniation and cervical spondylolysis. A C6 to C7 radiculopathy sends sensory symptoms in a dermatomal distribution to the thumb and index and middle finger as well as along the lateral aspect of the forearm, and occasionally along the radial aspect of the dorsum of the hand. This distribution pattern makes differentiation from CTS difficult without NCS and EMG testing. Radiculopathy patients may have exacerbation of radicular-type symptoms with coughing and sneezing and motor weakness or loss of reflexes in the upper extremity. The NCS/EMG result showed no cervical paraspinal muscle involvement, which is invaluable in differentiating cervical radiculopathy from CTS and other causes.

Peripheral Neuropathy

Peripheral neuropathy is a condition in which a peripheral nerve is affected by a systemic disorder such as diabetes mellitus, vitamin B_{12} deficiency, toxin exposure, alcohol abuse, or hypothyroidism. CTS may be an early sign of a diffuse polyneuropathy. A thorough history, physical examination, laboratory work-up, and electrodiagnostic studies may help with diagnosis. In this patient, results of history and physical examination and NCS/EMG studies did not support peripheral neuropathy.

Proximal Median Neuropathy (Pronator Syndrome and Anterior Interosseous Syndrome)

The pronator syndrome occurs when the median nerve is entrapped at the elbow by the pronator teres muscle or other structures. Symptoms and signs include volar forearm pain and numbness in the fingers, a positive Tinel test result in the forearm, negative result on Phalen test, pain during resisted pronation, and pain during resisted isolated flexion of the distal interphalangeal joints (DIP) of the long and ring fingers. Mrs. M. does not possess these typical features, and this is a very uncommon entrapment. Entrapment of the anterior interosseous nerve, a proximal branch of the median nerve 4 cm distal to the elbow, may cause pain in the midforearm with associated weakness in the flexor pollicis longus, flexor digitorum profundus to the index finger, and elbow flexion with no development of paresthesias. The patient did not have findings to support this diagnosis.

Thoracic Outlet Syndrome (TOS)

Compression of the neurovascular structures at the thoracic outlet region as a result of cervical ribs or a narrow interscalene space leads to symptoms very similar to those of CTS. The diagnosis is controversial and difficult to make, and there are many purported and disputed causes. In TOS, the lower portions of the brachial plexus are most likely involved.

Symptoms may include pain, paresthesias along the medial two digits and forearm worsened by activity, weakness in the thenar muscles, easy fatigue of the upper extremity with overhead activity, and skin pallor and coolness in the extremity. Physical examination provocative maneuvers such as Adson and Roos tests may help confirm the diagnosis. Rarely, EMG with NCS may show changes in the muscles innervated by the lower trunk of the brachial plexus.

Brachial Plexus Injury (Neuralgic Amyotrophy)

An injury to upper trunk nerve roots through stretching or some other mechanism leads to paresthesias and rather acute onset of weakness of the upper extremity. Diagnosis is made by documented muscle weakness and neurodiagnostic studies showing brachial plexopathy of upper trunk.

Idiopathic Arm Pain or Repetition Strain Injury (RSI)

Repetitive submaximal loading of the tissues of the lower extremity through occupational or sports activity may lead to arm pain. Some cases of wrist pain with paresthesias fall outside the traditional group of disorders known as *cumulative trauma disorders* (e.g., CTS, tendinitis, arthritis). Some investigators propose that unexplained wrist pain or upper limb regional pain in patients who are involved in repetitive movements may be included under a term such as *idiopathic arm pain*. This syndrome was formerly described as *repetition strain injury*. Once other causes of wrist pain have been ruled out and the cause remains unknown, one may consider calling this unknown diagnosis *idiopathic arm pain*. The condition responds to empiric conservative management that reduces activity. Treatment may include activity reduction, nonsteroidal drugs, and relative immobilization (splinting).

Multiple Sclerosis

The negative review of symptoms in the patient's history, coupled with a normal physical examination, may lower the likelihood. Bilateral symptoms increase the possibility.

Bony Fracture of Forearm, Wrist, or Hand

Fractures of the distal radius, hook of hamate, or scaphoid, and Kienböck disease (avascular necrosis of the carpal lunate bone) are all unlikely in this patient.

Osteoarthritis

Opposed to this diagnosis is the patient's lack of morning stiffness and absence of nodular involvement of the distal interphalangeal joints (Heberden nodes).

Tenosynovitis

De Quervain tenosynovitis and flexor or extensor wrist tendinitis are examples. Tenosynovitis results from overuse or trauma in which the normal motion of the tendon is disrupted by inflammation. De Quervain disease is diagnosed by first dorsal extensor compartment pain of the hand and a positive Finklestein test.

Less Likely Diagnoses

VASCULAR ABNORMALITIES. These include Raynaud phenomenon or an aneurysm of the distal radial and ulnar arteries presenting as a pulsatile mass over the artery.

GANGLION CYST OF THE RADIOCARPAL JOINT. Ganglion cysts are frequently seen as synovial outgrowths in the wrist, most commonly in the scapholunate area or adjacent to a tendon sheath.

RADIAL NERVE ENTRAPMENT. This condition presents as radial tunnel syndrome when nerve entrapment is distal to the elbow. Entrapment of the posterior interosseous branch of the radial nerve occurs with forearm compression. In radial tunnel disease, pain usually localizes at the brachioradialis roughly three fingerbreadths distal to the lateral epicondyle. This diagnosis is unlikely given the case study patient's lack of elbow pain. The resisted middle finger extension test reproduces symptoms of radial tunnel disease.

Posterior interosseous syndrome causes more proximal forearm pain, and patients are unable to extend the digits at the metacarpophalangeal joints.

ULNAR NEUROPATHY. Ulnar nerve entrapment at the wrist at the Guyon canal (ulnar tunnel syndrome) is characterized by intrinsic muscle weakness and decreased light touch sensation and two-point discrimination in the ulnar distribution. Entrapment at the elbow (cubital tunnel syndrome) features medial elbow pain and a positive Tinel sign over the ulnar nerve at the elbow. These symptoms were not present in the patient.

HAND-ARM VIBRATION SYNDROME AND RHEUMATOID ARTHRITIS AND CONNECTIVE TISSUE DISORDERS. These are two additional diagnoses.

DISCUSSION

Mrs. M.'s presentation is typical for CTS, an entrapment neuropathy of the median nerve at the wrist in the carpal tunnel. CTS is two to five times more common in women than in men. Some studies have demonstrated that it occurs most frequently between age 30 and 60 years. Dawson and David (1993) reported an incidence of 125 in 100,000. Other studies have reported that the industrial setting has the highest incidence.

Anatomy

The anatomic orientation of the various structures in the volar aspect of the wrist creates a "canal" or tunnel with clear boundaries. The carpal tunnel is bordered anteriorly by a flexor retinaculum with the transverse carpal ligament representing the roof of this canal. The posterior border of the canal is the carpal bones of the wrist. The median nerve is vulnerable to compression and increased intracompartmental pressure in the tunnel. Many other structures traverse the area: four tendons of the flexor digitorum superficialis, four tendons of the flexor digitorum profundus, and the tendon of the flexor pollicis longus. The muscles that the median nerve innervates, namely the abductor pollicis brevis, the opponens pollicis, and the superior head of the flexor pollicis brevis, may be affected by damage to the nerve.

Pathophysiology

Two theories of the pathophysiology of CTS include first, that it is a nonspecific flexor tenosynovitis caused by elevated intracarpal compartment pressures of 20 to 70 mm Hg above normal (Dawson and David, 1993). The result is ischemia to the nerve. The other theory is that chronic focal compression of the nerve trunk leads to focal demyelination due to mechanical stress. More study is needed to confirm the theories.

Causes

Potential causes of CTS abound in the literature. Any condition that limits the defined space of the carpal tunnel may result in significantly increased intracompartmental pressures and subsequent median nerve ischemia and symptoms. In addition, numerous associated medical conditions are described in the literature (see Table 51–1). Systemic disease frequently coexists with CTS. The relationship between occupational activity and CTS is controversial. CTS is a multifactorial problem. Associations have been found with age, wrist size measurements, body mass index, occupational repetitive activities, thyroid disease, and obesity. Studies have been unable to define what causal role certain occupational exposures may have on developing CTS due to confounding variables (Dawson and David, 1993).

Clinical Signs

A thorough clinical history and physical examination remain the mainstay of the prompt and accurate diagnosis of CTS. Patients frequently present complaining of "tingling" in the hands or wrists or the sensation that "their hands are going asleep." Paresthesias may be seen in other diagnoses, however, and these should be carefully excluded. Thus, the examiner must be diligent about accurately elucidating the anatomic location and any radiation of the paresthesias.

The following historical points typically seen in CTS may aid in further diagnosis:

- Nocturnal pain and awakening with numbness in the fingers
- Paresthesias or hypesthesia in a median nerve distribution (the fingers of the hand, possibly to the thumb, index and middle fingers)
- Pain may radiate into the forearm, shoulder, and neck. It may be present in the shoulder.
- Symptoms may be relieved by use of the hand or wrist ("shaking it out").
- Subjective sense of clumsiness or weakness of the hand
- Bilateral symptoms occur in 50 per cent of patients.
- Dry skin, color changes, or swelling of the hand

Physical Examination

This discussion highlights several of the physical findings, provocative manuevers, and tests that are routinely performed in assessing patients for wrist pain. First, the physical examination may be normal in CTS. Inspection of the hand may reveal thenar atrophy in long-standing cases of median nerve compression, which represents a sign of denervation and advanced disease. The skin over the thumb and index and middle fingers may be dry. Palpation may localize the source of pain to the carpal canal. Sensory testing for light touch and two-point discrimination at the median nerve distribution may give an abnormal result. Motor testing may demonstrate weakness in the thenar muscles, the abductor pollicis brevis, the opponens pollicis, and the superior head of the flexor pollicis brevis.

Standard provocative tests to determine the etiology of hand and wrist pain are not sensitive or specific for CTS. Common tests include Phalen, Tinel, and Durkan carpal compression. Despite the fact that Tinel and Phalen signs are reported to be positive in 45 per cent and 20 per cent of normal patients, respectively, they are clinically useful. (Table 51–2; see Provocative Tests.)

Electrophysiologic Testing for CTS

NCS/EMG testing is clearly the standard test for assessment of CTS and for denervation. A positive NCS test in a patient with suspected CTS is consistent with CTS 95 per cent of the time. In addition, this testing is valuable to rule out other possible causes of wrist and hand pain, and NCS/EMG plays a role in the standard work-up of more chronic symptoms of CTS. If median nerve demyelination has occurred, nerve conduction velocity is slowed, creating prolonged sensory latency.

Radiographic/Laboratory Evaluation

Carpal tunnel views of the wrist are rarely revealing in the absence of trauma. Computer tomography

TABLE 51–2.   Causes of Carpal Tunnel Syndrome

Increased canal volume
Nonspecific synovial proliferation
Rheumatoid tenosynovitis
Edema
Pregnancy
Postinjury
Hypothyroidism
Congestive heart failure
Renal failure
Acromegaly
Aberrant anatomy
Proximal lumbrical insertion
Distal extension of the flexor superficialis muscle
Persistent/thrombosed median artery
Abnormal palmaris longus tendon
Mass lesion
Benign tumor (lipoma, ganglion)
Hematoma
Gouty tophus
Calcium deposits
Amyloid
Malignant tumor
Multiple myeloma
Decreased canal volume
Acute fracture or callus from healing fracture
Arthritis or wrist malalignment
Congenitally small canal
"Sick" nerve with minimal compression (double crush)
Cervical radiculopathy
Thoracic outlet syndrome
Proximal median neuropathy

Adapted from Stevens JC, Beard CM, O'Fallon WM, Kurland LT. Conditions associated with carpal tunnel syndrome. Mayo Clin Proc 1992;67:541–548.

(CT) scans or magnetic resonance imaging (MRI) are reserved for cases in which a mass is suspected. Laboratory work may help confirm systemic causes such as rheumatoid arthritis, hypothyroidism, or diabetes.

Treatment

Carpal tunnel syndrome usually responds well initially to conservative nonsurgical treatment. Occasionally, early surgical referral is indicated. These cases include acute onset of CTS, severe electrodiagnostic abnormality, or progressive motor or severe sensory deficit. Decisions about treatment modalities are made by collaboration between patient and physician. A trial of conservative treatment should be used initially for 2 to 3 weeks. Standard conservative treatment consists of nonsteroidal anti-inflammatory medications such as Naproxen sodium and a wrist splint to hold the wrist in neutral position initially full time at night for 3 to 4 weeks. Patients should limit or modify activities that use the wrist. Administration of vitamin B_6 has had anecdotal success; however, no clinical trial has demonstrated its efficacy. Work station evaluations for ergonomic efficiency may prove beneficial. For 90 per cent of mild CTS cases, conservative treatment works within 3 weeks.

Invasive treatment is pursued if conservative treatment fails to improve quality of life or if there is a progressive motor or sensory deficit, or severe electrodiagnostic abnormality.

Whether surgery is chosen before trying an injection of steroid and local anesthetic is a mutually agreed upon quality-of-life decision made by the patient and physician. Invasive treatment includes an injection of a steroid and local anesthetic into the carpal canal by an experienced clinician. Studies have demonstrated a 60 to 70 per cent response rate to injection and a reasonable long-term cure rate (Katz, 1994). Certain patient groups are poor responders to conservative treatment. These include the following: age over 50 years at time of diagnosis, duration of disease for more than 10 months, and constant paresthesias.

Surgical treatment is considered if nonsurgical therapy fails, particularly if CTS is interfering with work or recreational activities and, consequently, quality of life. Surgery involves releasing by open technique the tense transverse volar carpal ligament that impinges upon the median nerve in the carpal canal. A Mayo Clinic study revealed good to excellent results in 80 per cent of patients who underwent the open procedure. No controlled trial has evaluated newer endoscopic surgical methods for success rates.

SUGGESTED READING

American Academy of Neurology, American Association of Electrodiagnostic Medicine, American Academy of Physical Medicine and Rehabilitation. Practice parameter for electrodiagnostic studies in carpal tunnel syndrome. Neurology 1993; 43:2404–2405.

Broderick J, Smith R, Cahill W, et al. Neurology in family practice. In Rakel RE. Textbook of Family Practice, 5th ed. Philadelphia, W.B. Saunders, 1995, pp 1422–1423.

Dawson DM. Entrapment neuropathies of the upper extremities. N Engl J Med 1993;329:70.

De Smet L, Steenwerckx A, Van Den Bogaert G, et al. Value of clinical provocative tests in carpal tunnel syndrome. Acta Orthop Belgica 1995;61:3.

Jardon OM, Matthews MS. Orthopedics. In Rakel RE. Textbook of Family Practice, 5th ed. Philadelphia, W.B. Saunders, 1995, p 933.

Katz, RT. Carpal tunnel syndrome: A practical review. Am Fam Physician 1994;49(6):1371–1379.

Kulick RG. Carpal tunnel syndrome. Orthop Clin North Am 1996;27:345–354.

QUESTIONS

For the following questions, select all the answers that may be correct.

1. The most common symptom(s) of carpal tunnel syndrome include(s):
   a. Paresthesias in the hand
   b. Night pain in the hand
   c. Sensation of having to shake hands out
   d. Dryness of the skin of the thenar eminence

2. Indications for possible surgical treatment of CTS include the following:

a. One-month history of mild CTS unresponsive to splints, nonsteroidals, and rest
b. Patient with previous history of contralateral CTS who presents with new-onset CTS of the other hand
c. Severe thenar atrophy on examination
d. Mild electrodiagnostic abnormality showing mildly prolonged sensory latency
3. Which of the following studies is routinely helpful in evaluating a patient for CTS?
a. Carpal tunnel radiographic views
b. MRI of the carpal canal
c. Serum rheumatoid factor

d. Tinel sign over the median nerve
4. Conservative nonsurgical treatment for CTS is indicated in which of the following situations?
a. Recent onset of wrist pain and paresthesias in fingers that is worse at night
b. Sudden onset of CTS symptoms following acute traumatic distal radius fracture
c. Duration of symptoms of over 6 months with impact on quality of life
d. Severe electrodiagnostic abnormality on initial NCS/EMG study

Answers appear on **page 606**.

Chapter 52

Lower Back Pain

Walter L. Calmbach, M.D.

INITIAL VISIT—SUBJECTIVE

PATIENT IDENTIFICATION. Tomas is a 42-year-old Hispanic male construction worker who presents with sudden-onset low back pain.

PRESENTING PROBLEMS. Tomas presents with a 2-day history of sharp low back pain.

PRESENT ILLNESS. Tomas is a slightly obese Hispanic male who developed sharp, right-sided low back pain that has worsened over the last 2 days. The pain began immediately after Tomas tried to lift a 50-lb bag of cement. He is experiencing neither paresthesias in his legs nor leg weakness. He has no bowel or bladder incontinence.

PAST MEDICAL HISTORY. Tomas has no previous history of back injury or back surgery and no previous motor vehicle accident (MVA). He has had no previous surgery or hospitalizations and has no allergies. He is taking no medications, except for occasional

acetaminophen (Tylenol) or aspirin for relief of his back pain (Table 52–1).

FAMILY HISTORY. His father is 62 years old and has a history of recent-onset hypertension, for which he takes no medications. His mother is 60 years old and has mild hypertension, type II diabetes mellitus, and a history of cholecystectomy for cholelithiasis "years ago." He has two older brothers and two younger sisters and is unaware of any medical problems they may have.

There is no family history of stroke, myocardial infarction, liver disease, renal disease, tuberculosis or bleeding disorders. The patient is unaware of the cholesterol status of any of his family members.

HEALTH HABITS. Tomas drinks about two beers each night, slightly more on weekends. He has never missed work or had medical problems related to alcohol abuse. He smoked about two packs of cigarettes per day for about 9 years but stopped smoking at age 25 years. He does not use any illicit drugs.

TABLE 52–1. History

Pain characteristics
    Onset
    Duration
    Severity
    Quality
    Radiation
    Aggravating factors
    Alleviating factors
Occupation
Mechanism of injury
Age
Fever
Weight loss
Adenopathy
Steroid use
Previous cancer
Leg weakness
Bowel or bladder incontinence
Menopausal status

SOCIAL HISTORY. Tomas has been married for 22 years and lives in a rented home with his wife and three of their four children.

REVIEW OF SYSTEMS. Tomas' ROS is essentially negative. In particular he has no history of polyuria, polyphagia, or polydipsia; no history of headache or epistaxis, and no urinary frequency or hesitancy.

OBJECTIVE

Physical Examination

Tomas' vital signs are normal: blood pressure is 136/84, pulse 68, respirations 12, temperature 98.6°F. Head is normocephalic, atraumatic. The eyes have extraocular muscles intact; pupils equal, round and reactive to light and accommodation; funduscopic examination showing sharp disk margins with mild "copper-wiring" of arterioles without A-V nicking or retinal hemorrhages or exudates. The ENT examination is normal. Neck examination shows full range of motion without tenderness, full carotid pulses without bruit, nonpalpable thyroid, trachea midline, and no adenopathy. Lungs are clear with normal breath sounds. Heart examination shows normal S^1 and S^2 sounds without murmur, rub, or gallop rhythm; there is no lift or leave, and PMI is not palpable. The abdomen is flat, without scars; bowel sounds are normal. There is no tenderness or guarding, no organomegaly, and no bruits. Liver span is approximately 8 cm (Table 52–2).

Back Examination

With the Patient Standing

The patient's stance shows splinting to the right side. Mild right paravertebral muscle tenderness is present in the lumbar area but there is no midline tenderness. The patient is able to flex the spine to 70 degrees; lateral bending and rotation are limited by pain in the right paravertebral lumbar area. The patient is able to toe-walk (walk on his toes), and heel-walk (walk on his heels), although this increases his right-sided pain (motor function—L4: knee extension; L5: foot dorsiflexion; S1: foot plantar flexion).

With the Patient Seated

With hips and knees flexed at 90 degrees, the knees are gently extended. The patient is able to extend the left knee to zero degrees without difficulty; however, extending the right knee to 20 degrees causes a sharp "electrical" pain to "shoot" from the right lumbar area, through the back of the leg, to the dorsum of the right foot. Sensation to light touch and pinprick is equal bilaterally. Deep tendon reflexes are normal at the knee and ankle, but dorsi-

TABLE 52–2. Physical Examination

Patient standing
    Stance
    Gait
    Tenderness
    Range of motion
    Flexion
    Lateral bending
    Rotation
    Heel-walk
    Toe-walk
    Squat-and-rise
    Romberg
Patient seated
    Distracted straight-leg-raising
    Sensation to light touch
    Resisted hip and knee flexion
    Deep tendon reflexes
        Knee jerk (L4)
        Ankle jerk (S1)
        Clonus
Patient supine
    Repeat straight-leg-raising test
    Cremasteric reflex
Patient prone
    Anal wink
    Anal sphincter tone

TABLE 52–3.   Indications for Plain Radiographs

Trauma
Fever
Anemia
Age > 50
Immunosuppression
 DM, ETOH, steroids, HIV
History of cancer
Pain at rest
Pain at night

DM = diabetes mellitus; ETOH = ethanolism; HIV = human immunodeficiency virus

flexion of the right first toe is slightly weak compared with the left.

With the Patient Supine

With the knee extended, the patient is able to flex the left hip to 80 degrees; he is able to flex the right hip to 45 degrees, which causes paresthesias to "shoot" to the posterior right thigh and the dorsum of the right foot. The cremasteric reflex is intact bilaterally.

With the Patient Prone

Rectal examination shows normal sphincter tone, no masses, normal prostate without tenderness or nodularity, and heme-negative stool.

Laboratory Tests

Lumbosacral radiographs are ordered (five views: anteroposterior [AP], lateral, right and left obliques, and a "spot" or close-up film of the L5-S1 interspace) (Table 52–3). These show normal alignment of the vertebral bodies, no spondylolysis (i.e., the pars interarticularis is intact) and no spondylolisthesis (i.e., the posterior aspect of the vertebral bodies is well aligned and does not encroach upon the spinal canal). The pedicles are intact and show no sign of infectious or metastatic disease. There is no vertebral body collapse or "wedging" of a vertebra; there are small osteophytes at L3, L4, and L5. Slight narrowing of the L5-S1 interspace is seen, compared with other disk spaces, but this may be the result of the relative angle at which this interspace is filmed.

ASSESSMENT

Working Diagnosis

At this point, the most likely diagnosis is lumbar disk herniation impinging on the L5 nerve root. Over time, there is degeneration of the intervertebral disk, leading first to protrusion of the disk into the spinal canal, and sometimes progressing to extrusion and sequestration of disk material. Ninety percent of disk herniations occur at the L4-L5 or L5-S1 interspaces (Figs. 52–1 to 52–3). The patient's description of paresthesias radiating from the back through the posterior thigh and to the dorsum of the foot are consistent with irritation of the L5

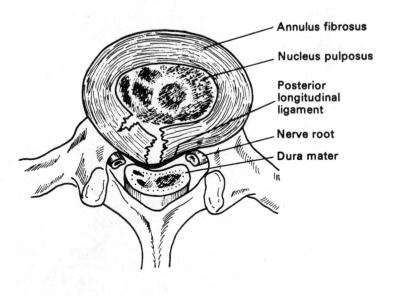

Annulus fibrosus
Nucleus pulposus
Posterior longitudinal ligament
Nerve root
Dura mater

Figure 52–1. The disk structure includes an outer fibrocartilaginous annulus fibrosus and an inner, more fluid nucleus pulposus. Either of these structures may rupture and produce sciatica. (From Cyriax J: Orthopaedic Medicine, vol. 1. London, Cassell Ltd, 1978.)

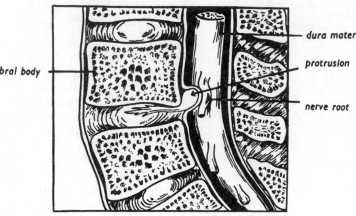

vertebral body

dura mater

protrusion

nerve root

Figure 52–2. Herniation of the nucleus pulposus through the tear in the annulus produces a collar stud abscess type of herniation that does not reduce spontaneously the way a moveable cartilaginous displacement reduces. (From Cyriax J: Orthopaedic Medicine, vol. 1. London, Cassell Ltd, 1978.)

nerve root. Motor function remains intact, which permits an attempt at conservative management.

Although musculoligamentous injury is by far the most common cause of low back pain, disk herniation should also be considered in a poorly fit 42-year-old male whose job includes heavy lifting.

Differential Diagnosis

Muscle Strain, Ligamentous Sprain

Many muscles and ligaments support the spine, and these can be injured through the same mechanism of heavy lifting. These patients also demonstrate splinting to one side and paravertebral muscle tenderness. Paresthesias consistent with dermatomal distribution of lumbar nerves, however, are not found in patients with musculoskeletal strain; motor function and deep tendon reflexes are intact (Table 52–4).

Degenerative Joint Disease (DJD) or Osteoarthritis (OA)

DJD of the lumbar spine is common, especially among older patients, those with a history of back trauma, or those with abnormalities of the spine (e.g., spondylolysis). In these selected cases, plain films of the lumbar spine may be helpful in diagnosing DJD. Degenerative changes in the lumbar spine are equally common among symptomatic and asymptomatic patients, however, and care must be taken to avoid ascribing pain to osteoarthritic changes when the pain may in fact be due to another cause.

Spondylolisthesis

Spondylolisthesis is defined as forward slippage of a vertebral body; it usually occurs in patients over 50 years of age. Hormonal and mechanical factors predispose older women, particularly black women, to this problem. In primary care settings, spondylo-

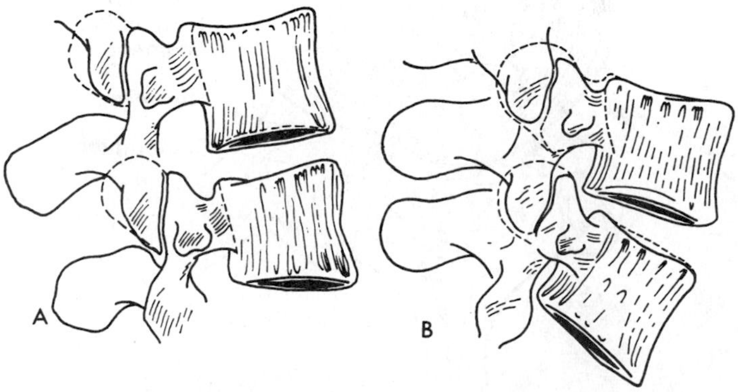

A

B

Figure 52–3. *(A)* Flexion of the lumbar spine produces most disk protrusions and herniations. When the spine is flexed forward in the standing position, the disk space is opened posteriorly and the cartilaginous portion of the annulus is pushed back toward the spinal canal. This may cause the lumbago associated with prolonged standing in this flexed position. *(B)* With the lumbar spine in lordotic position, the disk space closes posteriorly. Treatment for lumbago should be directed, therefore, at increasing lumbar lordosis. (From Cyriax J: Orthopaedic Medicine, vol. 1. London, Cassell Ltd, 1978.)

TABLE 52–4.   Differential Diagnosis

Musculoskeletal sprains and strains
Acute disk herniation
Degenerative joint disease
Spondylolisthesis
Spinal stenosis
Osteoporosis
Spondylolysis
Spondyloarthropathy
  Ankylosing spondylitis
Referred pain
  Hip
  Abdominal aortic aneurysm
Tumor
  Primary
    Multiple myeloma
  Metastatic
    Lung, breast, kidney, thyroid, prostate, gastrointestinal
Infection
  Diskitis
  Osteomyelitis
Psychogenic
  Hysteria
  Malingering
  Psychosomatic

listhesis complicates approximately 3 per cent of cases of acute low back pain. The posterior facet joints carry 3 to 35 per cent of the static compressive load of the lumbar spine, and DJD of the posterior facets leads to spondylolisthesis. Progression of this slippage occurs in approximately 30 per cent of patients, but only rarely does the slippage exceed 25 to 30 per cent of the width of the adjacent vertebrae. Patients may present with isolated back pain or back pain with pain in the hip or buttock as well. Symptoms are worsened by walking or by erect posture and are relieved by rest or flexion of the spine and hip. Spondylolisthesis most commonly occurs at the L4 to L5 level, with involvement of the L5 nerve root. Only 15 to 20 per cent of patients demonstrate muscle weakness, and the straight-leg-raising test result is usually negative. Among older patients, bladder problems are common but are usually unrelated to spondylolisthesis. Standing plain radiographs demonstrate the lesion, which can be further characterized by standing myelography, computed tomography (CT) scan, or magnetic resonance imaging (MRI). Initial treatment includes brief bed rest and anti-inflammatory medication, followed by physical therapy modalities, aerobic exercises, and back-strengthening exercises. Decompressive laminectomy with or without arthrodesis is indicated if pain persists despite a trial of conservative therapy or if there is presence of a progressive neurologic deficit.

Spinal Stenosis

This degenerative process can mimic vascular claudication symptoms. Patients report dull achy back pain and posterior thigh pain with standing or walking, which is relieved by rest or sitting down. This problem can be differentiated from vascular claudication by the lack of ischemic changes and the presence of full pulses. Symptoms of vascular insufficiency are more quickly brought on by activity, and more quickly relieved by rest, than are symptoms of spinal stenosis.

Posterior Facet Syndrome

The posterior facet joints are often overlooked in the evaluation of back pain, but they share the load of supporting the spine with the vertebral bodies and intervertebral discs. The facets are posterolateral zygapophyseal joints; the joint capsule is innervated by the posterior primary ramus of the dorsal nerve root. A tear in the capsule causes referred pain to the buttocks and posterior thigh. Treatment involves moist heat, non-narcotic analgesics, muscle relaxants, and facet nerve blocks. If conservative measures fail, spinal fusion or facet arthrodesis may be required.

Infection

Hematogenous spread of bacteria to the vertebral body is not uncommon, and vertebral osteomyelitis can be overlooked as a cause of back pain. Patients may initially present without fever or leukocytosis, and the diagnosis is delayed 3 months or more in as many as 50 per cent of cases. Tuberculosis, diabetes mellitus, intravenous drug abuse, alcohol abuse, steroid use, and disseminated malignancy are associated with an increased risk of vertebral osteomyelitis. Fever is usually present, but it may be absent in debilitated patients whose immune systems are impaired. An elevated erythrocyte sedimentation rate (ESR) is a nonspecific but confirmatory finding. Blood culture or bone biopsy can isolate the pathogenic organism, and bone scan or MRI can localize the lesion.

Tumor

MULTIPLE MYELOMA. This disease is the most common primary malignancy of the spine. It affects the vertebral bodies, predisposing the patient to pathologic fractures of the spine. The diagnosis can be confirmed by bone biopsy or by serum and/or urine protein electrophoresis.

CARCINOMATOUS METASTASES TO THE SPINE. Bony metastases are common among primary malignancies of the lung, breast, kidney, thyroid, prostate, and gastrointestinal (GI) tract. On plain radiographs of the spine, the pedicles are often obscured, and the vertebral bodies may show osteolytic or osteoblastic lesions. These lesions can cause vertebral body collapse and spinal cord injury. Pain at night, pain at rest, or pain in the recumbent position are clues to the presence of metastases.

SPINAL CORD TUMORS. Spinal cord tumors and nerve root tumors (neurofibroma, neurilemoma) are rare causes of back pain, and diagnosis requires a high index of suspicion. These lesions are best confirmed by MRI.

Psychogenic Causes

Most patients with back pain do not have a psychogenic cause for their pain. In some cases the pain is psychosomatic in origin, and treatment is aimed at the underlying cause of anxiety.

PLAN

Diagnostic Laboratory and Special Tests

Although the differential diagnosis outlined above must be kept in mind, the patient's presentation is fairly typical for L5 nerve root irritation due to a herniated intervertebral disk. Further characterization of the lesion is not necessary at this point, and the patient warrants a course of conservative therapy. If the patient's symptoms do not resolve with conservative therapy, or if they worsen, re-evaluation is required to direct further investigative studies.

Therapeutic Treatment Plan

Tomas' symptoms are of recent onset, and he demonstrates no muscle weakness or loss of bowel or bladder control. Therefore, an attempt at conservative management is warranted (Table 52–5).

In the acute phase, the patient benefits from a combination of physical and pharmacologic therapy. Brief bed rest on a firm surface is recom-

TABLE 52–5. Treatment for Low Back Pain

Brief bed rest (2–3 days) on a firm surface
Analgesics
  Time-limited prescription
  NSAIDs, 2–6 weeks
Muscle relaxants
  Time-limited prescription
  <1 week
Physical modalities
  Moist heat, 20 minutes, four times daily
  Ice packs, 15 minutes, three times daily
  Ultrasound
  Massage
Ambulation as tolerated
Exercise
  Extension exercises
  Aerobic fitness
  Flexion exercises (abdominal strengthening)
Weight loss
Back school
  Instruction on basic back biomechanics
  Proper sitting, standing, and lifting techniques

mended for 2 days, combined with non-narcotic analgesics, such as nonsteroidal anti-inflammatory drugs. There is some question as to the efficacy of muscle relaxants (e.g., carisoprodol, cyclobenzaprine), but these are often used. Physical modalities such as moist heat, ice packs, or massage are also helpful. Once the acute pain has resolved, the patient should be taught back extension exercises under the supervision of a physical therapist. Sending the patient to "back school" to learn simple measures to prevent reinjury is an important adjunct to education provided by the physician.

Patient Education

At this point, the patient is very concerned about his back pain, and care should be taken to explain to him how this occurred, what he can expect, what the treatment plan is, and a rough idea on when he might return to work. In particular, he should be instructed on the importance of brief bed rest on a firm surface for approximately 2 days. He should understand the usefulness of moist heat and its proper application, and how and when to use prescribed medications.

He should be told about possible surgical alternatives. In most cases, conservative therapy is sufficient. But if his symptoms do not resolve, or if they become worse, he may require referral to an orthopedist for possible surgery: standard diskectomy, microdiskectomy, laminectomy with or without fusion, or chemonucleolysis.

Disposition

Tomas is sent home to brief bed rest for 2 days, with instructions to apply moist heat to his back for about 20 minutes approximately four times a day. He is given a nonsteroidal anti-inflammatory drug and a muscle relaxant and is told to return for follow-up in 1 week or sooner, if symptoms worsen.

FIRST FOLLOW-UP VISIT—SUBJECTIVE

Tomas returns 1 week later feeling much better. He still reports occasional "electrical pains" that radiate from his back through the posterior thigh to the dorsum of the foot, but he denies any leg weakness or bowel or bladder incontinence. He says his back pain is much decreased.

OBJECTIVE

On physical examination, Tomas still has right-sided paravertebral muscle tenderness in the lumbar area but no midline tenderness. Heel-walking and toe-walking are intact, as are motor strength and deep tendon reflexes. In particular, dorsiflexion of the foot and first toe are intact. Straight-leg-raising capacity is still limited on the right side, but Tomas says that the pain is less severe than a week ago. The cremasteric reflex and rectal sphincter tone are intact.

ASSESSMENT

Tomas' symptoms seem to be decreasing and his physical signs are stable or improving. He probably has a small degree of disk herniation impinging upon the right L5 nerve root causing his current symptoms. The protruding disk material will probably degenerate further and cease to cause impingement and symptoms.

PLAN

Diagnostic Laboratory and Special Tests

Many tests are available, but are probably not indicated at the moment because Tomas' condition is improving. If his symptoms worsen, several options may be considered.

Computed Tomography

CT scan is especially useful in lesions involving the bone (e.g., spinal stenosis, facet joint disease, and bony lesions such as metastases or osteophytes). In particular, CT scan is 72 to 100 per cent sensitive in detecting disk herniation. Although it has the benefit of being a noninvasive test, it does expose the patient to a fair dose of ionizing radiation, and its use is usually restricted to the axial plane.

Magnetic Resonance Imaging

MRI is a noninvasive technique to examine soft tissues in multiple planes without the drawback of exposing the patient to radiation. It offers excellent differentiation among the several soft tissues of the spine and it is especially useful in visualizing epidural and extradural tumors or abscesses and spinal cord lesions and in differentiating scar tissue due to previous back surgery from disk herniation. Studies have shown that MRIs of the spine are abnormal in up to 64 per cent of asymptomatic patients; positive MRI findings must be interpreted in the context of the complete clinical presentation.

Myelogram

Myelogram using the water-soluble dye metrizamide is especially useful in diagnosing intradural and extradural masses, and it is indicated when tumor is suspected, when symptoms are referable to several different lumbar areas, when the cauda equina syndrome is present, when spinal stenosis is considered, and when the diagnosis is not clear or disk herniation is not suspected. Its diagnostic accuracy is in the range of 75 to 80 per cent, although the false-positive rate is about 10 per cent and the false-negative rate is about 16 per cent.

Electromyography and Nerve Conduction Velocity (EMG, NCV) Tests

These are helpful in differentiating the radiculopathy of nerve root impingement from peripheral neuropathy (e.g., irritation of the sciatic nerve in the obturator foramen, or the peripheral neuropathy of diabetes or heavy metal exposure).

Therapeutic Treatment Plan

1. Continue nonsteroidal anti-inflammatory drugs

2. Discontinue muscle relaxants

3. Continue moist heat therapy and refer patient to physical therapy for back extension exercises and additional modalities (e.g., ultrasound, diathermy, massage)

4. If available in the community, send the patient to "back school" to learn simple ways to avoid undue stress on the lumbar spine.

Patient Education

1. Instruct the patient on the importance of good back hygiene: how to lift properly with the back straight and the knees bent, how to relieve back strain during prolonged standing by placing one foot on a 6-inch footstool, other techniques.

2. If the patient is overweight, a diet and weight-loss program should be detailed. The patient should understand that maintenance of ideal body weight decreases the strain placed on the lumbar spine.

3. Aerobic exercise, most commonly walking, should be prescribed early in the recovery period (usually 7–14 days). Aerobically fit individuals report less low back pain, recover more rapidly, and suffer fewer episodes of recurrent low back pain. Patients should be instructed to begin a daily walking program with good foot gear on a regular and yielding surface (e.g., asphalt or running tracks). Walking on concrete, uneven pavement, or dangerously irregular surfaces should be avoided.

4. The patient should be encouraged to view back pain as a chronic problem that can be managed by close cooperation between the patient and physician. A "cure," that is, a totally pain-free spine, may not be possible and should not be an expectation. All attempts should be made to prevent the patient from becoming an invalid due to back pain. Patient education and active patient involvement in management of this chronic problem can greatly reduce the morbidity of back injury.

5. In cases of acute disk herniation, abdominal strengthening exercises (Williams flexion exercises) should not be started until all radicular symptoms and most back pain has resolved, which is probably 1 to 3 months. (In the setting of uncomplicated musculoligamentous low back pain, abdominal strengthening exercises can be initiated as soon as back pain symptoms allow, usually 3–7 days.) The patient performs these exercises while lying supine on a firm surface such as the floor, with the knees and hips slightly flexed. Williams flexion exercises include knee-to-chest stretches (to stretch the hamstrings and relieve lumbar lordosis), head-and-shoulder raises (i.e., abdominal "crunches"), elbow-to-opposite-knee raises (to strengthen the internal and external oblique muscles), and pelvic tilt (to strengthen the lower abdomen).

Disposition

The patient will implement the diet, weight-loss, and exercise regimens discussed, and return to clinic in 4 weeks to check on progress. The patient should return sooner if problems develop, such as worsening of back pain or appearance of new symptoms.

DISCUSSION

Tomas' presentation is fairly typical for lumbar disk herniation: acute onset of back pain, usually associated with an episode of heavy lifting, paresthesias consistent with nerve root irritation, and resolution of symptoms with conservative management. Most patients with low back pain do not present with radicular pain, however.

When abnormal compression or strain forces are applied to the intervertebral space, the annulus fibrosus may tear, allowing herniation of part or all of the nucleus pulposus. This defect can lead to protrusion of disk material, extrusion of disk material into the spinal canal, or even sequestration of disk material within the spinal canal.

Most patients with disk herniation enjoy resolution of symptoms spontaneously with conservative management, which consists of bed rest on a firm surface, use of non-narcotic analgesics, moist heat to help minimize muscle spasm, and physical therapy modalities such as ultrasound, diathermy, and massage. Although muscle relaxants are often prescribed, their effectiveness is not clear.

In the subacute phase, the patient can be counseled regarding weight loss and aerobic fitness exercises, both of which will decrease the amount of compression and strain forces applied to the lumbar spine. If a back school is available in the community, the patient will benefit from group discussion of back anatomy and causation of symptoms, as well as instruction on good back hygiene: proper techniques for sitting, standing, and lifting to help protect the back from further injury. The back school can reinforce weight loss counseling and the proper way to perform back extension exercises. If symptoms do not resolve or if they worsen, or if motor weakness or bowel or bladder incontinence are present, special diagnostic tests may be required to elucidate the pathogenic mechanism.

CT scan, MRI, and myelogram all have their place in diagnosis. These neuroradiologic tests should be reserved for a specific subset of patients—in the acute phase, patients with cauda equina syndrome or progressive neurologic deficit, and in the subacute phase, patients with radicular symptoms unresponsive to a 4- to 6-week trial of conservative therapy. CT scan of the lumbar spine is the single test that can provide the most information about the spinal canal, spinal cord, intervertebral disks, and soft tissue masses.

Surgical diskectomy can have up to a 95 per cent success rate in carefully selected patients. This procedure is not a therapy for low back pain alone but is indicated to relieve symptoms of radiculopathy unresponsive to conservative management.

Spinal fusion may be necessary for patients with unrelenting chronic low back pain, usually that due to degenerative changes at the intervertebral or facet joints. Decompressive laminectomy is reserved for patients with acute motor weakness or bowel/bladder dysfunction caused by disk material or other mass impinging on the canal.

Some cases of disk protrusion or extrusion can be treated by chemonucleolysis, or dissolution of disk material by chymopapain injected into the intervertebral disk space. Such therapy is successful in approximately 70 per cent of selected cases but is not effective if disk material is sequestered within the spinal canal. Chemonucleolysis is not without risks; anaphylaxis occurs in 0.5 to 1.0 per cent of cases, paraplegia in about one of every 3500 cases, and subarachnoid hemorrhage in about one of every 7000 cases.

SUGGESTED READING

Deyo RA, Koeser JD, Bigos SJ. Herniated lumbar intervertebral disk. Ann Intern Med 1990;112(8):598–603.

Deyo RA, Rainville J, Kent DL. What can the history and physical examination tell us about low back pain? JAMA 1992;268(6):760–765.

Deyo RA, Diehl AK, Rosenthal M. How many days of bedrest for acute low back pain? A randomized clinical trial. N Engl J Med 1986;315(17):1064–1070.

Frymoyer JW, Nachemson A. Natural history of low back disorders. In Frymoyer JW (ed). The Adult Spine: Principles and Practice. New York, Raven Press, 1991.

Gilette RD. A practical approach to the patient with back pain. Am Fam Physician 1996;53(2):670–676.

Jensen MC, Brand-Zawadzki MN, Obuchowski N, et al. Magnetic resonance imaging of the lumbar spine in people without back pain. N Engl J Med 1994;331(2):69–73.

Wheeler AH. Diagnosis and management of low back pain and sciatica. Am Fam Physician 1995;52(5):1333–1341.

Wipf JE, Deyo RA. Low back pain. Med Clin North Am 1995;79(2):231–246.

QUESTIONS

1. What motor function is impaired by nerve root injury at the L5 level?
   a. Hip flexion
   b. Knee flexion
   c. Knee extension
   d. Foot dorsiflexion
   e. Foot plantar flexion

2. Symptoms suggestive of infection or tumor as the cause of acute low back pain include
   a. Pain with walking
   b. Sharp pain with sudden onset
   c. Tearing pain with diaphoresis
   d. Paresthesias in the toes
   e. Pain at rest or pain at night

3. The optimal duration of bed rest for patients with mild to moderate low back strain is
   a. 2 days

b. 4 days
c. 6 days
d. 1 week
e. 2 weeks

4. The best test to confirm acute lumbar disk herniation in symptomatic patients unresponsive to conservative therapy is:

a. Plain radiograph
b. EMG/NCV
c. Myelogram
d. CT
e. MRI

Answers appear on **page 606**.

Chapter 53

Ankle Injury

Daniel S. Fick, M.D.

INITIAL VISIT

Subjective

PATIENT IDENTIFICATION. Linda F. is a 33-year-old woman who presents with acute right ankle pain.

PRESENTING PROBLEMS. The patient reports that earlier in the day when attempting to climb out of the pool after swimming she caught her ankle between the top step and the edge of the pool and twisted her ankle. She believes her foot got stuck and she could not stop in time. This had never happened to her ankle before. She felt a pop and the pain immediately. She was able to walk over to a chair on the pool deck where she was able to contact the lifeguard for assistance.

There was no medical supervision but the lifeguard was able to get ice for her to place on her right ankle. She kept the ice on her ankle for about 15 minutes. She noticed that her ankle seemed to swell up while she had the ice placed on the outside of the ankle. She did not notice any bruising. She needed to get to work so she limped without assistance to the showers where she reports the outside of her right ankle throbbed with pain while she was showering. The pain seemed to increase while she changed into her street clothes but it was somewhat better when she sat down and laid her leg out straight on the bench. She took two ibuprofen tablets that she keeps in her purse for headaches.

Linda is a schoolteacher whose job requires standing but she was able to sit some of the morning with her ankle on a chair. She decided to drive herself to the physician's office. Applying pressure to the pedals with her right foot was painful. The nurse said she requested a wheelchair to go into the examination room.

PAST MEDICAL HISTORY. The patient has had only one serious injury in the past. She suffered an open humerus fracture at age 10 from a gymnastic injury. She required 6 weeks of traction. Her only other hospital admissions were for two normal pregnancies. She takes oral contraceptives and an occasional ibuprofen for headaches. She has no allergies.

FAMILY HISTORY. Both her parents are alive and healthy. She has two younger sisters, who are both healthy.

SOCIAL HISTORY. Linda is married, a part-time elementary schoolteacher, and has a daughter and son. She does not smoke and consumes alcohol on rare occasions.

418

REVIEW OF SYSTEMS. She reports occasional headaches at the time of her menstrual flow.

Objective

PHYSICAL EXAMINATION. The patient sits on a chair with her foot elevated on an examination stool. She hopped over to the examination table and sat on the edge. She immediately requested that she be able to sit back and put her foot flat on the foot extension. On initial inspection she has obvious swelling around the lateral malleolus, with some erythema and loss of normal contour. There is no major deformity, bruising, or other discoloration or skin changes. She can actively plantar flex and dorsiflex but with discomfort and decreased range of motion. Attempts at active inversion and eversion are too painful. This pain appears located around the distal fibula.

Palpation reveals no tenderness of the anterior tibia or medial malleolus. The navicular tubercle and head of the talus are nontender. The medial collateral ligament and deltoid ligament just inferior to the medial malleolus are not tender. Posterior to the medial malleolus, the tibialis posterior, flexor digitorum longus, and flexor hallucis longus tendons are not tender and the posterior tibial pulse is strong. Moving to the dorsum of the foot, the tibialis anterior, extensor hallucis longus, and extensor digitorum longus tendons are not tender and the dorsal pedal pulse is also strong. Posterior examination of the Achilles tendon, gastrocnemius, and soleus muscles is normal.

Starting proximal on the fibula, pressure on the bone does not elicit tenderness until approximately 4 cm from the tip. The anterior and distal portion of the lateral malleolus are tender to palpation. The area corresponding to the anterior talofibular ligament and calcaneofibular ligaments is very tender. It is difficult to determine if the peroneus longus and brevis tendons are tender because of their close proximity to the swelling. The proximal fifth metatarsal is not tender.

Neurovascular testing reveals that the toes have brisk capillary refill in addition to the previously mentioned strong dorsalis pedis and posterior tibialis pulses. Sensation of the L4 dermatome (medial malleolus and the medial side of the foot), L5 (dorsum of ankle and foot), and S1 (lateral malleolus and foot) is normal.

Linda is asked to sit on the edge of the table and allow her feet to hang down in a normal sitting position. Passively she has 10 degrees of both plantar flexion and dorsiflexion. Attempts at strength testing cause too much discomfort to make an adequate assessment. Compared with the left side she has a normal right-sided posterior drawer test, but the anterior drawer test resulted in a 1- to 2-mm greater translation and she is again very tender with testing. She also is very tender on inversion stress of the calcaneofibular ligament but no laxity is noted.

Assessment

WORKING DIAGNOSIS. There are four injuries that can independently or in combination account for the patient's symptoms.

1. *Grade 2 anterior talofibular ligament sprain.* This ligament is the most common ankle ligament sprained. The patient gives a good history of an inversion ankle sprain, which places stress on the talofibular ligament. The physical examination with swelling, tenderness, and some laxity on anterior draw testing points to the talofibular ligament.

2. *Grade 2 calcaneofibular ligament sprain.* After the talofibular ligament, the calcaneofibular is the next most common ligament sprained. This ligament connects the talus with the distal fibula. It is often sprained along with the anterior talofibular ligament. The patient is also tender in the area of the calcaneofibular ligament.

3. *Distal fibular fracture.* Inversion injuries can also result in a fibular fracture together with or independent of a ligamentous sprain. The patient is tender over portions of the fibula and she cannot currently bear weight. A fracture needs to be ruled out.

4. *Distal fibular avulsion.* This is one type of distal fibular fracture but can be thought of separately. A severe calcaneofibular sprain may avulse a portion of the distal fibula. The patient has tenderness over the area where an avulsion would be expected.

DIFFERENTIAL DIAGNOSIS. There are several other diagnoses that need to be considered.

1. *Stress fracture.* The patient may have a stress fracture of the calcaneus or navicular. These are usually chronic injuries that hurt with activity and usually improve with rest but still may initially ache during inactivity. The examination reveals point tenderness over the fracture site. An x-ray film may reveal a fracture line with periosteal reaction if some healing has occurred, but this is unlikely given the acute nature of the patient's pain. A bone scan usually shows increased uptake at the fracture site. Computed tomography (CT) or magnetic resonance imaging (MRI) also reveals the fracture.

2. *Tendinitis.* Any one of a group of tendons that cross and manipulate the ankle may develop tendinitis. With Linda's symptoms, the peroneus brevis and peroneus longus tendons are the most likely tendons injured. The patient does have tenderness over the tendons but she also has tenderness over the distal fibula, which is not completely explained by tendinitis.

3. *Syndesmosis sprain.* The tibiofibular syndesmosis is made up of the anterior and posterior tibiofibular ligaments and the interosseous membrane. A sprain usually involves the interosseous membrane with or without the lateral ligaments involved. The mechanism of injury is external rotation, hyperdorsiflexion, or a combination of both. The talus impinges on the fibula and pushes the tibia and fibula apart. The interosseous membrane tears more distally and the tear may extend toward the knee. The presentation is usually painful weight bearing and lateral ankle swelling. The swelling is usually less prominent than typical lateral ankle sprains and more proximal, with ecchymosis at the level of the syndesmosis about 1 to 2 cm above the ankle joint. The patient has no proximal fibular pain or distal swelling, but attempts at external rotation are painful, so a syndesmosis sprain cannot be ruled out at this time.

4. *Fifth metatarsal fracture.* The fifth metatarsal may fracture in the proximal segment or the peroneus brevis tendon may avulse a segment of the bone. These fractures may be missed if the examiner does not specifically palpate in the area of the fifth metatarsal. The patient has diffuse swelling and tenderness in the area and a fifth metatarsal fracture cannot be ruled out.

Plan

DIAGNOSTIC. The first diagnostic decision that needs to be made is whether to obtain x-ray films of the affected ankle. Radiography usually includes standard anteroposterior (AP), lateral, and mortise views. Any pain or tenderness along the fibula, navicular, or fifth metatarsal requires extra views. Widening of the ankle mortise also requires the entire fibula to be viewed including stress views. Determining whether or not to radiograph an ankle sprain requires input from the history and physical examination. In addition, clinical guidelines known as the Ottawa ankle rules (Fig. 53–1) are helpful to determine the necessity of an x-ray series.

The clinical guidelines recommend an x-ray series if there is bone tenderness at the posterior edge or tip of the lateral or medial malleolus, or inability to bear weight both immediately and at the time of evaluation. In order to obtain radiographs of the foot the rules require bone tenderness at the base of the fifth metatarsal or at the navicular bone, or inability to bear weight both immediately and at the time of evaluation. The patient met the criteria with tenderness at the tip of the lateral malleolus and inability to bear weight during the examination. An x-ray series including AP, lateral, and mortise views are obtained in the office and are normal.

THERAPEUTIC. The patient has an anterior talofibular ligament sprain with perhaps a lesser calcaneofibular ligament sprain. This is a very common injury suffered after an inversion ankle sprain. The therapeutic mainstay of treatment initially involves the mnemonic PRICES. This stands for *p*rotection, *r*est, *i*ce, *c*ompression, *e*levation, and *s*upport.

Initially it is important to protect the ankle from reinjury, which usually involves keeping the patient from reproducing the mechanism of injury. Rest involves not walking for extended periods of time or distances during the first 2 to 3 days. Ice reduces the pain and brings down the swelling. It is important to not ice the affected area more than 15 minutes at a time because of the risk of superficial nerve damage. Circular motion with an ice cup provides maximum cooling. Compression also helps control swelling if used immediately and it can prevent a fair amount of swelling from reaccumulating. Elevation increases venous and lymphatic return. Support may be an elastic stocking, or for more severe sprains a pneumatic compression brace can be used. Nonsteroidal anti-inflammatory drugs (NSAIDs) are a common and accepted form of treatment for musculoskeletal injuries. They may help reduce inflammation and can relieve some of the discomfort from the inflammation.

PATIENT EDUCATION

1. The patient is instructed not to put excessive force on her ankle. She may use a crutch for the first 24 hours but it is important for her to keep her lower leg muscles from becoming weak from disuse. As soon as tolerated she should begin weight bearing on her ankle and slowly increase the percentage of pain-free weight she can place on her ankle.

2. She is instructed to ice the area of swelling with an ice cup for 15 minutes several times a day.

3. She also is given an elastic sleeve to wear over her ankle because she did not have the laxity neces-

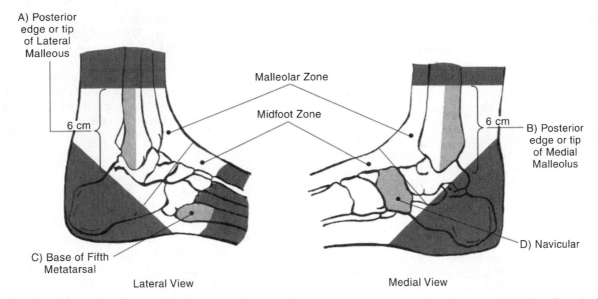

A) Posterior edge or tip of Lateral Malleous

Malleolar Zone

Midfoot Zone

6 cm

B) Posterior edge or tip of Medial Malleolus

6 cm

D) Navicular

C) Base of Fifth Metatarsal

Lateral View

Medial View

Figure 53–1. Ottawa ankle rules. An ankle radiologic series needed with malleolar pain and tenderness at A, B, C, or D, or inability to bear weight both immediately and in emergency department. (Modified from Stiell IG, Greenberg GH, McKnight RD, et al. Decision rules for the use of radiography in acute ankle injuries: Refinement and prospective validation. JAMA 1994;271:827–832.)

sary to warrant a more restrictive brace. The elastic sleeve also provides some compression.

4. A prescription for ibuprofen 600 mg three times a day is given. She is instructed that this may upset her stomach and sometimes it is better tolerated with a meal. She is instructed to stop the medication if she develops discomfort because of the medicine.

Disposition. She is instructed to return to the office in 4 days at which time her ankle will be reassessed and rehabilitation exercises prescribed at that time.

FIRST FOLLOW-UP VISIT

Subjective

The patient returned 4 days later. She reports that her ankle feels better but that it is still sore. She rates the pain as 50 per cent lessened, but she is concerned that her ankle is still swollen and there appears to be a bruise along the side of her foot. She has been using ice but not three times a day. She thinks the ibuprofen helps and has not had any stomach upset. At night she takes the elastic sleeve off but does wear it during the day. Work has not been a problem and she did not need to use crutches after the first day. Her main question is

when can she start exercising her ankle and get back to swimming.

Objective

The patient's ankle continues to be swollen; however, it is greatly improved from 4 days earlier. She now has obvious swelling anterior and distal to the lateral malleolus and some bruising distally on the foot over the calcaneus and fifth metatarsal. Actively she can almost fully plantar flex and dorsiflex, but has more limited inversion and eversion. These motions still elicit some discomfort. Palpation reveals tenderness anterior and distal to the lateral malleolus but none actually on the fibula. The bruising distally is also not tender. The remainder of the foot including the fifth metatarsal is not tender. She has no pain or laxity in testing the calcaneofibular ligament with the talar tilt, but still reports discomfort with anterior drawer testing of the anterior talofibular ligament. There is still 1 to 2 mm of laxity felt on the anterior drawer test compared with the unaffected left ankle.

Assessment

1. Grade 2 anterior talofibular ligament strain.
2. Grade 1 calcaneofibular ligament strain.

Plan

DIAGNOSTIC. Over the last 4 days the patient's symptoms and physical examination have improved. There is not any change on examination that would require any additional x-ray studies. No further diagnostic tests are necessary.

THERAPEUTIC. The patient has progressed to the point at which physical therapy can be started on the ankle without danger of promoting inflammation. During phase 1 of rehabilitation the emphasis is to control the patient's pain and inflammation, encourage early weight bearing, and provide protected mobilization of the ankle.

During phase 2 the aim is restrengthening appropriate muscles and re-educating the ankle's proprioceptive mechanism. Finally, during phase 3, the patient should be able to return to the former level of activity.

PATIENT EDUCATION

1. The patient is instructed to continue phase 1 of rehabilitation. This includes continued use of cryotherapy and the anti-inflammatory medication. She is to increase weight bearing to a normal gait as soon as she is pain free. She should continue wearing the elastic sleeve as long as she feels her ankle is still swollen. Early range of motion exercises include plantar flexion and dorsiflexion, and inversion and eversion movements in the pain-free range of motion, just stopping at the point of pain. Tracing out the letters of the alphabet with her big toe is an easy exercise to begin proprioceptive training.

2. She may begin phase 2 of rehabilitation once she can walk pain free and no longer feels pain or restriction with the active range of motion exercises previously described. The cryotherapy may be continued if she feels it helps reduce any remaining swelling. Usually 2 weeks of an anti-inflammatory drug is adequate for an uncomplicated ankle sprain. She may use a towel or flexible tubing to add resistance to the range of motion exercises. By the end of phase 2 the patient should have nearly full range of motion, minimal edema, and be fully weight bearing.

3. The patient may progress to phase 3 after successfully completing phase 2. She may return to the pool and gradually increase her distance in the pool. The flutter kick is actually difficult to perform with an acutely sprained ankle and may need to be avoided until other strokes are performed pain free.

DISPOSITION. The patient is instructed on the three phases of rehabilitation. She may progress through phase 2 as soon as phase 1 is successfully completed. It is up to the discretion of the patient whether to return for another visit before starting phase 3. Often, uncomplicated ankle sprains allow a patient to progress without difficulties through phase 3 without direct physician supervision.

DISCUSSION

Musculoskeletal complaints rank second only to respiratory complaints in terms of frequency of visits to family physicians' offices. Ankle injuries, and specifically ankle sprains, make up a large percentage of these complaints. In order to effectively treat ankle sprains some basic anatomy is worth reviewing. The ankle is a hinge joint composed of three bones: the tibia, the fibula, and the talus which form the ankle mortise. Plantar flexion and dorsiflexion are the movements of the ankle that permit ambulation. In dorsiflexion the talus is locked between the tibia and fibula and the joint is stable and strong. In plantar flexion the ankle is weak and unstable with less bony stability. Ligaments tightly bound by a retinaculum also stabilize the ankle and maintain the integrity of the ankle joint and limit the range of motion in any plane. The musculature of the lower leg, through its tendons, provides support and helps prevent injury by controlling the amount of shock that ligaments absorb. The muscles still provide sufficient support and stability to permit the patient some function and motion even if the ligaments are severely damaged.

Most ankle injuries tend to occur when the ankle is plantar flexed. These injuries are usually traumatic from a fall or twist and occur to an unsuspecting limb. Over 70 per cent of ankle sprains are inversion ankle sprains. The medial malleolus is more proximal than the lateral malleolus which allows a greater degree of inversion than eversion, putting stress on the lateral ligaments. The differences in length and position of the malleoli can be more readily appreciated if one places the fingers on the anterior portion of both malleoli.

The anterior talofibular ligament is the most frequently torn. The calcaneofibular ligament is the next most commonly involved in inversion sprain injuries. The posterior talofibular ligament is the strongest of the three and least likely to tear. Less than 1 per cent of the time are all three likely to tear; most of the time a tear occurs in only the anterior talofibular ligament. Since the lateral malleolus is more distal, when an eversion injury occurs the distal fibula frequently is broken along with a tear of the thick medial deltoid ligament.

It is important for family physicians to have a plan or clinical algorithm that they can implement when a patient presents to their office with the complaint of ankle sprain. The first order of business is often determining if the patient requires an x-ray study. Most ankle sprains seen in the clinic or emergency room are sustained by patients who are in pain and often expect an x-ray film. Accordingly, physicians often think an x-ray film is required either because of clinical or legal reasons. The Ottawa ankle rules have made determining the necessity of obtaining ankle radiographs much easier. Developed in Ottawa, Canada, these rules have attempted to identify the less than 15 per cent of patients with ankle fractures who present with ankle sprains. This would reduce the necessity of taking millions of radiographs a year.

In order to be useful clinical guidelines, the rules must be scientifically based, clear and relevant, concise, and easy to remember and use in a busy setting. After assessing 32 clinical variables, two clinical rules were developed that covered all malleolar and midfoot fractures. The rules require an ankle or foot x-ray series if there is bone tenderness at the posterior edge or tip of the lateral or medial malleolus, at the base of the fifth metatarsal, or at the navicular bone. A radiograph is also required if the patient is unable to bear weight both immediately and at the time of evaluation (Fig. 53–1). The sensitivity of diagnosing an ankle or foot fracture with the Ottawa ankles rules has been shown to be 100 per cent.

The next step after determining that the ankle is not broken is to determine which soft tissue structures are injured and how severe an injury the patient has suffered. The physical examination of a sprained ankle can usually narrow the diagnosis down to several ligaments or tendons. Inspection of the area of swelling and/or erythema is the best clinical clue to the soft tissues injured.

The ability of the patient to actively move the injured ankle also gives clues to injured tendons and ligaments. Normally the ankle has 20 degrees of dorsiflexion and 20 and 50 degrees of plantar flexion. There is 5 degrees of both subtalar calcaneal inversion and eversion. Forefoot adduction is 0 to 20 degrees, and forefoot abduction 0 to 10 degrees. If the patient reports pain and has decreased active range of motion, then there is a high probability of soft tissue damage. Palpating the precise areas for tenderness allows the family physician to match tenderness to ligament, tendon, and bony landmarks.

The physical examination should be performed when the patient is relaxed enough not to splint the ankle by contracting the entire lower leg musculature. The clinician can help relax the affected ankle by first examining the unaffected ankle. This gives the patient some idea of what to expect. The two ligaments that need to be tested for laxity in an inversion ankle sprain are the calcaneofibular ligament and the anterior talofibular ligament. The calcaneofibular ligament may be tested by the talar tilt test. One hand grasps the distal tibia while the other cups the posterior calcaneus and inverts and everts the ankle. This determines whether the ankle mortise is opening medially or laterally. A positive talar tilt test is a marked difference between the ankles or greater than 25 degrees or 10 mm of difference between ankles.

The second test is for anterior talofibular ligament laxity and is called the anterior drawer test. Again it is important to test the unaffected ankle first and keep the patient relaxed. When performing the anterior drawer test it is best to keep the knee bent 90 degrees. The foot is placed in the neutral position and the posterior calcaneus is cupped with the palm while the foot is supported on the hand and forearm. The distal tibia is stabilized with the other hand and the calcaneus is pulled forward. A positive drawer test is 4 mm or greater translation than the uninvolved foot. The end point can be compared, and any difference or absence indicates a tear.

Grading the ankle injury helps describe and standardize the extent of injury for the medical record and also helps guide rehabilitation. A grade 1 ankle injury has no or little hemorrhage at the ligament with no loss of function or strength, and the anterior drawer test is negative. Grade 2 shows swelling and hemorrhage, point tenderness over soft tissues such as ligaments or tendons, decreased motion, and some loss of function. The anterior drawer test is usually positive, but the ankle mortise is stable. Grade 3 is defined as diffuse swelling, hemorrhage, and extreme point tenderness. There is almost total loss of function and disruption of the ankle capsule. The anterior drawer test is positive and the mortise opens with stress.

Once the assessment is done and the ankle sprain is graded, then the focus is on controlling the pain and inflammation. This inflammation is the result of the acute injury of the soft tissues around the ankle. The pain, edema, and erythema are all accentuated by the release of histamines and bradykinins which cause vasodilation and enhance permeability of the peripheral capillaries. The transudate fluid then compounds the extent of tissue damage, and delays healing. Treatment should be focused on relieving pain, reducing swelling, and restoring normal function.

Pain can be readily controlled with the use of cryotherapy and NSAIDs. "Ice ever, heat never," is useful advice to patients who present with ankle sprains. Ice massage over the swollen and tender areas for 15 minutes at a time really decreases pain and swelling. The addition of oral anti-inflammatory medication has been shown to speed healing and recovery as well as decrease pain better than placebo. During the first several weeks of an ankle sprain this medication often helps the patient feel better and enhances compliance with rehabilitation exercises during later therapy.

Ankle support involves the application of an external structure to enhance the stability of the ankle joint. Tape is the most common support to use; it restricts range of motion and reduces the incidence of ankle sprains but loses its supportive characteristics within 10 to 20 minutes. The efficacy of high-top athletic shoes in reducing ankle sprains is controversial. Lace-up ankle stabilizers are popular, as they maintain range of motion and can be tightened during activity. Elastic slip-on ankle stabilizers provide compression and some minimal decreased range of motion. A semirigid orthosis that provides compression while allowing limited range of motion is popular.

The use of an elastic sleeve or rigid external support allows adequate range of motion for walking, which allows a more functional rehabilitation. It is important to allow movement along the uninjured axis (plantar flexion and dorsiflexion). Functional management allows a rapid return of mobility and function. This allows regeneration of tendons and ligaments parallel to the stress lines. Stress placed in a controlled fashion on ligaments as they heal allows them to regenerate in parallel lines and heal properly in their original form. Early return to function and weight bearing not only helps ligaments but also bones, tendons, and joint capsules to heal stronger and faster than results from prolonged immobilization.

The rehabilitation of ankle sprains needs to focus on returning range of motion, strength, and proprioception to normal. Any restriction from soft tissue tightness, scar tissue formation, or joint immobility disrupts normal biomechanical function. During the initial stage of rehabilitation, isometric strength exercises are tolerated well and can be performed to help strengthen the muscles without placing undue stress on compromised structures. In later phases of rehabilitation the patient can use endurance activities such as stationary bicycling, using stair machines, or treadmill walking before returning to more demanding physical activity.

Proprioception is the sense of movement and position in space. Compromised proprioception is a factor in functional ankle instability and it is difficult to prevent future sprains if a patient cannot tell in which position the ankle contacts the ground. A useful physical therapy exercise is a tilt board in which any type of sphere is cut in half and attached to a board that allows weight bearing. Initially the patient is in a seated position to minimize the stress at the ankle joint. A patient can progress to partial and then full weight bearing. Increasing the size of the sphere allows greater range of motion.

Chronic recurrent lateral ankle sprains may continue to demonstrate instability by the anterior drawer and talar tilt tests. Radiographic instability may also be present with stress views. This chronic instability may need a referral to an orthopedic surgeon. Other indications frequently seen by family physicians that are associated with ankle sprains include fractures with laxity of the ankle mortise, severe or total tearing of ligaments, and rupture of the Achilles tendon.

SUGGESTED READING

Bergfeld J, Halpern B. Sports Medicine: Functional Management of Ankle Injuries. Kansas City, MO, American Academy of Family Physicians, 1990.

Hoppenfeld S. Physical Examination of the Spine and Extremities. Norwalk, CT, Appleton-Century-Crofts, 1976.

Larkin J, Brage M. Ankle, hindfoot, and midfoot injuries. In Reider B (ed). Sports Medicine: The School-Age Athlete. Philadelphia, W.B. Saunders, 1991.

Ogilvie-Harris DJ, Gilbart M. Treatment modalities for soft tissue injuries of the ankle: A critical review. Clin J Sport Med 1995;5:175–186.

Rifat SF, McKeag DB. Practical methods of preventing ankle injuries. Am Fam Physician 1996;53:2491–2498.

Seto JL, Brewster CE. Treatment approaches following foot and ankle injury. Clin Sports Med 1994;13:695–718.

Stiell IG, McKnight RD, Greenberg GH, et al. Decision rules for the use of radiography in acute ankle injuries: Refinement and prospective validation. JAMA 1993;269:1127–1132.

1. True or false: The Ottawa ankle rules require an ankle series if
   a. The patient hears a pop and has immediate pain.
   b. Either malleolus is tender at the posterior edge or tip.
   c. The patient cannot walk immediately or at the time of evaluation.
   d. There is laxity on testing the lateral ligaments.

2. The most common ankle ligament sprained is the
   a. Calcaneofibular ligament
   b. Deltoid ligament
   c. Anterior talofibular ligament
   d. Posterior talofibular ligament

Answers appear on **page 606.**

Chapter 54

Joint Pain and Stiffness

John M. Heath, M.D.

INITIAL VISIT

Subjective

Harriet is a 77-year-old white woman complaining of worsening bilateral hip pain.

PRESENT ILLNESS. Harriet's complaint of pain with associated stiffness and mobility problems dates back to 3 years ago, when she noticed significant joint discomfort following weekly square dancing lessions. The pain, which she describes as a dull ache and most intense the day after prolonged weight-bearing exercise, mildly decreased in intensity when she was forced to give up square dancing after the death of her husband. It markedly worsened when she moved north to live in the same community as her daughter 3 months ago. Since that time the pain has been present constantly, but again it becomes much worse after walking two blocks or modest housecleaning. She localizes the discomfort to the anterior groin without radiation into the back or front of the leg and denies swelling about her hips or lower back discomfort. The marked difficulty she had getting out of her daughter's sports car last week precipitated the appointment today, both to establish primary care and to address her specific complaint. Occasional acetaminophen (Tylenol) has been modestly effective in reducing the discomfort the day following exertion, and she recently has been using a topical rub she purchased through a mail order catalog hoping to find some relief. She has no prior history of known fracture or bony trauma to her hips and denies prior x-ray studies of these or other joints. She has also noted her fingers becoming more stiff and "knobby" over this same time period.

SOCIAL HISTORY. Harriet continues to smoke half a pack of cigarettes a day, which she terms her "only vice." She drinks alcohol rarely and uses no other drugs or medications beyond the occasional Tylenol and laxative. She is a retired accountant and remains active in her college sorority social activities.

FAMILY HISTORY. Harriet has a younger sibling, Meg, with whom she has not spoken for years; she believes

Meg is using a walker, having undergone a knee joint replacement some years earlier. Her sister currently resides in the same community as Harriet and her daughter, whom she describes as in good health.

REVIEW OF SYSTEMS. Harriet reports a weight gain of approximately 15 lb since her husband's death 3 months ago that she attributes to reduced physical activity. Her vision and hearing remain unchanged. She denies that the hip pain affects her toileting, transferring, or other mobility skills, but does admit to having to "wince quite a bit" in pain when getting in and out of her daughter's sports car as well as on rising from the toilet in her apartment's bathroom. She awakens twice a night owing to pain in her hips for repositioning in bed. She remains independent in all instrumental activities of daily living.

Objective

PHYSICAL EXAMINATION. Harriet appears as a witty, somewhat obese white female; she stoops slightly forward in her chair. She is able to successfully stand from her sitting position on the third attempt and takes rather short, halting steps to climb on the examination table. Skin examination shows multiple plaquelike keratotic lesions on her upper back. Harriet is shocked to learn she is only 5 feet 2 inches tall, saying she was always 5 feet 5 inches, and blaming the "different gravity up here in the north!" Her weight is 149 lb. Blood pressure is 162/82 mm Hg in the left arm sitting; heart rate is 98 and irregular. Respirations are unlabored at 20 and she is afebrile.

Examination of the head is unremarkable, with modest hair thinning at the top. Dried earwax is noticed in both ear canals, although the tympanic membrane is visualized. Prominent cataracts are noted bilaterally. Nasal mucosa and septum are normal. Oral examination shows a number of fractured upper molars, with lower molars intact and receding gum lines. Thyroid gland and carotid pulses are normal. Breasts are symmetrical without palpable masses or nipple discharge, and skin appears unremarkable. Both axillae are clear of palpable mass. A soft sclerotic murmur of grade 2/6 is heard over the aortic area among the irregular rhythms. Lung auscultation shows moderately prolonged expiration with an expiratory wheeze heard bilaterally and clearing crackles in the bases. Modest kyphosis of the thoracic spine is noted. Abdominal examination shows active bowel sounds and poor anterior abdominal muscle tone with no organ enlargement.

Extremity examination shows prominent Heberden's node swelling over the distal phalangeal joints. Patient winces on adduction of both hips beyond 20 degrees and abduction beyond approximately 30 degrees. Shoulder, elbow, and ankle range of motion all appear normal without discomfort. On neurologic examination, Harriet shows depressed knee and ankle deep tendon reflexes, although biceps and triceps are symmetrical and intact. Cranial nerves II to XII seem symmetrical and intact, as is finger-to-nose coordination. Her gait is rather broad-based, short, and shuffling and she is unable to perform the Romberg test in part, being unable to bring both feet together. She has absent vibratory sensation from the midtibia distally, although superficial sensation to light touch and scratch seems intact. Cognitively she is well oriented temporally and spatially, shows intact registration and 5-minute recall of three objects, and is able to do simple math subtraction calculations appropriately.

Assessment

Progressive bilateral hip pain.

DIFFERENTIAL DIAGNOSIS

1. *Osteoarthritis.* The relatively gradual onset, progressive nature, prominent Heberden's nodes, and symmetrical distribution of complaints in weight-bearing joints all favor this diagnosis.

2. *Nonarticular rheumatologic disease.* Although Harriet has reported her problems as joint-related, the possibility of soft tissue inflammation should be considered. Given the modest stiffness and duration of her primary complaints, polymyalgia rheumatica might be a diagnostic consideration. The absence of distinct trigger points or tenderness palpated along the temporal artery and the time course of the complaints make this somewhat less likely. Fibromyalgia is also unlikely in the absence of significant fatigue and trigger points. Trochanteric bursitis is also a consideration.

3. *Lumbar spinal stenosis.* Harriet's initial symptom onset associated with upright sustained muscle activity could suggest neurogenic claudication, a condition in which progressive pain and discomfort occur in the proximal musculature associated with prolonged activity. It requires unloading of the lumbar spine by decompressing the spinal cord.

Diagnostic Plan

Harriet consents to have x-ray films taken of both hips and to undergo blood work to include erythrocyte sedimentation rate as well as a biochemical profile to include calcium, phosphorus, electrolytes, and renal function. She also agrees to take 650 mg of acetaminophen every morning before her most vigorous physical activities during the day and to return for a follow-up visit.

SUBSEQUENT VISIT

Harriet returns reporting that the routine use of acetaminophen has allowed her to travel with her daughter on a daily basis and to consider providing child care for her grandchildren. Symptoms about her fingers have modestly worsened, however, and she reports some difficulty in buttoning her clothing and fixing snaps on the children's clothing. Results of her bilateral hip x-ray studies show modest osteopenia about the femoral head and significant narrowing of the joint space with some sclerotic changes about the acetabulum and prominent osteophyte formation, consistent with a diagnosis of osteoarthritis. Laboratory studies show mild anemia with the hematocrit somewhat depressed at 32% and an elevated mean corpuscular volume of $102/\mu m^3$. Sedimentation rate is 24 mm per hour, and blood chemistry profiles are entirely normal.

Plan

A diagnosis of osteoarthritis is confirmed. Given the worsening upper extremity symptoms suggestive of mild inflammation, a short course of a nonsteroidal anti-inflammatory drug (NSAID) (e.g., ibuprofen 600 mg every 8 hours) is prescribed to be supplemented with the routine acetaminophen administration for 3 weeks. The need for weight loss through greater physical activity is emphasized. Harriet is encouraged to apply warm, moist heat to any involved painful fingers, is given literature to review about osteoporosis and postmenopausal estrogen replacement therapy, and is scheduled to return in a month. She is also encouraged to pursue a regularly scheduled walking program on flat surfaces with adequate shoe support and given a modest calorie reduction diet for weight loss. Because of the physical findings of absent vibratory sensation with the suggestion of a macrocytic anemia, vitamin B_{12} and folic acid levels are obtained.

DISCUSSION

Osteoarthritis represents the most common musculoskeletal form of morbidity and ranks only behind cardiovascular disease in overall disease burden and economic impact on the adult population seen in primary care settings. Although symptomatic presentations are most commonly seen in elderly women over age 55, early anatomic changes have been seen in over 60 per cent of pathologic specimens in individuals over age 35. This form of arthritis is characterized by articular cartilage deterioration associated with hypertrophic bony changes and is distinct from the more "atrophic" arthritic disorders, such as rheumatoid disease, which involves joint destruction. Historical evidence suggests that osteoarthritis affected the weight-bearing joints of early human ancestors in prehistoric times, as well as the large weight-bearing joints of early mammals. Its differentiation from other forms of joint disease was not achieved until the late eighteenth century, when it was distinguished from the more widely recognized gouty arthritis by the presence of bony changes surrounding the distal interphalangeal joints. This area of bony overgrowth is termed Heberden's nodes and remains a clinical hallmark of osteoarthritis.

Osteoarthritis is generally considered to be a noninflammatory state in which the anatomic and radiographic abnormalities of a joint may correlate poorly with the symptomatic and functional status of the affected individual. Clinical features include the presence of pain, most notably involving large weight-bearing joints of the knees and hips, morning stiffness, joint crepitation, and range of motion limitation. While the prevalence of Heberden's nodes in the United States, white population over the age of 75 is 70 per cent, less than 50 per cent of these individuals at any given time have the characteristic clinical presentation of symptomatic osteoarthritis. The association of symptoms localized to weight-bearing joints has historically led to consideration of osteoarthritis as being a "wear and tear" phenomenon linked to normal aging. More recent understanding has suggested that the loss of cartilage, felt to be the initial hallmark of osteoarthritis, may be associated with a normal joint being subjected to repeated abnormal range of motion stresses. Evidence suggesting this latter mechanism comes from the high association of osteoarthritic changes after identified knee meniscus injury or congenital abnormalities of the hip associated with misalignment. This theory views osteoarthritis as an imbalance of the normal, dynamic process of joint reabsorption and remodeling that goes throughout life, although associated with greater inelasticity and slower remodeling due to physiologic aging changes of the affected joints.

Clinical evaluation of osteoarthritic joints often includes radiographic imaging. Characteristic changes include loss of joint space associated with cartilage destruction, the presence of subchondral cysts due to synovial fluid intrusions into the ends of long bones, and the most characteristic finding, prominent osteophyte formation at the margins of joints. These lateral hypertrophic bone growths in effect increase the size of the overall joint by acting as a buttress. Although the overall extent of these radiographic changes correlates well with limitations in joint range of motion, the association with pain and stiffness is often poor, owing in part to the fact that cartilage destruction is not associated with pain perception, nor is significant synovitis present in most cases. If joint effusion is present, synovial fluid is often unremarkable, without significant evidence of inflammation or crystal deposition. This characteristic provides a valuable means to differentiate osteoarthritis from other arthritides in the differential diagnosis to include gout and chondral calcinosis (calcium pyrophosphate disease) (Table 54–1).

Research into the pathophysiology of osteoarthritis has focused most intensely on the degenerative process of the collagen and proteoglycan components of the cartilage, which gradually deteriorates in the osteoarthritic joint. The aging process in and of itself is associated with decreased water content in the cartilage as well as impairment of chondrocytes in effecting repairs of microinjuries. No unifying theory has been confirmed to satisfactorily explain the association between the cartilage degeneration and the hypertrophic bony changes.

Given the high prevalence of osteoarthritis, along with the relatively poor correlation between radiographic features and the actual clinical symptoms of pain and stiffness, consideration of alternative diseases is critical. Soft tissue processes such as fibromyalgia and polymyalgia rheumatica, both of which are relatively more common in older women than in men (as is osteoarthritis), can be differentiated on the basis of associated constitutional symptoms as well as broader distribution. Acutely inflamed joints warrant arthrocentesis both to eliminate crystal-induced arthritides and to rule out the possibility of infectious arthritides.

Once the diagnosis of osteoarthritis is established and its chronic nature is understood by the patient, one critical therapeutic aspect is to adopt a functional approach in assessing the effectiveness of subsequent interventions, both pharmaceutical and biochemical. Adequate pain management is an important initial feature and is best achieved through the use of routine analgesic preparations. While NSAIDs are commonly used for this purpose, there is no evidence to demonstrate their effectiveness over direct analgesics either in providing better pain relief or in modifying the outcome of the disease process. Corticosteroids, either given orally or injected directly into the affected joints, may play a specific role in crystal-induced osteoarthritic processes but have not been shown otherwise to be of any protective or enhanced therapeutic value. Future pharmacologic innovations involving strategies to enhance cartilage repair in affected joints may offer the hope of more targeted, specific interventions to alter disease progression.

Nonpharmacologic management has most frequently centered on techniques to relieve the weight-bearing load across the affected joint. The association between obesity and osteoarthritis has most clearly been demonstrated with osteoarthritis of the knees, hips, and, interestingly, the hands. Although weight reduction in itself can be anticipated to improve symptomatic osteoarthritis in such joints, an additional consideration to ensure better biomechanics and joint alignment may be necessary. The use of splinting and bracing and improved toning and conditioning of the periarticular muscles to allow a better balance of forces exerted against the joint that is also being "unloaded" are also important. The role of weight-bearing exercise in osteoarthritis has been examined in some detail. Although the therapeutic benefits of exercise itself, isolated from other interventions such as weight reduction and muscle reconditioning, are poorly understood, in no instance has the osteoarthritis been worsened by modest regimens of appropriately supervised exercise. Longitudinal studies of runners have not shown worsening osteoarthritis of knees or hips when compared with age-matched more sedentary cohorts. Thus, moderate weight-bearing exercise should be encouraged.

Heat is often applied to the osteoarthritic joint, either by direct heat application or through diathermy using ultrasound or microwave transmission. These latter techniques allow much deeper penetration of heat beyond the 1-cm depth provided by surface heat, although the evidence supporting the subjective improvement many individuals feel through such heat applications is limited. Topical irritant products rubbed over the affected joint have been receiving increased application in osteoarthritic therapies because of their value in improving pain tolerance through enhanced substance P excretion in the central nervous system as well as their

TABLE 54–1. Differential Diagnosis of Osteoarthritic Joint Pain

Characteristic	Osteoarthritis	Rheumatoid Arthritis	Gouty Arthritis	CPPD	Systemic Lupus
Age of onset >40 yr	**** (Unless traumatic)	**	***	**	**
Sites of involvement					
MCP joints	*	****	*	*	**
PIP joints	**	***	*	*	****
DIP joints	****	*	*	*	*
Knee	***	**	*	****	**
Hip	***	**	0	**	*
First metatarsal	*	*	****	*	*
Symmetrical joints involved	**	***	*	**	***
Symptoms					
Morning stiffness	*	****	*	**	**
Pain with motion	***	*	*	**	**
Signs					
Nodules	0	****	**(Tophi)	*	0
Joint effusion	*	****	****	**	**
Synovial fluid					
WBC count	*	****	***	**	*
Crystals	0	0	**** (−birefringent)	**** (+birefringent)	0
Laboratory findings					
+ Rheumatoid factor	0	****	0	0	*
+ ANA	*	*	0	0	****
ESR elevated	*	****	***	**	***
Hyperuricemia	0	0	***	*	*
Hypercalcemia	*	0	*	***	0
X-ray findings diagnostic	**	***	0	***	0

* = infrequent to **** = frequent; 0 = absent.

ANA = Antinuclear antibody; CPPD = calcium pyrophosphate dihydrate deposition disease; DIP = distal interphalangeal; ESR = erythrocyte sedimentation rate; MCP = metacarpophalangeal; PIP = proximal interphalangeal; WBC = white blood cell.

relatively greater safety margin in comparison with systemic nonsteroidal or opiate preparations.

Should a combination of such conservative measures fail to provide adequate pain relief, especially at nighttime, to the osteoarthritic joint, surgical approaches are then considered, generally in the form of joint replacement. Results with arthroscopic approaches to revise ongoing cartilage destruction in the osteoarthritic joint or, alternatively, to stimulate new cartilage matrix formation have been disappointing. Appropriate patient selection and review of concomitant medical conditions that might otherwise affect a successful long-term surgical outcome are critical steps in assessing an individual for potential joint replacement because of osteoarthritis.

SUGGESTED READING

Hamerman D. Clinical implications of osteoarthritis and aging. Ann Rheum Dis 1995;54:82–85.

Jones A, Doherty M. Osteoarthritis. Br Med J 1995;310:457–460.

Moskowitz RW, Howell DS, Goldberg BM, Manken HJ: Osteoarthritis: Diagnosis and Medical/Surgical Management, 2nd ed. Philadelphia, W.B. Saunders, 1994.

Puett DW, Griffin MR. Published trials of nonmedicinal and noninvasive therapies for hip and knee osteoarthritis. Ann Intern Med 1994;121:133–140.

Sack KE. Topics in primary care medicine: Osteoarthritis—a continuing challenge. West J Med 1995;163:579–586.

1. True or False: Osteoarthritis is characterized by the following initial pathologic findings in the joint space:
   a. Cartilage destruction
   b. Osteophytic "spurring" at the margins of the joints
   c. Gram-negative diplococcal microorganisms in the synovial space
   d. Birefringent crystals in the synovial fluid
   e. Extremely low glucose concentrations in the synovial fluid
2. The association between osteoarthritis and the normal aging process is best characterized as
   a. Normal aging of all joints inevitably involves osteoarthritis.
   b. Repetitive abnormal range of motion or stress of a joint, especially weight bearing, may contribute to the development of osteoarthritis.

c. Older men have a much greater incidence of osteoarthritis than older women.
d. Increasing inflammatory response associated with older age makes osteoarthritis more common.
3. In addition to the reduction in weight-bearing load across the osteoarthritic symptomatic joint, treatment of obesity may improve osteoarthritis by allowing:
   a. Better absorption of the crystal deposition within the synovium
   b. Improved joint alignment with better muscular tone
   c. Higher doses of nonsteroidal anti-inflammatory medications to be administered
   d. Better heat penetration of local warming into the joint capsule

Answers appear on **page 606.**

Chapter 55

Skin Papule

Shelley Roaten, Jr., M.D.

INITIAL VISIT

Subjective

PATIENT IDENTIFICATION. Marla A. is a 48-year-old white woman and homemaker who complains of a skin lesion.

PRESENTING PROBLEM. During a vacation to a beach resort on the Atlantic coast last month, Mrs. A. noticed a growth on the right side of her face after it bled when she washed her face. Two weeks ago, she applied hydrocortisone cream to the lesion for several days, with no apparent response.

PAST MEDICAL HISTORY. Mrs. A. has had no surgery or serious illnesses, and takes no medications rou-

tinely. About 6 years ago she had a forehead laceration repaired after a sailing accident. She had no acne in adolescence or adulthood.

FAMILY HISTORY. Mrs. A.'s father was a cattle rancher and real estate broker who died of injuries due to a tractor accident at age 60. She recalls that her father was treated for "skin cancers" several times before his death. Her mother is in good health at age 69. Her brother is an investment banker in good health at age 51, and she has two healthy children in college.

HEALTH HABITS. Mrs. A. drinks small amounts of alcoholic beverages occasionally and does not smoke. Two years ago, she and her husband began walking 2 miles each day and reduced dietary fat and cholesterol. Mrs. A. sometimes remembers to use a sunscreen during her summer vacation trips, but rarely wears a hat or gloves. She recalls a few episodes of blistering sunburn during childhood. Her last Pap smear and breast examination were performed about 8 months ago.

SOCIAL HISTORY. Mr. and Mrs. A. both enjoy outdoor activities including gardening and fishing. For many years they have met another couple for an annual summer vacation at the same beach resort, and they usually have a skiing trip in Colorado or Utah. They also play tennis and bridge with friends.

REVIEW OF SYSTEMS. Mrs. A. can recall no recent changes in the use of skin or hair products other than changing to a milder bath soap. She has a tendency to develop dry skin, particularly in the winter months, and uses a moisturizing cream as needed. She reports no changes in activities, appetite, weight, or sleep patterns.

Objective

PHYSICAL EXAMINATION. Mrs. A.'s vital signs are within normal limits. She is neatly dressed and has tanned skin. On her right face anterior to the pinna there is a solitary, firm, well-circumscribed, reddish-tan, nontender papule 5 mm in diameter with a smooth "pearly" margin and a 2-mm serous crust. Tiny superficial telangiectatic vessels are noted. Pigment variations on her forehead and malar areas and scattered telangiectasias on her nose and cheeks are suggestive of previous sun damage. There are no palpable lymph nodes in any location, and the remainder of the examination is normal.

LABORATORY TESTS. None were done at this visit. A chemistry profile obtained at the previous visit 8 months ago was entirely normal.

Assessment

WORKING DIAGNOSIS

Basal cell carcinoma.

DIFFERENTIAL DIAGNOSIS. The solitary nodule on her face could be any of several lesions, either malignant or benign. Features suggestive of nodular basal cell carcinoma include discrete borders, smooth pearly surface, crust, and superficial telangiectatic vessels. Squamous cell carcinoma often presents as a firm, erythematous papule or nodule in sun-damaged areas, typically with indistinct borders and hyperkeratotic scale but no telangiectasia. Bowen disease presents more often as a large plaque greater than 1 cm across than as a papule or nodule. Bowen disease on glabrous skin is probably best thought of as "squamous cell carcinoma in situ" and is thus distinguished histologically. A keratoacanthoma is a benign (although ugly and fast growing) tumor that may occur in this location, but it is typically bud-shaped or dome-shaped with a central keratinaceous plug, occasionally with ulceration. Sebaceous hyperplasia may resemble basal cell carcinoma, but closer examination should reveal multiple lobules emptying into a central dimple and a yellowish color. A pigmented basal cell carcinoma could be confused with a nevus or melanoma, especially in the absence of telangiectasia and ulceration.

Plan

LABORATORY AND SPECIAL TESTS. If a solitary skin tumor is not recognized as a benign lesion with certainty, the prudent response is complete removal of the lesion and histologic examination. Although other treatments can be used, complete excision of the lesion, followed by suture removal in about 3 to 5 days, is the method with which most family physicians are experienced. Excision is particularly important when the differential diagnosis includes melanoma. Properly done, excisional biopsy provides an excellent specimen for the pathologist and an acceptable cosmetic result. In most cases in which pathologic examination confirms that the entire tumor mass has been removed, the excisional biopsy results in diagnosis as well as cure for basal cell carcinoma. No additional diagnostic testing is necessary at this time.

PATIENT EDUCATION. At least the following issues should be discussed:

1. General wound care and suture removal, and discussion of the pending histologic examination.

2. Protection from sunlight and prompt attention to any new lesions or evidence of recurrence.

DISPOSITION. Sutures are removed 4 days later from a wound that appears to be healing well, and the biopsy confirmed the diagnosis of basal cell carcinoma and the absence of tumor cells at the margins of the specimen.

With her usual enthusiasm, Mrs. A. is eager to discuss options for protection from further sun damage. She expressed some embarrassment that this problem had never occurred to her in view of her other efforts to maintain good health habits. Since her usual outdoor activities are important to Mrs. A. and her husband, both have already begun using protective clothing and a topical sunscreen labeled with a sun protective factor (SPF) of 30. She is advised to use a waterproof sunscreen formula when swimming or exercising, and to limit the duration of sun exposure between 10:00 A.M. and 4:00 P.M.

DISCUSSION

Basal cell carcinoma (BCC) is a malignant tumor that arises from the epidermis and its appendages. It is the most frequently encountered cancer in humans, with an incidence about four times that of squamous cell carcinoma of the skin.

PATHOPHYSIOLOGY AND EPIDEMIOLOGY. Almost all victims of BCC are white, particularly fair-skinned individuals prone to sunburn. Higher incidence is noted in those of Scandinavian, Scottish, and Celtic origin. As occurs for squamous cell carcinoma, the incidence is directly related to exposure to ultraviolet radiation. Men are slightly more often affected than women, which may correlate with the relative likelihood of chronic sun exposure. Incidence increases sharply after age 40. Tumors are most common on the face and neck, with highest frequency on the nose.

While fair complexion and sunlight are the most significant predisposing factors, other causes are known. There is an association with prior injury at the site where a tumor arises, such as trauma, burns, vaccination, and x-irradiation. As with squamous cell carcinoma and Bowen disease, BCC is linked to prior exposure to inorganic arsenic in well water, insecticides, herbicides, and medicinal preparations. When related to arsenic exposure, the tumors tend to be multiple and truncal. Immunocompromised states also increase risk, although not as much as with squamous cell carcinoma. BCC is associated with several genetic syndromes including albinism, xeroderma pigmentosum, Rasmussen syndrome, and the basal cell nevus syndrome. Families with the basal cell nevus syndrome tend to have onset of BCC before age 20 and higher rates of other malignancies. Unlike the relationship between actinic keratoses and squamous cell carcinoma, there is no antecedent clinical lesion for BCC. Since causation is multifactorial, however, BCC is commonly found in the midst of actinic keratoses and other signs of ultraviolet light injury.

There are several types and subtypes of BCC described, based on clinical appearance and histology, but nomenclature is not standardized. The most common type is nodular BCC; other types include morpheaform BCC and superficial erythematous BCC, and variations. All contain both dermal and epidermal histologic elements on biopsy. Some subtypes have been shown to have higher rates of recurrence after surgical excision, which has been attributed to subclinical extension beyond the margins of the specimen.

Basal cell carcinoma is known for its capacity for local tissue destruction and propensity for recurrence after treatment. Distant metastasis, however, rarely occurs; one review reported fewer than 200 histologically proved cases of metastasis (Fitzpatrick et al., 1993). When it occurs, metastasis favors the lung.

CLINICAL FEATURES. Since clinical appearance and histology can vary, biopsy for pathologic examination is essential. The lesion most easily recognized by appearance is nodular BCC. This type of BCC presents as a waxy, pearl-colored or translucent nodule or papule with overlying tiny telangiectasias. Lesions are often found in an area where there is other evidence of sun damage, but that is not essential to the diagnosis. As the tumor grows, it has a tendency to develop ragged central ulceration, historically dubbed a "rodent ulcer." Growth patterns vary, and even small lesions can have significant depth and extension, especially when located around the nose, ears, or eyes. Mild erythema may be noted. Pigmentation may also occur, leading to potential difficulty in clinical distinction from melanoma or a nevus.

Superficial BCC appears as a nondescript (but persistent or growing) erythematous macule or patch. Pigmentation may be present, and there is sometimes a superficial fine scale. Distribution favors the trunk and extremities, rather than the face or neck, and this is the type of lesion often associated with arsenic exposure. Another variant of BCC is referred to as morpheaform or sclerosing, which has a scarlike appearance. These are difficult to treat owing to their indistinct borders and propensity for extensive tissue invasion.

The usual growth pattern of BCC is slow but persistent. This indolent behavior may lull the victim into delaying treatment, thus increasing the likelihood of subtle local extension and recurrence after treatment. The highest rate of recurrence after removal results from lesions on the nose, followed by other facial locations, with lowest risk on the trunk and extremities. Whether or not the relative risk relates to the degree of difficulty of aggressive treatment in facial locations is undetermined.

THERAPY AND PREVENTION. Goals in management of basal cell carcinoma include identification of risk factors, removal with a good cosmetic result, surveillance for additional lesions or recurrence, and reduction of future risk. History should be sought related to ultraviolet exposure, previous x-ray treatments (such as those once used for acne), arsenic exposure, immunosuppression, and genetic syndromes. Treatment options include sharp excision, cryosurgery, ionizing radiation, electrosurgery with curettage, and Mohs micrographic surgery. The choice is influenced by many factors, including location of the lesion, age and condition of the patient, desired cosmetic result, and access to health care providers trained in each of the procedures.

The highest likelihood of complete cure is obtained with Mohs microscopically directed surgery. Disadvantages of the Mohs technique are the expense, time requirements, and limited availability of those trained to do it. It is indicated for recurrent tumors, for primary lesions in difficult locations such as the nasolabial folds and orbital canthi, and for lesions greater than 1 cm in diameter on the head. Recurrence rates are approximately 1 per cent with the Mohs technique.

Skillful sharp excision is the method most familiar to family physicians and probably produces the best cosmetic result. Ionizing radiation, cryosurgery, chemosurgery, and electrosurgery with curettage are alternatives employed primarily by dermatologists. Rates of local recurrence with these techniques are similar, about 7 to 10 per cent after 5 years.

Patients should be advised about the possibility of recurrence or additional lesions, and should report any nodularity or other departures from the normal maturation of scar tissue at the site of removal. Since ultraviolet radiation is the most common modifiable risk factor, advice should be given regarding sun avoidance, chemical and physical sunscreens, and protective clothing. Fortunately, the use of arsenic in medicines, insecticides, and herbicides has declined in the United States, but remote past exposure or exposure in another country may still be pertinent. Advice about well water is appropriate in areas where arsenic contamination is known to exist. Individuals with one of the genetic syndromes may gain additional protection from regular surveillance, including periodic detailed skin photography.

SUGGESTED READING

Arndt KA, LeBoit PE, Wintroub BU. Cutaneous Medicine and Surgery. Philadelphia, WB Saunders, 1996, pp 1387–1391.

Fitzpatrick TB, Eisen AZ, Wolff K, et al. Dermatology in General Medicine. New York, McGraw-Hill, 1993, pp 840–847.

Friedman RJ, Rigel DS, Kopf AW, et al. Cancer of the Skin. Philadelphia, WB Saunders, 1991, pp 35–73.

Kruflik MD, Janniger CK. Basal cell carcinoma. Am Fam Physician 1993;48:1273–1276.

Weber RS, Miller MJ, Helmuth G. Basal and Squamous Cell Skin Cancers of the Head and Neck. Baltimore, Williams & Wilkins, 1996.

QUESTIONS

1. An actinic keratosis is an antecedent lesion of
   a. Basal cell carcinoma
   b. Melanoma
   c. Keratoacanthoma
   d. Squamous cell carcinoma
   e. Merkel cell carcinoma

2. Distant metastases are least likely to result from
   a. Basal cell carcinoma
   b. Squamous cell carcinoma
   c. Superficial spreading melanoma
   d. Intraductal breast carcinoma
   e. Hepatoma

3. True or false: Chronic sunlight exposure is a risk factor for the development of
   a. Melanoma
   b. Keratoacanthoma
   c. Actinic keratosis
   d. Basal cell carcinoma
   e. Squamous cell carcinoma

Answers appear on **page 606**.

Chapter 56

Eczema

Samuel T. Coleridge, D.O.

INITIAL VISIT

Subjective

PATIENT IDENTIFICATION. George C. is a 57-year-old white man and geology professor at the local university. He has been married for 32 years to the same spouse in a very supportive relationship with two grown children.

PRESENTING PROBLEM. George is concerned that a pruritic rash has developed over the dorsum of his right hand and fingers during the past 3 to 4 weeks. The skin has now become crusted, weeping, red, and infected.

He also explains that the skin overlying both knees is cracking and bleeding. He has applied petroleum jelly to both skin areas with minimal relief. He mentions that he has been more actively gardening during the past week while on vacation and that squatting and stooping on his knees have exacerbated the problem.

PAST MEDICAL HISTORY. George had surgery 12 years ago for a ruptured appendix and 5 years ago for an incarcerated right inguinal hernia. A precancerous skin lesion identified during this hospitalization was removed from his forehead by a dermatologist after discharge. He remembers being told that he had asthma as a child and took oral medication periodically with relief of symptoms until adolescence when he no longer required treatment. He recalls having recurrent episodes of dry, scaling skin as a child at various locations, including beneath his eyes, behind his ears, in his antecubital fossae, on his wrists, and in his popliteal fossae.

George describes no specific allergies but explains that he is sensitive to strong soaps and cannot tolerate antiperspirants.

FAMILY HISTORY. George's father was a garage mechanic who died of lung carcinoma at age 75. He smoked several packs of cigarettes per day for many years. He had no other known medical problems. His mother was a homemaker and died last year at age 74 from heart failure. George recalls that his mother always had problems with her hands and wore gloves when doing housework. Her skin would be red, scaling, and dry or crusted, oozing, and cracked. She only occasionally saw a physician and self-treated with hand cream, petroleum jelly, and applied dressings. She sometimes applied these same treatments to him.

HEALTH HABITS. George does not smoke and drinks two to three beers per week, usually with dinner. During the week, George tries to spend 1 to 2 hours per day in his 2-acre vegetable and flower garden and 4 to 8 hours per day on weekends. While gardening and when traveling, he usually wears a moderately rimmed hat, uses no sun protection, applies insect repellent, and is careful not to eat fresh, uncooked foods and local drinking water when traveling out of the country. George sometimes wears gloves when outdoors, but his hands are frequently in the soil or touching rocks, plants, or flowers. He does not have a family physician and has not had a complete physical examination, including digital rectal examinations, guaiac stool, electrocardiogram, chest x-ray study, or blood examinations for the past 5 years. Since George's parents did not see a physician regularly, he has not seen the necessity to make appointments with a physician when he had no significant medical complaints.

SOCIAL HISTORY. George loves being outdoors. He tries to work in his farm yard every day regardless of the weather. He feels he is very active and has no physical complaints except for his skin problems. He and his wife regularly enjoy annual 2-week vacations in the Southwest United States, Mexico, or

Central America hiking, exploring for rocks, and collecting mineral specimens for his university classes. George enjoys reading and maintaining his privacy. He does not make friends easily. His wife sells cosmetics outside the home by appointment and he describes her as more of an extrovert. Neither George nor his wife participates in any sport regularly, but they do dine at various restaurants once weekly either alone or with their next-door neighbors.

REVIEW OF SYSTEMS. George feels well and describes no changes in activity, appetite, weight, or sleep patterns. He identifies no changes in stool size, color or composition, but does note some terminal dribbling with urination. He has no respiratory symptoms, chest discomfort with activity, or musculoskeletal complaints.

Objective

PHYSICAL EXAMINATION. George's vital signs are within normal limits, including blood pressure 122/74 mm Hg, regular pulse 68, weight 134 lbs, and height 5 feet 6 inches. General examination is unremarkable, including a normal rectal examination and negative guaiac stool test. He is casually dressed, has dark brown and gray hair, cut short, with mild male-pattern baldness and thinning on his crown; his eyes are dark brown, and his skin is tanned. Inspection of the skin reveals a smooth, dark-tanned scalp; a forehead that is furrowed with two areas of ill-defined, light brown, slightly erythematous, scaly macules 3 × 6 mm and 4 × 7 mm above the left eyebrow and left temple, respectively. His eyelids are greasy and slightly scaly. Prominent on the dorsum of his right hand is an excoriated, crusted erythematous rash covering approximately one third of the surface with cracking at the index and middle proximal interphalangeal (PIP) joints, and slight warmth. There is excoriation of the web space between the index and middle as well as middle and ring fingers and some dry, scaling skin on the thenar eminence of the palm of the right hand. The palmar surface of his left hand also displays a mild scaling, dry, plaque-type rash overlying his hypothenar crease. His chest, abdomen, and back are untanned and show a definite tan line along his neck and upper arms. Of particular note were lichenification of both pretibial areas with cracking and crusting of his right knee with erythema and slight edema noted. The remainder of his skin examination was normal. His fingernails and toenails

were normal except for some apparent onychomycosis of his great toenails bilaterally.

LABORATORY TESTS. A urinalysis and prostate-specific antigen (PSA) level are obtained before the digital rectal examination, and a chemistry profile, electrocardiogram (ECG), and chest x-ray study are ordered because of the previously described family history.

Assessment

WORKING DIAGNOSIS. There are three presumptive diagnoses that may explain George's skin abnormalites:

1. *Actinic keratoses.* Irregularly shaped scaly macules that can be identified on sun-exposed areas (head, face, ears, dorsum of hands) are characteristic of active (solar) keratoses resulting from cumulative overexposure to ultraviolet light.

2. *Eczematous dermatitis (with secondary infection).* The clinical picture of recurrent and chronic scaling, serous exudates, excoriation, erythema, and fissures that is site dependent varying with age, best describes this disease spectrum. In infants, eczematous lesions can appear on the face, scalp, and extensor aspects of the extremities. In childhood, papules, erythema, and thickened skin usually appear on flexor surfaces including the wrists and neck. In adults, flexor surfaces, such as the neck, scalp and chest frequently have scaly, lichenified and erythematous lesions. The patient or family member often describes a history of hay fever, asthma, allergic rhinitis, or similar skin manifestations. Breaks in the skin at any stage can allow normal skin bacteria such as staphylococci or streptococci to cause a localized infection, which can progress to cellulitis if left untreated.

3. *Lichen simplex chronicus.* Well-circumscribed plaques with lichenified or thickened skin due to chronic scratching, rubbing or irritation, such as on the pretibial area, can become an end stage for chronic eczema or can be isolated to the posterior neck, dorsum of the feet, and ankles without the typical history of eczema.

DIFFERENTIAL DIAGNOSIS. The cause for the skin disruption on George's hands and knees is probably established by his history of atopy, long history of recurrent site-specific dermatitis, and response to treatment. This patient's disease could be confused with psoriasis, lichen planus, or contact dermatitis and he is at an increased risk for other skin manifestations and disease complications, such as impetigo or cellulitis, dermatophytoses, candidiasis, or some type of cutaneous drug reaction.

1. *Psoriasis.* One of the most common skin diseases, affecting 1 to 2 per cent of people, psoriasis is a chronic inflammatory disorder characterized by erythematous, sharply demarcated papules and rounded plaques, covered by a silvery scale. The most common areas involved are the elbows, knees, scalp, hands, and feet. On the hands, sterile pustules may be present and scaling is most marked on areas of pressure where painful fissuring can occur. Most patients eventually demonstrate nail thickening or punctate pitting. The characteristic sharp margination of these skin lesions with dry plaques that tend to fissure on slight pressure, the normal prolonged course of the psoriatic lesions, and the frequent nail changes differentiate this diagnosis from George's symptoms.

2. *Lichen planus.* An uncommon disorder frequently involving the mucous membranes, oral mucosa or genital area, as well as the skin, lichen planus is principally observed on the flexor surfaces of the wrist, arms, and trunk. The characteristic polygonal, flat-topped, violaceous papules are pruritic. The nails frequently show involvement and could be mistaken for this patient's apparent onychomycosis. Although George also experienced some pruritus in his hands, his skin lesions on the dorsum and palm of his right hand are slightly edematous, erythematous, vesicular and crusted, which distinguishes them from the isolated papules of lichen planus which demonstrate a characteristic purplish sheen when observed from a 45 degree angle.

3. *Contact dermatitis.* This is most frequently seen on exposed areas of the skin, for example, face, neck, hands, and forearms, and is due to contact with an external agent. Primary irritant contact dermatitis due to irritant compounds such as acids, alkalies, kerosene and other industrial agents demonstrates skin reactions within 24 hours. Allergic contact dermatitis normally occurs 48 hours or several days after sensitization and can result from contact with plants such as poison ivy, primrose, chrysanthemum, sap from trees, citrus fruits, or onions and other vegetables. The severity varies greatly from simple erythema and scaling to severe bullous erythematous eruptions and erosions. Pruritus can be severe and result in the linear excoriation so characteristic of poison ivy dermatitis. These episodes are usually identified by an attentive history, and the lesions persist for short periods of time and respond to appropriate drying agents and corticosteroids. They should not recur, as in George's case, unless the skin is reintroduced to the offending agent. Contact dermatitis that is not treated and becomes chronic can lead to eczema, which by definition is a chronic skin disorder often exacerbated by other acute and chronic skin eruptions.

4. *Impetigo.* Impetigo contagiosa due to streptococcus or staphylococcus organisms is a superficial skin infection highly contagious among newborns in nurseries and young children but less so in adults. The characteristic vesicopustule or bulla of impetigo ruptures to form the yellow-brown, honey-colored crust. Trauma due to rubbing or scratching can lead to deeper erosions or ulceration (ecthyma). George's eczema does indeed appear to demonstrate a complicating or secondary bacterial infection, which often is due to β-hemolytic streptococci or *Staphylococcus aureus.* Culture is usually not necessary for diagnosis before treatment with local débridement, soaks, and topical or oral antibiotics.

5. *Dermatophytosis.* Fungi that infect the skin, hair, and nails include members of *Trichophyton, Microsporum,* and *Epidermophyton.* The annular lesions of tinea corporis (ringworm) demonstrate peripheral erythema and a dry, central clearing with scales. Tinea manus can demonstrate variable erythema, edema, scaling, and pruritus in the web spaces of the fingers but would be unusual for this patient unless his hands were chronically exposed to a wet environment and a dermatophyte. George did not demonstrate the ringlike appearance of ringworm on his hands or knees. These locations would be very uncharacteristic for tinea unless the patient were severely immunocompromised, in which case he would be expected to demonstrate widespread lesions on his trunk and extremities.

6. *Cutaneous drug reactions.* The variety of morphologic patterns seen in drug eruptions includes widespread exanthematous reactions (32 per cent), urticaria and angioedema (20 per cent) as well as both widespread or localized fixed drug reactions (34 per cent), erythema multiforme (2 per cent), Stevens-Johnson syndrome (1 per cent) exfoliative dermatitis (1 per cent), and photosensitivity reactions (3 per cent). Fixed drug reactions can result in localized pruritus with a sharply demarcated, erythematous lesion that becomes hyperpigmented after repeated episodes of acute inflammation due to rechallenge by the allergen. Sulfonamides, tetracycline, and barbiturates are examples. Lichenoid

drug reactions, indistinguishable from lichen planus, are associated with gold, antimalarials, and antihypertensives including β-blockers and captopril. Although George traveled to Mexico and Central America, he never took prophylactic antimalarial medications.

DIAGNOSTIC. The small elevated, reddish scaling area on George's forehead, combined with a previous history of actinic keratoses in the same area, removed by a dermatologist 5 years previously, strongly suggests the same diagnosis. These areas could be treated with liquid nitrogen, or with topical applications of 5-fluorouracil (5-FU) cream. Biopsy is certainly an alternative if the depth of the skin lesion suggests a more serious diagnosis.

Scrapings of dried skin and debris from the hand and knees can be Gram stained for streptococci and staphylococci and a potassium hydroxide preparation can be tested for hyphae, which are often not present with inflammatory tinea corporis. A culture is often required for tinea if a definitive diagnosis is desired. Additionally, if treatment is entertained for the presumed mycotic toenail infection, small clippings or scraping of the affected nails placed in culture media can provide a more definitive diagnosis before beginning treatment with ketoconazole, griseofulvin, or the more expensive but more effective itraconazole.

THERAPEUTIC. Treatment and management of George's chronic eczema include eliminating irritants to his hands, treating the secondary infection with antibiotics, enhancing hydration to his hands and knees, treating acute flares with topical steroids and/or tar preparations, and providing antipruritics as needed to prevent further irritation to the already damaged skin.

George is given hydroxyzine (Atarax) 25 mg three times daily to reduce both his pruritus and anxiety about the chronicity of his disorder. He is also given oxacillin 500 mg three times daily to treat the early cellulitis of his right hand. Finally he is prescribed a jar of 1% triamcinolone in Aquaphor for both its anti-inflammatory and moisturizing effects. He is directed to apply this twice daily to his knees and three times daily to his hand after showering or soaking them in warm water for 15 to 20 minutes.

PATIENT EDUCATION. At least the following issues should be discussed with George and a patient handout or pamphlet provided. An excellent, comprehensive example is *Medfacts* on the Internet, which is also available by calling Lung Line (1-800-222-LUNG), or from the National Jewish Center for Immunology and Respiratory Medicine.

1. Avoid irritation to your hands and knees by minimizing the use of soaps, solvents, and other drying agents. Purchase inexpensive cotton garden gloves when working outdoors and wash them periodically.

2. Recognize that emotional stress may correlate with acute flares of your eczema and attempt to deal with these issues, as well as using the oral and topical medications provided to prevent more severe manifestations of the eczema.

3. Keep your hands clean but do not frequently wash your hands. Your skin is dry not because it lacks oil or grease but because it fails to retain water. After showering or soaking your hands in moderately warm water for 15 to 20 minutes, apply the triamcinolone with Aquaphor after mildly patting your hands dry. This retains the water in your skin and allows the steroid to decrease the inflammation and itching.

4. Realize that there are other treatments available if our current approach is not as successful as desired. Ultraviolet light therapy, oral corticosteroids, antibiotics, or other medications to control itching may be needed in the future.

5. Finally, this is a bothersome skin condition that can be managed effectively by you if you fully understand about eczema. I am willing and eager to assist you in managing this chronic skin disorder.

FOLLOW-UP VISIT

Subjective

George returned 1 month later and is very excited about the improvement of his eczema. He and his wife agree that he will pay more attention to his health. He accessed the Internet article and has written down several questions he would like answered. He has decreased his outdoor activities about 1 hour less per day but regularly wears cotton garden gloves (he purchased three new pair).

Objective

Nearly all the fissures, weeping, and crusting on George's hands are gone. He has only mild scaling on his left palm and dorsum of the right hand with mild to moderate scaling and mild erythema on his right palm. His knees are smooth but thickened. His facial and nail lesions remain unchanged. Findings on George's ECG, chest radiograph, and urine and blood chemistries are discussed. All are within normal limits.

Assessment

1. Eczema, marked improvement on both hands; mild improvement on both knees

2. Multiple actinic keratoses on forehead requiring treatment

3. Onychomycosis of both great toenails requiring treatment

Plan

DIAGNOSTIC. No further diagnostic measures are planned or requested by the patient.

THERAPEUTIC. A new prescription for Aquaphor is given as maintenance to be used twice daily. This hydrophobic base, when applied after the skin has been bathed, prevents further water loss and can replace the steroid mixture unless his symptoms become more acute. A topical preparation of 5-FU cream (Efudex) is selected for the actinic keratosis. George is instructed to apply a thin film twice daily to only the affected areas. George elects to delay treatment for his great toenails until he has resolution of his actinic keratoses.

PATIENT INSTRUCTION

1. The expected inflammatory response to 5-FU is discussed with George as well as caution to avoid his normal skin and mucous membranes. Other potential side effects are discussed.

2. Sunscreen protection is again discussed; employing more frequent work-rest cycles to protect from overuse of the hands in outdoor work is stressed; and repeated discussion is given to emphasize avoidance of irritant soaps and solvents with proper hygiene of the hands and hydration followed by application of the Aquaphor.

3. Switching to triamcinolone with Aquaphor for 3 to 5 days when scaling becomes more than double that seen in his current condition is also offered.

DISPOSITION. A follow-up visit is scheduled in 2 to 3 weeks to evaluate the response to 5-FU and to discuss the management strategy for the eczema.

Discussion and a handout regarding nail mycotic infections are planned for George's next visit.

DISCUSSION

Eczema is best described as the end stage of an unrelenting chronic dermatitis marked by reddening, epidermal thickening (acanthosis), scaling, and lichenification as opposed to an acute dermatitis that regresses rapidly. Eczema is a descriptive term for a variety of inflammatory diseases, including atopic dermatitis, allergic contact and irritant contact dermatitis, dyshidrotic eczema, nummular eczema, lichen simplex chronicus (neurodermatitis), asteatotic (xerotic or winter itch) eczema, and seborrheic dermatitis. All these conditions are associated with intraepidermal edema (spongiosis), demonstrated clinically as vesiculation.

The three stages of eczema include (1) *acute:* erythema, epidermal edema or vesiculation and oozing or crusting; (2) *subacute:* erythema, lichenification, patches, plaques, scaling, and signs of excoriation; and (3) *chronic:* erythema, marked lichenification and hyperkeratosis (scaling), epidermal thickening (acanthosis) and postinflammatory hypopigmentation or hyperpigmentation. These stages often overlap in the same patient but suggest the degree of progression of the inflammatory dermatosis.

When one is seeking a cause for the symptoms and manifestations of eczema, it is worthwhile to briefly review the history of atopic dermatitis, the acute disease most commonly associated with eczema. This disease was first named neurodermatitis to explain the pruritus as a nervous causation. Then the term "atopic dermatitis" was proposed to explain the frequency of patients demonstrating bronchial asthma, allergic rhinitis, eczema, some food or drug reactions, and occasionally gastrointestinal allergies and urticaria. Increased serum concentrations of IgE were noted in many of these patients.

The basic feature of atopic dermatitis is a pruritic dermatitis with a relapsing course. The distribution and morphology of the lesions vary with age. Eczematous lesions on the head and neck are prominent during infancy, whereas children and adults usually have lichenified lesions on the popliteal and antecubital areas. Other characteristics are xerosis of the skin, unusual lichenification, increased palmar markings, and Dennie-Morgan infraorbital folds. Many patients demonstrate one or more abnormal vascular markings such as pallor, white dermatographism following trauma to the epidermis, and occasionally abnormal response to heat and cold. The diagnosis is usually based on history, appearance, and distribution of skin lesions.

Genetic inheritance is clear. Between 50 and 75 per cent of atopic dermatitis patients have a family history of atopic eczema; 50 per cent have a history of respiratory allergy, 37 per cent have a history of allergic rhinitis, 17 per cent provide a history of bronchial asthma, and 13 per cent have a history of both rhinitis and asthma. Atopic dermatitis is separated into three age-related subgroups which include infantile (less than 2 years), childhood (2 to 12 years), and adult (greater than 12 years) eczema.

Infantile atopic dermatitis usually starts between 2 and 6 months of age with exudative papulovesicular eruptions, excoriations, and crusts on the cheek and forehead. Later the extensor aspects of limbs and sometimes the buttocks, thighs, and anogenital regions are involved. The irritant contact dermatitis from urine by-products (ammonia) in the infant's diaper can be differentiated from the *Candida* diaper rash with which it is often coexisting or confused. Childhood eczema is characterized by severe itching and papules or vesicles with secondary lichenification on the flexor folds at elbows and knees and often on both flexor and extensor surfaces of the wrists and neck. In adults, confluent

papules and large areas of lichenification can be identified anywhere on the body, particularly in the antecubital and popliteal fossae. Nummular distribution and localized hand eczema are common in adult eczema. The hands are affected in 20 to 60 per cent of all eczematous patients. Hand eczema is the most common dermatologic disorder encountered in occupational dermatology. Atopic skin appears to have a reduced resistance to irritants and consequently individuals with atopic dermatitis have a tendency to develop hand eczema. Aggravation of the eczema by wet and dirty work may force a job change. Hand lesions improve considerably in patients changing to clean, dry work.

Eczema encompasses a spectrum of disorders that begin as an acute inflammatory atopic dermatitis, often with a history of characteristic skin lesions in infancy and childhood plus childhood asthma or respiratory ailments leading to a chronic inflammatory lichenification and discoloration of the skin found in the adult stages.

Treatment through avoidance of irritants, stress reduction, and removal from allergies; application of hydrating lotions, tar preparations, and topical steroids; administration of antipruritics as well as antibiotics for secondary infection; and even utilization of ultraviolet light are available to be used separately or in combination to control this irritating and often disabling disease.

SUGGESTED READING

Altekrueger I, Ackerman AB. Eczema revisited: A status report based upon current textbooks of dermatology. Am J Dermatopathol 1994; 517–522.

Isselbacker KJ, Braunwald E, Wilson JD, et al. Harrison's Principles of Internal Medicine, 13th ed. New York, McGraw-Hill, 1994.

MedFacts. Treatment for eczema/atopic dermatitis [web page]. August 1996; http://www.njc.org/MFhtml/ECZ_MF.html

Oranje AP. Development of childhood eczema and its classification. Pediatr Allergy Immunol 1995; 6 (Suppl 7):31–35.

Rystedt A. Hand eczema and long-term prognosis in atopic dermatitis. Acta Derm Venereol Suppl (Stockh) 1985; 117:9–59.

Zug KA, McKay M. Eczematous dermatitis: A practical review. Am Fam Physician 1996; 54:1243–1250.

QUESTIONS

1. Match the following typical physical findings of eczema with the appropriate age-related subgroup in items (1) through (5).
   a. Infantile atopic eczema
   b. Childhood eczema

   c. Adult eczema
   (1) Severe pruritus and vesicles with thickening of skin on flexor surfaces of elbows and knees.
   (2) Confluent papules and multiple large areas of

lichenification especially in antecubital and popliteal fossae.

(3) Nummular distribution and localized hand eczema is common.

(4) Exudative papulovesicular eruptions, excoriations, and crusts on cheeks and forehead.

(5) Excoriations and papulovesicular eruptions on exterior aspects of limbs, buttocks, and anogenital area.

Answers appear on **page 606**.

Chapter 57

Acne

Michael A. Altman, M.D.

INITIAL VISIT

Subjective

PATIENT IDENTIFICATION. Rebecca L. is a 16-year-old white high school student who complains of longstanding complexion problems.

PRESENTING PROBLEM. Rebecca has experienced much emotional anguish about her facial complexion since the age of 12. She feels like a social outcast. She has otherwise enjoyed good physical health and identifies herself as a student in the top of her class academically. She admits to eating chocolate on occasion but otherwise watches a "strict diet." She says her "zits" make her feel dirty and washes her face with cosmetic astringents. She has tried a number of over-the-counter treatments without much improvement.

PAST MEDICAL HISTORY. Rebecca has had no surgery performed nor major illnesses. She remembers having skin problems as a child and was diagnosed with atopic dermatitis which cleared by 5 years of age.

FAMILY HISTORY. Rebecca's father is a chair manufacturer and is 52 years old. Her mother is a full-time homemaker and sells children's books. Rebecca has a sister 2 years younger who also has some trouble with skin complexion. No significant problems with acne or other skin problems run in the family. The rest of the family history is negative.

HEALTH HABITS. Rebecca is a nonsmoker. She denies any substance abuse and drinks only nonalcoholic beverages. She exercises and enjoys swimming. She always wears a sunscreen with a sun protection factor of 15 when outdoors.

MEDICATIONS. None.

SOCIAL HISTORY. Rebecca is a junior in high school in Houston, Texas. She enjoys school and plans to go to college. She has never been sexually active. Rebecca enjoys camping and skiing. She loves animals and helps out at a local veterinarian's office. She would like to have a boyfriend like her popular sister.

REVIEW OF SYSTEMS. Rebecca does not use cosmetics except "skin cleansers" for her face. She washes her skin with Dove soap. She describes her weight as average. She denies hair growth on her face. Menarche was at age 13 and her menstrual periods have been regular 26- to 28-day cycles.

Objective

PHYSICAL EXAMINATION. Rebecca's vital signs are all within normal limits. Her height is 65 inches and her weight is 115 lb. She is nicely dressed and has a fair-skinned complexion with brown eyes and long brown hair. She is wearing no makeup. Her face has multiple whiteheads with fewer blackheads involving her forehead and approximately 10 papules involving the malar and chin areas. No perioral involvement is identified. No nodules nor cysts are present. Some redness around one of the papules is identified and on questioning she admits trying to squeeze one of her pimples. Fortunately, no scarring is identified and her back and chest appear free of acne. The remainder of her examination is normal.

LABORATORY TESTS. None were done at this visit.

Assessment

WORKING DIAGNOSIS. Acne vulgaris. This is based on the characteristic appearance of open and closed comedones in addition to acne papules.

DIFFERENTIAL DIAGNOSIS

1. *Perioral dermatitis.* This is an eruption of discrete papules and pustules symmetrically distributed around the mouth. It is usually seen in women above the age of 20 and its cause is unknown.

2. *Acne cosmetica.* Cosmetics that contain lanolin, vegetable oils, lauryl alcohol, butyl stearate, and oleic acid are comedogenic. This form of acne slowly resolves with discontinuation of the offending agent.

3. *Rosacea.* This is a facial disorder characterized by telangiectasia, erythema, and papules/pustules. Comedones are *not* found. The nose, cheeks, and forehead are usually involved. It is a disease of adults involving more women than men and is most common between the ages of 30 and 50.

4. *Gram-negative folliculitis.* Usually present in long-time acne sufferers who have been treated with protracted courses of antibiotics. Most patients are men between the ages of 18 and 30. Diagnosis is by culture of the pustule and treatment is with a sulfa antibiotic, such as trimethoprim-sulfamethoxazole.

5. *Steroid acne.* This can be seen in individuals who use potent topical steroids. Patients taking oral steroids can develop acne 3 to 6 weeks after starting treatment and characteristically have papules and pustules on the trunk, shoulders, and arms.

6. *Underlying endocrinopathy.* Cushing disease, polycystic ovary disease, and hirsutism are often present with acne.

Plan

DIAGNOSTIC. In this case, the examination makes the diagnosis. No laboratory tests are needed. Since the differential diagnoses reflect the exceptions, our diagnosis of acne vulgaris is simple. Essentially all forms of acne (from minor whiteheads to disfiguring nodules and cysts) are forms of acne vulgaris. The terms acne and acne vulgaris are used synonymously in this chapter.

TREATMENT. Rebecca is started on a sequential regimen of tretinoin (Retin A) 0.05% cream and benzoyl peroxide 5% wash. She is instructed to use tretinoin alone the first 2 weeks. The first week she is advised to use tretinoin on alternate days and the second week to use it daily. Tretinoin should be restricted to bedtime use only. After tolerance to tretinoin is achieved, benzoyl peroxide 5% wash is added and Rebecca is to apply it to her face each morning before school and before dinnertime. She is advised to apply these topical medications to her entire face, not just on acne eruptions or acne-prone areas. She is advised to wash her face with water only to minimize skin dryness.

PATIENT EDUCATION

1. Acne skin eruptions afflict everyone at some time in their lives. Acne is an inflammatory condition and it is not anyone's fault for having it. It is not because a person is "dirty" or practices poor hygiene.

2. Frequent washing and scrubbing can do more harm than good.

3. Diet plays no known role in promoting acne—eating chocolate, drinking milk or sodas, and eating fried foods have nothing to do with acne.

4. Patients with oily skin should wash their skin with a mild, unscented soap (Dove, Neutrogena) and water.

5. Cosmetics can be comedogenic. When using them, select water-based makeup only. Heavy oils or dyes in cosmetics and hair sprays may worsen acne.

Cosmetics should be removed with gentle cleansing after use.

6. No medication is free of side effects. In Rebecca's case, Retin A is a photosensitive drug and is very drying to the skin. She is congratulated on using a sunscreen. A written calendar is also provided to show her how to use both medicines, with instructions to phone the nurse if she has any questions.

7. As Rebecca gets older, she will most likely find her acne to be much less of a problem and perhaps nonexistent with an occasional flare. It is important for her to avoid picking or squeezing her "zits," as it will only make her complexion problems worse and risk scarring.

DISPOSITION. Rebecca is advised to return to the office in 1 month to monitor medication compliance, answer any questions she might have from her last visit, and see how she is coping with her acne. She understands it will be too early to see marked improvement, which will take a total of 2 to 3 months before her treatment response can be assessed. We may spend more time on self-esteem issues than her acne, as this is an equally important issue.

FOLLOW-UP VISIT

Subjective

At her 1-month follow-up visit, Rebecca reports that she has not noticed any change except during the first days of tretinoin use, at which time she experienced a burning sensation to her skin. This got better over time. She is now using tretinoin and benzoyl peroxide.

We spent more time talking about issues of self esteem and feelings about herself, her sister, and her parents. She also admits to an "emotional roller coaster" with her body's changes (breast development, menstrual periods, skin complexion, and labile moods).

Objective

Rebecca's face has fewer whiteheads and blackheads. Papules are without change. No redness of the skin is present, and her skin appears to be tolerating the topical medicines well.

Assessment

Acne vulgaris with mild improvement.

Plan

DIAGNOSTIC. No laboratory screening is needed.

THERAPEUTIC. No change in treatment is made. Rebecca will begin oral tetracycline therapy next month if her papules show little or no change.

PATIENT EDUCATION. Acne can be successfully treated. Patience is the key to any satisfactory outcome. Realistically, cure takes months rather than weeks, depending on severity of the acne.

Physician comment. Acne interferes with social functioning such as sports, dating, and eating out. Understanding the negative impact of acne on social interactions is best achieved through the use of open-ended questions. Physicians treating acne should be sensitive to the psychological needs of these patients since their academic, social, and vocational needs may be adversely affected.

DISPOSITION. Rebecca is scheduled to return in 1 month with subsequent office visits at 2- to 3-month intervals. A referral is made for Rebecca to see one of our psychologists for additional counseling.

DISCUSSION

Rebecca's diagnosis of acne vulgaris is a very common problem. Acne is the most common skin disease of adolescents and is estimated to affect 80 per cent of individuals between 11 and 30 years of age (Bergfeld and Odom, 1995). It is more prevalent and severe in boys than girls, although acne seems to affect girls at an earlier age.

Acne can occur at any age. Newborns can develop acne—acne neonatorum—during the first 6 months, which can persist up to 12 months. This is thought to result from androgens made by the fetal gonads and adrenal glands. This is usually self-limiting and requires no treatment. Insufficient data are available to predict acne outcomes in later years based on the development of newborn acne alone (Thiboutot and Lookingbill, 1995).

Severe acne strikes most commonly in adolescence—a time when emotional, hormonal, and physical changes make the individual especially vulnerable to psychological distress. It is during adolescence that individuals expend large resources on doctors.

Acne may reflect a whole spectrum of disease. Misconceptions about acne are widespread and unfortunately are not limited to the public, but include primary care physicians and dermatologists. Acne vulgaris has long been thought to be a disease beginning at puberty; however, the basic lesion, the comedo, makes its appearance as early as 8 years old (Kligman, 1995a).

The pilosebaceous unit consists of sebaceous glands and a keratinized canal through which sebum may flow. If a sebaceous gland becomes plugged with sebum, duct obstruction follows. The tiniest form of acne vulgaris, the microcomedo, may go undetected without further investigation. Under androgenic hormonal influence (testis, ovary, adrenal), sebaceous glands enlarge and sebum production increases. Like a volcano, sebum moves up the follicular canal. Abnormal keratinization and hyperkeratosis of follicular epithelium also occurs and leads to duct obstruction. The "capped volcano" has its appearance as a "whitehead" or closed comedone. When the "cap" comes off, the exposed sebum is oxidized. The oxidized sebum together with melanin and densely packed keratinocytes gives it a black appearance (Nguyen and colleagues, 1994). This is the "blackhead" or open comedone. Thus the blackhead's color comes from oxidation of the sebum and is not dirt, as is popularly believed.

Complicating this dynamic process is the presence of an anaerobic diphtheroid bacterium, *Propionibacterium acnes*. Other microorganisms coexist either on the skin surface (e.g., *Staphylococcus epidermidis*) or just within the top portion of the follicle (e.g., the yeast *Pityrosporum*). However, only *P. acnes* plays a central role in the inflammatory component of acne. How does this happen? *P. acnes* survives in the duct by releasing lipases to break down sebum into glycerol and free fatty acids. The glycerol acts as fuel for the bacterium to grow. The free fatty acids along with other bacterial enzymes initiate destruction of the keratinized duct wall. *P. acnes* also releases neutrophil chemotactic factors which attract the body's neutrophils to engage in an all-out assault on the duct wall. Together, these forces result in the inflammatory and destructive form of acne: papules, pustules, nodules, cysts, and finally sinuses under the skin.

Treatment of acne is therefore based on understanding this disease process and attacking each of these components (Berson and Shalita, 1995; Leydon, 1995):

1. Overproduction of sebum

2. Abnormal degeneration and destruction of the sebaceous follicle

3. Proliferation of *P. acnes*

4. Inflammation

The pilosebaceous unit and the body's attack on the duct wall in acne is shown in Figure 57–1.

Treatment

Minor Acne

Blackheads and whiteheads, or acne vulgaris, is best treated with tretinoin (Retin A). Topical tretinoin is a preparation of vitamin A and is the *only* universally accepted topically applied comedolytic agent available. It works by loosening follicular impactions and reduces keratin-containing material trapped within the follicular duct (Sykes and Webster, 1994). Tretinoin is available in different strengths and vehicles—the mildest formulation is 0.025% cream, followed by 0.05% and 0.1%. Use the cream for those individuals with dry skin or who live in dry environments. The gel form (0.01% and 0.025%) should be reserved for individuals who have excessively oily skin or live in humid environments. Due to its irritating effect, it is advisable to use the least potent concentration to achieve desired results. At bedtime after washing the face, a fine film should be applied over the entire face, not just the areas where visible comedones exist.

Benzoyl peroxide is a potent bactericidal agent.

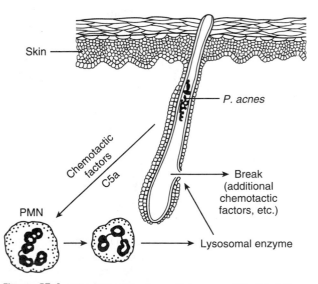

Figure 57-1. The pilosebaceous unit in acne. (Modified from Shalita AR, Lee WL: Acne. Dermatol Clin 1983;1:361–364.)

Its indication for comedones is not universally accepted, and it may actually be comedogenic (Kligman, 1995b). However, it is probably one of the most underrated acne-fighting drugs on the market due to its relatively cheap price and over-the-counter availability. It has the greatest bacteriostatic activity of compared antibiotics. Twice-daily application for 5 days reduced *P. acnes* populations by more than 95 per cent (Kligman, 1995b). Benzoyl peroxide preparations range between 2.5% and 10% concentrations and are found in creams, soaps, washes, and gels. Again, the lowest concentration should do well for most patients. Benzoyl peroxide also has the advantage of not sensitizing patients against antibiotics and contributing to the present problem of microbial drug resistance.

Inflammatory Acne

Benzoyl peroxide is indicated primarily for acne characterized by inflammatory lesions resulting from rupture of closed comedones. In addition, commonly available prescription antibiotics include erythromycin, and tetracycline or its derivative, clindamycin. The advantage of antibiotics is that not only do they provide antimicrobial activity against *P. acnes* but they also have anti-inflammatory properties. Therefore, combination therapy becomes the best defense against this form of acne.

Possible regimens may include:

1. Topical tretinoin and topical benzoyl peroxide

2. Topical tretinoin and topical antibiotic

3. Topical tretinoin, topical antibiotic, and topical benzoyl peroxide

TOPICAL ANTIBIOTICS

1. Clindamycin phosphate (Cleocin T) 1% gel, solution, or lotion

2. Erythromycin 2% gel, lotion, solution, pads (EryDerm, Emgel, Erycette)

3. Tetracycline 0.22% solution

4. Metronidazole 0.75% gel

5. Erythromycin 3% plus benzoyl peroxide 5% (Benzamycin) gel

All antibiotics are applied twice daily except for metronidazole, which is used once daily. Topical tetracycline and metronidazole are not commonly used for acne management. They are used mostly in the treatment of rosacea.

Benzoyl peroxide may be dosed either once or twice daily. *Very important*: benzoyl peroxide should not be applied simultaneously with topical tretinoin, as it will be ineffective.

Acne that is poorly responsive to topical therapy may show marked improvement with oral antibiotic therapy, especially with potent lipophilic antibiotics.

ORAL ANTIBIOTICS

1. Tetracycline in patients 12 years of age and older. Starting dose is 250 mg four times daily or 500 mg twice daily. Use should be avoided with dairy products, iron, or antacids, which decrease its absorption. This class of drugs increases susceptibility to sunburn, so a good sunscreen should be worn if outdoors.

2. Doxycycline, a tetracycline derivative, is more effective, and is dosed 100 mg once daily. It has greater anti-inflammatory activity but is a little more expensive.

3. Minocycline is the most costly tetracycline and is dosed 50 mg twice daily or 100 mg once daily. It has the ability to penetrate into the sebaceous gland and achieves higher follicle concentration in its class.

4. Erythromycin is dosed 500 to 1000 mg per day in divided doses. It enjoys the advantage of being nonphotosensitizing, but can cause gastrointestinal upset and therefore should be taken with food.

ISOTRETINOIN (ACCUTANE). Finally, one drug remains the best hope for cure in severe acne that is resistant to previously mentioned therapies. The drug is isotretinoin (Accutane) and in addition to the other acne drugs, it is indicated specifically for the treatment of nodulocystic acne and acne associated with scarring. It, however, is a double-edged sword: it is a known teratogen causing hydrocephalus, microcephaly, other neurologic impairments, and cardiovascular deformities. It is also very expensive to use (medication and laboratory costs). Accutane is a vitamin A derivative and is dosed at 0.5 to 1.0 mg/kg per day over 20 weeks. It may be used early on if scarring is present or if less than 50 per cent improvement is found after three consecutive courses of antibiotics.

If isotretinoin therapy is planned, initial laboratory screening should include a complete blood count, serum chemistries, liver enzymes, cholesterol, and triglycerides with monthly monitoring until treatment is discontinued. Women of childbearing age should have an initial serum pregnancy test

I.   Open or closed comedones - use tretinoin (Retin A). Can consider benzoyl peroxide, but it may be comedogenic.

II.   Inflammatory acne (everything else)

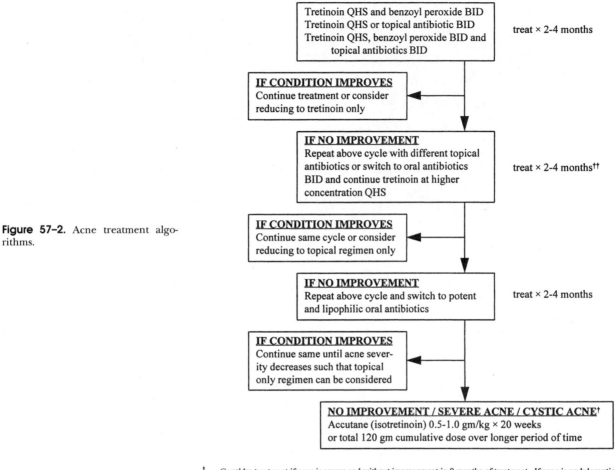

Figure 57–2. Acne treatment algorithms.

Tretinoin QHS and benzoyl peroxide BID
Tretinoin QHS or topical antibiotic BID
Tretinoin QHS, benzoyl peroxide BID and topical antibiotics BID

treat × 2-4 months

IF CONDITION IMPROVES
Continue treatment or consider reducing to tretinoin only

IF NO IMPROVEMENT
Repeat above cycle with different topical antibiotics or switch to oral antibiotics BID and continue tretinoin at higher concentration QHS

treat × 2-4 months[††]

IF CONDITION IMPROVES
Continue same cycle or consider reducing to topical regimen only

IF NO IMPROVEMENT
Repeat above cycle and switch to potent and lipophilic oral antibiotics

treat × 2-4 months

IF CONDITION IMPROVES
Continue same until acne severity decreases such that topical only regimen can be considered

NO IMPROVEMENT / SEVERE ACNE / CYSTIC ACNE[†]
Accutane (isotretinoin) 0.5-1.0 gm/kg × 20 weeks
or total 120 gm cumulative dose over longer period of time

[†] Consider treatment if acne is severe and without improvement in 9 months of treatment. If acne is nodulocystic or with the presence of scarring - initial treatment with Accutane may be indicated. Referral to a dermatologist may be appropriate at this time. Also, before reaching this point, consideration of drug resistance should be entertained with possible culture of pustule for gram negative folliculitis.

[††] Oral antibiotics should be tried 4 to 6 months prior to calling them a treatment failure.

that *must* be negative before treatment is begun. Pregnancy tests should be performed monthly to ensure safety of continued treatment. In addition, a woman should provide both verbal and written consent to the use of this drug as a potent teratogen before its use. The drug should be started on the second day of a woman's menstrual cycle. Women should not try to conceive until they have been off isotretinoin for at least 1 month. Abortion is strongly recommended if accidental pregnancy occurs during this month.

The most common side effect is cheilitis, which can be managed with lip balm application. Other less common side effects are nasal irritation, dry skin, photosensitivity, headaches, and arthralgias. Pseudotumor cerebri may also occur.

Special Circumstances

On occasion, you will find a patient with an underlying endocrinopathy presenting initially as acne. Examples include Cushing disease, in which there is overproduction of the steroid cortisol and adrenal

TABLE 57–1. Costs of Acne Therapy*

Agent	Cost
Topical	
Tretinoin (45-gm tube × 2)†	$94.56‡
Clindamycin (60 ml × 6)†	$114.24‡
Erythromycin (60 ml × 6)†	$26.76‡
Benzoyl peroxide (42.5 gm × 2)†	$21.58‡
Benzoyl peroxide/erythromycin (23 gm × 4)†	$94.04‡
Systemic	
Tetracycline (500 mg × 2)§	$45.04‡
Erythromycin (500 mg × 2)§	$174.00‡
Minocycline (100 mg × 2)§	$1445.50‡
Isotretinoin	
Agent (70 mg × 1)§	$1326.75‖
Laboratory studies¶	
CBC/differential blood count	$150.00‡ ($25.00 × 6)#
Liver function tests	$186.00‡ ($31.00 × 6)#
AST	$111.60‡ ($18.60 × 6)#
Lipid profile tests	$116.40‡ ($19.40 × 6)#
Urine pregnancy tests (women)	$113.40‡ ($16.20 × 7)#
Consultation fees**	
Initial	$65.00‡ ($65.00 × 1)#
Follow-up	$250.00‡ ($50.00 × 5)#
Additional tests	
DHEAS	$72.50
Testosterone	$90.50
Androstenedione	$77.50

AST = aspartate aminotransferase; CBC = complete blood cell count; DHEAS = dehydroepiandrosterone sulfate.
*Pricing of pharmaceutical agents based on average wholesaler price listed in Red Book Update, Montvale, NJ, Medical Economics Co., June 1994.
†Unit size/no. units used per year.
‡One-year cost.
§Dose/times given per day.
‖Twenty-week cost.
¶Prices of laboratory studies based on national supplier of such services, June 1994.
One-time cost × no. of times performed during treatment.
** Consultation fees based on personal survey of clinicians, reporting to the average of the responses.
From Bergfeld W, Odom RB: Introduction. J Am Acad Dermatol 1995;32(5 Pt 3):S1.

androgens. In women, polycystic ovary disease (PCOD) may elaborate ovarian androgens. These women may exhibit obesity, menstrual irregularity, and hirsutism as clues to their underlying disorder. Hormonal therapy is currently restricted to women with either PCOD or simple virilization. Additional clues to these disorders include adult onset in women, acne flares before menses, excessive facial oiliness, and acne predominantly below the malar areas and jaw. These patients mandate screening for elevated levels of dehydroepiandrosterone sulfate (DHEAS) and serum testosterone (Berson and Shalita, 1995).

Hormonal therapy works at different sites, depending on the drug used. Birth control pills suppress ovarian androgen production by means of estrogen (50-μg doses of ethinyl estradiol or mestranol and low progesterone doses). Combination oral contraceptives that contain androgenic progesterone (e.g., norgestrel) should be avoided since these can worsen acne. Prednisone in low doses (5 to 10 mg every other morning) can also be employed for adrenal androgen suppression and for reduction of acne-associated inflammation. This drug is best used in women with elevated DHEAS levels but who are not hirsute (Sykes and Webster, 1994). The antiandrogens spironolactone and cyproterone may be new treatments for acne and hirsutism (Jurzyk et al., 1992). They work by blocking androgenic effects on target cells within the sebaceous glands and subsequently reduce sebum production. However, these drugs have not received Federal Drug Administration approval for this indication and are hampered by their side effects.

Figure 57–2 contains a flow diagram summarizing the treatment process for acne.

Cost of Treatment

Table 57–1 displays cost comparisons of various treatment modalities. Health care plans and diminishing health care dollars have forced us to examine cost considerations in acne treatment.

Prevention

Early intervention may save children at risk from the ravages of acne. One dermatologist (Kligman, 1995a) looks for:

1. One or both parents having seborrhea

2. One or both parents having shallow or deep acne scars

3. One first-degree relative having had adolescent acne

It is possible to screen for potentially severe acne before its visible appearance. One technique uses an adhesive tape (Sebutape) that is applied for 1 hour to the cleaned forehead, cheek, and chin and then removed. The representative strips trap sebum droplets and display a pore pattern which under the microscope reveals low or high sebum-producing skin. Those in the high sebum-producing group may benefit from treatment before the development of visible acne in the prepubertal patient (ages 7 to 8). Treatment consists of tretinoin (Retin A cream or gel), and treatment success is based on close follow-up and periodic Sebutape screens.

SUGGESTED READING

Bergfeld WF, Odom RB. Introduction. J Am Acad Dermatol 1995;32(5 Pt 3):S1.

Berson DS, Shalita AR. The treatment of acne: The role of combination therapies. J Am Acad Dermatol 1995;32(5 Pt 3):S31–41.

Jurzyk RS, Spielvogel RL, Rose LI. Antiandrogens in the treatment of acne and hirsutism. Am Fam Physician 1992;45:1803–1806.

Kligman AM. Acne vulgaris: Tricks and treatments. Part I: Cutis 1995a;56:141–143.

Kligman AM. Acne vulgaris: Tricks and treatments. Part II: The benzoyl peroxide saga. Cutis 1995b;56:260–261.

Layton AM, Cunliffe WJ. Guidelines for optimal use of isotretinoin in acne. J Am Acad Dermatol 1992;27(6 Pt 2):S2–7.

Leydon JJ. New understandings of the pathogenesis of acne. J Am Acad Dermatol 1995;32(5 Pt 3):S15–25.

Nguyen QH, Kim YA, Schwartz RA. Management of acne vulgaris. Am Fam Physician 1994;50:89–96, 99–100.

Sykes N, Webster G. Acne: A review of optimum treatment. Drugs 1994;48:59–70.

Thiboutot DM, Lookingbill DP. Acne: Acute or chronic disease? J Am Acad Dermatol 1995;32(5 Pt 3):S2–5.

QUESTIONS

1. True or false: Inflammatory acne includes
   a. Papules
   b. Pustules
   c. Cysts
   d. Open and closed comedones

2. True or false:
   a. Acne is caused by dirty skin or dirt particles entrapped in pores.
   b. Chocolate and milk worsen acne.
   c. Hair sprays may worsen acne.
   d. Acne only occurs in adolescence.
   e. Topical antibiotics are more effective in treating the organism *P. acnes* than benzoyl peroxide.
   f. The basic lesion of acne is the comedo.

Answers appear on **page 606.**

Chapter 58

Rash and Fever

Walter D. Leventhal, M.D.

FIRST VISIT

Kathy T. is 33-year-old white woman from Chicago who presents to her family physician in May with a 1- to 2-day history of flulike illness—headache, myalgia, nausea, and a temperature that has ranged between 100° to 101°F. About 10 days earlier, she and her husband went to their mountain cabin in North Carolina to clear out the underbrush. There she found a tick on her abdomen one evening, which she removed. The patient is briefly examined and antipyretics and antiemetics are prescribed. Over the next several days, her condition changes with the development swollen cervical glands and continued nausea and vomiting.

SECOND VISIT

Kathy returns to her physician. Examination fails to show any signs of pulmonary, cardiovascular or abdominal infection, and there is no hepatosplenomegaly. A diagnosis of a viral syndrome is made. A complete blood count (CBC) shows a hemoglobin of 11.3 gm/dl and a white blood cell (WBC) count of 9500/mm³; 65 per cent polymorphonuclear leukocytes, 30 per cent lymphocytes, and 5 per cent monocytes. Platelets are noted to be 90,000/mm³. The patient mentions the tick bite again but only supportive therapy is prescribed.

Within 36 hours Kathy's condition has worsened and her musculoskeletal pain has increased. The fever has persisted and she has developed a reddish–purplish macular rash on her forearms and legs. Overnight, Kathy's level of consciousness has diminished to the point that she does not respond to verbal stimuli. The rash has developed into purpura, some parts of which are palpable, spreading centrally to involve her thighs and trunk.

Kathy is immediately admitted to an intensive care unit with a presumptive diagnosis of sepsis of

uncertain cause. Her platelet count now is 9000/mm³, and her WBC count has risen to 26,500/mm³. Cultures are drawn and intravenous chloramphenicol and gentamicin are administered. She has begun to have seizures and has developed renal and hepatic failure. The patient became hypotensive and all resuscitative efforts failed. She died within 24 hours after admission.

An autopsy has determined her death to be due to disseminated intravascular coagulation (DIC), probably caused by rickettsial disease or meningococcemia. Cultures for meningococcus are negative and complement fixation titers and indirect fluorescent antibodies are negative for *Rickettsia* infection, but the diagnosis is later confirmed as *Rickettsia* by immunofluorescent staining of skin biopsies.

DIFFERENTIAL DIAGNOSIS

The combination of fever and rash present the practitioner with a difficult and common problem. Although many conditions may present initially with fever and rash, one can subdivide these by considering their potential severity, for example, life threatening or minor.

Life-threatening conditions associated with fever and rash include:

1. *Rocky Mountain spotted fever.* See diagnosis of Kathy's case in Discussion section.

2. *Meningococcemia.* Meningococcemia tends to occur in late winter and early spring and often in crowded conditions, for example, barracks or schools. The patient may present with petechiae initially on the trunk and extremities, but in fulminating cases petechiae can spread visibly over several hours. Shock and disseminated intravascular coagulation are associated clinical manifestations. Diagnosis is confirmed by Gram stain of skin lesions, blood

cultures, and spinal fluid examination. A chronic form of meningococcemia associated with rash has also been described.

3. *Disseminated gonococcemia.* There is a much higher incidence in women. The rash consists of pustules on an erythematous base, usually over the extremities. It is often associated with migratory polyarthralgia, arthritis, and pelvic inflammatory disease. Diagnosis can be confirmed by a Gram stain of the lesions, as well as culture and sensitivity of the blood, joint fluid, or cervical secretions.

4. *Toxic shock syndrome.* Toxic shock syndrome occurs in women predominantly, with the rash preceded by a flulike illness and diarrhea associated with mucus. The rash is macular, giving a sunburned appearance, and occurs over the whole body, but is seen predominantly on the hands and feet. The clinical presentation is that of multisystem involvement. The diagnosis is confirmed by history, physical examination, and isolation of a toxin-producing strain of *Staphylococcus aureus.*

5. *Bacterial endocarditis.* Bacterial endocarditis is often associated with a history of valvular heart disease, prosthetic valves, and recent dental or surgical procedures. The rash is petechial and associated with Osler nodes and Janeway lesions. The rash is found in the palate and upper chest, and may be present on the palms, fingers, soles, and toes. Presence of a heart murmur, splenomegaly, hematuria, and metastatic abscesses may be present. Diagnosis is by echocardiogram and serial blood cultures.

6. *Lyme disease.* Lyme disease is caused by exposure to ticks in endemic areas—Northeast, Midwest, or West—in the summer. The rash classically manifests as erythema migrans, often on the thigh, groin, or axillae. Clinically, the patient presents with a flulike syndrome, later developing central nervous system, cardiac, or joint involvement. The diagnosis is confirmed by history and serology.

The preceding differential diagnosis does not include many other minor conditions associated with fever and rash often found in children, that is, the viral exanthems associated with measles, chickenpox, roseola, rubella, and fifth disease (erythema infectiosum). One should also consider in this category the rashes associated with drug reactions, which also may be associated with fever.

DISCUSSION

This case illustrates many of the characteristics of Rocky Mountain spotted fever. Unfortunately, it also demonstrates the rapid course of the infection from the time of first exposure to the tick to prodrome and ultimately to fulminating multiorgan failure and shock when not recognized and treated.

The patient lived in Chicago, but had vacationed in North Carolina, and this particular area typifies the most common area of cases reported, that is, the South Atlantic, Southeastern, and South Central states. The name, Rocky Mountain spotted fever, is misleading because even though the condition has been reported in every state besides the Carolinas and Tennessee, Oklahoma is the state with the most other cases reported. A clue to the etiology is that the majority of these cases appear between April and late September, that is, the spring and the summer, which is when ticks are most prevalent. It also coincides with a period of time when people are active outdoors and, therefore, are more prone to exposure. The main vector for this condition is the American dog tick which transmits the offending organism, *Rickettsia rickettsii.*

After the tick has bitten its human host, organisms are usually disseminated through the blood stream during the first 6 to 12 hours when the tick is attached to the host. Attachment by the tick to the host is usually painless, and the tick is often only discovered accidentally at the end of the day when the patient undresses.

This patient also showed the initial symptoms, a flulike illness, fever, headache, myalgia, and sometimes vomiting within 4 to 20 days after being bitten.

Usually, the rash occurs on the fourth to the sixth day after the patient first complains of the systemic symptoms and begins on the wrist and ankles. It can then involve the palms and soles and later becomes more generalized. Initially, the rash is erythematous and macular but can become petechial if untreated. The rash is difficult to see in African Americans. It is also important to note that in approximately 15 per cent of cases, the rash does not develop. The infection is then referred to as Rocky Mountain spot*less* fever. The spotless type appears to be more common in adults.

The fact that systemic symptoms frequently develop before the rash is important in considering preventive and early treatment modalities. Rocky Mountain spotted fever should be suspected in any patient who presents with a flulike illness with headache and has been in the endemic areas, especially during the summer. When the patient gives a history of removing a tick, it should heighten the physician's suspicions even more. Unfortunately, in the case presented, despite the fact that the history of the tick bite was given repeatedly, it was ignored, with deadly consequences. The overall mortality for an untreated individual may be as high as 30 per cent. The mortality is usually higher for individuals who are 40 years or older and in African Americans. Most of the delays in initiating appropriate treatment result from failure to recognize the significance of the history of a tick bite in an endemic area.

The diagnosis must rely on a high degree of suspicion and on familiarity with the clinical presentation and the epidemiologic criteria for the area. This case also illustrates the importance of asking about and paying attention to a patient's history of travel and insect bites, especially when patients present with flulike illnesses in the summer. When this patient presented to her physician with a flulike illness, thrombocytopenia was noted but no intervention was initiated.

Laboratory diagnosis is usually confirmed serologically with fourfold increases or decreases in antibody titer between acute and convalescent sera by indirect immunofluorescence, complement fixation, indirect hemagglutination, or latex agglutination.

In practical terms, the decision to treat the patient with suspected Rocky Mountain spotted fever should not await the result of a laboratory test. Only on the very rarest of occasions is culture from blood or tissue obtained. Complement fixation and microagglutination tests are specific for the disease, but lack sensitivity especially if the patient has received antibiotic treatment. In the case described, confirmation of the diagnosis was obtained by immunofluorescent staining of the skin biopsy specimen.

Treatment in the early phases of the suspected illness is very effective. Drugs of choice are tetracycline, doxycycline, and chloramphenicol. In children younger than 9 years of age, it is generally recommended that tetracycline not be given routinely. The choice of using chloramphenicol for pregnant women and for children less than or equal to 8 years of age is generally recommended although some would argue that in weighing the benefits and risk, tetracycline would be the drug of choice for all children. Therapy is usually given for 6 to 10 days, or until the patient has been afebrile for 2 to 3 days. Given the widespread range of illnesses that can result from tickborne diseases, including Lyme disease, relapsing fever, ehrlichiosis, tularemia, tick fever and babesiosis, this case also provides an opportunity to consider the control of all tickborne infections.

Both physicians and the local communities should be aware of the prevalence of tickborne infections in their areas. The onset of spring should provide a reminder on an annual basis to promulgate precautions through the summer. Some specific suggestions include the following:

1. Widespread education especially in endemic areas by all the media from early spring through summer.

2. The avoidance of known tick-infested areas.

3. Use of protective clothing to cover the arms, legs, and other exposed areas.

4. Permethrin spray to decrease tick attachment may be employed and tick repellents containing diethyltoluamide (DEET) may also be used to limit exposure to ticks. Great care especially with children should be employed in using DEET-containing repellents.

5. Regular body checks for tick attachment by people who have been possibly exposed in endemic areas should be performed. Adults should inspect themselves and their children's bodies regularly for potential tick exposure. The more frequently this is done, the better. It is generally felt that the longer the tick remains attached, the higher the inoculum will be.

6. Tick removal should also be taught with an emphasis on removing all the mouthparts with curved forceps or tweezers and avoidance of squeezing tick body parts. A simple plastic tool called Ticked Off is now available. It consists of a small plastic spoon-shaped instrument with a V-shaped notch cut into the distal part of the spoon. If the mouthparts are placed in the notch, the tick and all its body parts may be removed with careful pressure and traction.

This case of Rocky Mountain spotted fever embodies many of the basic principles of modern family medicine, for example, the prevention of a serious illness, the ability to make an early, accurate diagnosis and provide effective treatment, and the opportunity to educate our patients and community.

SUGGESTED READING

American Academy of Pediatrics. 1994 Redbook: Report of the Committee on Infectious Diseases, 23rd ed. (Peter G [ed]) Elk Grove, IL: American Academy of Pediatrics, 1994, pp 114, 399–404.

Ferri F. The Internal Medicine Companion. St. Louis, Mosby–
Year Book, 1994.

Gubler D, Koster F, Legters L, et al. A Field Guide to Animal-
Borne Infections. Patient Care 1994;28(16):23–44.

Habif T. Clinical Dermatology, 3rd ed. St. Louis, Mosby–Year
Book, 1996.

Isselbacher K, Braunwald E, Wilson J, et al. Harrison's Principles
of Internal Medicine. Companion Handbook, 13th ed. New
York, McGraw-Hill, 1995.

QUESTIONS

1. Match each of the following rashes with the diseases
   in items (1) through (5).
   a. Erythematous macular papular lesions spreading
      centripetally (from feet to hands)
   b. "Slapped face," lacy reticular rash on forearms
      and trunk
   c. Sunburned rash with palmar and sole desquamation
   d. Pustules in an erythematous base, mainly on ex-
      tremities
   e. Expanding annular lesion with reddish outer ring
      and central clearing
      (1) Gonococcemia
      (2) Fifth disease (erythema infectiosum)
      (3) Staphylococcal toxic shock syndrome
      (4) Lyme disease
      (5) Rocky Mountain spotted fever

2. Appropriate treatment for a 10-year-old boy with presumed Rocky Mountain spotted fever would be:
   a. Chloramphenicol 250 mg four times daily for 10
      days
   b. Clarithromycin 250 mg twice daily for 10 days
   c. Tetracycline 250 mg four times daily for 7 to 10 days
   d. Amoxicillin 250 mg and clavulanic acid 125 mg
      every 8 hours for 10 days
   e. Cefalexin 250 mg four times daily for 7 to 10 days
      or until afebrile for 6 days

Answers appear on **page 606.**

Chapter 59

Obesity

Tomas G. Lumicao, Jr., M.D.

INITIAL VISIT

Subjective

Lloyd Z. is a 40-year-old white man, married and a
janitor; he is obese and first came to the clinic
because of pain in both knees that he has experienced for about 1 year.

PRESENT ILLNESS. Lloyd has had progressive pain in
both knees since 1 year ago. The pain is worse on
the left; he describes it as sharp and nonradiating,
as "if the bones are rubbing against each other."
He has morning stiffness and the pain gets worse
during the day. The pain is precipitated by putting
pressure on both knees and is relieved by rest. Ibuprofen (Advil) and aspirin provide temporary relief.
There is no recent history of trauma. He denies
fever, swelling, or redness of the knees. With his
job as a janitor, he has found it harder to do his
routine work.

PAST MEDICAL HISTORY. Lloyd had an uncomplicated appendectomy as a child. At about the age of 35, he was told by a physician that his blood pressure was high. He did not return for follow-up and very seldom saw a physician. He claims he is generally in good health and takes ibuprofen or aspirin for his knee pain.

FAMILY HISTORY. Lloyd's mother died at the age of 45 from ovarian cancer. His father died of a heart attack at the age of 55. He describes his parents as heavy-set. He is the eldest and has one sister. His sister is likewise heavy-set and has been diagnosed with adult-onset diabetes mellitus. His paternal grandfather died of a stroke in his seventies.

SOCIAL HISTORY. Lloyd has been a janitor in a firm for 10 years working usually on the night shift. He has been married for 14 years with two daughters ages 12 and 10. His wife works in a clothing factory during the day. He describes his family as a regular family, healthy and hard-working.

HEALTH HABITS. Lloyd has smoked a half to one pack of cigarettes per day for 15 years. He usually smokes at night to keep him awake. He occasionally drinks one to two beers on weekends while watching basketball or football games on television. On weekdays, he sleeps during the day. His family teases him about falling asleep easily and snoring loudly while "watching" television. He does not exercise, claiming that his work is exercise enough.

REVIEW OF SYSTEMS. He has occasional headaches and feels fatigue most of the time. He gets short of breath after one flight of stairs. He denies urinary or bowel problems.

Objective

PHYSICAL EXAMINATION. Lloyd's initial vital signs include heart rate of 86, blood pressure 150/104 mm Hg, respiratory rate of 22. His weight is 280 lb with a height of 5 feet 10 inches. Funduscopic examination shows no hemorrhages or papilledema. No carotid bruits are noted. The thyroid gland is not enlarged. Examination of the heart is unremarkable. Lung examination shows occasional rhonchus that disappears with coughing. Abdomen is soft, flat, obese, and nontender. There are no musculoskeletal deformities. Examination of the knees shows no swelling and no erythema, with equivocal effusion bilaterally. There is crepitation and tenderness underneath the patellae but he has full range of motion. Ligaments are intact. Gait is normal.

LABORATORY TESTS. A multiple-panel blood analysis is significant for the following: total cholesterol is 260 mg/dl, low-density lipoprotein (LDL) cholesterol is 165 mg/dl, high-density lipoprotein (HDL) is 30 mg/dl γ-glutamyltransferase (GGT) is 80 U/L; and random blood glucose (RBG) 170 mg/dl. The rest of the electrolytes and liver function tests are normal. Complete blood count (CBC) and urinalysis are likewise normal.

Bilateral knee series shows degenerative changes of the tibial tubercle bilaterally left greater than right, with osteophyte formation.

Plans on follow-up include fasting blood sugar (FBS), chest radiograph, electrocardiogram (ECG), and pulmonary function test.

Assessment

WORKING DIAGNOSIS

1. *Degenerative joint disease.* Osteoarthritis has increased prevalence with obesity. The knee seems to be the most frequently involved joint, most likely due to its weight-bearing function.
2. *Moderate obesity.* Lloyd's body mass index (BMI) is 38. Health risks related to obesity are elucidated further on in the Discussion section.
3. *Multiple coronary risk factors:*

   a. Hypertension.
   b. Hypercholesterolemia.
   c. Diabetes mellitus. Will confirm diagnosis with fasting blood sugar level. Sister with history of diabetes mellitus.
   d. Father died of heart attack at the age of 55.
   e. Smoking.

DIFFERENTIAL DIAGNOSIS

1. Other causes of bilateral knee pain

   a. Rheumatoid arthritis
   b. Gout

2. Secondary causes of obesity

   a. Neuroendocrine disorders
   b. Genetic disorders
   c. Drug induced

3. Secondary hypertension

   a. Cushing disease
   b. Renovascular hypertension

Plan

DIAGNOSTIC. The diagnosis of obesity is easy to make and does not usually require laboratory tests. Secondary causes of obesity are rare and screening tests are obtained only when clinically indicated.

The combined effects of smoking and obesity-related obstructive sleep apnea or restrictive defects increase Lloyd's risk of developing pulmonary disease. Polysomnography, pulmonary function test, and chest x-ray studies are in order. Case discussions of hypertension, arthritis, diabetes mellitus, hypercholesterolemia and obstructive pulmonary disease are covered as separate subjects in this text.

THERAPEUTIC. Lloyd is given a nonsteroidal anti-inflammatory drug (NSAID) to alternate with acetaminophen (Tylenol) for pain relief. Long-term treatment is weight reduction.

The therapy of obesity is challenging to both the patient and physician. It involves major lifestyle changes on the part of the patient. The different modalities are fraught with complications as well as limitations. There is no qualm as to the health benefits of reducing weight, but it is also clear that the majority of people who lose weight will regain it. Hence, reasonable goals and expectations should be laid out. A small (5 to 10 kg) to moderate weight loss is associated with health benefits related to a reduction in blood pressure, improvement of dyslipidemia, and better control of type II diabetes mellitus.

Before initiating a strict dietary program or regular aerobic exercise, it is important to check CBC, obtain a multiple electrolyte panel to check levels of magnesium and calcium, and to test for uric acid, glucose, and lipid profile. ECG with careful attention to QT interval is recommended. It may also serve as a baseline examination for Lloyd, who has multiple coronary risk factors.

Diet. Net loss of 3500 calories is equivalent to a 1-lb weight loss. A *Low-calorie diet* provides 1200 kcal per day. This is best suited to mildly obese patients and does not require close medical supervision. A *very low caloric diet (VLCD)* supplies only 500 to 800 kcal per day. Strictly followed, it results in an average weight loss of 3 to 5 lb per week regardless of exercise. Initiation of a VLCD should be preceded by a detailed medical evaluation. Close monitoring and at least weekly visits are recommended.

Behavior Modification. Behavior modification involves applying the principles of psychology to implement changes directed to reduce calorie intake and increase exercise. Self-instructional techniques, relaxation training, environmental programming (reducing the urge to eat by making food less accessible), assertiveness, and self-rewarding acts are behaviors that the patient learns to use to reduce food intake. Furthermore, psychotherapy is most helpful when obesity is related to emotional problems leading to overeating.

Activity. Regular aerobic exercise burns calories as well as reduces cardiovascular risk. It is a useful predictor of weight loss maintenance in conjunction with the other modalities. Swimming or biking are probably the best exercises for Lloyd, considering the problem he has with his knees.

Medication. The patient most likely to benefit from the use of appetite suppressant drugs are those with body mass indexes greater than 30, or greater than 27 if the patient has comorbid conditions such as diabetes, dyslipidemia, or hypertension and in whom nonpharmacologic measures were not successful.

Different drugs are used to suppress appetite. Amphetamine analogues and central serotonergic drugs have been shown to produce weight loss in short-term studies. The University of Rochester and Strong Memorial Hospital study on weight loss (1992) has concluded that a combination of two prescribed appetite suppressant medications has enabled obese patients to lose weight as well as maintain weight loss.

Primary pulmonary hypertension (PPH) has been associated with the use of all types of prescription weight loss drugs. The risk of PPH is estimated to be about 28 cases per 1,000,000 users of prescription weight loss drugs per year. The annual incidence of PPH in the general population estimated from one study is 1 case per 500,000 people. The corresponding risk for obese persons who use anorectic agents for more than 3 months is more than 30 times higher than for nonusers. In addition, tachyphylaxis associated with the use of many of these drugs develops, necessitating an increase in dose to achieve anorectic effect.

Dexfenfluramine is an important new drug, but it is not free from risks. Physicians and patients need to be informed that the possible risk of PPH associated with dexfenfluramine is small but real. Surveillance is necessary and patients are advised to report new or progressive dyspnea, chest pain, leg edema, or other symptoms of pulmonary hypertension.

A recent article by Connolly et al. at the Mayo Clinic reported 24 women who were found on echocardiogram to have unusual valvular disease after an average 12 months of therapy with fenfluramine and phentermine. The patients presented with signs and symptoms of dyspnea, palpitation, chest pain, and cardiac murmur. The histopathologic characteristics were identical to valvular heart diseases caused by carcinoid, ergotamine, or methylsergide. It is believed that the mechanism of valve injury is related to serotonin. The same article reported eight women who had newly documented pulmonary hypertension.

Fenfluramine and dexfenfluramine were voluntarily withdrawn from the market by their producers in September 1997. The true association between valvular disease and fenfluramine-phentermine will be further elucidated by prospective studies using control group or case-control studies.

Other drugs used to achieve weight loss are thyroid hormone preparations, which increase metabolic rate. They may, however, increase appetite and produce signs and symptoms of hyperthyroidism.

Ephedrine is an over-the-counter drug that may suppress appetite, but definitely increases heart rate and blood pressure and causes nervous system stimulation.

Surgery. Obese patients who manifest serious comorbid risks and have failed medical therapy are ideal candidates for surgical intervention. Only two procedures were recommended at the recent National Institutes of Health consensus conference on obesity, namely, vertical banded gastroplasty and roux-en-Y gastric bypass operation.

PATIENT EDUCATION

1. Lloyd is educated about the pathophysiology of obesity, its consequences, and the different modalities of treatment. He is initially concerned about his painful knees. He seems to accept his 'destiny' to be obese like the rest of his family. On discussion, he had a better understanding of the different complications of obesity as well as treatment options.

2. Assess Lloyd's motivation and commitment to

TABLE 59–1. Age-Specific Weight-for-Height Tables (Gerontology Research Center)*

Height	Weight Range for Men and Women by Age (years)†				
	25	35	45	55	65
ft-in	lb				
4-10	84–111	92–119	99–127	107–135	115–142
4-11	87–115	95–123	103–131	111–139	119–147
5-0	90–119	98–127	106–135	114–143	123–152
5-1	93–123	101–131	110–140	118–148	127–157
5-2	96–127	105–136	113–144	122–153	131–163
5-3	99–131	108–140	117–149	126–158	135–168
5-4	102–135	112–145	121–154	130–163	140–173
5-5	106–140	115–149	125–159	134–168	144–179
5-6	109–144	119–154	129–164	138–174	148–184
5-7	112–148	122–159	133–169	143–179	153–190
5-8	116–153	126–163	137–174	147–184	158–196
5-9	119–157	130–168	141–179	151–190	162–201
5-10	122–162	134–173	145–184	156–195	167–207
5-11	126–167	137–178	149–190	160–201	172–213
6-0	129–171	141–183	153–195	165–207	177–219
6-1	133–176	145–188	157–200	169–213	182–225
6-2	137–181	149–194	162–206	174–219	187–232
6-3	141–186	153–199	166–212	179–225	192–238
6-4	144–191	157–205	171–218	184–231	197–244

*Values in this table are for height without shoes and weight without clothes. To convert inches to centimeters, multiply by 2.54; to convert pounds to kilograms, multiply by 0.455.

†Data from Andres R. Gerontology Research Center, National Institute of Aging, Baltimore, Maryland.

Adapted from Pi-Sunyer FX. Obesity. In Wyngaarden JB, Smith LH Jr, Bennett JC (eds). Cecil Textbook of Medicine, 19th ed. Philadelphia, W.B. Saunders, 1992, p 1163.

institute and maintain treatment. Lloyd is averse to exercise and loves to eat. However, he is willing and motivated to undergo major lifestyle changes related to diet and exercise to alleviate his present health problems for himself and his family. He is anxious about a life-long "struggle" to improve and maintain a reasonable weight. At this point, he is not resolved to quit smoking.

3. The physician should suggest to the patient an appointment with other professionals, or a psychologist to lay out a clearer plan regarding diet, behavior modification, emotional problems, or exercise. Lloyd's continued support from his primary care physician is likely all he needs to lose some weight.

DISCUSSION

Obesity is defined as an excess of body fat that poses a health risk. Ideal weight for height is that weight at which longevity is the greatest (Table 59–1). The Framingham study demonstrated that a 20 per cent excess over desirable weight clearly increases health risks.

Several methods are used for classifying obesity (Table 59–2). Simple anthropometric measurements such as body mass index (BMI) (Table 59–3) and percentage overweight are commonly used. BMI is the ratio of body weight in kilograms to height in meters squared. Due to limited availability, tediousness and expense, body composition studies such as underwater weighing, dual photon absorptiometry, or dual x-ray absorptiometry are seldom performed in routine clinical practice.

Obesity is a challenging disorder often fraught with frustrations for both the patient and the physi-

TABLE 59–3. Classification of Severity of Obesity

Class	Body Mass Index	Percentage Overweight
Mild	27–30	20–40
Moderate	30.1–35	41–100
Severe	>35	>100

From Smith LG. Obesity. *In* Rakel RE (ed). Saunders Manual of Medical Practice. Philadelphia, W.B. Saunders, 1996, P 693.

cian. This is probably born of the multifactorial etiology of obesity ranging from the genetic to the environmental, socioeconomic, and psychological. Successful therapy is based on the patient's motivation to institute and maintain major lifestyle changes as well as continued support from his or her physician, nutritionist, physical fitness trainer, psychologist, and family members.

The prevalence of obesity increased by 8 per cent in the United States during the past decade. From 1980 to 1991, the nation's obesity rates have gone up from 25 to 33.4 per cent in adults over the age of 20, and it continues to rise. Data show that

TABLE 59–2. Classification of Obesity

Anatomic Methods
Size and number of
    adipocytes—hypertrophic, hyperplastic
Per cent body fat
Distribution of body fat—gynoid, android

Etiologic Methods
Neuroendocrine disorders
Excessive dietary intake
Obesity syndromes
Pharmacologic agents

From Apaorian CM, Jensen GL. Overnutrition and obesity management. In Kirby DF, Dudrick SJ (eds). Practical Handbook of Nutrition in Clinical Practice. Boca Raton, FL, CRC Press, 1994.

TABLE 59–4. Medical Complications Associated with Obesity

Gastrointestinal	Cardiovascular
Cholecystitis	Coronary artery
Cholelithiasis	disease
Hepatic steatosis	Congestive heart
Delayed orocecal	failure
transit time	Systemic hypertension
Endocrine/Reproductive	Malignancy
Type II diabetes	Colon
mellitus	Prostate
Hirsutism	Endometrium
Dyslipidemias	Gallbladder
Menstrual disorders	Cervical
Pre-eclampsia	Ovarian
Endometrial disorders	Musculoskeletal
Respiratory	Osteoarthritis
Sleep apnea	Gout
Obesity hypoventilation	
syndrome	
Erythrocytosis	
Respiratory tract	
infections	

Adapted from Apaorian CM, Jensen GL. Overnutrition and obesity management. In Kirby DF, Dudrick SJ (eds). Practical Handbook of Nutrition in Clinical Practice. Boca Raton, FL, CRC Press, 1994.

the average general weight of an individual in the general population in the United States gradually increases with age, and it is more marked in women than men. The prevalence of obesity is almost twice as high in black women than in white women. It is strongly related to a lower socioeconomic stratum. Obesity is the second leading cause of preventable death in the United States, exceeded only by cigarette smoking. The medical complications associated with obesity are enumerated in Table 59–4.

Obese patients usually seek consultation due to problems other than obesity. Lloyd's main reason for seeking medical help is his painful knees. Good history, however, unravels his other health risks. Lloyd's fatigue, excessive daytime sleepiness, and lack of energy are probably due to obesity-related obstructive sleep apnea. He has multiple coronary risk factors as mentioned in the assessment. The goals of successful therapy are to decrease food intake and increase physical exercise. These are important nonpharmacologic means for the control of obesity, hypertension, diabetes mellitus, and hypercholesterolemia.

It should be emphasized that even small amounts of weight loss are consistently associated with improvements in blood pressure, serum lipid values, and glucose tolerance.

The economic cost of obesity is likewise enormous. A recent study estimated the yearly costs of obesity and its complications at $40 billion or 5.5 per cent of total health care expenditures.

PREVENTION. The primary prevention for obesity has yet to be clearly defined. However, it is clear that such programs should begin at an early age. Children with a strong family history of obesity should learn good dietary habits and exercise at the family level. Secondary prevention of the health risks associated with obesity starts with the early recognition of being "overweight." The different modalities previously discussed, especially behavior modification, are recommended. In conclusion, increasing the public's awareness of obesity—its prevalence, health risks, and economic drain—is a worthwhile national project that may be beneficial in the prevention of this costly disease.

SUGGESTED READING

Apaorian CM, Jensen GL. Overnutrition and obesity management. In Kirby DF, Dudrick SJ (eds). Practical Handbook of Nutrition in Clinical Practice. Boca Raton, FL, CRC Press, 1994, pp 32–43.

Connolly HM et al. Valvular heart disease associated with fenfluramine-phentermine. N Engl J Med 1997;337:581.

Manson JE, Faich GA. Pharmacotherapy for obesity—do the benefits outweigh the risks? N Engl J Med 1996;335:659–660.

Pi-Sunyer FX. Obesity. In Wyngaarden JB, Smith LH Jr, Bennett JC (eds). Cecil Textbook of Medicine, 19th ed. Philadelphia, W.B. Saunders, 1992, pp 1158–1169.

Smith LG. Obesity. In Rakel RE (ed). Saunders Manual of Medical Practice. Philadelphia, W.B. Saunders, 1996, pp 693–695.

Wolfe GR, Trozzolino LA, Kern PA. Exogenous obesity: What actually works? Hosp Med 1993;29:112–119.

QUESTIONS

1. The following are health risks associated with obesity *except:*
   a. Cholelithiasis
   b. Prostatic cancer
   c. Gout
   d. Menstrual disorder
   e. Hepatic cancer

2. The following are acceptable therapeutic modalities for obesity *except:*
   a. Roux-en-Y gastric bypass operation
   b. Behavior modification
   c. Aerobic exercise
   d. Thyroid hormone

3. The most dreaded complication of anorectic medications is
   a. Hypertension
   b. Habituation
   c. Myocardial infarction
   d. Primary pulmonary hypertension
   e. Pedal edema

Answers appear on **page 606.**

Chapter 60

Type II Diabetes

Martin S. Lipsky, M.D.

INITIAL VISIT

Subjective

PATIENT IDENTIFICATION. Robert W., a 52-year-old African American auto mechanic, requests a routine checkup and treatment for hypertension.

PRESENT ILLNESS. Robert has not seen a physician since he lost his health insurance about 1 year ago. He recently started a new job and now that he has health insurance he is requesting a checkup. He takes hydrochlorothiazide for high blood pressure but ran out of his last refill about a month ago. In addition to his hypertension, his previous physician told him he was a borderline diabetic. Although he occasionally "cheats," he feels that he follows a healthful diet and is proud that he has kept off the 15 lb, that he lost after being told that his blood sugar was high. His only complaint is occasional fatigue, which he attributes to work and running out of his blood pressure medication.

PAST MEDICAL HISTORY. Robert has had no surgical procedures performed other than sutures for a hand laceration about 2 years ago. He denies any hospitalizations and his only medication is hydrochlorothiazide and an occasional ibuprofen for headaches. He has no known allergies to medications.

FAMILY HISTORY. Robert's father died in his sixties about 10 years ago of unknown causes. His mother is in her eighties and according to Robert gets around fairly well. He has one brother, age 59, who takes a "sugar pill" but is otherwise healthy.

SOCIAL HISTORY. Robert does not smoke. He drinks two beers about once a week during football season and denies ever using illicit drugs. He has been happily married for 30 years with three grown chil-

dren and six grandchildren. His wife does most of the shopping and cooking. Robert does not exercise regularly and although he gets a fair amount of exercise at work he would like to start an exercise program.

REVIEW OF SYSTEMS. Robert feels well except for occasional aches and pains that he attributes to aging. He denies any chest pain, shortness of breath, polyuria, or polydipsia. Before losing his insurance, Robert had regular checkups and routine health maintenance, including a normal flexible sigmoidoscopy. He wears glasses but has not seen his ophthalmologist for years.

PHYSICAL EXAMINATION. A general examination reveals a well-developed, well-nourished black male. Vital signs are blood pressure 140/100 mm Hg, pulse 72, respirations 12, and an oral temperature of 98.1°F. Pertinent funduscopic findings include arteriovenous nicking, exudates, and copper-wiring. Cardiac examination reveals a regular rate and rhythm. S_1 and S_2 heart sounds are within normal limits and no murmur is appreciated. A faint S_4 heart sound is heard in the left lateral decubitus position. There is no evidence of edema and the peripheral pulses are easily palpable. The remaining physical examination is within normal limits.

LABORATORY TESTS. A fasting finger-stick blood sugar taken in the office is 177 mg/dl. A dipstick urine analysis and electrocardiogram are within normal limits.

Assessment

1. *Probable type II diabetes mellitus.* Robert gives a history of borderline diabetes and has an elevated fasting blood sugar level. Any one of three criteria is sufficient to diagnose diabetes mellitus: (1) a

random plasma glucose greater than 200 mg/dl associated with classic symptoms; (2) two fasting plasma glucose levels greater than 125 mg/dl; and (3) two plasma glucose levels greater than 200 mg/dl at either 1/2 or 1 hour and 2 hours during an oral glucose tolerance test. For whole blood glucose levels, these values are 10 to 15 per cent lower.

2. *Essential hypertension.* Robert's blood pressure level is consistent with mild hypertension. Typically, three separate elevated blood pressure readings above 140/90 mm Hg are needed to establish the diagnoses of hypertension. However, given Robert's previous diagnosis and treatment for hypertension, along with the presence of end-organ damage, it seems reasonable to accept Robert's previous diagnosis of hypertension.

DIFFERENTIAL DIAGNOSIS

1. *Type II diabetes mellitus.* Most often patients with type II diabetes are easily identified by routine glucose testing. A glucose tolerance test (GTT) is rarely necessary. The two most common indications for a GTT are to test pregnant patients and to establish the diagnosis in patients with clinical manifestations suggestive of diabetes such as a neuropathy who have plasma glucose levels that do not meet the diagnostic criteria for diabetes. Although most patients with elevated glucose levels meeting the criteria for diabetes have type II diabetes mellitus, secondary and reversible causes of hyperglycemia should be considered before establishing a permanent diagnosis of diabetes. Generally a thorough history and physical examination are sufficient to eliminate these considerations.

2. *Secondary diabetes.* Secondary diabetes results from hyperglycemia due to an underlying condition. Examples include pancreatitis or an infiltrative pancreatic process such as hemochromatosis. Hyperglycemia may also occur in association with endocrine diseases such as Cushing syndrome, pheochromocytoma, or acromegaly. In selected patients it may be worth pursuing these rare diagnoses. For example, a patient with hypertension, central obesity, muscle weakness, and striae merits an overnight dexamethasone suppression test to rule out Cushing disease. In Robert's case, there is no evidence to support testing for these uncommon illnesses.

3. *Reversible hyperglycemia.* Reversible factors such as infection, stress, or trauma may transiently cause hyperglycemia. Correcting these conditions may normalize or improve the glucose level. Patients undergoing the stress of surgery may also show transient blood sugar elevations that resolve postoperatively. An important reversible factor to consider is drug therapy. Some drugs that can cause hyperglycemia are the glucocorticoids, phenytoin, thiazide diuretics, oral contraceptives, and nicotinic acid.

Plan

DIAGNOSTIC. Fasting blood work including a fasting plasma glucose, complete blood count, glycosylated hemoglobin (HbA_{1c}), general chemistry panel, thyroid-stimulating hormone and lipid profile are ordered. In addition, since Robert wants to start an intensive exercise program he elects to undergo an electrocardiographic (ECG) stress test to screen for occult coronary artery disease.

PATIENT EDUCATION. Patient education materials discussing diabetes and hypertension are given and reviewed with the patient. In particular, the importance of diet and exercise are stressed.

THERAPEUTIC. Robert plans to be even more conscientious about watching his diet. A diet consisting of 50 to 60 per cent of calories from carbohydrates, 20 to 30 per cent of calories from fat with less than 10 per cent of calories from saturated fat, and 12 to 20 per cent of calories from protein is reviewed with the patient. Robert wants to see a dietitian to plan a diet that incorporates his own food preferences. Since his wife does the shopping and cooking for the household, Robert arranges for her to accompany him to this appointment.

Robert wants to resume hydrochlorothiazide for his blood pressure since this worked well previously. However, he is willing to try another medication once he learns that hydrochlorothiazide can elevate cholesterol and glucose levels. Angiotensin converting enzyme (ACE) inhibitors are the antihypertensive medication of choice in diabetes because of their benefits in preventing diabetic nephropathy. Robert is started on lisinopril (Prinivil, Zestril), an ACE inhibitor 5 mg once daily, and is scheduled back in 2 weeks for re-evaluation and a review of his laboratory results.

FOLLOW-UP VISIT

Robert returns 2 weeks later for follow-up and to review his test results. He reports no side effects from his new blood pressure medication and is following his diet carefully. Today Robert's blood pressure is 140/95 mm Hg. The physical examination is otherwise unchanged.

TEST RESULTS. Test results include the following: fasting plasma glucose 170 mg/dl, HbA$_{1c}$ 8.4 per cent, total cholesterol level 230 mg/dl, high-density lipoprotein (HDL) cholesterol 56 mg/dl, and low-density lipoprotein (LDL) cholesterol 159 mg/dl. The remaining blood tests are within normal limits. The ECG stress test shows an average exercise tolerance with no associated chest pain or ischemic changes. A random blood sugar level today is 208 mg/dl.

Assessment

1. *Type II diabetes.* With two elevated fasting plasma glucose levels, Robert meets the diagnostic criteria for diabetes. His elevated glycosylated hemoglobin is consistent with chronic hyperglycemia. Since he already watches his diet carefully and is not overweight, it seems likely that Robert needs pharmacologic intervention to normalize his blood sugar level even if he increases his exercise level.

2. *Essential hypertension.* Robert's blood pressure improved but is still suboptimally controlled. The synergistic effects of diabetes and hypertension merit aggressive blood pressure control and the plan is to lower his blood pressure further.

3. *Diabetic complications.* Diabetic complications can be divided into two groups: microvascular and macrovascular disease. Although poor glycemic control correlates strongly with an increased risk of microvascular disease, hyperglycemia is less strongly associated with developing macrovascular complications. These complications are more influenced by smoking, blood pressure, and hyperlipidemia. Since Robert's evaluation for macrovascular disease showed no evidence of coronary artery disease or peripheral vascular disease, one goal is to lessen Robert's chance of developing clinically significant macrovascular complications. This goal requires optimal management of his hypertension and LDL cholesterol count. Microvascular complications include retinopathy, nephropathy, and neuropathy. Since microvascular complications appear to correlate more closely with glycemic control, normalizing glucose levels is valuable both for primary and secondary prevention of microvascular disease. Clinically Robert's examination reveals evidence of diabetic retinopathy and he needs further evaluation by an ophthalmologist.

4. *Borderline cholesterol.* A low-fat diet is reinforced and a gradual exercise program is planned for Robert with an eventual goal of 30 to 45 minutes of vigorous exercise three to four times a week.

Plan

Robert's dose of lisinopril is increased to 10 mg each morning and he is to start glipizide (Glucotrol), 5 mg, taken 30 minutes before breakfast. He is monitored closely over the next few weeks until his blood sugar and blood pressure are under good control. Dosages of the oral hypoglycemic agents should generally not be increased more frequently than about every 5 to 7 days. More rapid dosage adjustments may cause low blood sugar levels once a steady state is reached. Sometimes the dosage of these agents may need to be reduced or even discontinued in patients who become more active and/or change their eating habits. Optimally, blood sugar levels should be maintained as close to normal as possible. Values suggesting good control are a fasting plasma glucose level less than 140 mg/dl, postprandial glucose level less than 180 mg/dl, and an HbA$_{1c}$ level of less than 7.5 per cent. Although treatment should be individualized, most experts recommend improving glycemic control for glucose above these levels. Examples in which more moderate control might be acceptable are in patients who are frail, elderly, have a limited life expectancy, or are at high risk of hypoglycemia.

A referral to Robert's ophthalmologist is made for a thorough funduscopic examination. Also, a spot urine test to detect microalbuminuria is needed since a typical urine dipstick is not sensitive enough to detect low levels of urinary albumin.

DISPOSITION. Robert's ophthalmologic examination shows an early nonproliferative diabetic retinopathy that does not require intervention at this time. The ophthalmologist plans follow-up in 6 months. A spot urine test for microalbuminuria is normal and will be repeated in 1 year. Over the next several months, Robert's blood sugar levels become controlled better through the combination of diet, exercise, and a sulfonylurea medication.

DISCUSSION

Approximately 6 per cent of the American population has type II diabetes mellitus, although only about one half of these patients are aware of their condition. The prevalence is even greater in African Americans, Hispanics, Native Americans, and those having a first-degree relative with diabetes. Although many people think of type II diabetes as a "mild" illness, it is a serious condition associated with an average loss of 5 to 10 years of life. Morbidity and mortality can be reduced by aggressive glycemic control and treatment of associated conditions such as hypertension and dyslipidemias.

Management goals are to eliminate acute symptoms, reduce morbidity and mortality from macrovascular disease, and to prevent or minimize microvascular complications. Maintenance of a fasting glucose level less than 200 mg/dl generally alleviates classic symptoms such as polyuria and polydipsia. Glucose levels less than 150 mg/dl are sufficient to promote a sense of well-being and prevent acute complications. Prevention of chronic complications is best achieved by normalizing blood sugar levels. Although treatment goals must be individualized, fasting glucose levels less than 140 mg/dl and an HbA_{1c} level less than 7.5% are suggested targets.

Diet and exercise are the cornerstones of therapy. Exercise improves glucose metabolism, decreases insulin resistance, and heightens a patient's sense of health. Exercise also helps reduce weight, lower blood pressure, and improve lipid levels. Physical activity for diabetics requires careful planning. Since many patients already have established coronary artery disease when first diagnosed with type II diabetes, many authorities recommend that diabetic patients undergo screening ECG stress testing before initiating a vigorous exercise program. Exercise programs should also take into account the presence of peripheral vascular disease.

Although initially hyperglycemia may improve significantly with diet and exercise, this approach ultimately fails to control hyperglycemia in up to 90 per cent of patients. Generally drug therapy is indicated in patients who fail to show reasonable improvement after 6 weeks to 3 months of diet and exercise.

Suitable drugs to initiate are the sulfonylureas and metformin. The sulfonylureas work primarily by stimulating the beta cells to produce insulin and to a lesser extent by decreasing insulin resistance. Sulfonylureas tend to be more effective in patients over the age of 40, those who have had diabetes for less than 5 years, and those who are not overweight. Sulfonylurea therapy lowers fasting plasma glucose levels by 36 to 54 mg/dl and the HbA_{1c} level by 1.5 to 2.0 per cent. Studies indicate that about 7 of 10 patients may respond to these drugs at first; however after 5 years, less than 40 per cent of the initial responders maintain adequate control as the patient's ability to endogenously produce insulin worsens. The principal side effect of sulfonylureas is hypoglycemia, which can be life threatening, particularly in older patients. However, most hypoglycemic episodes are mild and caused by erratic eating.

Metformin (Glucophage), a biguanide that is now available in the United States, is similar in effectiveness to the sulfonylureas. Metformin lowers the fasting plasma glucose level by 36 to 54 mg/dl and the HbA_{1c} level by 1.5 to 2.0 per cent. It is effective in about 75 to 80 per cent of patients with type II diabetes.

Metformin is associated with weight loss and can lower lipid levels. These qualities make it a good first choice in overweight patients without contraindications to the medication. The most serious side effect is the development of lactic acidosis. Lactic acidosis can be fatal but is rare if the drug is avoided in patients with impaired renal function, congestive heart failure, chronic obstructive pulmonary disease, or chronic liver disease. Less severe but more common are gastrointestinal symptoms such as nausea, bloating, diarrhea, and cramping. Initiating therapy at a low dose and increasing the dosage slowly minimize these side effects. Unlike the sulfonylureas, hypoglycemia is not a side effect of metformin.

Another new class of oral agent, the α-glucosidase inhibitors, is also available. Acarbose (Precose) is an α-glucosidase inhibitor that prevents the breakdown and absorption of carbohydrates by the gut. These agents are less effective than either metformin or the sulfonylureas, and lower the HbA_{1c} by 0.5 to 1 per cent. Their major clinical role is to decrease postprandial hyperglycemia and as adjunctive therapy along with another agent.

One essential aspect of successful diabetic management is to routinely follow and monitor patients. Patients with type II diabetes mellitus should be seen in the office at least three to four times per year. Visits should focus on glucose control, patient education, reinforcement of diet and exercise, and prevention of complications. Aggressive treatment of hypertension, dyslipidemia, and promotion of smoking cessation are of prime importance for avoiding macrovascular disease. Giving careful in-

TABLE 60–1. Foot Care Recommendations for Diabetic Patients

1. Wash feet daily in lukewarm water. Check water temperature with hand before immersing feet.
2. Inspect feet daily.
3. Apply moisturizing cream daily to prevent dry cracking skin.
4. Seek medical evaluation for any signs of infection or skin abnormality.
5. Break shoes in carefully and slowly.
6. Alternate shoes daily.
7. Clip toenails straight across.
8. Wear cotton socks.
9. Try to keep feet clean and dry.

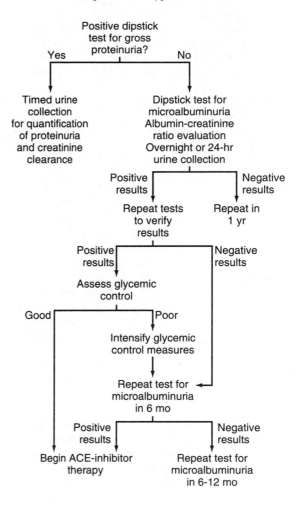

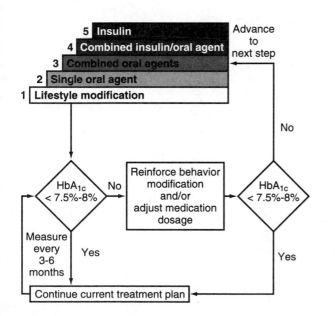

Figure 60–1. Screening algorithm for diagnosis of diabetic nephropathy. ACE = angiotensin-converting enzyme. (From Hirsch IB. Surveillance for complications of diabetes. Postgrad Med 1996;99:147–162.)

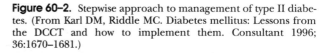

Figure 60–2. Stepwise approach to management of type II diabetes. (From Karl DM, Riddle MC. Diabetes mellitus: Lessons from the DCCT and how to implement them. Consultant 1996; 36:1670–1681.)

structions to patients with peripheral vascular disease can prevent ulceration and infection (Table 60–1). A careful foot examination, including peripheral pulses, sensation, and searching for skin lesions or deformities is important at each visit for both detecting disease and reinforcing the importance of good foot care.

Monitoring patients for a microvascular complication is also important. Signs of neuropathy can be detected clinically, by a careful history and neurologic examination. The three main types of diabetic neuropathy are focal neuropathy such as footdrop, distal symmetrical polyneuropathy, often associated with paresthesias, and autonomic neuropathy. Symptoms of autonomic neuropathy are impotence, gastrointestinal dysmotility, and orthostatic hypotension. Generally, an ophthalmologist should assess a patient for diabetic retinopathy unless the primary care physician feels confident in his or her own ability to screen for retinopathy. Patients with retinopathy need careful follow-up. Laser surgery, especially if done in an appropriate and timely fashion, reduces the risk of visual loss.

Measuring the urine for microalbuminuria is important to detect incipient nephropathy. Although a 24-hour urine collection is the gold standard, most clinicians use a spot urine test which measures the protein:creatinine ratio. This test has about a 95 per cent sensitivity compared with a 24-hour urine collection. The presence of microalbuminuria is a signal to intensify glycemic control and to add an ACE inhibitor to the patient's treatment regimen (Fig. 60–1). ACE inhibitors reduce intraglomerular filtration pressure and help preserve renal function. Serum creatinine levels should be obtained annually. Many experts also recommend a creatinine clearance for patients with an elevated creatinine level or microalbuminuria.

Finally, the family physician needs to provide psychological support. The demands that diabetes places on patients can frustrate and anger them. The skilled family physician individualizes treatment and works cooperatively with the patient. Developing short-term goals that are readily achievable are important for developing the patient's self-confidence. For example, overweight patients may benefit from setting incremental goals to lose weight rather than focusing on achieving their ideal weight. Even a modest weight loss of 10 to 20 lb can produce significant metabolic improvement and reinforce a healthful lifestyle. Encouragement and reinforcement of treatment goals are also an important part of care.

For patients who do not achieve glycemic control with a single drug, using a stepped-care approach may be beneficial (Fig. 60–2). In the case described, Robert is fortunate to achieve hyperglycemic control with a single drug. Unfortunately, in about 5 to 10 per cent of patients per year the sulfonylureas lose their effectiveness. Stepped care using a combination of agents may help avoid insulin therapy. The mechanisms of action for the various classes of oral agents are different and their effects are additive. Alternatively, some clinicians use the combination of a daytime sulfonylurea medication and a small dose of insulin at night.

SUGGESTED READING

Cefalu WT. Treatment of type II diabetes. Postgrad Med 1996;99:109–122.

Goo A, Carson DS, Bjelajoc A. Metformin: A new treatment option for non–insulin dependent diabetes mellitus. J Fam Pract 1996;42:612–618.

Hirsch IB. Surveillance for complications of diabetes. Postgrad Med 1996;99:147–162.

Karl DM, Riddle MC. Diabetes mellitus: Lessons from the DCCT and how to implement them. Consultant 1996;36:1670–1681.

Lebovits HE, Lipsky MS. Management of Type II Diabetes Mellitus. Kansas City, Mo, American Academy of Family Practice, 1995.

QUESTIONS

1. The single most important cause of excess mortality in type II diabetes is:
   a. Coronary artery disease
   b. Cerebral vascular disease
   c. Renal failure
   d. Ketoacidosis
   e. Infections

2. Which of the following medications can cause an elevated blood sugar?

a. Hydrochlorothiazide
b. Nicotinic acid
c. Lisinopril
d. Nifedipine
e. Phenytoin

3. The reason for using ACE inhibitors in managing hypertension in diabetic patients is:

a. To prevent diabetic nephropathy
b. To reduce cost
c. To avoid osmotic diureses
d. To prevent diabetic neuropathy
e. To prevent diabetic retinopathy

Answers appear on **page 606.**

Chapter 61

Weight Loss

Barbara A. Majeroni, M.D.

INITIAL VISIT

Subjective

PATIENT IDENTIFICATION AND PRESENTING PROBLEM. Mrs. Sheila P. is a 53-year-old married white woman, who was in her usual state of good health until about 6 months ago. At that time she noticed that she was losing weight. She began to pay more attention to her eating habits, and feels she has a good appetite and eats a well-rounded diet, but she has continued to lose weight. By her scale at home, she has lost 30 lb over the last 6 months. She initially attributed the problem to nervousness and stress at work, where she is in a supervisory position at a nursing home, but the problem has continued despite her efforts to delegate work to her subordinates. Now she is experiencing excessive fatigue and difficulty sleeping as well as continued weight loss. Her sister was recently diagnosed with breast cancer, and she worries that this might be the problem, although she hasn't noted any changes on her monthly breast self-examination.

PAST MEDICAL HISTORY. Mrs. P. has been in good health. She had a tubal ligation at age 32, and cholecystectomy at age 48. Her two pregnancies resulted in normal spontaneous vaginal deliveries.

She stopped menstruating 2 years ago. There is no history of diabetes, heart disease, hypertension, cancer, gastrointestinal, or psychiatric illness. She has no known allergies. Her only medication is an over-the-counter multiple vitamin and mineral supplement, which she started about 4 months ago. Her last Pap smear was 5 years ago. She has never had a mammogram.

FAMILY HISTORY. Sheila's father died at age 76 of prostate cancer. Her mother is living and well at age 74. One older sister had surgery for breast cancer. Another sister and brother are well. There is no family history of cardiovascular, respiratory, renal, hematologic, gastrointestinal, or endocrine disease. Her children and grandchildren have no medical problems.

SOCIAL HISTORY. Mrs. P. lives with her husband, who works as a computer consultant. One daughter lives upstairs. The other is married and lives with her husband and two children about an hour away. Sheila has never smoked and denies any past or present use of alcohol or illicit drugs. She enjoys her work as a nursing supervisor, and is able to take some time off now and then to travel with her husband to various cities in the United States. She has always been physically active, biking or swimming several times a week. Her husband is her only sexual partner, and she feels sure that he doesn't see anyone else.

REVIEW OF SYSTEMS. Sheila P. has no headaches, visual disturbances, hearing problems, or dizziness. She denies chest pain, but admits to occasional palpitations, not necessarily associated with activity. There is no shortness of breath, or productive cough or sputum; no abdominal pain, diarrhea, or constipation; no blood in stools. She has soft bowel movements two or three times a day. She has had no vaginal bleeding or discharge. She notes some vaginal dryness and complains of excessive sweating, which she attributes to hot flashes. There are no rashes or skin changes, no jaundice or pruritus. She denies feeling hopeless or suicidal, but states she has felt very tense and anxious lately. She has had no hallucinations or delusions.

Objective

PHYSICAL EXAMINATION. Mrs. P. is well groomed, pleasant, and cooperative. She appears tense and worried. Her height is 5 feet 8 inches, weight 120 lb. Weight at last visit, 1 year ago was 158 lb. Blood pressure is 128/80 mm Hg, pulse 100, respirations 16, oral temperature 37.6°C. Hair is normal. Head is normocephalic. Her eyes are normal in configuration. Sclerae are clear, extraocular movements are intact. Pupils are equally round and reactive to light and accommodation; fundi show no hemorrhages or vascular changes. Tympanic membranes are clear. Pharynx is clear. Teeth are in good condition. There is no lymphadenopathy; thyroid is diffusely enlarged, with no nodules or tenderness. Heart is regular with normal S_1 and S_2 heart sounds and no murmur. Lungs are clear to examination. Breasts are symmetrical, with no masses, skin changes, or nipple discharge. There is no axillary adenopathy. Her abdomen is soft and nontender with no organomegaly. Bowel sounds are active in all quadrants. On pelvic examination, the vaginal mucosa is atrophic; there are no skin lesions. The cervix has no lesions or discharge. Pap smear is taken from the cervix. There are no masses or tenderness of the uterus or adnexae. Rectal examination shows normal tone and no lesions; Hemoccult stool test is negative; soft brown stool. Extremities show no edema, clubbing, or cyanosis. Hands are warm and moist. Distal pulses are normal. Neurologic examination reveals no focal abnormalities except for a symmetrical fine tremor of the hands. Deep tendon reflexes are brisk and symmetrical. Cranial nerves II through XII are intact. Gait and station are normal. There are no deficits in strength or sensation. Memory, thought processes, and speech patterns are normal.

Assessment

Unexplained weight loss results from either decreased intake (or absorption) or increased output (or metabolism) of caloric energy. A loss of more than 5 per cent of total body weight within a 6- to 12-month period suggests underlying pathology.

DIFFERENTIAL DIAGNOSIS (Table 61–1)

1. *Decreased intake.* Common causes of weight loss that result from social isolation, such as problems with finances, dentition, inability to shop, or loneliness, are unlikely in this woman who has a job and family support. She is on no drugs that would cause nausea or anorexia.

2. *Psychiatric disorders.* Because of Sheila's age and her history of good appetite, the diagnosis of anorexia nervosa is unlikely. Loss of appetite due to mood disorders occurs in depression and in bipolar disorder. Psychotic patients may stop eating because of delusions, such as fear of being poisoned. This patient has been worried, and is concerned about her sister, but denies feeling sad or hopeless, and continues to take pleasure in activities, such as traveling with her husband. She does not fulfill criteria for a diagnosis of depression.

3. *Cancer.* The most common cause of unexplained weight loss is malignancy, for which it may be the presenting complaint. In a woman of this age, common cancers would include lung, breast, and gastrointestinal cancers. Since the patient never smoked, lung cancer is less likely, although not impossible. The absence of productive cough or sputum is reassuring. A first-degree relative with breast cancer increases Sheila's risk for this cancer. A mammogram is indicated despite a normal examination. A single heme-negative stool does not rule out colon cancer, and if no other cause is found for the weight loss colonoscopy would be appropriate.

4. *Infection.* Chronic infectious processes such as subacute bacterial endocarditis, tuberculosis, or acquired immunodeficiency syndrome (AIDS) can result in weight loss. This patient has no lifestyle risk factors for AIDS. Because she works in a health care facility, she has an annual tuberculin test (purified

TABLE 61–1. Differential Diagnosis of Involuntary Weight Loss

Reduced intake
  Social isolation
  Financial limitations
  Problems with dentition
  Inability to obtain food, mobility, transportation
    restrictions
  Alcohol or drug abuse
Drugs that alter appetite, cause nausea, or affect taste
Psychiatric disorders
  Anorexia nervosa
  Depression, anxiety, bereavement
  Dementia
  Psychosis
Cancer
  Gastrointestinal tract is most common site for
    occult tumors
Infection
  Tuberculosis
  Fungal disease
  Amebic abscess
  Subacute bacterial endocarditis
  Human immunodeficiency virus
Endocrine/metabolic diseases
  Diabetes mellitus
  Hyperthyroidism
  Apathetic hypothyroidism
Gastrointestinal disorders
  Peptic ulcer disease
  Gastroesophageal reflux
  Pancreatitis
  Sprue
  Short bowel syndrome
  Inflammatory bowel disease
Chronic illnesses
  Congestive heart failure
  Renal disease
  Hepatic disease
  Connective tissue disease
  Pulmonary disease
Idiopathic (25%)

protein derivative [PPD]), and all have been negative. There are no physical signs of infection.

5. *Endocrine diseases.* Diabetes mellitus causes weight loss initially due to osmotic diuresis, and in insulin-dependent forms, weight loss occurs from caloric wastage. Weight loss in diabetes is frequently associated with increased food intake. Increased metabolism resulting in weight loss can be caused by hyperthyroidism. Signs and symptoms are variable and may be subtle. This patient's symptoms of nervousness, weight loss, palpitations, increased sweating, and fatigue could be secondary to hyperthyroidism even in the absence of exophthalmos and heat intolerance. Although more commonly associated with weight gain, patients with hypothyroidism sometimes present with apathy and weight loss. This is more common in patients over age 65.

6. *Gastrointestinal disorders.* Upper gastrointestinal tract disorders such as reflux, gastritis, and peptic ulcer disease may result in reduced caloric intake. Decreased absorption of calories can occur with chronic pancreatitis, short bowel syndrome, sprue, inflammatory bowel disease, or parasitic infection. Mrs. P. has no symptoms to suggest an intestinal disorder. If no cause for her weight loss is found in her initial evaluation, further gastrointestinal evaluation will be considered.

7. *Chronic disease.* In addition to cancer, other chronic disease can result in loss of appetite and weight loss. Some examples are congestive heart failure, renal failure, cirrhosis, and chronic obstructive pulmonary disease. This patient's physical examination does not point to any of these.

8. *Idiopathic.* In approximately 25 per cent of patients evaluated for weight loss, the problem remains unexplained despite extensive evaluation and prolonged follow-up (Reife, 1995).

Plan

Since the cause of Sheila's weight loss has not been clearly defined by the history and physical, further evaluation is indicated (Table 61–2). Laboratory tests ordered include a complete blood count (CBC), glucose, electrolytes, blood urea nitrogen (BUN), creatinine, amylase, liver enzymes, albumin, thyroxine (T_4), and thyroid-stimulating hormone (TSH). A mammogram and chest x-ray study are scheduled. Further testing will be determined based on these results.

TABLE 61–2. Evaluation for Unexplained Weight Loss

Complete history and physical examination
Laboratory tests: Complete blood count, electrolytes,
  blood urea nitrogen, creatinine, glucose, thyroxine,
  thyroid-stimulating hormone, liver function tests,
  amylase, urinalysis
Stool Hemoccult test (three tests)
Chest x-ray study
Further studies based on symptoms: upper
  gastrointestinal studies, barium enema, or
  colonoscopy
If the above do not reveal a cause, and social factors
  have been corrected, close follow-up is
  recommended rather than extensive undirected
  testing

FOLLOW-UP VISIT

On return visit, Sheila's laboratory tests are reviewed. A normal CBC made infection unlikely. Glucose is 100 mg/100 ml. Normal electrolytes, BUN, and creatinine suggest normal renal function. Amylase and liver enzymes are also in the normal range. Albumin is 2.5 gm/100 ml (normal: 3.5–4.8 gm/100 mL) suggesting chronic malnutrition. T_4 is elevated at 19.5 µg/100 ml (normal: 1.0–11.0 µg/100 ml); sensitive TSH is 0.03 mU/L (normal: 0.5–6.0 mU/L. Chest radiograph shows no lung disease. The heart appears mildly enlarged. Mammogram and Pap smear are normal.

DIAGNOSIS. The combination of low TSH with an elevated T_4 is diagnostic of thyrotoxicosis. This is consistent with the patient's symptoms of weight loss with nervousness, palpitations, fatigue, and sweating, and the physical findings of enlarged thyroid and a higher than expected heart rate. A radioactive iodine uptake scan is ordered and blood is drawn for antithyroglobulin and antimicrosomal antibodies.

DISCUSSION

Most common in white females, hyperthyroidism affects up to 2 per cent of women and 0.2 per cent of men. Over age 60, prevalence increases to 3 per cent. Although signs and symptoms are variable, the most common signs of thyrotoxicosis include thyroid gland enlargement, a thyroid bruit, exophthalmos, lid lag, tremor, tachycardia, hyperkinetic muscular activity, and warm, moist hands. More than 50 per cent of patients exhibit some of the common symptoms, which include nervousness, increased sweating, heat intolerance, palpitations, dyspnea, fatigue, weight loss, and eye complaints. Causes of thyrotoxicosis are summarized in Table 61–3. The most common cause of thyrotoxicosis is Graves disease, a disorder of unknown cause that includes primary hyperthyroidism. Most common in the third and fourth decades, Graves disease is seen more frequently in women than men. Genetic factors are important. The classic triad of Graves disease includes thyrotoxicosis with goiter, ophthalmopathy, and dermopathy, but the three major manifestations need not appear together.

Appropriate evaluation for thyrotoxicosis includes a radioimmunoassay for total serum concentrations of T_4 and a sensitive TSH. When alterations of thyroxine-binding globulin are suspected, free T_4 should be measured directly. If free T_4 is not avail-

TABLE 61–3. Causes of Thyrotoxicosis

Graves disease (most common)
Iatrogenic
  (Overtreated hypothyroidism)
Thyroiditis
  Hashimoto thyroiditis, subacute thyroiditis, silent
    thyroiditis, postpartum thyroiditis
Toxic nodular goiter
Toxic adenoma
Factitious hyperthyroidism
  (Patient taking excess thyroid hormone)
Excess exogenous iodine
Rare causes
  TSH producing tumor
  Trophoblastic tumor
  Struma ovarii
  Thyroid cancer

TSH = Thyroid-stimulating hormone.

able, it can be estimated using the free thyroxine index (FTI), which is calculated by measuring the triiodothyronine resin uptake (T3U) and multiplying this by the total serum T_4.

$$FTI = T_4 \times T3U$$

If TSH is low, T_4 and T_3 are normal, but the patient is clinically hyperthyroid, a thyrotropin-releasing hormone (TRH) test may be helpful. The lack of TSH response to intravenous TRH indicates excessive T_4, and treatment is indicated. In middle-aged women with a firm goiter, antithyroglobulin antibodies and antimicrosomal antibodies are measured to evaluate for Hashimoto thyroiditis.

Misleading laboratory results may occur. For example, in chronic liver disease or nephrotic syndrome, thyroxine-binding globulin is low, resulting in a low serum T_4, but free T_4 and TSH are normal. Drugs such as glucocorticoids, levodopa, and dopamine can cause a low TSH in patients who are euthyroid. Estrogen in pregnancy, hormone replacement therapy, or oral contraceptives may cause an increased T_4, but free T_4 is normal, and the patient is euthyroid.

The usual pattern in hyperthyroidism is a high T_4 and free T_4 with a low TSH. A thyroid scan with radioactive iodine uptake (RAIU) can help differentiate the causes of thyrotoxicosis. Factitious or iatrogenic thyrotoxicosis can be differentiated by the RAIU, which is suppressed to less than 5 per cent in the presence of excess exogenous thyroid hormone. The RAIU is also reduced, at times to zero, in patients with hyperthyroidism due to excess iodine (Jod-Basedow disease). These patients have goiter, but no image on thyroid scan. In endogenous hyperthyroidism, the RAIU is elevated. Toxic adenoma or toxic multinodular goiter concentrates the radioisotope in one or more areas, whereas Graves disease causes diffuse uptake throughout the gland. With thyroiditis, the RAIU may be reduced when T_4 is high and increased when T_4 is low, in a patchy nonhomogeneous pattern. Trophoblastic tumors, which are rare, can cause a low TSH due to tumor secretion of excess β-human chorionic gonadotropin (βhCG), which interacts with TSH receptors in the thyroid. Another rare cause of hyperthyroidism is struma ovarii, in which thyroid rests in the ovary become hyperplastic and produce thyroxine. If no other cause for the hyperthyroidism is found, focusing the gamma camera on the ovaries at the thyroid scan may reveal increased radioactive iodine uptake in this condition.

RESULTS. Mrs. P.'s thyroid scan showed diffuse increased uptake, suggestive of Graves disease. Although the classic triad of Graves disease includes hyperthyroidism with diffuse thyroid enlargement, ophthalmopathy, and dermopathy, some patients exhibit only one of the three.

TREATMENT. Hospitalization is required only in the case of serious arrhythmias, congestive heart failure, or impending thyroid storm. Sheila can be treated as an outpatient. Symptoms of nervousness and palpitations may be controlled with a β blocker while awaiting definitive treatment. In acute thyroiditis, symptomatic treatment may be used alone in anticipation of spontaneous remission. Graves disease may be treated with propylthiouracil, methimazole, or carbimazole in the hope of remission or to achieve a euthyroid state before ablative treatment with radioactive iodine. In Sheila's case, the history suggested a long duration of hyperthyroidism. Definitive treatment with ^{131}I is administered. The patient is informed before the treatment that as many as 40 to 70 per cent of patients treated with this modality will develop hypothyroidism within 10 years, requiring lifelong hormone replacement therapy.

FOLLOW-UP. After her treatment with radioactive iodine, Mrs. P. will be followed by her family doctor, watching carefully for signs of hypothyroidism and monitoring her T_4 and TSH to determine whether she has obtained a euthyroid state. The β blocker will be tapered as symptoms permit. Health maintenance issues that continue to be addressed include the advisability of annual mammograms, regular Pap smears, and consideration of calcium supplementation and hormone replacement therapy.

SUGGESTED READING

Franklin JA. The management of hyperthyroidism. N Engl J Med 1994;330:1731–1738.

Knudson PB. Hyperthyroidism in adults: Variable clinical presentations and approaches to diagnosis. J Am Board Fam Pract 1995;8:109–113.

Rabinovitz M, Pitlik SD, Leifer M, et al. Unintentional weight loss, a retrospective analysis of 154 cases. Arch Intern Med 1986;146:186–187.

Reife CM. Involuntary weight loss. Med Clin North Am 1995;79:299–313.

Smith SA. Concise review for primary care physicians: Commonly asked questions about thyroid function. Mayo Clin Proc 1995;70:573–577.

QUESTIONS

1. The most common cause of unexplained weight loss is
   a. Hyperthyroidism
   b. Cancer
   c. Peptic ulcer disease
   d. Alcoholism
   e. Social isolation

2. Which set of laboratory values is most consistent with primary hyperthyroidism?
   a. High T_4; high TSH
   b. High T_4; normal TSH
   c. Normal T_4; high TSH
   d. High T_4; low TSH
   e. Normal T_4; low TSH

3. The classic triad of Graves disease includes which of the following:
   a. Diffuse thyroid enlargement
   b. Thinning of the hair
   c. Ophthalmopathy
   d. Constipation
   e. Dermopathy

Answers appear on **page 606**.

Chapter 62

Malnutrition in the Elderly

Jane V. White, Ph.D., R.D.

INITIAL VISIT

Subjective

Hilary B. is a 76-year-old white woman; her family physician has referred her to a registered dietitian (RD) for dietary counseling regarding an involuntary weight loss of approximately 30 lb. History and physical examination information from her referring physician are summarized.

PRESENTING PROBLEM. Weakness and decreased appetite.

PAST MEDICAL HISTORY. Hilary has chronic obstructive pulmonary disease. She has a history of chronic angina and had a myocardial infarction 6 years ago. Mild hypertension has been treated for the past 30 years and despite compliance with medication has resulted in chronic congestive heart failure. Hypothyroidism in her thirties was controlled by daily medication. A hiatial hernia was repaired 10 years ago.

FAMILY/SOCIAL HISTORY. Mrs. B. is a widowed, retired food service worker who lives alone. She smoked three packs of cigarettes per day but quit 20 years ago; Hilary consumes no alcoholic beverages. She is in good compliance with all her prescription medications.

CURRENT MEDICATIONS. Albuterol (Proventil) inhaler, two puffs three times a day; aspirin, 81 mg (baby aspirin), once daily; amlodipine besylate (Norvasc), 2.5 mg once daily; beclomethasone dipropionate (Vanceril) inhaler, two puffs four times a day; cimetidine, 300 mg three times a day; digoxin, 0.125 mg once daily; furosemide, 40 mg twice a day; isosorbide mononitrate (Ismo), 20 mg twice a day; levothyroxine sodium, 0.1 mg once daily; metolazone (Zaroxolyn), 2.5 mg every other day; nitroglycerin tablet, 0.4 mg as needed for pain; and propoxyphene (Darvocet-N 100) every 8 hours for pain.

Objective

PHYSICAL EXAMINATION. Blood pressure is 100/52 mm Hg, oral temperature 97.6°F, heart rate 60 beats per minute, respiratory rate 16, weight 120 lb (down from 148 lb approximately 1 year ago). Head, eyes, ears, nose, and throat examinations are unremarkable. Thyroid not palpable. Lungs are clear. Cardiovascular examination demonstrates regular rate and rhythm; no murmur; no complaints of pain. Abdomen is soft, nontender; no organomegaly; positive bowel sounds. Extremities: minimal edema, warm and dry. Neurologic signs: alert, oriented; no focal findings. Limited ambulation.

LABORATORY DATA. Albumin 2.9 gm/dl; fasting glucose 68 mg/dl; cholesterol 205 mg/dl; triglycerides 93 mg/dl. Digoxin level is adequate. Thyroid, renal, and liver function studies normal; urinalysis normal. Chest radiograph is normal.

INITIAL DIETITIAN VISIT

Subjective

PRESENTING PROBLEM. In addition to weakness and decreased appetite, Hilary complains of increased fatigue and dyspepsia which she describes as a vague feeling that the food "just doesn't sit well in her stomach." She has problems sleeping, and feels of little value to her family and friends. Widowed for the last 10 years, she is usually alone at mealtimes and feels no desire to cook or to eat. She becomes increasingly "uneasy" as the day progresses. She is seated in a wheelchair today because her daughter reports that the patient was "too tired" to walk into the office from the parking lot. Hilary states that she doesn't have the energy to answer questions, and that her daughter "knows what she eats."

SOCIAL HISTORY. Mrs. B.'s six children are married with families of their own. Until this last year, one of her two daughters ate meals with her daily. Since both daughters have begun full-time jobs, neither is available to spend mealtimes with her mother. They continue to send her cooked meals on a weekly basis.

DIET HISTORY. A review of Mrs. B.'s food intake over the last 24 hours shows consumption of approximately 500 calories per day. Breakfast is her "best" meal. She does not care for unflavored milk or other dairy products and has stopped eating meats because she is unable to chew them with ease. She states that the salt-free, low-fat, low-cholesterol diet she is supposed to eat is tasteless. The foods prepared by her family contain no salt, fat, or other seasonings. She refuses to eat them. She prefers to eat in her own home and rarely accepts invitations from family or friends to eat out. Hilary states that her typical weight at age 50 was between 135 to 145 lb.

Objective

PHYSICAL FINDINGS. Mrs. B.'s weight today is 118 lb (down from 120 lb at her visit to her family physician 2 weeks ago and down 30 lb over the past year). Height is 64 inches (when last measured 15 years ago, her height was 66 inches.) She appears thin, weak, and pale. There is some evidence of temporal wasting. Upper and lower dentures are present but ill-fitting; her gums are bright red and very sore under the lower plate. Extremities are nonedematous.

Assessment

DIFFERENTIAL DIAGNOSIS

1. *Protein-calorie malnutrition.* Hilary has experienced a 30-lb involuntary weight loss during the last year. Temporal wasting is evident. She is thin, pale, and tires easily. Her serum albumin is 2.9 gm/dl, indicative of malnutrition of moderate severity. She exhibits a number of risk factors that place her at increased risk for poor nutritional status: *poor food intake, multiple chronic diseases, multiple medication use, poor oral health, social isolation, physical limitations, implementation of an overly restrictive dietary prescription.*

2. *Depression.* Inability to sleep, poor appetite, fatigue, and feelings of low self-esteem are suggestive of depression. Her "uneasiness" might suggest that her depression may be compounded by an anxiety component.

3. *Dyspepsia.* This condition is associated with both hiatial hernia and extraintestinal diseases such as congestive heart failure. A variety of drugs such as aspirin, glucocorticoids, digoxin (Lanoxin), and propoxyphene can contribute to gastrointestinal distress.

4. *Chronic obstructive pulmonary disease (COPD).* Hilary uses supplemental oxygen as needed and inhalers as prescribed. She is in no acute respiratory distress. However, anorexia, early satiety, fatigue, and bloating are common complaints voiced by 60 to 90 per cent of patients with COPD.

5. *Atherosclerotic cardiovascular diseases.* Preliminary lipid values appear reasonable for a woman of this age. Hilary has not smoked in 20 years. She reports no chest discomfort at this time.

6. *Hypertension with congestive heart failure.* Blood pressure seems well controlled at this time. No obvious edema is present.

7. *Hypothyroidism.* Thyroid studies are within normal limits at this time.

Plan

PATIENT EDUCATION

1. Stop weight loss within the next week.

- Liberalize the diet by placing Mrs. B. on a no-added-salt diet (3 to 4 gm sodium per day) for hypertension and congestive heart failure.
- Monitor body weight (fluid status) closely. Contact physician or RD if weight gain exceeds 1 lb per day.
- Encourage family members providing food to prepare menu items based on Mrs. B.'s individual food preferences and tolerances and to be more liberal in their use of herbs, spices, and fat to flavor foods.
- Modify food textures as needed to ensure appropriate food intake.
- Consult a dentist regarding oral health problems identified.

2. Promote a weight gain of 0.5 to 1.0 lb per week.

- Switch to a three-meal–three-snack-a-day regimen. Smaller, more frequent meals tend to reduce abdominal distention and aid in the reduction of cardiac and pulmonary workloads.
- Assess Mrs. B.'s functional status. Should her physical status limit her ability to access food or to manage other aspects of independent living, consider the limited use of homemaker services to prepare meals, to be present at mealtimes, and to perform other functions that Mrs. B. is unable to do regularly.
- Increase consumption of calorically dense foods. Increase the fat content of Mrs. B.'s diet by encouraging increased use of mono- and polyunsaturated fats in the form of oils, margarines, salad dressings, commercial mayonnaise (egg yolks are not used in its preparation), sandwich spreads, sauces or gravies, and fried foods. Offer sweets as snacks between meals. Offer flavored milks, juices, fruit aides, and sugar or a carbohydrate supplement (Polycose) added to beverages.
- Encourage Mrs. B. to use a timer or to set an alarm clock as an eating reminder.
- Keep nonperishable foods out on counters and tabletops where they are more likely to be seen and eaten.

- Supplement meals and snacks with commercial medical nutritional products (e.g., Ensure, Sustacal, Carnation Instant Breakfast) if food intake remains inadequate.

3. Increase socialization at mealtimes.

- Have Mrs. B. eat in front of the television set to provide the illusion that others are present at mealtimes.
- Encourage family members to establish a "dinner at grandma's" rotation. Instead of simply dropping food off, have the family or family member who delivers the food spend 30 minutes conversing with Mrs. B. as she eats.
- Consider the use of home-delivered meals (Meals-on-Wheels) since the volunteers who deliver the meals frequently spend time conversing with meal recipients. The social interaction aspects of this program are as valuable to meal recipients as the food provided.

4. Ensure food safety.

- Check to see that the food being delivered is eaten. Date food offerings and discard those not consumed within 3 to 4 days.

5. Record actual food intake.

DISPOSITION. Mrs. B. is scheduled to return to the dietitian's office in 3 to 4 weeks for follow-up so that success in implementing the recommended nutrition interventions can be assessed. Her daughter has agreed to bring her to the office.

RECOMMENDATIONS TO THE REFERRING PHYSICIAN

In providing a written summary of the nutrition consultation to the referring physician, the following issues should be raised for consideration:

1. Consider evaluation for depression/anxiety and the prescription of an antidepressant/anxiolytic agent if indicated.

2. Evaluate current medications to see if any might be reduced or stopped, particularly those with the potential to negatively impact nutritional status.

3. Consider a formal assessment of functional status using the activities of daily living—instrumental activities of daily living (ADL–IADL) format.

4. Consider the prescription of a vitamin-mineral and/or calcium supplement since Mrs. B. has limited food and calcium intake.

FIRST DIETITIAN FOLLOW-UP VISIT

Subjective

Mrs. B. returns to the RD's office 4 weeks later with food records. She saw her family physician 3 weeks ago, at which time he stopped her prescriptions for Norvasc, Darvocet-N 100, and Ismo, and placed her on lorazepam, 0.5 mg twice a day; trazodone HCl (Desyrel), 50 mg at bedtime; nitroglycerin ointment 2%, 1/2 inch every 8 hours; and nitroglycerin tablet, 0.4 mg sublingually as needed for chest pain. Her family has implemented the dietary revisions suggested when preparing Hilary's meals and her food intake has improved. Eating meals in front of the television during the day and implementation of the family eating rotation for the evening meal three times a week makes Mrs. B. feel less lonely. Because six of her children live in the area, the burden on each family is not too great. Mrs. B. is snacking between meals one to two times per day. She feels that her appetite has improved. A dental consult is scheduled for next week.

Objective

Mrs. B.'s weight is now 123 lb, a gain of 5 lb in the last month. Her vital signs were stable at her last physician visit. Extremities are nonedematous. She did not require a wheelchair today.

Assessment

A review of Hilary's food records show her average daily intake to be approximately 1200 to 1400 calories, distributed over three meals and two snacks. During the last week her food intake has increased to between 1300 and 1600 calories per day. She states that her food tastes better and her appetite has improved. She is taking a multivitamin tablet daily, and drinks a glass of chocolate- or strawberry-flavored low-fat milk twice a day with snacks. The more liberal sodium and fat prescription allows Mrs. B. to incorporate low-fat cheeses and eggs into her diet weekly.

Plan

Mrs. B. is to follow through with a dental consult. She is to continue her present eating regimen and return to the RD in 1 month to re-evaluate her caloric and other dietary needs. As she approaches her usual weight, caloric and nutrient intake may need to be adjusted to allow her to maintain a reasonable weight. She is referred back to her family physician for recommendations regarding an exercise program that would allow her to improve her physical conditioning so that independent living can be maintained.

DISCUSSION

Malnutrition is a major risk factor for increased morbidity and mortality in the elderly. The prevalence of malnutrition in older Americans is quite high with significant nutritional deficits estimated to range from 10 to 51 per cent in community-dwelling elderly, 20 to 60 per cent in hospitalized elders, and up to 85 per cent in long-term care elderly populations (Mion et al., 1994). In Western nations, malnutrition is not due to widespread food shortages but coexists with acute or chronic disease and psychosocial factors such as poor food intake, depression, poor oral health, isolation, physical impairments that limit access to food or make food preparation difficult, poverty, and the chronic use of multiple medications (Mion et al., 1994; White, 1994). Many of these factors are modifiable or easily reversed.

Contributors to Malnutrition in the Elderly

1. *Inadequate or inappropriate food intake* places a substantial number of older persons at increased nutritional risk. Those who are unable or unwilling to eat and must depend on others to purchase or prepare food, and those who have limited financial resources with which to obtain food are particularly vulnerable. In the United States, approximately 12 per cent of households with a person in their seventies, and 17 per cent with an elder age 80 or older, report incomes of less than $5000 annually (White, 1994). Significantly more women than men subsist on this poverty level. Few elderly households receive Supplemental Security Income (less than 8 per cent) and less than 6 per cent receive food stamps. Basic needs such as utilities, phone, medication, and transportation compete for food dollars and are often perceived by older persons as more important than are food needs. Hilary B.'s family provided food; however, many elderly women retired from menial jobs have insufficient economic resources to buy nutritious food. General questions regarding the type and quantity of food eaten and the regularity with which food is consumed should be asked of

all persons 65 years of age and older. Factors indicative of limited economic resources, such as reliance on economic assistance programs to meet basic needs, is a potential sign of increased nutritional risk. *Overly restrictive dietary prescriptions* are a frequent contributor to poor food intake in older persons (Gamble, 1994). Physician recommendations are often implemented more stringently than was originally intended for an elderly individual. Food restriction, the reason for it, level of compliance with dietary prescriptions, and their impact on total food intake should be routinely assessed.

In Mrs. B.'s case, her inability to eat was compounded by depression and poor oral health. Recent studies in older people show that leading causes of involuntary weight loss are depression and poor oral health; occult neoplastic disease is seen with less frequency (NSI, 1994; White, 1994).

2. *Depression.* Subtle deficits in vitamin status can contribute to depression and to impaired mental status in older adults. Vitamins B₁₂, folate, and pyridoxine intake are of concern, as is thiamine status in those elderly who drink alcoholic beverages. Preventable causes of cognitive decline in older persons in addition to nutritional factors include inactivity, isolation, sensory impairment, alcohol or drug abuse, thyroid dysfunction, and overmedication (White, 1994). Abnormal attitudes toward eating and body image occur in older women and men. The family physician should be aware of the potential for chronic anorexia nervosa or anorexia tardive to present in this age group. Diet-related diseases that may contribute to cognitive decline in older persons and that are amenable to nutritional therapy include the lipid disorders, hypertension, and diabetes mellitus.

3. *Isolation.* Isolation is a significant contributor to poor nutritional status in the elderly. Living alone has been shown to contribute to poor nutritional status through apathy, depression, and lack of motivation to provide self-care. In Mrs. B.'s case although her family provided food, they spent little time interacting with her in ways that would facilitate food consumption. Diet-related problems diminish, and independent living is maintained, in elderly persons who perceive the frequency of visits from family and friends as adequate. Although Mrs. B.'s response to participation in outside activities was initially negative, questions regarding social contact and a discussion of food-oriented community services designed to facilitate social interaction among older persons could be reintroduced once her mental status improves.

4. *Oral health problems.* Dental neglect is a com-

mon cause of poor eating habits in older adults. Although the incidence of edentulism is declining in this country, approximately 35 to 40 per cent of Americans currently 65 years of age and older have no teeth (Baum, 1993). Thus for the foreseeable future, many older patients will present with a myriad of dental prostheses that have the potential to seriously impair their ability to eat. The oral cavity of an elderly person should be examined routinely. The incidence of common problems such as leukoplakia, lichen planus, herpes zoster, benign mucous membrane pemphigoid, and epulis fissuratum is much greater in those over age 60 than in younger adults. The incidence of oral cancer peaks in persons ages 65 to 74, and is more common in men and in African Americans (Baum, 1993). The patient should be asked to remove dentures so that the oral structures on which the dentures rest can be adequately examined. Ill-fitting or broken dentures are a common complaint of the elderly and should be referred for appropriate treatment. Denture-associated candidiasis is the most common oral candidal infection (Baum, 1993). The oral mucosa appears bright red and corresponds to the denture outline. Symptoms of burning mouth and taste abnormalities are often reported by patients with oral candidal lesions. Topical treatment of the mouth with an antifungal rinse or troche and soaking the dentures in an antifungal solution during long periods when they are not being worn (i.e., at night) are effective treatment strategies for this problem. Angular cheilitis is common in elderly edentulous patients, particularly in those who wear their dentures infrequently since the teeth are no longer there to support the cheeks and lips. Occasionally, a deficiency of the B-complex vitamins is associated with its occurrence (Baum, 1993; White, 1994).

5. *Acute or poorly controlled chronic illness.* Recent surgery, significant trauma or infection, recent hospitalization, or the initiation or withdrawal of nutritional support suggests increased nutrient demands and potential nutritional risk. Familiarity with subtle physical or biochemical signs and symptoms of malnutrition is critical. In this case, Mrs. B. had very gradually lost a considerable amount of weight, her height had decreased, her serum albumin level was quite low, and evidence of temporal wasting was apparent. In adults, body weight usually varies by not more than 0.1 kg per day. Weight loss of greater than 0.5 kg per day suggests a significant caloric deficit, fluid deficit, or combination of the two. Body weight shows a U- or J-shaped relationship to mortality with highest survival rates found in individuals who maintain a stable weight at or

slightly above that deemed desirable (Casper, 1995). Table 62–1 shows the degree of involuntary weight loss over time that is considered significant and that should trigger a nutritional status evaluation.

It is well known that height tends to decrease with age. In younger adults, therefore, height should be measured at least every 5 years. In those age 65 and older, height should be measured annually. If the patient's physical status makes obtaining a reliable height or weight difficult, formulas for estimating height using leg or arm span measurements and the use of wheelchair or bed scales can facilitate obtaining this information (NSI, 1994). Edema, if present, should be noted.

Serum albumin is a fairly reliable indicator of baseline nutritional status (see Table 62–1). Although it can be influenced by a number of factors such as hydration status, impaired renal or liver function, thyroid disease, protein-losing enteropathies, and by advanced age itself, it is information that is obtained when most routine laboratory procedures are ordered and when combined with measures of body weight, offers reasonable insight regarding the adequacy of macronutrient intake. Because serum albumin has a half-life of approximately 18 to 20 days, it is not particularly helpful in the re-evaluation or modification of enteral or parenteral nutrition interventions once they have been instituted. Serum proteins such as prealbumin, with a half-life of approximately 2 to 3 days, are more useful in this circumstance (see Table 62–1).

6. *Dependence or disability.* Inability to perform the usual activities of daily living can hamper an elder's efforts to obtain an adequate diet. Irrespective of cause, functional impairment reduces independence, negatively impacts self-esteem, and reduces the elderly person's ability to maintain interpersonal relationships, provide self-care, and enjoy other pursuits important to an integrated ego. Determination of functional status using the activities of daily living

(ADLs) assessment tool, which measures ability to complete basic self-care activities such as bathing, dressing, and eating; and the instrumental activities of daily living (IADLs) assessment, which measures home management skills such as telephone use, food purchasing, conduct of personal affairs should be performed routinely, especially in patients who begin to exhibit failure to thrive. Although Mrs. B. wants to remain in her own home, at times she is so fatigued that ambulation is difficult. Her need for supplemental oxygen is variable, but certainly contributes to her immobility. As her nutritional status improves with a more consistent and appropriate food intake, an assessment of functional status and the implementation of an exercise regimen designed to meet physical mobility needs will facilitate her ability to live independently.

7. *Multiple medication intake.* It is estimated that 76 to 92 per cent of older persons take at least one or more prescription or nonprescription drugs daily (White, 1994). In the elderly, three out of four office visits to family physicians relate to the continuance or initiation of drug therapy. Antihypertensive agents, antiarrythmics, cardiac glycosides, diuretics, and sedatives or hypnotics are the classes of drugs most commonly prescribed for this age group. Over-the-counter drugs most commonly consumed by the elderly include analgesics, laxatives, and nutritional supplements. A review of clinically important drug–food interactions of which family physicians should be aware has been published recently (e.g., Trovato et al., 1991, and Kirk, 1995).

SUMMARY

Hilary B.'s case is representative of the types of nutritional problems frequently encountered by family physicians in the delivery of medical care to geriatric patients. Only 5 to 6 per cent of our

TABLE 62–1. Selected Indicators of Nutritional Depletion in Adults

Indicator	Degree of Depletion		
	Mild	*Moderate*	*Severe*
Weight loss	5–15%	15–25%	>25%
Serum albumin level	2.8–3.5 mg/dl	2.1–2.8 mg/dl	<2.1 mg/dl
Serum prealbumin level	10–15 mg/dl	5–10 mg/dl	<5 mg/dl

Adapted from Chicago Dietetic Association, South Suburban Dietetic Association. American Dietetic Association Manual of Clinical Dietetics. Chicago, American Dietetic Association, 1992.

The Warning Signs of poor nutritional health are often overlooked. Use this checklist to find out if you or someone you know is at nutritional risk.

Read the statements below. Circle the number in the yes column for those that apply to you or someone you know. For each yes answer, score the number in the box. Total your nutritional score.

DETERMINE YOUR NUTRITIONAL HEALTH

	YES
I have an illness or condition that made me change the kind and/or amount of food I eat.	2
I eat fewer than 2 meals per day.	3
I eat few fruits or vegetables, or milk products.	2
I have 3 or more drinks of beer, liquor or wine almost every day.	2
I have tooth or mouth problems that make it hard for me to eat.	2
I don't always have enough money to buy the food I need.	4
I eat alone most of the time.	1
I take 3 or more different prescribed or over-the-counter drugs a day.	1
Without wanting to, I have lost or gained 10 pounds in the last 6 months.	2
I am not always physically able to shop, cook and/or feed myself.	2
	TOTAL

Total Your Nutritional Score. If it's —

0-2   **Good!** Recheck your nutritional score in 6 months.

3-5   **You are at moderate nutritional risk.** See what can be done to improve your eating habits and lifestyle. Your office on aging, senior nutrition program, senior citizens center or health department can help. Recheck your nutritional score in 3 months.

6 or more You are at high nutritional risk. Bring this checklist the next time you see your doctor, dietitian or other qualified health or social service professional. Talk with them about any problems you may have. Ask for help to improve your nutritional health.

These materials developed and distributed by the Nutrition Screening Initiative, a project of:

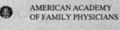

AMERICAN ACADEMY OF FAMILY PHYSICIANS

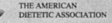

THE AMERICAN DIETETIC ASSOCIATION

NATIONAL COUNCIL ON THE AGING, INC.

sponsored in part through a grant from Ross Products Division, Abbott Laboratories.

Remember that warning signs suggest risk, but do not represent diagnosis of any condition. Turn the page to learn more about the Warnings Signs of poor nutritional health.

The Nutrition Screening Initiative • 1010 Wisconsin Avenue, NW • Suite 800 • Washington, DC 20007

Figure 62–1. Self-assessment tool for nutritional screening in the elderly. (Reprinted with permission by the Nutrition Screening Initiative, a project of the American Academy of Family Physicians, the American Dietetic Association, and the National Council on the Aging, Inc., and funded in part by a grant from Ross Products Division, Abbot Laboratories.)

nation's elderly reside in institutional settings (NSI, 1994). On any given day, less than 1 per cent of all elderly persons are hospitalized. Thus most elderly patients presenting to family physicians for care are seen in the ambulatory care setting. In both long-term and acute-care institutional settings, the federally mandated Minimum Data Set and revised Joint Commission on Accreditation of Healthcare Organizations guidelines mandate minimal nutrition screening with further assessment and intervention as indicated. These types of nutrition-related activities are encouraged, but are not currently mandated in ambulatory care settings. It is imperative, therefore, that family physicians be aware of the myriad of factors that contribute to malnutrition in the elderly and that a routine system of screening and intervention be implemented as an integral component of health care services to the elderly provided by them regardless of setting.

A number of simple self-assessment tools and other screening devices have been developed to assist physicians in the nutritional evaluation of the elderly (NSI, 1994). The Determine Your Nutritional Health Checklist (Fig. 62–1) is particularly suited to routine use in ambulatory care settings. It consists of a set of key statements or questions to which the older person or his or her caregiver can respond. Written at a fourth- to sixth-grade reading level, the average reading level of American adults, it allows the caregiver or elderly individual to identify risk factors in the elder's daily environment that may jeopardize nutritional well-being. Low-cost interventions such as nutrition education or counseling, congregate or home-delivered feeding programs, shopping assistance, homemaker services, medication review and revision, physical exercise, a

dental evaluation, and so forth can then be implemented to improve or to stabilize nutritional health.

More sophisticated screening tools have been developed to aid in the diagnosis and quantification of moderate to severe malnutrition in older persons, particularly those residing in institutional settings (NSI, 1994). These screening devices, which include assessment of functional, cognitive, and emotional status as well as anthropometric and laboratory assessments of nutritional health, can be implemented at the discretion of the family physician and serve as an initial step in the provision and monitoring of more sophisticated forms of nutritional support.

Consultation with a Registered Dietitian

Registered dietitians (RDs) are eager to work with physicians to ensure the nutritional health of America's older population. Both recognize the integral role nutrition plays in the maintenance of health and quality of life, and its positive impact on health care costs. RDs are well versed in the screening and assessment of nutritional status and in the development of cost-effective nutritional care plans to provide for the diversity of nutritional needs that members of this age group have.

When referring an elderly patient for nutritional care, it is critical that the RD be provided with the medical information relevant to the nutritional status of the patient being referred. It is equally necessary for the RD to convey back to the referring physician a complete summary of all relevant information gleaned during the interview and counseling session that follows. Suggestions regarding care of the patient can be offered to the physician for consideration and implementation as deemed appropriate.

SUGGESTED READING

Casper RC. Nutrition and its relationship to aging. Exp Gerontol 1995;30:299–314.

Gamble CL. Lipid disorders: Tailoring diet and drug therapy for individual needs. Geriatrics 1994;49:55–58.

Kirk JK. Significant drug-nutrient interactions. Am Fam Physician 1995;51:1175–1185.

Mion LC, McDowell JA, Heaney LK. Nutritional assessment of the elderly in the ambulatory care setting. Nurse Pract Forum 1994;5:46–51.

Nutrition Screening Initiative (NSI). Incorporating Nutrition Screening and Interventions into Medical Practice: A Monograph for Physicians. Washington, DC, NSI, 1994.

Oral and dental problems in the elderly. Clin Geriatr Med 1992;8:447–692.

Trovato A, Nuhelieck D, Midtling J. Drug-nutrient interactions. Am Fam Physician 1991;44:1651–1658.

White JV. Risk factors for poor nutritional status. Prim Care Clin 1994;21:19–32.

1. True or false: Objective signs of protein-calorie malnutrition include
   a. Involuntary weight loss of greater than 10 per cent of body mass in 6 months
   b. A serum cholesterol greater than 240 mg/dl
   c. Temporal muscle wasting
   d. A serum albumin less than 3.5 gm/dl
   e. A fasting glucose of less than 70 mg/dl

2. Which of the following diseases or conditions is most frequently associated with involuntary weight loss in the elderly?
   a. Diabetes mellitus, poorly controlled
   b. Chronic obstructive pulmonary disease
   c. Depression
   d. Congestive heart failure
   e. Hypercholesterolemia

3. True or false: The following dietary suggestions are appropriate for older individuals who are trying to gain weight:
   a. Add sugar to beverages.
   b. Drink only low fat or skim milk.
   c. Eat a bedtime snack.
   d. Fry foods.
   e. Avoid gravies and sauces.

Answers appear on **page 606**.

Chapter 63

Eating Disorders

Lawrence H. Miller, M.D.

INITIAL VISIT

Subjective

PATIENT IDENTIFICATION. Nancy P., a 34-year-old white woman, is an elementary school teacher who presents with continuous cough, constipation alternating with diarrhea, and abdominal pain.

PRESENTING PROBLEM. Nancy gives a 3-year history of cyclic constipation, requiring laxatives to correct, followed by protracted episodes of diarrhea and abdominal pain. She also is concerned about fatigue, insomnia, crying spells, and a recently acquired continuous cough.

PRESENT ILLNESS. Nancy has described herself as a lifelong perfectionist who has never succeeded in gaining her desired degree of perfection. She has been previously diagnosed with anorexia. Over 3 years ago, after an intentional weight loss of 21 lb in 3 months, she became obsessed with her weight. She took diuretics to control fluid retention, which resulted in severe constipation. She then resorted to numerous laxatives to correct the constipation, which resulted in diarrhea and cramping abdominal pain. More recently, she has started inducing vomiting after binge eating in reaction to marital discord. Nancy admits to feelings of depression, guilt associated with eating or weight gain, and great pride in her thinness and ability to control her weight.

PAST MEDICAL HISTORY. Nancy had a fractured arm at age 13. She has no drug or other allergies. Her only medication is birth control pills.

476

FAMILY HISTORY. Nancy is the eldest of three children. Her father is age 57 and in good health except for hypertension. She describes him as extremely strict, overprotective, and judgmental, frequently teasing her about weight fluctuations. Her mother is age 55, works as a relief special-education teacher, and has always had to watch her weight. Siblings are ages 30 and 28 and are in good health.

SOCIAL HISTORY. Nancy has recently filed for divorce from her husband after 9 years of marriage. She has two children—a daughter age 7, and a son age 5. She describes her husband as emotionally and physically abusive, frequently making degrading comments about her appearance, claiming that no other man would ever find her desirable.

HEALTH HABITS. Nancy works as a schoolteacher and tutors students after school to support herself and her children during the divorce process. She smokes half a pack of cigarettes per day and has smoked since she was 17 years old. She denies drinking. She walks at least 2 miles every day. Nancy eats one meal a day and drinks juices and water for her remaining meals. She proudly reports that she has the lowest fat diet of anyone she knows.

REVIEW OF SYSTEMS. Nancy is concerned about a recent 2-lb weight gain. She associates her cough with a persistent throat irritation which coincides with her frequent purging. She has noticed a discoloration of her teeth. Her hair and skin are drier than usual. Her menses are irregular. Her last menstrual period was 4 months ago.

Objective

PHYSICAL EXAMINATION. Nancy is a pleasant, thin white woman who is alert and cooperative. She is 66 inches tall and weighs 102 lb. Her blood pressure is 98/60 mm Hg in the left arm (sitting), pulse 78 and regular, respirations 16, temperature 98.2° F. Her physical examination is significant for the following. Skin: She has dry skin generally, no scars. Hair is dry, brittle, and with split ends. Head, eyes, ears, nose, and throat: Dry, erythematous oropharynx. Halitosis. Etched enamel on teeth with discoloration. Lungs: Clear to auscultation. Cardiovascular: Sinus rhythm without murmur. Abdomen: Scaphoid. No masses or organomegaly. Hyperactive bowel sounds. Rectal: Normal tone, no masses, negative fecal occult blood. Pelvis: Normal parous female, no masses or tenderness. Extremities: Thin, no edema or joint swelling. Neurologic: Cranial

nerves II to XII intact. Deep tendon reflexes 2–3+ and symmetrical. No tremor. Normal sensory, balance, and proprioceptions.

Assessment

WORKING DIAGNOSIS

1. *Anorexia nervosa.* Nancy meets numerous criteria—weight 15 per cent below ideal, fear of gaining weight, amenorrhea, dry skin, constipation.

2. *Bulimia nervosa.* Purging, diuretics, self-induced vomiting.

DIFFERENTIAL DIAGNOSIS

1. *Somatization disorder.* Characterized by recurrent somatic complaints over several years, usually involving several organ systems.

2. *Depression.* Usually involves a disturbed sleep-wake cycle, depressed mood, suicidal ideation, weight loss, poor concentration.

3. *Irritable bowel syndrome.* Symptoms are primarily focused on abdominal complaints, such as bloating, cramping, constipation, diarrhea, and flatulence, all of which are frequently associated with life stressors. The patient's focus on weight control is inconsistent with this diagnosis.

Plan

LABORATORY AND SPECIAL TESTS. The focus is on diagnostic modalities for general physical health: blood chemistry tests, thyroid profile, complete blood count (CBC), urinalysis, and electrocardiogram (ECG).

THERAPEUTIC. The focus must be on weight restoration by way of a balanced diet and reduction of excessive exercise. This includes dealing with issues of self-esteem, self-control, and reaction to stressors.

PATIENT EDUCATION. Accurate instruction on appropriate caloric intake coordinated with basic metabolic needs is essential. Education balancing energy consumption with caloric intake while maintaining self-image is crucial.

DISPOSITION. Nancy is placed on a regular, scheduled program of physical assessment with her family physician as well as instructional, limited physical therapy and insight-oriented psychotherapy. Bulking agents are used to avoid episodic constipation and her former abuse of laxatives.

DISCUSSION

Eating disorders constitute a spectrum moving in both directions from the median we call normal. If we consider the actuarial tables from insurance companies as accurately representing normal weight ranges for height and age, then deviations in either direction constitute being over or under one's ideal weight. The spectrum runs from morbid obesity to obesity to overeating to normal to dieting to partial syndrome eating disorder to full syndrome anorexia and/or bulimia nervosa. For the purpose of this case study, eating disorders on the underweight side of normal are considered. Obesity is considered separately (see Chapter 59).

In the DSM-IV (American Psychiatric Association, 1994) are published diagnostic criteria for anorexia and bulimia (Table 63–1). Unfortunately, health care professionals have focused on these criteria and lost sight of the fact that the general societal emphasis on dieting has resulted in an eightfold rise in the risk of later development of an eating disorder. Prevalence rates for the partial syndrome are about 3 per cent, for bulimia about 1 per cent, and for anorexia about 0.5 per cent.

There are predictive behaviors in early childhood of later developing eating disorders. Pica and problems at mealtime in early childhood are related to later bulimia, whereas picky eating and digestive problems are related to later anorexia.

Surveys of adolescents reveal that 60 per cent of girls and 15 per cent of boys are dieting at any point in time. Many youth are dieting to lose weight even though their weight is normal or less than normal at the time. Five to 15 per cent of adolescent girls use unhealthy practices to control weight, such as self-induced vomiting, laxatives, and diuretics.

TABLE 63–1. DSM-IV Diagnostic Criteria for Anorexia and Bulimia

DSM-IV criteria for the diagnosis of anorexia include the following:
1. Refusal to maintain body weight over minimal normal weight for age or height
2. Body weight being 15% below expected
3. Body image distortion (patient sees herself as fat)
4. Absence of three consecutive menstrual cycles
5. Excessive exercises and hyperactivity
6. Social and sexual withdrawal
7. Constipation, bradycardia, electrolyte imbalance

DSM-IV criteria for the diagnosis of bulimia include the following:
1. Recurrent episodes of binge eating, with minimum of two episodes a week for three months
2. Purging behaviors: self-induced vomiting, laxative and diuretic abuse
3. Body image distortion (patient sees herself as fat)
4. Excessive exercise and hyperactivity
5. Social and sexual withdrawal

From American Psychiatric Association. Diagnostic and Statistical Manual of Mental Disorders, 4th ed (DSM-IV). Washington, DC, American Psychiatric Association, 1994, pp 251–254. By permission of the publisher.

Anorexics see themselves as fat—despite their actual size or weight. Their goal is a "perfect" body, not just good or close to great. Being fat, or consuming or approaching fat creates a sense of terror. They are obsessed with food, diets, exercise, and metabolism. Denial of emaciation, despite the obvious, is normal because they see themselves differently than others see them. Underlying psychological features include intense awareness of body image, a desire for perfection, and a sense of lack of control.

Treatment approaches cannot be limited to caloric balance and actuarial reports. Restructuring of self-image and a broadened approach to control issues are critical to achieving therapeutic goals.

SUGGESTED READING

Lemberg R. Controlling Eating Disorders with Facts, Advice, and Resources. Phoenix, AZ, Oryx, 1992.

Low BL. Eating disorders. Singapore Med J 1994;35:631–634.

Orr D, McAnarney E, Comerci G, Kreipeeds R (eds). Textbook of Adolescent Medicine. Philadelphia, W.B. Saunders Company, 1992.

Traweger C, Kinzl JF, Guenther W, Biebl W. Family background and sexual abuse associated with eating disorders. Am J Psychiatry 1994;151:1127–1131.

Yager J, Andersen A, Devlin M, et al. Practice guideline for eating disorders. Am J Psychiatry 1993;150:212–228.

1. True or False:
   (a) Most adolescents with eating disorders develop them while dieting.
   (b) Anorexia nervosa has a mortality rate of 2 to 8 per cent.
   (c) Families of anorexics are typically physically and sexually abusive.
   (d) Control and autonomy are underlying goals to anorexics.
   (e) Pica behavior in infants is related to later bulimic behavior.
   (f) Anorexic patients, although underweight, perceive themselves as fat.
   (g) Repeated vomiting may result in acid damage to the teeth.
   (h) Hospitalization and parenteral nutrition may be necessary in severe cases of anorexia and bulimia.
   (i) Patients with anorexia are obsessed with the caloric value of foods.
   (j) Hyperthyroidism causes anorexia nervosa.
   (k) Irritable bowel syndrome leads to bulimia nervosa.

Answers appear on **page 607.**

Chapter 64

Heartburn

William MacMillan Rodney, M.D.

INITIAL VISIT

Subjective

PATIENT IDENTIFICATION AND PRESENTING PROBLEM. Mr. Steve W. is a married, 35-year-old white father of two. He is a registered nurse who works rotating shifts in the hospital. He is a reliable historian and a compliant patient who has been in the practice for 5 years. His index complaint is continuing epigastric and substernal pain over the past 3 months.

PATIENT ILLNESS. Steve has experienced mild "heartburn" related to large meals sporadically over the past few years. He has self-medicated with over-the-counter (OTC) products, and these episodes were self-limited.

Three months ago after "all-you-can-eat-night"

at the hospital cafeteria, the gradual onset of a severe burning discomfort extending from the xiphoid to the jaw kept Steve awake for 15 to 30 minutes past his normal sleep time. Although not as severe, these attacks have persisted at the rate of three to four times per week since then. By reading in his nursing textbooks, he has implemented several clinical strategies which include no meals after 8:00 P.M. and raising his head by using two extra pillows. This seemed to help a little.

Two weeks ago, he noted the gradual onset of diffuse upper abdominal pain during the day in contrast to his other pain, which occurs in the evening and at bedtime. Although the pain occurs 1 to 2 hours after meals, it also comes at other times. He has started a regular antacid routine of 1 tablespoon of Maalox with each meal. The pain has continued. One week ago, it radiated to his back, but not to his shoulders or jaw. Two days ago, Steve was awakened by his worst pain ever. He was going to come to the office as an emergency work-in, but by morning, the pain was gone.

SYMPTOM ANALYSIS

Provoked: By going to bed (supine posture), but the pain is not pleuritic.
Palliated: By getting up and swallowing some antacids. The pain seems to go away with time.
Quality: Sharp, burning.
Quantity: At its worst, it is 9 on a scale of 10. Now it is 0 to 1.
Region: Diffuse upper abdomen and midchest.
Radiation: Radiation to the shoulders or jaw, but patient stated the pain has radiated through to his back on several occasions.
Severity: By morning, Steve feels well enough to go to work. He worked the full day without further problems.

Temporal factors:

(1) Previous *onsets* were gradual; this one was sudden.

(2) Pains are *constant*, lasting 30 to 120 minutes.

(3) Pains have been *recurrent* over months, but this was *the first time* he was awakened.

PAST MEDICAL HISTORY. Surgeries: None. Allergies: None. Hospitalizations: None. Illnesses: Early A.M. insomnia and dysphoria diagnosed as depression 4 months ago. Medications: (1) Prescription medications: nortriptyline, 75 mg and (2) OTC medications: Antacid preparations (Tums, Alka-Seltzer tablets) P.M. Average consumption of two Alka-Seltzer tablets after a meal once in a while; and a generic antacid (Maalox, Mylanta, Gelusil, and others) taken 1 tablespoon before each meal during the past week; this has not relieved his worsening pain.

FAMILY AND SOCIAL HISTORY. Steve grew up as the only child of a divorced registered nurse who raised him lovingly. His father died at age 60 of a sudden "heart attack." Among bloodline relatives, there is no report of diabetes, high blood pressure, or tuberculosis. A maternal aunt has had breast cancer, but is still alive. The father's side of the family is known for "bad nerves," including a "nervous stomach."

Steve was a corpsman in the Army for 4 years after high school. By working shifts in a nursing home, he was able to put himself through college obtaining his nursing degree at age 28. His wife works as an accountant and they have two healthy children, ages 7 and 5. He does not smoke. He drinks alcohol rarely. He jogs on weekends whenever he can.

REVIEW OF SYSTEMS. He denies any new headaches, change in vision, dyspnea, wheezing, exercise-related chest pain, diaphoresis, night sweats, cough, syncope, palpitations, numbness, tingling, arthralgia, myalgia, weakness, or rash. He has experienced some nausea, but no actual vomiting. In particular, there has been no hematemesis, melena, diarrhea, or constipation. His appetite is good, but recently there has been some pain associated with eating. He has lost 5 lb. He is sexually active with his wife. He denies dysuria and penile discharge.

Objective

PHYSICAL EXAMINATION. Steve's height is 70 inches, weight 235 lb, and he has the following vital signs: blood pressure 140/88 mm Hg, pulse 80 regular, respirations 14, temperature 37°C by mouth. He is alert, cooperative, and overweight. Integument: Normal distribution and quality. Head, eyes, ears, nose, and throat: Unremarkable. Chest: Mild pectus excavatum; no point tenderness; lungs are clear. Bowel sounds can be heard on the left anterior, inferior chest wall. Heart: The point of maximal impulse is localized to the fourth intercostal space within the left midclavicular line. There are no heaves, gallops, or murmurs. Pulses are appropriately strong and equal (carotid, brachial, femoral, and dorsalis pedis). Abdomen: The abdomen is convex, and bowel sounds are present. No bruits are heard. Although the abdomen is soft, examination is suboptimal secondary to the patient's increased girth. No masses are palpated. The liver percusses to a vertical span of 12 cm in the right midclavicular line. Moderate palpation creates reproducible discomfort in the upper abdomen, generally most prominent in the midline. Murphy sign (simultaneous palpation to the right costal margin in the midclavicular line while the patient takes a deep breath) is positive. Abdominal and inguinal hernias are absent. Testicles are normal in size, shape, and consistency. Mild external hemorrhoids are present without fissures, fistulas, or sinus tracts. Sphincter tone is normal, and digital rectal examination produces soft, dark brown stool which tests "trace" positive for occult blood. The musculoskeletal and neurological examinations are normal. The patient appears appropriately concerned regarding his condition. He responds in a guarded, but appropriate fashion to humor. He feels his family is supportive.

His job is difficult, but fulfilling. He is hopeful regarding his illness and optimistic regarding his future.

FOLLOW-UP EXAMINATION AND LABORATORY TESTS. Blood pressure and pulse are remeasured in the supine and standing position. Supine blood pressure is 140/90 mm Hg, pulse 82; standing after 2 minutes, blood pressure 126/80, pulse 92. The results of tests in the office laboratory are as follows: hemoglobin 14.1 gm/dl (normal 14 to 18 gm/dl), white blood cell count (WBC) 8000/mm³ (normal 4200 to 10,000/mm³), aspartate aminotransferase (AST) 31 U/L (normal 1 to 36 U/L), alanine aminotransferase (ALT) 47 U/L (normal 1 to 45 U/L), total bilirubin 0.9 mg/dl (normal 0.5 to 1.1 mg/dl), amylase 44 U/L (normal less than 240 U/L), prothrombin time, activated partial thromboplastin time, and creatine phosphokinase (CPK) all normal. Urinalysis reveals pH 5.0 and specific gravity 1.014. The dipstick chemistries and the microscopic examination are normal.

The electrocardiogram (ECG) reveals a normal sinus rhythm of 84 with an axis of -30 degrees. The intervals are measured as follows: PR, 200 msec; QRS, 100 msec; QT, 340 msec. There are no signs of cardiomegaly or ischemia. The posteroanterior and lateral chest films are negative for effusions, infiltrates, and cardiomegaly. There is no air under the diaphragm.

Assessment

WORKING DIAGNOSIS. The working diagnosis is *undifferentiated peptic disease* of the upper gastrointestinal system. This category of disease includes ulcer, gastritis, duodenitis, and esophagitis. Each of these distinct entities exists on a continuum which ranges from mild to severe.

Interpretation of the medical literature requires a common definition of terms. "Peptic ulcer disease" is a traditional catch-all diagnosis; however, "peptic disease syndrome" more accurately describes the variety of these conditions. In one series from the offices of family physicians, less than 10 per cent of dyspeptic patients actually had ulcers (Rodney et al., 1993).

"Dyspepsia" is the preferred general term which encompasses all others (i.e., heartburn, indigestion, reflux, upper abdominal pain, meal-related epigastric pain.) Patients may describe it partially or totally with terms like, "gas," "bloating," or even "food allergy."

Dyspepsia can reflect a single peptic disease or the concurrent existence of several. For example, a duodenal ulcer and esophagitis can exist simultaneously. Dyspepsia can occur in nonpeptic conditions such as cancer, cholelithiasis, pancreatitis, pneumonia, depression, and others. Commonly prescribed drugs such as erythromycin, nonsteroidal anti-inflammatory drugs (NSAIDs), ampicillin, theophylline, and others can cause dyspepsia.

Describing the diagnostic dilemma that faces the clinician of first contact, a widely respected gastroenterologist has said, "It has been taught that there are classic symptoms which differentiate types of peptic ulcer diseases with regard to meals, types of pain, and other symptoms. With endoscopy, all of these concepts have been dramatically revised. We have detected patients with large ulcers who had minimal, if any, symptoms. Other patients have had disabling symptoms with a totally normal endoscopic examination" (Rogers, 1988).

DIFFERENTIAL DIAGNOSIS

1. *Gastric or duodenal ulcer.* A gastric or duodenal ulcer can perforate, requiring immediate hospitalization. These patients usually present with unrelenting abdominal pain which can radiate to the back and/or shoulder. When the condition advances to generalized peritonitis, the abdomen becomes rigid and bowel sounds usually disappear. Less advanced cases may be detectable only by the appearance of free air under the diaphragm. A chest radiograph is ordered for Steve to rule out the possibility of silent perforation.

2. *Bleeding secondary to peptic disease.* This can range from subclinical to life-threatening. A positive fecal occult blood test (FOBT) is consistent with peptic disease, colorectal cancer, intestinal arteriovenous malformations, coagulopathy, hemorrhoids, and others. Normal coagulation chemistries are reassuring, but these laboratory tests are not mandatory when the patient does not bleed excessively with normal activities (e.g., brushing of teeth).

Although the age of 35 does not exclude colorectal cancer, it is reasonable to pursue the more probable diagnosis of peptic disease. This decision is based on the strong history. Similarly, the finding of hemorrhoids is not sufficient to explain and dismiss a positive FOBT in this setting.

Immediate analysis of the FOBT includes a hematocrit or hemoglobin (Hb) along with orthostatic measurements. A Hb of less than 10 and/or significant orthostatic changes require close observation in the hospital.

3. *Upper gastrointestinal neoplasia.* Cancer is always

a consideration; however, Steve exemplifies the clinical situation in which a thoughtful analysis and empirical therapy precede full-scale technological investigations designed to "rule out cancer." Immediate endoscopy, computed tomography (CT) scans, and upper gastrointestinal x-ray studies are *not* indicated at this time. Consider other possibilities and return to this one if the patient becomes increasingly ill or unstable.

4. *Emotional disorder.* Depression and/or anxiety can be expressed as a chronic nervous, painful stomach. Severe depression may include anorexia, weight loss, and insomnia. Steve has been recently diagnosed with this depression. His appetite has been unchanged although some episodes of eating have become more painful.

The awakening with severe pain is not characteristic of depression. Depression may exhibit early A.M. insomnia with difficulty getting back to sleep. Anxiety may lead to difficulty initiating sleep. Neither are usually associated with severe burning substernal pain. This pattern is consistent with severe esophagitis. Furthermore, sitting up, swallowing, and antacid ingestion can palliate a severe attack within 30 to 120 minutes. Pain at bedtime is common among patients with gastroesophageal reflux disease (GERD).

Patients with GERD may have difficulty initiating sleep. In contrast to the poorly defined symptoms of anxiety-related insomnias, GERD patients know exactly why they cannot sleep. It is because of epigastric-substernal pain. Ironically, strong sedatives can produce sleep which overrides the symptom while the underlying esophageal pathology continues unabated. Steve's symptoms are *not* characteristic of depression or anxiety.

5. *Side effects from drugs.* Dyspepsia can be initiated or exacerbated by a variety of widely prescribed medications. Steve does not take aspirin or NSAIDs. Antidepressants are notorious for their anticholinergic effects. Theoretically, the antisecretory effects of well-known tricyclic antidepressants (TCADs) should palliate peptic disease. Before the arrival of the H_2 receptor antagonists, several studies demonstrated this helpful effect of TCADs on peptic ulcer patients. This line of investigation was discontinued after successful introduction of cimetidine and other more specific medications.

Could nortriptyline be a problem? Appetite stimulation, sedation, and weight gain may be TCAD side effects which promote GERD. Decreased gastric motility is a possible side effect. However, these are unlikely given the current subtherapeutic dose of nortriptyline.

6. *Cardiovascular problems.* Cardiac and pericardial conditions can present as atypical substernal pain with or without dyspepsia. Risk factors include male sex, family history, and overweight. The ECG demonstrates a PR interval of 200 msec and a QRS axis of 300 msec. Thoracic aortic aneurysm can present as crushing pain which radiates to the back. However, there are no signs of ischemia, and these isolated findings are not sufficient to displace peptic disease syndrome as the working diagnosis.

7. *Hiatal hernia.* Mechanical possibilities include trauma, hernias, and anatomic variations (congenital, iatrogenic, and naturally occurring). There is no history of trauma, chest surgery, abdominal surgery, or caustic ingestion. Pectus excavatum has been associated with atypical chest pains, palpitations, and mitral valve prolapse. The presence of pectus excavatum in Steve is an incidental finding which cannot explain his symptoms. An echocardiogram and/or CT of the chest is not indicated.

Hiatal hernia is prevalent in 20 to 50 per cent of U.S. and western European adults. Diaphragmatic hernias are rare. This patient has auscultable bowel sounds in the left lower chest. Should this finding be heavily weighted? These sounds can be heard at the edge of the left lower chest in 10 to 15 per cent of normal adults. Therefore, the positive predictive value of this finding for diaphragmatic hernia is very low.

However, incarcerated diaphragmatic hernias can present acutely in adults. Continuous pain and dyspnea are characteristic. A normal chest radiograph and the history are not consistent with this possibility. Hiatal hernia is a strong possibility, particularly with the patient being 40 to 50 lb overweight. Hiatal hernia is an anatomic feature which promotes reflux and esophageal inflammation. Weight loss through diet and exercise should be recommended for Steve.

8. *Gastroesophageal reflux disease (GERD).* This can occur in the presence or absence of hiatal hernia. Esophageal inflammation can be painful or painless. The mucosal integrity is protected by the lower esophageal sphincter (LES). LES dysfunction can be associated with hiatal hernias, or it can be idiopathic. In infants, chalasia describes the condition in which LES relaxation permits reflux and pseudo-regurgitation of meals.

In adults, this phenomenon bathes the esophageal mucosa with acidic gastric contents. Small amounts of reflux are well tolerated, but once an injury breaches the mucosal integrity, a vicious cycle begins. The wet environment, continued acid irritation, and the periodic passage of food make healing of esophageal lesions more difficult than healing of peptic lesions elsewhere. As peptic esophagitis advances, swallowing of food can become painful and difficult. Steve does not exhibit overt dysphagia (mechanical difficulty with swallowing, such as food sticking), but his symptoms could be consistent with a mild dysphagia secondary to esophagitis. Chronic esophagitis can produce strictures. Usually these patients describe more difficulty swallowing solids than liquids, but this is also true with some cases of esophagitis. Pain avoidance can lead to severe or mild weight loss. Steve has lost 5 lb.

Steve has accurately self-diagnosed at least part of his problem as esophageal. The heartburn has been present for years, but this condition has dramatically worsened in the last few months. As adults age and girth increases, reflux can become more severe. Discontinuation of evening meals should be expanded to an overall diet plan which includes an explicit weight loss goal, an exercise plan, calorie restriction, and dietary awareness.

Fat, chocolate, and alcohol are notorious LES relaxants. Caffeine is probably not. Under normal conditions, small amounts (and even excesses) are tolerated. Once esophagitis begins, these foods and others should be monitored closely. Positional therapy for GERD has traditionally included placement of 4- to 6-inch blocks under the legs supporting the head of the bed. This has not been proved in clinical trials, but seems prudent. Extra pillows should be discontinued because clinical studies have demonstrated that pillow-supported reclining postures can even increase the amount of reflux.

Antacids should be selected to achieve maximal effect. One tablespoon is not sufficient to neutralize normal stomach acid. However, standing upright and swallowing fluids can produce relief in patients who have been awakened or unable to sleep. A neutralizing equivalent of antacid is 140 mEq. This requires 30 ml of Mylanta, Maalox TC, Gelusil TC, and other high-potency antacids. Gaviscon may be an especially helpful option because the alginate component may create an additional barrier of protection for GERD patients. Patients need explicit, written instructions advising them to take 1 oz ("a shot glass" or "2 tablespoons," but not "a swig") 1 and 3 hours after meals and at bedtime. Therapy is 30 ml orally 1 and 3 hours after meals and again at bedtime. Steve has not fully maximized the potential effect of antacids. This antacid regimen is a fundamental cornerstone of conservative therapy for all the peptic diseases, but ulcers, diet, weight loss, and risk reduction are equally important cornerstones. A low cholesterol diet is also indicated for Steve's elevated cholesterol levels and high-risk cardiovascular profile.

9. *Duodenal ulcer.* Steve's complaints have gone beyond garden variety heartburn and indigestion. Radiation of pain to the back and midcycle sleep awakening suggest more advanced disease that is less likely to respond to conservative measures. Additionally, upper abdominal pain occurring 1 to 2 hours after meals is characteristic of gastric and duodenal lesions rather than lesions limited to the esophagus.

Although pain can radiate to the back with esophageal lesions, this pain can also represent an ulcer on the posterior duodenal wall, gallbladder disease, pancreatitis, perforation, aneurysm, and others. The physical findings of epigastric tenderness and an ambiguous Murphy sign can be found with inflammation of the liver, gallbladder, duodenum, stomach, and esophagus. These physical findings are consistent with several diseases, but not pathognomonic for any one disease in particular.

Laboratory findings reveal elevations of amylase and ALT. These elevations are minuscule and insufficient to displace the working hypothesis of peptic disease syndrome with probable simultaneous involvement of the esophagus, stomach, and duodenum.

Plan

DIAGNOSTIC. When the physician has considered and discounted those conditions requiring hospitalization, investigation and management commonly proceed in the office and by telephone. No further diagnostic tests are needed before the initiation of medical therapy.

Prior to 1985, there was controversy regarding the value of immediate radiologic contrast studies and/or esophagogastroduodenoscopy (EGD). An upper gastrointestinal series with a small bowel follow-through (UGI/SBFT) was frequently ordered when EGD was not available. Similar to the controversy regarding air contrast barium enema (ACBE) versus colonoscopy in lower gastrointestinal lesions, test selection depends on the patient's risk, the community's resources, and the physician's preference.

In contrast to ACBE versus colonoscopy, EGD has emerged as generally superior to UGI/SBFT (Table 64–1). There are exceptions (i.e., motility disorders) and clinical judgment is necessary. Generally the sensitivity of UGI/SBFT is 35 to 60 per cent that of EGD. On the other hand, EGD detects histologically confirmed gastritis in 15 to 20 per cent of healthy, asymptomatic controls. Other than this, EGD has very good sensitivity (75 to 98 per

TABLE 64–1. Comparison of Diagnostic Methods for Peptic Disease Syndromes

Variable	Upper GI X-Ray Series	Esophagogastroduodenoscopy (EGD)
Operator-dependent?	Yes	Yes
Average charge	$140–$240	$470–$970
Continuity of care possible?	No	By family physician: Yes
		By consult: No
Biopsy possible on same visit?	No	Yes
Sedation used?	No	Yes
Portable to the bedside?	No	Yes
Usable in the office?	No	Yes
Usable in the nursing home?	No	Yes
Hard copy of diagnostic images routinely retained?	Yes	By video: Yes
		By photography: Yes
Sensitivity under ideal conditions		
Cancer	30%–40%	60%–80%
Ulcer	40%–60%	90%–98%
Esophagitis	30%–50%	90%–95%
Motility disorder	60%–90%	10%–20%

Note: High specificity and a definite edge in sensitivity for peptic disease lesions favor EGD as the diagnostic test of choice except in suspected motility disorders of the esophagus. Complications are rare with both tests.

GI = Gastrointestinal.

cent) and high specificity (95 to 99 per cent) for peptic disease lesions. Specificity figures are confirmed by biopsy and brushing.

In 1985, the Health and Public Policy Committee of the American College of Physicians published a thoughtful and widely accepted consensus statement advocating empirical therapy for probable peptic disease syndrome. Further diagnostic tests are delayed pending the results of this therapy. This consensus concluded that "if all dyspeptic patients are treated empirically, considerable diagnostic resources will be saved."

Upper gastrointestinal cancers are relatively uncommon, and the collective survival rate for these cancers is not improved significantly by universal detection 6 to 8 weeks earlier. Endoscopy should be reserved for two subsets of patients: (1) those who have no or minimal response to therapy after 7 to 10 days; and (2) those patients (30 per cent) whose illness improves but does not resolve after 6 to 8 weeks.

By 1995, *Helicobacter pylori* was a proved cofactor in peptic ulcer disease. The eradication of *H. pylori* became an essential factor in the treatment of patients with ulcer disease. Since *H. pylori* could be diagnosed by rapid urease testing (formerly known as the *Campylobacter*-like organism [CLO] test) available to family physicians performing EGD in the office, this diagnostic advantage even more firmly established EGD as the diagnostic modality of choice (Conwell et al., 1995).

THERAPEUTIC. Short-term therapeutic goals include prevention of complications, pain relief, and mucosal healing. Simultaneously, there is hypothesis testing with empirical therapy. Peptic disease is notoriously recurrent at an annual rate of 44 to 70 per cent. A secondary therapeutic goal is the long-term prevention of recurrence.

Placebo-controlled studies of duodenal ulcers have demonstrated that one third of patients have spontaneous resolution of disease over 8 weeks. Rigorous administration of 15 to 30 ml of antacids significantly increases the healing rate to 85 to 87 per cent. If the response is favorable, the 15-ml dose may decrease some of the side effects.

The inconvenience and bulk of liquids is a barrier to compliance. Dosage schedules requiring seven daily doses are difficult to maintain. For these reasons, a variety of more convenient tablets have emerged as the drugs of choice (Table 64–2). These drugs are all effective and safe. The H_2 receptor antagonists can be prescribed in split doses, such as cimetidine 400 mg twice daily or 300 mg four times daily, ranitidine 150 mg twice daily, famotidine 20 mg twice daily, and nizatidine 150 mg twice daily. Alternatively, the entire daily dose can be given at bedtime.

TABLE 64–2. Comparison of Healing Rates in Duodenal Ulcer Using Various Medications

Drug	Dosage	Per Cent Ulcers Healed	
		4 Weeks	*8 Weeks*
Cimetidine (Tagamet)	800 mg h.s.	80–85	90–95
Ranitidine (Zantac)	300 mg h.s.	80–85	90–95
Famotidine (Pepcid)	40 mg h.s.	80–85	90–95
Nizatidine (Axid)	300 mg h.s.	80–85	90–95
Sucralfate (Carafate)	1 gm q.i.d.	75	86
Misoprostol (Cytotec)	200 μg q.i.d.	70	80
Omeprazole (Prilosec)	20 mg daily	90–95	90–95
Lansoprazole (Prevacid)	30 mg daily	90–95	90–95

All of these medical therapies in dosages listed are probably equally effective for empirical therapy of dyspepsia. Therefore, where available, generic drugs are the best first choice.

For shift workers, a twice-daily dosing schedule may be better than a strict bedtime-only dosage. Most patients notice improvement in 24 to 72 hours with these medications. Based on the cumulative millions of patient-years experience with H_2 receptor antagonists, long-term usage is probably safe. They cannot be used in pregnancy.

Sucralfate, a cytoprotective agent, can be given 2 g twice daily. It is an agent that preferentially binds to ulcerated mucosa. Since it does not act systemically, it probably is safe during pregnancy. Onset of effect may require 2 to 7 days.

Misoprostol is a cytoprotective agent and prostaglandin analogue that promotes bicarbonate and mucus secretion by gastric mucosa. Omeprazole and lansoprazole are potent antisecretory agents that inhibit the H^+/K^+ ATPase proton pump. This pump is the final step in gastric acid secretion by the parietal cell. Bismuth agents may promote duodenal and gastric ulcer healing by a bactericidal effect on *H. pylori*. These various agents are effective, but their properties and long-term benefits are not as well studied.

When ulcers are present, *H. pylori* should be eradicated with antibiotic therapy. Effective eradication requires acid suppression with an H_2 receptor antagonist or a proton pump inhibitor. Simultaneously, antibiotics with or without bismuth are given for 7 to 14 days. Multiple possible permutations of equally effective *H. pylori* eradication regimens exist. The author currently recommends a low-cost generic protocol for the vast majority of these patients. One example would be cimetidine or ranitidine coupled with amoxicillin 1 gm orally twice a day and metronidazole 500 mg orally three times daily.

The antibiotics are given for 7 to 14 days, while acid suppression is continued for at least 8 weeks total.

Esophageal lesions require a special treatment plan. Placebo trials confirm a 30 to 40 per cent spontaneous improvement in erosive GERD. Sucralfate also assists in healing. Those episodes that do not resolve may require larger doses and longer periods of traditional H_2 receptor antagonists (e.g., cimetidine 800 mg twice daily or ranitidine 300 mg twice daily). Despite 12 weeks of therapy, only 70 to 75 per cent of patients may be healed.

Omeprazole has produced complete healing in 85 to 95 per cent of esophagitis patients. However, once the omeprazole is stopped, there may be an 82 per cent recurrence rate. Long-term maintenance up to 12 years with omeprazole has been studied, and it has been found safe.

In summary, high-dose H_2 receptor antagonist therapy should be chosen as first-line treatment of common gastric, duodenal, and esophageal diseases, but omeprazole 20 mg twice daily or lansoprazole 30 mg daily are the likely agents of choice for severe esophageal disease. Additional prokinetic agents such as cisapride 10 mg twice daily or four times daily are recommended by some authorities. Previously used prokinetic agents such as metoclopramide and/or bethanechol are no longer recommended by this author.

PATIENT EDUCATION. The patient is encouraged to consider a therapeutic contract for initiation and maintenance of lifestyle changes including weight loss, exercise, avoidance of specific foods, and a calorie/fat diary. Alcohol should be avoided. The head of the bed can be elevated, but no more than one pillow should be used for sleeping.

Chewable or liquid antacids can be used as needed, but should not be taken to interfere with absorption of the primary therapy—high-dose H_2 receptor antagonists twice a day. Antacids taken within 2 hours of these pills may interfere with absorption.

Chewing gum may enhance esophageal clearance, thereby decreasing the amount of time that irritating substances are in contact with damaged mucosa. This is particularly useful for pregnant patients.

DISPOSITION. Re-evaluate in 7 to 14 days. The patient is requested to bring his calorie/fat content diary, which includes a record of daily weight. The diary will report exercise compliance also. Steve is told to anticipate a repeat cholesterol measurement.

Steve is given a prescription for 2 weeks without refills. A phone call will be made by the office nurse at 7 to 10 days to determine if symptoms remain unchanged, have worsened, or improved. Without improvement, Steve will be prepared for EGD in the office by the family physician. Family physicians without EGD skills may request consultation.

FIRST FOLLOW-UP VISIT

Subjective

Steve reports only mild improvement in the dull epigastric pain that had been occurring 1 to 2 hours after meals. However, substernal pain has awakened him nightly for the past three nights. This pain does not radiate to the back, jaw, or shoulders. With upright posture and antacids, the pain gradually dissipates allowing a return to sleep in 30 to 60 minutes.

Steve has initiated the diet/exercise diary, with a loss of an additional 2 lb. He admits difficulty following the diet and misses the camaraderie of "all-you-can-eat-night" at the hospital cafeteria. However, he is determined to succeed at weight and dietary control. He has come to the office NPO since midnight in anticipation of early morning EGD in the office. He has read and signed an informed consent.

Objective

Steve's weight is 233 lb, and his vital signs are stable. Bowel sounds are present, and the epigastric pain to palpation is now gone. Otherwise the abdominal examination is unchanged. Twilight sedation is achieved with the gradual administration of diazepam 7 mg and mepcridine 100 mg intravenously. The endoscopy report states, "Duodenal ulcer, gastritis, and erosive esophagitis. No bleeding noted."

Several biopsies are taken from the edge of the duodenal and esophageal ulcerations. Biopsies are taken from the gastric antrum and fundus. After an hour of observation, normal vital signs, and a return to clear sensorium, Steve is driven home.

Assessment

Based on signs and symptoms, healing of the probable gastritis and the probable duodenal ulcer is proceeding. However, the esophagitis is severe and symptoms are worsening. In summary, high-dose H_2 receptor antagonist therapy could be chosen for simultaneous treatment of probable gastric, duodenal, and esophageal disease, but omeprazole 20 mg twice daily or lansoprazole 30 mg daily are the likely agents of choice for severe esophageal disease. Additional prokinetic agents such as cisapride 10 mg twice daily or four times daily are recommended by some authorities. Previously used prokinetic agents such as metoclopramide and/or bethanechol are not recommended by this author.

Plan

Because of the ulcer, acid suppression is to be continued and *H. pylori* eradication is initiated. Ordinarily an H_2 receptor antagonist could be continued, but because of the severe esophagitis, a proton pump inhibitor is started. Specifically, Steve will receive omeprazole 20 mg twice daily for at least 8 to 12 weeks. For the initial 10 days, he will also receive amoxicillin 2 gm orally twice a day and metronidazole 500 mg twice daily. Recently there has been approval of the regimen that uses omeprazole 20 mg twice daily and clarithromycin 500 mg three times a day. Otherwise, Steve is to continue with all other elements of the previously described management plan. If overt dysphagia develops, stricture formation would be suspected and dilation could be necessary.

A report on the biopsies will be available in 3 to 5 days, but Steve is reassured that malignancy is unlikely. A minimum of an 8-week course of therapy is predicted and maintenance therapy with an H_2 receptor antagonist or a proton pump inhibitor will be necessary for at least an additional year.

SUGGESTED READING

Conwell C, Lyell R, Rodney WM. Prevalence of *Helicobacter pylori* in family practice patients with refractory dyspepsia: A comparison of tests available in the office. J Fam Pract 1995;41:245–249.

DeGowin EL, De Gowin RL (eds). Bedside Diagnostic Examination. New York, Macmillan, 1985.

Dooley CP, Larson AW, Stace NH, et al. Double contrast barium meal and upper gastrointestinal endoscopy: A comparative study. Ann Intern Med 1984;101:538–545.

Rodney WM: Gastrointestinal disorders in the "family physician." In Rakel RE (ed). Textbook of Family Practice, 5th ed. Philadelphia, W.B. Saunders Company, 1995, pp 1192–1227.

Rodney WM, Hocutt JE, Coleman WH, et al. Esophagogastroduodenoscopy by family physicians: A national multisite study of 717 procedures. J Am Board Fam Pract 1990;3:73–79.

Rodney WM, Weber JR, Swedberg JA, et al. Esophagogastroduodenoscopy by family physicians. Phase II: A national multisite study of 2,500 procedures. Fam Pract Res J 1993;13:121–131.

Rogers A. A clinician's approach to dyspepsia. Pract Gastroenterol 1988;12:21–23.

Sall AH. Selection and timing of diagnostic studies for dyspepsia. JAMA 1996;275:624.

Silen W. Cope's Early Diagnosis of the Acute Abdomen. New York, Oxford University Press, 1979.

QUESTIONS

1. Which of the following statements is accurate regarding antacid prescriptions for peptic disease?
   a. Should be taken before meals.
   b. Different OTC brands are equally potent.
   c. Can interfere with absorption of H_2 receptor antagonists.
   d. Do not help esophageal lesions.
   e. An ounce per dose is too much.

2. Nonulcerated gastritis is one histologic manifestation of the peptic disease syndrome. This entity:
   a. Is painful in over 90 per cent of cases.
   b. Can be detected with equal power by either EGD or UGI/SBFT x-rays.
   c. Commonly presents with epigastric pain radiating to the back.
   d. Exists in up to 20 per cent of asymptomatic healthy controls.
   e. All of the above.
   f. None of the above.

3. Esophagogastroduodenoscopy (EGD) as a primary care diagnostic procedure is:
   a. Excessively expensive to place into office practice.
   b. Offers no diagnostic advantage among dyspepsia patients as compared with the less expensive barium meal (upper gastrointestinal x-ray study).
   c. Is the diagnostic method of choice for dyspeptic patients who fail a trial of empirical therapy.
   d. All of the above.
   e. None of the above.

Answers appear on **page 607**.

Chapter 65

Constipation

George A. Nixon, M.D.

INITIAL VISIT

Subjective

PATIENT IDENTIFICATION. Priscilla B., a 61-year-old junior high school principal, retired 1 year ago at the urging of her family after experiencing a myocardial infarction and subsequent cardiac revascularization. After surgery she kept two appointments with her cardiologist, but has seen no other health providers.

PRESENTING PROBLEM. Priscilla has come today complaining of constipation. This problem is associated with recurrent abdominal swelling and vague discomfort in her left side. She is accompanied by her daughter who is pregnant.

PRESENT ILLNESS. Priscilla reports that since her coronary artery bypass surgery 1 year ago she has been unable to get her bowels regulated. Previously, one bowel movement per day was her customary pattern, and she rarely took a laxative. Now she regularly uses laxatives to achieve two to three bowel movements per week. She states, "If I do not take something to keep regular I develop swelling and bloating in my abdomen which make me feel miserable, and I look more pregnant than my daughter." These symptoms are at times associated with mild cramping across the abdomen with radiation of this discomfort into her left side. When this occurs she often anticipates a bowel movement, but usually without results. Priscilla complains that she must strain even when she feels the urge and "when I do go I do not feel fully relieved." She denies any rectal pain or discomfort, but does mention that on two occasions she noticed blood in her stool.

PAST MEDICAL HISTORY. Usual childhood illnesses without sequelae. Menarche at age 13. No history of dysmenorrhea. Menopause at age 50. Previously

took estrogen for perimenopausal symptoms for 8 months, then decided to discontinue therapy. She now takes a calcium supplement for osteoporosis prevention. No history of significant medical illnesses other than the myocardial infarction. Surgical history is that of coronary bypass grafting 1 year ago following her myocardial infarction, and subtotal thyroidectomy for a thyroid adenoma 28 years ago. Other surgeries include cholecystectomy 21 years ago, and a cesarean section for fetal distress after two term vaginal deliveries. No history of significant accidents or trauma.

FAMILY HISTORY. Priscilla's father died at the age of 73 of colon cancer; he had a history of skin cancer and elevated cholesterol. Her mother, age 80, has coronary artery disease and early Alzheimer disease. Her siblings are a brother age 55 in good health except for hypertension and obesity, and a sister age 63 with chronic obstructive pulmonary disease. Priscilla thinks her grandmother died with breast cancer. She does not know the cause of death of her grandfather, but believes it might have been from cancer also.

HEALTH HABITS. Before her heart attack Priscilla had more than a 30 pack-year smoking history. Since her illness she and her husband have both quit. She denies alcohol use, illicit drug use, or drug dependence. She admits to a sedentary lifestyle and to the usual indiscretions of the American diet to which she attributes her excess weight.

SOCIAL HISTORY. Priscilla began her career as a math teacher, before becoming a middle school principal. She had anticipated retiring at the age of 65 years, but reluctantly had now done so at the urging of her spouse and children who convinced her that she had given enough of her time and life to the school system. She and her husband have been happily married for 36 years. They are proud of their children, who have all started families and careers of their own. Priscilla's youngest daughter accompanies her today.

REVIEW OF SYSTEMS. Priscilla reminisces that her heart attack was a surprise to her. She had previously felt fine and enjoyed her job as principal of a local junior high. The job had become more stressful than when she had assumed the position 14 years ago, but she thoroughly enjoyed the students and held the admiration and respect of the school's teachers as well as most parents. Priscilla is disappointed in her recovery from heart surgery. She was informed by her cardiologist that she did not suffer any significant loss of cardiac function, but she has not experienced a return of the mental or physical vitality she had previously known. She denies chest discomfort, shortness of breath, and faithfully takes her prescribed medications: enteric-coated aspirin 325 mg every day and a calcium channel blocker, diltiazem, 180 mg per day. Priscilla's daughter is concerned about what she sees as a change in her mother's behavior. She describes her mother as sitting around the house all day. She states, "When Mom was working she managed to keep up with housework and friends. Now she seems not only to have retired from her job, but also from life. Last month she overdrew her checking account after making a subtraction error in her checkbook. This did not seem to bother Mom, who before would have been highly embarrassed because she was a math teacher. Dad bought her some vitamins and I have given her some of my iron pills, hoping that they might perk her up."

Objective

PHYSICAL EXAMINATION. Vital signs: Blood pressure 138/88 mm Hg, afebrile, heart rate 58, respirations 16, weight 174 lb, and height 67 inches. Priscilla complains about a cold examination room, but is in no acute distress. Her dress is neat; missing, however, is the gregariousness which had before been a hallmark of her personality. Examination of the abdomen revealed it to be protuberant, but not distended. Bowel sounds are present, but hypoactive. No mass or organomegaly is noted. There is an indistinct fullness and mild discomfort in the left lower quadrant to deep palpation, but no guarding or rebound tenderness. A hard dark hemoccult stool is negative on the rectal examination. No impaction is present. Rectal sphincter tone is normal and no prolapse of rectal mucosa is noted on Valsalva maneuver. No hemorrhoids are noted exter-

nally or by anoscopic viewing. The remainder of the examination is otherwise normal except for xeroderma, and notation of previous thyroidectomy and cesarean section surgical scars.

LABORATORY TESTS. A complete blood count reveals a hemoglobin of 13.6 gm/dl with normal white blood cell and red blood cell indices. A urinalysis is normal. A multiple-panel blood analysis shows normal liver function, renal function, electrolytes, glucose, total protein and albumin, but a moderate elevation of triglycerides and a high cholesterol count with a low high-density lipoprotein (HDL) fraction. Thyroid tests revealed an elevated thyroid-stimulating hormone (TSH) and low thyroxine. One of three Hemoccult tests on separate stools is positive.

Assessment

The cause of constipation is often multifactorial, and a comprehensive investigation to identify primary and contributing causes should be the initial step in its evaluation (Table 65–1). The majority of patients do not need extensive diagnostic tests, but those with more severe and chronic symptoms warrant a thorough diagnostic work-up.

TABLE 65–1. Causes of Constipation

Dietary causes: Deficiency of dietary fiber, poor fluid or caloric intake
Gastrointestinal disorders
  Congenital: Hirschsprung disease, irritable bowel syndrome, idiopathic megarectum and megacolon, slow transit syndrome
  Acquired: Carcinoma, diverticulitis, postsurgical or postinflammatory adhesions, volvulus, hernias
Rectal disorders: Hemorrhoids, anal fissures, perirectal abscess, rectocele, rectal prolapse
Genitoreproductive: Pregnancy, hernias, large fibroids, or ovarian masses
Neurologic: Stroke, spinal cord lesions, Parkinson disease, tabes dorsalis, multiple sclerosis
Musculoskeletal: Immobility, debilitated states, weak abdominal muscles
Metabolic/endocrine: Hypothyroidism, hypokalemia, hypercalcemia, diabetes mellitus, uremia, volume contraction
Psychiatric: Depression, social or environmental inhibition, acute emotional disturbance
Systemic conditions: Advanced age, scleroderma, amyloidosis
Medications: See Table 65–2.

WORKING DIAGNOSES. The most likely diagnoses explaining Priscilla's symptoms are:

1. *Side effects of medications.* Constipation is an adverse effect of numerous prescribed and over-the-counter medications (Table 65–2). Review of Priscilla's medications reveals several current and possibly past medications that may have initiated or are presently contributing to her complaints. Calcium channel blockers, used in the treatment of hypertension and coronary artery disease, slow intestinal transit by their effects on the autonomic nervous system and smooth muscle. The calcium antacids that Priscilla takes for osteoporosis prevention, and the iron supplement given to her by her daughter, have constipation as a side effect. Since these complaints date back to Priscilla's myocardial infarction and subsequent bypass surgery, anticholinergics and narcotics likely received at that time may have been inciting agents. Paradoxically, prolonged use of stimulant laxatives (bisacodyl, cascara, phenolphthalein, senna) which may have been taken by Priscilla to address the adverse effects of these medications may now be contributing to the persistence of current symptoms. Stimulant laxatives are associated with melanosis coli (a harmless darkening of the colonic mucosa), injury to the myenteric plexus, development of laxative dependence, and malabsorption of fats, calcium, and potassium.

2. *Hypothyroidism.* Constipation can be a side effect of hypothyroidism. Priscilla has a history of thyroid disease, and her complaint about the room being cold and her dry skin are a symptom and sign of this condition.

3. *Obstruction.* Constipation may result from obstructive lesions in the intestinal lumen (colon carcinoma), within the intestinal wall (diverticular disease), or from external compression (adhesions or extrinsic mass). Clinical signs and symptoms that make it necessary to exclude an obstructive lesion include an abrupt worsening of constipation, abdominal distention, weight loss, stools positive for occult blood or a report of rectal bleeding by the patient. Priscilla has several of these symptoms as well as a family history of cancer.

CONTRIBUTING DIAGNOSES. Likely diagnoses contributing to Priscilla's symptoms are the following:

1. *Low fiber diet.* You should not presume the cause of constipation to be the result of a low fiber diet. A diet low in fiber is, however, a frequent contributor to the severity of the complaint of constipation when it presents. On average, constipated patients are ingesting less than the recommended intake of 25 to 50 gm of dietary fiber. The majority of the processed and fast foods that form the bulk of the American diet add little to the stool bulk. Fiber increases stool weight and improves stool consistency, reduces colonic transit time, and increases the frequency of defecation. Priscilla suggests in the review of her health habits that her diet is lacking in fiber. It is unlikely that diet alone is an encompassing explanation for her abdominal complaints, but it is a probable significant comorbid factor in her presentation.

2. *Physical inactivity.* Priscilla's lack of physical activity may be contributing to her difficulties. She led a sedentary lifestyle, which has become more so since retiring. The relationship between a lack of physical activity and the occurrence of constipation is not conclusively established, but exercise is believed to be of benefit.

3. *Depression.* Depression is thought to inhibit the intestinal muscular activity which controls the release of intestinal contents through neurophysiologic pathways. If Priscilla is depressed, then an antidepressant may improve her symptoms. One must use caution in selecting an antidepressant, as many have anticholinergic effects that may be constipating.

DIFFERENTIAL DIAGNOSIS

1. *Patient misdiagnosis.* Constipation is difficult to define because it is a symptom and not a diagnosis. It therefore has different meanings for individual patients. Some patients expect a bowel movement each day, but there are many for whom one every second or third day is natural. Others define constipation not in terms of frequency, but in terms of stool consistency and size, or the effort needed to defecate. It is important to understand what the patient is defining as constipation as it relates to his

---

TABLE 65–2. Medications Causing Constipation

Prescription Drugs
Pain medications (especially narcotics), anticholinergics, anticonvulsants, antidepressants (especially tricyclics), monoamine oxidase inhibitors, phenothiazines, antiparkinson agents, calcium channel blockers, central α agonists, diuretics, ganglionic blocking agents, barium, many others

Nonprescription Drugs
Aluminum- or calcium-containing antacids, chronic use of stimulant laxatives, iron supplements, bismuth

or her perception of what is normal bowel function. This is useful in guiding assessment and management. Current clinical criteria for defining constipation describe it as two or fewer bowel movements per week when patients are not taking laxatives. There are two distinct syndromes recognized: (1) functional constipation (slow transit) associated with the sensation of incomplete evacuation, and (2) rectosigmoid outlet delay associated with prolonged defecation and periodic occurrence of impaction. Priscilla's symptoms represent a dramatic change from her usual pattern. Her description of decreased frequency, increased straining, and the feeling of incomplete evacuation meet clinical criteria for presence of functional constipation and warrant evaluation.

2. *Metabolic-hormonal abnormalities.* Chronic constipation is associated with endocrine and metabolic diseases such as diabetes, hyperparathyroidism or other hypercalcemic states, and uremia. Diabetics with neuromuscular symptoms of gastroparesis are more apt to complain of constipation. Poorly controlled diabetics may have an osmotic diuresis with lumpy or hard stool secondary to intestinal water reabsorption.

Potassium serum value is of special importance. Gut motility is decreased when potassium is low. Hypokalemia is associated with use of diuretics and also may occur as a consequence of protracted vomiting or diarrhea. Patients who have symptoms of bloating or who are overweight may take diuretics hoping to relieve their discomfort or reduce their weight. They are often reticent in this practice. Although Priscilla gives no history suggesting this behavior, hypokalemia occurs often enough that a determination of serum potassium is a standard part of the work-up of chronic constipation.

3. *Neurogenic causes.* Diseases of the central nervous system, the spinal cord, and the neurophysiologic pathways of the intestine can result in constipation. Priscilla has no evidence of neurologic disease except for possible clinical depression. A differential of neurogenic causes to be considered includes *tabes dorsalis, congenital megacolon (Hirschsprung disease),* and *idiopathic megarectum* or *megacolon.* Syphilis would have other neurologic symptoms if it were the cause. Patients with congenital megacolon usually have symptoms of constipation that date back to childhood, but this condition, in which a section of colon is aganglionic, may not present clinically until much later in life. Absence of any earlier history of recurrent constipation makes it a doubtful explanation in this case. Idiopathic megarectum or megacolon for similar reasons ranks low on the list

of differential diagnoses. As a group, these conditions present with symptoms of constipation and pseudo-obstruction. Barium contrast studies are diagnostic.

4. *Mechanical causes.* Rectal examination while the patient strains can reveal those with *rectal prolapse* or *rectocele.* These patients complain that they sense frequently the urge to defecate but are unable to do so, despite long periods of straining. Patients with *hemorrhoids* or *anal fissures* experience but ignore the call to defecate because of pain on defecation.

Plan

DIAGNOSTIC. Evaluation of constipation in older persons begins with a search for a specific obstructive or medical cause (Table 65–3). The abdomen should be examined for evidence of surgical scars, incisional hernias, distention, and masses. A genitorectal examination should be performed entailing a survey for hernias, rectocele, rectal mass, and assessment of sphincter tone and Hemoccult status. Important medical conditions to exclude include anemia, hypokalemia, hypercalcemia, hypothyroidism, diabetes mellitus, and uremia. A complete blood cell count, fasting blood glucose level, serum chemistry panel, and TSH level should be obtained. Flexible sigmoidoscopy with barium enema or co-

---

TABLE 65–3. General Management of Constipation

1. Rule out other causes of constipation in addition to the irritable bowel syndrome and habitual constipation by a thorough history and physical examination, an extensive medication history, routine blood studies, stool Hemoccult determination, sigmoidoscopy, barium enema, and upper gastrointestinal tract x-ray studies.
2. Discontinue all laxatives.
3. Eliminate fecal impaction, if present, by digital disintegration and saline or soapsuds enema.
4. Treat any irritating local lesions of the anus and rectum.
5. Increase fluid intake.
6. Increase bulk in the diet and supplement with bulk-forming laxatives such as psyllium hydrophilic mucilloid (Metamucil, Konsyl).
7. Re-establish a regular time for bowel movement—have the patient sit at stool in a leisurely fashion for 10 to 15 minutes after breakfast each day to retrain the bowels.
8. Reassure the patient that this is a benign condition and this type of management requires many weeks before beneficial effects will be noticed.

Boydston JS, Barker JD, Lawhorne LW. Gastrointestinal disorders. In Rakel RE. Textbook of Family Practice, 3rd ed. Philadelphia, W.B. Saunders, 1984, p 1006.

lonoscopy is indicated in the presence of weight loss, anemia, positive Hemoccult stool test, or a family history of colon cancer.

Special Tests. Measures of *colon transit time* using ingested stool markers or *anorectal manometry* to measure rectal tone may be helpful in patients with chronic constipation for whom the work-up for obstructive or medical causes remains elusive.

THERAPEUTIC. Priscilla is instructed to discontinue all unnecessary medications (laxatives, iron and calcium tablets). Consider possibly the risk versus benefit of discontinuing the calcium channel blocker and replacing it with a β blocker. A synthetic fiber supplement, increased fluid intake, and daily exercises are recommended. Thyroid hormone replacement (levothyroxine, 25 μg orally daily) is started after thyroid function tests are diagnostic of hypothyroidism.

PATIENT EDUCATION. Priscilla is informed that a change in bowel habits of more than 2 to 3 weeks' duration as well as any occurrence of undiagnosed rectal bleeding should be promptly reported to the physician. A list of high-fiber foods is provided (fresh fruits, vegetables, and cereal grains). She is informed that it may take several weeks for a high-fiber diet to work, to increase her intake of fluids, and that she may initially experience a transient increase in bloating. Increased physical activity is recommended. Finally she is instructed to avoid prolonged use of laxatives, but to follow the urge to defecate.

DISPOSITION. Priscilla will implement the instructions received during patient education and return in 2 to 3 weeks. In the interim, flexible sigmoidoscopy and air contrast barium enema studies are scheduled.

FIRST FOLLOW-UP VISIT

Subjective

Priscilla reports increased softness in her stools and less straining. The cramping and bloating have lessened and the frequency of bowel movements has increased. She also denies any symptoms of angina, which would possibly indicate too rapid correction of her hypothyroidism.

Objective

Priscilla's affect remains somewhat depressed, but is more animated than on the initial visit. Flexible sigmoidoscopy and barium studies revealed dark discoloration of the colonic mucosa (melanosis coli) and the presence of moderate diverticula, but no obstruction, masses, or functional impairment. Repeat thyroid function tests reveal progression toward a euthyroid status. Other laboratory studies are within normal limits.

Assessment

1. Chronic constipation secondary to the adverse effects of medications and untreated hypothyroidism

2. Contributing factors: low-fiber diet, lack of exercise, and possible depression

Plan

Prescribe an antidepressant once thyroid levels are normal if evidence of clinical depression remains. If an antidepressant is needed, select an agent with low anticholinergic properties. Consider referral to a local chapter of Mending Hearts for group psychotherapy. Restart calcium supplements for osteoporosis prevention and observe tolerance.

SUGGESTED READING

Gattuso JM, Kamm MA. Review article: The management of constipation in adults. Ailment Pharmacol Ther 1993;7:487–500.

Krevsky B. A practical approach to managing constipation. Fam Pract Recertif 1995;17(4):41–53.

Marshall J. Chronic constipation in adults. Postgrad Med 1990;88(3):49–60.

Read N, Celik A, Katsinclos P. Constipation and incontinence in the elderly. J Clin Gastroenterol 1995;20:61–70.

Romero Y, Evans J, Fleming K, Phillips S. Constipation and fecal incontinence in the elderly population. Mayo Clin Proc 1996;71:81–92.

Wald A. Constipation and fecal incontinence in the elderly. Gastrointest Disord Elderly 1990;19:405–418.

1. Nonpharmacologic measures recommended in the prevention of constipation include which of the following?
   a. A diet containing at least 25 to 30 gm of fiber daily
   b. A program of regular physical exercise
   c. Responding to the urge to defecate
   d. Reducing to ideal body weight
   e. Maintaining liberal fluid intake

2. Pharmacotherapy of which of the following conditions may have constipation as a side effect?
   a. Treatment of iron deficiency anemia
   b. Prolonged management of constipation with stimulant laxatives
   c. Medical management of acute or chronic pain syndromes
   d. Achieving tighter control of glycemia in diabetics
   e. Treatment of osteoporosis with calcium supplements

3. Definite indications for radiographic or endoscopic examination in the evaluation of chronic constipation include which of the following?
   a. Discovery of a rectocele on physical examination
   b. The presence of concurrent weight loss
   c. A previous history of abdominal surgery
   d. Detection of a positive Hemoccult stool test
   e. A family history of colon cancer

Answers appear on **page 607**.

Chapter **66**

Fatigue and Anemia

William MacMillan Rodney, M.D.

INITIAL VISIT

Subjective

Mrs. Candace L. is a 70-year-old white widow who lives alone with two cats for which she cares faithfully. She takes the bus to scheduled visits with the doctor, and she is a reliable historian. Although she values the doctor's advice, she does not always follow it. For example, she has chosen not to accept referral for mammography.

Recently she has noted a decrease in her energy. She feels it is increasingly difficult to maintain her one-story, well-lit, one-bedroom bungalow. She fears that she may have to give up her home and independence.

PAST MEDICAL HISTORY. She has been well without hospitalization during the 10 years she has been in the family practice. There are no allergies. She underwent hysterectomy 25 years ago for unknown reasons, and old records are not available. She believes her ovaries and appendix were removed at the same time. Her gallbladder was removed 5 years ago for symptomatic cholelithiasis.

Illnesses include mild osteoarthritis for which she receives a nonsteroidal anti-inflammatory drug (NSAID), Naprosyn, 375 mg orally twice per day, and idiopathic essential hypertension which has responded to 40 mg of propranolol twice daily. She has coronary artery disease, having sustained a silent inferior wall myocardial infarction of indeterminate age. This was noted on her first electrocardiogram 10 years ago. she carries sublingual nitroglycerin 0.3 mg in her purse as a prophylactic measure. She receives estrogen replacement therapy, and she suffers from hemorrhoids.

FAMILY HISTORY. As an adoptee, her biological parents are unknown. She has a 30-pack-a-year smoking history, but she quit 25 years ago. She watches her diet, but acknowledges being 30 lb over her "ideal weight." Before delivering her three children, she weighed 137 lb. She does not drink alcohol.

She is gravida 4, para 3 with one miscarriage. Her three living children have moved to a neighboring state. Whenever possible, she visits at Christmas or Thanksgiving by bus travel. She worries that this may no longer be possible.

SOCIAL HISTORY. Her husband died 10 years ago, leaving her with a modest pension and Social Security. She has Medicare health insurance without supplementation. She has a tenth grade education, and remains an avid reader of mystery novels.

REVIEW OF SYSTEMS. Her review of systems is negative for a new headache, change in vision, localized weakness, paresthesias, fainting, cough, dyspnea, palpitations, dysuria, frequency, change in bowel habit, and bright red blood per rectum.

She states that she has experienced some mild, intermittent, poorly localized cramping abdominal pains which have not been associated with meals. There is no memorable pattern and these pains do not awaken her from sleep. She feels her appetite is coming under control, and acknowledges a 10-lb weight loss since a visit of 3 months ago. She reports "watching what I eat." This week she has felt lightheaded when she gets up.

She denies melena, but on closer questioning comments on the anesthetic nature of examining one's own bowel movement. She has been unwilling to retrieve stool specimens from the toilet bowl for fecal occult blood testing (FOBT). She agrees to attempt a bowel movement at the office today. If successful, nursing staff will obtain a specimen for FOBT.

Objective

PHYSICAL EXAMINATION. On physical examination, Candace is a well-developed, well-nourished, cooperative, white female who appears slightly younger than her stated age.

Vital signs include blood pressure 145/88 mm Hg, pulse 92 and regular, respiratory rate 16 per minute, and oral temperature 37.0°C.

On further examination, pertinent positive findings include mild arteriovenous nicking, dentures, and diffusely scattered 2- to 4-mm nonpigmented skin tags on the upper torso and neck. Rales which clear on deep inspiration occur at both posterior lung bases. There is a 2/6 midsystolic murmur at the left sternal border. The point of maximal impulse is localized to the fourth intercostal space in the midcavicular line.

The abdomen is normal to inspection and auscultation. Deep palpation produces slight discomfort more on the left than the right. Nonpulsatile masses are not felt, but the aorta is palpable midline above the umbilicus. Pelvic examination is normal, and the digital rectal examination is normal. Inspection reveals a left lateral skin tag near the anus. There are no fissures, fistulas, sinus tracts, or external hemorrhoids.

LABORATORY TESTS. A chest x-ray reveals no evidence of acute heart failure, although cardiomegaly is noted. Blood is drawn for thyroid, renal, and liver function studies. Electrolytes, glucose, urinalysis, and a hemogram are ordered.

Serendipitously, Candace successfully produces an in-house natural bowel movement which tests positive for occult blood.

Assessment

WORKING DIAGNOSIS. In this age group, positive FOBT suggests the possibility of, but is not pathognomonic for, colorectal cancer. Based on prevalence alone, secondary cancer prevention programs target breast, colorectal, and cervix/uterine cancers for these patients. Lung cancer is a primary prevention project through smoking cessation. Because of signs and symptoms noted earlier, further investigation will proceed. However, as it relates to colorectal cancer, this process is literally defined as a "case-finding" investigation (fully covered by Medicare) as contrasted with "asymptomatic screening" (not always covered by Medicare).

DIFFERENTIAL DIAGNOSIS

1. *NSAID-induced gastrointestinal bleeding.* Since NSAIDs are well-known causes of gastric irritation and subclinical bleeding, it would be tempting to attribute the positive FOBT to the NSAID effect. Do not send these patients home with additional FOBT cards, because a positive test is likely to be a true positive. Although it is recommended to discontinue NSAIDs 7 days before FOBT, this is not always

possible. Furthermore, in a study of FOBT among rheumatoid arthritis patients, true-positive results outnumbered false-positive findings seven to one. A positive FOBT requires further investigation.

2. *Hemorrhoids.* Hemorrhoids are present in over 70 per cent of women this age. Most of these are subclinical and are only seen on retroversion (the J-maneuver, or turnaround maneuver) of the flexible sigmoidoscope or colonoscope. Instrumentation of the anus by digital examination or endoscopy can produce a false-positive FOBT.

However, this patient has mild abdominal pain, a 10-lb weight loss, and recent lightheadedness. If the patient could not have produced a natural bowel movement, digital examination for FOBT would have been indicated. The presence of hemorrhoids is not sufficient to explain Candace's signs and symptoms.

3. *Acute gastrointestinal bleeding.* Specifically, acute bleeding is a possibility. Orthostatic measurements are taken: supine blood pressure 143/88, pulse 92; standing after 2 minutes, blood pressure 130/80 mm Hg, pulse 98. An in-office hematocrit is obtained (Hct 40). These values must be normal to continue the work-up as an outpatient. For acute gastrointestinal bleeding of unknown cause, hospitalization is recommended when the patient is hemodynamically unstable.

4. *Diverticulitis.* Bleeding diverticulosis, also known as diverticulitis, can cause brisk and/or chronic lower gastrointestinal bleeding. These patients usually present with left lower quadrant abdominal pain, low-grade fever, and leukocytosis. Abdominal guarding occurs and, in severe cases, perforation can lead to peritonitis. These patients should be hospitalized. Candace does not fit this picture. Based on age and prevalence, it is likely that Candace's diverticulosis is unrelated to her major problem.

5. *Angiodysplasia.* During the 1980s, angiodysplasia emerged as a frequent cause of painless lower gastrointestinal bleeding among seniors. Candace does not have the anemia or aortic stenosis associated with angiodysplasia. Nevertheless, these ectatic vessels of the bowel wall remain a possibility. Only colonoscopy detects these lesions, unless bleeding is so brisk that they can be detected angiographically. Angiodysplasia is not highly probable as the cause, but it is possible.

6. *Thyroid dysfunction.* The loss of energy remains unexplained, although it could be related to the working diagnosis of occult colorectal cancer. Thyroid dysfunction should be considered.

7. *Cardiac failure.* Based on the physical findings and the chest radiograph, cardiac failure is unlikely although the cardiomegaly and previous myocardial infarction are ongoing separate problems.

8. *Abdominal aneurysm.* An in-office ultrasound is immediately performed, revealing a 4×3.5 cm aneurysm. Although this is of importance, it does not explain all of the signs and symptoms. For this size aneurysm, outpatient management and further imaging studies can proceed once a definitive diagnosis of the major problem is found. This aneurysm is *not* a contraindication for colonoscopy or air contrast barium enema.

9. *Upper gastrointestinal tract disease.* If examination of the lower gastrointestinal tract is negative, upper tract disease may be sought. The weight loss and abdominal pain could be early indicators of esophageal, gastric, or pancreatic disease. In this patient, the uterus, ovaries, appendix, and gallbladder have been surgically removed, but not all of the old records are available. Organs mistakenly retained and/or poorly remembered should be kept in mind when the work-up does not proceed to a logical conclusion.

10. *Colitis.* Colitis does occur among seniors, although Candace does not relate the more severe abdominal pain and markedly abnormal bowel movements consistent with infectious colitis. Idiopathic inflammatory bowel disease (ulcerative colitis, or Crohn disease) would be a rare possibility. Radiation colitis can affect patients who have received radiation therapy for pelvic tumors. This would not apply to Candace. A normal colonoscopy excludes these possibilities in over 90 per cent of cases.

Finally, ischemic colitis can be as difficult a diagnosis of exclusion among the elderly as irritable bowel syndrome (IBS) is among young and middle-aged adults. The patient has no abdominal angina related to meals. Although it is likely that Candace suffers from widespread atherosclerotic cardiovascular disease, it is not a likely cause of her pain, weight loss, and positive FOBT.

11. *Miscellaneous and rare possibilities.* Follow-up on the hemogram and other tests would be mandatory to exclude rarer diseases such as leukemia, diabetes, polymyalgia rheumatica, coagulopathy, and others.

Plan

DIAGNOSTIC. Given the possibilities and probabilities, a plan for the detection of colorectal cancer is suggested. Many possible permutations and combinations of flexible sigmoidoscopy, air contrast barium enema, and/or colonoscopy exist (Table 66–1). There are several valid investigation pathways which have different strengths and weaknesses. Endoscopy techniques and barium enema techniques are both operator-dependent with varying degrees of sensitivity and specificity. Under ideal conditions, false-negative rates can be minimized to 5 to 10 per cent for both modalities. In some cases, both techniques are required when the first technique is inconclusive.

All things being equal, patient access to the technique should be considered. If colonoscopy is unavailable, flexible sigmoidoscopy (FS) may be synergistic with air contrast barium enema (ACBE). This approach is frequent in Great Britain and some American communities. When available, colonoscopy offers the advantage of high specificity (almost zero false-positive results) and the ability to obtain tissue through biopsy. Polypectomy at the time of colonoscopy can be curative, although some lesions are not resectable by endoscopy.

On the other hand, colonoscopy is more expensive ($500 versus $250 for ACBE). Perforation of the intestine can require immediate surgery, although some perforations can be managed conservatively by antibiotics and close observation. Perforation occurs more frequently (1:500 to 1:1000 persons) with colonoscopy than it does with ACBE. Complications are rare with both techniques.

Patient comfort is operator-dependent. Controlled studies suggest a patient preference for colonoscopy over barium enema. Probably this is due to the use of intravenous sedation and analgesia for colonoscopy. Meperidine (25 to 125 mg) and/or diazepam (1 to 12 mg) are slowly administered under controlled conditions to produce twilight sedation and analgesia. Therefore, informed consent must include the possibilities of drug reaction and phlebitis. These are rare. With ACBE, the risk of phlebitis is nonexistent. Bowel preparation is critical to the success of both techniques.

In the case of Candace, the family physician performed colonoscopy in the office. She received a 24-hour clear liquid diet and a mixed-electrolyte purge solution (e.g., GOLYTELY, Colyte, others) as bowel preparation. Multiple lesions were detected. At 15 cm of insertion depth, a pale, sessile, hemispheric, nonfriable lesion 5 mm in diameter was biopsied and sent to the laboratory. Pathology reports usually return 2 to 5 working days later.

At 35 cm, a pedunculated polyp (measuring 12 to 15 mm across its head) was found. This was left undisturbed while examination proceeded to the cecum. The bowel preparation was excellent, and 97 per cent of the mucosal surface was directly visualized. Haustrae, sharp turns, and isolated fecal debris make 100 per cent visualization a conceptual "ideal" that is rarely attained. Therefore, a negative examination can never be viewed as a "guaranteed clean bill of health."

At the hepatic flexure, an irregularly contoured, friable, asymmetrical, sessile lesion describing 120 degrees of arc was found. Two biopsies were taken with minimal bleeding. The scope was withdrawn atraumatically. On withdrawal, multiple sigmoid di-

TABLE 66–1. Comparison of Diagnostic Methods for Colorectal Cancer

Variable	Flexible Sigmoidoscopy (35 cm)	Short Colonoscopy (65 cm)	Full Colonoscopy (180 cm)	Air Contrast Barium Enema
Operator dependent?	Yes	Yes	Yes	Yes
Average patient charge	$90–$240	$90–$240	$500–$900	$250–$400
Doable in the office?	Yes	Yes	Yes	No
Continuity of care possible?	Yes	Yes	By FP–Yes	No
			By GE consult–No	No
Biopsy possible on same visit?	Yes	Yes	Yes	No
Equipment cost (average)	$4000–$7000	$4000–$7000	$10,000–$20,000	Hospital $40,000
Intravenous sedation used?	No	No	Yes	No
Hard copy of diagnostic images routinely retained?	No	No	Video Fiberoptic	Yes No
Sensitivity under ideal conditions	40%–50%	60%–65%	90%–95%	90%–95%

These are the most commonly used and the most diagnostically powerful methods currently available for the early detection of colorectal cancer. Accessibility and community standards vary. It is not uncommon for physicians to use more than one technique in pursuit of diagnostic certainty.

FP = family physician; GE = gastroenterologist.

verticuli were noted. The turnaround maneuver examined the pectinate line. Mild internal hemorrhoids with no active bleeding were seen.

The patient tolerated the procedure well. Vital signs were observed until stable and the patient was alert. She was driven home by a friend from church, with a return appointment scheduled for 1 week.

THERAPEUTIC. Prior to leaving, Candace is told of the findings and the probable need for removal of the polyp in the hospital. The lesion at the hepatic flexure would require surgical consultation. A videotape of the lesion would be shared with the surgeon when the pathology reports are returned.

The next day, the pathologist called with a preliminary report. The lesion at 15 cm is a hyperplastic polyp. The hepatic flexure lesion is "moderately well-differentiated adenocarcinoma." In consultation with a surgeon, hospitalization was scheduled for the next day. A metastatic survey is negative. At laparotomy 2 days later, a Dukes B colonic adenocarcinoma was resected. Nodes were negative and a primary reanastomosis of the remaining bowel segment was successful. The patient was discharged 10 days later. Removal of the remaining polyps by the family physician was accomplished 2 months later.

PATIENT EDUCATION. During the hospitalization, the patient is visited daily. During that time, she has received information regarding the high likelihood of a "cure." Nevertheless, the need for surveillance is explained. The pedunculated polyp is felt to be a benign risk with good surgical margins possible on endoscopic removal. Although data are limited regarding the safest time for subsequent removal following open laparotomy, a 1- to 2-month interval is felt to be safe. Once removed, the colon was felt to have been cleared of disease. A surveillance protocol is established. The patient underwent colonoscopy 1 year later. At that time, no additional lesions were found. The patient understands that she is at "above average" risk for additional lesions. She agrees to report any additional new symptoms and follow-up on a 3-year colonoscopy surveillance protocol as long as she is asymptomatic.

DISPOSITION. The patient remains under the care of her family physician for her other illnesses and continuing support.

SUGGESTED READING

Blackstone MO. Endoscopic Interpretation: Normal and Pathologic Appearances of the Gastrointestinal Tract. New York, Raven Press, 1984.

Gillett E, Thomas S, Rodney WM. False-negative endoscopic biopsy of colonic adenocarcinoma in a young man. J Fam Pract 1996;43:178–180.

Rodney WM. Gastroenterology. In Rakel RE (ed). Textbook of Family Practice, 5th ed. Philadelphia, W.B. Saunders Company, 1996.

Rodney WM (ed). Flexible Sigmoidoscopy and Colonoscopy for the Family Physician. Kansas City, MO, American Academy of Family Physicians, 1997.

Rodney WM, Dabov G, Orientale E, Reeves W. Colonoscopy in FP: Sedation as associated with a more complete exam. J Fam Pract 1993;36:394–400.

Rodney WM, Felmar E: Why flexible sigmoidoscopy instead of rigid sigmoidoscopy? J Fam Pract 1984;19:471–476.

Smith CW (ed). Gastrointestinal disease in primary care. Primary Care 1988;15(1):79–91.

QUESTIONS

1. A 63-year-old man presents with hemorrhoidal bleeding and a hematocrit of 36. Endoscopic examination confirms the presence of mild internal hemorrhoids. No bleeding is seen. Colonoscopy is not available. You would recommend:
   a. Air contrast barium enema (ACBE)
   b. Flexible sigmoidoscopy and ACBE
   c. Referral for hemorrhoidal surgery
   d. Iron replacement therapy, anorectal ointment (Preparation H), and warm sitz baths
   e. None of the above

2. Which of the following is not associated with lower gastrointestinal bleeding?
   a. Ischemic colitis
   b. Cancer
   c. Hemorrhoids

d. Diverticulosis
e. Pancreatitis

3. Regarding fecal occult blood testing, which of the following statements are true?
   a. A positive test in a patient taking nonsteroidal anti-inflammatory drugs can be disregarded.
   b. Screening fecal occult blood testing can be performed by digital rectal examination.
   c. Under screening conditions described by most medical societies, fecal occult blood testing is appropriately performed on stool specimens that result from a natural bowel movement.
   d. All of the above.
   e. None of the above.

Answers appear on **page 607**.

C h a p t e r 67

Anemia

Paul M. Paulman, M.D.

INITIAL VISIT

Subjective

Patient Identification and Presenting Problem

Lorine H. is a 39-year-old African American woman who presents to the clinic for an annual physical examination and a complaint of "fatigue."

Present Illness

Lorine complains of mild fatigue gradually worsening for the past 6 months. She notes no sleep or appetite disturbance, change in mood, or difficulty concentrating. No major upheavals have occurred in her home life, work, or social life. She has noted a gradual decrease in her work tolerance and feels "washed out" at the end of her work day. No changes have occurred in her diet; she eats "a typical American diet." She denies nausea, vomiting, and diarrhea and has not noticed any dark stools or blood in her stools. She has had an occasional mild nosebleed and has noticed that her menstrual flow has been "a bit heavier than usual" for the past several months. She has had no cold intolerance, muscle weakness, fever, chills, or joint pain. She began to take over-the-counter vitamins (with iron), one tablet a day, 2 weeks ago and has felt somewhat better since she started the vitamins.

Past Medical History

OPERATIONS. Laparoscopic tubal ligation at age 35 years.

ALLERGIES. None.

ILLNESSES. History of depression treated 10 years previously, no recurrences; hypertension.

HOSPITALIZATIONS. Normal vaginal delivery 16 years ago and tubal ligation 4 years ago.

MEDICATIONS. Prescription medications: Vasotec 10 mg, one every day. Over-the-counter medications: multivitamin with iron, one every day; aspirin 325 mg, one tablet every other day.

Family and Social History

Lorine was born in the United States. Her parents are natives of Algeria. No family history exists of sickle cell disease, diabetes, kidney disease, hypertension, malignancy, or thyroid disease. Her parents are college professors. Her husband owns a retail business and their son (an only child) attends a local high school. Lorine works in a clerical position at a local insurance company. She is a nonsmoker and nondrinker, and she denies illicit drug use.

Review of Systems

Lorine denies change in diet, nausea, vomiting, diarrhea, melena, or bright red blood in her stools. She has had no chest or abdominal pain, weight loss, night sweats, cough, muscle aches, joint pain, lymphadenopathy, fever, or dyspnea. She denies any history of thyroid disease. Lorine denies any polydipsia, polyuria, or polyphagia. She has noticed an occasional mild nosebleed and an increase in menstrual flow for the past several months. She has not been exposed to tuberculosis or other infectious diseases.

Objective

PHYSICAL EXAMINATION. Height 64 in; weight 135 lb; vital signs: BP 110/86 mm Hg; pulse 82 and regular; temperature 37.1° C (tympanic); respirations 13 per min. General: alert, well-oriented × 3, well-nourished, and in no acute distress. Integument: normal distribution and quality with no rashes. Lymph nodes: no adenopathy. HEENT: palpebral conjunctivae are pale bilaterally; otherwise normal. Lungs clear. Heart: regular sinus rate and rhythm, no murmurs. Breasts: no masses, tenderness, or nipple discharge. Neurologic: normal. Extremities: normal. Abdomen: soft; normal bowel sounds; no tenderness, masses, or organomegaly. Pelvic: normal external genitalia, cervix and vagina normal, uterus and ovaries of normal size and nontender; rectovaginal examination reveals no masses, normal sphincter tone, stool negative result for blood.

LABORATORY TESTS. Office laboratory hemoglobin level is 10.1 gm/dl. Office laboratory urinalysis result is normal. A CBC specimen drawn at the hospital laboratory showed a hemoglobin level of 9.9 gm/dl, WBC level of 9400/μl, adequate platelets, and hypochromic microcytic red cell indices.

Assessment

MICROCYTIC HYPOCHROMIC ANEMIA. In a woman of reproductive age, with monthly blood loss due to menses, iron deficiency is the most likely cause of her anemia. Iron deficiency is the most common cause of anemia in every country in the world. Because of the microcytic hypochromic indices, the megaloblastic anemias can be ruled out at this time.

Differential Diagnosis

1. Anemia of chronic disorders. Microcytic anemia is seen in association with various infections, connective tissue diseases, and malignancies. Lorine has no signs or symptoms of chronic illness.

2. Thalassemias. The thalassemias are genetic disorders that result in a reduced rate of globin (alpha or beta) chain synthesis. Because Lorine's parents are from the "thalassemia belt" in northern Africa, this diagnosis must be considered as a possible cause of Lorine's anemia.

3. Sideroblastic anemia. Sideroblastic anemia is associated with a defect in heme synthesis and is characterized by the sideroblast, an erythroblast with a ring of iron granules surrounding the nucleus. This condition is most commonly seen as an acquired form of myelodysplasia.

4. Lead poisoning. Lead inhibits both heme and globin synthesis. Lorine has no risk factors for lead exposure.

Plan

Diagnostic laboratory tests are to be undertaken. Ferritin, iron, and total iron binding capacity levels are ordered. Three guaiac cards are sent home with the patient to screen for gastrointestinal blood loss.

Treatment

Lorine is given a prescription for ferrous sulfate 325 mg orally three times daily for 14 days.

Patient Education

The patient was educated about foods high in iron and the pathophysiology and treatment of iron deficiency anemia.

Disposition

The patient was asked to return for follow-up in 2 weeks.

FIRST FOLLOW-UP VISIT

Subjective

Lorine reports no improvement in her symptoms. She complains of constipation. She has been taking her ferrous sulfate as prescribed.

Objective

No change has occurred in findings on physical examination. All three guaiac cards were returned and results are negative. Her ferritin level is 224 ng/ml (normal for premenopausal women is 10 to 100 ng/ml), serum iron 60 ng/dl (normal 50–90 ng/dl), total iron binding capacity 312 ng/dl (normal 230–400 ng/dl).

Assessment

Lorine has microcytic anemia, not iron deficiency anemia.

Plan

1. Discontinue ferrous sulfate.

2. Order reticulocyte count, haptoglobin, and hemoglobin electrophoresis.

3. Return to clinic in 1 week.

SECOND FOLLOW-UP VISIT

Subjective

Lorine returns as requested for follow-up. She notes no change in her symptoms. She had her laboratory samples drawn as requested.

Objective

No change has occurred in her physical examination. Her haptoglobin is 110 mg/dl (normal 100–300 mg/dl), reticulocyte count is 3.9×10^3/mcl (normal $3.8–5.2 \times 10^3$/mcl), reticulocyte percentage 2.6 per cent (normal 0.4–2.7%), absolute reticulocyte count 120,000/mm³ (normal 25,000–125,000/mm³). Hemoglobin electrophoresis reveals a pattern consistent with alpha thalassemia.

Assessment

Lorine has a diagnosis of alpha thalassemia.

Plan

Lorine is referred to the hematology specialist for development of a treatment and monitoring plan.

DISCUSSION

Anemia is a common problem in primary care practice. The leading cause of anemia is iron deficiency. Lorine had some symptoms (heavy menses, nosebleeds) and laboratory findings (hypochromia and microcytosis) that are suggestive of iron deficiency anemia. It was only after iron therapy failed that the proper diagnosis of alpha thalassemia was made.

Anemia refers to an absolute or relative reduction of hemoglobin or red blood cells (RBCs). Normal hemoglobin values by age are listed in Table 67–1. Anemia can be caused by decreased RBC production, increased RBC destruction, increased plasma volume, or a combination of these causes (Table 67–2). The signs and symptoms of anemia are caused by decreased delivery of oxygen to peripheral tissues.

Signs and Symptoms of Anemia

The patient with mild anemia is often asymptomatic. The most common symptoms of anemia are dyspnea with exertion, weakness, headache, lethargy, and palpitations. Older patients may experience angina pectoris, heart failure, claudication, or confusion. Decreased vision due to retinal hemorrhage has been reported as a symptom of severe anemia. Physical signs include pallor of the mucous membranes (if the hemoglobin level is less than 9–10 gm/dl), tachycardia, systolic heart murmur,

TABLE 67–1. Normal Hemoglobin Values

Age	Male	Female
Newborn	15.0–21.0 gm/dl	15.0–21.0 gm/dl
3 months	9.5–12.5 gm/dl	9.5–12.5 gm/dl
1 year to puberty	11.0–13.5 gm/dl	11.0–13.5 gm/dl
Adults	13.5–17.5 gm/dl	11.5–15.5 gm/dl

TABLE 67–2. Common Causes of Anemia

Decreased RBC Production	Increased RBC Destruction	Increased Plasma Volume
Iron deficiency (microcytic)	Hemolytic anemias (normocytic)	Pregnancy (normocytic)
Sideroblastic (microcytic)		
Thalassemias (microcytic)		
Lead poisoning (microcytic)		
Anemia of chronic disorders (normocytic or microcytic)		
Vitamin B_{12} or folate deficiency (macrocytic)		
Bone marrow failure (normocytic)		

and jaundice. The severity of signs and symptoms depends on the degree and rapidity of onset of the anemia and the age and general medical condition of the patient. Lorine exhibited fatigue and pale mucous membranes as manifestations of her anemia.

Causes of Anemia

Anemia Due to Decreased Production of RBCs

IRON DEFICIENCY. Iron deficiency anemia owes its high prevalence to the body's limited ability to absorb iron from the gastrointestinal tract. The average Western diet contains 10 to 15 mg of iron daily; only 5 to 10 per cent of this is normally absorbed. Absorption increases to 20 to 30 per cent in cases of iron deficiency or high iron demand. Ordinarily, iron absorption is just enough to replace iron loss. Iron is found in RBCs, in muscle cells, and in iron-containing enzymes. Animal products, particularly meat and liver, are good dietary sources of iron. Anemia is the final expression of iron deficiency and occurs only after body iron stores are depleted and RBCs have become hypochromic and microcytic.

The causes of iron deficiency include chronic blood loss, increased iron demand (prematurity, pregnancy, or growth), malabsorption, and poor diet. Diet is the leading cause of iron deficiency in developing countries but is rarely the sole cause of anemia in developed countries.

The diagnosis of iron deficiency is made by examination of the peripheral blood smear, which reveals hypochromic microcytic RBCs, and determination of a low serum iron level, elevated total iron binding capacity (TIBC), and a low serum ferritin level.

Treatment consists of oral iron. Ferrous sulfate is the least expensive preparation. Oral iron should be taken in a fasting state with doses separated by at least 6 hours. The daily dose of ferrous sulfate is 10 mg per kg, up to 300 mg, bid to qid as tolerated.

Parenteral iron preparations are available for patients unable to tolerate oral iron. Therapy should be given long enough to replete body iron stores (4–6 months). An increased reticulocyte count is usually seen within 7 days of initiation of therapy, and the hemoglobin level should rise at a rate of 2 gm/dl every 3 weeks. Prophylactic iron dosing should be considered for pregnant patients, those receiving regular hemodialysis, and premature infants. Lorine's normal iron level and TIBC and high ferritin levels ruled out iron deficiency anemia.

SIDEROBLASTIC ANEMIA. Sideroblastic anemia is characterized by hypochromic RBCs, increased marrow iron, and ringed sideroblasts in the bone marrow. Ringed sideroblasts are abnormal erythroblasts with iron granules surrounding the nucleus. Sideroblastic anemia can be hereditary, caused by a defect in heme synthesis, or acquired from bone marrow dysfunction or replacement. Some patients with hereditary sideroblastic anemia respond to pyridoxine therapy. Folic acid therapy is also recommended. In acquired sideroblastic anemia, treatment is aimed at correcting the cause of the bone marrow failure. For some patients, the only treatment is repeated blood transfusions, sometimes resulting in iron overload requiring chelation therapy. Erythropoietin has been used in some cases of sideroblastic anemia.

THALASSEMIA. The thalassemias (alpha and beta) are a group of genetic disorders characterized by a reduced rate of production of alpha or beta globin chains. The severity of the disease is dependent on the number of genes affected. Thalassemia is seen most commonly in patients from the "thalassemia belt" (southern Europe, northern Africa, the Middle East, Indian subcontinent, and Southeast Asia, including Indonesia). Patients with thalassemia present with microcytic hypochromic RBCs with or without anemia, depending on the severity of genetic defect. Hemoglobin electrophoresis is usually required to make the diagnosis. Treatment depends on the severity of the illness and is aimed at maintaining the hemoglobin at 10 g/dl or more. Treatment modalities include regular blood transfusions (with iron chelation if iron overload occurs), folic acid supplementation, splenectomy if hemolysis is a problem, and bone marrow transplantation in very severe cases.

Lorine's hemoglobin electrophoresis results confirmed the diagnosis. Because she has been hematologically stable, no specific treatment has been recommended for her.

LEAD POISONING. Lead causes a microcytic hypochromic anemia by inhibiting heme and globin synthesis. Children are at highest risk for lead poisoning from various sources including ingestion of lead-containing paint chips. Signs and symptoms of lead poisoning include pallor, abdominal pains, irritability followed by lethargy, anorexia, ataxia, slurred speech, and convulsions. Laboratory findings include basophilic stippling of RBCs, elevated lead level, and elevated free erythrocyte protoporphyrin level. The treatment of lead poisoning consists of removing the source of exposure and removal of lead through chelation when clinically indicated. Because lead poisoning is very widespread, screening is recommended for any child at risk for lead exposure or any child who demonstrates cognitive, language, or learning deficits.

ANEMIA OF CHRONIC DISORDERS. A number of chronic infections, connective tissue diseases, and malignancies can cause a microcytic hypochromic anemia by blocking erythropoietin response, decreasing RBC life span, and decreasing iron release from macrophages. The characteristics of anemia of chronic disorders include mild anemia (hemoglobin level rarely less than 9.0 gm/dl), decreased serum iron and TIBC levels, and normal or raised ferritin level. Treatment of the anemia usually depends on treatment of the underlying cause. Erythropoietin has been successfully used in some cases of anemia of chronic disorders.

B$_{12}$ AND FOLATE DEFICIENCY. Deficiencies of both vitamin B$_{12}$ and folate can cause a macrocytic anemia. The most common cause of B$_{12}$ deficiency is malabsorption (including that due to pernicious anemia). The most common causes of folate deficiency include dietary deficiency, malabsorption, excessive folate demand, and drugs (including alcohol and chemotherapeutic agents). The diagnosis can be made via blood levels of vitamin B$_{12}$ and/or folate, and replacement therapy can be instituted. Vitamin

B$_{12}$ is usually replaced by the parenteral route (500–1000 μg per month) because malabsorption is the leading cause of vitamin B$_{12}$ deficiency. Folate can usually be replaced via the oral route (5 mg per day). Signs and symptoms include mild jaundice, glossitis, angular stomatitis, and peripheral sensory neuropathy. Folate deficiency does not cause neurologic symptoms. Laboratory findings include macrocytic RBCs, hypersegmented neutrophils, and elevated bilirubin level. The Schilling test is valuable in assessing the absorption of vitamin B$_{12}$ from the gastrointestinal tract.

BONE MARROW FAILURE. Replacement or an intrinsic defect of bone marrow usually is the cause of normocytic anemia. Treatment is aimed at correcting the cause of the marrow replacement or defect, if possible, or maintaining an acceptable hemoglobin level via transfusion.

Anemia Due to Increased RBC Destruction

A number of intrinsic and acquired illnesses including splenomegaly, hemoglobinopathies (e.g., sickle cell disease), infections, drug effects, collagen vascular diseases, and tumors can cause an increase in RBC destruction. Laboratory findings include an elevated reticulocyte count, abnormal RBC morphology, increased unconjugated bilirubin level, decreased haptoglobin level, and increased plasma hemoglobin level. Treatment is aimed at correcting the cause of hemolysis or at maintaining an acceptable hemoglobin level thru transfusion.

Anemia Due to Increased Plasma Volume

A relative anemia due to hemodilution from increased plasma volume can be seen in various conditions including pregnancy. This disease responds to treatment of the underlying condition.

Initial Evaluation of Anemia in the Office

A cause for most cases of anemia can be determined by a thorough history and physical examination and judicious use of the clinical laboratory. Patients with anemia from suspected underproduction of RBCs should be screened for gastrointestinal blood loss; iron studies are indicated if RBC indices are microcytic. Vitamin B$_{12}$ and folate levels should be obtained in patients with macrocytic RBC indices, with or without anemia. Bone marrow examination may be helpful in some patients with anemia from RBC underproduction, especially those who fail standard treatment protocols. If hemolysis is suspected, a reticulocyte count, haptoglobin level, and examination of the peripheral blood smear for abnormal cell forms are reasonable screening tests. Lead screening is recommended for children with micro-cytic anemia. Other tests are indicated based on the history and results of screening laboratory evaluations. Further testing may be indicated to evaluate uncommon causes of anemia.

In Lorine's case, the hemoglobin electrophoresis study was ordered because of the high incidence of thalassemia in her parents' country of origin.

SUGGESTED READING

Beutler E. Red Cell Metabolism. New York, Grune & Stratton, 1984.

Brittenham GM. Hematology: Basic Principles and Practice. New York, Churchill Livingstone, 1991.

Fairbanks VF, Beutler E. Hematology. New York, McGraw-Hill, 1990.

Holtbrand AV, Pettit JE. Essential Haematology. Oxford, Blackwell Scientific Publications, 1993.

Jacobs A. Iron deficiency and iron overload. Crit Rev Oncol Hematol 1985;3:143–186.

QUESTIONS

1. The leading cause of iron deficiency in the United States is
   a. Diet
   b. Hematuria
   c. Bone marrow failure
   d. Uterine or gastrointestinal blood loss
   e. Epistaxis

2. Which of the following are found in patients with hemolytic anemia?
   a. Low reticulocyte count, normal haptoglobin level
   b. Normal reticulocyte count, high haptoglobin level
   c. High reticulocyte count, low haptoglobin level
   d. Normal reticulocyte count, normal haptoglobin level

3. At what age does hemoglobin reach its lowest level?
   a. At birth
   b. 5 years
   c. Variable
   d. 65 years
   e. 3 months

Answers appear on **page 607.**

Chapter 68

Vomiting and
Low Back Pain

Daniel J. Derksen, M.D.

INITIAL VISIT

Subjective

PATIENT IDENTIFICATION AND PRESENTING PROBLEM. Sally C. is a 60-year-old Hispanic female who presents to the Family Practice Center complaining that "I've been sick for 2 days." Her complaints include "a bad cold" associated with nausea, vomiting, low back pain, trouble breathing, chills, and fever.

PRESENT ILLNESS. Other than controlled hypertension, Sally had been well until 2 days before her office visit. Her illness started with severe bilateral low back pain associated with nausea, vomiting, and fever. The back pain improved but did not completely resolve. Sally became worried when she discovered that her temperature the morning of her office visit was 104.6°F. She also was concerned because she had shaking chills, she was urinating less frequently than normal, and the urine had a foul odor.

Sally had not noticed any hematuria or pain with urination. She could not remember any back trauma or intense physical exertion before the present illness. Her bowel movements were normal. She was anorexic, and when she tried to eat, she vomited after intake of both solids and liquids.

PAST MEDICAL HISTORY. Sally has been a patient in the Family Practice Center for 1 1/2 years. During this time, she has been treated for hypertension, which was diagnosed 5 years ago. Four months ago her treatment was changed from hydrochlorothiazide to verapamil, a calcium channel blocker, to better control her hypertension and to correct hypokalemia. She has been on estrogen replacement

therapy since her hysterectomy and bilateral salpingo-oophorectomy 6 years ago for "heavy bleeding." Other surgeries included a cholecystectomy for cholelithiasis with incidental appendectomy 5 years ago. Eight years ago she had a stone in the left kidney that required surgical removal.

FAMILY HISTORY. No family history of diabetes, myocardial infarction, kidney disease, hypertension, or breast cancer exists. Sally's mother is still living, at age 81 years, and is in good health. Her father died a few years ago at age 78 of "natural causes."

SOCIAL HISTORY. A few years ago Sally was divorced. Presently she lives with her 30-year-old mentally retarded daughter and relies on a small alimony payment and her daughter's disability income. She owns her house and her car. Since her divorce, Sally has not been sexually active.

HEALTH HABITS. Sally has never smoked, rarely drinks alcoholic beverages, and denies the use of illicit drugs. She eats a diet high in saturated fat and cholesterol. During a typical week she eats six to eight eggs, beans cooked in lard, cheese, whole milk, pork, green chiles, tortillas fried in animal fat, and fried red meat. Results of her last cholesterol test 3 months ago, however, were normal. Sally rarely exercises. Her Pap test and mammogram results were normal less than 1 year ago. She cannot remember when her last tetanus shot had been given.

REVIEW OF SYSTEMS. Sally has not lost any significant amount of weight over the last year. Since her present illness, she has felt a little lightheaded on standing up suddenly. She has not experienced abdominal pain, nor has she noticed bloody or black tarry stools. She has no known allergies and is not taking over-the-counter medications or vitamin or mineral supplements.

Objective

Physical Examination

Sally's vital signs are as follows: temperature is 101.5°F, respiratory rate 22, pulse 92, and blood pressure 110/80 mm Hg; there are no orthostatic changes in pulse and blood pressure, and her weight is 65 kg. General: Sally looks tired but is alert and seems to be a reliable historian. She is in mild to moderate distress with her back pain. Mouth: dry mucous membranes. Lungs: clear to auscultation and percussion. Cardiovascular: the heart point of maximal impulse (PMI) is not displaced; the rate and rhythm are normal; there is a grade II/VI early systolic murmur heard best in the supine position in the lower left sternal border, but the murmur does not radiate. Abdomen: a midline scar in the lower abdomen and a scar in the right upper quadrant are noted. Bowel sounds are present but diminished. The abdomen is soft and nontender. The liver and spleen are of normal size, and the kidneys are not palpable. Back: there is mild to moderate left costovertebral angle (CVA) tenderness to fist percussion and normal range of motion. Extremities: Sally's two-point discrimination, vibratory sense, and deep tendon reflexes are normal. The peripheral pulses are also normal. Breasts: no masses palpated. Pelvic: no external lesions are noted. The vagina is atrophic, and no cervix is visible. The uterus and ovaries are not palpable. There are no adnexal masses, and the pelvic support is good without evidence of cystocele. Rectal: no masses are found. The stool is negative for occult blood.

Assessment

Working Diagnoses

Several possible diagnoses can explain Sally's symptoms.

1. Urinary tract infection. Sally's history of fever, malaise, back pain, nausea and vomiting, shaking chills, decreased urination, and foul-smelling urine is suggestive of an infection of the upper urinary tract. Sally's risk factors include her age (postmenopausal) and her history of surgery for a kidney stone.

2. Nephrolithiasis or ureterolithiasis. Sally's history and physical examination are suggestive of a stone in the upper urinary tract. The CVA tenderness to fist percussion on the left, fever, past history of nephrolithiasis, nausea and vomiting, shaking chills, and foul-smelling urine suggest that a stone and a secondary infection may be present. The recent discontinuation of her thiazide diuretic may have contributed to stone formation.

The nausea and vomiting and the physical examination finding of diminished bowel sounds suggest that stones may be obstructing the upper urinary tract (ureterolithiasis with obstruction of the ureter) and causing gastric and small bowel ileus. Sally's history of a temperature of 104.6°F at home is of concern for bacteremia or early sepsis.

Differential Diagnosis

1. Lower urinary tract infection. This diagnosis seems less likely, because Sally does not complain of pain, frequency, urgency, or burning during urination. In addition, the patient reported a temperature of 104.6°F at home; a high fever is uncommon in lower urinary tract infections.

2. Lower urinary tract stone (ureterolithiasis). Sally's presentation makes this diagnosis less likely. Her pain was vague, in the lower back, with mild to moderate CVA tenderness. Patients with ureterolithiasis more often present with excruciating pain radiating from the flank down to the labia, scrotum, or inner thigh in association with diaphoresis and difficulty finding a comfortable position.

3. Musculoskeletal injury. Without a history of extreme exertion, heavy lifting, or trauma, this diagnosis seems unlikely. The associated findings of fever, shaking chills, and foul-smelling urine do not support this diagnosis.

4. Pancreatitis. Although Sally's history of nausea, vomiting, and back pain may suggest this diagnosis, findings of foul-smelling urine, fever and chills, history of nephrolithiasis, and lack of epigastric tenderness point to the genitourinary tract rather than the pancreas. A common bile duct stone with pancreatic inflammation, however, is a consideration in a patient with a history of cholelithiasis and this symptom complex.

5. Gastrointestinal tract problem. The diminished bowel sounds, nausea, vomiting, fever and chills, and back pain can be consistent with an acute abdominal process. Sally's past medical history, how-

ever, reveals that she had an appendectomy and cholecystectomy in the past. Diverticulitis or gastrointestinal tract cancer must be considered, but the stool is negative for blood and Sally has no weight loss, history of melena, change in caliber of stool, or passage of bright red blood per rectum. No masses are palpated on rectal or abdominal examination. Sally has no abdominal tenderness or guarding.

6. Pelvic inflammatory disease. This diagnosis is very unlikely considering Sally's history of hysterectomy and salpingo-oophorectomy, age, and lack of sexual activity.

7. Urinary tract tuberculosis. This is a rare disease that is unlikely in this patient because of the acuity of the presentation and high-grade temperature.

8. Mesenteric infarction. Usually, infarction presents more suddenly, with rapid decline and death without surgical intervention. The time course (2 days), lack of peritoneal findings (rebound tenderness, guarding, or rigidity), and absence of blood in the stool make this diagnosis unlikely.

Plan

Patient Education

Sally was told that she needed to be admitted to the hospital for treatment of her kidney infection and for further tests to determine whether she had developed another kidney stone. Although she realized that she was seriously ill, she was extremely concerned about who would pick up her retarded daughter from the day care facility and tend to her at home. Her anxiety was considerably decreased when Sally's sister was reached by telephone and agreed to care for her niece during the hospitalization. Sally demonstrated an understanding that the type of infection she had required treatment with parenteral antibiotics. She also realized the possibility of another kidney stone.

Diagnostic

1. Urinalysis with culture (catheterized specimen); blood cultures; CBC with differential; determination of serum sodium, potassium, chloride, carbon dioxide (CO_2), calcium, phosphorus, uric acid, amylase, lipase, and creatinine and blood urea nitrogen (BUN) levels; and a plain film of the abdomen.

2. Renal ultrasound. A renal ultrasound can help determine if obstruction of the upper urinary tract has occurred by detecting the presence of hydronephrosis. In addition, a better localization of the stone in the urinary tract can be ascertained.

3. Intravenous pyelogram (IVP). An IVP is often used in the work-up of a patient with a suspected stone, but the history of decreased urine output, evidence of dehydration, possibility of pyelonephritis, and obstruction make renal ultrasound a reasonable alternative with fewer possible complications.

4. Other imaging procedures—computed tomography (CT) or magnetic resonance imaging (MRI)—can be used to narrow the differential diagnosis. Had the history or physical examination been more suggestive of a pancreatic problem or abdominal tumor, these modalities might have been chosen.

Therapeutic

1. Admission. Sally's problem requires hospital admission because of the possibility of two emergency conditions: pyelonephritis and obstructive ureterolithiasis with early sepsis. In addition, Sally was not able to tolerate oral fluids or medications.

2. Culture. Appropriate cultures were obtained before treatment and included samples of the urine (catheterized specimen) and blood to check for sepsis.

3. Intravenous administration of antibiotics. Because of Sally's inability to tolerate liquids or solids by mouth and the difficulty obtaining serum concentrations of antibiotic sufficient to treat pyelonephritis by oral antibiotics, intravenous (IV) administration of antibiotics was ordered. Ampicillin and an aminoglycoside were chosen to cover the most likely organisms in pyelonephritis. Ampicillin 1 gm every 6 hours IV and a loading dose of gentamicin equal to 2 mg per kg IV (65 kg × 2 mg/kg = 130 mg gentamicin) were given. Sally was placed on a maintenance dose of 3 mg per kg IV gentamicin (65 kg × 3 mg/kg = 195 mg ÷ 3 = 65 mg every 8 hours) to begin 8 hours after the loading dose. Peak (6–8) and trough (<2) gentamicin levels were ordered to be drawn 30 minutes before and 30 minutes after administration of the third dose of gentamicin. In addition, Sally's creatinine level is to be followed closely while she receives gentamicin.

4. Intravenous hydration. The nausea, vomiting, and evidence of mild dehydration on examination

(dry mucous membranes) make IV fluid for maintenance necessary. Sally was designated NPO except sips of water or chips of ice and started on D5NS with 30 mEq potassium chloride (KCl) per liter at 150 ml per hour. Urine output, daily weight, and electrolyte determinations were ordered.

5. Renal ultrasound. Because of the severity of the illness and the possibility of obstruction of the upper urinary tract, an emergency renal ultrasound study was ordered.

6. Treatment of chronic conditions. Sally's estrogen (0.625 mg daily) and verapamil sustained-release (240 mg daily) regimens were discontinued until she could take medication by mouth. Vital signs, including blood pressure, were ordered to be checked every 4 hours.

FIRST FOLLOW-UP VISIT (LATER IN THE DAY AT THE HOSPITAL)

Subjective

Sally reports that she "feels about the same."

Objective

PHYSICAL EXAMINATION. The physical examination is unchanged from the outpatient examination 4 hours previously. Sally is still febrile (102.5°F) and has moderate CVA tenderness and diminished bowel sounds.

LABORATORY TESTS. The results of the laboratory tests are as follows: sodium 128 (normal 135–145 mEq/L), potassium 2.8 (normal 3.5–5.0 mEq/L) chloride 93 (normal 100–110 mEq/L), CO_2 25 (normal 25–30 mEq/L), calcium 9.2 (normal 8.6–10.4 mg/dl), phosphorus 3.3 (normal 2.7–4.5 mg/dl), uric acid 5.4 (normal 2.5–6.5 mg/dl), creatinine 0.6 (normal 0.8–1.2 mg/dl), BUN 13 (normal 10–25 mg/dl), glucose 108 (normal 80–130 mg/dl), WBC 20 (normal 5–11 $\times 10^3$), Hct 38.4 (normal 37–47 gm/dl), neutrophils 85 (normal 31–71%), bands 1, lymphocytes 9.7 (normal 15–50%), amylase 37 (normal 23–115 IU/L), lipase 54 (normal 46–208 IU/L), urine sodium less than 15, and urine osmolality 314. The chest radiographs (PA/LAT) are normal. The abdominal film shows calcified densities within the kidney outline on the left. The ECG shows evidence of left ventricular hypertrophy and nonspecific ST-T wave changes. Urinalysis: Specific gravity 1.020, pH 6.0, positive assay for leukocyte

esterase, and RBCs and WBCs too numerous to count. The renal ultrasound study was reviewed with the radiologist. The left kidney was enlarged and showed evidence of three to four stones (0.5–2.2 cm) in the calyx with marked hydronephrosis of the left ureter. The right kidney was normal.

Assessment

The working diagnoses were correct—hydronephrosis due to ureteral obstruction resulting from upper urinary tract ureterolithiasis and nephrolithiasis. The patient's urinalysis, elevated WBC count, fever, and chills suggest a complicating pyelonephritis. The high fever at home suggests bacteremia or early sepsis.

Plan

Therapeutic

1. Evidence of obstruction on the renal ultrasound with associated pyelonephritis necessitated immediate urologic consultation and intervention.

2. Co-management with the urologist. The urologist recommended immediate placement of a nephrostomy tube to relieve the obstruction and continued treatment with IV antibiotics until Sally's condition was medically stable. During the procedure the urologist performed a retrograde pyelogram, which demonstrated obstruction and justified the placement of a stent. When the WBC count, fever, pain, and electrolyte abnormalities were corrected, the urologist would then perform percutaneous removal of the stones. Because one of the stones was greater than 2 cm in diameter and multiple stones were present, percutaneous removal was chosen over extracorporeal shock-wave lithotripsy (ESWL). Sally agreed with the recommendations.

Disposition

Sally underwent placement of a nephrostomy tube that evening. Once the tube was placed, pus was drained from the left renal calyx. Within 48 hours of nephrostomy tube placement and treatment with IV antibiotics, Sally had defervescence and felt better. Her WBC count and electrolyte concentrations returned to normal with IV hydration, replacement of sodium and potassium, and parenteral antibiotics. Sally was taken back to the operating room, and multiple small stones were removed by percutaneous extraction through the nephrostomy site. The stones were sent for analysis. Two days later a nephrostogram was done, revealing no evidence of residual stones. The nephrostomy tube was clamped and then removed the next day. Urine culture done the day of admission grew out of 10^5 *Escherichia coli* sensitive to ampicillin; blood cultures were negative for growth.

Sally was discharged on oral antibiotics (ampicillin), and she did well postoperatively. She was seen frequently in the postoperative period, including visits 2 days and 2 weeks after discharge to have a follow-up urine culture. Sally returned 4 weeks later to obtain a 24-hour urine collection. The specimen was sent for analysis, including calcium, citrate, oxalate, uric acid, and creatinine levels, to determine renal function, to decide whether metabolic work-up would be necessary, and to better advise Sally on how to prevent further stone formation.

DISCUSSION

Upper urinary tract stones are encountered commonly in Western countries. In the United States, calcium oxalate stones are the type most frequently found, especially in the arid Southwest. Other types of renal calculi include calcium phosphate stones; struvite stones (magnesium ammonium phosphate), which are the result of urinary tract infections caused by urea-splitting organisms (*Klebsiella, Pseudomonas, Proteus*); uric acid stones, which are usually associated with gout; and cystine stones, which result from a congenital defect in the metabolism of cystine. Although nephrolithiasis affects less than 1 per cent of the population, the recurrence rate is quite high in patients with a history of a previous stone (50%–80%). Because more than 80 per cent of the stones contain calcium, most are visible on a plain film of the abdomen.

The pathogenesis of nephrolithiasis may be related to hypercalciuria. The cause of hypercalciuria may be excess absorption from the gut or excess leak of calcium from the renal tubules. Other causes of hypercalciuria include hypervitaminosis D, type I renal tubular acidosis, prolonged immobilization, drugs such as acetazolamide, sarcoidosis, and excess resorption of calcium from bone due to hyperparathyroidism.

Patients suspected of having a stone need a rapid assessment, including location of the stone, the degree of obstruction, determination of whether infection is present, and assessment of renal function. Stones greater than 6 mm in size are unlikely to be passed spontaneously. Obstruction and upper urinary tract infection (pyelonephritis) are emergency conditions that require immediate attention, including IV antibiotics and removal of the stone. Removal of the stone can be undertaken percutaneously with a grasping instrument or basket (percutaneous nephrolithostomy), by ESWL, or with stone dissolution (alkalinizing the urine in patients with uric acid stones).

The most important issues to consider in the management of patients with urolithiasis include the following:

1. Stone analysis is important in all patients with urolithiasis.
2. Medical prevention of stones is important to reduce recurrence.
3. Spontaneous passage of ureteral stones is optimal (if possible).
4. Increased hydration is important in managing and preventing urolithiasis.
5. ESWL is effective for stones less than 2 cm in diameter.
   a. Medical follow-up is necessary after ESWL treatment.
   b. ESWL does not replace medical prevention.
   c. ESWL can be used in combination with the percutaneous technique.
   d. For asymptomatic stones less than 0.5 cm diameter, ESWL is controversial.

SUGGESTED READING

Coe FL, Parks JH, Asplin JR. The pathogenesis and treatment of kidney stones. N Engl J Med 327:1141–1152, 1992.

Jacobson EJ, Fuchs G. Nephrolithiasis. Am Fam Physician 1989;39(3):233–245.

Kupin WL. A practical approach to nephrolithiasis. Hosp Pract 1995;30(3):57–66.

Levin FL, Adams-Huet B, Pak C. Ambulatory evaluation of nephrolithiasis: An update of a 1980 protocol. AJR 1994; 163(6):1309–1313.

NIH Consensus Development Conference in the Prevention and Treatment of Kidney Stones. J Urol 1989;141:705–808.

1. Match the following.
   a. IVP
   b. Ultrasound
   c. Both
   d. Neither
      (1) Should be avoided in renal failure
      (2) Should be avoided in dehydrated elderly patients
      (3) Localizes kidney stones
      (4) Associated with allergic reactions

2. The most common type of kidney stone is
   a. Struvite
   b. Calcium oxalate
   c. Calcium phosphate
   d. Cystine
   e. Uric acid

Answers appear on **page 607.**

Chapter **69**

Hematuria

Lori Anne Whittaker, M.D., Ph.D.

INITIAL VISIT

Subjective

PATIENT IDENTIFICATION. Henry is a 62-year-old Native American male who makes his living hunting and trapping.

PRESENTING PROBLEM. While on a hunting trip, Henry noted a reddish discoloration to his urine that lasted for 1 day. He also experienced mild low back pain.

HISTORY OF PRESENT ILLNESS. Henry's hunting cabin lies some distance from the village in which he lives. During the winter, it takes 6 hours by snowmobile, over rough terrain, to reach it. On the morning following such a trip to his cabin, Henry noted that his urine was a reddish color. He had no fever or chills, but he did note mild nonradiating lower back pain. He had experienced similar back pain in the past when he overexerted himself. He therefore attributed it to chopping firewood the evening before. The discolored urine lasted for approximately 1 day, and the low back pain resolved after several days.

Henry returned to town a week later, again by snowmobile, and on his arrival noted that his urine was once more a reddish color. He had no recurrence of the low back pain. He went to the local nurses' station for evaluation, and the nurses performed a dipstick urinalysis, which showed 4+ blood and 1+ protein, but the result was negative for leukocytes and nitrates. Concerned that the low back pain and the blood in the urine signified a kidney infection, the nurses treated him empirically with oral trimethoprim-sulfamethoxazole (Bactrim, Septra), and sent off a urine culture. Henry was instructed to return for follow-up urinalysis when he completed the course of antibiotics, but he left town to go hunting again before doing so.

When he returned, a repeat urine dipstick analysis showed 3+ blood, although at that time his urine was normal in appearance. The patient re-

509

ported no further discolored urine, and his back pain had not returned. On two more occasions when the patient was back in town after hunting trips, urine dipstick analyses were positive for blood. The original urine culture report came back negative for bacterial growth. Because of the persistently abnormal dipstick analyses, the nurses sent the patient to the regional health center in another town for further evaluation.

PAST MEDICAL HISTORY. Henry is generally in good health. He has mild hypertension for which he takes 25 mg hydrochlorothiazide once daily. He had a tonsillectomy at age 8 years, an appendectomy at age 45 years, and an open reduction and internal fixation of a right tibial ankle fracture at age 52 years. He has no known drug allergies and uses no medications other than his blood pressure pills and occasional acetaminophen or ibuprofen given to him by the nurses in the station.

FAMILY HISTORY. Henry's mother died of colon cancer at the age of 69 years. His father had hypertension and ethanol-induced hepatic cirrhosis. He died of accidental causes at age 56 years. Several of his six brothers have hypertension, and two are diabetic. His one sister is diabetic and was recently diagnosed with breast cancer at age 72 years. One uncle has died of lung cancer and another is suffering from throat cancer. Both were heavy smokers. Last year there was a small outbreak of tuberculosis (TB) in Henry's village, and two people, including Henry's uncle, were found to have active TB. Testing with purified protein derivative (PPD) was performed on all members of the village who were not known to be PPD-positive, and Henry's PPD result was negative at that time. There is no known history of kidney disease in Henry's family.

HEALTH HABITS. Henry has smoked over two packs of cigarettes a day for the past 40 years. He currently does not drink alcohol but was a heavy drinker in the past. He quit drinking approximately 5 years ago at the insistence of his wife. His hunting and trapping keep him physically active.

SOCIAL HISTORY. Henry lives with his wife, daughter, and three grandchildren in a two bedroom house in a small rural village in Alaska. One son lives with his wife and children in the same village, and another son lives in a larger town several hours away. Henry has a large extended family of siblings, aunts, uncles, and cousins living in his village.

Objective

Physical Examination

Henry is a small, lean man, looking somewhat older than his 62 years. His blood pressure is 140/85, pulse 68, respirations 18, and temperature 98.5°F. He weighs 145 lb and is 66 in tall. He has poor dentition, but otherwise head, ear, eye, nose, and throat examinations are within normal limits. On chest examination there are a few basilar crackles but good air entry bilaterally. Heart sounds are normal. Abdominal examination reveals no masses or tenderness, although the liver edge is smooth and palpable 1 cm below the costal margin. A well-healed right lower quadrant abdominal scar is noted. Back examination reveals mild kyphosis of the thoracic spine. No tenderness is elicited in the costovertebral angles or lumbosacral areas. The patient has good range of motion of the back. Upper and lower extremity reflexes are symmetrical and within normal limits. The patient has normal gross motor strength in upper and lower extremities. Rectal examination reveals a normal-sized smooth prostate and no rectal masses. Fecal occult blood testing is negative.

Laboratory

Urinalysis revealed normal-appearing urine with 2+ blood but no protein, leukocytes, glucose, or other abnormalities, and a specific gravity of 1.025. On microscopic analysis there were 10 to 20 red blood cells per high power field. The urine sediment was examined under phase contrast microscopy, which showed red cells of normal morphology. No casts or white blood cells were present. A complete blood count showed a hemoglobin level of 13.5, hematocrit level of 45, a mean cell volume (MCV) of 88, and a normal white blood cell count and differential. Prothrombin time (PT) and partial thromboplastin time (PTT) were within normal limits. Electrolytes, glucose, blood urea nitrogen (BUN), and creatinine levels were all within normal limits. A PPD was placed and the result read as negative 48 hours later.

Assessment

Working Diagnosis

The patient is experiencing recurrent gross and microscopic hematuria, a diagnosis based on the finding of red blood cells in the urinary sediment. It is useful to note that Henry's presenting complaint, that of red-colored urine, can be due to various factors, including hematuria, hemoglobinuria, myoglobinuria, porphyria, hyperbilirubinemia, or the ingestion of certain drugs or dyes. Urine dipstick analysis can help to narrow the diagnosis, but the dipstick reagent orthotolidine will show a positive reaction in the presence of red blood cells, free hemoglobin, or myoglobin. Thus, the diagnosis of hematuria relies on microscopic evaluation. Red blood cells may lyse spontaneously if the urine is hypotonic or left standing for extended periods of time, and in such cases the urinalysis should be repeated on a fresh urine specimen to avoid confusion over the diagnosis.

Small numbers of erythrocytes may be excreted in the urine under normal circumstances, but they usually do not exceed two to three per high power field (HPF) in urinary sediment. Values greater than this constitute hematuria and warrant investigation. Hematuria may be either gross or microscopic, de-

pending on the amount of blood loss. Although patients with specific conditions causing hematuria are more or less likely to bleed heavily, a definitive diagnosis cannot be ruled in or out based on the amount of bleeding.

Hematuria is caused by blood loss anywhere within the urinary tract, and the list of possible causes is extensive (Table 69–1). Clues to the source of the blood loss may be determined by a careful history and physical examination, paying particular attention to a history of trauma, strenuous exercise, medications or drug use, family history of renal disease, systemic symptoms, associated pain and, on examination, pain or tenderness; bleeding at other sites; palpation of abdominal, renal, or prostatic masses; and evidence of systemic disease.

Differential Diagnoses

1. *Renal parenchymal disease.* Further clues as to the cause of hematuria can be gained by careful

---

TABLE 69–1.   Causes of Hematuria

Renal Parenchymal Lesions
Glomerular Disease
Primary glomerulopathy: IgA nephropathy, minimal change disease, cresenteric glomerulonephritis, membranous glomerulopathy, membranoproliferative glomerulonephritis, poststreptococcal glomerulonephritis
Systemic disease: Systemic lupus erythematosus, Wegener granulomatosis, Henoch-Schönlein purpura, Goodpasture syndrome, hemolytic-uremic syndrome, Alport syndrome
Tubulointerstitial Disease
Interstitial nephritis: toxins, acute hypersensitivity, gout, hypercalcemic
Papillary necrosis: analgesic use, diabetes mellitus, ethanol abuse, sickle cell disease or trait, obstructive uropathy
Hereditary: Polycystic kidney disease, medullary sponge kidney
Vascular Lesions
Malignant hypertension
Renal artery embolism or thrombosis
Renal vein thrombosis
Arteriovenous malformations
Renal Tumors
Infection
Acute bacterial pyelonephritis
Renal tuberculosis
Trauma

Lesions of the Urinary Tract
Renal Pelvis
Severe hydronephrosis
Calculi
Transitional cell carcinoma
Trauma

Ureters
Calculi
Transitional cell carcinoma
Ureterocele
Periureteritis
Bladder
Infection: bacterial cystitis, tuberculosis, *Shistosoma haematobium*
Chronic interstitial cystitis
Foreign bodies
Trauma
Exercise-induced hematuria
Bladder calculi
Radiation-induced cystitis
Diverticuli
Endometriosis
Malignancy: transitional cell carcinoma, squamous cell carcinoma, adenocarcinoma
Urethra
Infection: condyloma acuminatum, acute or chronic urethritis
Carcinoma of the penis or urethra
Foreign bodies or other trauma
Strictures
Prostate
Prostatitis
Carcinoma
Benign prostatic hypertrophy

Systemic Coagulopathies

examination of the urinary sediment. The presence of red blood cell casts suggests a renal parenchymal origin (usually glomerulonephritis or interstitial nephritis), whereas the absence of casts suggests bleeding from elsewhere in the urinary tract. Renal parenchymal bleeding may be either glomerular or nonglomerular. Examination of red cell morphology, which is best done using phase contrast microscopy, can aid in distinguishing between these two possibilities. Fragmented and dysmorphic red cells are associated with glomerular lesions, whereas nor-

mal red cell morphology suggests a nonglomerular origin. The presence of significant proteinuria (greater than 100–300 mg/dl or greater than 1 g in a 24-hour collection) further points to glomerular disease. Blood itself contributes protein to the urine but is unlikely to cause the presence of greater than 1 g of protein in 24 hours unless the bleeding is massive. These distinctions can help to direct further investigations into the cause of the hematuria (Fig. 69–1).

In this case, microscopic evaluation of Henry's

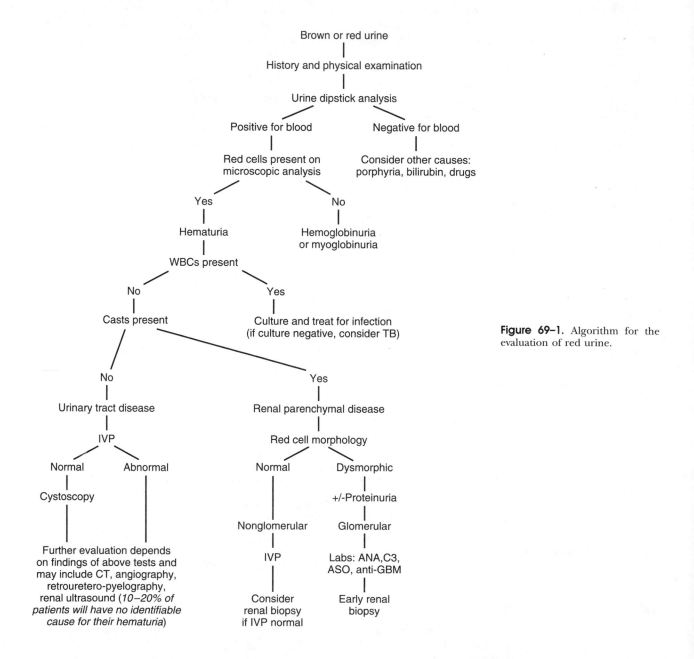

Figure 69–1. Algorithm for the evaluation of red urine.

urine did not reveal any casts and did show normal red cell morphology. Dipstick analyses failed to show significant proteinuria. Thus, the evaluation so far suggests bleeding in the urinary tract outside the renal parenchyma. These findings are not absolute, however, and they do not completely exclude the possibility of renal disease, which should be borne in mind as the investigation proceeds.

2. *Exercise-induced hematuria.* Of particular note in this case is the fact that the episodes of documented hematuria occurred following prolonged snowmobile trips, suggesting a diagnosis of exercise-induced, or stress, hematuria. This is a benign condition frequently seen in athletes. It can be brought on by any repetitive jarring or bouncing motion. It is a diagnosis of exclusion, however, and should not be made in a patient of this age without ruling out more serious causes.

3. *Infection.* Acute bacterial infection, either cystitis or pyelonephritis, is unlikely given the absence of associated symptoms and laboratory findings. The patient had no complaints of suprapubic tenderness, dysuria, or frequency to suggest cystitis, nor did he complain of costovertebral angle tenderness, fever, or chills characteristic of pyelonephritis. In addition, urinalysis and urine culture showed no evidence of infection. Prostatitis is unlikely given the lack of symptoms and the normal prostate examination. Urinary tuberculosis is a consideration given the presence of the disease in Henry's community, but the negative PPD result makes this diagnosis unlikely.

4. *Renal calculi.* Another common cause of hematuria is renal calculi. Severe back and flank pain may be expected during passage of a calculus through the ureters or urethra. Henry did complain briefly of low back pain, but this was mild and nonradiating. The discomfort was more characteristic of musculoskeletal pain from overexertion than of renal colic. A calculus confined to the renal pelvis is usually painless, however, and cannot be ruled out based on the patient's symptoms.

5. *Malignancy.* Malignancy of the urinary tract is always a concern when evaluating hematuria, especially in the older age group. Henry's risk factors for malignancy include his age, a fairly strong family history of cancer, and smoking. Tumors may occur in the kidney, renal pelvis, ureter, bladder, prostate, and urethra. The most common cancer of the urinary tract in men is prostate cancer, but a prostate tumor large enough to cause gross hematuria is likely to be detected on rectal examination. Henry's strong smoking history is a risk factor for both bladder cancer and renal cell carcinoma, and both have an average age of onset in the 60s. Thus, malignancy of the urinary tract is a definite consideration in this patient.

6. *Other urinary tract causes of hematuria.* Various rarer causes of bleeding in the urinary tract outside the renal parenchyma are listed in Table 69–1 and should be considered during evaluation.

7. *Systemic coagulopathy.* A normal PT and PTT essentially rule out systemic coagulopathy as a cause of bleeding in this case.

8. *Essential hematuria.* It should be noted that in 10 to 20 per cent of patients who present with hematuria, no specific diagnosis can be made. In these cases, once potentially serious but treatable causes, such as infection or malignancy, have been ruled out, observation with follow-up as needed for recurrent symptoms is a reasonable approach.

Plan

1. Serial urinalyses over several days to determine if the red blood cells clear when the patient has not engaged in any recent snowmobile trips.

2. Intravenous pyelogram (IVP). An IVP helps visualize the upper urinary tract and aids in the detection of lesions (seen as filling defects or obstructions to dye flow) in the kidney, renal pelvis, ureters, and, to a lesser extent, the bladder.

3. Renal ultrasound. In patients with decreased urine output or elevated BUN or creatinine level, a renal ultrasound may be a safer, but less sensitive, option to IVP. Renal ultrasound is also helpful in distinguishing cystic from solid renal masses seen on IVP.

4. Cystoscopy. If the IVP or renal ultrasound studies fail to identify a cause of bleeding, the next step in evaluation is cystoscopy to evaluate the lower urinary tract. Direct visualization of the urethra, bladder, and ureteral orifices is possible. Urine from each ureter may be collected separately and examined for the presence of blood.

5. Other tests. Depending on the results of the above studies, other tests may be warranted. A renal mass should be further imaged by computed tomography (CT) scanning. Bleeding from ureteral orifices may be evaluated by angiography to identify arteriovenous malformations or fistulas, and retro-

grade ureteropyelography can be performed if the ureter was not completely visualized on IVP. Renal biopsy is primarily indicated in the evaluation of suspected glomerular or other renal parenchymal disease.

FIRST FOLLOW-UP VISIT

Subjective

Henry remained at the regional health center for 3 days while undergoing tests, and he reported no further episodes of discolored urine.

Objective

Serial urinalyses performed over several days showed decreasing numbers of red blood cells, and by the third day the urine was clear. Results of an IVP were within normal limits. Cystoscopy showed mild erythema of the posterior bladder wall, but no ulceration, active bleeding, or malignancy was noted. No further testing was undertaken.

Assessment

Exercise-induced hematuria caused by the jarring motion associated with prolonged snowmobile trips was the diagnosis.

Plan

Because hunting is his livelihood, it is not feasible to recommend that Henry discontinue his snowmobile rides. Therefore, it was suggested that he use a well-padded seat, have the suspension of his snowmobile examined and optimized, and that he not completely empty his bladder before his trips.

DISCUSSION

In this case, a diagnosis of exercise-induced hematuria was made on the basis of history and the exclusion of other pathology by appropriate diagnostic testing. Exercise-induced hematuria, also known as "marathon-runners' hematuria" or "stress hematuria," is a common cause of gross or microscopic hematuria in physically active individuals. It occurs following strenuous exercise or repetitive physical jarring and resolves spontaneously with rest.

The source of bleeding in exercise-induced hematuria has not been clearly delineated but is likely not a single entity (Gambrell and Blount, 1996). One common postulate is that the flaccid posterior wall of the bladder strikes against the fixed trigone area, resulting in contusions. In studies of marathon runners following a race, cystoscopy revealed ecchymosis of the bladder wall that resolved rapidly over 48 hours. It is thought that the condition is aggravated by an empty bladder, when the bladder walls are more likely to rub against each other. Bleeding may also occur from the prostate or urethra, especially in sports such as cycling that can cause mild trauma to these structures. It has also been suggested that renal trauma, either in the form of a direct blow in heavy-contact sports, or from repetitive jarring, may cause bleeding from damaged small blood vessels in the kidney. Furthermore, in very strenuous activity, renal blood flow may decrease and renal vasoconstriction may occur, causing hypoxic damage to the nephron and leakage of blood through the glomerular membrane. This process has been suggested as a cause of hematuria observed in long distance swimmers, who are not exposed to the trauma or jarring motions seen in other sports. This hypothesis also helps to explain the red cell casts and dysmorphic red cells sometimes observed in exercise-induced hematuria.

Regardless of the source of bleeding, exercise-induced hematuria is seen as a benign, self-limited condition. In a young, otherwise healthy athlete, when the hematuria can be shown to occur in temporal relationship to strenuous physical activity and to resolve spontaneously with rest, the diagnosis can be made without further evaluation. A more extensive work-up is recommended to rule out urinary tract pathology, however, when one of the following conditions is present: (1) gross hematuria; (2) microscopic hematuria that does not clear within 48 to 72 hours; (3) recurrent episodes of hematuria; (4) the patient is a male over 40 years old; or (5) the patient has not engaged in prolonged or intense physical activity (Gambrell and Blount, 1996).

Some controversy remains over the long-term affects of exercise-induced hematuria, but most indications are that it causes no permanent damage. It is generally recommended that individuals refrain from strenuous exercise until urinary findings return to normal, but patients may then resume their usual activity.

SUGGESTED READING

Benson GS, Brewer ED. Hematuria: Algorithms for diagnosis. JAMA 1981;246:993–995.

Bicknell SL, McCallum O, Wright LF. Urinary tract disorders. In Rakel RE (ed). Textbook of Family Medicine, 5th ed. Philadelphia, W.B. Saunders, 1995.

DeGowin RL. The genitalia. In DeGowin's and DeGowin's Bedside Diagnostic Examination. New York, Macmillan, 1987.

Gambrell RC, Blount BW. Exercise-induced hematuria. Am Fam Physician 1996;53(3):905–911.

Glassock RJ. Hematuria and pigmenturia. In Massry SG, Glassock RJ (eds). Textbook of Nephrology, 3rd ed. Baltimore, Williams & Wilkins, 1995, pp 557–562.

QUESTIONS

1. True or False: The urine dipstick test for blood will be positive in the presence of
   a. Hemoglobin
   b. White blood cells
   c. Red blood cells
   d. Myoglobin
   e. Protoporphyrins

2. The presence of red cell casts in the urine suggests
   a. A bladder tumor
   b. Calculi
   c. Renal parenchymal disease
   d. Cystitis

3. True or False: Exercise-induced hematuria may be caused by
   a. The posterior wall of the bladder striking the fixed trigone area
   b. Long-distance swimming
   c. Hypoxic damage to nephrons
   d. Direct trauma to kidneys or bladder in contact sports
   e. Walking
   f. Cycling

Answers appear on **page 607**.

Chapter 70

Dysuria

Karen M. Bolton, M.D.

INITIAL VISIT

Subjective

PATIENT IDENTIFICATION AND PRESENTING PROBLEM. Callie S. is a 20-year-old college student who presented with the complaint of dysuria for the past several days. She also noted urgency, frequency, vaginal discharge, and low back discomfort. The vaginal discharge had been present for 1 week before the onset of dysuria.

PAST MEDICAL HISTORY. Callie takes low-dose birth control pills for contraception. A rash was associated with penicillin when she was an infant. She denies prior genitourinary tract infections.

FAMILY HISTORY. Callie's mother and father are both in their mid-50s and are healthy. She has two brothers in good health. Grandparents have heart disease, adult-onset diabetes, and hypertension.

HEALTH HABITS. Callie has never used tobacco. She occasionally drinks alcohol and denies drug use. She jogs 4 miles at least four times per week and tries to follow a low-fat diet.

SOCIAL HISTORY. Callie lives in an apartment near campus with two female roommates. She is heterosexual and sexually active with a new male partner. She has a part-time job in a research laboratory.

REVIEW OF SYSTEMS. Callie denies fever, chills, nausea, or diarrhea. Her last menstrual period was 2 months ago; however, she frequently skips a period since she began using birth control pills. It is possible she skipped some of the pills in the last few packs. She denied anorectal intercourse or intercourse with a partner with known sexually transmitted disease (STD).

Objective

PHYSICAL EXAMINATION. Callie is a healthy-appearing thin white female. Her temperature is 98.2°F, blood pressure is 106/60, respiratory rate is 12, heart rate is 62, weight is 110 lb, and height is 64 in. She has no costovertebral angle (CVA) tenderness but has mild suprapubic tenderness. Pelvic examination reveals no vulvar lesions, the vagina is normal in color with a creamy discharge, and there is no mucopurulent discharge from the cervix, which appears to have a significant ectropion. The bimanual examination is normal. There is no urethral discharge or inflammation and no inguinal adenopathy.

LABORATORY TESTS. Midstream clean catch urine dipstick test is negative for protein, blood, and glucose but positive for nitrites and leukocyte esterase. Microscopic examination of the urine reveals significant pyuria (10–20 WBC/high power field [HPF] spun urine) and bacteriuria. *Gonorrhoeae* and *Chlamydia* cultures were taken of cervix and urethra. Test result for urinary chorionic gonadotropin (UCG) was negative. Wet prep showed occasional leukocytes, no clue cells, negative whiff test, and rare hyphae.

Assessment

Differential Diagnosis

1. Acute bacterial cystitis is the most likely etiology of her dysuria associated with pyuria and bacteriuria.

2. Urethritis from *Chlamydia* or *Gonorrhoeae* is possible.

3. Vaginitis is unlikely.

4. Herpes urethritis is unlikely because no characteristic lesions were found on examination.

Plan

DIAGNOSTIC. Send cultures for *Gonorrhoeae* (GC) and *Chlamydia*.

THERAPEUTIC. Trimethoprim 160 mg and sulfamethoxazole 800 mg (Bactrim DS) are prescribed to be taken every 12 hours for 3 days.

PATIENT EDUCATION. Methods to prevent cystitis and STDs were discussed.

FOLLOW-UP. Follow-up was not prearranged. Callie is to be notified if the pending culture results are positive.

FIRST FOLLOW-UP VISIT

SUBJECTIVE. Callie was notified that the *Chlamydia* culture was positive two days after her initial visit. She was feeling somewhat better with improved symptoms of dysuria, frequency and urgency. Her vaginal discharge was unchanged. She was quite upset that the culture showed a *Chlamydia* infection.

OBJECTIVE. Vital signs were normal, negative GC culture, positive *Chlamydia* culture results.

ASSESSMENT. Diagnosis is cystitis, which is improving; *Chlamydia* urethritis/cervicitis.

PLAN. Doxycycline 100 mg twice daily for 7 days was prescribed.

FOLLOW-UP. Follow-up was arranged for 2 to 4 weeks to perform a follow-up *Chlamydia* culture to verify eradication of the organism.

PATIENT EDUCATION. She was encouraged to refrain from intercourse with her current partner until eradication of the organism in both partners is achieved.

SECOND FOLLOW-UP VISIT

SUBJECTIVE. Callie presented 4 weeks later for follow-up *Chlamydia* culture. She reported that her partner had been treated for urethritis by the student health clinic. Her last menstrual period (LMP) was 1 week before. She complains of pruritus and vaginal discharge.

OBJECTIVE. Cervix was normal with ectropion again noted. Vaginal discharge was white and curdy. Vulva was quite red with satellite lesions noted. Wet prep revealed fungal elements and pseudo-hyphae. *Chlamydia* culture was taken of her urethra and cervix.

ASSESSMENT. Yeast vulvovaginitis; *Chlamydia* urethritis/cervicitis treated.

PLAN. Fluconazole 150 mg tablet once and check *Chlamydia* culture.

FOLLOW-UP. Follow-up as needed.

DISCUSSION

Dysuria and other symptoms of genitourinary tract infection account for several million primary care office visits per year, especially in the young sexually active female population. The complaint of dysuria in this population is most likely from acute bacterial cystitis; urethritis from *Gonorrhoeae, chlamydia,* or herpes simplex virus; or vulvovaginitis from candidiasis or trichomoniasis (Table 70–1). Patients with acute bacterial cystitis present with dysuria, urgency, frequency, and suprapubic and/or lower back discomfort. The onset of symptoms is usually short-lived and can be associated with hematuria. The diagnosis of cystitis in the office can be made by a positive result on urine culture, which grows 100 or more colony-forming units per milliliter of a uropathogenic species. Demonstrating pyuria by dipstick for leukocyte esterase or presence of nitrites or microscopic examination of urine for WBCs with typical symptoms of cystitis can be sufficient for diagnosis, however. If pyuria is not present and cystitis is suspected, a culture should be performed.

Antibiotic treatment of acute bacterial cystitis is based on the result of a culture if it is available.

Empirical therapy is usually aimed at the predictable uropathogenic species most likely to cause acute cystitis. *Escherichia coli* has been demonstrated in 80 per cent of such infections followed by *Staphylococcus saprophyticus* (in summer months), *Proteus mirabilis, Klebsiella pneumoniae,* and *Enterobacter.*

One-, three-, and seven-day treatment regimens of antibiotics have been studied. Three-day regimens have been found to be comparable to the 7-day regimen in effectiveness, and are less costly with fewer side effects (Stamm and Hooton, 1993). It is reasonable to choose trimethoprim, trimethoprim-sulfamethoxazole combination, nitrofurantoin, a quinoline, or amoxicillin-clavulanic acid for empirical antibiotic therapy. An appropriate 7-day regimen should be considered when the patient is pregnant, has diabetes, has had a recent urinary tract infection (UTI), uses a diaphragm or spermicidal jelly, or is older than 65 years (Stamm and Hooton, 1993).

Patients with urethritis usually present with a milder and more insidious onset of dysuria than that of cystitis. It frequently is associated with cervicitis or vulvar lesions, a history of a new sexual partner, or history of previous herpes infection. *C. trachomatis, Neisseria gonorrhoeae,* and herpes simplex virus are the usual causative agents of urethritis.

Gonorrheal urethritis is suspected in patients having exposure to a sexual partner with gonorrhea, expression of a urethral discharge, inflammation of skene's glands, bartholinitis, mucopurulent cervicitis, or proctitis. The diagnosis is confirmed with a positive result on urethral or cervical culture, or reliable nonculture detection method. Treatment options include ceftriaxone sodium (Rocephin), 125 mg IM once or cefixime (Suprax), 400 mg po once or ciprofloxacin (Cipro), 500 mg po once or ofloxacin (Floxin), 400 mg po once followed by treatment for *C. trachomatis.* The patient should be cautioned about further sexual exposure and encouraged to have her partner treated as well.

Chlamydial urethritis is suspected with exposure to a partner with *Chlamydia,* longer duration of dysuria usually more than 1 week, the same physical findings as gonorrheal urethritis, and pyuria and a sterile urine culture or pyuria with absent bacteriuria in microscopic examination of urine. Verification of *C. trachomatis* requires a positive culture result or reliable demonstration by a nonculture method such as DNA amplification, indirect fluorescent antibody (IFA) or enzyme immunoassay test. Treatment regimens include doxycycline (Vibramycin), 100 mg po bid for 7 days or azithromycin (Zithromax), 1 g po once. Her partner should be examined and treated as well.

Herpes simplex urethritis is almost always ac-

TABLE 70–1. Differentiating Dysuria in Women

	Symptoms	Signs	Lab	Etiology
Cystitis	Internal dysuria Urgency Hematuria Frequency <4 days of symptoms Onset <24 hr after intercourse	Suprapubic tenderness	Pyuria Bacteriuria Hematuria Culture ≥100 cfu/ml urine	*E. coli* *S. saprophyticus* *Proteus, Klebsiella*
Urethritis	Internal dysuria New sex partner	Urethral discharge Endocervical exudate	Pyuria Culture <100 cfu/ml urine + GC culture	*Neisseria gonorrhoeae*
	Internal dysuria ≥7 days of symptoms New sex partner	Urethral discharge Endocervical exudate	Pyuria Culture <100 cfu/ml urine + *Chlamydia* culture	*Chlamydia trachomatis*
	Difficulty urinating Dysuria History of herpes	Characteristic lesions on vulva	Positive herpes simplex virus culture	Herpes simplex
Vulvovaginitis	External dysuria Curdy vaginal discharge Pruritus	Red vulva and vagina Curdy discharge Satellite lesions	Wet prep—pseudohyphae or budding yeast	*Candida*
	Malodorous vaginal discharge Irritated vulva	Frothy green discharge Rarely strawberry cervix	Wet prep—trichomonads	*Trichomonas*

companied by characteristic herpes lesions of the vulvovaginal region and inguinal adenopathy. Herpes culture of a lesion can be obtained. Treatment with acyclovir can help but does not necessarily prevent further outbreaks.

Patients with candidal or trichomonal vulvovaginitis usually present with external dysuria and vaginal discharge. Pyuria is rarely demonstrated. Other suspicious symptoms include vaginal odor, pruritus, dyspareunia, but no frequency or urgency.

Candidal vaginitis is accompanied by vulvar and perivaginal itching and a curdy white discharge. Examination can show erythema of the vagina, vulva, or cervix; satellite papules or pustules on the vulva; and usually budding yeast and/or pseudohyphae on a wet prep of the vaginal discharge. Predisposing conditions include diabetes, previous antibiotic treatment, high estrogen states such as pregnancy or oral contraceptive use, and immunosuppression. Treatment can be oral fluconazole (Diflucan), 150 mg po once or any one of several topical regimens of miconazole, clotrimazole, terconazol, tiocinazole, or butoconazole.

Trichomonal vulvovaginitis is a sexually transmitted protozoan infection that can be asymptomatic or accompanied by copious malodorous discharge and irritation. An examination reveals thin yellow or green frothy discharge. The vaginal walls are erythematous, and rarely a strawberry cervix (punctate hemorrhages) can be observed. A wet prep of the discharge can show motile trichomonads and a large number of leukocytes. Trichomonal infection is treated with metronidazole (Flagyl), 2 gm po once. Partners should also be examined and treated.

Dysuria as a presenting symptom in men is a much less frequent occurrence than in women. Men are usually found to have urethritis and occasionally cystitis or irritative symptoms of prostatitis or prostadynia. Urethritis is characterized by urethral discharge, dysuria, or itching at the end of the urethra. Physical examination usually reveals a urethral discharge, and laboratory confirmation finds an increased number of leukocytes on Gram stain of the urethral smear or in the sediment of the first-voided urine.

Urethritis is classified into gonococcal or nongonococcal. Gonococcal urethritis is diagnosed when *Neisseria gonorrhoeae* is identified by Gram stain, culture, or reliable nonculture technique. Nongonococcal urethritis is caused by several other entities including *C. trachomatis* (30%–50% of the time), *Ureaplasma urealyticum* (10%–40% of the time), and rarely *Trichomonas*, yeasts, herpes simplex virus, adenoviruses, and *Haemophilus* (Bowie, 1990). Treatment of men with gonococcal urethritis is the same as treating women. Nongonococcal urethritis in men is similarly treated as women with *Chlamydia* infection with tetracycline or doxycycline for seven days.

Men with cystitis present with dysuria, urgency, and frequency, but occasionally they may have symptoms of urethritis as well. Risk factors for cystitis include homosexuality (anal intercourse and exposure to *E. coli*), uncircumcised penis, sexual exposure to a vagina colonized with pathogenic bacteria, and immunosuppression (Stamm and Hooton, 1993). Diagnosis is advisedly confirmed with a pretreatment urine culture. Young healthy men with cystitis can be treated with trimethoprim, trimethoprim-sulfamethoxazole, nitrofurantoin, a quinolone, or amoxicillin-clavulanic acid for 7 days. A urologic evaluation may be indicated after treatment, especially with a complicated treatment course.

Dysuria in children can represent a urinary tract infection, rarely a pinworm infestation, or irritation of the genital region. Children can also present with other symptoms such as urgency, frequency, fever, abdominal pain, nausea, or vomiting. Physical findings can include CVA and bladder tenderness. Office urine studies for pyuria, hematuria, and bacteriuria help in the clinical diagnosis, but diagnosis is confirmed with a positive result on urine culture. Treatment is begun empirically before the culture result is received, then switched to an appropriate antibiotic. Eighty per cent of childhood UTIs are caused by *E. coli*, followed by *Pseudomonas, Klebsiella*, and *Proteus* (Lerner, 1994). A UTI can be a marker for significant vesicoureteral reflux requiring close follow-up or even surgery. Therefore, urologic evaluation should be considered once UTI is identified.

SUGGESTED READING

Bowie WR. Urethritis in males. In Holmes KK, Mardh P, Sparling PF, Wiesner PJ (eds). Sexually Transmitted Diseases, 2nd ed. New York, McGraw-Hill, 1990, pp 627–637.

Colleen S, Mardh P. Prostatitis. In Holmes KK, Mardh P, Sparling PF, Wiesner PJ (eds). Sexually Transmitted Diseases, 2nd ed. New York, McGraw-Hill, 1990, pp 653–670.

Fox KK, Behets FM. Vaginal discharge. Postgrad Med 1995;98(3):87–104.

Holmes KK. Lower genital tract infections in women: Cystitis, urethritis, vulvovaginitis, and cervicitis. In Holmes KK, Mardh P, Sparling PF, Wiesner PJ (eds). Sexually Transmitted Diseases, 2nd ed. New York, McGraw-Hill, 1990, pp 527–545.

Lerner GR. Urinary tract infections in children. Pediatr Ann 1994;23(9):463–473.

Stamm WE, Hooton TM. Management of urinary tract infections in adults. N Engl J Med 1993;329(18):1328–1334.

QUESTIONS

1. Match each of the following conditions with its characteristic presentations, diagnostic entities, or treatment plan.
   a. Acute bacterial cystitis
   b. Gonococcal urethritis
   c. Chlamydial urethritis
   d. Candidal vulvovaginitis
   e. Trichomonal vaginitis

   f. Herpes simplex urethritis/vulvovaginitis
      (1) Dysuria, urgency, frequency, pyuria, onset usually short-lived
      (2) Insidious onset of dysuria, sterile pyuria
      (3) Pruritus, curdy vaginal discharge, vulvar satellite lesions
      (4) Treated with Rocephin 250 mg IM followed by doxycycline 100 mg po bid for 7 days
      (5) Inguinal adenopathy can be present

Answers appear on **page 607.**

Chapter 71

Nocturia

Joseph C. Konen, M.D., M.S.P.H.

INITIAL VISIT

Subjective

PATIENT IDENTIFICATION AND PRESENTING PROBLEM. Mary called last week and scheduled a visit for her 70-year-old husband, Bob. Both she and Bob have been having difficulty sleeping. For the last several months he has been waking up to urinate two or three times a night. When he awakens, she awakens also. They arrive together for an early morning appointment.

PRESENTING ILLNESS. For many years Bob has occasionally needed to arise once during the night to urinate. About 3 years ago this became a nightly occurrence. But, for the last 6 months, he voids as much as three times each night. Initially his arising seemed to disturb his wife more than it did him. Over the last month, however, he has begun to complain of fatigue. His wife also complains of his occasional snoring, but she does not seem to think that he holds his breath while sleeping.

PAST MEDICAL HISTORY. For the past 10 years Bob has had mild hypertension, non–insulin dependent diabetes, and hypercholesterolemia. These conditions had been well controlled when he carefully followed his diet and exercise routine. After retiring 5 years ago, however, he became more sedentary and his weight increased. He has no past history of renal or urologic problems. His current medications include hydrochlorothiazide 50 mg and glipizide 5 mg, both of which he takes each morning.

FAMILY HISTORY. Bob's mother died at age 85 years from congestive heart failure. She also had diabetes mellitus. Bob's father died at age 86 years from a myocardial infarction. He also had prostate cancer detected the year before he died. Bob has one sibling, a brother who is 5 years younger and is alive and well.

HEALTH HABITS. Bob has never used tobacco. He routinely has a cup of coffee each evening after dinner. Most evenings he has a mixed alcoholic drink before retiring. He and his wife retire together at about 10 P.M. and usually arise for the day about 6 A.M. He used to walk 2 miles a day but abandoned this exercise a year ago.

SOCIAL HISTORY. Bob is married. He retired 5 years ago after working for nearly 30 years as a repairman for a telephone company. He has two children who have families of their own and do not live at home. He is sexually active and usually attempts intercourse less than once a month.

REVIEW OF SYSTEMS. Except for his sleep and urinary problems, Bob has no health complaints. He initially denies increased urinary frequency other than the nocturia, but on close questioning realizes that his voiding every 2 hours during the afternoon is more frequent than it was a few years ago. He denies urinary hesitancy, urgency, and dysuria. He believes that nightly voids seem to be of a smaller volume than those that occur during the day. Although he sometimes snores, this is not a nightly occurrence, and his wife does not notice any apnea. Bob acknowledges that he usually awakens in the morning feeling refreshed but finds that he desires to take a nap most afternoons.

Objective

Physical Examination

Bob's blood pressure is 160/100 mm Hg; he weighs 205 lb; his height is 70 in; and his temperature is 98.4°F. The examination of his head, eye, ears, neck, and oral cavity is normal. No jugular venous distention or carotid bruits is seen. The chest is clear to percussion and auscultation. Examination of the heart reveals regular rhythm without murmurs, rubs, or clicks. His abdomen and costovertebral angles are soft and nontender, but obese. No masses are palpable. The bladder does not appear to be enlarged by percussion. He is circumcised; there are no penile lesions or discharge. Testes are moderately soft, nontender, and descended. He has no inguinal masses. The prostate is nontender, only slightly enlarged, and slightly asymmetric. The gland is firm, but there are no distinct nodules. Stool is guaiac negative. Extremities are warm and have good color. Pulses are symmetric and full except for reduced impulses in both dorsalis pedal areas. A slight trace of pedal edema is found in both ankles.

Laboratory Tests

Fasting serum chemistry studies reveal a glucose level of 160 mg/dl, creatinine level of 1.8 mg/dl, and a blood urea nitrogen (BUN) level of 20 mg/dl. Electrolytes and liver chemistry study results are normal. Total cholesterol level is 240 mg/dl with a high-density lipoprotein (HDL) cholesterol level of 35 mg/dl. A glycosylated hemoglobin level is 10.2 per cent. A prostatic specific antigen (PSA) level is 5.5 ng/ml. A dipstick urinalysis of an early morning specimen shows no protein but trace glucose. No hemoglobin or leukocyte esterase is detected. Microscopic examination of the urine does not show any red or white blood cells nor any bacteria.

Bob completes an International Prostate Symptom Score sheet (IPSS), which is a semi-quantitative measure of his urinary symptoms and receives a score of 12 (normal 0–7). Inspection of individual items reveals mostly obstructive but little irritative symptoms. He acknowledges mixed feelings about the impact his urinary symptoms have on the quality of his life.

Assessment

Working Diagnosis

Benign prostatic hypertrophy is diagnosed. Hypertension and diabetes mellitus are not well controlled.

Differential Diagnosis

Many conditions besides prostatic hypertrophy cause nocturia. The more common causes of nocturia that may fit Bob's symptoms include:

1. Caffeine and alcoholic beverages. The consumption of these beverages even several hours before retiring commonly causes if not aggravates nocturia.

2. Glucosuria. Although the urinalysis from an early morning specimen is relatively unremarkable and a morning fasting serum glucose level suggests reasonable glycemic control, the elevated glycosylated hemoglobin level suggests significant hyperglycemia at other times during the day. Evening hyperglycemia may be accompanied by significant glucosuria, resulting in nocturia.

3. Primary renal disorder. A history of hypertension and diabetes is a strong risk factor for nephropathy. In spite of a normal urinalysis, an elevated serum creatinine level, and early pedal edema may suggest renal compromise, in this case most likely from diabetic nephropathy. "Silent" prostatism through slowly progressive urinary obstruction can cause an obstructive nephropathy.

4. Other edematous states including congestive heart failure, liver disease, venous stasis, and others can also result in nocturia. History, physical, and laboratory findings do not support congestive heart failure or significant liver disease. Age, hypertension, diabetes, and dyslipidemia are risk factors for systemic atherosclerosis, which is further suggested by decreased peripheral pulses. This condition may explain Bob's trace pedal edema.

5. Other causes of urinary obstruction. Prostate cancer, bladder tumor, or genitourinary stones may also cause urinary obstruction and nocturia. Although most laboratories use a PSA level of 4.0 ng/ml as the upper limits of normal, values from 0 to 6.5 ng/ml are considered normal in men ages 70 years and above. The patient's family history of prostate cancer is a significant additional risk factor and warrants either a repeat PSA in a few months or transrectal ultrasound.

6. Obstructive sleep apnea syndrome. This syndrome (OSA) commonly causes fatigue, and may cause nocturia. In this case, however, there are no reports of apnea, and the snoring is intermittent and not nightly. Bob usually awakens refreshed, which also does not suggest significant OSA.

Plan

Diagnostic

Without the history of diabetes and the finding of a slightly elevated serum creatinine level, no other diagnostic tests at this time usually are warranted. In this case, however, a negative dipstick analysis for protein is not sensitive enough to detect microalbuminuria—a finding that would confirm early nephropathy. A determination of creatinine clearance is warranted if a repeat serum creatinine level shows any further deterioration. A renal ultrasound may be useful to rule out silent obstructive nephropathy.

Therapeutic

Bob's diabetes and hypertension are not well controlled. He is instructed to increase his glipizide (Glucotrol) dose to 5 mg twice a day. The hydrochlorothiazide is discontinued because it does not seem to be controlling the blood pressure and there is a concern that it may be contributing to his hyperglycemia and dyslipidemia. Terazosin (Hytrin) 1 mg at bedtime is initiated with instructions to increase the dose to 2 mg each evening after a week and a week later to 5 mg each evening. He is advised to return to the office each week before increasing his dose to have his blood pressure measured by the office nurse.

Patient Education

Bob and his wife are informed about the differential diagnostic possibilities. He prefers to return in a month for another office visit and a repeat PSA before further considering a transrectal ultrasound or further renal studies, although he agrees to a urinary determination for microalbumin. Literature explaining the natural history of benign prostatic hypertrophy and nocturia is given. He is advised to avoid caffeinated and alcoholic beverages in the evening and over-the-counter cold remedies.

Disposition

Instructions are given for obtaining an overnight urine collection for microalbuminuria. Bob is advised to return his sample when he comes next week for a nurse blood pressure check. He is scheduled to return in 1 month for additional evaluation including an IPSS and PSA.

DISCUSSION

Nocturia is simply the need to urinate at night, or more exactly, after retiring because those who sleep during the day after working at night may experience a daytime version of the need to urinate while sleeping.

The normal capacity of the adult bladder is approximately 400 ml. Whether one sleeps through the night without the need to urinate depends on a diurnal rhythm and the fact that the volume of urine formed while recumbent must not exceed bladder capacity. Increased urinary volume may be the result of reduced osmotic concentration, increased sodium excretion, solute diuresis, or reduction in bladder capacity. Any disease process that results in an increased solute or osmotic load to the kidney can result in nocturia, as can any polyuria state.

Nocturia may be a symptom of renal disease related to a relative decrease in renal parenchymal function. Even in the earliest stages of most renal diseases, the ability to concentrate urine is compromised, and overnight urinary volume can easily exceed bladder capacity. In the absence of overt daytime polyuria, nocturia may be the first signal of renal disease. Nocturia commonly accompanies edema-forming diseases and is frequently experienced in those with congestive heart failure, nephrotic syndrome, and cirrhosis with ascites.

Nocturia may also occur in the absence of disease. Commonly nocturia is experienced by those who consume excessive amounts of fluids late in the evening or before retiring. Caffeinated and alcoholic beverages have specific diuretic effects either directly (caffeine) or indirectly through suppression of antidiuretic hormone (alcohol) and commonly cause or aggravate nocturia.

In older ambulatory individuals, some degree of fluid retention is common. This retention may be the result of a relative decline in cardiac output with aging or increased venous stasis or venous varicosities. On becoming recumbent, this excess fluid is stored in perivascular and tissues. The excess is reabsorbed and is presented to the kidneys for excretion (Tanagho and McAninch, 1988). Renal perfusion is also increased in the recumbent position, further facilitating mobilization of fluid retention. Nocturia may be the presenting symptom of those with congestive heart failure because of these very mechanisms, reflecting the decreased functional status of the cardiovascular system during the day. Nocturia is often compounded by therapies that include diuretics.

Urinary frequency at night may be an important disrupter of sleep. Hence, patients presenting with complaints of fatigue or difficulty sleeping should be evaluated for common causes of nocturia including urinary tract infection, diabetes, and prostatism, or poor timing of diuretic use. Often nocturia and disturbed sleep are the complaints that bring patients, especially men with prostatic hyperplasia, or their sleeping partners to seek medical assistance (Gorol and colleagues, 1995). Obstructive sleep apnea syndrome may also commonly cause nocturia. It is believed that increased secretion of atrial natriuretic factor produced during sleep in affected individuals causes increased natriuresis and diuresis (Brown, 1996).

Reduced bladder capacity may also cause nocturia. Infection, bladder stones, or tumor may produce an inflammatory reaction and increased bladder irritability. Prostatic hyperplasia, urethral stricture, stones, or neoplasms may also cause chronic partial urinary outflow obstruction, initiating frequent voiding and a thickening of the bladder wall, which can reduce bladder compliance and hence reduce bladder capacity. Often early in obstructive processes nocturia may appear only as a single nocturnal voiding of reasonable volume, whereas later in more advanced degrees of obstruction, multiple nocturnal voidings of smaller volumes become the rule (Isselbacher, 1994).

Benign prostatic hypertrophy (BPH) is predominantly a quality-of-life problem. Whereas almost every male living into his eighth decade has histologic evidence of BPH, only half develop palpable prostatic enlargement, and only half of these men develop sufficient symptoms to undergo surgical resection. Although BPH is considered a mostly benign condition, for many men the condition is not benign in terms of disruption of daily activities and altered sleep patterns for them and their bed partners when urinary obstruction causes symptoms.

Symptoms are generated from increased prostatic tissue and resulting pressure on the prostatic urethra and capsule, prostatic enlargement, bladder contributions from increased muscle tone and contractility, and alterations in smooth muscle of the prostate and bladder neck. The tough prostatic capsule is relatively resistant to distention. Hence, prostatic cellular hyperplasia results in increased intraprostatic pressure, which is transmitted to the prostatic urethra, causing obstruction.

The quality-of-life problem for men with BPH arises from the need to balance the bothersomeness of symptoms with the potential complications of untreated disease versus unintended side effects of pharmacologic and surgical treatments. It is also clear that each man has a different threshold for how bothersome symptoms need to become before

he seeks professional advice or treatment. Therefore, the patient must be lead partner in guiding further investigations or suggesting therapy. Except for when the health provider discovers asymptomatic signs of obstructive nephropathy that infrequently accompany "silent prostatism," the patient's perceived seriousness of symptoms should drive the decision process.

Giving control over treatment strategies to the patient is essential because the natural history of BPH is very variable. Whereas BPH occurs in nearly all men as they age, only 25 per cent are bothered enough to have a procedure performed to relieve the problem. In general, even without therapy, symptom progression is uncommon. Stabilization and even improvement of symptoms constitute the normal course of events. Progression to complications such as acute urinary obstruction, urinary tract infection, obstructive uropathy, or renal failure rarely occurs. Because symptoms often wax and wane, and risk of serious complications is relatively low, an initial "wait and see" management approach is often in the man's best interest.

Assessing a man's IPSS may be useful in screening for BPH. It is often surprising to see what proportion of middle-aged men purporting to be asymptomatic have significant scores when asked to complete the instrument. Just as important to the total score and irritative and obstructive subscores, however, is the consideration whether symptoms detected by this screening tool are associated with a significant enough dissatisfaction with altered urinary function to pursue further evaluation and treatment.

Because the examiner cannot feel the entire prostate gland in three dimensions, digital rectal examination (DRE) is a poor estimator of gland size. Sixty per cent of the normal gland is inaccessible to examining finger. The DRE results in palpation only of the posterior aspects of the prostate. Whereas detection of nodules, consistency, and tenderness may be important for other diagnostic considerations, by itself DRE is a poor screening tool for either BPH or prostate cancer.

The differential diagnosis for BPH depends on the nature of symptomatology. Purely irritative symptomatology may accompany urinary tract infections, prostatitis, bladder cancer, bladder calculi, interstitial or radiation-induced cystitis, and uninhibited bladder contractions that may result from cerebrovascular accidents. Pure obstructive symptoms may be due to urethral stricture, urethral valves, prostate cancer, bladder neck contracture, or a poorly contracting bladder in response to paraplegia. Mixed obstructive and irritative symptoms may result from neurologic insults such as spinal cord injury, multiple sclerosis, or Parkinson disease. Patients with prostatitis, just as those with BPH, may also present with mixed symptomatology.

Evaluation for BPH should begin with a careful recorded history supplemented by use of the IPSS to semiquantitate urinary symptomatology. The prostate should be evaluated by a DRE, realizing that significant BPH may exist despite the appearance of a normal DRE result. In most cases of BPH, however, the gland is enlarged, symmetric, elastic, and firm. The abdomen should also be palpated and percussed for signs of bladder distention, which is a finding often missed.

Laboratory evaluation should include a urinalysis with at least a qualitative measurement for blood and leukocyte esterase activity if not microscopic examination. If the urinalysis result is abnormal, the urine should be cultured. If culture results are negative and hematuria is detected, a work-up to rule out carcinoma and stones should continue. Serum creatinine levels should also be measured at the initial evaluation and repeated along with periodic urinalysis in symptomatic men, especially those undergoing "watchful waiting" protocols. In the absence of abnormal urinalysis results and serum creatinine level, other studies are not likely to contribute significantly to management decisions.

Unless complications are suspected, there is no clear value for performing an intravenous pyelogram, renal ultrasonography, cystometrics, or cystoscopy. Measuring post–residual volume and urine flow rates have poor reproducibility and for the most part add little to the diagnosis. Pressure flow studies may be useful in differentiating neurogenic and decompensated bladder conditions from BPH. Transrectal ultrasound may have value in measuring large glands and in consideration of surgery.

Measuring PSA levels in the initial evaluation of BPH is controversial and problematic for three reasons. First, there is great overlap between values seen for BPH and prostate cancer. Second, there is presently no consensus on the protocol to evaluate minimally elevated PSA levels. Third, there is presently no evidence that knowledge of PSA levels decrease either the morbidity or mortality associated with BPH or prostate carcinoma. Before implementing hormonal manipulation for BPH, as discussed later, however, baseline PSA measurements may be useful in measuring compliance with hormonal therapy.

Decisions regarding management options are ideally made with the interests of the patient clearly expressed. The primary goal should be toward the reduction of symptoms to a level where the patient

and sleeping partner are no longer dissatisfied. Comparing serially performed IPSSs is useful in evaluating response to therapy.

In general, watchful waiting should be the treatment of choice for men who are not moderately to severely dissatisfied by their symptoms. Men should be instructed to report increases in severity or frequency of symptoms between evaluations. In the absence of progression of symptoms, men with BPH should be re-evaluated at least yearly with the IPSS, DRE, urinalysis, and serum creatinine level if results of all of these were initially normal.

Alteration in lifestyle should be recommended to all men with significant BPH symptomatology regardless of other treatment options they may select. In particular, they should avoid alpha-adrenergic stimulants such as decongestants and cough syrups that can increase prostatic muscular tone. Avoidance of anticholinergic and antihistaminic medications may also be helpful. Reduction in late evening fluids and caffeine after dinner may be effective in reducing the frequency of nocturia. Cold, immobility, and excessive alcohol ingestion may also precipitate acute urinary retention in men with significant BPH and should be avoided.

After patient education, pharmaceutical approaches should be considered as a second line of intervention. Useful medications include alpha-adrenergic blockers for treatment of dynamic and obstructive components of BPH and hormonal strategies for the static obstructive components of the symptom complex.

Alpha-adrenergic blockers such as terazosin, doxazosin, and prazosin relax bladder neck and prostatic smooth muscle. Although these drugs are antihypertensive agents, they do not appear to significantly lower blood pressure in normotensive men. To avoid first-dose hypotension severe enough to cause syncope or orthostasis, first and preferably all doses should be given on retiring. Efficacy of alpha blockers can usually be apparent in a few weeks with marked reduction in dynamic symptomatology. Improvements can be monitored with the IPSS in as little as 2 to 4 weeks after initiating therapy. The use of alpha blockers may be appropriately considered as a first line of therapy in men who have BPH symptoms and require an antihypertensive agent.

Hormonal manipulations may also be useful in selected patients, especially those with large glands (>50 gm). 5-Alpha reductase inhibitors such as finasteride block the conversion of testosterone to dihydrotestosterone (DHT) and cause an involution of the prostate and reduction of static obstructive forces. Patients usually notice significant improvement in symptomatology within 3 to 4 months of initiating therapy when reductions in prostate size begin to become apparent. Improvements in symptoms can also be measured using the IPSS.

Invasive or surgical treatments should be considered when other strategies have failed, when estimates of prostate gland size are markedly high (i.e., greater than 60 gm), or the patient has expressed a preference for a urologic opinion. Referral to an urologist is also appropriate for refractory urinary retention after a trial of catheterization or for men who experience recurrent urinary tract infections, hematuria, or signs of renal insufficiency, all of which suggest significant obstruction that may be a condition other than BPH.

FIRST FOLLOW-UP VISIT

Subjective

Bob returned 1 month after his initial visit. In the interim he returned to the office for blood pressure checks by the nurse as instructed. He tolerated well the increases in doses of terazosin. Bob had complied with taking his glipizide twice a day. He was successful in reducing his caffeinated and alcoholic beverages after dinner. He and his wife were pleased with his marked reductions in nocturia from three times a night to approximately once every other night. Both felt more rested and have both restarted a walking program they used to enjoy.

Objective

Bob's blood pressure is 140/82 mm Hg. His weight is 195 lb. The rest of his physical examination is unchanged except that the trace pedal edema is now nearly nonexistent. A repeat IPSS is 7. Bob readily acknowledges that the quality of his life related to his nocturia has improved. An overnight urine collection for microalbuminuria was normal at 0.015 gm albumin per gram creatinine (normal range 0–0.020 gm albumin per gram creatinine). Fasting serum chemistry studies reveal a glucose level of 120 mg/dl, a creatinine level of 1.2 mg/dl, and BUN level of 18 mg/dl. Total cholesterol level is 220 mg/dl with an HDL-cholesterol level of 45 mg/dl. A glycosylated hemoglobin level is 8.8 per cent. PSA is 4.9 ng/ml. A dipstick urinalysis of an early morning specimen shows no protein, no glucose. No hemoglobin or leukocyte esterase is detected.

Assessment

1. Benign prostatic hypertrophy, improved

2. Non–insulin dependent diabetes mellitus, improved

3. Hypertension, improved

4. Mild renal insufficiency, improved

Plan

DIAGNOSTIC. No further diagnostic work-up is warranted at this time.

THERAPEUTIC. The prescriptions for terazosin and glipizide were renewed.

PATIENT EDUCATION. The patient was congratulated on the many lifestyle changes he had made. The natural history of BPH was again briefly reviewed.

DISPOSITION. Bob agreed to return in 2 to 3 months for a brief recheck. He was reminded to report changes in his symptomatology. Because of his family history of prostate cancer and the finding of slight prostatic asymmetry on the initial examination, he agreed to return for a follow-up PSA in 6 months.

SUGGESTED READING

Brown LK. Sleep apnea. In Rakel R (ed). Saunders' Manual of Medical Practice. Philadelphia, W. B. Saunders, 1996, p 199.

Goroll AH, May LA, Mulley AG (eds). Primary Care Medicine: Office Evaluation and Management of the Adult Patient, 3rd ed. Philadelphia, J. B. Lippincott, 1995, pp 1062–1063.

Isselbacher, KJ (ed). Harrison's Principles of Internal Medicine, 13th ed. New York, McGraw-Hill, 1994, pp 239–240.

Konen, JC. Men's Health Issues: Prostate Disorders in Adult Health: Multidisciplinary Approaches to Wellness. Bala Cynwyd, PA, Meniscus Educational Institute, 1997, pp 18–26.

Tanagho EA, McAninch JW (eds). Smith's General Urology, 12th ed. Norwalk, CT, Appleton & Lange, 1988, p 34.

1. Which of the following is the most reasonable method for following the progression of benign prostatic hypertrophy?
   a. Cystometrics and urine flow velocities
   b. International Prostate Symptom Scores
   c. Prostate-specific serum antigen
   d. Transrectal ultrasonography

2. Avoidance of the following substances is likely to reduce symptoms of prostatic hypertrophy?
   a. Alcohol
   b. Caffeine
   c. Antihistamines
   d. Decongestants

3. Measuring prostatic specific antigen (PSA) levels in the initial evaluation of BPH is controversial and problematic because there is
   a. A significant overlap between values seen for BPH and prostate cancer
   b. There is no consensus on the protocol to evaluate minimally elevated PSA levels.
   c. There is no evidence that knowledge of PSA levels decrease either the morbidity or mortality associated with BPH or prostate carcinoma.
   d. The upper limit of normal values for PSA is 4.0 ng/ml in all age groups.

Answers appear on **page 607.**

Chapter **72**

Urinary Incontinence

Richard W. Demmler, M.D.

SUBJECTIVE

Mr. S., an 84-year-old gentleman, is admitted to the nursing home because of the inability of his wife to care for him. Mr. S. has a 7-year history of Parkinson disease. He presently receives carbidopa/levodopa (Sinemet) 10/100, one orally qid, selegiline (Eldepryl) 5 mg bid, trihexyphenidyl (Artane) 2 mg bid, and bromocriptine (Parlodel) 5 mg tid. He experienced a significant reduction in his mobility over the last several months and most recently became incontinent of urine. He says he just cannot get to the bathroom soon enough when he feels the need to urinate. He notes that when he coughs, he occasionally spontaneously urinates, and he reports a decreased urinary flow over the last 2 or 3 years.

PAST MEDICAL HISTORY. Mr. S. underwent a transurethral resection of the prostate 10 years ago for benign prostatic hypertrophy, a left herniorrhaphy 15 years ago, and an appendectomy while in the service during World War II. Three years before admission, he suffered a stroke. He has no previous history of hypertension, diabetes, asthma, cancer, or cardiac disease. He has no reported drug allergies or reactions. He is a social drinker. He quit smoking in 1968 after smoking two packs a day for 20+ years.

FAMILY HISTORY. Mr. S.'s father died of a myocardial infarction at age 86 years. His mother died of breast cancer at age 94 years. He has two brothers in relatively good physical health, and one brother was recently diagnosed with prostate cancer. No other relative has had Parkinson disease, but there are several with dementia on his mother's side of the family.

SOCIAL HISTORY. Mr. S. has been married for 60 years to the same woman, and they are clearly dedicated to one another. They have two children, a boy and a girl, who live 2 hours away by commercial jet. Mrs. S. has been in declining health over the past 2 years. She underwent a mastectomy for breast cancer 6 months ago and now receives megestrol (Megace). She has been less able to care for Mr. S. since the diagnosis. Mr. S. has been attending a day care center three times per week. In addition, a visiting nurse's aide assists with activities of daily living (ADL) 3 days a week.

REVIEW OF SYSTEMS. HEENT: Mr. S. uses glasses and has noticed of late that the vision in his right eye is blurry. He has well-fitting dentures and reports no limitations with different food consistencies. He wears a hearing aid in his left ear that he finds satisfactory. He breathes through his nose without difficulty. Cardiopulmonary: he denies chest pain, orthopnea, or paroxysmal nocturnal dyspnea. He also denies chest pain or dyspnea on exertion but admits that his Parkinson disease significantly limits his walking speed and he is unable to climb stairs. He does not remember a history of pneumonia or night sweats but had a positive result on purified protein derivative (PPD) testing by the time he left the service. Gastrointestinal: he denies dyspepsia or history of ulcers. He has occasional gastrointestinal upset relieved with aluminum hydroxide–magnesium hydroxide, simethicone (Mylanta). He suffers from occasional constipation but also has trouble with episodes of diarrhea. Genitourinary: Mr. S. had benign prostatic hypertrophy that required transurethral resection of the prostate 10 years ago. Subsequently, he has been unable to have an erection. Recently, he became incontinent of urine. Six months before admission, he had a prostate specific antigen (PSA) test, with a normal result. He states that he urinates within seconds after he feels the urge. He does not describe large amounts of urine when he urinates and has not noted any blood in his urine. Neurologic: Mr. S. suffered a left medial cerebral artery embolic stroke 3 years ago requiring a short stay in a skilled nursing facility (SNF). He was able to ambulate with a walker until recently. His Parkinson disease began as a tremor in his right hand 7 years ago and steadily progressed, requiring appropriate modifications of his medication regimen. Neuroendocrine: no significant history suggesting any difficulties.

OBJECTIVE

His BP is 140/76, pulse 82, respiration 14 per minute. General appearance: well-developed male in no acute distress. He has a flattened affect, speaks slowly, deliberately, and in a whisper. HEENT: flat facies, he wears dentures. No fasciculation of his tongue is noted. He has cataracts in both eyes, more in the right than the left. Neck: supple, no masses, no bruits, and a normal palpable thyroid. Chest: moves symmetrically with no retractions. The lung sounds are clear but with diminished breath sounds in all lung fields. Heart: Normal S_1, S_2, with no S_3, S_4, or murmurs.

Abdomen: increased abdominal tone, no masses are noted but some tenderness is noted in the left lower quadrant. The liver is normally palpated and percussed. Bowel sounds are audible. Genitourinary: normal external genitalia. There is evidence of a previous left inguinal herniorrhaphy. Rectal: there is a large amount of stool in the rectal vault. The prostate feels flattened, consistent with previous prostatectomy, and there are no masses palpable. Testing for fecal occult blood is negative.

Neurologic: cranial nerves are intact except for somewhat less ability to raise the left mouth in a grin. The face has a flattened affect. Gross motor examination demonstrates a rigidity of all extremities and cogwheeling more on the right than the left. Position sense for standing and sitting is normal. His gait with a walker is slow and shuffling. Mini-mental status examination shows a score of 24 with 1/3 recall, 3 of 5 subtraction, and missed day and date.

ASSESSMENT

Mr. S. is an 84-year-old gentleman with multiple problems, but he is admitted to the nursing home because of the onset of urinary incontinence and because his wife can no longer care for him at home. He had a stroke 3 years ago and has a 7-year history of Parkinson disease requiring multiple medications. His rehabilitation from the cerebrovascular accident (CVA) went well; he returned home after a short stay in a SNF. He now has some cognitive impairment with recent memory loss. The onset of incontinence made it impossible for his wife to care for him even with in-house help and day care. In addition, Mrs. S. has significant medical problems of her own that diverted some of her attention from Mr. S.

Mr. S.'s urinary incontinence presents a very interesting dilemma for the physician. He has every condition for urinary incontinence including urinary tract infection, hyperglycosuria, and detrusor instability (a result of the CVA). Overflow incontinence from urethral obstruction due to prostate cancer is a possibility but doubtful with a low PSA and a normal prostate examination. In addition, the presence of rectal impaction and the possibility of strictures from previous prostate surgery may also result in urethral obstruction. Stress incontinence is another possibility because of the previous prostate surgery. One must not forget functional incontinence because of decreased mobility, decreased mentation, and decreased assistance from others.

PLAN

Mr. S. is admitted to the nursing home and he will remain on his usual medications consisting of carbidopa/levodopa, selegiline, trihexyphenidyl, and bromocriptine. Laboratory tests will be obtained including a fasting blood sugar and a catheterized urine for urinalysis and culture and sensitivity. The fecal impaction must be properly treated. After resolution of the impaction, Mr. S. must have a urinary catheterization for a post–voiding residual volume. If the urine volume is less than 100 ml and the urinalysis and fasting glucose level results are normal, the patient will be assessed for detrusor instability.

RESULTS OF TESTS

The urinalysis revealed a specific gravity of 1.020, negative protein, glucose, nitrates, and leukocyte esterase levels. One to two RBCs/high power field (HPF) and two to four WBC/HPF were seen with 1+ bacteriuria. The fasting blood sugar was 109 mg/dl. The post–voiding residual urine was 75 ml, and the catheter passed easily into the bladder.

Cystometric examination demonstrated an uninhibited detrusor contraction consistent with detrusor instability.

As a result of these tests, oxybutynin 5 mg bid was administered. Follow-up in 2 weeks found the urinary incontinence resolved. In addition, Mr. S.'s face appeared to have considerably more expression and his gait was quicker but still shuffling. The amount of rigidity was decreased, and cogwheeling was manifested only after many repeated flexion/extension repetitions.

The patient had repeat cystometric examination that demonstrated no change in previous findings. The oxybutynin was discontinued and the patient continued to be continent of urine; however, the frequency of urination was unchanged.

DISCUSSION

Mr. S. demonstrates the presence of detrusor instability compounded by functional incapacity. This condition was a result of his inability to remember his medications because of his dementia and his wife's declined physical condition that limited her caregiver ability to ensure that he received his medications. Once he was admitted, he received his medications in the prescribed manner, and his functional ability improved. The detrusor instability remained, but the patient was now able to modify his behavior to maintain continence. As a result, oxybutynin was discontinued without ill effect and thus allowed for a reduction in medicine in a patient already on multiple drugs. It is appropriate to review the needs for the anti-parkinsonian medications (carbidopa/levodopa, selegiline, trihexyphenidyl, and bromocriptine) because some may have been added more because of nonutilization than ineffectiveness of treatment.

Understanding the conditions that predispose to incontinence makes the diagnosis and treatment straightforward. The bladder is an expandable storage container dependent on anatomic structures and neurologic feedback that involves the interplay of sympathetic, parasympathetic, and somatic innervation. The neurologic innervation is represented in Figure 72–1. The sympathetic nervous system maintains sphincter tone (alpha receptors) and relaxation of the bladder (beta receptors). The parasympathetic tone remains basically constant through filling and contraction. Micturition occurs with a reduction in sympathetic tone that reduces the sphincter tension, and the detrusor contracts. Incontinence results from disruption of the anatomic, neurologic, and functional interplay and is divided into four categories.

Detrusor instability results in evacuation at low filling volumes and is the most common condition resulting in incontinence. Early detrusor contraction results from local irritation such as infection or tumor. The permanent condition of detrusor instability, however, is because of decreased sympathetic nervous system tone resulting in the unopposed parasympathetic nervous system tone that leads to spontaneous contractions at small volumes of urine. Sympathetic tone emanates from central nervous system (CNS) centers, and thus this condition is the result of primary CNS diseases. The most common of these are Alzheimer disease and stroke. But other diseases, such as Parkinson disease, play a role in this entity. This disorder is referred to as detrusor hyper-reflexia, spastic bladder, urge incontinence, or unstable bladder. At this time, in the

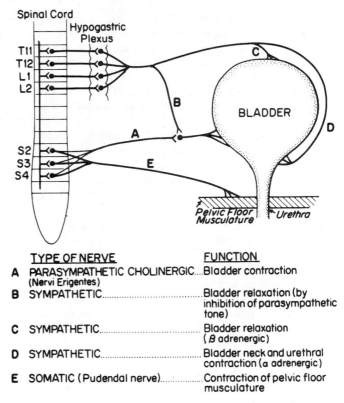

Figure 72-1. Peripheral nerves involved in micturition. (From Kane RL, Ouslander JG, Abrass IB [eds]: Essentials of Clinical Geriatrics, 3rd ed. New York, McGraw-Hill, 1994, with permission.)

	TYPE OF NERVE	FUNCTION
A	PARASYMPATHETIC CHOLINERGIC (Nervi Erigentes)	Bladder contraction
B	SYMPATHETIC	Bladder relaxation (by inhibition of parasympathetic tone)
C	SYMPATHETIC	Bladder relaxation (β adrenergic)
D	SYMPATHETIC	Bladder neck and urethral contraction (α adrenergic)
E	SOMATIC (Pudendal nerve)	Contraction of pelvic floor musculature

presence of a degenerative CNS disease, this condition is referred to as *detrusor hyper-reflexia*.

Stress incontinence results from the loss of the cystourethral angle following childbirth or pelvic surgery. This anatomic disruption reduces the effectiveness of the sphincter, resulting in episodes of incontinence when there is increased intra-abdominal pressure, as seen with coughing or the Valsalva maneuver.

Overflow incontinence is the result of an obstruction or a neurogenic bladder. Obstruction results from prostatic hypertrophy, urethral stricture, or fecal impaction. Neurogenic bladder results from paraplegia or degenerative neurologic disorders such as multiple sclerosis or diabetes. Overflow incontinence is the inability of the bladder to contract until it is significantly dilated and usually when it contains more than 500 ml.

Functional incontinence results from the inability of an individual to toilet properly. It is the result of an immobility from physical restraints, drowsiness from tranquilizing medications, or immobility resulting from disease or end-stage dementing illnesses.

The most efficient method of diagnosing a patient presenting with incontinence is to evaluate for overflow incontinence by obtaining a post-voiding residual volume. One hundred milliliters of urine strongly suggests the presence of the condition. Obstruction from urethral stricture or prostatic hypertrophy must be considered if there is an inability to pass a 20 French catheter into the bladder. One should be mindful that the catheter can coil distal to the prostate and give a false sense of passing into the bladder without urine return.

Rectal impaction also results in overflow incontinence even though a catheter is passed easily. Persons prone to impaction (those with dementia, paraplegia, or quadriplegia; those who are bed bound; or those with hypothyroidism or hypercalcemia) need an appropriate bowel program to mitigate the occurrence of impaction. Hydration and correction of metabolic abnormalities resolve temporary states that lead to impaction. If the patient suffers from chronic recurring impaction, continuous use of lactulose or sorbitol should be considered. It is sometimes necessary to provide rectal stimulation with either glycerin or medicated suppository after a meal to obtain adequate evacuation. Hypothyroidism and hypercalcemia should be appropriately managed to minimize the associated constipation and impactions. In addition, drugs with anticholinergic properties such as antihistamines, tricyclic antidepressants, antispasmodics, and trihexyphenidyl may lead to bowel hypomotility, which leads to impaction. Sympathomimetic drugs such as pseudoephedrine and phenylpropanolamine may increase the sphincter tone in the presence of subtotal obstruction of the urethra to result in urinary retention.

The treatment of neurogenic bladder is clean intermittent catheterization every 4 hours in competent, noninstitutionalized patients. The clinician should evaluate the utility of intermittent catheterization in the nursing home setting. An indwelling Foley catheter should be employed only if necessary because of the frequent morbidity associated with its use. A person with an indwelling Foley catheter will be hospitalized twice per year on average. In addition, the urethra adapts to the foreign object by dilating more and requiring ever increasing catheter size.

Stress incontinence can be diagnosed by having the patient stand, hold a gloved hand below the urethral aperture, and cough or perform a Valsalva maneuver. The treatment begins with Kegel exercises to increase the tone of the perineal floor musculature. If exercises fail or if the patient is unable to perform these exercises, estrogen vaginal cream or oral estrogen can be used. In addition, pseudoephedrine (Sudafed) or phenylpropanolamine (Ornade) increases the sympathetic tone of the bladder neck and thus increases resistance to voiding. If these measures fail to correct the problem and the patient finds the condition unacceptable, a Marshall-Marchetti-Kranz procedure or anterior repair can be performed to surgically restore the cystourethral angle.

Functional incontinence should always be considered by clinicians caring for elderly patients. The case of Mr. S. demonstrated the effect of inadequate treatment for a condition that resulted in immobility. Most frequently, however, functional incontinence is the result of sedatives (benzodiazepines and neuroleptics) and/or physical restraints used by physicians to treat agitation. Thus, review of current therapies may reveal immediate steps to alleviate incontinence. The physician must maximize the functional status of the patient to minimize the possibility of incontinence.

Multiple agents have been used for detrusor instability, but oxybutynin (Ditropan) is the most commonly used. Others include propantheline (Pro-Banthine), dicyclomine (Bentyl), flavoxate (Urispas). These medications block the parasympathetic stimulation and therefore allow for continued dilation of the bladder. Imipramine appears to be a good drug because of its dual action to increase the capacity of the bladder and increase the sphincter tone. This drug results in agitation, apprehension, sleeplessness, tremulousness, and weight loss however, which limits its effectiveness in this age group.

Many investigators now believe that the diagnosis of detrusor instability is assured after excluding the other entities associated with urinary incontinence. I believe, however, that because this condition requires a new medication in an elderly patient, confirmatory testing is mandatory. Testing includes the cystometric examination for capacity of the bladder before it contracts. In this procedure, a Foley catheter is placed in the patient's bladder and a steady rate of gas or water is administered. Significant events during the recording are at the point when the person first experiences discomfort, usually around 150 to 250 ml, difficulty resisting urination, usually 250 to 400 ml, and uncontrolled urination, usually occurring at 350 to 600 ml. These values differ by laboratory, and the clinician should know the criteria used at each urodynamic laboratory. The patient with detrusor instability usually begins experiencing discomfort early, around 50 ml, and usually is incapable of holding a volume past 75 ml.

In conclusion, urinary incontinence is voiding at times when the patient does not wish to do so. Patients are usually embarrassed. Urinary incontinence is a frequent precipitating factor that leads to admission to a nursing home, as was the case reported here. By understanding the interaction of anatomy, neural mediation, functional abilities of the patient, and social situation, a management plan can be easily implemented to greatly benefit the patient.

SUGGESTED READING

Kane RL, Ouslander JG, Abrass IB. Essentials of Clinical Geriatrics, 3rd ed. New York, McGraw-Hill, 1994.

Kegel AH. Stress incontinence of urine in women: Physiologic treatment. J Int Coll Surg 1956;24(4):487–499.

Ouslander JG. Incontinence. In Hazzard WR, Bierman EL, Blass JP, et al. (eds). Principles of Geriatric Medicine and Gerontology, 3rd ed. New York, McGraw-Hill, 1994.

Raz S. Pharmacological treatment of lower urinary tract dysfunction. In Urol Clin North Am 1978;5(2):323–334.

Williams ME, Fitzhugh CP. Urinary incontinence in the elderly: Physiology, pathophysiology, diagnosis, and treatment. Ann Intern Med 1982;97:895–907.

QUESTIONS

1. True or false: Functional incontinence is the result of
   a. Oversedation of the patient
   b. Undertreatment of the patient
   c. Physically restraining the patient
   d. Dementia

2. True or False: Detrusor instability is
   a. An early reactive response to minimal dilation stimulation
   b. An increased sympathetic tone
   c. Seen in paraplegics
   d. The result of a rectal impaction

3. True or False: Stress incontinence can be treated with
   a. Surgery
   b. Oxybutynin
   c. Pseudoephedrine
   d. Imipramine

Answers appear on **page 607**.

Chapter **73**

Headache

Robert Smith, M.D.

INITIAL VISIT

Subjective

A new patient, a 48-year-old white female who had recently moved into the area with her family, presented with daily headaches. She reported that otherwise she was healthy.

She had had headaches for years, but they were now occurring on a daily basis and had become more severe. Initially she was treated by her family doctor. Because there was no improvement she had been referred to an ear, nose, throat (ENT) specialist, an allergist, and a neurologist, who ordered a computed tomography (CT) scan of the head. The scan had been reported as normal. The neurologist diagnosed "mixed headache" and prescribed propranolol (Inderal), Fiorinal (aspirin, butalbital, caffeine), and sumatriptan (Imitrex). He explained that the Inderal was to be taken as a preventive on a daily basis, the Fiorinal to relieve the headache pain, and the Imitrex injections to be taken for the severe attacks. He also advised the patient to avoid stress as much as possible. Initially these medications helped, but the effects appeared to be wearing off because she was finding she was using greater amounts of medication. She was now using Fiorinal with codeine capsules, which she thought helped her to use less Imitrex. It was difficult for her to avoid stress because of the move.

About a year ago she was involved in a rear-end auto accident and sustained a "whiplash" injury to her neck. A radiograph of her neck was normal. She wore a cervical collar for some weeks. She still had some pain in her neck. Physical therapy had given some relief. She believed her headaches had been worse since the accident. A court case against the other driver had been satisfactorily concluded.

The family had moved into the area because her husband's firm had relocated there. They had two teenage daughters and overall they were happy with the move. Her husband, who accompanied her, was appropriately supportive, but both were increasingly frustrated because of the worsening of the headaches. The patient was seeking work as a part-time secretary and worried about absenteeism due to her headaches. She requested a refill prescription for her pain medication and Imitrex, which she pointed out she would require on a regular basis. She had stopped taking the Inderal because she did not think it now helped. She lived in the hope that some better treatment would soon become available. Her prescriptions were refilled on this occasion and she readily agreed to return for a second longer visit.

SECOND VISIT

Subjective

When questioned, the patient was able to recognize that she experienced two different types of headache. One she described as a mild everyday sort of headache, the second as severe and the main cause of her seeking medical help.

MILD HEADACHE. This occurred every day and was felt more like pressure than pain. The headache was usually present when she awoke in the morning or it developed soon afterward. It began as a pressure at the back of her head and neck and gradually spread forward over the top of her head to her forehead and both temples. She took two ibuprofen (Motrin) tablets and carried on with her everyday activities. She usually repeated the Motrin every 3 or 4 hours. This headache was becoming more difficult to control; and when it was advancing, she took one or two Fiorinal with codeine capsules. If the mild headaches were not controlled they frequently developed into a severe headache. This development occurred more often since the move. For

the past month she had been taking as many as six Fiorinal with codeine capsules a day.

SEVERE HEADACHE. About twice a week she developed a severe headache with nausea and vomiting. This headache was usually concentrated on the left side behind the eye and in the left temple. She described the pain as throbbing, and any movement made it worse. Noise and bright lights also aggravated it. She usually lay down in a darkened room and tried to sleep. An Imitrex injection helped, but her use of this drug had doubled in the past few months. To avoid using too much Imitrex, two Fiorinal with codeine capsules every 4 hours and a phenergan 25 mg suppository helped her to cope with the attack.

For some years she had avoided eating chocolate and food containing monosodium glutamate (MSG), such as that from Chinese restaurants. She was not aware of any other trigger factors. Her most severe recent headache occurred on the day of the move.

Objective

As requested, the patient brought copies of her previous medical records, which included a report of a CT scan of the head. The data confirmed her long history of headaches and the multiple medications prescribed by various physicians in the past. The CT scan with contrast reported "small foci of high intensity scattered in the white matter, seen in migraine, early multiple sclerosis, and small-vessel vasculitis." The neurologist had reassured her that this finding in her case was of no concern. Results of recent renal and hepatic screens as well as an electrocardiogram (ECG) were all normal.

Physical Examination

Vital signs were BP 120/80 mm Hg, pulse 72 per min and regular, respirations 12 per minute, weight 130 lb. Chest was clear and heart sounds were normal. There were no carotid bruits. The temporalis and trapezius muscles on the left were tender on palpation; pressure over the left temporomandibular joint caused pain. There was marked dental overbite. Flexion, extension, and lateral movements of the neck were not restricted, but there was ache on lateral rotation to the left.

Nervous System

Cognition, speech, and hearing were normal. The patient wore glasses for reading only. Pupils were equal in size and reacted normally to direct and indirect light and accommodation reflexes. There was no strabismus. Fundi were normal, and the optic disc margins were sharply defined. There was no papilledema; no signs of facial palsy were seen. Tongue protrusion was central and no tongue tremor was present. Hand grips were normal. No hand tremor was present, and results of the finger-nose test were normal. Upper and lower limb movements were normal, as were their tendon reflexes. Plantar reflexes were normal; tests for Kernig and Brudzinski signs showed normal results, as did the Romberg test. No skin sensory deficits were detected.

Assessment

It was concluded that the patient had coexisting migraine and tension-type headache (International Headache Society Classification) and migraine without aura combined with chronic tension-type headache, also known as chronic daily headache (Broderick and colleagues, 1995).

Plan

The treatment of chronic daily headache required an approach to deal with both migraine and chronic tension-type headache, treated together.

Common Treatment

HEADACHE EDUCATION. It was explained to the patient that she had a significant role to play in the control of her headaches. She was advised to join the local headache patient support group and to obtain information on headache educational materials from the American Council on Headache Education (Telephone 1-800-255-ACHE).

STRESS REDUCTION. The patient was advised to postpone starting a new job until the headaches were under better control. She and her spouse were counseled on the need for stress reduction, and she was advised on listening to relaxation tapes and learning about biofeedback. It was explained that stress was likely to be contributing to her neck and jaw pain, which in turn were adding to her headaches, both migraine and tension-type. She had seen an orthodontist in the past who had prescribed a bite plate, which she no longer wore. She was advised to consult him again because of her jaw

pain, which may require further orthodontic treatment.

The patient was instructed on ways in which to maintain a headache diary and chart to monitor response to treatment and to identify possible trigger factors. Particular attention was to be paid to having regular meals and a regular sleep pattern.

DISCONTINUATION OF NARCOTIC ANALGESICS. The patient's recent increase in the use of narcotic analgesics indicates probable misuse, in that the medications are being used to prevent headaches and not to abort the pain. It is likely that the patient has become habituated to the drugs, and rebound headache was contributing to the increase in headache (Mathew and colleagues, 1990). Because the patient appeared well motivated, a gradual tapering program was started. Withdrawal symptoms such as restlessness, sleeplessness, excessive sweating, and increase in headache was avoided by using a 0.2 mg clonidine (Catapres) skin patch. Written instructions were given to the patient on ways in which over a period of 1 month the pain medication would be systematically changed, eliminating first the codeine, then the barbiturate, then the caffeine, aiming eventually at using small amounts of simple analgesics. If it becomes apparent that this patient is not succeeding in controlling her drug intake within 1 month, a more intensive inpatient treatment plan would be recommended (see Discussion).

PREVENTIVE PHARMACOTHERAPY. Both elements of the headache can benefit by the daily use of a tricyclic antidepressant such as amitriptyline (Elavil). The patient was started on 10 mg at night, and she was warned about sedation, dry mouth, and weight gain. If the drug is well tolerated the dose can be increased to 25 mg daily in 2 weeks. If not tolerated, an alternative tricyclic such as nortriptyline or desipramine can be introduced.

The beta blocker nadolol (Corgard) was prescribed 10 mg daily as a migraine preventive. In 1 week, after monitoring for hypotension and bradycardia, the dose can be gradually increased to 20 to 40 mg daily. The patient was warned that the full effect of the beta blocker in reducing the frequency and intensity of the migraine can take 2 months.

ACUTE ATTACKS. With the initiation of the preventive measures, a reduction in acute attacks of migraine and their severity should occur. Milder headaches should be treated with nonsteroidal analgesics after elimination of the narcotic analgesics has been achieved. Because the patient had found ibuprofen in the past not to have reduced her headaches, naproxen (Naprosyn, Anaprox) 550 mg was prescribed, to be used one to four times daily on an as-needed basis.

Residual acute attacks of migraine were to be treated by Imitrex injections, which had worked effectively in the past. As the migraine attacks lessened, replacement of sumatriptan with acetaminophen, dichloralphenazone, isometheptene mixture (Midrin) was planned, and this combination, in turn, was to be replaced by nonsteroidal analgesics. It was explained that the level of headache control likely to be achieved depends on identification and elimination of trigger factors, effectiveness of the preventive medication, and ongoing continuity of care, with appropriate adjustments in therapy being made when necessary. Headache education of the patient would play a major role in her achieving control of her headaches.

DISCUSSION

Differential Diagnosis

History is the cornerstone of headache diagnosis. Because of constraints in a busy practice, a new patient with a complicated headache history may require two visits initially, as was the case with this patient. Table 73–1 lists the information required of all new patients with headache.

Severe recurrent headaches negatively affect family and social functioning, which in turn may aggravate the headaches. Noise, dust and smells in the workplace, disturbed sleep patterns due to shift work, and prolonged exposure to work with com-

TABLE 73–1. Data Required of Headache Patients at First Visit*

- General health status
- Family history of headache
- Age when first headache occurred
- Characteristics and location of headache
- Frequency of headache
- Duration of headache
- Progressive worsening of headache
- Factors that trigger headache
- Symptoms that precede or accompany headache
- Aggravation of headache by exertion, light, or sound
- Severity of headache
- Psychosocial history

*Adapted from Differential diagnosis. In Davidoff RA. Migraine: Manifestations, Pathogenesis, and Management. Contemp Neurol 1995;42:108.

TABLE 73–2. Migraine and Tension-type Headaches

Feature	Migraine	Tension-type Headache
Pain	Moderate to severe, throbbing	Slight to moderate pressure
Effect of movement	Worsens	Unaffected
Location	Unilateral	Bilateral
Duration	4–72 hours	Minutes to days
Photophobia, phonophobia	Present	Occasionally present

puters are some of the many factors that should be kept in mind when headache history is taken. If both parents have migraine there is a 70 per cent chance that a child will inherit the condition. The risk is 45 per cent if one parent has migraine and 30 per cent if a near relative is involved (Davidoff, 1995). Migraine is commonly associated with menstruation, use of birth control pills, estrogen therapy, and endometriosis. Migraine in pregnancy is usually quiescent during the second and third trimesters and during breast feeding.

The same patient may present with either migraine or tension-type headache on different occasions, or one may present with tension-type headache leading to migraine. In the latter instance, an increase in the frequency of these headaches eventually may produce chronic daily headache, especially when narcotic analgesics are used, resulting in rebound headaches (Manzoni and colleagues, 1987) (Table 73–2).

Headache and the Temporomandibular Joint

Tension-type headache is frequently associated with temporomandibular joint (TMJ) pain, especially if there is also a bite problem present, as was the case with this patient. TMJ pain is associated with two different clinical conditions.

OROMANDIBULAR DYSFUNCTION. This condition consists of pain in the joint on chewing hard food or on prolonged talking, jerky jaw movements, lateral deviation of the mandible from the midline on opening the mouth, and teeth grinding during sleep (bruxism). Radiographs of the joint are normal. Patients are often anxious and depressed and complain of tension-type headaches associated with tenderness of the pericranial muscles. Treatment includes stress management and referral to an orthodontist. The patient under consideration fell into this category of TMJ dysfunction.

TEMPOROMANDIBULAR JOINT DISEASE. Symptoms are similar to those of oromandibular dysfunction but joint pathology is present, such as rheumatoid arthritis, osteoarthritis due to an old fracture, or derangement of the intra-articular disk. Intense joint pain and persistent headache may require surgical treatment and, if necessary, replacement with a joint prosthesis.

Whiplash Headache

Twenty five per cent of patients who sustain a whiplash headache caused by a rear-end collision develop chronic headache (Balla and Karnaghan, 1987). Those who already suffer from migraine report an increase in frequency of attacks (Winston, 1987). Whiplash headache is usually frontal and occipital and in most patients disappears in weeks or months. Less commonly, headaches may last years due to compression injury to the C1 and C2 nerve roots or shearing injuries to nerve pathways resulting in migraine-like headaches (Edwards and Soyka, 1993). Lack of objective findings and associated injury litigation may color the clinical picture. It does not follow that such headaches disappear after successful litigation, as was the case with this patient.

When the C2 nerve root is damaged, an area of paresthesia is found over the distribution of the greater occipital nerve. A CT-guided C2 nerve block is sometimes used as a diagnostic procedure, followed by surgical decompression. No area of paresthesia of the scalp was noted in the area of distribution of C2 in this patient, and thus surgical intervention was not considered.

Further Investigations

Imaging studies (Table 73–3) have become widely available. Many patients with chronic headache expect to have this type of expensive investigation performed on demand. Nonspecific abnormalities such as mild ventricular enlargement or, as in the case being presented, white matter foci suggesting multiple sclerosis or cerebral vasculitis can delay appropriate management and cause endless anxiety and additional cost. Scattered bilateral cerebral white matter foci are common findings on CT scans in patients with migraine in whom neurologic findings are absent.

TABLE 73–3. Indications for Imaging Studies in Headache Patients

- First headache in patient over 50 years
- Intense headache without a history of significant headache
- Marked change in headache pattern, including precipitous onset, unusual severity, or increased frequency
- Neck rigidity with positive Kernig or Brudzinski signs
- Diplopia, papilledema, or retinal hemorrhage
- Persistent or new neurologic deficits
- Headache with unexplained vomiting
- Head trauma
- Headache with history of malignancy or coagulopathy
- Excessive elevation of blood pressure
- Persistent headache precipitated by exertion
- Headache increasing as patient's general condition worsening under observation

Adapted from Headaches as emergencies. In Davidoff RA. Migraine: Manifestations, Pathogenesis, and Management. Contemp Neurol 1995;42:84.

Choice of Imaging Method

CT scanning is the method of choice for identifying bone abnormalities in the skull and early subarachnoid hemorrhage. It is more widely available than magnetic resonance imaging (MRI), is less costly, and is faster, which may be a significant factor when dealing with a clinically unstable condition. MRI provides greater detail, especially of abnormalities in the brain stem, cerebellum, and medulla. It is the method of choice for identifying subarachnoid hemorrhage 1 or 2 days after the bleeding episode has occurred.

Magnetic resonance angiography (MRA) is a noninvasive method for identifying aneurysms and arteriovenous malformations and other vascular abnormalities. The more accurate method of carotid angiography is required if surgery is contemplated.

Preventive Medication

Beta blockers (nadolol, propranolol) are the most widely used preventive medications for migraine control. Contraindications include asthma, congestive heart failure, and diabetes. Side effects are common, especially when first used.

Initial dosage should be low, and increases should be made gradually. Side effects are bradycardia and hypotension, weight gain, depression, insomnia, impotence, and decreased tolerance for physical exercise. Calcium channel blockers (verapamil, nifedipine, diltiazem) are used as alternatives to beta blockers but are usually less effective. Contraindications include heart block, sick sinus syndrome, atrial flutter, and atrial fibrillation. Side effects are hypotension, skin rash, hair loss, and diarrhea. Clearly, such medications are used only in disabling migraine occurring on two or more occasions per month.

Antidepressants are particularly useful in mixed headaches. In this patient amitriptyline was indicated because of her sleep problems. If a less sedating medication is indicated, desipramine or nortriptyline may be used. Fluoxetine (Prozac), a selective serotonin inhibitor, is particularly valuable in the treatment of patients with migraine and depression.

Anticonvulsants

Divalproex sodium (Depakote 250 mg, 1500 mg daily) has been shown to have a preventive effect in migraine. In the case presented, it will be used to replace the beta blocker if this drug is shown not to be effective after 2 months' treatment. Depakote is contraindicated if liver damage is present. An adequate therapeutic blood level is required which should be monitored during the early stages of treatment. Four to eight weeks' treatment may be required before any beneficial effect is noted. Side effects include gastrointestinal upset, sedation, tremor, and ataxia. In tapering barbiturate analgesics, where there is risk of seizure due to barbiturate withdrawal, treatment with Depakote is valuable because of its antiseizure action.

Relaxation Therapy and Biofeedback

Relaxation therapy and biofeedback are widely used in the treatment of migraine, tension-type headache, and mixed headache. Success is reported as more likely in female patients, where there is strong motivation to practice at home and where success has been demonstrated during the training sessions (Farmer, 1995). Thermal biofeedback, a learned technique of autogenic hand-warming induced by relaxation and imagery, is commonly used. Benefits from such methods are unpredictable and insurance coverage may not always be available, as was the case with this patient.

Inpatient Treatment for Chronic Daily Headache

Persistent chronic daily headache that does not respond to outpatient therapy should be considered

for more intensive inpatient treatment. This consists of intravenous dihydroergotamine (DHE 45) 0.5 mg to 1.0 mg every 8 hours preceded by intravenous metoclopramide (Reglan) 10 mg to control nausea. Treatment is continued for 2 to 3 days (Raskin, 1986). Breakthrough headache, if it occurs, is best treated with a non-narcotic analgesic such as ketorolac (Toradol) 30 to 60 mg IM. Metoclopramide is discontinued after 24 hours to avoid the risk of tardive dyskinesia. When the headache ceases, the DHE is tapered over 24 hours. The patient is then discharged, and ongoing care is continued on an outpatient basis. Hospitalization is needed to monitor DHE side effects, such as chest pain, nausea and vomiting, and other withdrawal symptoms.

Headache Specialists and Headache Clinics

Chronic daily headache is a major reason for referral to a headache specialist (Smith, 1995). Other indications for referral include:

- Inadequate level of physician comfort in treating headache patients or patient request for a referral
- Uncertainty in diagnosis or fear of possible underlying pathology
- Failure to respond to treatment

Headache specialization is a relatively new field. Headache clinics and centers now provide multidisciplinary treatment programs for patients with intractable headaches who have so far been nonresponsive to treatment. A list of such programs is available from the American Association for the Study of Headache (AASH), 875 Kings Highway, Suite 200, Woodbury NJ 08096.

CONCLUSION

Headache is a special area of responsibility for family physicians because they are the practitioners most often consulted for this problem. They are well suited to treat headache because of its chronic nature.

Six months following the initial consultation, this patient's headaches were greatly reduced in frequency and intensity. She was still maintaining her records because she claimed it gave her a sense of control over her headaches. She was sleeping better and was no longer taking amitriptyline. She continued to take nadolol 40 mg daily and used Imitrex injections about twice monthly. She attributed her improvement to her increased knowledge about headache as a result of reading and attending the local headache support group. She was now able to control her milder headaches without the use of narcotic analgesics. She no longer had guilt feelings about her headaches, and she was now back at work.

SUGGESTED READING

Balla J, Karnaghan J. Whiplash headache. Clin Exp Neurol 1987;23:179–182.

Broderick J, Smith R, Cahill W, et al. Neurology in Family Practice. In Rakel RE (ed). Textbook of Family Practice, 5th ed. Philadelphia, W. B. Saunders, 1995, pp 1380–1437.

Davidoff RA. Migraine: Manifestations, pathogenesis, and management. Contemp Neurol 1995:42.

Edwards J, Soyka D. Headache association with disorders of the skull and cervical spine. In Olesen J, Tfelt-Hensen P, Welch KMA (eds). The Headaches. New York, Raven Press, 1993, pp 741–743.

Farmer K. Biofeedback and the treatment of headache. In Cady RK, Fox AW (eds). Treating the Headache Patient. New York, Marcel Dekker, 1995, pp 287–303.

Manzoni GC, Micieli G, Granella F, et al. Daily chronic headache: Classification and clinical features. Observation of 250 patients. Cephalalgia 1987;7[Suppl 6]:169–170.

Mathew NT, Kurman R, Perez F. Drug induced refractory headache: Clinical features and management. Headache 1990;30:634.

Raskin NH. Repetitive intravenous dihydroergotamine as therapy for intractable migraine. Neurology 1986;36:995–997.

Robbins LD. Management of Headache and Headache Medications. New York, Springer Verlag, 1944.

Smith R. Headache specialists and headache clinics. In Cady RK, Fox AW (eds). Treating the Headache Patient. New York, Marcel Dekker, 1995, pp 305–315.

Smith R. Headache. Monograph 203. Home study, self-assessment program. Kansas City, MO, American Academy of Family Physicians, April, 1996.

Winston KR. Whiplash and its relationship to migraine. Headache 1987;27(8):452–457.

QUESTIONS

1. At the time of a whiplash injury a patient had no immediate pain or loss of consciousness. The next day she had headache and neck pain. There were no neurologic abnormalities. Recommended initial management is
   a. Nonsteroidal anti-inflammatory drugs
   b. Radiograph of neck
   c. CT scan of the neck
   d. Physical therapy

2. Migraine aura without headache is most likely to occur in
   a. A 6-year-old child
   b. A woman in the second trimester of pregnancy
   c. A 42-year-old man
   d. An 81-year-old woman with a history of migraine

3. A 45-year-old woman recently developed sudden one-sided frequent severe stabbing head pains of short duration. Response to which of the following is diagnostic as well as therapeutic?
   a. Ergotamine tartrate
   b. Nadolol
   c. Indomethacin
   d. Butorphanol nasal spray

Answers appear on **page 607.**

Chapter 74

Tremors

Eduardo C. Gonzalez, M.D.

INITIAL VISIT

Subjective

PRESENT ILLNESS. John is a 62-year-old male with a history of benign prostatic hypertrophy (BPH) with an elevated prostate specific antigen (PSA) for which he is being followed by his urologist. He has had recent biopsies of the prostate, all read as benign. He is being treated with doxazosin (Cardura), which has improved his symptoms significantly. He believes that his BPH is doing well and he presents today for a complete physical examination (CPE). He has not had a CPE in some time and is concerned about a slight hand tremor that has recently been affecting his tennis game.

John has remained very active throughout his life. He is currently working full time, playing tennis twice a week, and working out with gym equipment. Over the past year he has noted a slight tremor in his left hand and leg. The tremor initially began in his left leg and then moved to his left hand. It appears worse when sitting and remains constant unless he gets up and does something. John has noted that anxiety also appears to worsen the symptoms. He has noted some muscle soreness and stiffness in his legs, which he has attributed to "getting older." He denies any previous history of similar symptoms. He has not had any weakness, tingling, headaches, dizziness, or visual changes. Other than the doxazosin, he has not been on any other medications. He does admit to having four to five glasses of red wine per week but denies any history of alcohol abuse. The wine does not make his tremor any better. He has no knowledge of being exposed to any toxic substances. There is no family history of neurologic problems or tremors. He has not noted any weight change, and his appetite remains good. John is concerned that the tremor is slowly worsening and wants to know if there is anything he can do to prevent further worsening.

PAST MEDICAL HISTORY (PMH). As mentioned previously, John's PMH is significant only for a history of BPH. He denies a history of coronary artery disease, diabetes mellitus, tuberculosis, hepatitis, hypertension, or thyroid disease. He has no drug allergies.

FAMILY HISTORY. John's family history is noncontributory. His mother died at the age of 86 years of natural causes and his father is still alive and well at 91 years. He has one brother who is alive and healthy. The family has no history of heart disease or cancer. No family history of neurodegenerative illnesses or tremors exists. He has a daughter who is 36 years of age and in good health.

HEALTH HABITS. John denies any history of smoking and drinks wine only with dinner. He has four to five glasses of red wine per week with dinner. He exercises regularly and is a good tennis player.

SOCIAL HISTORY. John has been married for 42 years. He has worked in radio broadcasting for some time. Over the past 2 to 3 years he has been doing less in anticipation of retirement.

REVIEW OF SYSTEMS. Other than the complaints already mentioned, John is doing well. He denies recurrent headaches, visual disturbances, or changes in speech or swallowing. He has no complaints of lung, cardiac, or gastrointestinal disease. His bowel movements are regular with no history of melena or hematochezia.

Objective

Physical Examination

John's height is 67 in; weight is 157 lb; pulse is 51; and blood pressure is 141/77. HEENT examination shows male pattern alopecia. Eyes have full range of motion in all quadrants with no gaze abnormality. Nose and ears are clear. Hearing is intact bilaterally. Mouth has good dentition. Neck examination shows the thyroid normal, no bruits, no thyromegaly. Lungs are clear to auscultation. Heart examination shows sinus bradycardia without murmur. Abdomen is soft, nontender, nondistended, no hernias, no organomegaly. Genital/rectal examination reveals normal external male genitalia, uncircumcised. Testicles are descended bilaterally, no masses, no hernias. Rectal tone is normal, 60-g prostate, smooth, symmetrical without nodules; Hemoccult tests negative. Extremities show muscle tone normal; full range of motion in all extremities; no cyanosis, edema, clubbing, or joint deformities; peripheral pulses 2+ and equal bilaterally. Skin reveals no rash nor pigment changes. Neurologic examination reveals he is oriented to person, place, and time. Affect is appropriate. Cranial nerves II to XII are grossly intact. There is no focal motor or sensory deficit. At rest there is a noticeable tremor in his left hand and leg. The hand tremor is fine with a pill-rolling appearance. The tremor disappears with movement and picking up a magazine. The hand tremor is of slow frequency and is best noted when John is resting his hands in his lap. There is no rigidity in the larger joints, but noticeable cogwheeling in his left wrist. John shows no difficulty in arising from the examining room chair when asked to sit on the examining table. His gait is appropriate, but he shows decreased arm swing with his left arm. Rapid alternating movements reveal slight bradykinesia on his left side as compared with his right. Romberg test result is negative. Reflexes are 2+ in upper and lower extremities bilaterally, with no Babinski sign nor clonus. The tremor disappears when he is asked to touch the physician's fingers.

Laboratory Tests

Office laboratory analyses ordered with the first visit included a normal complete blood cell count (CBC), chemistry profile, and thyroid stimulating hormone level.

Assessment

Working Diagnoses

1. Tremor. The differential diagnosis includes various causes of tremor. Because the patient's tremor is resting, unilateral, progressive, and associated with some rigidity, the diagnosis of *idiopathic Parkinson disease* is more likely.

2. BPH. Controlled with current medication. Followed by a urologist

Plan

Diagnostic

1. Rediscuss key symptoms and signs in John's history and examination to help rule in or rule out a diagnosis of Parkinson disease versus benign tremor.

2. Serum chemistry laboratory work to include liver function tests to evaluate for Wilson disease and creatine phosphokinase levels to evaluate for muscle disease. A serum copper level to evaluate for Wilson disease should not be necessary because John's symptoms and signs developed in his sixth decade.

3. Magnetic resonance imaging (MRI) of the brain to evaluate for other neurodegenerative processes, although MRI is not of benefit for making the diagnosis of Parkinson disease

4. Cerebrospinal spinal fluid (CSF) analysis to evaluate for other neurologic disorders manifesting with parkinsonism (optional)

Therapeutic

A full explanation of the diagnosis and treatment of Parkinson disease is given to John and his wife. John is begun on selegiline (Eldepryl) at 5 mg twice a day by mouth. He is told to take it with breakfast and lunch, to limit its amphetamine-like stimulation that can interfere with sleep, and always to take it with food to limit nausea.

Patient Education

1. John is asked to maintain a symptom diary and to bring it with him to all future visits.

2. John is encouraged to maintain a program of exercise and social activity to keep physically and mentally healthy, yet to balance these activities with the necessary rest and precautions required of patients with this disease.

Disposition

John is asked to complete the diagnostic testing, initiate the medication previously discussed, and return in 4 weeks.

FIRST FOLLOW-UP VISIT

Subjective

John has noted no difficulty with the medicine. Initially there was some nausea, but this has resolved. His tremor is no worse and at times appears better. He continues playing tennis twice a week and remains active at work.

Objective

PHYSICAL EXAMINATION. No change from the previous physical findings. John's resting tremor is still present, but it is less visible. The elbow and wrist joint rigidity are still present and slightly decreased.

LABORATORY TESTS. Results of the serum chemistry studies, including liver function tests, and creatine phosphokinase levels, were all normal. The MRI of the brain shows mild cerebral atrophy, not unusual for his age; otherwise normal. CSF studies were not obtained.

Assessments

1. Idiopathic Parkinson disease, in early stages. Patient's daily activities not yet affected by symptoms. Tolerating selegiline (Eldepryl) well. John's history, essentially normal laboratory results, and MRI help support this diagnosis.

2. BPH symptoms are stable.

Plan

The selegiline (Eldepryl) is now at the maximum recommended dose. Because John's symptoms are not affecting his activities of daily living (ADLs), no further medication is prescribed. He is encouraged to continue with his work and routine exercises and to report any worsening of symptoms.

PATIENT EDUCATION. John and his wife are given the phone number and address of the local Parkinson disease support group to contact for further education and social support.

DISPOSITION. John is scheduled to return for office follow-up in 1 month (sooner if there is any deterioration in his condition).

DIFFERENTIAL DIAGNOSIS OF TREMOR

The purpose of this case study is to discuss the differentiation of tremors and, in particular, Parkinson disease (PD). No laboratory or imaging tests at this time can be used to make a diagnosis of PD. Instead, these tests help rule out other neurodegenerative disorders. The diagnosis of Parkinson disease is purely clinical and is largely based on the symptoms of tremor and other factors. The type, onset, duration, frequency, progression, ameliorating, and aggravating factors are all important in helping to distinguish between a parkinsonian tremor and other tremors. To aid in the diagnosis of a patient with a tremor, the tremor must first be classified. Classifications can be either based on a description or on the pathophysiology. Classification of tremor by description includes:

1. Resting tremor. This type occurs only at rest. It may worsen when the patient is engaged in mental tasks or moving an unaffected body part. It disappears quickly with muscle contraction, and thus the patient's performance is rarely affected. Clinically, this type of tremor is associated with idiopathic Parkinson disease and secondary parkinsonism. Secondary parkinsonism is constituted of those conditions that mimic PD clinically but are caused by known agents. These include:
   a. Postinfectious. This is seen primarily during the convalescent phase of viral encephalitis.
   b. Toxin-induced. This includes exposure to carbon monoxide, carbon disulfide, manganese, cyanide, methanol, and the synthetic heroin analogue (1-methyl-4-phenyl-1,2,3,6-tetrahydropyridine) (MPTP).
   c. Hereditary diseases, especially Wilson disease, involving a defect in copper metabolism that first appears in the second or third decade and is treatable with chelating agents and diet.
   d. Drug-induced. Those drugs that block dopamine receptors, especially the neuroleptic agents, as well as metoclopramide (Reglan) and reserpine.

2. Postural tremors. These are tremors that are provoked by isometric contraction of the affected

body segment. They can be seen involving almost all body parts (i.e., head, neck, trunk, upper extremities, and lower extremities). They are the most common type of tremors and include both physiologic and pathologic tremors.

a. Physiologic tremors (normal or enhanced). These are normal tremors that occur in most individuals. The tremor is continuous but with an irregular rate. It is usually not visible. The enhanced physiologic tremor is a more pronounced type. It is provoked by fatigue, anxiety, hypoglycemia, caffeine, dopaminergic agonists, beta-adrenergic agonists, valproic acid (Depakene), lithium, and tricyclic antidepressants.

b. Essential tremor. This is the most prevalent pathologic postural tremor. Onset is commonly in the second to sixth decades. There is a family history in over 50 per cent of patients with this disorder, whereas family history is uncommon with PD. It primarily affects the hands, followed by the head, voice, tongue, lower extremities, and trunk. In severe instances, it can appear as a resting tremor. Its progression is slow, and usually no significant change is noted for years. Usually patients have noted that alcohol appears to ameliorate the tremor. Beta blockers and primidone are also effective in treatment.

c. Tremor with basal ganglia disease. Postural tremor is also visible in conditions affecting the basal ganglia. Therefore, conditions such as Parkinson disease, Wilson disease, and dystonia are associated disorders in which this type of tremor is seen.

d. Cerebellar tremor. Along with a postural tremor, conditions causing a cerebellar tremor also have symptoms of dysmetria and kinetic tremor. The most common cause of cerebellar postural tremor is multiple sclerosis, but brain stem tumors, strokes, and paraneoplastic cerebellar degeneration can also be responsible.

e. Tremor with peripheral neuropathy. These are postural tremors that occur concomitantly with a peripheral neuropathy, either acquired or hereditary. Motor conduction velocities are slow in these patients, and beta blockers have little benefit.

f. Post-traumatic tremor

g. Alcoholic tremor

3. Kinetic tremor. These tremors are action (kinetic) and goal-oriented (intention). They are usually the most incapacitating, and their appearance may indicate disorders of the cerebellum and related pathways. The tremors usually involve proximal muscles. They can be evoked through goal-oriented movements such as finger-to-nose or heel-to-shin testing. As the patient's finger or heel approaches the target, the tremor increases. Other signs can include disruptions in gait, coordination, ocular movements, proprioception, and slurred speech. Kinetic and intention tremors can develop in patients with heavy metal poisoning (lead, mercury, bismuth, thallium), carbon tetrachloride exposure, and metal chelator intoxication.

4. Task-specific tremors. These tremors encompass both primary writing tremor and vocal tremor. These tremors have only recently been recognized. They appear with only specific tasks. Primary writing tremor appears only with handwriting or a few other skilled manual tasks, and in general is not produced by posture or goal-directed movement. Vocal tremors are apparent only when speaking. Both these types of tremors are similar to essential tremor, but differ in that they are not always responsive to beta blockers, and there is no family history.

The type of tremor thus aids in the diagnosis. In John's case, the resting, unilateral tremor in a 62-year-old patient with evidence of rigidity and no other evidence of neurologic disease is most indicative of PD.

DISCUSSION

Parkinson disease is the second most common neurodegenerative disorder (Alzheimer-type dementia is more common), affecting more than 500,000 Americans. Parkinson disease usually manifests itself clinically in patients aged 55 to 70 years, after 75 per cent of the dopaminergic neurons in the substantia nigra are destroyed by mechanisms not fully understood at this time. It is a difficult disease to diagnose because many of its signs and symptoms are characteristic of several other disease entities. The classic symptoms and signs of PD include a resting tremor (most commonly of the hands but not limited to or necessary for the diagnosis); rigidity, especially of the upper extremities, which is called "cogwheel rigidity" if there are superimposed tremors; bradykinesia or akinesia (reduced or absent muscle movement); and postural reflex impairment causing patients to be unstable and to fall. Very importantly, the diagnosis of PD does not require all four of these symptoms and signs to be present. In fact, early PD is often without balance problems. The diagnosis, however, is a clinical one, because there are no specific reliable laboratory or radiologic studies that confirm the diagnosis of PD. Laboratory and radiologic studies are performed, however, to help rule out other disease entities that can cause similar symptoms and signs. Other more subtle signs and symptoms of PD include drooling due to impairment of swallowing and increased salivation; hypophonia (a soft, monotonous voice due to the loss of the ability to vary speech intensity); micrographia (very small handwriting, probably a component of bradykinesia); depression (either endogenous or reactive); and autonomic nervous system dysfunction with orthostatic hypotension.

The treatment of PD includes not only medications but also patient and family education, as well as physical therapy to help keep the patient mobile. There are various national PD organizations available to assist patients and their families in dealing with the social and physical implications of this illness.

The treatment of PD has become much more controversial over the past 10 years. Although the initiation of physical and occupational therapy, good nutrition, and education of patient and family is not argued, when medicine should be initiated is. The disagreement revolves around two basic concerns: (1) whether selegiline (Eldepryl) acts as a neuroprotector; and (2) whether the delay of levodopa therapy reduces the occurrence of late treatment complications such as wearing off of the drug's effectiveness or motor fluctuations. In any event, the goal of treatment should be to extend and improve the quality of life and maintain function.

For the patient with newly diagnosed PD whose symptoms have not affected his or her ADLs, treatment with selegiline is now preferred. Before selegiline, medications were not begun if ADLs were not affected. This approach was taken to avoid the side effects and expense of PD medication. With the introduction of selegiline, this approach changed. Studies have shown that selegiline appears to slow down the progression of PD as well as providing a useful symptomatic therapy adjunct to levodopa.

Selegiline is a monoamine oxidase B inhibitor that limits the breakdown of dopamine, which results in a higher level of dopamine at the receptors to control symptoms. Selegiline also slows the oxidative metabolism of dopamine. This effect is believed to limit the formation of free radicals, which can further damage substantia nigra cells (i.e., neuro-

protective effect). Although the Federal Drug Administration (FDA) approval for selegiline is for combination use only with carbidopa/levodopa (Sinemet), most movement disorder experts are prescribing it alone in early PD for neuroprotection before the need for symptom control with carbidopa/levodopa therapy. Recommended dosing of selegiline is 5 mg twice a day by mouth. It should be given with food to limit nausea. It is recommended that it be taken with breakfast and lunch, to limit its amphetamine-like stimulation that can interfere with sleep. A reduced dosage of simultaneous carbidopa/levodopa therapy by 10 to 30 per cent is often recommended, because inhibition of dopamine metabolism occurs, potentially inducing clinical manifestations of dopamine toxicity. The concern with monamine oxidase type A inhibitors inducing hypertensive crises with the ingestion of dietary tyramine is not similar to the concern with the recommended treatment doses of selegiline for PD. Selegiline's side effects include nausea, dyskinesia, hallucinations, and confusion when used with carbidopa/levodopa. Very few side effects with selegiline are noted when used alone; however, fatal reactions have been reported when monoamine oxidase inhibitors type A or B and meperidine (Demerol) are used simultaneously.

Concern over the concomitant use of selegiline and levodopa has arisen from the United Kingdom Parkinson's Disease Research Group. One study by this group revealed that concomitant use of selegiline and levodopa conferred no clinical benefit over levodopa alone in the treatment of early PD. The study also showed a higher mortality rate in those patients on the combination therapy. Further research is required to support this finding.

Levodopa therapy continues to be the most effective symptomatic drug therapy for PD. More recent information suggests that utilization of levodopa early in the course of PD does not risk more rapid progression of symptoms, and it has a beneficial effect on life expectancy.

Although dopamine deficiency is the primary abnormality in PD, dopamine itself cannot be given to patients because it is not able to cross the blood-brain barrier. Levodopa, however, is converted in the brain to dopamine, although it also can be converted to dopamine outside the blood-brain barrier. If significant conversion of levodopa to dopamine occurs outside the blood-barrier, side effects, especially nausea, can be a significant problem. Carbidopa was therefore combined with levodopa, because it is able to effectively block much of the conversion of levodopa to dopamine outside the brain. A minimum of 75 mg carbidopa per day is usually necessary to block the peripheral conversion of levodopa.

Currently there are two formulations of carbidopa/levodopa. The older version carbidopa/levodopa (Sinemet) is a fast-release agent. The newer version, controlled-release carbidopa/levodopa (Sinemet-CR) provides a slower sustained release of medication. PD patients taking the older, faster release preparations are often frustrated with the short duration of action causing motor fluctuations, such as "wearing off" and "on-off" effects. The addition of controlled-release carbidopa/levodopa (Sinemet-CR) provides more stable plasma levodopa levels, helping to limit dyskinetic motor fluctuations in patients with more advanced PD. Dosing intervals can often be lengthened, although not dramatically, when PD treatment is initiated on this formulation. A drawback encountered with this formulation is that achieving levodopa peak plasma levels is likewise lengthened. Use of the older, faster-acting preparations early in the morning followed by use of the newer, controlled-release formulation has been employed as an answer to this therapeutic concern. Another benefit of the controlled-release formulation is its use at bedtime, which appears to improve sleep patterns in the majority of PD patients. This sustained-release preparation is usually initiated as a dose of carbidopa/levodopa 50/200 mg. Often, it is initially prescribed twice a day, but it has been utilized as often as five to six times a day.

Early in PD, carbidopa/levodopa can be initiated with either the 25/100 mg or 50/200 mg sustained-release formulation orally twice a day early in the morning and early to mid-afternoon. To limit nausea, it is best to give carbidopa/levodopa with food. It is best to maintain a relatively low dose of 200 to 400 mg of levodopa until progressive disabling symptoms require an increase in dosage or dosing frequency. Upon reaching a daily dose of 600 mg of levodopa, the addition of a dopamine agonist is usually favored over further increases in levodopa. If there is a delayed onset of effect or lack of sufficient peak effect, fast-release carbidopa/levodopa may be added to the regimen. Excessive levodopa most often manifests itself as dyskinesia (involuntary nonperiodic hyperkinetic movements) and confusion.

Limiting the protein in both the breakfast and noontime meals and maximizing protein in the evening meal and taking carbidopa/levodopa on an empty stomach after the first couple of weeks of levodopa therapy are adjuncts to maximize levodopa absorption in the gastrointestinal tract. Nausea can also be limited by starting with low doses of carbidopa/levodopa combinations and building up to therapeutic doses gently.

In the majority of PD patients on long-term levodopa therapy, the response to therapy eventually deteriorates. After 5 years of carbidopa/levodopa therapy, approximately 50 per cent of patients develop unstable, fluctuating response patterns to levodopa. The two most common types of levodopa response deterioration that are noted are the wearing-off effect and dyskinesia. The wearing-off effect (often called end-of-dose failure) is characterized by the symptomatic benefits of each carbidopa/levodopa dose becoming more short-lived than in the past, lasting only a few hours or less. This type of response is believed to be the result of progressive loss of dopaminergic nigrostriatal neurons. As the disease progresses, the remaining nigrostriatal neurons are slowly depleted, limiting the brain's capacity to metabolize and store dopamine, causing a shorter response to levodopa therapy. The initial therapeutic adjustment often beneficial in limiting the wearing-off effect is to increase the frequency of doses, sometimes as often as every 2 to 3 hours.

The other common type of levodopa response deterioration is dyskinesia. Dyskinesia is involuntary, nonperiodic hyperkinetic movements. Several varied forms of dyskinesia can be noted as complications of levodopa therapy and include peak-dose, end-of-dose, and biphasic pattern dyskinesias. Peak-dose dyskinesia occurs at the peak plasma drug levels or time of maximal levodopa effect. Hyperkinetic movements about 1 hour after the first daily morning levodopa dose are usually manifestations of peak-dose dyskinesia. This type of dyskinesia can be limited by reducing the levodopa dose. End-of-dose dyskinesia occurs when the levodopa effect wears off. Hyperkinetic movements, especially dystonia, before the first daily morning levodopa dose are usually manifestations of end-of-dose dyskinesia. This type of dyskinesia is best approached by shortening the interval between each dose. Biphasic pattern dyskinesia occurs as levodopa plasma levels increase and decline. This pattern is the least common form of dyskinesia and is more commonly associated with chorea-type dyskinesia. Biphasic pattern dyskinesias are often difficult to treat, but they may improve by shortening the dosing intervals. In addition to the levodopa dosage and interval adjustments discussed earlier, the addition of a dopaminergic agonist may help stabilize the response to levodopa therapy in patients with dyskinesia.

Anticholinergic drugs have been widely used for the symptomatic treatment of PD. Their benefit is based on the balance that exists between acetylcholine and dopamine in the brain. PD patients with a depletion of dopamine have a relative excess of acetylcholine. The anticholinergic medications help limit this relative excessive influence of acetylcholine. These agents are most helpful as early monotherapy in patients younger than 60 years of age with tremor-predominant PD. Their effect is minimal, with bradykinesia, gait problems, or postural reflex impairment. The most commonly used anticholinergic agents are benztropine (Cogentin), trihexyphenidyl (Artane), ethopropazine (Parsidol), and procyclidine (Kemadrin). Their usefulness is limited by their common and significant side effect profiles, especially in the elderly and in patients with more advanced disease. The side effects consist of dry mouth, constipation, urinary retention, blurred vision, hallucinations, and confusion. Anticholinergic treatment should be initiated at low doses and increased very slowly to limit these side effects.

Amantadine (Symmetrel), which was used for years as drug prophylaxis against influenza A, has some therapeutic benefits for patients with early PD. Amantadine's therapeutic benefits seem to be derived from its ability to increase dopamine release, block dopamine reuptake, and stimulate dopamine receptors and possible peripheral anticholinergic properties. Its use appears most effective in reducing rigidity and bradykinesia. The normal starting dose is 100 mg two to three times a day, but it must be adjusted to lower doses if renal function is impaired. The dose can be increased as needed up to 300 mg per day. Side effects seen with other PD medications, including dystonia, nausea, confusion, are also seen with amantadine.

Dopamine agonists are ergotamine compounds that are most useful when given in combination with carbidopa/levodopa when levodopa requirements exceed 600 mg per day, but they may also be administered alone. The two products currently available are bromocriptine (Parlodel), which stimulates dopamine (D-2) receptor sites, and pergolide (Permax), which stimulates dopamine (D-1 and D-2) receptor sites. Bromocriptine therapy is begun with a dose of 1.25 mg/day for 1 week and then the dose is increased by 1.25 mg every week until symptoms are controlled or side effects occur. Bromocriptine can be given to a total effective dose of 15 to 30 milligrams per day, although doses up to 60 mg per day have been utilized to limit severe response fluctuations. The daily dose is usually administered three times a day, but it may be given more frequently in smaller doses. Pergolide mesylate is longer acting and more potent. Therapy is begun with a single 0.05-mg dose daily and increased very slowly during the next several weeks up to a total dosage of 3 mg daily, which is usually administered on a three-times-a-day regimen or more frequently. Side effects of these dopamine agents include gastrointestinal distress, dyskinesia, and orthostatic hypotension.

Surgical procedures for the treatment of difficult to manage PD has been an area of renewed interest. Surgical procedures have ranged from cortical resection, to creating lesions of areas in the internal capsule, to thalamotomy and ventral pallidotomy, to thalamic stimulation, to fetal tissue transplantation. Although some of the procedures such as pallidotomy and thalamotomy have seemed to improve bradykinesia, rigidity, and tremor, fetal tissue transplantation still remains unstandardized and fraught with legal and ethical debates.

SUGGESTED READING

Ahskog JE, Wilkinson JM. New concepts in the treatment of Parkinson's disease. Am Fam Physician 1990;41(2):574–584.

Consensus Conference. An algorithm for the management of Parkinson's disease. Neurology 1994;44[Suppl 10]:S9–S52.

Hallett M. Classification and treatment of tremor. JAMA 1991;266(8):1115–1117.

Hopfensperger K, Koller WC. Recognizing early Parkinson's disease. Postgrad Med 1991;90(1):49–59.

Sandroni P, Young RR. Tremor: Classification, diagnosis and management. Am Fam Physician 1994;50(7):1505–1512.

Stacy M, Brownlee HJ. Treatment options for early Parkinson's disease. Am Fam Physician 1996;53(4):1281–1287.

Sweeney, Patrick J. Considerations in the diagnosis and management of Parkinson's disease. Fam Pract Recertification 1996;18(4):27–45.

1. Which one of the following is a common characteristic of tremor of Parkinson disease?
   a. A family history of tremor
   b. A head tremor
   c. Alcohol reduces the tremor
   d. A resting tremor

2. The four classic symptoms and signs of Parkinson's disease include all the following *except*
   a. Dystonias
   b. Tremor
   c. Rigidity
   d. Bradykinesia
   e. Postural reflex impairment

3. Essential tremor can be characterized by all of the following *except*
   a. Improves with alcohol
   b. A family history is usually present 50 per cent of the time
   c. Although more commonly postural, it can also appear at rest
   d. It is usually isolated only to the voice and head
   e. Its progression is slow and usually is not noticed

4. Amantadine's therapeutic benefits seem to be derived from its ability to
   a. Increase dopamine release
   b. Block dopamine reuptake
   c. Stimulate dopamine receptors
   d. All of the above

Answers appear on **page 607.**

Chapter **75**

Child with Fever and Lethargy

Dawn Schissel, M.D.

INITIAL VISIT

Subjective

John is a 20-month-old white male who has been a patient in the clinic intermittently since birth.

PRESENTING PROBLEM. John had been in good health until 3 days ago when he developed a fever. Mother has also noticed increasing lethargy.

PRESENT ILLNESS. Three days before his appearance in the clinic, John developed a fever to 102°F that was controlled initially fairly well with oral acetaminophen. Mother now reports that John is becoming increasingly lethargic. He has had a decreased appetite and over the past 12 hours has had poor fluid intake. She has also noted increasing irritability and inconsolability over the past 24 hours. John has had normal bowel movements, but the mother does report fewer wet diapers.

PAST MEDICAL HISTORY. John is the product of an uncomplicated term pregnancy. He has had three episodes of otitis media since birth and has needed no surgical intervention for these. He has no known

545

drug allergies and takes no long-term medications. He uses over-the-counter acetaminophen as needed for fever.

FAMILY HISTORY. John's maternal grandmother has hypertension. Both of John's parents are alive and well. No other chronic illnesses run in the family.

SOCIAL HISTORY. John is an only child and lives with his parents. He is exposed to secondhand smoke in his home, since both parents smoke. They have no pets. John attends a day care center daily with eight other children. Several of the other children in the day care center have upper respiratory infections.

REVIEW OF SYSTEMS. John had a viral upper respiratory infection with nasal congestion 1 week ago. He has not had a cough. He has not had any changes in bowel habits and has had decreased urinary output. He has had lethargy and irritability as described earlier. Immunizations include diphtheria, pertussis, and tetanus (DPT) and *Haemophilus influenzae* type B (Hib) at 2, 4, and 6 months; oral polio vaccine at 2 and 4 months. He has received no further immunizations, and hepatitis B series has not been given.

Objective

Physical Examination

John is a well-nourished white male who is lying very still in his mother's arms. He moans intermittently with movement. Temperature (rectal) is 103°F, pulse 120, respirations 40. Skin is warm and moist without rash. There is decreased skin turgor. HEENT:PERRL shows no papilledema, no tears; tympanic membranes bilaterally are erythematous with decreased motion. Nose is congested. There is mattering noted in the eyelashes bilaterally. Throat is clear with slightly dry mucous membranes. Neck is tender with anterior and posterior cervical adenopathy. There is pain with flexion of the neck, and a positive Kernig sign is present. Chest reveals tachypnea without rales, rhonchi, or wheezes. Cardiovascular examination shows tachycardia without murmur, gallop, or rub. Abdomen is soft with mild diffuse tenderness; no masses. Normal bowel sounds are present. There is no guarding or rebound tenderness. Genitourinary examination reveals a circumcised male with bilateral descended testes. Extremities have no deformity; a positive Brudzinski sign is present. On neurologic examination, John is lethargic, but arousable. He does not resist examina-

tion; he has a weak cry. Cranial nerves are grossly intact. He moves all extremities equally; sensory is intact to touch throughout.

Diagnostics

Chest radiograph shows no infiltrate. CBC results are white blood cell (WBC) count 25,000 with a predominance of neutrophils and 10 bands, hemoglobin level 11.5, platelets 450,000. Electrolyte levels are within normal limits. Urinalysis is within normal limits. Blood cultures are pending. A lumbar puncture was done: opening pressure is 120 mm H_2O (normal to 85), 2000 WBC/mm³ with 90 per cent polymorphonuclear cells (PMNs), glucose level 30 mg/dl (low), and protein level 80 mg/dl (high).

Working Diagnosis

1. Bacterial meningitis—a febrile illness with meningismus and abnormal cerebral spinal fluid findings strongly indicates a central nervous system source of infection that is likely bacterial.

2. Otitis media—fever and erythematous tympanic membranes are diagnostic. Mattering eyes suggest that the etiology is *H. influenzae*.

3. Immunization deficiency—child has not had measles, mumps, rubella (MMR) or fourth DPT/Hib and oral polio vaccine (OPV), or hepatitis B vaccine (HBV), all due at 15 to 18 months.

Differential Diagnosis

1. Viral meningitis—although physical signs make this a possibility, the cerebral spinal fluid (CSF) WBC count of 2000 with predominantly PMNs suggests a bacterial source and makes viral etiology less likely.

2. Viral syndrome with dehydration—this child's original upper respiratory infection may have been viral, but increased WBC count with a left shift suggests bacterial etiology.

3. Pneumonia—although the child is febrile and tachypneic, the lung sounds are clear and the chest radiograph is normal, making this an unlikely diagnosis.

4. Sepsis—a child with fever and lethargy may be septic from many sources—lungs, gastrointestinal tract, or meningitis. A high WBC count with fever, chills, and lethargy are a part of the sepsis syn-

drome. Blood cultures confirming bacteremia would prove the diagnosis.

Plan

John was admitted to the hospital emergently with the diagnosis of meningitis. Latex agglutination studies done on the CSF were positive for *H. influenzae*, negative for *Streptococcus pneumoniae* and *Neisseria meningitidis*. Before the administration of antibiotics, John received dexamethasone at 0.6 mg per kg per day in four divided doses to decrease the inflammatory response. John received ampicillin 50 mg per kg every 6 hours IV and ceftriaxone 50 mg per kg every 12 hours IV. Fluids were replaced at a maintenance rate. The antibiotics were continued for a total of 10 days and the steroids for 2 days. John showed a marked improvement throughout the hospital course. The electrolyte levels were monitored closely because there is an increased incidence of syndrome of inappropriate antidiuretic hormone (SIADH) in cases of *H. influenzae* meningitis. John was discharged home fully recovered without oral antibiotics.

FOLLOW-UP

John will need his hearing tested approximately 1 month after discharge when the clinical picture has completely become normal. Subsequent well child visits will entail thorough assessment of John's behavioral and motor development.

DISCUSSION

Bacterial meningitis is a life-threatening pediatric infection with long-term sequelae occurring in 30 per cent of all infected children, including neurologic and learning disorders and sensorineural deafness. Most cases occur in children younger than 2 years of age. Annual mortality rates range from 5 to 20 per cent, depending on the age group. The disease is spread through a hematogenous route and is often preceded by a viral illness. Risks for the disease include young age, male gender, urban dwelling, and inadequate immunizations. Children with a more gradual onset and longer history of illness tend to have better outcomes (Ashwal, 1995).

Presentations of bacterial meningitis are many, and a high index of suspicion is necessary to diagnose the disease. Fever, nuchal rigidity, headache, and altered states of consciousness are present in 85 per cent of adults (Ashwal, 1995), but children often lack the classic symptoms. Seizures with a febrile illness may be the presenting problem. Nausea, vomiting, myalgias, weakness, and photophobia may also accompany the process. Pneumonia and otitis media frequently are seen in conjunction with bacterial meningitis. Kernig sign, wherein extension of the child's knee when the hip is flexed 90 degrees elicits pain in the thigh and knee, is positive in 43 per cent of the cases (Lipton, 1995). Brudzinski sign, wherein flexion of the child's neck causes flexion of the knees, is present 66 per cent of the time in children with meningitis (Lipton and Schafermeyer, 1995).

Laboratory diagnosis of meningitis lies mainly in the evaluation of the CSF. Any child in whom meningitis is suspected must undergo a lumbar puncture. A lumbar puncture is performed once signs of increased intracranial pressure (i.e., papilledema) are ruled out. Normal CFS is clear without turbidity and contains less than 5 WBC/mm^3. The vast majority of patients with bacterial meningitis have CSF WBC counts in excess of 1000 WBC/mm^3 with predominantly PMNs. CSF glucose and protein levels are also measured. A CSF protein level greater than 50 mg/dl and/or CSF glucose level less than 40 mg/dl suggest meningeal infections. Gram stain of the CSF can be done to identify the causative bacteria, and the result is positive in 60 to 90 per cent of all cases (Ashwal, 1995). Detection of bacterial antigens by latex agglutination is more specific and is 90 to 100 per cent sensitive. These latex agglutination studies are now performed routinely on CSF and are able to identify *N. meningitidis, S. pneumoniae,* and *H. influenzae*.

Causative agents of bacterial meningitis vary in predominance by age of the child. Neonates exhibit pathogens related to the fetal environment; therefore group B streptococci *Escherichia coli,* and *Listeria monocytogenes* are most prevalent. After the neonatal period, or in children older than 3 months of age, *H. influenzae, N. meningitidis,* and *S. pneumoniae* are the predominant organisms with *H. influenzae* present in 65 per cent of all cases (Pohl, 1993). This predominance is expected to change as use of the *H. influenzae* vaccine becomes more widespread. After 12 years of age and into adulthood, *S. pneumoniae* and *N. meningitidis* are the predominant causes of bacterial meningitis.

Bacterial meningitis requires immediate therapy. Initial therapy with ampicillin and a third-generation cephalosporin (i.e., ceftriaxone or cefotaxime) has been shown to be effective empirically. Once the Gram stain and latex agglutination results are available, therapy may be narrowed. Intravenous antibiotics are continued for a 10- to 14-day course. Initial fluid management is directed toward the treatment of hypovolemia and dehydration with care to avoid over-rehydration and cerebral edema. Outpatient therapy is not recommended.

Corticosteroid therapy for meningitis is controversial. Although no change in mortality is seen with steroid therapy, it has been postulated that long-term sequelae may be reduced if steroids are given before antibiotics. Through their anti-inflammatory properties, corticosteroids can neutralize the response to bacterial death by the host. The decreased inflammatory response may reduce the chance of poor audiologic and neurologic outcome (Lipton and Schafermeyer, 1995).

Long-term sequelae of bacterial meningitis include deafness, seizure disorders, paralysis, or other CNS abnormalities. Close follow-up to assess developmental milestones and audiologic function is recommended. Contacts of children with documented meningococcal meningitis must be prophylactically treated with rifampin to prevent the spread of the potentially fatal disease. Contacts include members of the child's household, day care providers, and other children in the day care center.

Aseptic meningitis, which is usually of viral etiology, presents itself in much the same manner as bacterial meningitis, thus complicating the clinical picture. It is most common in children ages 1 to 10 years. Children usually present with fever, headache, nausea, and vomiting occasionally preceded by a nonspecific febrile illness. The child may be irritable, but profound changes in mental status are uncommon. Older children report myalgias and photophobia, but less than 50 per cent has nuchal rigidity. The causative agent is usually viral with enteroviruses accounting for over 80 per cent of identifiable causes. Herpes virus, fungal infections, tuberculosis, and adenovirus are infrequent etiologies of aseptic meningitis.

Diagnosis of viral meningitis depends on the clinical picture and CSF findings. As in bacterial meningitis, any child with a suspicion of meningeal disease warrants a lumbar puncture. Typically, the CSF WBC count is between five and 500 WBC/mm^3 and consists of predominantly lymphocytes. The CSF protein is elevated approximately 50 per cent of the time, and the CSF glucose level is usually normal. The Gram stain shows no organisms, and results of all latex agglutination studies are negative. Bacterial cultures should always be performed, with cultures for fungal entities and acid-fast bacilli done as indicated. Viral cultures are difficult to obtain and may not add to the diagnosis. The peripheral WBC count may be normal or slightly elevated, and it rarely shows immature or band cells.

Treatment of viral meningitis depends on accurate diagnosis. Patients are often treated with intravenous antibiotics empirically until CSF studies fail to diagnose a bacterial etiology. If the diagnosis is unclear, intravenous antibiotics should be continued until all cultures are negative after 3 days. Once bacterial meningitis has been excluded, antibiotics can be discontinued, and care is generally supportive. Fluids, rest, and pain medications are appropriate therapy with expectant management. Any patient whose condition deteriorates should be evaluated for an alternative cause of the aseptic meningitis (i.e., fungal, tuberculous, or herpetic). The prognosis of viral meningitis is usually benign, and less than 1 per cent has a complicated course. Two weeks is the average duration for symptoms. Full recovery can be expected.

Tuberculous meningitis is becoming more prevalent. It is found most commonly in children younger than 4 years of age and is uncommon in children younger than 4 months old. The disease progresses insidiously in three stages. Stage I is characterized by fever, headache, and malaise. It generally lasts 1 to 2 weeks. Stage II shows classic meningeal signs with nuchal rigidity and seizures. This represents cerebral edema. The brain stem is the site most commonly affected, and abnormalities in cranial nerves can be seen. Stage III consists of high fever and coma and generally culminates in death. CSF evaluation is similar to other forms of aseptic meningitis except that the CSF glucose is generally very low with a blood glucose:CSF glucose ratio of greater than 2:1. Other diagnostic criteria include a history of exposure to tuberculosis, an abnormal chest radiograph and a CSF culture positive for acid-fast bacilli.

Treatment for tuberculous meningitis consists of antibiotics directed toward *Mycobacterium tuberculosis*. Isoniazid and rifampin are major components of the treatment, with a third agent often added. Patients are treated for a total of 12 months. Dexamethasone therapy for 2 to 4 weeks has also been shown to increase the survival rates and decrease neurologic complications and sequelae. Mortality from tuberculous meningitis is approximately 50 per cent (Lipton and Schafermeyer, 1995).

Children and immunocompromised adults are at the highest risk for all forms of meningitis. With a high index of suspicion for the disease; accurate and prompt evaluation of the CSF; and appropriate, timely treatment, meningitis can result in fewer long-term sequelae, and mortality from the disease can be decreased.

SUGGESTED READING

Ashwal S. Neurologic evaluation of the patient with acute bacterial meningitis. Neurol Clin 1995;13:549–577.

Feigin RD, McCracken GH, Klein JO. Diagnosis and management of meningitis. Pediatr Infect Dis J 1992;11:785–814.

Klein NC, Cunha BA. Bacterial meningitis. Emerg Med 1994;2:14–18.

Lipton JD, Schafermeyer RW. Central nervous system infections. Emerg Med Clin North Am 1995;13:417–443.

Pohl CA. Practical approach to bacterial meningitis in childhood. Am Fam Physician 1993;5:1695–1703.

QUESTIONS

1. The most likely causative agent in bacterial meningitis in children less than 3 months old is
   a. Group B streptococcus
   b. *H. influenzae*
   c. *S. pneumoniae*
   d. *L. monocytogenes*

2. Aseptic meningitis is most frequently caused by
   a. Tuberculosis
   b. Enteroviruses
   c. Herpes
   d. Arboviruses

3. Match each set of laboratory values with the most likely diagnosis.
   a. Viral meningitis
   b. Bacterial meningitis
   c. Tuberculous meningitis
   d. Normal CSF
      (1) WBC 2500, protein 70, glucose 25
      (2) WBC 300, protein 70, glucose 50
      (3) WBC 0, protein 40, glucose 90
      (4) WBC 50, protein 40, glucose 10

Answers appear on **page 607.**

Chapter 76

Chronic Anxiety

Michael G. Kavan, Ph.D.

INITIAL VISIT

Subjective

PATIENT INFORMATION. Sarah B. is a 20-year-old married white woman who works as a secretary. She currently complains of a headache, which is causing her to worry excessively about her health. The patient presents for the first time at this clinic.

PRESENTING PROBLEM. Sarah reports that she has been experiencing a modest headache for the past several days that "just won't go away." She describes this as a "dull, pressure feeling" around her head.

She also reports that she has been experiencing occasional low back pain, stomach aches, and diarrhea, recently. Sarah indicates that these problems have "drained me physically and emotionally." The patient complains about difficulties with sleep and fatigue, which have resulted in occasional performance problems at work.

PRESENT ILLNESS. The patient initially voiced concern that her headaches were indicative of a more serious medical problem. After discussing her headaches and possible antecedents to these, the patient was able to show fairly good insight into the relationship between various stressors (e.g., work, marriage, and family issues) and the onset of her headaches. Her other physical complaints seemed to follow a similar pattern. As a result of these findings, the interview focused on the patient's tendency to worry about various life issues.

Sarah reports a history of worrying that dates to "as long as I can remember." She describes herself as "a worrier just like my mom." The patient indicates that she has tried various ways to control her stress and worrying including distraction, avoidance, deep breathing, and the occasional use of alcohol. Although all of these methods have been somewhat effective, she is unable to use them consistently and persistently.

PAST MEDICAL HISTORY. Sarah reports a history of respiratory infections and stomach problems. A review of medical records, which were forwarded to the clinic before this initial visit, indicates recurrent pharyngitis, sinusitis, tonsillitis, bronchitis, upper respiratory infections, headaches, low back pain, and gastrointestinal complaints since the age of 16 years. The upper respiratory infections were treated with antibiotics. Her gastrointestinal complaints were worked up with esophagogastroduodenoscopy (EGD) and pelvic ultrasound, both of which were negative. She was being considered as having irritable bowel syndrome at that time. Sarah has recently taken cisapride (Propulcid), ranitidine (Zantac), and cimetidine (Tagamet) for stomach distress. The patient also reported that she gave birth 3 years ago and gave the baby up for adoption. Although she was not married at the time, she did subsequently marry and is currently married to the father of this child. Sarah reports past involvement in individual counseling for depression and family counseling for "communication problems."

FAMILY AND SOCIAL HISTORY. The patient has been married for the past year. She reports a variety of stressors within the marriage, including opposing work schedules and alcohol abuse (possibly dependency) by her spouse. She admits to "getting on" her spouse about his drinking, which has further served to alienate him from her. The patient currently works as a secretary, but is worried about her job due to problems with a coworker. Her parents are divorced. Both her natural father and mother are described as chemically dependent. Her mother lives out of town and has custody of her 14-year-old sister. The patient describes her relationship with her mother as strained since the mother "uses" the opportunity for visitation with the sister to manipulate the patient. The patient reports that she experiences increased worrying, gastrointestinal complaints, and headaches when she approaches occasions that require visitation with her mother. Sarah lived with her father, stepmother, and stepsister from the time she was 13 years old until her marriage. The patient's father and step-family recently left town without notifying the patient and left no forwarding address or phone number for the patient. No other information is offered or available from the medical records regarding any history of family illnesses or diseases.

HEALTH HABITS. Sarah denies the use of nicotine and illicit drugs. She admits to the rare use of alcohol with no associated social or occupational problems. Sarah reports eating a "bland" diet. She indicates that she is tired of this diet, but it seems to moderate her stomach distress. Sarah admits to minimal caffeine use. Whereas the patient was exercising regularly before her pregnancy, she has not engaged in any type of regular exercise since that time.

REVIEW OF SYSTEMS. The patient denies significant weight changes. She does report a current bandlike headache, but denies any other musculoskeletal pain at this time. Sarah admits to experiencing some lightheadedness recently. In addition, she reports left lower quadrant cramping pain with diarrhea occurring several times per week. Her stomach distress is often precipitated by work or familial stress. The patient denies any shortness of breath, cardiac complaints, or paresthesias. She has no known allergies.

Objective

PHYSICAL EXAMINATION. On physical examination, Sarah is a well-developed, well-nourished, cooperative, and friendly white female. The patient is 5 feet 4 inches tall and weights 136 lb. Blood pressure is

130/78, respiration 16, oral temperature 98.2°F. The patient demonstrated mild distress during the examination. Heart is regular rate and rhythm. Lungs are clear to auscultation. Breast examination is normal. Abdominal examination reveals positive bowel sounds. The abdomen is soft and slightly tender over the left lower quadrant. No rebound, peritoneal signs, or masses noted. Pelvic examination is normal. Rectal examination is refused by the patient. Patient demonstrates appropriate affect.

LABORATORY TESTS. Initial laboratory tests included thyroid function, serum glucose and electrolytes, and a complete blood count (CBC). These test results are within normal limits.

Assessment

WORKING DIAGNOSIS. The original working diagnosis for Sarah's presenting complaint is: (1) headache, tension type, since she does describe the sensation of dull, bandlike discomfort around her head, and (2) Generalized Anxiety Disorder (GAD), since she reports excessive worrying about her work, marriage, and family, associated physical complaints (e.g., headaches, sleep disturbance, fatigue), and performance problems at work (American Psychiatric Association, 1994).

Plan

The plan for Sarah is to provide her with education on her tension-type headaches and the role that stress and worrying play in their development and exacerbation. She is told to use naproxen (Aleve) as needed for her headaches. In addition, she is written a prescription for buspirone (BusPar) 5 mg three times daily with instructions to increase this to 10 mg three times daily after 1 week. The patient is also provided with brief education and a handout on stress management. The patient is asked to return to the clinic in 2 weeks.

FOLLOW-UP VISIT

The patient returned several times over the course of treatment. During these sessions, Sarah is provided with additional information on stress management techniques. Specifically, she is instructed on the importance of exercise as a method to reduce anxiety and stress. She is also instructed on the use of an audio relaxation tape and cognitive tech-

niques (e.g., thought stopping) to deal with her worrying and subsequent physiologic responses to it. In addition, Sarah is continued on buspirone 10 mg three times daily, since it seems to "take the edge off" of her worrying.

DIFFERENTIAL DIAGNOSIS. The preceding information would result in the consideration of several possible diagnoses by the physician. These include:

1. *Generalized anxiety disorder.* Since the patient is reporting excessive anxiety and worrying about a variety of issues, the physician must consider anxiety disorders in the differential. Sarah reports excessive anxiety and worrying for several years, which has been difficult to control. This has resulted in sleep disturbance, muscle tension, and fatigue. Her fatigue has caused occasional performance problems at work, whereas her irritability has caused additional strain within the marriage. These symptoms are characteristic of GAD (see Table 76–1) (American Psychiatric Association, 1994).

TABLE 76–1. DSM-IV Diagnostic Criteria for Generalized Anxiety Disorder

---

A. Excessive anxiety and worry (apprehensive expectations), occurring more days than not for at least 6 months, about a number of events or activities (such as work or school performance).
B. The person finds it difficult to control the worry.
C. The anxiety and worry are associated with three (or more) of the following six symptoms (with at least some symptoms present for more days than not for the past 6 months).
   Note: only one item is required in children.
   (1) restlessness or feeling keyed up or on edge
   (2) being easily fatigued
   (3) difficulty concentrating or mind going blank
   (4) irritability
   (5) muscle tension
   (6) sleep disturbance (difficulty falling or staying asleep, or restless, unsatisfying sleep)
D. The focus of the anxiety or worry is not confined to features of a DSM-IV Axis I disorder (i.e., related to Panic Disorder, Social Phobia, Obsessive-Compulsive Disorder, Separation Anxiety Disorder, Anorexia Nervosa, Somatization Disorder, Hypochondriasis, or Post-traumatic Stress Disorder).
E. The anxiety, worry, or physical symptoms cause clinically significant distress or impairment in social, occupational, or other important areas of functioning.
F. The disturbance is not due to the direct physiologic effects of a substance or a general medical condition and does not occur exclusively during a Mood Disorder, a Psychotic Disorder, or a Pervasive Developmental Disorder.

From American Psychiatric Association. Diagnostic and Statistical Manual of Mental Disorders, ed 4 (DSM-IV). Washington, DC: American Psychiatric Association, 1994.

2. *Panic disorder.* When patients present with complaints of anxiety, Panic Disorder should be considered in the differential. Panic Disorder is defined as the occurrence of unexpected panic attacks (i.e., a discrete period of intense fear or discomfort accompanied by symptoms such as palpitations, sweating, trembling, chest pain, nausea, dizziness, paresthesias, and fears of dying) that peak in intensity within 10 minutes (American Psychiatric Association, 1994). Such episodes are typically followed by persistent worry about future attacks and their consequences, and significant behavioral change in response to the attacks. Whereas Sarah describes anxiety and worrying, her symptoms do not occur with the sudden intensity typically associated with Panic Disorder. Also, she only admits to two physical symptoms (i.e., lightheadedness and abdominal distress) characteristic of panic disorder.

3. *Somatization disorder.* In order to be given a diagnosis of Somatization Disorder, the patient must have a history of many physical complaints for which she has sought medical care over the past several years beginning before age 30 years. The following symptoms must be present: (a) four pain symptoms, (b) two gastrointestinal symptoms, (c) a sexual symptom, and (d) a pseudoneurologic symptom (American Psychiatric Association, 1994). Sarah reports two pain symptoms (i.e., headaches, low back pain), two gastrointestinal complaints (i.e., cramping, diarrhea), and a pseudoneurologic symptom (i.e., lightheadedness). However, she reported no sexual symptoms. Since she does not meet all of the above criteria, a diagnosis of Somatization Disorder is not likely.

4. *Adjustment disorder with anxiety.* For a diagnosis of Adjustment Disorder with Anxiety, a patient must experience emotional or behavioral symptoms within 3 months of the onset of the stressor(s). There must also be excessive distress or significant impairment in functioning (American Psychiatric Association, 1994). Sarah reports experiencing multiple stressors in her life, which have resulted in feelings of anxiety and some impairment in her relationships and at her work setting. However, her response is not necessarily considered excessive. Also, this diagnosis should not be used when the pattern of symptoms presented by a patient is better accounted for with another DSM-IV Axis I diagnosis, in this case GAD (American Psychiatric Association, 1994).

5. *Hypochondriasis.* Hypochondriasis involves a preoccupation with fears of having a serious illness based on the patient's misinterpretation of symptoms (American Psychiatric Association, 1994). Although Sarah presents with multiple physical complaints and is concerned about her physical functioning, she is not likely to be diagnosed with this disorder, since she is not *preoccupied* with fears of having a serious disease and she *does* appear to be comforted by medical evaluation and reassurance, both of which are not characteristic of someone with hypochondriasis. Also, there is some physiologic basis for her complaints of headaches and stomach distress. Therefore, a diagnosis of GAD better accounts for her symptoms.

6. *Anxiety disorder due to a general medical condition.* In order for Sarah to be diagnosed with this disorder, there must be direct evidence from history, physical findings, and/or laboratory data that her anxiety is due to a physiologic consequence of a general medical condition (American Psychiatric Association, 1994). As noted within the *Objective* section, Sarah's physical examination and laboratory work were negative.

7. *Substance-induced anxiety disorder.* This diagnosis is considered when there is evidence that the patient's anxiety is due to the direct physiologic effects of substance intoxication or withdrawal, the anxiety is etiologically related to substance use, the anxiety is not better accounted for by another anxiety disorder, the anxiety must not occur exclusively during the course of delirium, and the anxiety must cause significant functional impairment (American Psychiatric Association, 1994). Although the patient has a strong family history for substance dependency, she admits to only the rare use of alcohol and denies the use of any other substance that could account for her anxiety. Therefore, this diagnosis is not likely.

8. *Major depressive disorder.* Depression should be considered whenever symptoms of anxiety are present due to their high degree of comorbidity. Sarah presents with several complaints that may be indicative of depression. These include fatigue, multiple, vague physical complaints, and sleep difficulties. In addition, the patient reports marital problems, which are often related to depression. However, in order to have a diagnosis of Major Depressive Disorder, the patient must have at least five of the following nine symptoms nearly every day for at least 2 weeks: (a) depressed mood; (b) markedly diminished interest or pleasure in activities; (c) significant decreases or increases in appetite or weight; (d) insomnia or hypersomnia; (e) psychomotor agitation or retardation; (f) fatigue; (g) feelings of worthlessness or excessive or inappropriate feelings of

guilt; (h) diminished ability to think or concentrate, or difficulties with decision making; and (i) recurrent thoughts of death or suicide (American Psychiatric Association, 1994). As noted previously, Sarah admits to insomnia and fatigue, but denies other symptoms characteristic of depression.

9. *Medical conditions.* A variety of medical problems can result in symptoms of anxiety, and thus should be considered in the differential diagnosis and subsequently ruled out. These include (a) endocrine conditions such as hyperthyroidism, hypothyroidism, hypoglycemia, and hyperadrenocorticism; (b) cardiovascular problems such as congestive heart failure, pulmonary embolism, and arrhythmia; (c) respiratory conditions such as chronic obstructive pulmonary disease and pneumonia; (d) metabolic conditions such as vitamin B_{12} deficiency; (e) neurologic conditions such as neoplasms, vestibular dysfunction, and encephalitis; (f) intoxication associated with caffeine, alcohol, amphetamines, cannabis, cocaine, hallucinogens, inhalants, phencyclidine, and sympathomimetics; and (g) withdrawal from alcohol, cocaine, sedatives, hypnotics, and anxiolytics (American Psychiatric Association, 1994; Katon and Geyman, 1995) (Table 76–2). As noted previously, history, physical examination, and laboratory testing ruled out medical conditions as a cause of Sarah's anxiety.

DISCUSSION

Prevalence of Disorder

Anxiety is a common problem in the United States and in primary care settings (Katon and Geyman, 1995). The 1-month prevalence rate for all anxiety disorders in U.S. adults is 7.3 per cent (4.7 per cent for men; 9.7 per cent for women). For GAD, the 1-year prevalence rate is approximately 2 to 3 per cent, whereas the lifetime prevalence rate is estimated at 5 per cent (American Psychiatric Association, 1994). In clinical settings, women are diagnosed with GAD somewhat more frequently than men (American Psychiatric Association, 1994). The National Ambulatory Medical Care survey found that anxiety and nervousness accounted for 11 per cent of physician visits.

Diagnostic Criteria and Clinical Presentation

General anxiety disorder is characterized by excessive anxiety and worry (apprehensive expectation), which occurs fairly persistently for a 6-month period, about a number of events. Persons with GAD find it difficult to control such worry. In addition, the anxiety and worry is associated with various psychological and physical symptoms including restlessness, fatigue, concentration difficulties, irritability, muscle tension, and sleep disturbance. These symptoms produce functional impairment at home, work, and/or school (see Table 76–1) (American Psychiatric Association, 1994).

Clinically, patients with anxiety disorders often present to their family physician with nonspecific or vague somatic complaints such as headaches, low-back pain, gastrointestinal distress, upper respiratory infections, cardiovascular symptoms, sleep difficulties, fatigue, and diminished appetite. One must rule out medical problems through history, physical examination, and laboratory tests (see Table 76–2).

Sarah presented to the family practice clinic with the main complaint of headaches. Other physical complaints included a history of gastrointestinal complaints (e.g., stomach aches, diarrhea), low-back pain, upper respiratory infections, sleep problems, and fatigue, all of which are characteristic of the clinical presentation for GAD. On further history

TABLE 76–2. Medical Differential Diagnosis in Patients with Anxiety

Endocrine
Hyperthyroidism
Hypothyroidism
Hypoglycemia
Hyperadrenocorticism

Cardiovascular
Congestive heart failure
Pulmonary embolism
Arrhythmia
Mitral valve prolapse
Myocardial infarction

Respiratory
Chronic obstructive pulmonary
  disease
Pneumonia
Hypoxia

Metabolic Conditions
Acidosis
Electrolyte abnormalities
Pernicious anemia

Neurologic
Neoplasms
Vestibular dysfunction
Encephalitis

Intoxication
Caffeine
Alcohol
Amphetamines
Cannabis
Cocaine
Hallucinogens
Inhalants
Phencyclidine
Sympathomimetics

Withdrawal
Alcohol
Cocaine
Sedatives
Hypnotics
Anxiolytics

Nutritional Deficiencies
Vitamin B_{12}
Pyridoxine
Folate

taking, she was noted to have a pattern of excessive worrying regarding her marriage, job, and family that occurred for several years. Sarah has had difficulty controlling her worrying. This, in combination with her physical complaints, has caused her to experience problems at work such as decreased performance and increased absenteeism. Although she reports the occasional use of alcohol and caffeine, she denies any other substance use. In addition, physical examination and laboratory testing rule out any medical explanation for her anxiety. As a result, she meets the DSM-IV criteria for GAD (American Psychiatric Association, 1994).

Management of Generalized Anxiety Disorder

Therapeutic management of the patient with GAD should be catered to those factors thought to be responsible for its onset. Organic disease as well as psychosocial and personality factors all must be considered and appropriately ruled in or out before the development of a treatment plan (Katon and Geyman, 1995). Once this occurs and hypotheses are generated regarding the cause of the patient's anxiety, the physician must work closely with the patient to educate him or her about the cause of the anxiety and develop a mutually agreed-on treatment plan for the problem. Physician interventions typically include two approaches: (a) psychosocial management and/or (b) pharmacologic management.

PSYCHOSOCIAL MANAGEMENT. In terms of psychosocial management, several therapeutic interventions are available to the physician. A helpful way of thinking about these is to use the *REST* mnemonic (Table 76–3), which cues the physician to address several issues in regard to psychosocial interventions. First, *R* represents reassurance/support. The patient with anxiety is typically worried about his or her health and other factors, symptoms characteristic of GAD. Because of this, it is helpful to provide reassurance to the patient that an appropriate history, physical examination, and laboratory tests will be conducted to rule out medical disease. This, combined with support, is often enough to reduce some anxiety, especially in those patients with cardiac symptoms. The *E* stands for education. A patient may feel anxious due to a lack of understanding about his or her symptoms, which may lead to misperceptions about his or her mental and physical health. The physician should take time to define anxiety, the factors that may cause it, and how the body responds to such events. A simple explanation of the

TABLE 76–3. Psychosocial Management of Anxiety: REST Mnemonic

R   **Reassurance** and support provided to patient regarding the physician's ability to conduct appropriate tests to rule out serious medical problems.

E   **Education** provided to the patient on anxiety, its etiology, the neuroendocrine response (i.e., "fight or flight" response), and how these may lead to physiologic symptoms.

S   **Stress management** techniques discussed and taught to the patient. These include:
  Exercise
  Relaxation training
  Positive thinking (e.g., use of thought stopping strategies)
  Time management
  Social support
  Habit reduction

T   **Therapy** may be necessary for patients who do not respond well to the above interventions. For these patients, referral to a psychologist for formal psychotherapy for anxiety reduction may be warranted.

neuroendocrine response to stress (e.g., the "fight or flight" response) and how this can lead to physiologic symptoms provides the patient with information, and thus increased control over the problem. The *S* represents stress management strategies. A host of these are available to the patient and include (a) exercise, (b) relaxation techniques, (c) positive self-talk, (d) time management, (e) social support, and (f) habit reduction. The physician should supplement this information with patient education handouts and/or self-help resources (e.g., Davis et al., 1995) on these techniques. Often, these strategies prove useful for the patient and no further interventions are necessary. However, in more severe cases of GAD, *T*, which stands for therapy (both psychological and pharmacologic), may be necessary.

As in the case of Sarah, psychosocial factors appeared to precipitate her anxiety. Once her physician ruled out medical factors, she was provided with reassurance and support, and then educated on how problems with her spouse, marriage, and family likely resulted in her worrying and subsequent physical symptoms. Emphasis was then placed on teaching her the importance of various stress management techniques, including "thought stopping" (i.e., catch, stop, and replace negative thinking/worrying with rational thinking), exercise (i.e., Sarah was encouraged to exercise aerobically three times a week for 20 minutes each time), and relaxation strategies (i.e., she was taught deep breathing techniques and provided with a relaxation tape to practice daily). She was also encouraged to consider marital counseling. Sarah initiated a walking program, practiced relaxation regularly, and began to use thought stopping techniques; however, she was unable to persuade her spouse to participate in counseling.

PHARMACOLOGIC MANAGEMENT. There are two major pharmacologic agents available for the management of GAD. These include the nonbenzodiazepines (e.g., azopirones) and benzodiazepines.

Nonbenzodiazepines. The only nonbenzodiazepine anxiolytic currently available is the azopirone, buspirone (Buspar) (see Table 76–4). Buspirone is thought to exert its influence by acting as an agonist at presynaptic 5-hydroxytryptamine (serotonin) 1A (5-HT_{1A}) sites. It has a slow onset of action, which usually requires several days to 2 weeks or longer to reach its full therapeutic effect. Thus, buspirone appears to be most effective in patients experiencing chronic stress and/or anxiety who do not necessarily need the immediate relief associated with the benzodiazepines. Buspirone lacks the sedative, muscle relaxant, and anticonvulsant qualities of the benzodiazepines. In addition, it does not impair psychomotor performance, which is advantageous in elderly persons and those operating vehicles or heavy equipment. Buspirone has no significant abuse potential or withdrawal effects. There is negligible overdose toxicity, no serious drug interactions, and no anticholinergic, cardiotoxic, or respiratory depression effects. It should be noted that patients with a substantial history of benzodiazepine use may respond less well to buspirone. Patients should be educated about the delayed onset of effect and lack of euphoria associated with its use. Buspirone has also been noted to have some antidepressant uses.

It is recommended that the starting dose of buspirone be 7.5 mg twice daily. It may be increased 5 mg daily every 2 to 3 days. In clinical trials, the most common dose was 20 to 30 mg daily in divided doses. The maximum dose is 60 mg per day. Few side effects are associated with the use of buspirone and are noted to include dizziness (12 per cent), drowsiness (10 per cent), nausea (8 per cent), headaches (6 per cent), nervousness (5 per cent), lightheadedness (3 per cent), and agitation (2 per cent).

Sarah was prescribed buspirone 5 mg three times daily, which was increased to 10 mg three times daily after 1 week. She reported that it was effective for her, and thus she remained at this dose. Sarah reported no untoward side effects associated with its use.

Benzodiazepines. The second major class of medications available for the management of anxiety are the benzodiazepines (Table 76–4). These are the most commonly used medications for anxiety disorders. The benzodiazepines are believed to exert their influence on the γ-aminobutyric acid ($GABA_A$) receptors in the central nervous system. Their half-lives and dosages vary considerably; however, all benzodiazepines have relatively equal efficacy. Therefore, selection is often based on half-lives and side effect profiles. In addition to being useful for the management of GAD, benzodiazepines have been shown to be beneficial with panic disorder and alcoholic withdrawal.

Benzodiazepine side effects include sedation, slowed psychomotor performance, and amnesia. However, these are typically transient and disappear as tolerance to these effects develops. Although there is potential for abuse and dependency, it has been found that most community patients do not abuse benzodiazepines prescribed to them. Persons taking benzodiazepines may experience withdrawal symptoms on their abrupt discontinuation. Therefore, gradual dosage reduction before discontinuation is recommended to limit this effect.

Other Medications. Other medications have also been used for the management of anxiety (see Table 76–4). These include the selective serotonin reuptake inhibitors (e.g., fluoxetine and fluvoxamine for obsessive-compulsive disorder), tricyclic antidepressants (e.g., imipramine for panic attack, clomipramine for obsessive-compulsive disorder), β blockers (e.g., propranolol for social phobias such as speech anxiety), and monoamine oxidase inhibitors (e.g., phenelzine for patients with symptoms of both anxiety and depression).

SUMMARY

Generalized anxiety disorder is a common problem in family practice settings. It is characterized by chronic, excessive anxiety and worrying about a variety of issues, difficulty controlling worrying, related physical symptoms, and functional impairment. Patients with GAD often present with vague, physical complaints such as headaches, low-back pain, gastrointestinal disorders, and fatigue. These patients should have a thorough work-up, including full history and physical examination and laboratory testing to rule out physical disease.

Once physical problems are ruled out, the physician must assist the patient in the management of his or her stress through strategies outlined by the

TABLE 76–4. Pharmacologic Agents Used in the Management of Anxiety

Agent	Usual Starting Dose (mg)	Total Dosage Range (mg/day)	Half-life (hr)
Nonbenzodiazepines			
Buspirone (Buspar)	7.5 b.i.d.	15–60	2–3
Benzodiazepines			
Alprazolam (Xanax)	0.25–0.5 t.i.d.	0.75–4	6–27
Chlordiazepoxide (Librium)	5 b.i.d., t.i.d., or q.i.d.	10–100	6–20
Clonazepam (Klonopin)	0.5 t.i.d.	1.5–20	18–50
Chlorazepate (Tranxene)	7.5–15 q.d.	7.5–60	48
Diazepam (Valium)	2 b.i.d.–q.i.d.	4–40	>20
Lorazepam (Ativan)	1–3/day in divided doses	1–10	12–18
Oxazepam (Serax)	10 t.i.d.	30–90	6–11
Selective Serotonin Reuptake Inhibitors			
Fluoxetine (Prozac)	20 q.d.	20–80	72–360*
Fluvoxamine (Luvox)	50 q.d.	100–300	15.6
Tricyclic Antidepressants			
Clomipramine (Anafranil)	25 q.d.	25–250	20–40
Imipramine (Tofranil)	75 q.d.	75–300	12–34
β Blockers			
Propranolol (Inderal)	10 q.d.–q.i.d.	10–40	4
Monoamine Oxidase Inhibitors			
Phenelzine (Nardil)	15 t.i.d.	15–90	†

*Includes both fluoxetine and norfluoxetine.
†Variable half-life related to acetylator phenotype.

REST mnemonic (see Table 76–3). Whereas the physician may be able to assist the patient with reassurance, education, and training in basic stress management techniques, more formal psychological therapy may require a referral to a psychologist. In addition to psychosocial interventions, pharmacologic agents have been shown to be efficacious in the management of GAD. In particular, the nonbenzodiazepine buspirone (Buspar) and benzodiazepines have proved effective in ameliorating symptoms associated with GAD. As in the case of Sarah, the family physician can maximize therapeutic efficacy by using both psychosocial and pharmacologic interventions.

SUGGESTED READING

American Psychiatric Association. Diagnostic and Statistical Manual of Mental Disorders, 4th edition (DSM-IV). Washington, DC, American Psychiatric Association, 1994.

Barlow DH (ed). Clinical Handbook of Psychological Disorders, 2nd ed. New York, Guilford, 1993.

Davis M, Eshelman ER, McKay M. The Relaxation and Stress Reduction Workbook, 4th ed. Oakland, CA: New Harbinger, 1995.

Kayton W, Geyman JP. Diagnosis and treatment of anxiety disorders. In Rakel RE (ed). Textbook of Family Practice, 5th ed. Philadelphia, W.B. Saunders Company, 1995.

Schatzberg AF, Nemeroff CB (eds). Textbook of Psychopharmacology. Washington, DC, American Psychiatric Association, 1995.

1. The anxiolytic likely to cause the least sedation is:
   a. Alprazolam
   b. Chlordiazepoxide
   c. Oxazepam
   d. Buspirone
   e. Diazepam

2. Match the symptoms with the disorder that best fits.
   a. Excessive worrying
   b. Intense fear accompanied by intense physical complaints
   c. Chronic history of physical complaints

   d. Development of emotional symptoms in response to an identifiable stressor
   e. Anxiety that is a physiologic response to a disorder such as hyperthyroidism
      (1) Adjustment disorder with anxiety
      (2) Generalized anxiety disorder
      (3) Anxiety disorder due to a general medical condition
      (4) Somatization disorder
      (5) Panic disorder

Answers appear on **page 607.**

Chapter **77**

Sleep Disturbance

Thomas L. Schwenk, M.D.*

INITIAL VISIT

Subjective

Karen E. is a 35-year-old female nurse who works at University Hospital and presents at a routine office visit with concerns about fatigue and poor sleep. The patient describes general good health until the past 3 months when she experienced increasing fatigue. She does not initially express concern about other symptoms or mood alterations. She says she has a long history of iron deficiency anemia and wants a blood count done.

HISTORY OF PRESENT ILLNESS. Karen describes the fatigue manifesting as hypersomnolence that has led to her sleeping 10 to 12 hours per day. Despite this excessive sleeping, the patient reports morning fatigue and difficulty getting through her workday. She is concerned about anemia as noted previously, and is somewhat obsessed about this potential diagnosis and doing appropriate laboratory tests to investigate it. She also asks about testing for hypothyroidism. She initially denies mood disturbance or other neurovegetative complaints such as change in appetite or weight, or decreased sexual interest. She also denies anxiety or suicidal intent.

On further questioning, the patient describes the fatigue as a decreased enthusiasm for her usual activities and an inability to maintain her usual family and personal responsibilities. She describes her usual day as feeling tired on awakening, going to work and performing satisfactorily but without much energy, and coming home without any interest or energy to exercise or pursue other pleasurable activities. She is accustomed to a moderate

---

*The author wishes to acknowledge the help of James C. Coyne, Ph.D., in the preparation of this chapter.

exercise program, running 3 to 4 miles three times per week. She is not involved in an active sexual relationship, but when questioned more closely, her answers suggest that she has minimal sexual interest. She also reports some emotional lability with occasional episodes of crying for unexplained reasons.

Karen denies other problems, except for a mild intermittent tension-type headache. She denies other pain, cardiac, metabolic, skin, or gastrointestinal symptoms. She says her work performance is good and she is not suffering from cognitive dysfunction, such as memory loss or difficulty making decisions.

PAST MEDICAL HISTORY. The patient reports a long history of anemia for which she was told in the past to take iron supplements, but cannot provide details or specific blood values. She denies other chronic illnesses or hospitalizations except one uncomplicated obstetric delivery. The patient reports an episode of severe "breakdown" in her late teens or early twenties but cannot be more specific and does not seem to relate her current illness to this episode.

FAMILY HISTORY. The patient is divorced and does not have custody of her teenage daughter, who lives with her father in a city several hours' drive away. The patient sees her daughter occasionally but the relationship is strained and a source of considerable stress. The patient was raised as one of four children in a family she describes as strict in its discipline but without sexual or physical abuse. She reports that one brother and one sister are currently being treated with antidepressants, but she does not know specific details about their diagnoses. She knows of no psychiatric diagnoses in her parents or other relatives. There is no hereditary disease in the family otherwise.

HEALTH HABITS. The patient used to exercise regularly but has lost interest in exercise in the last few months. She does not smoke and drinks alcohol very occasionally. She takes no illicit or prescription drugs and is very wary of taking any medication, especially psychotropic medication, due to fears about possible addiction.

SOCIAL HISTORY. Karen works on an inpatient surgical unit at University Hospital as a registered nurse (RN). She lives alone and does not have a current sexual relationship. She has few close personal friends, but has lost contact with a couple of close friends in the last few months.

REVIEW OF SYSTEMS. Negative for other symptoms.

Objective

PHYSICAL EXAMINATION. The patient's vital signs are within normal limits. The patient's weight has increased 10 lb from 140 to 150 lb over the past 6 months, according to chart records. A brief physical examination with an emphasis on neurologic, cardiac, and metabolic systems is negative, including an absence of focal neurologic findings and no vascular or skin abnormalities.

LABORATORY TESTS. No tests are done at the time of the visit but a complete blood count (CBC) and thyroid function studies are ordered.

Assessment

WORKING DIAGNOSIS. The most likely diagnosis for Karen is major depressive disorder (MDD). She does not fully fit the DSM-IV criteria (Table 77–1) based on the information available at this visit. She reports anhedonia plus three additional criterion-based symptoms (fatigue, weight change, and sleep disturbance). On further investigation at the next visit there is a high likelihood that she will provide additional information that will bring her into a full fit with these criteria (such as psychomotor retardation or feelings of worthlessness or guilt). The patient's report of fatigue includes an element of moderately severe anhedonia, or loss of pleasure and involvement in usual daily activities such as exercise. Patients frequently do not comprehend more abstract phrasing of questions about loss of interest or pleasure, but Karen is able to identify this loss specifically in relation to her interest in running and exercise. While her sleep is excessive, it is usually of poor quality, resulting in morning fatigue.

Karen exhibits a weight gain of 6 to 7 per cent but is not aware of an associated appetite disturbance, so the weight change may be due to decreased exercise. Her mood as well as psychomotor and cognitive function are apparently not disturbed and the length of the routine office visit does not allow much exploration of feelings of worthlessness or guilt. The presence of these feelings would bear closer questioning and scrutiny, particularly in regard to her relationship with her daughter. She does describe significant emotional lability with occasional crying for no apparent reason. She has experienced these symptoms for several months, during

TABLE 77–1.   DSM-IV Criteria for Major Depressive Episode

A. At least five of the following symptoms have been present during the same 2-week period and represent a change from previous functioning; at least one of the symptoms is either (1) depressed mood or (2) loss of interest or pleasure.
  1. Depressed mood most of the day, nearly every day, as indicated by either subjective report (e.g., feels sad or empty) or observation made by others (e.g., appears tearful). *Note:* in children and adolescents, can be irritable mood.
  2. Markedly diminished interest or pleasure in all, or almost all, activities most of the day, nearly every day (as indicated either by subjective account or observation made by others).
  3. Significant weight loss or weight gain when not dieting (e.g., more than 5 per cent of body weight in a month), or decrease or increase in appetite nearly every day. *Note:* in children, consider failure to make expected weight gains.
  4. Insomnia or hypersomnia nearly every day.
  5. Psychomotor agitation or retardation nearly every day (observable by others, not merely subjective feelings of restlessness or being slowed down).
  6. Fatigue or loss of energy nearly every day.
  7. Feelings of worthlessness or excessive or inappropriate guilt (which may be delusional) nearly every day (not merely self-reproach or guilt about being sick).
  8. Diminished ability to think or concentrate, or indecisiveness, nearly every day (either by subjective account or as observed by others).
  9. Recurrent thoughts of death (not just fear of dying), recurrent suicidal ideation without a specific plan, or a suicide attempt or a specific plan for committing suicide.
B. Symptoms cause clinically significant distress or impairment in social, occupational, or other important areas of functioning.
C. Not due to the direct effects of a substance (e.g., drugs of abuse, medication) or a general medical condition (e.g., hypothyroidism).
D. Not occurring within 2 months of the loss of a loved one (except if associated with marked functional impairment, morbid preoccupation with worthlessness, suicidal ideation, psychotic symptoms, or psychomotor retardation).

Adapted from American Psychiatric Association: Diagnostic and Statistical Manual of Mental Disorders, 4th ed (DSM-IV). Washington, DC, American Psychiatric Association, 1994, with permission.

which she had several periods of consistent symptoms exceeding 2 weeks. Her functioning is clearly disturbed, and there is no obvious superseding diagnosis at this time.

Her positive past history and family history increase the likelihood of the diagnosis of MDD. The details of the "breakdown" episode in her past are unclear, but it likely was a first episode of MDD, which is common in the third or fourth decade of life. The fact that the patient did not relate the current illness to this earlier episode is not uncommon, since depressed patients often have distorted recall about past depressive events. The fact that two siblings are currently taking antidepressants strongly suggests that they have a diagnosis of MDD, but that would require further elaboration. Her family and social history are otherwise not particularly remarkable, especially for the lack of physical or sexual abuse, but a divorced, single mother (even without child custody) has an increased risk for MDD. A history of physical or sexual abuse is increasingly identified as a risk factor for the development of MDD, possibly due to the associated poor self-esteem involved.

A lack of other physical complaints or chronic illness tends to draw attention away from other biomedical illness, particularly metabolic or hematologic diseases, which are usually multisymptom in presentation.

In summary, Karen shows evidence of anhedonia and three additional criteria of MDD, present for more than 2 weeks.

DIFFERENTIAL DIAGNOSIS. Karen's symptoms suggest several other diagnostic possibilities, although none is nearly as likely as MDD.

1. *Dysthymia.* The patient's emotional disturbance could be characterized as a less severe depression, such as dysthymia (Table 77–2) except that the symptoms have been present for only a few months. Her symptoms of tearfulness and possible social withdrawal are criteria for dysthymia, but the intensity of the vegetative symptoms and their presence for a shorter length of time argue against dysthymia.

2. *Adjustment disorder.* The constellation of symptoms could fit a diagnosis of adjustment disorder, except that no obvious precipitating event can be identified.

3. *Hypothyroidism.* The patient shows no additional stigmata of hypothyroidism, and has neurovegetative symptoms beyond simple fatigue.

4. *Anemia.* The history of anemia is pertinent, but the patient shows no pallor or weakness in support of this diagnosis. This diagnosis is easily confirmed or refuted with a hematocrit/hemoglobin determination.

5. *Chronic fatigue syndrome.* Fatigue is the presenting complaint for this patient, but on further questioning her complaint is really a lack of motivation to pursue usual activities. She is functional in her work and home roles, but has no pleasure in usual recreational activities. She also reports no initiating illness or event.

TABLE 77–2. DSM-IV Criteria for Dysthymia

A. Depressed mood (or can be irritable mood in children and adolescents) for most of the day, for more days than not, as indicated either by subjective account or observation made by others, for at least 2 years (1 year for children and adolescents).
B. Presence, while depressed, of at least three of the following:
   1. Low self-esteem or self-confidence, or feelings of inadequacy.
   2. Feelings of pessimism, despair, or hopelessness.
   3. Generalized loss of interest or pleasure.
   4. Social withdrawal.
   5. Chronic fatigue or tiredness.
   6. Feelings of guilt, brooding about the past.
   7. Subjective feelings of irritability or excessive anger.
   8. Decreased activity, effectiveness, or productivity.
   9. Difficulty in thinking reflected by poor concentration, poor memory, or indecisiveness.
C. During the 2-year period (1 year for children or adolescents) of the disturbance, the person has never been without the symptoms in A and B for more than 2 months at a time.
D. No major depressive episode during the first 2 years of the disturbance (1 year for children and adolescents).
E. Has never had a manic episode or an unequivocal hypomanic episode.
F. Does not occur exclusively during the course of a chronic psychotic disorder, such as schizophrenia or delusional disorder.
G. Not due to the direct effects of a substance (e.g., drugs of abuse, medication) or a general medical condition (e.g., hypothyroidism).

Adapted from American Psychiatric Association: Diagnostic and Statistical Manual of Mental Disorders, 4th ed (DSM-IV). Washington, DC, American Psychiatric Association, 1994, with permission.

6. *Generalized anxiety disorder.* Many patients with depression present with anxiety and vice versa. This patient shows none of the psychological, physical, or autonomic hyper-reactivity symptoms or findings required for a diagnosis of anxiety.

Plan

FURTHER TESTING. As noted earlier, a CBC and thyroid-stimulating hormone (TSH) level were ordered.

PSYCHOTHERAPY AND PATIENT EDUCATION. The interview helps to clarify for Karen the full constellation of symptoms that suggested the diagnosis of MDD, and helped to de-emphasize the possibility of anemia or hypothyroidism as an explanation for her symptoms. Significant discussion ensues regarding the consequences of this possible diagnosis, the pertinence of her past and family history, the ways in which MDD can cause her symptoms, and the potential treatments.

Karen is given a detailed pamphlet from the National Institute of Mental Health to read, and is encouraged to purchase additional reading material such as the book *Feeling Good*, by David Burns, M.D. or the book *How to Heal Depression* by Harold Bloomfield, M.D. and Peter McWilliam.

The patient is encouraged to resume at least a portion of her previous exercise program at a reduced intensity and length, perhaps performing 20 to 30 minutes of aerobic exercise three times per week. She is also asked to consider which relatives or friends are potential sources of support not yet tapped. Karen suggests a friend who lives in another city, with whom she has not had contact recently, due primarily to her own lack of initiative. She agrees to consider calling her friend in the next week to tell her how she is feeling and discuss the possibility of depression as an explanation for her illness. She is also asked if she has any significant decisions to make in the coming week, and reports that she has been avoiding writing or calling her daughter but wishes to do so. She is encouraged to follow through with this plan.

Above all, the patient is told that several possible diagnoses are being explored and that a resolution of her fatigue is likely. She is also told that if depression is the eventual diagnosis, her prognosis is reasonably good, given that she has experienced relatively few recurrences and has been symptomatic a relatively short time for this episode. She is also encouraged to consider pursuing specific psychotherapy related to her family stress, irrespective of subsequent diagnoses.

MEDICATIONS. Because of the uncertainty of a firm diagnosis of MDD, and the patient's reluctance to take psychoactive medication, no medication is offered at the first visit, but Karen is told that medications will be discussed at the next visit after a further exploration of symptoms and criteria for MDD, and a review of the laboratory tests.

DISPOSITION. Karen is asked to return in 1 week after completing the various reading, exercise, and personal assignments. She is asked to consider the possibility of additional counseling in the future and to contact the physician should any significant suicidal ideation develop.

FIRST FOLLOW-UP VISIT
Subjective

Karen returns in 1 week and reports that she is somewhat more receptive to the diagnosis of MDD after reading the assigned material. She has also called her sister with questions about her sister's illness and finds that she is taking a seritonergic antidepressant at therapeutic doses for MDD, as is her brother. This information appears to make the patient more receptive to the diagnosis of MDD, especially after she admits to looking up her laboratory values on the hospital computer system and finding them to be normal. Karen continues to report no actual mood disturbance but describes considerable guilt and feelings of helplessness regarding her relationship with her daughter, and a stressful relationship with her husband. She was unable to reach her friend from another city for other support but is relatively satisfied with how she has felt during the past week. She has exercised twice in the past week, to her considerable satisfaction.

Objective

The patient's vital signs are normal, and she has lost 1 lb. Her mood appears stable without evidence of lability, and she manifests no suicidal ideation. Her hematocrit is 40.2% and her TSH level is 3.5 mU/L, both of which are normal.

Assessment

The patient now meets the criteria for MDD and is deserving of treatment, despite the transient improvement in her ability to exercise. She has responded to the hope and support offered at the previous visit, and was compliant with most assignments. She is more receptive to the use of an antidepressant due to discussions with her sister. No other biomedical cause for her symptoms has been found, nor are there other symptoms to suggest that further testing should be done. No other causes for a secondary MDD have been found (Table 77–3).

Plan

Karen is started on fluoxetine, 20 mg in the morning, due to fluoxetine's appetite suppression and likely resultant weight loss, although this side effect is true to some extent for all seritonergic antidepressants (Table 77–4). She is encouraged again to contact her friend, and is asked to contact her daughter as a way to clarify the impact of the ongoing estrangement and conflict on her current illness. She is encouraged to increase her exercise consistent with her energy level. The patient is asked again to

TABLE 77–3. Organic Illnesses and Drugs Associated with Depression

Rheumatologic: systemic lupus erythematosus, rheumatoid arthritis
Cardiac: mitral valve prolapse, myocardial infarction, hypertension
Endocrine: hyperthyroidism and hypothyroidism, diabetes mellitus, hypercalcemia, Cushing syndrome, postpartum state
Gastrointestinal: cirrhosis, inflammatory bowel disease, pancreatitis, intestinal bypass
Hematologic: sickle cell anemia
Nutritional deficiencies: vitamin B_{12}, folate, iron, thiamine, niacin
Infectious: encephalitis, hepatitis, influenza, infectious mononucleosis, pneumonia, tuberculosis
Renal: renal transplant, uremia
Neoplastic: intracranial, leukemia, pancreatic, lymphoma
Neurologic: subdural hematoma, multiple sclerosis, CVA, Parkinson disease, uncontrolled epilepsy
Miscellaneous: psoriasis, sarcoidosis, drugs such as:
    Amphetamines, other CNS stimulants
    Barbiturates
    Benzodiazepines
    Cimetidine
    Clonidine
    β Blockers
    Corticosteroids
    Indomethacin
    α-Methyldopa
    Oral contraceptives, estrogens
    Reserpine, guanethidine
    Sulfonamides

CVA = Cerebrovascular accident; CNS = central nervous system.

consider pursuing outside psychotherapy, particularly concerning her family relationships.

SUBSEQUENT FOLLOW-UP VISITS

The patient is seen weekly for two more visits during which the dose of fluoxetine is held constant. The side effects of seritonergic antidepressants are dose-dependent, and increasing doses are usually not needed for moderate MDD. Karen reports sleep normalization and markedly increased energy levels. Her exercise program is continuing to develop. As her knowledge about depression increases, from reading and talking to friends, she becomes very accepting of the diagnosis of MDD and adds additional buttressing evidence to support the criteria for MDD, particularly more pronounced feelings of guilt related to her daughter. She is accepting of a referral for counseling in this regard, particularly focused on her feelings of poor self-worth due to a perception of having failed in her relationship with

TABLE 77–4. Side Effect Profiles and Therapeutic Dosage Ranges of Antidepressant Medications

Drug	Anticho-linergic*	CNS Effects		Cardiovascular Effects			Weight Gain (over 6 kg (13 lb))	Therapeutic Dosage Range (mg)
		Drowsi-ness	Insomnia/ Agitation	Ortho-static Hypo-tension	Cardiac Arrhyth-mia	GI Distress		
Amitriptyline (Elavil, Endep)	4+	4+	0	4+	3+	0	4+	75–300
Desipramine (Norpramin, Pertofrane)	1+	1+	1+	2+	2+	0	1+	75–300
Doxepin (Adapin, Sinequan)	3+	4+	0	2+	2+	0	3+	75–300
Imipramine (Tofranil)	3+	3+	1+	4+	3+	1+	3+	75–300
Nortriptyline (Aventyl, Pamelor)	1+	1+	0	2+	2+	0	1+	40–200
Protriptyline (Vivactil)	2+	1+	1+	2+	2+	0	0	20–60
Trimipramine (Surmontil)	1+	4+	0	2+	2+	0	3+	75–300
Amoxapine (Asendin)	2+	2+	2+	2+	3+	0	1+	100–400
Maprotiline (Ludiomil)	2+	4+	0	0	1+	0	2+	100–225
Trazodone (Desyrel)	0	4+	0	1+	1+	1+	1+	150–600
Nefazodone (Serzone)	0	3+	0	2+	1+	2+	1+	200–600
Bupropion (Wellbutrin)	0	0	2+	0	1+	1+	0	225–450
Venlafaxine (Effexor)	1+	0	2+	1+	1+	3+	0	75–375
Fluoxetine (Prozac)	0	0	2+	0	0	3+	0	10–60
Paroxetine (Paxil)	0	0	2+	0	0	3+	0	20–50
Sertraline (Zoloft)	0	0	2+	0	0	3+	0	50–200
Mirtazapine (Remeron)	3+	2+	1+	4+	2+	2+	2+	15–45
Monoamine oxidase inhibitors	1	1+	2+	2+	0	1+	2+	Varies (usual dose 30–50)

0 = absent or rare; 2+ = in between; 4+ = relatively common.
*Dry mouth, blurred vision, urinary hesitancy, constipation.
Adapted from Depression Guidelines Panel. Vol 1: Treatment of Major Depression. (AHCPR Publication No. 93-0550. Rockville, MD, U.S. Department of Health and Human Services, Public Health Service, Agency for Health Care Policy and Research, 1993.

her daughter. Over several visits the patient denies suicidal ideation.

Karen improves in function, mood, and energy level over the course of several months. She continues at the same dosage of fluoxetine. She continues in therapy and is seen every 3 months by the physician to monitor the fluoxetine treatment. After 12 months of being functional and relatively symptom-free the fluoxetine is discontinued, and she continues to feel good.

DISCUSSION

This patient demonstrates several characteristic features of patients with MDD seen by family physicians, including the following: (1) presentation with a somatic emphasis for the chief complaint and related symptoms, including an actual denial of mood disturbance and an interpretation of anhedonia as fatigue for which a biomedical explanation is sought; (2) a past history of probable MDD in the late teens or early twenties; (3) being a divorced woman with significant family and child relationship disturbances; and (4) a rapid and productive response to standard doses of an antidepressant. Overall, 70 to 80 per cent of patients with MDD respond to antidepressant therapy, but a higher percentage of primary care MDD patients probably respond because of a decreased severity of the disease compared with patients seen by psychiatrists.

The patient was somewhat atypical but not rare due to the presentation with hypersomnia. The most common sleep problem in depression is insomnia, which is usually mild. About 15 to 30 per cent of depressed patients report hypersomnia, and it is usually part of a picture that includes increased appetite and weight gain rather than the more common decreased appetite and weight loss. Depressed patients with hypersomnia are more likely than those with insomnia to report depression in a first-degree relative, agitation, earlier age of onset, and headaches.

There are several indications for referral of MDD patients to a psychiatrist (Table 77–5) for more specialized psychopharmacology, electroconvulsive therapy, or associated psychotherapy. However, patients with these indications for referral constitute only about 10 per cent of the MDD patients in a typical family practice. A majority of patients have relatively uncomplicated presentations and respond well to usual treatment. The biggest challenge for the family physician is to uncover the MDD diagnosis in the face of a strong bias (on the part of both the patient and physician) toward a biomedical explanation of somatic symptoms, particularly chronic pain and neurovegetative problems.

With severe depression some combination of medication and psychotherapy is usually indicated.

TABLE 77–5. Indications for Referral to a Psychiatrist

1. Moderate or high suicidal risk
2. Severe cognitive dysfunction with difficulty in daily living or nutritional deficiencies
3. Psychotic or delusional symptoms
4. Lack of family support for observation or care
5. Significant physical illness complicating antidepressant treatment
6. Uncertain diagnosis or complicating psychiatric diagnosis such as alcoholism
7. Bipolar disease
8. Lack of response to antidepressants (combined with severe neurovegetative symptoms, suggesting need for electroconvulsive treatment)

With mild to moderate MDD, the choice of one or the other treatment, or a combination, depends somewhat on the presentation of the patient and the preferences of the patient and physician. When vegetative symptoms predominate and patients do not give evidence of significant stresses in their lives, treatment with antidepressant medication may prove sufficient. However, depression tends to occur in a stressful interpersonal context, and there are several reasons for considering psychotherapy or counseling. Many patients want the opportunity to discuss their psychosocial problems, and an opportunity to participate in psychotherapy increases their adherence to medication and allows them to focus more specifically on the effectiveness and side effects of their medication during physician office visits. Also, medication has limited effect on the psychosocial problems that precipitate or accompany depression, and its effect on vegetative symptoms and mood may be diminished when these problems persist. Psychotherapy may thus be indicated to resolve problems not affected by the medication, increase the effectiveness of the medication, and reduce the probability of a relapse or recurrence.

Psychotherapists are increasingly recognizing the efficacy of relatively brief, structured, problem-focused therapy sessions for depression. That a patient presents with depression and serious psychosocial problems does not necessarily indicate the need for long-term, insight-oriented therapy. Myths about the incompatibility of psychotherapy and medication are also being discarded. Family physicians would do well to identify psychotherapists who are prepared to work in a brief, collaborative, goal-oriented manner.

The indication for antidepressant therapy is primarily the presence of neurovegetative symptoms suggesting an underlying neurotransmitter abnormality. The selection of a specific antidepressant is somewhat dependent on matching the side effect profile of a specific medication to the patient's symptoms (see Table 77–4), although some evidence suggests that even patients with psychomotor retardation and fatigue respond to sedating antidepressant owing to the correction of the underlying neurotransmitter deficiencies. However, patient acceptance and compliance are very low in these situations. Therefore, selection of an antidepressant that complements the patient's symptoms is helpful.

Specific guidance includes avoiding medications with strong orthostatic effects in elderly patients, being careful about the anticholinergic effects of some medications (leading to prolonged

QT intervals and decreased heart rate variability in patients with cardiac disease), choosing medications with an anorectic effect (such as fluoxetine) in patients who are trying to lose weight, and avoiding the use of trazodone in male patients due to the risk, albeit small, of priapism. Newer agents, such as nefazodone, are helpful if patients suffer significant sexual dysfunction with a seritonergic agent.

SUGGESTED READING

American Psychiatric Association. Diagnostic and Statistical Manual of Mental Disorders, 4th ed (DSM-IV). Washington, DC, American Psychiatric Association, 1994.

Depression Guidelines Panel. Depression in Primary Care. Vol 1: Treatment of Major Depression. Vol 2: Clinical Practice Guideline. (AHCPR Publication No. 93-0550 and 93-0551). Rockville, MD, U.S. Department of Health and Human Services, Agency for Health Care Policy and Research, 1993.

Schwenk TL, Coyne JC. Depression. In Rakel RE (ed). Textbook of Family Practice, 5th ed. Philadelphia, W.B. Saunders, 1996.

Sturm R, Wells KB: How can care for depression become more cost-effective? JAMA 1995;273:51–58.

QUESTIONS

1. Which of the following statements about the treatment of major depressive disorder is true?
   a. Joint psychotherapy and antidepressant treatment are contraindicated due to mutually exclusive objectives and occasional confounding interactions between these two approaches to depressed patients.
   b. An antidepressant should be started even if the physician has only a strong suspicion of major depressive disorder, before the diagnosis is fully explored.
   c. Matching the side effect profile of a specific antidepressant to the somatic complaints of a patient may improve the patient's compliance with therapy.
   d. Antidepressant therapy should be withdrawn as soon as the patient improves so as to decrease the risk of medication tolerance.
   e. Since depressed patients often suffer from feelings of worthlessness and low self-esteem, they should not be asked to complete specific assignments, such as contacting supportive friends, exercising, or reading about depression.

2. Drugs or substances commonly associated with depression include all of the following *except*:
   a. Oral contraceptives
   b. β blockers
   c. Alcohol
   d. Benzodiazepines
   e. Angiotensin converting enzyme inhibitors

Answers appear on **page 607**.

Chapter 78

Motor Vehicle Accident–Related Anxiety

Patrick O. Smith, Ph.D.

INITIAL VISIT

Subjective

PRESENTING PROBLEM. Lee E. is a 36-year-old divorced, state penal system inmate, African American man presenting to the inpatient Family Medicine Service (FMS) with a chronic open ulcer on the lower right leg.

PRESENT ILLNESS. The penal system staff has recognized Mr. E.'s chronic open ulcer on his lower right leg. The ulcer and an elevated glucose measurement have led to his admission. The ulcer has resulted from complications following a motorcycle accident at age 19; multiple orthopedic procedures led to the current chronic ulcer. Mr. E. complains of polydipsia and polyuria, and experiences numbness and paresthesia in his right leg. Diagnoses at the time of admission include hypertension, major depressive disorder, and schizophrenia. Initial insomnia, middle insomnia, nocturnal polyuria, unwanted awakenings, and nightmares have resulted in chronic sleep disturbance and poor sleep hygiene. With abrupt awakenings, he is frequently fearful and diaphoretic. After each awakening, a minimum of 45 minutes passes before sleep onset. When awakened by a nightmare, Mr. E. is frequently "crying and hollering." The content of his nightmares varies; however, he reports dreaming about his motorcycle accident. Mr. E. averages three awakenings per week with accident-related nightmares. During waking hours, Mr. E. experiences accident-related memories at least once per day. His accident memories are uninterruptable and lead to feelings of

worthlessness. He attributes his unemployment, polysubstance abuse, illegal activities, relationship problems, and subsequent prison sentence to his accident 17 years ago. Mr. E. reports no significant relationships in prison and that people make him nervous. One to two times a year, Mr. E. feels as though he is not part of this world. When reading, Mr. E. gets confused easily and must review the same material several times. Irritability and angry outbursts are his predominant emotions. Mr. E. has difficulty in showing loving feelings and feels close only to his mother. Mr. E. is very "jumpy" and is constantly fearful of being approached from behind. Loud unexpected noises really bother him. Thus, he constantly feels on guard and anxious.

PAST MEDICAL HISTORY. Mr. E. reports incurring severe injuries to both legs during a 1979 motorcycle accident with multiple subsequent orthopedic procedures and complications. Mr. E. describes unintentionally drinking a toxic chemical 2 years after his 1979 accident, resulting in unconsciousness and a several-day hospital stay. Mr. E. reports having a motor vehicle accident in 1983 resulting in minor abrasions. His diagnostic history includes hypertension, schizophrenia, and depression. Presently the ulcer on his lower leg is not healing and his glucose is significantly elevated.

FAMILY HISTORY. Mr. E.'s immediate family includes his mother, father, two brothers, and three sisters. All immediate family members are healthy, except his father, age 60, who is diagnosed with hypertension. Mr. E. is divorced with no children and considers his divorce a consequence of his polysubstance abuse.

HEALTH HABITS. Mr. E. smokes 6 to 7 cigarettes per day, is sedentary due to his leg injuries, and has a polysubstance (i.e., alcohol, marijuana, and crack cocaine) abuse history. He reports abstinence over the last 10 months, which is how long he has been in prison.

SOCIAL HISTORY. Mr. E. grew up in a small southern town while working in the logging industry for his father. He married at age 19 and moved to New Orleans where he worked as a truck driver. In 1979 while driving a motorcycle on an interstate highway, he recounts being struck by a car. The force of the impact threw him over an overpass bridge, severely injuring both legs. The leg injuries required surgery and chronic complications with his right leg continue to date. In his description of the accident, Mr. E. believes he is going to die as he flies over the overpass bridge. He describes severe depression and anxiety following the accident as he continued his employment. Eventually his physical and emotional difficulties led him to move back to his hometown and subsequent employment with his father. Mr. E.'s feelings of worthlessness have grown since he is not able to do his job because of his lower leg problems. Often Mr. E.'s leg prevents him from some activity, which leads to recurrent intrusive thoughts, which he finds difficult to interrupt. As a truck driver for his father he began using marijuana and alcohol to "feel better." Drinking alcohol and smoking marijuana relax him, reduce his initial insomnia, and help his "nerves." During this period his orthopedic complications worsened and led to a heel amputation. Subsequent rehabilitation led to a further reduction in his employment income and an increase in depression and anxiety. Mr. E. relates attempting to increase his income by handling stolen goods. While participating in this activity, he began smoking crack cocaine daily. He participated in illegal activities to support the habit. His spouse left him and he quit his job. Using cocaine and alcohol daily, Mr. E.'s lifestyle further complicated his physical problems. He reports that smoking crack alleviated the depression and the alcohol allowed uninterrupted sleep. Mr. E. points out that his combination of polysubstance abuse was expensive. Following three felony convictions, he was captured, prosecuted, and sentenced to 10 years in prison for shoplifting and receiving stolen goods. He is just completing 10 months of his 10-year sentence, which has recently been reduced to 5 years. Throughout his history following the motorcycle accident, Mr. E. reports continual sleep disturbances, motorcycle accident–based memories, nightmares, anxiety, depression, and chronic complications related to his lower leg. In the state penal environment he has no friends, but enjoys a spiritual component to his life and attends weekly church services. He looks forward to a release from prison, finding employment, studying the Big Book, and continuing involvement with Narcotics Anonymous for relapse prevention.

Objective

PHYSICAL EXAMINATION. Mr. E.'s vital signs are normal: temperature 98.1°F, pulse 90, respiration 18, blood pressure 140/60 mm Hg. Mr. E. is alert, oriented, and in no apparent distress. His head, neck, heart, lungs, and abdomen examinations are unremarkable. There is no cyanosis or swelling of his lower extremities. His leg lesion has good granulation tissue. His neurologic examination showed no focal deficits, but he did have decreased sensation to light touch and pain on the bottoms of both feet (signs of peripheral neuropathy). Motion and sensory examinations are otherwise normal.

LABORATORY TESTS. Mr. E.'s complete blood count is normal: white blood count 6.4 10^9/L, hematocrit 47.6%, and platelet count 214 10^9/L. Acetone is negative. His sodium 133 mEq/L, chloride 99 mEq/L, blood urea nitrogen 12 mg/dl, potassium 4.4 mEq/L, bicarbonate 21 mEq/L, and creatinine 1.1 mg/dl are normal. His urinalysis indicates glucose greater than 1000 mg/dl with no ketones.

Assessment

In synthesizing this presentation, consideration is given to several diagnoses to explain Mr. E.'s symptoms, signs, and laboratory assessment.

DIFFERENTIAL DIAGNOSIS

1. *Diabetes mellitus.* Mr. E.'s laboratory result of a glucose level greater than 1000 mg/dl confirms a diagnosis of diabetes mellitus. No evidence of ketones suggests adult (type II) diabetes, or non–insulin dependent diabetes.

2. *Hypertension.* Mr. E. presents with the diagnosis of hypertension controlled with nifedipine (Procardia). His blood pressure falls within the normal range and the FMS team maintains this diagnosis and the medication regimen.

3. *Schizophrenia.* Mr. E. is carrying a diagnosis of schizophrenia made 10 months ago following his incarceration. He is receiving two common drug types for the treatment of schizophrenia: dopamine receptor antagonist (perphenazine [Trilafon]) and an anticholinergic agent (trihexyphenidyl [Artane]). It is important to identify characteristic symptoms (namely, delusions, hallucinations, disorganized speech, disorganized or catatonic behavior, and negative symptoms) of schizophrenia in clinical interviewing to verify this diagnosis for treatment continuation. Mr. E. demonstrates no disorganization in speech or behavior. He reports a gradual and recent onset (i.e., several months) of numbing and tingling in his feet and legs. This could be mistaken as a distortion or exaggeration of perception (i.e., delusion); however, his newly developed diagnosis of diabetes mellitus rules out this self-report as a delusion. He describes infrequent (i.e., 1 to 2 per year) dissociative experiences over the last 10 or more years, in which he does not feel as if he is in touch with reality and is experiencing something other than reality. Commonly confused with hallucinations or bizarre delusions, dissociative experiences are qualitatively different in duration, frequency, intensity, and onset. He appears to have a flattening of affect, a common negative symptom of schizophrenia, but does not demonstrate a constricted range of affect. He reports a variation of mood from depressed to very depressed ever since his motorcycle accident. His report of constant alertness and fearfulness that something is going to happen to him may have been mistaken as a paranoid delusion. This report does not have the common delusional qualities. He is socially isolated and this can be construed as a negative symptom. Also, the neuroleptic medication can produce side effects that mimic negative symptoms of schizophrenia. Overall, Mr. E. believes his symptoms are related to his motorcycle accident and subsequent polydrug abuse. Mr. E's age at the time of initial diagnosis of schizophrenia (age 35 to 36) is unusually old. Additionally, 60 to 70 per cent of individuals with schizophrenia do not marry and Mr. E. has been married. An additional diagnostic clue for schizophrenia regards family history; Mr. E. has no confirmed first-degree relative with schizophrenia. From his symptom self-report, his accident history, and age of onset, it does not appear that Mr. E. suffers from schizophrenia. He does not clearly experience the characteristic symptoms for schizophrenia provided in the *Diagnostic and Statistical Manual of Mental Disorders*, fourth edition (DSM-IV), and other nonpsychotic diagnoses should be considered to explain his present chronic mood and anxiety symptoms.

4. *Major depressive disorder (MDD).* An obvious diagnostic consideration given Mr. E.'s self-report is major depressive disorder. Mr. E. reports receiving a diagnosis of MDD simultaneously with his schizophrenia diagnosis. He is currently receiving the tricyclic antidepressant amitriptyline (Elavil). In the examination Mr. E. presents some information relevant to the typical symptoms of a major depressive episode (namely, depressed mood, diminished interest in pleasurable activities, change in weight and appetite, insomnia/hypersomnia, psychomotor retardation or agitation, fatigue, feelings of worthlessness or guilt, diminished concentration abilities, and suicidal ideation). Mr. E. is frequently irritable and angry, but relates these emotions to anxiety, not sadness. He rates his mood as depressed more days than not since age 19. This duration is unusually long as a symptom of MDD and is more common in dysthymic disorder, for which the duration criterion for depressed mood is at least 2 years. His affect is not constricted (i.e., a reduction of experience within each emotion) but restricted in range (i.e., a reduction in the different moods experienced), and he experiences difficulty in having pleasurable moods. Typically, clinically depressed patients indicate a lack of affect range, rather than a restriction of affect experienced. Mr. E. does not seek previously enjoyable activities and attributes this symptom to his physical limitations and incarceration. Mr. E.'s present somatic complaints clearly relate to his medical conditions (open ulcer, diabetes mellitus, and hypertension) rather than to the typical body aches and pains reported by clinically depressed persons. Mr. E. reports no significant change in weight or his sexual or food appetites. He does confirm a sleep disturbance (initial and middle insomnia). Typically, in major depressive disorder middle and early insomnia are more common than initial insomnia. He denies hypersomnia. Mr. E. describes a jumpiness feeling which is unlike descriptions of agitated psychomotor symptoms, nor does he describe psychomotor retardation. Mr. E. complains of decreased energy/fatigue in association with his sleep disturbance. He does not report feelings of guilt, and does not have unrealistic evaluations of himself. He does complain of feelings of worthlessness, impaired concentration, and immediate and short-term memory difficulties. He denies suicidal ideation. Mr. E. reports some clear symptoms of a major depressive episode (namely, depressed mood, diminished interest in pleasurable activities, middle insomnia, feelings of worthlessness, and diminished concentration abilities); however, he does not meet the minimum number of symptoms to meet diagnostic criteria for MDD.

We do not consider Mr. E. to be suffering predominantly from a mood disturbance. Thus, we have ruled out psychotic or mood disturbances as our primary multiaxial diagnosis and consider the possibility of an anxiety disorder.

5. *Post-traumatic stress disorder (PTSD)*. The most important feature of Mr. E.'s self-report for our differential diagnosis of psychosocial problems is the description of his motorcycle accident 17 years ago. From this clue the FMS team considered a diagnosis of PTSD (Table 78–1). Mr. E. describes himself as experiencing extreme fear and being horrified that he was going to die during his motor-cycle accident. This event is characterized as traumatic (i.e., Criteria A, Table 78–1). Following this accident he persistently re-experienced the event through dreams, intrusive thoughts, and dissociative states (i.e., Criteria B, Table 78–1). During his description of the accident, Mr. E. demonstrates visible signs of anxiety and attempts to hurry the description, leaving out details. He reports extreme anxiety when riding or driving over interstate bridges and avoids motorcycles. He actively attempts to avoid thinking or talking about his accident to prevent having accident-related memories. Mr. E. tries distraction techniques to interrupt accident-related memories such as watching television, listening to

TABLE 78–1. Diagnostic Criteria for Post-traumatic Stress Disorder

A. The person has been exposed to a traumatic event in which both of the following were present:
    1. The person experienced, witnessed, or was confronted with an event or events that involved actual or threatened death or serious injury, or a threat to the physical integrity of self or others.
    2. The person's response involved intense fear, helplessness, or horror. *Note:* In children, this may be expressed instead by disorganized or agitated behavior.
B. The traumatic event is persistently re-experienced in one (or more) of the following ways:
    1. Recurrent and intrusive distressing recollections of the event, including images, thoughts, or perceptions. *Note:* In young children, repetitive play may occur in which themes or aspects of the trauma are expressed.
    2. Recurrent distressing dreams of the event. *Note:* In children, there may be frightening dreams without recognizable content.
    3. Acting or feeling as if the traumatic event were recurring (includes a sense of reliving the experience, illusions, hallucinations, and dissociative flashback episodes, including those that occur on awakening or when intoxicated). *Note:* In young children, trauma-specific re-enactment may occur.
    4. Intense psychological distress at exposure to internal or external cues that symbolize or resemble an aspect of the traumatic event.
C. Persistent avoidance of stimuli associated with the trauma and numbing of general responsiveness (not present before the trauma), as indicated by three (or more) of the following:
    1. Efforts to avoid thoughts, feelings, or conversations associated with the trauma.
    2. Efforts to avoid activities, places, or people that arouse recollections of the trauma.
    3. Inability to recall an important aspect of the trauma.
    4. Markedly diminished interest or participation in significant activities.
    5. Feeling of detachment or estrangement from others.
    6. Restricted range of affect (e.g., unable to have loving feelings).
    7. Sense of a foreshortened future (e.g., does not expect to have a career, marriage, children, or a normal life span).
D. Persistent symptoms of increased arousal (not present before the trauma), as indicated by two (or more) of the following:
    1. Difficulty falling or staying asleep.
    2. Irritability or outbursts of anger.
    3. Difficulty concentrating.
    4. Hypervigilance.
    5. Exaggerated startle response.
E. Duration of the disturbance (symptoms in Criteria B, C, and D) is more than 1 month.
F. The disturbance causes clinically significant distress or impairment in social, occupational, or other important areas of functioning.

Specifiy if:
Acute: if duration of symptoms is less than 3 months.
Chronic: if duration of symptoms is 3 months or more.
Specify if:
With delayed onset: if onset of symptoms is at least 6 months after the stressor.

From American Psychiatric Association. Diagnostic and Statistical Manual of Mental Disorders, 4th ed (DSM-IV). Washington, DC, American Psychiatric Association, 1994, with permission.

music, and reading. He describes a general feeling of "numbness" (i.e., a diminished responsiveness to the external world) and a diminished interest in previously pleasurable activities. He says he is unable to show loving feelings and feels as though he is detached from others. The range of emotions he feels is reduced and the emotions he experiences are negative (namely, anger, fear, and sadness). Hypervigilance is expressed by being constantly on guard and feeling uncomfortable in situations that he cannot control. He has initial and middle insomnia and nightmares related to his accident. Loud noises or surprises lead to an exaggerated startle response. He describes himself as irritable and this leads to angry outbursts. He has difficulty concentrating. Overall, these symptoms meet diagnostic criteria for PTSD, which was subsequently considered his primary multiaxial diagnosis, having ruled out schizophrenia and major depressive disorder.

Plan

DIAGNOSTIC. The FMS team continues treatment of Mr. E.'s hypertension and begins active treatment intervention for his diabetes mellitus. After ruling out Mr. E.'s previous diagnoses of schizophrenia and depression, he is diagnosed with PTSD.

THERAPEUTIC. Because Mr. E. is incarcerated, the FMS team expects his inpatient admission to be short and we do not expect to continue his outpatient care. Thus, we are treating his diabetes, hypertension, and tapering his neuroleptic and antiseizure medications. For his PTSD we are providing an intensive short-term patient education program and will make specific recommendations for a PTSD treatment regimen.

PATIENT EDUCATION. The FMS team is providing Mr. E. with information regarding the cause and course of his PTSD. We are using the two-factor model of learning to facilitate Mr. E.'s understanding of PTSD so he can realize what to expect with future treatment. We are supplying Mr. E. with clinical case examples similar to his to enhance his insight into PTSD. We are furnishing him with role-play experiences for clearly stating his symptoms to future clinicians to prevent misdiagnosis.

DISPOSITION. Mr. E. leaves the FMS with hypertension controlled and a diagnosis of diabetes mellitus. His ulcer is healing and he expresses an understanding of his present PTSD symptoms.

DISCUSSION

PTSD is very easy to misdiagnose due to avoidance by those who suffer from the disorder. Mr. E.'s case highlights the fact that, other than acute stress disorder, there is no other DSM-IV diagnosis that considers traumatic events as a diagnostic criterion. There are a variety of event categories that can be characterized as traumatic (i.e., combat, civilian combat, motor vehicle accidents (MVA), physical assault, sexual assault, and natural disasters). This case is an example of untreated PTSD resulting from an MVA which has gone undiagnosed or misdiagnosed for 17 years.

Motor vehicle accidents represent one of the most prevalent and underdiagnosed human-origin traumas. The costs related to MVA are staggering ($137 billion for 1992), and unfortunately, there was a scarcity of research reported on the relationship between MVA and PTSD until the 1980s. The growing body of MVA–PTSD research addresses psychophysiologic correlates, predictors, prevalence, treatment recommendations, and subcategories of PTSD.

In Mr. E.'s case, we conceptualized his PTSD and our treatment recommendations on Mowrer's two-factor model. Fundamentally, Mowrer's two-factor model proposes that anxiety/fear is classically conditioned and maintained by means of operant conditioning. Mr. E.'s MVA represented an unconditioned stimulus (UCS), which evoked an unconditioned response (UCR: namely, fear). A strong association (classical conditioning) was learned between the UCS and incidental stimuli (conditioned stimuli [CS]: interstate highway, overpass bridge, motorcycle, and driving conditions). Following the event, Mr. E. experienced the conditioned response ([CR] i.e., fear) in relation to exposure to the CS. He learned that fear could be reduced by avoidance or escape. He developed several strategies for using avoidance or escape to prevent prolonged exposure to the CS and subsequent fear. Polysubstance abuse, constricted affect, and dissociative states are common examples of avoidance or escape strategies to reduce cue-reactive anxiety in persons with PTSD.

Several investigators have attempted to elucidate predictors for who will develop PTSD following an MVA. At present, severity of stressor, degree of stressor exposure, perception of bodily injury, severity of bodily injury, prior trauma, and prior diagnosable depression are predictors being considered; however, no agreement has been reached about these variables. There are some researchers who suggest that unconsciousness and amnesia during the traumatic event may provide protection from development of PTSD. Mr. E. was not unconscious during his accident and remembers the accident in vivid detail.

In our assessment of Mr. E., he provided a thorough history in which we used a semi-structured mental health examination given his previous diagnosed conditions (depression and schizophrenia). Mr. E.'s case highlights the importance of effective interviewing techniques in gathering a detailed history. Often, patients with PTSD prefer to avoid discussion of traumatic events owing to the arousal associated with those verbal discussions. Thus, as in Mr. E.'s case, it was critical to establish an effective patient–physician rapport to assess trauma history. Mr. E. had revealed his dissociative experiences, hypervigilance, sleep disturbance, mood variations, paresthesias, and polysubstance abuse to clinicians who interpreted his descriptions as clusters of negative and positive symptoms of schizophrenia with a secondary diagnosis of major depressive disorder.

The first step in PTSD treatment for Mr. E. included intensive patient education, including an explanation of the conditioning factors that led to his present signs and symptoms. We provided the referring facility with a recommendation of exposure-based therapy in combination with pharmacotherapy. We emphasized the importance of selecting a clinician who is skilled in deconditioning techniques. Exposure-based therapy is the systematic delivery of fear-evoking stimuli (i.e., in vivo or imaginal) without allowing escape or avoidance from the feared stimuli. This form of therapy is based on extinction or deconditioning and is particularly effective for the reduction of re-experiencing symptoms (i.e., Criteria B in Table 78–1). In some cases the symptoms of Criteria C (Table 78–1), which are more treatment resistant, typically require pharmacotherapy. Selective serotonin reuptake inhibitors or tricyclic antidepressants are recommended for this treatment component.

Prognosis

Mr. E. may experience a significant reduction in re-experiencing and avoidance symptoms provided that he receives a systematic multimodal intervention while incarcerated.

SUGGESTED READING

Blanchard EB, Hickling EJ, Taylor AE, et al. Who develops PTSD from motor vehicle accidents? Behav Res Ther 1996;34:1–10.

Bryant RA, Harvey AG. Initial posttraumatic stress responses following motor vehicle accidents. J Traum Stress 1996;9:223–234.

de L Horne, DJ. Traumatic stress reactions to motor vehicle accidents. In Wilson JP, Raphael B (eds). International Handbook of Traumatic Stress Syndromes. New York, Plenum Press, 1993 pp 499–506.

Mowrer OH. On the dual nature of learning: A reinterpretation of "conditioning" and "problem-solving." Harvard Educ Rev 1947;17:102–148.

Solomon SD, Gerrity ET, Muff AM. Efficacy of treatments for posttraumatic stress disorder: An empirical review. JAMA 1992;268:633–638.

Taylor S, Koch WJ. Anxiety disorders due to motor vehicle accidents: Nature and treatment. Clin Psychol Rev 1995;15:721–738.

QUESTIONS

1. What is the major difference between post-traumatic stress disorder and chronic anxiety disorders?
   a. Delayed onset
   b. Evidence of a traumatic event
   c. Evidence of a horrific traumatic event and flashbacks
   d. Hallucinations and hypervigilance
   e. Dissociative states and sleep disturbance

2. Which combinations of treatment are effective with post-traumatic stress disorder?

   a. Systematic desensitization and direct exposure therapy
   b. Direct exposure therapy and operant conditioning
   c. Antidepressant pharmacotherapy and systematic desensitization
   d. Neuroleptic pharmacotherapy and direct exposure therapy
   e. Direct exposure therapy and antidepressant pharmacotherapy

3. Which group of events best represents potentially traumatic events?

a. Motor vehicle accidents, funeral, tornado, being held up at gunpoint
b. Combat, flood, motor vehicle accidents, rape, mid-air explosion kills loved one
c. Physical assault, sexual assault, bankruptcy, motor vehicle accidents, hurricane

d. Motor vehicle accidents, long-term illness, incest victim, armed robbery
e. Sexual assault, physical assault, motor vehicle accident, natural disaster, combat

Answers appear on **page 607.**

Chapter **79**

Domestic Violence

L. Kevin Hamberger, Ph.D.

INITIAL VISIT

Subjective

Marietta P. is a 33-year-old white, married woman. She comes to the clinic for help with a "stress problem" which adversely affects her work as a file clerk. Adverse effects include tardiness, excessive absenteeism, and inefficiency and friction with co-workers. In addition, the patient states that her marriage is also suffering. In particular, the patient states she does not enjoy sexual relations, and is afraid her husband will leave her if she does not "get a grip."

Assessment of stress symptoms revealed the following picture: sleep-onset insomnia, with occasional sleep-interruption insomnia, the patient averaging about 5 hours of sleep per night. Marietta reports feeling little energy, and a poor appetite, although she forces herself to eat. She reports feeling "shaky inside," difficulty sitting still, feeling "nervous a lot," and frequently concerned that something bad is about to happen. She denies suicidal plans, but at times wishes she could just "go to sleep and not wake up." She reports feeling irritable and having frequent arguments with her coworkers and husband. At work, she is often tired and has difficulty performing her duties, resulting in criticism from her supervisors, complaints from

coworkers, and threats of disciplinary action. Arguments with her husband focus primarily on disagreements about sex, particularly frequency. Frequency of sexual intercourse is estimated as once every 4 months. She states that her husband has at times threatened to "go elsewhere for sex," and to end the relationship if she does not give him sex. In addition, she stated that, on occasion, he just "takes it."

PAST HISTORY. The patient states that her symptoms have persisted for about 2.5 years. They are not associated with any specific stressor that she can identify. The symptoms have steadily gotten worse over time. She has been married for 6 years. She describes her marriage as "difficult," due to sexual incompatibility. Relationship stress has been getting worse over the past 3 years, with occasional severe fights and one separation which lasted for 3 months. Her husband has threatened to leave her if she does not "get more interested in sex." Frequency of forced sex was reported to be about two times per year. At other times, their fights have "become physical." Frequency of physical fights is estimated at about three times per year, and includes throwing food, pushing, slapping, punching. Frequency has been stable over time, but severity is estimated to have increased. Alcohol and drugs are not viewed

571

as contributory factors, as neither partner is reported to drink or use street drugs.

Objective

PHYSICAL EXAMINATION. Marietta is a well-nourished female; height 5 feet 3 inches, weight 123 lb, respiratory rate 60, blood pressure 120/75 mm Hg, temperature 98.6°F. Physical examination and laboratory studies revealed no abnormalities.

Assessment

DIFFERENTIAL DIAGNOSIS. The most likely diagnosis for this patient is that she is a domestic violence victim. The correct International Classification of Diseases, ninth edition, (ICD-9) code is Adult Maltreatment Syndrome (995.81). Subcategories include Battered Person Syndrome, NEC (not elsewhere classifiable); Spouse, Woman. The most obvious reason for this diagnosis is the fact that the patient reports being forced to have sex with her partner, both physically and through psychological coercion. These assaults occur at a rate of two per year. In addition, she reports physical assaults at a rate of three times per year. Therefore, violence in the life of this young woman must be seen as fundamental to all other symptoms she reports. All other diagnoses, no matter how classically correct (and assuming no pathophysiology), must be viewed as secondary to the traumatic victimization.

Marietta has many symptoms of dysthymic disorder and generalized anxiety disorder. Symptoms of dysthymic disorder include sleep disturbances, appetite problems, inhibited sexual desire, and feelings of hopelessness accentuated by intermittent desires to die (although no active suicidal ideation). Duration of symptoms and the lack of a specific precipitating event also are consistent with a diagnosis of dysthymic disorder. On the other hand, duration of violence history appears to coincide with duration of symptoms. In addition, victims of ongoing trauma frequently exhibit symptoms of depression. Therefore, such a diagnosis should be entertained, but only with caution.

Generalized anxiety disorder also involves symptoms consistent with those presented by the patient. These include tremulousness, easy fatigability, difficulty sleeping, feeling on edge and apprehensive. In addition, Marietta feels worried about two life circumstances, namely, her job and her marriage. However, in this case, her fears are not unrealistic, nor necessarily excessive, as would be required for a diagnosis of generalized anxiety disorder. Her fatigue and preoccupation with abuse and trauma may actually interfere with her ability to perform her job functions adequately. In addition, her husband's physical and sexual abuse, coupled with threats to leave her, poses a real threat to the integrity of her marriage.

Hypoactive sexual desire disorder or sexual aversion disorder may also be part of the diagnostic picture. The patient appears to have very little interest in sexual activity and, indeed, seems to avoid virtually all sexual contact with her partner. Given the relationship context of sexual and physical violence to which this patient is subjected, these diagnoses would be inappropriate. The lack of sexual desire is a reasonable response to her husband's aggression.

Plan

1. *Offer support.* Tell Marietta that the physical and sexual abuse is not her fault, that abuse is always wrong and she does not deserve it, and that help is available.

2. *Conduct safety planning.* Given the severity of violence, which appears to be increasing, concern is expressed to the patient about her safety. The patient reports feeling safe going home today, but is fearful of violence recurring at some point in the near future. She is provided information about a local resource, the Domestic Abuse Project (DAP), including where to locate its number in the phone book. DAP services, including emergency shelter, legal advocacy, and support meetings, are described. Marietta refuses to take a pamphlet home, but does agree to read it in the office before leaving. She also states that she will call the DAP to inquire further about its services. In addition, she is assured that information provided by her will not be disclosed to her partner, unless she specifically requests and authorizes such release.

3. *Identify an emergency escape plan.* Marietta is informed of the state mandatory arrest law for domestic violence. She states that she will call police in the event of another physical or sexual assault. She does not have friends or family in the area she can go to for emergency shelter. If needed, she will use DAP services.

4. *At 1-week follow-up.* Review safety concerns, refine safety plan, and complete assessment of violence history.

5. *Physical examination.* Obtain follow-up information to complete the physical examination.

DISCUSSION

The present case illustrates case-finding for partner violence. Marietta did not directly communicate that she has been battered. Instead, she presented symptoms related to anxiety and depression. In addition, she presented evidence of relationship problems because of sexual avoidance. In research, battered women, compared with nonbattered women in a family medicine practice, were significantly more likely to be diagnosed as depressed. This finding is consistent with the often-stated "profile" of battered women as likely to present with vague somatic complaints, insomnia, irritability, and musculoskeletal pain. Taken as a whole, these symptoms could add up to a diagnosis of depression or anxiety. In addition, the pattern of sexual avoidance and aversion suggests that the relationship may be distressed. Research has shown that, compared with nonbattered women, battered women rate their marriages as significantly more distressed.

Marietta also presented important clues, through her statements to the physician, that her relationship is severely distressed and that her partner is coercive, both sexually and physically. Specifically, she stated that her partner threatened to go elsewhere for sexual activity if she did not provide it to him. In addition, she described physical coercion when she stated that on some occasions he would "just take it." These statements are clear indicators that the patient is at risk, and demand further inquiry.

When given information in small, seemingly unconnected chunks by patients, the task of the family physician is to pull these pieces of information together into a coherent conceptualization. In the present case, although the patient exhibited symptoms of anxiety, depression, and sexual dysfunction, a comprehensive conceptualization of her situation requires the further step of exploring what may underlie these dysphoric symptoms. Specifically her physician used knowledge of domestic violence in medical settings to cue further consideration and inquiry about partner violence in assessing the patient. Areas of knowledge relied on in this case include the facts that (1) rates of partner violence in family medicine clinics are around 25 per cent; (2) violent relationships are frequently highly stressed; (3) battered women frequently present a number of vague somatic complaints reminiscent of depression and anxiety; and (4) battered women rarely directly report their victimization.

To maximize the probability of a positive patient response to inquiry about abuse, the physician presented the conceptualization in a manner that included all of the relevant information provided by the patient herself. In this case, such an inquiry would appear as follows: "When I hear you tell me your partner 'just takes' sex, and at other times uses threats to get you to have sex, I've learned to be concerned. In addition to forcing sex, are you currently in a situation where your partner uses other types of force to get you to do things that you otherwise would not? For example, has he ever laid a hand on you in any other way, such as a push, shove, or slap?"

The diagnostic plan, as used in the case study, should include the following elements.

1. *Offer support.* Positive responses to the inquiry in the previous paragraph led to five important interventions. First, the patient was told, unequivocally, that she did not deserve to be abused in any way, and that she deserved to feel safe in her home. This exoneration and statement of support is important because it may be the first time anyone has told her that it was not her fault to be physically and sexually assaulted. In most violent relationships, the abusive partner repeatedly tells the victim that the violence is her fault, avoidable if only she would change her behavior. To be exonerated and supported by an important outside helper begins emotional healing and identifies the physician as a credible potential helper. Another supportive communication from the physician was the assurance that Marietta's concerns would not be disclosed to her partner. Secrecy and isolation are very important to abusive men to facilitate maintenance of control and domination. Inappropriate disclosure of the "secret," for example confronting the abuser, may result in more violence against the victim. Therefore, confidentiality, particularly from the abusive partner, is of paramount importance.

2. *Conduct safety planning.* The physician began the process of evaluating safety by soliciting the patient's concerns about returning home that day. In addition, the physician understood from prior training that a number of factors have been associated with highly dangerous and potentially lethal relationship violence. These include history of attempted or actual sexual assault, increasing violence severity, high violence frequency, use of intoxicants by the abuser, threats by the abuser to kill the woman, and suicidal ideation and attempts by the woman. Although Marietta did not exhibit all of these lethality indicators, those she did express caused appropriate concern, leading to preliminary safety planning.

3. *Identify resources.* In addition, the physician dis-

cussed local resources for battered women. These included identification of the local battered women's shelter and its many services, how to find the shelter number in the phone book, the availability of legal advocacy services, and the local mandatory arrest law in the event of future violence. The DAP was also identified as a resource for continuation of safety planning and problem solving in an emotionally supportive, safe, and confidential setting. Battered women greatly value the ability of their physician to provide them with resource information. Therefore, it is important for physicians to know about local resources, as well as laws regarding partner violence.

4. *Schedule follow-up visits.* The patient was scheduled for follow-up. The follow-up interval was brief—1 week—owing to the serious nature of the violence in this case. Cases of less severe violence may warrant follow-up intervals of longer duration, but should not exceed 1 month. During the follow-up interval, the patient should be encouraged to follow through on referrals, work on safety plans and any other mutually agreed-on activity. Follow-ups should continue until the patient has developed other supportive resources.

5. *Document findings.* The physician should document findings, such as the victim's report of the violence, including quotes where possible. Physician observations of injuries, behavior, and mental status as related to the violence should be included. Also, assessment of danger, safety planning, and follow-up plans are part of documentation. The documented medical record may be the only official record of her history of victimization. Such a record may be valuable in subsequent legal proceedings validating her claims of abuse.

Women victims of partner violence are not rare in family practice settings. Our research has determined that about one in four adult female patients reported an incident of partner violence in the past year. Nearly 40 per cent reported victimization at some time in their adult life. Therefore, family physicians must be prepared to identify partner violence and assist victims, once identified. Historically, many barriers have prevented adequate response to partner violence. These barriers include those originating with patients and those originating from physicians.

Patient barriers include denial, fear, shame, and a sense of futility that disclosure of their situation will result in meaningful assistance. With respect to denial, many battered women do not view the violence against them as "abuse" or "violence." Reasons for this are many, but often are related to stereotypes about "battered" or "abused" women that a particular patient may not accept within herself. She may also feel ashamed of what is happening to her, as she has been told by her abusive partner that the violence is her fault. Therefore, the partner's admitting violence against her is tantamount to his exposing all the "faults" he has convinced her she possesses. Further, she must overcome the belief that she does not deserve to be helped, since the violence is accepted as her fault. In addition, although many battered women reach out for help, they are often met with disbelief, indifference, or blame for their plight, and are encouraged to patch things up with their abusive partner. Therefore, battered women often develop a sense that physicians and others are unwilling or unable to help them. These factors may combine to keep the woman from directly reporting battering.

Physician barriers include lack of time, lack of skill in handling the problem of partner violence, feelings of powerlessness to immediately resolve the problem, and adherence to a biomedical model of health care. These barriers are all related, in various ways, to lack of education about the dynamics of partner violence, how to ask about and assess partner violence, and what to do after violence has been identified.

For example, in the present case, adherence to a biomedical model and failure to uncover factors underlying Marietta's anxiety, depression, and sexual avoidance led to less than complete, and even dangerous, intervention for the patient. In particular, diagnosing the patient as anxious and depressed may result in prescribing medications only. Such medications may reduce the patient's coping capacity by reducing reaction time and clear thinking. She may be less able to think out safety plans and other escape strategies to avoid further violence. Using medication for her anxiety about violence also communicates the subtle but powerful message that her symptoms represent a deficit within herself rather than being caused by an abusive partner who has created a terrifying environment. Further, diagnosing her report of sexual avoidance as a sexual dysfunction could lead to referral for marital or sex therapy. Under such a scenario, she also becomes diagnosed and conceptualized as having the problem. The traditional marital therapy approach is to assign equivalent levels of responsibility for problems to both partners, and frequently conceptualizes violence as a symptom of the communication problems in the relationship. Marital and sex therapy would therefore reinforce her responsibility for relationship problems, including the violence against her. She would be encouraged to engage in exercises designed to increase her "communication" and amenability for sex, without adequately addressing her safety or her partner's abusive and controlling tendencies.

The biopsychosocial model of family medicine is ideally suited to facilitate appropriate identification and intervention into partner violence among women victims who are also patients. The model goes beyond simple diagnosis and treatment of illnesses and requires assessment of contextual and underlying factors. Conversely, as this case illustrates, physicians are not required to solve all the patient's problems. Rather, the physician's responsibility is to ask appropriate questions, provide appropriate information and support, encourage the patient to take steps to increase her safety, and allow the patient to ultimately choose her own course of action. Such an approach is consistent with ethical principles of doing good for our patients, as well as doing no harm.

SUGGESTED READING

Ambuel B, Hamberger LK, Lahti J. Partner violence: A systematic approach to identification and intervention in outpatient health care. *Wis Med J* 1996;95:292–297.

Elliott BA, Johnson MMP. Domestic violence in primary care settings: Patterns and prevalence. *Arch Fam Med* 1994;4:113–119.

Hamberger LK, Saunders DG, Hovey M. Prevalence of domestic violence in community practice and rate of physician inquiry. *Fam Med* 1992;24:283–287.

Saunders DG, Hamberger LK, Hovey M. Indicators of woman abuse based on a chart review at a family practice center. *Arch Fam Med* 1993;2:537–543.

Sugg NK, Inui T. Primary care physicians' response to domestic violence: Opening Pandora's box. *JAMA* 1992;267:3157–3160.

QUESTIONS

1. Research in family practice settings has found that the rate of partner violence in the 1990s among women patients is:
   a. 15%
   b. 7%
   c. 45%
   d. 25%

2. Research has shown that compared with nonbattered women, battered women are more likely to be diagnosed with:
   a. Generalized anxiety disorder
   b. Alcoholism
   c. Depression
   d. Tobacco abuse

3. One major barrier to disclosure experienced by battered women is:
   a. Shame
   b. Masochism
   c. Depression
   d. Lack of skill

Answers appear on **page 607.**

Chapter 80

Memory Loss

Richard E. Finlayson, M.D.

INITIAL VISIT

Subjective

PATIENT IDENTIFICATION. Martha T. is a 66-year-old single, white, retired public schoolteacher accompanied by a concerned friend.

PRESENTING PROBLEM. Memory problems have developed after the death of Martha's mother 6 months ago. In addition, she has continued to grieve and feel "very depressed" about her loss.

PRESENT ILLNESS. Martha's mother had come to live with her 16 years ago after Martha's father died. Her mother died at age 86 as the result of a myocardial infarction. In the days after the funeral, Martha had much difficulty with sleep and her brother, a physician, wrote a prescription for lorazepam (Ativan), a benzodiazepine, taken as a single 2-mg tablet at bedtime as needed. One tablet nightly was enough initially, but she later took two once or twice a week. At this time, she is using the lorazepam five to six nights per week. Her sleep is still interrupted by waking periods and it is difficult for her to get back to sleep. She has anorexia without weight loss, lacks energy, and is withdrawn, but she says that she has some interest in doing things if she can "just get going." She denies feeling anger about her mother's death, hostility toward her mother, guilt feelings, or suicidal thoughts.

A collaborative history is very helpful in assessing psychopathology, especially in the elderly. Martha's friend, Catherine stated that a few days ago the telephone company shut off Martha's service because she forgot to pay the bill. Catherine said that she had noted these memory problems for about a year before Martha's mother died, but they are "much worse now." Catherine also noted that Martha had difficulty in "finding the right words to say" in everyday conversation.

Martha told her friend that she had fallen at home twice within recent weeks, but Catherine said that Martha did not strike her head or seem to have a serious injury.

PAST MEDICAL HISTORY. Martha has enjoyed generally good health. She has essential hypertension, diagnosed at age 42, for which she takes a thiazide diuretic daily and follows a no-salt-added diet.

FAMILY HISTORY. Her mother had maturity-onset diabetes mellitus, hypertension, and memory problems. Her grandmother died in a public mental institution because of "senility" caused by "hardening of the arteries." Her father died at age 72 as a result of prostate cancer. Martha's brother is well at age 64, but he was treated for depression after his first wife died.

HEALTH HABITS. Martha has been moderate in her approach to activity, diet, and recreation. She likes to go for daily walks, but she has done little of this since her mother died. Alcohol use is minimal. She does not use tobacco.

SOCIAL HISTORY. Martha likes to care for her small yard and vegetable garden. Her neighbors are friendly, but she has not been particularly close to any of them. She belongs to and attends a church, but she is not active in any of its organizations or special activities. Her nearest relative, her brother, lives about 200 miles away.

REVIEW OF SYSTEMS. Martha has a dull discomfort in her head and says that thinking is difficult. The discomfort is not relieved by analgesics such as aspirin. She is also constipated because, as she explains, "I just do not eat right these days."

Objective

PHYSICAL EXAMINATION. Martha's height is 66 inches, weight 132 lb, blood pressure (sitting) 164/92 mm Hg, pulse rate 84 with regular rhythm. The positive findings on the physical examination include a grade 1 hypertensive retinopathy and a faint bruit over the left carotid bifurcation. Resolving ecchymoses were noted over the right elbow and forearm and left hip area. The lung fields are clear, and heart sounds and rhythm are within normal limits. The results of neurologic examination are normal.

LABORATORY TESTS. Results of blood tests and urinalysis are normal. The chest radiograph reveals mild cardiomegaly.

MENTAL STATUS EXAMINATION. Martha's posture is somewhat slumped and eye contact is fair. Her speech is slurred (dysarthria). She seems to have difficulty finding words to express her thoughts (anomia). Her affect is moderately flat. The underlying mood is depressed. Psychomotor activity is moderately slowed. Depressive themes are noted in her thinking, but she is not psychotic or suicidal.

The Mini-Mental Status Examination (Folstein et al., 1975) was scored as 23/30, with deficiencies being noted in orientation to time, arithmetic, short-term memory, and naming objects.

Assessment

DIFFERENTIAL DIAGNOSIS. This elderly woman presents with symptoms common to several disorders that are frequently seen alone or in combination in her age group.

1. *Dementia.* Of persons this age who have dementia, dementia of the Alzheimer type (DAT) represents 50 to 60 per cent, whereas vascular dementia (VAD) (formerly multi-infarct dementia) occurs in about 15 per cent (estimates vary greatly), and the remaining persons have various, less common conditions (Table 80–1). In Martha's case, VAD must be considered because of the history of hypertension, although it is unusual for the syndrome to occur apart from evidence of past or current cerebrovascular accidents. Table 80–2 describes a basic dementia work-up, to be supplemented by specialty consultation and additional tests, as recommended.

2. *Depression.* Martha's symptoms also suggest major depression. It is well to remember that it is common for persons with bereavement such as

TABLE 80–1. Categories of Dementia Based on Reversibility: Some Causes and Disorders

Causes That Can Be Removed or Reversed
Intoxications
　Prescription drugs
　Illicit drugs
　Carbon monoxide
　Heavy metals
　Drug combinations
Infections
　Any agent capable of affecting brain
Metabolic disorders
　Endocrinopathies
　Encephalopathy of renal or hepatic failure
　Wilson disease
Nutritional disorders
　Thiamine deficiency
　Folate deficiency
　Niacin deficiency
Vascular disorders
　Hypertension
　Atherosclerosis
　Vasculitis
　Embolic disease
　Cardiac disease
Space-occupying lesions
　Chronic subdural hematoma
　Brain tumor
　Affective disorders

Progressive Degenerative Diseases
Without important neurologic findings other than dementia
　Alzheimer disease
　Pick disease
With important neurologic findings, with or without dementia
　Parkinson disease
　Huntington disease
　Progressive supranuclear palsy
Many others

From Finlayson RE. Dementia. In Rakel RE (ed). Textbook of Family Practice, 5th ed. Philadelphia, W.B. Saunders Company, 1995, pp 1531–1536.

Martha's to develop a depressive illness. The history of her brother having had a depressive illness in response to similar loss suggests a possible familial vulnerability for affective illness. The diagnosis of depression should not be seen as excluding dementia because it has been reported that about 30 per cent of persons with DAT also develop a syndrome of depression. In most practice situations, the diagnosis of depression is based on the history and mental status examination.

3. *Pathologic grief.* Although this should be considered in any case in which psychopathology accompanies bereavement, the history in this case does not suggest this diagnosis. Symptoms consistent with this condition are hostility toward the deceased or other

TABLE 80–2. Standard Diagnostic Studies for New-onset Dementia

---

Complete blood cell count
Electrolyte panel
Screening metabolic panel
Thyroid function tests
Vitamin B_{12} and folate levels
Tests for syphilis and, depending on history, for human
    immunodeficiency virus
Urinalysis
Electrocardiogram
Chest radiograph

From Finlayson RE. Dementia. In Rakel RE (ed). Textbook of Family Practice, 5th ed. Philadelphia, W.B. Saunders Company, 1995, pp 1531–1536.

person closely related to the death, overidentification with the deceased, having symptoms like those of the deceased's final illness, failure to mourn or process feelings (seeming to be too happy or euphoric), and giving away possessions in a reckless or foolish fashion. Pathologic grief usually requires active intervention with grief counseling and sometimes psychotherapy.

4. *Drug intoxication.* Drug intoxication is suggested as a possibility by the history of the patient having taken a benzodiazepine for much of the course of her recent illness. Even though Martha may not have misused this drug in a major way, it would have the potential for causing a depressed mood, memory difficulty, and falls. A toxicology screen would not be particularly helpful in Martha's case unless other drug or alcohol use is not acknowledged but suspected.

Plan

DIAGNOSTIC

1. Chemistry panel, Pap smear, thyroid function tests, vitamin B_{12} and folate levels, tests for syphilis, and electrocardiogram.

2. Minnesota Multiphasic Personality Inventory.

3. Neurologic and psychiatric consultation.

THERAPEUTIC

1. Martha's friend, Catherine, who is a widow, offered to stay with her to provide domestic help and psychological support.

2. Lorazepam will be tapered with medical supervision during 2 weeks.

PATIENT EDUCATION

1. The symptoms are possibly the result of many factors (e.g., bereavement, depression, medication, possibly an undiagnosed medical disorder).

2. Possible complications of the lorazepam taper include tremors, fast pulse or palpitations, excessive sweating, diarrhea, and a feeling of anxiety and insomnia. In severe cases of withdrawal, seizures or delirium (or both) may be experienced.

DISPOSITION. Martha will return every 3 to 4 days for assessment of the progress of the drug taper, monitoring of her mental status, vital sign checks, and supportive counseling. The next full visit for summarization of diagnostic studies and additional treatment recommendations is in 4 weeks.

FOLLOW-UP VISIT

Subjective

Martha returns in 4 weeks for a follow-up visit. She has tolerated the drug withdrawal fairly well. She has, however, experienced a worsening of her insomnia and her mood is more depressed. She continues to process her grief quite well.

Objective

Martha's blood pressure is 172/96 mm Hg. The only laboratory abnormality is a creatinine value of 1.2 mg/dl. The electrocardiogram reveals left-axis deviation. The neurologic and psychiatric consultations, supported by magnetic resonance imaging of the head, electroencephalography, and psychological testing, suggest the presence of generalized organic cerebral impairment (e.g., as evidenced by deficits in memory, language, abstract reasoning, and constructional ability). No evidence of focal neurologic disease is found. A depressive disorder does not adequately explain the extent of her cognitive problems. The psychiatric consultant, however, recommended a trial of an antidepressant and ongoing psychosocial support.

Assessment

Martha's affective state has worsened. This is not explained by normal grief. A drug abstinence syndrome seems unlikely. Her blood pressure has increased and better control is needed. The work-up to date has not revealed another medical disorder to explain her symptoms. VAD seems unlikely because of the clinical course and laboratory findings. DAT is the most likely primary explanation for her cognitive problems. Depressive symptoms are common in DAT, but some persons may also have major depression as a primary illness occurring in combination with DAT. Both are commonly distributed in the general population.

Plan

DIAGNOSTIC. No additional tests are planned at this time.

THERAPEUTIC

1. Start on the selective serotonin reuptake inhibitor (SSRI) antidepressant sertraline (Zoloft), 25 mg daily (one half of a 50 mg tablet). A tricyclic antidepressant is best avoided in this case because of the risk of confusion and postural hypotension complicating Martha's cardiovascular status. Discuss potential side effects of sertraline. Add trazodone (Desyrel) 25 to 75 mg at bedtime if sleep does not improve on sertraline.

2. Salt restriction is increased and the dose of the thiazide diuretic is increased.

3. Have Martha report her initial response to sertraline by telephone in 2 days.

DISPOSITION. A conference with Martha, her brother, and a social worker from county social services is arranged. The goal of the meeting is to discuss the implications of Martha's diagnoses and what community resources are available to her and her family in coping with illness and aging issues. The next visit to the clinic is in 2 weeks.

DISCUSSION

The elderly, compared with younger persons, are more likely to present to a physician with diverse symptoms that do not lead to a specific diagnosis or define a "case." This is particularly so with the syndrome of dementia, as Martha's history illustrates. Her very earliest symptom, as reported by her friend, was memory loss and language difficulty. It may be difficult to differentiate the early stages of dementia from "age-associated memory impairment" (Crook et al., 1986). This latter phenomenon is experienced by most people as they age and is accepted as normal because the frequency and intensity of memory lapses do not seriously interfere with life.

Affective symptoms may be the first observed evidence of a dementing illness. This is particularly true with so-called subcortical dementia (Albert et al., 1974). This syndrome has been linked to various diseases (including progressive supranuclear palsy, Huntington disease, Jakob-Creutzfeldt disease, Parkinson disease, lacunar state, human immunodeficiency virus dementia, and others). The earliest symptoms may include apathy, slowed thinking, depressive moods, restlessness, insomnia, and somatic complaints that may reflect a disturbed affective state. DAT has been identified as a "cortical dementia" but this distinction from subcortical is controversial. The important point is that affective symptoms arising from various causes may contribute in a significant way at any stage to the manifestations of dementia. Because of their diverse characteristics, affective symptoms alone do not easily lead to or provide a basis for a diagnosis of dementia. Affective symptoms may of course represent a psychological response to stress, a primary affective disorder, or an affective disorder secondary to another medical illness.

The scope of personality changes seen in dementia is broad. Personality traits that seemed adaptive, or at least were well tolerated by others, may become exaggerated and cause considerable social tension. Sometimes one observes what seems to be a complete reversal of personality. In Martha's case it was noted that she had been a rather private person, close to her mother, but with little interaction with the community. This became exaggerated during her illness.

The clinical history is the single most important source of information in the diagnosis of dementia. An awareness of the wide range of psychobehavioral disturbances and diverse causes is essential to accurate diagnosis. For example, in an older person treatment of a psychological disturbance or pain with benzodiazepines, barbiturates, narcotics, or other central nervous system depressants occasionally unmasks an underlying, previously unrecognized dementia. There were clues in this case study for affective illness and for dementia. Both disorders may be present. Major depression, when accompanied by overt cognitive problems, may mimic dementia. The history that the brother had been treated for depression in similar circumstances should raise that diagnostic possibility. There is evidence of genetic vulnerability for some types of affective illness and dementia. The history that Martha's grandmother had died as a result of

TABLE 80–3.   DSM-IV Diagnostic Criteria for Dementia of the Alzheimer Type

A. The development of multiple cognitive deficits manifested by both
  1. Memory impairment (impaired ability to learn new information or to recall previously learned information)
  2. One (or more) of the following cognitive disturbances:
      a. Aphasia (language disturbance)
      b. Apraxia (impaired ability to carry out motor activities despite intact motor function)
      c. Agnosia (failure to recognize or identify objects despite intact sensory function)
      d. Disturbance in executive functioning (i.e., planning, organizing, sequencing, abstracting)
B. The cognitive deficits in Criteria A1 and A2 each cause significant impairment in social or occupational functioning and represent a significant decline from a previous level of functioning.
C. The course is characterized by gradual onset and continuing cognitive decline.
D. The cognitive deficits in Criteria A1 and A2 are not due to any of the following:
  1. Other central nervous system conditions that cause progressive deficits in memory and cognition (e.g., cerebrovascular disease, Parkinson's disease, Huntington's disease, subdural hematoma, normal-pressure hydrocephalus, brain tumor)
  2. Systemic conditions that are known to cause dementia (e.g., hypothyroidism, vitamin B_{12} or folic acid deficiency, niacin deficiency, hypercalcemia, neurosyphilis, HIV infection)
  3. Substance-induced conditions
E. The deficits do not occur exclusively during the course of a delirium.
F. The disturbance is not better accounted for by another Axis I disorder (e.g., Major Depressive Disorder, Schizophrenia).

    Code based on type of onset and predominant features:
    With Early Onset: if onset is at age 65 years or younger
        290.11 With Delirium: if delirium is superimposed on the dementia
        290.12 With Delusions: if delusions are the predominant feature
        290.13 With Depressed Mood: if depressed mood (including presentations that meet full symptom criteria for a Major Depressive Episode) is the predominant feature. A separate diagnosis of Mood Disorder Due to a General Medical Condition is not given.
        290.10 Uncomplicated: if none of the above predominates in the current clinical presentation
    With Late Onset: if onset is after age 65 years
        290.3 With Delirium: if delirium is superimposed on the dementia
        290.20 With Delusions: if delusions are the predominant feature
        290.21 With Depressed Mood: if depressed mood (including presentations that meet full symptom criteria for a Major Depressive Episode) is the predominant feature. A separate diagnosis of Mood Disorder Due to a General Medical Condition is not given.
        290.0 Uncomplicated: if none of the above predominates in the current clinical presentation
  Specify if:
    With Behavioral Disturbance
    Coding note: Also code *331.0 Alzheimer's disease on Axis III.*

HIV, human immunodeficiency virus.
From Diagnostic and Statistical Manual of Mental Disorders, 4th ed (DSM-IV). Washington, DC, American Psychiatric Association, 1994, pp 142–143. By permission of the publisher.

"senility" due to "hardening of the arteries" should be questioned unless this was confirmed by a tissue diagnosis. Many persons so diagnosed years ago probably had DAT.

Once a physician suspects the dementia syndrome from the history, it is important to document (or eliminate as a possibility) the presence of cognitive impairment. A structured mental status examination such as the "mini-mental state," as was given in Martha's case, is very useful and much preferred over a hit-or-miss attempt at bedside assessment of mental status. This examination helps to identify cognitive impairment but is not sufficient to make a diagnosis of dementia. The historical search for

clues leading to an explanation for cognitive impairment must cover a wide variety of conditions (see Table 80–1). Some of these are reversible causes of dementia.

The physical examination of the older patient should be performed with a knowledge of findings that are related to aging per se. In the case presented for discussion, the findings related to hypertension suggested a possible cerebrovascular source for cognitive loss. Other physical findings were quite unremarkable, except for the bruising related to her falls. Some examples of physical findings that might reflect an illness causing dementia are hypoactive deep tendon reflexes in hypothyroidism, a gait disturbance in subdural hematoma, and hepatomegaly in alcoholism.

A standard laboratory diagnostic study for new-onset dementia is indicated (see Table 80–2). Beyond this basic work-up one might consider neurologic and psychiatric consultation, especially when the question of depression or dementia arises. Neuropsychological assessment is most useful when the history and examination results are equivocal and for providing a baseline estimation of cognitive performance. The diagnosis of dementia is based on all available evidence, but not infrequently it remains tentative. In those special settings in which advanced brain imaging is available (e.g., positron emission tomography), very early evidence of brain dysfunction may be obtained, but even then specific diagnosis is unlikely.

Table 80–3 provides the diagnostic criteria for dementia according to the *Diagnostic and Statistical Manual of Mental Disorders-IV.* Observation during a period of months may be necessary to make a reasonably firm diagnosis. Martha's case presentation ends with a strong suspicion of DAT.

Once a dementia is moderately advanced, it is readily discernible to those living and working in close association with the person that cognition is impaired. The person may get lost on the way home. Self-care diminishes to varied degrees, resulting in poor hygiene and inappropriate dress. A steady progression is characteristic of DAT. Patients eventually require assistance in being clothed, fed, and bathed and in excretory functions. Language is lost. The person can no longer sit up and finally becomes comatose.

The typical course of VAD is one of abrupt onset (usually in conjunction with a stroke), and the deterioration is stepwise. Personality is relatively spared, but emotional lability can be intense. Focal neurologic findings are common. There may be prolonged stable periods.

The primary focus of this case study has been on the early manifestations of dementia and the conditions that may overlap and interact with its symptoms. The wise physician will keep in mind the possibility of multiple causes of dementia in a given patient. A program that addresses the obvious medical disorders that are treatable and provides psychosocial management from the outset is most desirable. The involvement of Martha's brother and the social agency early in the course of her illness provided a good starting point for long-term management.

SUGGESTED READING

Albert ML, Feldman RG, Willis AL. The 'subcortical dementia' of progressive supranuclear palsy. J Neurol Neurosurg Psychiatry 1974;37:121–130.

American Psychiatric Association. Diagnostic and Statistical Manual of Mental Disorders, 4th ed. Washington, DC, American Psychiatric Association, 1994, pp 123–163.

Crook T, Bartus RT, Ferris SH, et al. Age-associated memory impairment: Proposed diagnostic criteria and measures of clinical change—report of a National Institute of Mental Health work group. Dev Neuropsychol 1986;2:261–276.

Finlayson RE. Dementia. In Rakel RE (ed). Textbook of Family Practice, 5th ed. Philadelphia, W.B. Saunders, 1995, pp 1531–1536.

Folstein MF, Folstein SE, McHugh PR. "Mini-mental state": A practical method for grading the cognitive state of patients for the clinician. J Psychiatr Res 1975;12:189–198.

QUESTIONS

1. Which statement is most correct with reference to the relationship between affective symptoms and dementia?
   a. Affective symptoms usually develop late in the course of dementia.
   b. About one third of cases of Alzheimer disease develop depression.
   c. Huntington disease is generally considered as a type of cortical dementia.
   d. Depression and dementia are likely to present as clear-cut syndromes in older people.

2. The finding of focal neurologic abnormalities on physical examination is least characteristic of:
   a. Vascular dementia
   b. Brain tumor
   c. Dementia of the Alzheimer type
   d. Stroke

3. Based on the information provided in this case history and discussion, what treatment modality would you think is most likely to alter the course of vascular dementia?
   a. High-dose vitamin therapy
   b. Use of choline precursors
   c. Antibiotics
   d. Antihypertensive therapy
   e. Physical therapy

Answers appear on **page 607.**

Chapter 81

Alcoholism

Scott H. Frank, M.D.

INITIAL VISIT

Subjective

Donna B. is a 38-year-old African American woman who presents as a new patient for a 40-minute visit seeking routine well-woman care. Her only complaints are of increasing fatigue, insomnia, and mild dyspepsia. On questioning, she relates some difficulty with lethargy during her workday, but is able to accomplish all of her tasks without a drop-off in her productivity as an executive secretary. She experiences nightly waking around 2:00 A.M., with difficulty returning to sleep. Donna complains of mild epigastric pain, relieved by food, worse several hours following a meal. The pain does not wake her from sleep, but while awake, she is aware of the same epigastric discomfort. She relates no change in bowel movements, including no melena or rectal bleeding. Because of her fatigue and difficulty sleeping, a detailed, structured depression history is taken, using the "Dark Clouds" mnemonic described as follows:

- **D**ysphoria: Admits to feeling "down and blue" more often than not over the past 3 months. She has had an increase in tearful episodes during that time. She can relate no life changes contributing to her sadness, although she relates that family relationships have deteriorated during the past few months. She attributes these changes to her "moodiness."
- **A**nhedonia: Relates that she had difficulty recalling the last time she felt happy. Has experienced a loss of interest in usual activities.
- **R**educed energy: Troubled by fatigue and lethargy.
- **K**inesis: Appears sluggish, slowed speech, poor eye contact. Describes feeling "stuck in the mud."
- **C**oncentration/**C**ognition: Mildly impaired, but able to function at work and home without others noticing problems.
- **L**ow self-esteem: Feels lowered sense of self-worth, preoccupied with ill-defined feelings of guilt.
- **O**ral intake: No increase or decrease in appetite or weight.
- **U**ncertainty: Strong sense of uncertainty about what the future holds. Denies feelings of hopelessness, but admits feeling helpless at times.
- **D**eath or suicide: Denies feeling preoccupied with thoughts of death or suicide. No family history of suicide.
- **S**leep: Sleep disturbance described in the presenting complaints.

DEPRESSION HISTORY SUMMARY. The Dark Clouds mnemonic encompasses the nine criteria for major depression, with one additional item (uncertainty) that does not represent one of the criteria, but leads to queries about hopelessness, an important predictor of suicidality. One of the first two criteria (dysphoria or anhedonia), plus a total of five of nine criteria must be present in order to make the diagnosis. Donna is positive on six of nine criteria for the diagnosis of major depression. Duration of symptoms (greater than 2 weeks) is also consistent with this diagnosis. Underlying medical conditions must be considered as possible sources of depressive symptoms before a final diagnosis.

FAMILY HISTORY. Donna has been married for 15 years and has two children, ages 14 and 11 years. She describes her husband (a "factory worker") as supportive and understanding. She is concerned about the behavior of her 14-year-old son. She relates frequent conflict with her 11-year-old daughter. Despite these concerns, she describes her family as dependable and as a source of comfort. She feels distant from her extended family, although they live in town. There is a family history of hypertension and heart disease (father); diabetes and alcoholism (mother).

BEHAVIORAL HEALTH RISK INTERVIEW. Donna is a nonsmoker, with substantial exposure to secondary smoke as a child from both parents, and now from her husband. She describes a varied, low-fat diet, claims regular seatbelt use for herself and her family. There is a handgun in her home, kept unloaded with ammunition stored away from the weapon. Donna has been monogamous for the 15 years of her marriage and believes her husband has as well. She has no history of sexually transmitted disease and has had three lifetime sexual partners.

ALCOHOL USE INTERVIEW. One of Donna's presenting physical symptoms is used to introduce the alcohol history, in this case, "Have you found yourself drinking more alcohol in order to help you sleep?" Donna admits that she had begun to use vodka before bed to help her sleep. On initial questioning, she acknowledges drinking one 12-oz beer each day in addition to the nightly vodka. When asked what is the most alcohol she has consumed during the past year, she relates six "screwdrivers" (vodka and orange juice). When asked to quantitate how much vodka she uses per glass, she guesses that it was "at least a double." She relates "beginning to feel high" with the fifth or sixth drink. When asked how often she consumes six or more drinks in a day, she replies "weekends." After alcohol consumption great enough to cause concern has been estab-

lished, alcohol-related behaviors are assessed using the simple CAGE mnemonic, an effective screen for alcoholism:

- **C**ut down: "Have you ever felt you ought to cut down on your drinking?" Donna answered that she is becoming concerned about her drinking and on several occasions has tried to quit without success.
- **A**nnoyed: "Have you ever felt angered or annoyed by people criticizing your drinking?" Donna responds that she feels the criticisms are valid and therefore does not feel annoyed by them. Although on the surface Donna's answer is a "No," the fact that she is receiving criticism at all is important information and can be considered a "soft positive" response.
- **G**uilty: "Have you ever felt bad or guilty about your drinking?" Donna replies that she is heavily burdened by guilt about her drinking behavior.
- **E**ye-opener: "Have you ever had a drink first thing in the morning to steady your nerves or get rid of a hangover?" This item reveals Donna's most surprising response. She admits in response to this question that for the past several months she has started each day with a vodka double to relieve hand tremor. Asked when her next drink came, she relates that she also greets her arrival home from work each day with a drink. A clarifying statement is made, "So, on workdays, you drink at least when you wake, when you return home, and before bed." She added, "with dinner and after dinner." When asked whether she ever drinks at work, she breaks down in tears, admitting that she has begun hiding vodka at work and around the home, "drinking whenever I can get away with it." When asked when her last drink was, she admits that she has had a drink the morning of the visit, about 6 hours before our encounter.

DRUG USE INTERVIEW. Because drug use generally carries a strong stigma, making patients less likely to be reliable in reporting drug behaviors, approaching the topic routinely, nonjudgmentally, and firmly is more likely to result in valid responses. "Many patients with alcohol problems also use other drugs [bridging statement]." Have you ever experimented with street drugs?" Donna replies that she has experimented with marijuana use as a teen but had not enjoyed it and had not used any drug in several decades. "What would I find today if I were to do a urine drug screen?" She first responds,

"Nothing," then adds, "except alcohol. You can check!" she says proudly and firmly. The physician confirms, "I think it would probably be in your best interest to do so, just to prove to others that this isn't a concern." This simple query is highly effective at eliciting important information about drug use. With many patients the need for the urine drug screen may be obviated by admission of recent drug use when faced with the prospect of a urine drug screen. The nondefensiveness of her response predicted a negative urine drug screen, which was in fact the result. The documentation of this negative result in the alcoholic patient is important because of the very high incidence of multidrug dependence. This "proof" of negative result is important in decisions about treatment and may be helpful in advocating for the patient with her employer. If the result is positive, it is far better for the patient to find out in the physician's office than through drug testing which may be performed at the work site.

Objective

"I realize that you came in today expecting a complete physical examination, but with your permission, I'd like to do a brief examination only, then focus on your alcohol use and its effect on your health." The patient eagerly agrees to this plan, allowing a focused examination that attends to vital signs, looking for autonomic hyperactivity, and to examination of the abdomen primarily to assess liver size. Blood pressure is 150/94 mm Hg, pulse 80, afebrile. Liver is enlarged to 4 cm below the right costal margin (liver span 14 cm) and is mildly tender. There is no other tenderness or organomegaly and no sign of ascites. The remainder of her physical examination is deferred to compensate for the extra time taken during the interview, and the anticipation of the time necessary for presentation of the diagnosis to the patient.

Assessment

1. Alcoholism with physiological dependence. While the CAGE questionnaire is a screening tool, not a true diagnostic instrument, the information gathered during its administration clearly identifies Donna as an alcoholic. The differential diagnosis of alcoholism (used interchangeably with alcohol dependence) includes alcohol abuse (heavy drinking) and multidrug dependency. Although many definitions of alcoholism exist, it is best defined by its *cardinal features*.

- *Impaired control:* The patient clearly demonstrates loss of control over alcohol with the progressively increasing course of her drinking behavior. Alternatively, the clinician may ask, "How often do you find yourself unable to stop drinking once you've started?" It is important to understand that escalating alcohol use is not a necessary component of impaired control. Impaired control may also be characterized by the consistent need to drink "to a level" consuming at least a certain number of drinks a day to "feel normal." Periods of abstinence and relapse or a persistent desire to quit or cut down on alcohol use are other expressions of impaired control.

- *Tolerance:* Tolerance is characterized by the need for increasing quantities of alcohol to achieve the same effect, or by a marked diminishment in the effect of a substance in the face of continued use. Development of neuroadaptation to alcohol as expressed through tolerance or alcohol withdrawal confirms that physiological dependence on alcohol is present. To many, this represents the defining difference between alcohol dependence and alcohol abuse. The diagnosis of alcoholism, however, may be made without withdrawal or tolerance being present in a significant minority of patients. Ideally, the diagnosis of alcoholism should specify if it is with or without physiological dependence. Donna has evidence of tolerance in the recent escalation of the quantity of alcohol consumed and when she relates that it took five or six drinks before she felt the euphorogenic effects of alcohol. It is important to note that acute intoxication is not necessary to the diagnosis of alcoholism, since tolerance may diminish any appearance of intoxication.

- *Alcohol withdrawal:* Alcohol withdrawal symptoms may begin as early as 4 hours and as late as 12 hours following a sharp decline in alcohol use. The major consequences of alcohol withdrawal peak at 24 to 48 hours, and generally disappear by 5 to 7 days. Symptoms include autonomic hyperactivity such as tachycardia, blood pressure elevation, and diaphoresis; tremor; insomnia; anxiety; and psychomotor agitation. The most serious consequences of alcohol withdrawal, that is, delirium tremens (DTs) and seizures, occur only in a minority of patients (5 per cent and 3 per cent respectively). Delirium tremens are characterized by visual, tactile, or auditory hallucinations. Anxiety, insomnia, and autonomic hyperactivity may persist for months following cessation of alcohol use. Donna's use of alcohol in the morning to relieve hand tremor is characteristic withdrawal-related behavior.

- *Blackouts:* Alcoholic blackouts are characterized by a waking amnesia to behaviors performed while intoxicated. They are not equivalent to passing out while intoxicated. Blackouts are not necessary or sufficient for the diagnosis of alcoholism, but provide important supportive evidence. Continued drinking despite a recurrent pattern of blackouts is characteristic of alcohol dependence. This is not a prominent feature of Donna's presentation.

- *Substance-seeking behavior:* Alcoholic patients are preoccupied with consumption of alcohol and tend to take great risks or go to great lengths in an effort to obtain the alcohol. Donna's practice of hiding alcohol at work and home is an example of such behavior.

- *Ambivalence:* Most alcoholics have a "love-hate" relationship with alcohol. This feature is well characterized by the following quote from "The Drinker's Dilemma" (S. Frank, unpublished data, 1983): "I don't want to drink, but I don't want to quit. I do want to quit but I do want to drink. I know I must quit but I feel I must drink. I feel out of control but must be in control. I hate that I drink, yet love when I drink. I can't imagine myself without alcohol for the rest of my life. I don't want to drink but I don't want to try to quit and fail. What scares me more is that I might succeed, then be left without my alcohol."

- *Functional impairment:* Continued alcohol use despite a known, persistent pattern of functional impairment is perhaps the single most important defining characteristic of alcohol dependence. Functional impairment also occurs in patients with alcohol abuse, with the major difference being the persistence of the impairment over time. Such impairments may occur related to role obligations, legal problems, excessive risk taking while intoxicated, and social or interpersonal problems. Continued alcohol use despite known health problems caused or contributed to by alcohol use is generally associated with alcoholism rather than alcohol abuse.

- *Denial:* Denial is invariably present at some level in alcoholism. Donna certainly displayed denial in hiding her drinking behavior from her family and coworkers. Components of denial include:

Subconscious self-delusion

Conscious lying or distortion

Euphoric recall: remembering only the good parts about the substance use

Wishful thinking: the belief that "normal" drinking is possible for the alcoholic

Rationalization: blaming alcohol use on other causes such as job stress, nagging spouse, or misbehaving kids

Social comparison: comparing oneself to others who drink more or who seem healthy despite drinking in order to justify one's own behavior

"Dry drunk syndrome": periods of abstinence intended to convince others that there isn't a problem, despite full intention to return to previous behavior as soon as possible. This term also involves attempts to quit drinking while ignoring the need for other life changes, thus setting the stage for the failure that part of the alcoholic desires anyway.

2. Alcohol-induced mood disorder. On further questioning it becomes clear that Donna's depressive symptoms began well after the onset of her escalating alcohol use, which she dates to about 2 years before her visit. Depression and alcoholism are frequently comorbid conditions. The label of dual diagnosis is given to patients who demonstrate persistent symptoms of depression 3 to 6 months following abstinence from alcohol, or who had depressive symptoms clearly preceding their alcoholic drinking pattern. There has been some success in the use of antidepressants in the treatment of depressive symptoms as part of the recovery process whether or not depressive symptoms preceded the alcohol use.

Plan

DIAGNOSTIC. Whereas in this patient the diagnosis of alcoholism appears clear, several additional diagnostic steps should be considered. First, laboratory tests investigating hepatic dysfunction secondary to alcohol use should be undertaken. The gamma-glutamyltransferase (GGT) is the liver enzyme most sensitive to alcohol and is generally the earliest laboratory sign of alcoholism. Although this liver enzyme may support the diagnosis of alcoholism, it is neither sensitive nor specific when examined in research settings. In addition, the ratio of aspartate aminotransferase (AST) to alanine aminotransferase (ALT) has been demonstrated to be helpful in supporting the diagnosis of alcoholism. AST should be elevated to a greater extent than ALT, often approaching a ratio of 2:1. This patient has a GGT of 372, AST of 138, and ALT of 76, highly consistent with alcohol-induced liver damage. A complete blood count may also reveal a macrocytosis in 40 per cent of alcoholics, again allowing this test to offer supportive confirmation to the clinical picture. Donna's MCV was 106 μm³ (normal values 80 to 100 μm³).

THERAPEUTIC

Presentation of the Diagnosis. Perhaps the most important part of the therapeutic process in the treatment of alcoholism is to present the diagnosis to the patient in a manner that he or she can understand and accept. Presentation of the diagnosis should move the patient toward treatment and change rather than creating conflict between the patient and the physician or cause a sense of despair, stigma, or hopelessness in the patient. The approach described below uses components of the "patient-centered medical approach" and a technique referred to as "motivational interviewing."

Suggested Steps in Presentation of the Diagnosis of Alcoholism

- *Therapeutic assessment:* A thorough history is essential to effectively present the diagnosis. If the interview process makes it clear to the patient that the clinician understands the problem of alcoholism, there is a simultaneous enhancement of the patient's feelings of hopefulness and diminishment of patient denial with recognition that this physician would more be difficult to deceive than others.

- *Self-assessment:* Ask patients to self-assess whether believe they are alcoholic. If the patient admits to this belief, time spent convincing him or her of the diagnosis is wasted. If patients do not recognize this diagnosis in themselves, the physician is prepared for a more difficult task.

- *Determine patient explanatory model:* Regardless of the self-assessment, ask the patient to offer a personal definition of alcoholism. Personal definitions are generally based on one's particular experience with the phenomenon of alcoholism, and therefore vary widely. Understanding the patient's "explanatory model" for alcoholism allows the physician to directly address areas of misunderstanding and misperception.

- *Offer the physician's explanatory model:* Present a simple, straightforward medical definition of alcoholism so that the patient understands the medical view of alcohol dependence. My own definition follows:

Alcoholism is a medical disease characterized by

impaired control over drinking, preoccupation with alcohol, and continued use of alcohol despite a pattern of compelling reasons to stop. Alcoholism is a primary disease. By primary, I mean that alcoholism is not caused by other illnesses (though it may cause other illnesses), and is not caused by life problems (though it may cause life problems). Because genetic, psychosocial and environmental factors affect the development of alcoholism, other illnesses or life problems may contribute to the onset of the disease, but they do not cause it, and simply taking away the illness or life problem would not cure alcoholism. Alcoholism is a chronic disease. By chronic, I mean that alcoholism is treatable, but not curable. Just as with other chronic diseases like diabetes or hypertension, if the treatment is withdrawn, the disease comes back. The fact that we in medicine consider alcoholism a disease implies that it is an involuntary disability. The alcoholic does not deliberately pursue alcoholism. While the alcoholic is not to blame for his illness, he is responsible to pursue treatment, and responsible for the consequences of his drinking.

- *Redefinition:* Ask the patient whether the *medical* definition of alcoholism fits him or her. Ask for concrete examples to support this point of view.

- *Physician assessment:* Offer your assessment of whether and why you believe the patient does or doesn't fit the medical definition. Use concrete examples taken from the history to support your point of view. This strategy of "negotiating" between the patient's understanding of alcoholism and yours allows expression of empathy for his or her plight. You are not *judging* the patient to be alcoholic. You are *diagnosing* the condition.

- *Avoid argumentation:* It is not necessary to coerce the patient into immediate acceptance of the diagnosis of alcoholism. It is necessary to engage the patient to the degree that it is likely that he or she will return, or at least will benefit at some later time from the assessment you offer today.

- *Develop a discrepancy:* Point out the discrepancy between the patient's current behaviors and his or her values and goals in life. This key precept of motivational interviewing dramatizes the need for change, provokes meaningful introspection, and encourages action.

- *Support self-efficacy:* Self-efficacy refers to patients' belief in their ability to move toward effective change. The physician can enhance patient self-efficacy by pointing out positive prognostic factors, by relating anecdotes of others who have successfully changed, and by implying through his or her concern that the patient is worth changing.

■ *Roll with resistance:* There is more than one way to move toward recovery from alcoholism. If the patient shows strong resistance to the approach you suggest, offer other options.

Donna accepted the diagnosis of alcoholism and treatment suggestions eagerly. She declined inpatient treatment, desiring to "handle this on my own" first. She accepted the suggestion to contact the employee assistance plan at her workplace and the telephone number for Alcoholics Anonymous. She declined the physician's offer to join her as she informed her family of the problem, stating that telling them would be difficult, but something she felt capable of handling herself.

Outpatient Detoxification. Because she declined admission for alcohol treatment, an outpatient "detox" program is necessary to ensure her safety as she discontinues her alcohol use. The point of alcohol detoxification is to protect the patient from the sequelae of withdrawal and decrease the incidence of relapses resulting from "self-treatment" of withdrawal symptoms with alcohol. Many protocols have been described, including the one detailed next.

1. *Patient selection.* The patient should be motivated for home withdrawal and have a reliable person present during the first 72 hours of withdrawal. He or she should have access to a phone and someone in the physician's office to check in with for assessment of daily progress. Presence of other illnesses such as diabetes or hypertension is a relative contraindication to home withdrawal. The patient should see a nurse or physician daily during the first 72 hours of treatment.

2. *Home monitoring.* Warning signs indicating need for emergency care should be described to the patient and withdrawal partner and include fever greater than 38.1°C, pulse over 140, marked agitation, chest pain, persistent shortness of breath, severe abdominal pain or protracted vomiting, recurring hallucinations, and delirium.

3. *Pharmacotherapy.* Clonidine has been demonstrated to be useful in diminishing the autonomic hyperactivity of alcohol withdrawal. Clonidine may be given in a dose of 0.2 mg for the initial dose, then 0.1 mg every 4 hours during the first 48 hours, tapering to 0.1 mg every 6 hours, then every 8 hours, then every 12 hours on a daily basis for 1 week.

It is ideal to avoid use of psychotropics in home detoxification. Certainly, because of the abuse potential, it is inadvisable to administer benzodiazapines at home, although they work well in the inpatient setting. On the other hand, for a patient such as this, with a high likelihood of substantial withdrawal symptoms, use of a phenobarbital detoxification program carries far less risk of cross addiction. Phenobarbital provides excellent seizure protection and helps decrease anxiety, agitation, insomnia, and hallucinations. Phenobarbital can be administered orally, 60 mg every 6 hours for 72 hours, then every 12 hours for 48 hours.

4. *Follow-up.* Donna is seen daily during home detoxification, then weekly for a month, then every other week for a month, then monthly. Her family responded to her admission supportively, stating they knew "something was wrong," but not understanding exactly what. There were no complications with home detoxification. She entered an outpatient treatment program through her job, and attends Alcoholics Anonymous three to five times a week. Her husband and children attend Alanon and Alateen, respectively, once a week. Her depression has persisted and she was started on sertaline 50 mg a day after 2 months of sobriety. Her mood has lifted and she remains abstinent from alcohol 1 year after her presentation to the office.

SUGGESTED READING

Flavin DK, Morse RM. The definition of alcoholism. JAMA 1992;268:1012–1014.

Fleming MF, Barry KL. Addictive Disorders. St. Louis, Mosby–Year Book, 1992.

Frank SH, Graham AV, Zyzanski SJ, White S. Use of the family CAGE in screening for alcohol problems in primary care. Arch Fam Med 1992;1:209–216.

Mason BJ, Kocsis JH, Ritvo EC, Cutler RB. A double-blind, pla-cebo-controlled trial of desipramine for primary alcohol dependence stratified on the presence or absence of major depression. JAMA 1996;275:761–767.

Miller WR, Rollnick S. Motivational Interviewing: Preparing People to Change Addictive Behavior. New York, Guilford Press, 1991.

Stewart M, Brown JB, Weston WW, et al. Patient-Centered Medicine: Transforming the Clinical Method. Thousand Oaks, CA, Sage, 1995.

1. Which of the following laboratory tests of liver enzymes shows the earliest and most dramatic rise with alcoholic liver disease?
   a. Alkaline phosphatase
   b. γ-Glutamyl transferase
   c. Aspartate aminotransferase
   d. Alanine aminotransferase
   e. Lactate dehydrogenase

2. True or false: The following characteristics contribute to the diagnosis of alcoholism:

   a. The appearance of intoxication
   b. Tolerance
   c. Impaired control over alcohol intake
   d. Withdrawal
   e. Continued alcohol use despite a known, persistent pattern of functional impairment

Answers appear on **page 608.**

Chapter 82

Approaches to Patients Who Smoke

Alan Blum, M.D.

Robert W., a 31-year-old firefighter and father of four, visits the family practice center because of abdominal pain 1 week ago that lasted 20 minutes. Apart from three previous episodes in the past 2 months, he states that he has been in good health. He drinks four cups of coffee and three cans of Lite beer daily. He admits to financial worries and fears of being laid off from work, and he has recently increased his consumption of cigarettes from one and a half to two packs per day of Marlboro Mediums. "But my chest x-ray was normal in the preemployment physical exam last year," he adds.

At the same time, Andy B., a 50-year-old executive at a major corporation, has come to the center at the insistence of his wife. She is extremely concerned about her husband's increasing shortness of breath over the past 3 months. In addition to being in a sedentary occupation, he is 40 lb overweight and has smoked a pack of Kent cigarettes each day for 32 years. "I guess for my New Year's resolution, I'll try that stop-smoking patch," he muses.

Jane L., a 28-year-old psychologist, is also waiting to see her family physician for her annual well-woman examination. In addition, she is concerned about an article in the *Woman's Home Magazine* that she has just read in the waiting room. The author warned of dangers associated with the use of oral contraceptives by women who smoke. Accordingly, she is interested in stopping the pill and in being fitted for a diaphragm.

Another young lady, 15-year-old Paula D., has just arrived at the center, having been referred by the high school nurse because of constant coughs and colds that have led to frequent absences. She has a hoarse voice and stained teeth and notes on the health questionnaire that she has smoked a pack a day of Virginia Superslims for 2 years.

Paula had received a ride from a fellow patient, Jeannie W., a 48-year-old food service supervisor at the high school, who has recently been diagnosed as having essential hypertension and has come for a check of her blood pressure. She is on her feet all day long, gets no exercise, and is 50 lb overweight. Her mother died at age 50 from a stroke. Since being told she has high blood pressure, she has switched from Salem Longs cigarettes to Carlton Menthol Lights 100s and continues to smoke at least a pack a day. "But I do chew nicotine gum when I go to church or the movies," she proudly points out.

Sitting next to her is Bess T., age 24, who is in the 16th week of her first pregnancy. She has an unremitting, nonproductive cough; moreover, she has gained only 1 lb in the past 2 months. She has assured her physician that she would never buy a brand of cigarettes with the label that warns of injury to the fetus; rather, she seeks out the brands with the label that says only that cigarette smoke contains carbon monoxide.

Ted K., a 62-year-old disabled Korean War veteran suffering from Buerger disease, has just been added to the schedule because of a worsening of his condition and the possibility of gangrene in his right foot. Since basic training in the army more than 40 years ago, he has smoked two packs a day of Camel regular cigarettes.

Regardless of the additional history and physical findings that the family physician would glean in the examining room, the cessation of smoking is the most crucial action that can be taken to improve the health of each of these seven patients. Cigarette smoking is the major preventable cause of numerous fatal diseases, including cancer of the lung, larynx, nasopharynx, and esophagus; emphysema; coronary heart disease; Buerger disease; and cerebrovascular disease. It is also associated with cancers of the pancreas, bladder, kidney, stomach, and uterine cervix; indeed, 40% of all deaths from cancer are caused by smoking. Smoking is almost synonymous with chronic bronchitis and is frequently found in association with peptic ulcer disease. The common factor in the three leading causes of death—coronary heart disease, cancer, and cerebrovascular disease—is cigarette smoking. In short, cigarette smoking is the chief avoidable cause of death in our society.

Although it may come as a shock to the firefighter, Robert W., detection of a lung cancer on an x-ray study does not improve the survival rate. Many benefits from stopping smoking can be demonstrated at all ages, even in the case of Ted K., the older man with Buerger disease. And while several factors may be contributing to Robert W.'s abdominal pain, removing cigarettes from the picture is the most elemental, economical, and sensible measure that may afford relief. Granted, it may not be easy to stop smoking, much less to motivate a patient to do so, but therein lies a creative intellectual challenge far exceeding that of refilling a prescription for an antibiotic for chronic bronchitis or a regimen of antibiotics and an acid pump inhibitor for peptic ulcer disease with *Helicobacter pylori* infection. Most gratifyingly, in retrospective studies, patients report that the physician's active involvement in motivating them to stop smoking was a significant impetus. Such informative dialogue may well be what patients are seeking when they criticize physicians for not listening to them. A variety of factors may inhibit the physician from addressing this issue, such as the perceived lack of time or lack of reimbursement by insurance carriers for such counseling. Nonetheless, the physician may well find that an enhanced role in promoting smoking cessation, regardless of the minimal extra income, helps build a practice as word spreads about the doctor who cares.

None of these patients presents with a primary concern about smoking, and none of them expects a lecture on smoking at this time. However, in each case, the family physician has an opportunity to lead the patient to make the connection between the improvement of the predominant health problem and the cessation of smoking. The physician's active role in encouraging patients to stop smoking—akin to his or her role in the prevention of smoking among teenagers—can be the determining factor in the patient's success. In only a few minutes, there is much the physician can do to motivate patients to stop using cigarettes, in lieu of relegating this task to ancillary personnel, a smoking cessation clinic, or a pamphlet off the shelf.

LOOKS, SEX, AND MONEY

The key to successfully enhancing the motivation of patients to stop smoking is a positive approach. Although admonitions about the diseases caused by smoking and the harmful constituents of tobacco smoke are important, the benefits of not *buying* cigarettes must be emphasized at least as strongly.

As with any patient encounter, the overall approach must be individualized, taking into account social, cultural, and ethnic factors. Different methods will be needed for a blue-collar worker beginning to show symptoms of a cigarette-related illness, a seriously ill executive, a health professional who acknowledges the hazards of smoking but continues her habit, and a high school girl who is relatively new to smoking.

Solely educating patients about the facts of smoking in a single office visit is unlikely to result in behavioral change. On the other hand, the family physician can, through the use of creative analogies related to the patient's hobbies, romantic interest, or occupation, succeed in changing the patient's entire attitude toward smoking. For example, listing the toxic gases in tobacco smoke, such as cyanide, formaldehyde, carbon monoxide, and ammonia, may mean little at first, but by noting that ammonia causes the odor in urine and cat litter, the physician is likely to cause the patient to think about smoking a bit differently.

The use of an everyday, nonmedical vocabulary is essential for patient education in general and smoking cessation efforts in particular. Instead of the medical term "pack-year history," which merely refers to the approximate number of packs per day multiplied by the number of years the patient has smoked, a more relevant term for the patient is the "inhalation count." A 20-cigarette (pack-a-day) smoking patient will breathe in upward of 1 million doses of poisonous fumes in less than 15 years, not including the inhalation of the smoke of coworkers and family members. Another nonthreatening way to emphasize the enormous waste of smoking is to restate the amount smoked in financial terms: A pack-a-day cigarette buyer will spend in excess of $800 a year or in excess of $10,000 in a decade.

INDIVIDUALIZE AND DEMYTHOLOGIZE

Thus, whereas smoking cessation rests on the knowledge of the deleterious aspects to health, the cognitive component alone is insufficient. Both the physician and the patient must be motivated to succeed. The three keys to motivating the patient are to individualize, personalize, and demythologize. Individualizing the message to the patient is the cornerstone of success. The same words cannot be used for a high school girl, a firefighter, or an executive already showing signs of emphysema. The teenager, perhaps more anxious about her self-image than any of the other patients (and therefore more susceptible to the glamorous images in cigarette advertisements and promotions), may or may not respond to a discussion about lung cancer and heart disease; it is usually more helpful to focus on the cosmetic unattractiveness of yellow teeth and bad breath, as well as the diminution of athletic ability

and the drain on the pocketbook. Rather than acknowledging that smoking is an adult custom, the physician should refer to it as a childish and silly-looking habit like picking one's nose. The most important comment the physician can make to an adolescent is, "You still smoke? Come on, that's for little kids."

The psychologist who diligently reports for an annual Pap smear may seem well-motivated about maintaining her health, yet she chooses to give up the pill rather than stop smoking. She has been misinformed about the relative risks involved. A straightforward presentation of the facts should occur before any cervical smear is taken, to clarify the proper health priorities.

For the firefighter, the best approach might be to talk about the chances of increased fitness for work, athletic ability, and even an improved sex life were he to stop smoking. Money saved and the reduced risk of fire at home are worth mentioning.

In talking with Andy B., the executive, it is especially important to explode various myths about smoking, such as that the low-tar cigarettes he is smoking are safer. To the contrary, use of so-called low-tar brands, which should be referred to as "low-poison" by the physician, results in compensatory deeper inhalation of greater concentrations of poisonous gases and chemical additives that increase the risk of heart attack and emphysema. One way to highlight the absurdity of the belief that low-tar cigarettes are safer is to ask rhetorically, "Safer than what? Fresh air?" or to wonder aloud if it is safer to jump from the 50th floor of a skyscraper instead of the roof. Another analogy is to point out that one would never buy a loaf of bread that was advertised as containing only "2 mg of cancer causers." Similarly, Jeannie W., the food service worker, might be intrigued, if not astonished, to learn that menthol is an anesthetic agent that deadens the throat and creates the impression that the cigarette is not as irritative. An additional analogy is that paying $2.50 for a pack of cigarettes (which costs less than 15¢ to manufacture) is like spending $100 for a pound of baloney.

The physician must learn to personalize approaches to smoking cessation by reviewing existing pamphlets and other audiovisual aids, as one would with a new drug or medical device. Personally handing a brochure to a patient while underlining certain points or illustrations provides an important reinforcing message.

EXPLODING CONSUMER MYTHS

The most important myth surrounding smoking is that it relieves stress. This can be debunked by pointing out that the stress that is relieved is that which resulted from being dependent on cigarettes; this is the essence of addiction. At the same time, it is important to point out that deep breathing in and of itself has a relaxing effect. An equally sad myth, reinforced in advertisements for Virginia Superslims and other brands of long, thin cigarettes aimed at young women, is that smoking keeps weight off. On hearing this rationalization from a patient, the famous chest surgeon Dr. Alton Ochsner would reply, "So who wants to be a svelte corpse?" Aside from pointing to all the overweight women who smoke, one must emphasize that smoking is a far greater health risk. Smoking inhibits appetite by damaging taste buds and other digestive tract cells, and one may well start to gain weight on stopping smoking as the body feels better. Weight gain does not follow, however, if one will learn to enjoy walking or other exercise.

Once the physician has succeeded in enhancing the patient's motivation to stop smoking, it must be pointed out that accomplishing this may not be as difficult as the patient believes. Too much sympathy and coddling of the patient concerning the challenge of breaking the power of nicotine addiction serves only to reinforce the obstacles to change. The patient should be encouraged to transfer the guilt and anger over smoking away from oneself and onto those who are pushing the cigarettes, namely, the manufacturers. In this way, the physician is no longer a finger-wagging lecturer on the dangers of smoking but rather a consumer advocate who points out the cheap and defective nature of the product that has been purchased in good faith by the consumer/patient. Unfortunately, the medical profession has been slow to put aside its authoritarian image on this issue, and virtually all other published or promoted methods for smoking cessation focus on "the smoker" and "nicotine addiction" without even mentioning the product itself or its promoters. There is scant science in the field of smoking cessation, the result of which has been to witness 95% of persons who smoke today switching to low-tar filter brands in the misguided belief that these are safer. (The tobacco advertisers could be called our leading health educators.)

Unfortunately, too, despite little evidence to back up their claims, expensive commercial aids for smoking cessation abound. These include acupuncture, hypnotherapy, aversive conditioning with electric shock, special filters, pocket calculators for tracking cigarette consumption, and a host of pharmacologic agents, including antihypertensive medications, minor tranquilizers, nicotine substitutes, and nicotine itself in the form of chewing gum, skin patch, or nasal spray. The nicotine-based products are designed to ease abstinence from tobacco by partially replacing the drug of dependence in the absence of the other harmful chemicals in the smoke. Most manufacturer-funded studies report enhanced rates of smoking cessation among users of nicotine replacement products. Yet even the manufacturers acknowledge that they can be of help only in concert with a comprehensive behavior modification effort such as can be facilitated by the physician. At the same time, the pharmaceutical companies successfully lobbied the Food and Drug Administration to permit these products to be sold over the counter.

Before recommending a pharmacologic adjunct for smoking cessation, the clinician should suggest starting with a simpler, inexpensive method. It is essential to review various situational modifications that can postpone or otherwise inhibit the times at which one is most likely to light up (e.g., after meals, while driving, with coffee). In lieu of smoking, one can learn to take 5-minute breaks at work and at home for slow, deep breathing while sitting with eyes closed and the mind free of intrusive thoughts (the "relaxation response" introduced by Herbert Benson, M.D. in the treatment of hypertension). Cinnamon, mint, or lemon candies are helpful oral substitutes, as is iced tea or club soda. The goal to keep in mind is to smoke as few cigarettes as possible, and the key teaching point is that low-tar filter cigarettes are not safer than other cigarettes.

Notwithstanding the earnestness of recent clinical guidelines on smoking cessation, as well as of ubiquitous television commercials for nicotine replacement drugs, tobacco use is not a straightforward chemical addiction with a pharmacologic solution. Time, commitment, and encouragement on the part of the family physician are essential components to successful smoking cessation, and can result in a tremendous feeling of satisfaction on the part of doctor and patient alike.

SUGGESTED READING

Blum A. Cancer prevention: preventing tobacco-related cancers. In DeVita VT, Hellman S, Rosenberg SA (eds). Cancer: Principles and Practice of Oncology, 5th ed. Philadelphia, Lippincott-Raven, 1997, pp 545–557.

Blum A (ed). The Cigarette Underworld. Secaucus, NJ: Lyle Stuart, 1985.

Blum A. Consumer advocacy: a crafty approach to counseling. Patient Care, Feb 28, 1993, pp 80–83.

Blum A, Solberg E. The role of the family physician in ending the tobacco pandemic. J Fam Pract 1992;34:697–700.

Smith S, Smith J (eds). Medical Activism: DOC's Approach to Countering the Tobacco Pandemic. Houston: DOC (Doctors Ought to Care, 5013 Kirby Drive, Houston, TX 77005), 1992.

QUESTIONS

1. Cigarette smoking is a causative factor in each of the following conditions EXCEPT:
   a. Bladder cancer
   b. Esophageal cancer
   c. Stroke
   d. Ulcerative colitis
   e. Buerger disease

2. The following myths are widely believed by people who smoke EXCEPT:
   a. Smoking relieves stress
   b. Smoking reduces weight
   c. Low-tar cigarettes are safer
   d. Light cigarettes are safer
   e. Smoking kills bacteria in the mouth

3. Essential components of effective health education include each of the following EXCEPT:
   a. Individualize
   b. Personalize
   c. Demythologize
   d. Chastise
   e. Re-emphasize (on each visit)

Answers appear on **page 608**.

Chapter **83**

Terminal Cancer and Pain

Robert E. Rakel, M.D.
Porter Storey, M.D.

INITIAL VISIT

Objective

PATIENT IDENTIFICATION AND PRESENTING PROBLEM. Thelma B. is a 63-year-old woman who presents in the emergency room with severe pain in her chest, abdomen, and low back.

PRESENT ILLNESS. Two years ago Thelma was diagnosed with cancer of the left breast and underwent a radical mastectomy followed by radiation therapy. Since then she has been taking tamoxifen, 20 mg daily. One year ago she developed back pain and was found to have bone metastases. She was placed on acetaminophen with codeine (Tylenol No. 3) every 4 hours but this did not control the pain, so she was changed to hydromorphone (Dilaudid), 4 mg orally every 4 to 6 hours. She fell asleep after taking the first hydromorphone tablet and then felt drowsy and confused when she awoke. She is reluctant to take the hydromorphone because she wants to remain more alert and has taken only one every other day. She is now moaning and complaining of pain "all over" although it is most severe in the back. The abdominal pain is cramping in nature. Her last bowel movement was 4 days ago.

PAST MEDICAL HISTORY. Aside from an appendectomy at age 11, there have been no other hospitalizations or serious illnesses until the breast cancer was diagnosed on a routine mammogram 2 years ago.

FAMILY HISTORY. Thelma's mother died from carcinoma of the breast at age 68 and her father died at age 72 after his second heart attack. She has one brother, age 61, in good health and a sister, age 59, who has had carcinoma of the cervix. Her grandparents on both sides died in their seventies and eighties of natural causes.

SOCIAL HISTORY. For the past 20 years Thelma has had a stable sexual relationship with Louise who, because of arthritis, is having increasing difficulty caring for her. Louise reports that the pain became much worse after Thelma discovered that her brother Harry was filing a petition with the court for legal guardianship. Harry has never accepted Thelma's sexual preference or lifestyle and Thelma is extremely upset that he is attempting to take her away from her life partner. Louise currently has durable power of attorney. She reports that Thelma is very afraid of dying and that she feels guilty that she has not attended church for the past 20 years because of the church's disapproval of her sexual preference.

REVIEW OF SYSTEMS. Unremarkable except for vaginal itching recently. There is a history of occasional monilial vaginitis that always responded to treatment with vaginal cream. Her Pap smears have been consistently negative.

Objective

PHYSICAL EXAMINATION. Physical examination reveals an underweight white female who is in acute distress due to pain. Vital signs are within normal limits with blood pressure 110/70 mm Hg, pulse 86 and regular, respiratory rate 18, and temperature 98°F. Head, eyes, ears, nose, and throat examination is normal, thyroid is normal size, and there is no cervical lymphadenopathy. The chest is clear to auscultation except for bilateral basilar rales that clear with deep inspiration. The left breast is surgically absent, the scar is well healed, and no abnormal lymph nodes are palpable in either axilla. There is moderate tenderness to palpation of the left anterior chest wall over the ribs but no abnormal masses are noted. No lesions are palpable in the right breast. The heart tones are normal and no murmurs or cardiomegaly are noted. No carotid or epigastric bruits are heard.

The abdomen is slightly distended and tympanitic to percussion. The liver edge is palpable two fingerbreadths below the right costal margin. The spleen and kidneys are not palpable. Firm stool is palpable in the left lower quadrant. There is no tenderness to palpation and no other masses are palpable. Pelvic examination reveals a small amount of white vaginal discharge and slides are obtained for a wet mount examination. A parous cervix appears normal and nontender on motion. A Pap smear was taken. Bimanual examination reveals a normal-size uterus and no abnormal adnexal masses or tenderness. Rectovaginal examination confirms these findings.

LABORATORY TESTS. Wet preparation of the vaginal discharge shows normal epithelial cells and some yeast cells that are more evident on the potassium hydroxide preparation. A complete blood count shows hemoglobin of 8.0 gm/dl, hematocrit 23, white blood cell (WBC) count 8600/mm^3. Serum chemistries are normal except for a potassium of 3.1 mEq/L, sodium 129 mEq/L, and calcium 12.0 mg/dl. Radiographs of the chest, abdomen, and back are obtained showing a pleural effusion on the left side of her chest and signs of osteolytic metastases in her left rib cage. The abdominal film shows bowel full of stool but no air-fluid levels, and the lumbosacral spine radiographs show osteolytic lesions in L3 and L4.

Assessment

1. Carcinoma of the breast with metastases to bone

2. Constipation secondary to narcotics

3. Anemia

4. Hypokalemia

5. Hypercalcemia

6. Hyponatremia

Plan

1. Admit to the hospital.

2. Discontinue the hydromorphone and start oxycodone, 5 mg every 4 hours until pain control is achieved. Add ibuprofen, 400 mg every 8 hours to assist with control of bone pain.

3. Start 5% dextrose in normal saline with 20 mEq of potassium.

4. Furosemide (Lasix), 20 mg orally daily.

5. Enemas until clear, then start a daily stool softener and mild stimulant.

6. Transfuse with two units of packed red blood cells.

7. Discuss with the patient and her partner the value of joining a hospice.

FOLLOW-UP VISIT

After institution of the prescribed measures, Thelma is substantially improved. She has less bone pain and her bowels are moving. She is in an active dialogue with her social worker and chaplain about her social problems. One day when she is transferring from the bed to the commode she falls and sustains a pathologic fracture of the left femur. Louise consents to surgery when she is told it is the only way to get the pain under adequate control. Thelma undergoes internal fixation of her left femur and has difficulty recovering after surgery. She is quite confused most of the time, is unable to turn in bed, and does not resume eating more than a teaspoon or two of soft food. She is unable to swallow oral agents and her condition seems to be deteriorating. A continuous infusion of morphine is given to provide adequate comfort. Consideration is given to transferring Thelma to the local hospice as soon as possible.

DISCUSSION

The essential feature of managing Thelma is to maximize the quality of the life she has remaining. Since the cancer cannot be cured, attention must be given to controlling her symptoms and allowing her to remain as alert and in control of her life as much as possible.

Pain Control

Analgesics should be given in adequate amounts to provide comfort. The approach to analgesic medication in which doses are given as needed should be abandoned in the treatment of dying patients, since it contributes to a lower pain threshold and a need for increasing doses of medication to relieve the pain. When medication is given regularly in adequate doses, the anxiety and fear that accentuate pain are avoided and lower doses of the drug are effective, since the patient no longer fears pain recurrence or "breakthrough."

High doses of opioids may be necessary to obtain initial pain control in a patient with severe pain. Dependence is rarely a problem in patients who receive appropriate opioid doses for chronic severe cancer pain. When medication is given *prior* to the recurrence of pain, craving for medication does not occur. There should be no more than a 20 per cent reduction in dosage in any 2-day period; otherwise, withdrawal symptoms may occur.

OPIOIDS. A symptom-oriented history and careful examination may reveal a number of different sources of pain. Oral candidiasis, decubitus ulcers, constipation, and infected wounds all have specific remedies. Most patients with pain from cancer (and many patients with pain from non-neoplastic illnesses) require an opioid analgesic. Opioids are often the safest analgesics available, usually causing only temporary sedation and increased need for laxatives.

Concerns about addiction, respiratory depression, and tolerance are usually unwarranted in these patients. If the dose is carefully titrated, the patient's pain (or dyspnea) can usually be completely controlled and the patient still be alert and mentally clear on even hundreds of milligrams of oral morphine given every 4 hours.

A number of effective oral opioid preparations are available (Tables 83–1 and 83–2). If hydrocodone, 5 to 10 mg every 4 hours is not adequate, oxycodone 5 to 10 mg every 4 hours should be used. Oral morphine beginning with 10 to 15 mg every 4 hours is usually the next step, but hydromorphone is a good alternative. The morphine dose should be titrated upward until analgesia lasts the full 4 hours, even if a dose of 300 mg every 4 hours is required.

The particular drug used is less important than the method of administration. In order to *prevent* pain and end the cycle of uncontrolled pain followed by oversedation, an oral narcotic should be administered on a regular schedule, around the

TABLE 83–1.   Selected Oral Opioids

	Oral Morphine Equivalent (mg)
Codeine 30 mg and acetaminophen 300 mg (Tylenol No. 3)	1–2
Hydrocodone 5 mg + homatropine (Hycodan)	1–2
Hydrocodone 5 mg + acetaminophen 500 mg (Vicodin)	1–2
Oxycodone 5 mg + aspirin 325 mg (Percodan)	5
Oxycodone 5 mg + acetaminophen 325 mg (Percocet)	5
Oxycodone 5 mg per 5 ml (Roxicodone)	5 mg/5 ml
Hydromorphone 2 mg (Dilaudid)	10
Morphine slow release 30 mg (MS Contin 30 mg Oramorph SR)	10 mg q 4 hr × 3
Fentanyl patches (Duragesic) 50 ng/hr	15 mg q 4 hr
Morphine	
Tablets (Lilly, Roxane, Purdue-Frederick)	10, 15, or 30 mg
Syrup (Roxane, Purdue-Frederick)	10 or 20 mg/5 ml
Solution (Roxane, Purdue-Frederick)	20 mg/ml
MS Contin 30 mg Oramorph SR	10 mg q 4 hr × 3
Fentanyl patches 50 μg/hr (Duragesic)	15 mg q 4 hr

clock. "Booster" doses equal to about half of the regular 4-hour dose can be used as needed for breakthrough pain. Long-acting drugs like methadone (half-life 48 to 72 hours) can be prescribed every 6 to 8 hours, but are unsuitable for "booster" doses. They accumulate over several days and are difficult to titrate, especially in patients who have fluctuating levels of pain or deteriorating renal or hepatic function. Slow-release morphine preparations like MS Contin or Oramorph SR can provide excellent analgesia for 8 to 12 hours but are unsuitable for "booster" doses. These tablets may be given rectally when the patient cannot swallow. Small, soluble tablets or concentrated solutions of morphine or hydromorphone can be given sublingually when the patient is too weak to swallow, and can be used for both 4-hour and booster doses. Transdermal fentanyl patches (Duragesic) are now available in 25, 50, 75, and 100 μg per hour strengths. Since they are very expensive and deliver a wide variation of plasma levels (a 25-μg patch delivers 4 to 11 mg of oral morphine every 4 hours), they should be reserved for patients who cannot use the oral or subcutaneous routes. There is no need to use injections when an adequate dose by mouth will

work as well. Table 83–3 provides a checklist of items to remember when prescribing an opioid.

Two opioid agents that are also available orally are not recommended for cancer pain. Meperidine (Demerol) has a very low oral potency, a short duration of action, and a toxic metabolite that can cause tremors or even seizures. Pentazocine (Talwin, Talacen) is an agonist-antagonist agent that is no more potent than aspirin with codeine and has a high incidence of psychotomimetic effects (hallucinations, confusion) in cancer patients.

CO-ANALGESICS. Co-analgesics or adjuvants are drugs that potentiate the analgesic effects of opioids for particular types of pain (Table 83–4). Nonsteroidal anti-inflammatory drugs are quite helpful in the alleviation of pain from lesions in bones or skeletal muscles. The nonacetylated salicylates (e.g., salsalate [Disalcid], choline magnesium trisalicylate [Trilisate]) may be less toxic to the gastric mucosa and do not inhibit platelet function but are less potent analgesics. The newer nonsalicylate nonsteroidal anti-inflammatory drugs are more potent, more convenient, and less toxic than aspirin. Although no single agent has been shown to be consistently more efficacious, particular patients do seem to favor one drug over another. If swallowing large tablets becomes a problem, piroxicam (Feldene) capsules, naproxen (Naprosyn) suspension, or indomethacin (Indocin) rectal suppositories may be used.

For the burning, stabbing, or shooting pain caused by nerve damage, a tricyclic antidepressant or an anticonvulsant may be a useful addition. Amitriptyline, in doses smaller than those used to treat depression (10 to 100 mg at bedtime), is often effective. If swallowing problems arise, doxepin (Sinequan) solution should be used. The addition of carbamazepine (200 to 400 mg three times daily) or valproate (Depakene 250 to 500 mg three times daily) should be considered if the tricyclic agent alone is not adequate. Both doxepin and carbamazepine can be administered rectally in gelatin capsules (Storey and Trumble, 1992). A short course of steroids has also been helpful in treating some difficult, opioid-resistant types of pain.

Visceral or Bladder Spasms

These spasms are best treated with an anticholinergic agent like dicyclomine (Bentyl) or oxybutynin (Ditropan). For more severe cases, the addition of 0.4 to 1.0 mg of glycopyrrolate (Robinul) to a 24-

TABLE 83–2. Dosing Data for Opioid Analgesics

Drug	Approximate Equianalgesic Oral Dose*	Approximate Equianalgesic Parenteral Dose*	Recommended Starting Dose (Adults > 50 kg Body Weight)		Recommended Starting Dose† (Children and Adults < 50 kg Body Weight)‡	
			Oral	Parenteral	Oral	Parenteral
Opioid Agonist						
Morphine§	30 mg q 3–4 hr (around-the-clock dosing) 60 mg q 3–4 hr (single dose or intermittent dosing)	10 mg q 3–4 hr	30 mg q 3–4 hr	10 mg q 3–4 hr	0.3 mg/kg q 3–4 hr	0.1 mg/kg q 3–4 hr
Codeine‖	130 mg q 3–4 hr	75 mg q 3–4 hr	60 mg q 3–4 hr	60 mg q 2 hr (intramuscular/subcutaneous)	1 mg/kg 3–4 hr¶	Not recommended
Hydromorphone§ (Dilaudid)	7.5 mg q 3–4 hr	1.5 mg q 3–4 hr	6 mg q 3–4 hr	1.5 mg q 3–4 hr	0.06 mg/kg q 3–4 hr¶	0.015 mg/kg q 3–4 hr
Hydrocodone (in Lorcet, Lortab, Vicodin, others)	Equivalence data not substantiated	Not available	10 mg q 3–4 hr	Not available	0.2 mg/kg q 3–4 hr¶	Not available
Levorphanol (Levo-Dromoran)	4 mg q 6–8 hr	2 mg q 6–8 hr	4 mg q 6–8 hr	2 mg q 6–8 hr	0.04 mg/kg q 6–8 hr	0.02 mg/kg q 6–8 hr
Meperidine (Demerol)	300 mg q 2–3 hr	100 mg q 3 hr	Not recommended	100 mg q 3 hr	Not recommended	0.75 mg/kg q 2–3 hr
Methadone (Dolophine, others)	20 mg q 6–8 hr	10 mg q 6–8 hr	20 mg q 6–8 hr	10 mg q 6–8 hr	0.2 mg/kg q 6–8 hr	0.1 mg/kg q 6–8 hr
Oxycodone (Roxicodone, also in Percocet, Percodan, Tylox, others)	30 mg q 3–4 hr	Not available	10 mg q 3–4 hr	Not available	0.2 mg/kg q 3–4 hr¶	Not available
Oxymorphone§ (Numorphan)	Not available	1 mg q 3–4 hr	Not available	1 mg q 3–4 hr	Not recommended	Not recommended
Opioid Agonist–Antagonist and Partial Agonist						
Buprenorphine (Buprenex)	Not available	0.3–0.4 mg q 6–8 hr	Not available	0.4 mg q 6–8 hr	Not available	0.004 mg/kg q 6–8 hr
Butorphanol (Stadol)	Not available	2 mg q 3–4 hr	Not available	2 mg q 3–4 hr	Not available	Not recommended
Nalbuphine (Nubain)	Not available	10 mg q 3–4 hr	Not available	10 mg q 3–4 hr	Not available	0.1 mg/kg q 3–4 hr
Pentazocine (Talwin, others)	150 mg q 3–4 hr	60 mg q 3–4 hr	50 mg q 4–6 hr	Not recommended	Not recommended	Not recommended

*Note: Published tables vary in the suggested doses that are equianalgesic to morphine. Clinical response is the criterion that must be applied for each patient; titration to clinical response is necessary. Because there is not complete cross tolerance among these drugs, it is usually necessary to use a lower than equianalgesic dose when changing drugs and to retitrate to response.

†Caution: Recommended doses do not apply to patients with renal or hepatic insufficiency or other conditions affecting drug metabolism and kinetics.

‡Caution: Doses listed for patients with body weight less than 50 kg cannot be used as initial starting doses in babies less than 6 months of age. Consult the *Clinical Practice Guideline for Acute Pain Management: Operative or Medical Procedures and Trauma* section on management of pain in neonates for recommendations.

§For morphine, hydromorphone, and oxymorphone, rectal administration is an alternate route for patients unable to take oral medications, but equianalgesic doses may differ from oral and parenteral doses because of pharmacokinetic differences.

‖Caution: Codeine doses above 65 mg often are not appropriate due to diminishing incremental analgesia with increasing doses but continually increasing constipation and other side effects.

¶Caution: Doses of aspirin and acetaminophen in combination opioid/NSAID preparations must also be adjusted to the patient's body weight.

From Agency for Health Care Policy and Research: Acute Pain Management in Adults: Operative Procedures (Quick Reference Guide for Clinicians) (AHCPR Publication No. 92-0019). Rockville, MD, Agency for Health Care Policy and Research, 1992.

596

TABLE 83–3. Physician's Checklist When Prescribing Opioids

1. Has an appropriate starting dose been determined?
2. Is a co-analgesic needed?
3. Is an antiemetic needed?
4. Has a laxative been prescribed?
5. Is the drug regimen written out in sufficient detail?
6. Has the patient been warned about possible side effects that might occur initially?
7. Do the patient and family know what to do if the pain remains uncontrolled?
8. Have arrangements been made for follow-up after 1, 3, and 7 days—either by the physician or a trained hospice nurse?
9. Does the patient know what to do if he or she needs help or advice before the next follow-up visit?
10. Is the patient confident that the pain will improve considerably, probably within a few days, certainly within 1 or 2 weeks?

Modified from Twycross RG. Symptom Control in Far Advanced Cancer: Pain Relief, 2nd ed. London, Pitman, 1993.

hour subcutaneous infusion of opioid should be used.

Anxiety

If anxiety is severe enough to require drug therapy use a benzodiazepine, or if pain remains a problem, consider hydroxyzine (Atarax or Vistaril) 10 to 50 mg every 4 to 8 hours. This drug has also been shown to potentiate morphine in large doses. If a parenteral agent is needed, use methotrimeprazine (Levoprome). This is the only phenothiazine with analgesic activity, and it is a potent sedative and antiemetic as well. An intramuscular injection of 20 to 50 mg usually calms a crisis, and 50 to 300 mg per day can be used by subcutaneous infusion. Orthostatic hypotension and irritation at the injection site are possible side effects.

Dyspnea

Like pain, dyspnea can have a multitude of causes. When anemia, bronchospasm, and heart failure have been excluded or treated, the focus should be on symptom control. Oxygen can be helpful but is much less effective than opioids for controlling this distressing symptom. When the dose of opioid is carefully titrated to control the pain and the narcotic is administered on a regular schedule with "booster doses" available, the patient can get excellent relief without significant respiratory depres-

sion. Careful consideration should be given to the use of antibiotics for pneumonia in the terminally ill patient. Since dyspnea can be well controlled without antibiotics, the physician must decide whether the antibiotics will improve the quality of life or just prolong the dying.

Constipation

When gastrointestinal motility and oral intake decrease and narcotic analgesics are required, virtually every patient will require regular doses of laxatives to avoid distressing constipation. The laxative should be given once or twice *every* day and the amount increased until an effective dose is found. Bulk laxatives are poorly tolerated and are rarely adequate for these patients. If docusate (Colace), 100 to 200 mg twice daily, is not effective, add senna (Senokot) or bisacodyl (Dulcolax), 1 to 4 tablets twice daily. Sorbitol 70% should be added in doses of 15 to 45 ml two or three times per day if the tablets are inadequate or cause excessive cramping. If a patient has gone several days without a bowel movement or is having small, frequent, liquid stools, an impaction may require manual removal. Bisacodyl suppositories or enemas may be needed occasionally until an effective oral regimen is found.

Nausea and Vomiting

In patients with nausea and vomiting, first look for a reversible cause such as constipation or gastritis from nonsteroidal anti-inflammatory drugs. If increased intracranial pressure is the cause, then the patient may require steroids. Overfeeding may be the problem if a nasogastric or gastrostomy tube is in place. Metoclopramide (Reglan) is the agent of choice when an enormous liver limits gastric emptying. Many patients whose nausea and vomiting have not responded to prochlorperazine (Compazine) or promethazine (Phenergan) are relieved by haloperidol (Haldol), 0.5 to 2 mg orally or subcutaneously every 8 hours.

Like persistent pain, persistent nausea should be treated with regularly scheduled doses. Combinations of antiemetics that have different modes of action may be needed. A combination of haloperidol with metoclopramide or hydroxyzine (Vistaril) may be effective. When oral antiemetics cannot be tolerated, rectal suppositories can be tried but rarely provide adequate control for persistent nausea and vomiting. Continuous subcutaneous infusions of metoclopramide, haloperidol, and/or methotri-

TABLE 83–4. Co-analgesics

Pain Source	Pain Character	Drug Class	Examples	Comments
Bone or soft tissue	Tenderness over bone or joint Pain on movement	NSAIDs	Ibuprofen, 400 mg q 4 hr	Inexpensive; *large* pills
			Sulindac (Clinoril), 200 mg q 12 hr	Well tolerated; preferred in renal impairment
			Naproxen (Naprosyn susp., 125 mg/5 mL), 15 mL q 8 hr	Liquid preparation
			Indomethacin (Indocin 50 mg capsules *or* suppository), q 8 hr	Suppository; more gastritis?
			Piroxicam (Feldene 20 mg capsules), 1 q day	Easiest to swallow; more gastritis?
			Choline magnesium trisalicylate (Trilisate susp., 500 mg/5 mL), 15 mL q 12 hr	No platelet dysfunction; less problem with gastritis; less effective
Nerve damage or dysesthesia	Burning or shooting pain radiating from plexus or spinal root	Tricyclic antidepressant	Amitriptyline (Elavil), 10–50 mg q hs	Best studied; sedating; start with low dose
			alone or with Doxepin (Sinequan), 10–50 mg q hs	10 mg/mL susp. available
			or Trazodone (Desyrel), 25–150 mg q hs	Less anticholinergic effect; one third as potent as amitriptyline
		Anticonvulsant	Carbamazepine (Tegretol), 200 mg q 6–12 hr)	Absorbed from rectum, unlike phenytoin
Smooth muscle spasms	Colic—cramping, abdominal pain, bladder spasms	Anticholinergic	Dicyclomine (Bentyl), 10 mg q 4–8 hr	Capsules
			Oxybutynin (Ditropan), 5–10 mg q 8 hr	Tablets
Anxiety	Generalized restlessness and discomfort	Antihistamine	Hydroxyzine (Atarax or Vistaril), 10–50 mg q 4 hr	PO or by SQ infusion only
		Phenothiazine	Methotrimeprazine (Levoprome), 50–300 mg/day	IM or SQ infusion only

IM = Intramuscular; PO = orally; SQ = subcutaneous; susp. = suspension.

meprazine are more effective. Even vomiting associated with complete bowel obstruction can usually be controlled *without* a nasogastric tube or gastrostomy with a continuous subcutaneous infusion of opioids, antiemetics, and anticholinergic agents.

Hiccup

Persistent hiccuping can be caused by any lesion affecting the phrenic nerve and by gastric distention or systemic problems such as uremia. Treatment can consist of chlorpromazine (Thorazine), 25 to 50 mg orally every 4 to 6 hours; metoclopramide (Reglan), 10 to 20 mg orally every 6 to 8 hours; or haloperidol (Haldol), 1 to 2 mg orally every 4 to 6 hours.

Subcutaneous Infusions

When oral narcotics or antiemetics cannot be tolerated because of nausea, vomiting, stupor, or extreme weakness, parenteral medications may be needed. Frequent intramuscular injections or frequently restarting intravenous infusions can be painful and difficult to manage at home. Up to 50 ml of medication per day can be infused through a small-gauge butterfly needle under the skin of the upper chest, arms, abdomen, or thighs using a miniature pump. Morphine and hydromorphone (Dilaudid) have been shown to be safe and effective when administered by this route (Bruera et al., 1988). Metoclopramide (Reglan), 20 to 90 mg per day; methotrimeprazine (Levoprome), 50 to 300 mg per day; and glycopyrrolate (Robinul), 0.4 to 1.0 mg per day, can be combined with an opioid for control of nausea, colic, and secretions. Haloperidol can also be combined with the opioid and infused by this route, but a white crystalline precipitate of pure haloperidol sometimes forms in the syringe at higher (greater than 1.5 mg per ml) concentrations. This infusion is often started in the hospital or hospice inpatient unit to ensure proper dose selection. The family can be taught to maintain the infusion and give "booster" doses as needed either with the pump or sublingually.

Hospice Care

"Hospice" originally meant a way station for pilgrims and travelers where they could be replenished, refreshed, and cared for. The Irish Sisters of Charity viewed death as one stage of a journey. They opened hospices for dying patients in Dublin in 1879 and in London in 1905. These were places where dying people could be cared for when they could not be managed at home.

Cicely Saunders was trained as a nurse and social worker in London in the 1940s. She cared for a dying cancer patient who made a £500 donation to "be [used for] a window" in the special home for the dying they both knew was needed. Saunders went to medical school and then worked in St. Joseph's Hospice in London from 1958 to 1965. She discovered the effectiveness of interdisciplinary team support, scheduled doses of oral opioid, and other methods to relieve the symptoms and stresses of her patients and their families. When she opened St. Christopher's Hospice in south London in 1967, the modern hospice movement was born.

A hospice program consists of palliative and supportive services that provide physical, psychological, social, and spiritual care for dying persons and their families. Services are provided by a medically supervised interdisciplinary team of professionals and volunteers and are available both in the home and in an inpatient setting. Home care is provided as necessary—on a part-time, intermittent, regularly scheduled, or around-the-clock on-call basis. The hospice concept is directed toward providing "support and care for persons in the last phases of incurable diseases so that they might live as fully and as comfortably as possible . . . (and) that, through appropriate care and the promotion of a caring community sensitive to their needs, patients and families may be free to attain a degree of mental

and spiritual preparation for death that is satisfactory to them" (National Hospice Organization, 1979).

Hospice care is not focused only on the patient; the unit of care is the patient and family. The physical, psychological, and interpersonal needs of both the patient and the family are addressed.

Admission to a hospice program requires that a person have an inevitable fatal illness with a prognosis of weeks or months, that a request be made for the services, and that the attending physician consent to and cooperate with the hospice care. Table 83–5 lists the standards of a hospice program as developed by the National Hospice Organization (NHO).

The interdisciplinary hospice team consists of a patient care coordinator, a nurse, a physician, a counselor, a volunteer coordinator, and spiritual support. Medical services are on call 24 hours a day, 7 days a week. Continuity of care by the same group of team members provides a familiarity that is comforting to the patient. Volunteers are an integral part of the program and provide many helpful services.

Support for the Family

Following a patient's death, family members experience increased morbidity and mortality, emphasizing the need for greater family support from the physician. Unfortunately, most physicians do not routinely contact the family following a patient's death, so this need often goes unrecognized.

The hospice team provides follow-up bereavement care to the family up to 1 year after the patient's death. Family members who experience grief following the death of a loved one are more vulnerable to physical and other emotional disturbances than at any other time in their lives. They need help dealing with the grief, guilt, and symptoms associated with this emotional turmoil. The bereavement services of a hospice team can minimize these problems and can help family members cope with the pain of memories that arise from time to time, especially at holidays, birthdays, and other stressful occasions.

One man who was dying of cancer kept it a secret from family and friends in order to spare them having to suffer with him. After his death some admired his ability to suffer in silence but many were angry and hurt, interpreting his actions to mean that he did not feel they were strong enough to suffer with him. The survivors were angry not only because he did not appear to need them,

TABLE 83–5. NHO Standards of Hospice Program of Care

1. Appropriate therapy is the goal of hospice care.
2. Palliative care is the most appropriate form of care when cure is no longer possible.
3. The goal of palliative care is the prevention of distress from chronic signs and symptoms.
4. Admission to a hospice program of care is dependent on patient and family needs and their expressed request for care.
5. Hospice care consists of a blending of professional and nonprofessional services.
6. Hospice care considers all aspects of the lives of patients and their families as valid areas of therapeutic concern.
7. Hospice care is respectful of all patient and family belief systems, and will employ resources to meet the personal philosophic, moral, and religious needs of patients and their families.
8. Hospice care provides continuity of care.
9. The hospice care program considers the patient and the family together as the unit of care.
10. The patient's family is considered to be a central part of the hospice care team.
11. Hospice care programs seek to identify, coordinate, and supervise persons who can give care to patients who do not have a family member available to take on the responsibility of giving care.
12. Hospice care for the family continues into the bereavement period.
13. Hospice care is available 24 hours a day, 7 days a week.
14. Hospice care is provided by an interdisciplinary team.
15. Hospice programs will have structured and informal means of providing support to staff.
16. Hospice programs will be in compliance with the Standards of the National Hospice Organization and the applicable laws and regulations governing the organization and delivery of care to patients and families.
17. The services of the hospice program are coordinated under a central administration.
18. The optimal control of distressful symptoms is an essential part of the hospice care program requiring medical, nursing, and other services of the interdisciplinary team.
19. The hospice care team will have:
    a. a medical director on staff
    b. physicians on staff
    c. a working relationship with the patient's physician
20. Based on the patient's needs and preferences as determining factors in the setting and location for care, a hospice program provides inpatient care and care in the home setting.
21. Education, training, and evaluation of hospice services is an ongoing activity of a hospice care program.
22. Accurate and current records are kept on all patients.

From the NHO Standards Document, National Hospice Organization, Arlington, VA, 1993. Reprinted with permission.

but also were hurt because he did not even say good-bye.

The most remarkable contribution of the hospice movement is not that it provides a special and compassionate setting in which terminally ill persons can die without heroic measures being applied to them, but that the family becomes involved and comfortable in caring for the ill member.

With the rapid increase of scientific and technological competence in the field of medicine, families feel increasingly incompetent and impotent to deal with dying. The hospice movement has reversed that trend and helps family members to work with community support services to provide home care for many of these patients. When symptoms cannot be controlled at home, the hospice inpatient unit can provide medical and nursing expertise in a "homelike" setting.

The hospice concept can benefit patients and families wherever death takes place. What is important is a network of support for all concerned. However, there should not be an arbitrary judgment as to what is best for all people. Some patients do not want to be a burden to their family and pride themselves on being able to afford hospitalization or nursing home care. For some of these patients, the gradual withdrawal from family may be an emotional "letting go" that is necessary for all concerned in their particular family and circumstances. On the other hand, there may be a spouse of a perfectly good marriage who is simply not equipped either physically or psychologically to deal with the loved one dying right there in the house over a 2-month period. The family physician will be sensitive to the style of living and the style of dying that seems most appropriate in a given case once the options have been explained to the family.

SUGGESTED READING

AMA Council on Scientific Affairs. Good care of the dying patient. JAMA, 1996;275;6:474–478.

Bruera E, Brenneis C, Michaud M, et al. Use of the subcutaneous route for the administration of narcotics in patients with cancer pain. Cancer, 1988;62:407–411.

National Hospice Organization. Hospice Philosophy, Arlington, VA, 1979.

Rakel RE, Storey P. Care of the dying patient. In Rakel RE (ed). Textbook of Family Practice, 5th ed. Philadelphia, W.B. Saunders, 1995, pp 134–152.

Storey P, Hill HH, St. Louis RH, Tarver EE. Subcutaneous infusions for control of cancer symptoms. J Pain Symptom Manage, 1990;5:33–41.

Storey P, Trumble M. Rectal doxepin and carbamazepine therapy in patients with cancer. N Engl J Med, 1992;327:1318–1319.

Twycross RC: Principles and practice of pain relief in terminal cancer. In Corr CA (ed). Hospice Care—Principles and Practice. New York, Springer Publishing, 1983, pp 55–72.

Wilkinson TJ, Robinson BA, Begg EJ, et al. Pharmacokinetics and efficacy of rectal versus oral sustained-release morphine in cancer patients. Cancer Chemother Pharmacol, 1992;31:251–254.

QUESTIONS

1. If codeine is not adequate to control pain in a terminally ill patient, the next choice should be:
   a. Oral morphine
   b. Oxycodone
   c. Hydrocodone
   d. Hydromorphone

2. Which of the following co-analgesics would be most appropriate for a patient with burning, nerve root pain?
   a. Naproxen
   b. Amitriptyline
   c. Hydroxyzine
   d. Glycopyrrolate

3. Which of the following is not an opioid?
   a. Dolophine
   b. Robinul
   c. Vicodin
   d. Tylox

Answers appear on **page 608.**

Answers

Chapter 1   The Family Physician

1. a   2. d   3. (1) d; (2) e; (3) a; (4) b; (5) d

Chapter 2   Ethics in Family Medicine

See text and references for discussions of these questions.

Chapter 3   Family Dynamics and Health

1. b   2. c   3. c

Chapter 4   Patient Compliance

1. Retrieving patients who fail to attend appointments. Keeping patients in care is essential to all compliance interventions, and it is easier to do and more successful than virtually all other interventions.

2. (1) Stimulus control. (2) Contingency management. (3) Goal setting. (4) Self-monitoring. (5) Development of self-efficacy. (6) Relapse prevention.

Chapter 5   Disease Prevention

1. c
2. e
3. (a) true; (b) false; (c) false; (d) true; (e) true; (f) true
4. (1) d; (2) d; (3) c; (4) e; (5) b; (6) a; (7) d

Chapter 6   The Consultation Process

1. a   2. a, b, d, e   3. e   4. b

Chapter 7   The Problem-Oriented Medical Record

1. b   2. a, c, d   3. a, b, d   4. b, c, d

Chapter 8   Problem Solving in Family Medicine

1. b   2. c   3. d   4. b

Chapter 9   Interpreting Laboratory Tests

1. a   2. a   3. c   4. d   5. d   6. c

Chapter 10   Selecting Radiographic Tests

1. e   2. b   3. c   4. d

Chapter 11   Managed Health Care

1. (1) c; (2) d; (3) a; (4) b   2. c   3. d

Chapter 12   Basics of Prescription Writing

1. b   2. c   3. d

Chapter 13   Immunizations

1. c   2. a   3. c   4. c

Chapter 14   Weight Loss and Diarrhea

1. b, c, d   2. b, c, d   3. f   4. c

Chapter 15   Chronic Cough

1. a   2. (1) c; (2) a; (3) d; (4) b; (5) d

Chapter 16   Fever and Chest Pain

1. (a) false; (b) false; (c) true; (d) true

Chapter 17   Dyspnea

1. d   2. c   3. a

Chapter 18   Acute Bronchitis

1. (a) false; (b) true; (c) true

Chapter 19   Blurring of Vision

1. (1) d; (2) b; (3) c; (4) e; (5) a
2. c

Chapter 20   Ear Pain

1. (a) true; (b) true; (c) false; (d) false; (e) false
2. b
3. e

Chapter 21   Sinus Congestion

1. b   2. b   3. e

Chapter 22   Dizziness

1. (a) true; (b) false; (c) true; (d) true
2. (a) true; (b) true; (c) false; (d) true
3. (a) true; (b) true; (c) true; (d) true
4. (a) true; (b) false; (c) true; (d) false

Chapter 23   Sore Throat

1. (a) true; (b) true; (c) true; (d) true; (e) true
2. (a) true; (b) true; (c) true; (d) true; (e) false

Chapter 24   Oral Leukoplakia

1. b   2. c   3. b

Chapter 25   Nasal Congestion

1. (1) d; (2) c; (3) b; (4) a

Chapter 26   Wheezing

1. c;   2. (a) false; (b) true; (c) false;   3. b

Chapter 27   Diarrhea

1. c

2. d.
    The literature clearly shows that diarrhea is the major presenting symptom in 90 to 100 per cent of the cases. This is followed by fatigue (72–97%), abdominal pain (61–83%), foul stool (75–79%), bloating (63–79%), and weight loss (59–73%).

3. b.
    Chronic giardiasis is characterized by flatulence (94%), upper abdominal pain (84%), epigastric gnawing (75%), nervousness (72%), and weight loss (53%). It is important to recognize that diarrhea represents only 41% of the cases.

Chapter 28   Pregnancy

1. (a) false; (b) true; (c) false; (d) false; (e) true
2. b
3. (a) false; (b) true; (c) false; (d) true
4. (a) true; (b) false; (c) false; (d) true

Chapter 29   Newborn Care

1. e
2. (a) true; (b) false; (c) false; (d) true; (e) false
3. All

Chapter 30   Hyperactivity

1. (a) true; (b) true; (c) false; (d) true; (e) true
2. (a) true; (b) false; (c) true; (d) true; (e) false
3. (a) true; (b) false; (c) true; (d) false

Chapter 31   Short Child

1. (c); a 5-year-old's speech should be entirely understandable.
2. (c)
3. (1) c; (2) a; (3) b; (4) b

Chapter 32 Preschool Physical Examination

1. (a) true; (b) false; (c) true; (d) true

2. (a) true; (b) true; (c) true; (d) true

3. (a) true; (b) false; (c) true; (d) true

Chapter 33 Abdominal Pain

1. c   2. b

Chapter 34 Breast Lump

1. a, b, d, f   2. b   3. b, c

Chapter 35 Laceration Repair

1. b   2. (1) c; (2) a; (3) b

Chapter 36 Vaginal Discharge

1. b   2. d   3. a

Chapter 37 Amenorrhea

1. b   2. e   3. a

Chapter 38 Postmenopausal Vaginal Bleeding

1. (a) 2; (b) 3; (c) 1   2. c

Chapter 39 Contraception

1. a

The most effective barrier method is the male condom; see Table 39–2. Periodic abstinence methods on average are less effective than the male condom. However, effectiveness of periodic abstinence varies with the type of method used. The postovulation method is the most effective periodic abstinence method.

2. (a) true; (b) false; (c) true; (d) false

Combined oral contraceptives (COCs) are contraindicated in women with estrogen-dependent cancer. Breast cancer, endometrial cancer, and ovarian cancer are estrogen-dependent cancers. PID (pelvic inflammatory disease) is considered a contraindication to the use of an IUD (intrauterine device). Cardiovascular disease is a contraindication to the use of combined oral contraceptives. Risk factors for cardiovascular disease are relative contraindications to the use of COCs. The presence of these relative contraindications should make the physician weigh the benefits and risks of COC use carefully. These should always be discussed with the patient. If more than one relative contraindication is present, as in answer D, alternatives should be considered. See Table 39–3.

3. (a) false; (b) true; (c) true; (d) false

The combined oral contraceptive pill and the progestin-only pill require good patient compliance to be effective. Patients need to remember to take the pill at the same time each day. Barrier methods such as condoms, diaphragms, caps, and sponges require strong motivation to use the method each time intercourse takes place. For patients for whom compliance is difficult, an injectable or implantable progestin, an intrauterine device, or sterilization may be considered. These methods require little in the way of patient compliance. Patients using injectable progestin as a method of contraception need to remember to attend for repeat injections at regular intervals. Doctors can help their patients by issuing computer-generated reminders that are mailed to patients before repeat injections are due.

Chapter 40 The Abnormal Pap Smear

1. a   2. a   3. c

Chapter 41 Menopause

1. b   2. a   3. c

Chapter 42 Chest Pain

1. (1) b; (2) c; (3) d; (4) a

Chapter 43 Shortness of Breath

1. (a) true; (b) true; (c) false; (d) true

2. (a) true; (b) true; (c) false; (d) true

Chapter 44 Hypertension

1. a   2. c   3. e

Chapter 45   Hypercholesterolemia

1. a   2. e   3. d   4. c

Chapter 46   Atrial Fibrillation

1. (a) false; (b) true; (c) true; (d) true; (e) false
    Only the classes IA, IC, and III antiarrhythmic agents have been shown to be effective in converting atrial fibrillation to a sinus rhythm. Digoxin and propranolol are effective only in slowing the ventricular response rate.

Chapter 47   Knee Injury

1. e   2. f   3. b

Chapter 48   Neck Pain

1. c   2. d   3. c

Chapter 49   Shoulder Pain in a Recreational Athlete

1. (a) true; (b) true; (c) false; (d) true; (e) true—think Marfan's syndrome
2. d
3. (a) true; (b) false; (c) false; (d) true; (e) true

Chapter 50   Elbow Pain

1. (1) c; (2) a; (3) d; (4) b

Chapter 51   Wrist and Hand Pain

1. a, b, c, d   2. c   3. d   4. a

Chapter 52   Lower Back Pain

1. d   2. e   3. a   4. e

Chapter 53   Ankle Injury

1. (a) false; (b) true; (c) true; (d) false
2. c

Chapter 54   Joint Pain and Stiffness

1. (a) true; (b) true; (c) false; (d) false; (e) false
2. b
3. b

Chapter 55   Skin Papule

1. d   2. a   3. (a) true; (b) false; (c) true; (d) true; (e) true

Chapter 56   Eczema

1. (1) b; (2) c; (3) c; (4) a; (5) a

Chapter 57   Acne

1. (a) true; (b) true; (c) true; (d) false
2. (a) false, (b) false; (c) true; (d) false; (e) false; (f) true

Chapter 58   Rash and Fever

1. (1) d; (2) b; (3) c; (4) e; (5) a   2. c

Chapter 59   Obesity

1. e   2. d   3. d

Chapter 60   Type II Diabetes

1. a   2. a, b, e   3. a

Chapter 61   Weight Loss

1. b   2. d   3. a, c, e

Chapter 62   Malnutrition in the Elderly

1. (a) true; (b) false; (c) true; (d) true; (e) false
2. c
3. (a) true; (b) false; (c) true; (d) true; (e) false

Chapter 63   Eating Disorders

1. (a) true; (b) true; (c) false; (d) true; (e) true; (f) true; (g) true; (h) true; (i) true; (j) true; (k) false

Chapter 64   Heartburn

1. c   2. d   3. c

Chapter 65   Constipation

1. a, b, c, e   2. a, b, c, e   3. a, d, e

Chapter 66   Fatigue and Anemia

1. b   2. e   3. c

Chapter 67   Anemia

1. d   2. c   3. e

Chapter 68   Vomiting and Low Back Pain

1. (1) a; (2) a; (3) c; (4) a
2. b.
    Calcium oxalate stones make up 75 per cent, struvite 15 per cent, and the other types each 5 per cent or less. Cystine stones are the least common type of kidney stone at < 1 per cent.

Chapter 69   Hematuria

1. (a) true; (b) false; (c) true; (d) true; (e) false
2. c
3. (a) true; (b) true; (c) true; (d) true; (e) false; (f) true

Chapter 70   Dysuria

1. (1) a; (2) c; (3) d; (4) b; (5) f

Chapter 71   Nocturia

1. b
2. (a) true; (b) true; (c) true; (d) true
3. (a) true; (b) true; (c) true; (d) false

Chapter 72   Urinary Incontinence

1. (a) true; (b) true; (c) true; (d) true
2. (a) true; (b) true; (c) false; (d) false
3. (a) true; (b) false; (c) true; (d) true

Chapter 73   Headache

1. a   2. d   3. c

Chapter 74   Tremors

1. d   2. a   3. d   4. d

Chapter 75   Child with Fever and Lethargy

1. a   2. b   3. (1) b; (2) a; (3) d; (4) c

Chapter 76   Chronic Anxiety

1. d   2. (1) d; (2) a; (3) e; (4) c; (5) b

Chapter 77   Sleep Disturbance

1. c   2. e

Chapter 78   Motor Vehicle Accident–Related Anxiety

1. b   2. e   3. e

Chapter 79   Domestic Violence

1. d   2. c   3. a

Chapter 80   Memory Loss

1. b   2. c   3. d

Chapter 81   Alcoholism

1. b   2. (a) false; (b) true; (c) true; (d) true; (e) true

Chapter 82   Approaches to Patients Who Smoke

1. d   2. e   3. d

Chapter 83   Terminal Cancer and Pain

1. c   2. b   3. b

Index

Note: Page numbers in *italics* refer to illustrations; page numbers followed by t refer to tables.